Volume Two

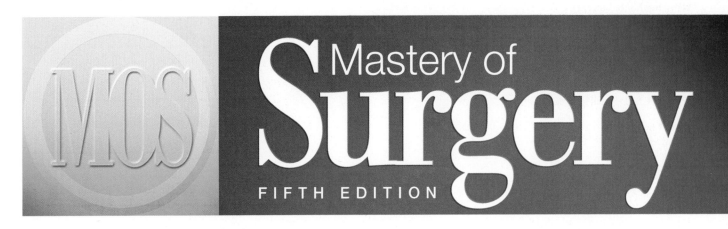

Mastery of Surgery
FIFTH EDITION

Editor

Josef E. Fischer, M.D.

Mallinckrodt Professor of Surgery
Harvard Medical School;
Chairman, Department of Surgery
Beth Israel Deaconess Medical Center
Boston, Massachusetts

Associate Editor

Kirby I. Bland, M.D.

Fay Fletcher Kerner Professor
Chairman, Department of Surgery
University of Alabama at Birmingham School of
Medicine
Birmingham, Alabama

Section Editors

Mark P. Callery, M.D.

Associate Professor
Department of Surgery
Harvard Medical School;
Chief, Division of General Surgery
Beth Israel Deaconess Medical Center
Boston, Massachusetts

G. Patrick Clagett, M.D.

Jan and Bob Pickens Distinguished Professor
Division of Vascular Surgery
Department of Surgery
University of Texas Southwestern Medical
Center
Dallas, Texas

Daniel B. Jones, M.D.

Associate Professor
Department of Surgery
Harvard Medical School;
Chief, Section for Minimally Invasive Surgery
Beth Israel Deaconess Medical Center
Boston, Massachusetts

Frank W. LoGerfo, M.D.

William McDermott Professor of Surgery
Harvard Medical School;
Director, Division of Vascular and Endovascular
Surgery
Beth Israel Deaconess Medical Center
Boston, Massachusetts

James M. Seeger, M.D.

Professor and Chief
Division of Vascular Surgery
Department of Surgery
University of Florida College of Medicine
Gainesville, Florida

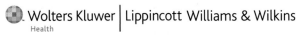

Wolters Kluwer | Lippincott Williams & Wilkins
Health

Philadelphia · Baltimore · New York · London
Buenos Aires · Hong Kong · Sydney · Tokyo

Acquisitions Editor: Brian Brown
Managing Editor: Julia Seto
Associate Director of Marketing: Adam Glazer
Project Manager: Bridgett Dougherty
Manufacturing Manager: Kathleen Brown
Creative Director: Doug Smock
Designer: Karen Quigley
Compositor: TechBooks
Printer: R.R. Donnelley, Willard

Library of Congress Cataloging-in-Publication Data
    Mastery of surgery / editor, Joseph E. Fischer ; associate editor, Kirby
I. Bland ; section editors, Mark P. Callery . . . [et al.]. – 5th ed.
        p. ; cm.
    Includes bibliographical references and index.
    ISBN-13: 978-0-7817-7165-8 (alk. paper)
    ISBN-10: 0-7817-7165-X (alk. paper)
    1. Surgery. I. Fischer, Josef E., 1937- II. Bland, K. I.
    [DNLM: 1. Surgery. 2. Surgical Procedures, Operative. WO 100 M423
                                                2007]
RD11.M29 2007
617–dc22

                                2006035127

Care has been taken to confirm the accuracy of the information presented and to describe
generally accepted practices. However, the authors, editors, and publisher are not responsible for
errors or omissions or for any consequences from application of the information in this book
and make no warranty, expressed or implied, with respect to the currency, completeness, or
accuracy of the contents of the publication. Application of this information in a particular situation remains the professional responsibility of the practitioner.

    The authors, editors, and publisher have exerted every effort to ensure that drug selection
and dosage set forth in this text are in accordance with current recommendations and practice at
the time of publication. However, in view of ongoing research, changes in government regula-
tions, and the constant flow of information relating to drug therapy and drug reactions, the
reader is urged to check the package insert for each drug for any change in indications and
dosage and for added warnings and precautions. This is particularly important when the recommended agent is a new or infrequently employed drug.

    Some drugs and medical devices presented in this publication have Food and Drug
Administration (FDA) clearance for limited use in restricted research settings. It is the responsibility of the health care provider to ascertain the FDA status of each drug or device planned for
use in their clinical practice.

    To purchase additional copies of this book, call our customer service department at (800)
638-3030 or fax orders to (301) 223-2320. International customers should call (301)223-2300.

    Visit Lippincott Williams & Wilkins on the Internet: at LWW.com. Lippincott Williams &
Wilkins customer service representatives are available from 8:30 am to 6 pm, EST.

10 9 8 7 6 5 4 3 2

Contents

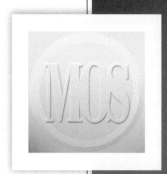

 Chapters with icon are web-only

Volume I

B. The Stomach and Duodenum

C. Morbid Obesity

VIII. NONGASTROINTESTINAL TRANSABDOMINAL 1649

A. The Spleen

B. Surgery of the Urinary Tract and Bladder

C. Gynecologic Surgery

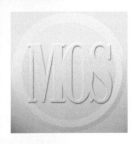

Contributors

John J. Aiken, MD
Associate Professor of Surgery
Medical College of Wisconsin
Children's Hospital of Wisconsin
Milwaukee, Wisconsin

Robert J. Allen, MD
Chief, Section of Plastic Surgery
Louisiana State University Health Sciences
    Center
Chief, Section of Plastic Surgery
Memorial Medical Center;
Consultant in Plastic surgery
Veterans Administration Hospital
New Orleans, Louisiana

Maraya Altuwaijri, MD
Division of Vascular Surgery
Mayo Clinic
Rochester, Minnesota

Parviz K. Amid, MD
Faculty member
Department of Surgery
Harbor University of California
Los Angeles, California

J. Kyle Anderson, MD
Assistant Professor
Department of Urology
University of Minnesota
Minneapolis, Minnesota

John A. Androulakis, MD, FACS
Professor and Chairman of Surgery (Retired)
Department of Surgery
University of Patras Medical School
Patras, Greece

Enrico Ascher, MD, FACS
Director, Division of Vascular Surgery
Department of Surgery
Maimonides Medical Center
Brooklyn, New York

Salman Ashruf, MD
Indiana Hand Insitute
Indianapolis, Indiana

Bernadette Aulivola, MD, RVT
Assistant Professor of Surgery and Radiology
Division of Peripheral Vascular Surgery
Loyola University Medical Center
Maywood, Illinois

Mary T. Austin, MD, MPH
Resident Physician
Department of Surgery
Vanderbilt University Medical Center
Nashville, Tennessee

Samir S. Awad, MD
Associate Professor
Michael E. DeBakey Department of Surgery
Baylor College of Medicine;
Acting Chief of Surgery
Chief and Medical Director of Surgical Intensive Care
    Unit
Veterans Affairs Medical Center
Houston, Texas

Ziad T. Awad, MD, FRCSI
Instructor in Clinical and Laparoscopic Surgery
New York Presbyterian Hospital
Columbia University Medical Center
New York, New York

Richard G. Azizkhan, MD, PHD (HON)
Professor of Surgery and Pediatrics
Director of Division of Pediatric Surgery
Departments of Surgery and Pediatrics
College of Medicine
University of Cincinnati
Surgeon in Chief
Lester Martin Chair of Pediatric Surgery
Department of Pediatric Surgery
Cincinnati Children's Hospital Medical Center
Cincinnati, Ohio

Ali Azizzadeh, MD
Assistant Professor
Vascular Surgery Section
Department of Cardiothoracic and Vascular Surgery
Memorial Hermann Hospital
The University of Texas at Houston
Houston, Texas

Gopal H. Badlani, MD
Vice Chairman
Department of Urology
Long Island Jewish Medical Center
New Hyde Park, New York

Robert W. Bailey, MD, FACS
Professor of Clinical Surgery
University of Miami School of Medicine
Division of Laparoendoscopic and Bariatric Surgery
Miami, Florida

Robert J. Baker, MD
Professor of Surgery
Department of Surgery
Pritzker School of Medicine
University of Chicago
Chicago, Illinois

William H. Baker, MD
Professor Emeritis
Department of Surgery
Loyla University Medical Center
Maywood, Illinois

Glen W. Barrisford, MD
Department of Surgery
Division of Urology
Brigham and Women's Hospital
Harvard Medical School
Boston, Massachusetts

Robert H. Bartlett, MD
Department of Surgery
University of Michigan Medical School
Ann Arbor, Michigan

Robert W. Beart, Jr., MD
Professor and Chairman
Department of Colorectal Surgery
Keck School of Medicine
University of Southern California
Los Angeles, California

Samuel W. Beenken, MD
Associate Professor
Department of Surgery
Section of Surgical Oncology
University of Alabama School of Medicine
Birmingham, Alabama

Hans G. Beger, MD, MD Hon, Prof. em of
   Surgery
Professor em of Surgery
Department of Surgery
University Hospital
Ulm, Germany

Michael Belkin, MD
Division Chief
Division of Vascular and Endovascular
   Surgery
Brigham and Women's Hospital
Harvard Medical School
Boston, Massachusetts

Richard H. Bell, Jr., MD
Professor
Department of Surgery
Northwestern University
Feinberg School of Medicine
Chicago, Illinois

Robert Bendavid MD, FACS
Shouldice Hospital
Toronto, Ontario
Canada

Henri Bismuth, MD, PHD
Emeritus Professor
Department of Surgery
University Paris-South
Hospital Paul Brousse
CHB
Villejuif, France

George L. Blackburn, MD, PHD
S. Daniel Abraham Associate Professor of
   Nutrition
Associate Director, Division of Nutrition
Harvard Medical School
Director, Center for the Study of Nutrition
   Medicine
Department of Surgery
Beth Israel Deaconess Medical Center
Boston, Massachusetts

Kirby I. Bland, MD
Fay Fletcher Kerner Professor and Chair
Department of Surgery
University of Alabama at Birmingham
Birmingham, Alabama

Seth B. Blattman, MD
Beth Israel Deaconess Medical Center
Boston, Massachusetts

Joseph G. Borer, MD, FACS, FAAP
Assistant Professor
Harvard Medical School
Department of Urology
Children's Hospital Boston
Boston, Massachusetts

Philippus C. Bornman, MMed (SA), FRCS
   (Ed), FCS (SA), FRCS (Glasg)
Professor
Department of Surgery
University of Cape Town Health Sciences Faculty and
   Surgical Gastroenterology
Groote Schuur Hospital
Cape Town, South Africa

Loren J. Borud, MD
Instructor In Surgery
Department of Surgery
Harvard Medical School
Attending Surgeon
Department of Surgery
Beth Israel Deaconess Medical Center
Boston, Massachusetts

Richard D. Branson, MSC, RRT
Associate Professor
Department of Surgery
University of Cincinnati
Cincinnati, Ohio

Murray F. Brennan, MD
Chairman
Department of Surgery
Memorial Sloan-Kettering Cancer Center
New York, New York

Stacy Alan Brethauer, MD
Fellow, Advanced Laparoscopic and Bariatric
   Surgery
Department of General Surgery
Cleveland Clinic Foundation
Cleveland, Ohio

David C. Brewster, MD
Clinical Professor of Surgery
Massachusetts General Hospital;
Harvard Medical School
Boston, Massachusetts

L. D. Britt, MD, MPH
Brickhouse Professor and Chair
Department of Surgery
Eastern Virginia Medical School
Norfolk, Virginia

Kellie R. Brown, MD
Assistant Professor
Division of Vascular Surgery
Medical College of Wisconsin
Zablocki VA Medical Center
Milwaukee, Wisconsin

L. Michael Brunt, MD
Department of Surgery
Institute for Minimally Invasive Surgery and Section of
   Endocrine and Oncologic Surgery
Washington University School of
   Medicine
St. Louis, Missouri

Henry Buchwald, MD, PHD
Department of Surgery

University of Minnesota
Minneapolis, Minnesota

Kelli M. Bullard, MD
Assistant Professor
Department of Surgery
University of Minnesota
Minneapolis, Minnesota

Rudolf Bumm, MD
Technische Universitat Munchen
Munich, Germany

Iliya M. Buriev, MD
Russia

Robert M. Byers, MD
University of Texas M. D. Anderson Cancer
   Center
Houston, Texas

Jeffrey A. Cadeddu, MD
Associate Professor
Department of Urology and Radiology
University of Texas Southwestern Medical Center
Dallas, Texas

Kristine E. Calhoun, MD
Assistant Professor
Department of Surgery
University of Washington School of Medicine
Seattle, Washington

Mark P. Callery, MD, FACS
Associate Professor of Surgery
Department of Surgery
Harvard Medical School
Chief, Division of General Surgery
Department of Surgery
Beth Israel Deaconess Medical Center
Boston, Massachusetts

Sir Roy Calne, FRS
Professor
Department of Surgery
Cambridge, United Kingdom
Retired NUK
Professor of Surgery NUS
Singapore

David J. Caparrelli, MD
Fellow
Division of Vascular Surgery
The Johns Hopkins Medical Institutions
Baltimore, Maryland

Denise M. Carneiro-Pla, MD
Fellow
Endocrine Surgery
Jackson Memorial Medical Center
University of Miami
Miami, Florida

Nadine R. Caron, MD
Department of Surgery
University of British Columbia
Northern Medical Program
Prince George, British Columbia, Canada

William R. Carroll, MD
Associate Professor
Department of Surgery–Otolaryngology
University of Alabama
Birmingham, Alabama

Jerry R. Castro, MD
Fellow
Department of Head and Neck Surgery

Memorial Sloan-Kettering Cancer Center
New York, New York

Santiago Chahwan, MD
Jobst Vascular Center
The Toledo Hospital
Toledo, Ohio

Benjamin B. Chang, MD
Associate Professor
Department of Surgery
Albany Medical College
Albany, New York

Bernard W. Chang, MD
Department of Plastic and Reconstructive Surgery
Mercy Medical Center
Baltimore, Maryland

Eugene Y. Chang, MD
Research Fellow
Department of Surgery
Oregon Health and Science University
Portland, Oregon

David S. Chapin, MD
Assistant Professor of Obstetrics, Gynecology and
   Reproductive Biology
Beth Israel Deaconess Medical Center
Boston, Massachusetts

Irshad H. Chaudry, MD
Department of Surgery
University of Alabama School of Medicine
Birmingham, Alabama

William G. Cheadle, MD
Professor
Department of Surgery
University of Louisville
Associate Chief of Staff for Research and Development
Veterans Affairs Medical Center
Louisville, Kentucky

Kenneth Cherry, Jr. MD
Department of Surgery
University of Virginia Health System
Charlottesville, Virginia

David K.W. Chew, MD
Division of Vascular and Endovascular Surgery
Brigham and Women's Hospital;
Harvard Medical School
Boston, Massachusetts

W. Randolph Chitwood Jr., MD, FACS, FRCS
Senior Associate Vice Chancellor
Professor of Surgery
Chief, Division of Cardiothoracic and Vascular Surgery
Brody School of Medicine
East Carolina University
Greenville, North Carolina

Emily R. Christison-Lagay, MD
Children's Hospital Boston
Boston, Massachusetts

Ram Chuttani, MD
Director of Endoscopy
Beth Israel Deaconess Medical Center;
Assistant Professor of Medicine
Harvard Medical School
Boston, Massachusetts

G. Patrick Clagett, MD
Chairman, Vascular and Endovascular Surgery
Department of Surgery

University of Texas Southwestern
Dallas, Texas

Orlo H. Clark, MD
Department of Surgery
University of California, San Francisco
UCSF Comprehensive Cancer Center at Mount Zion
   Hospital
San Francisco, California

William S. Cobb, IV, MD
Department of Surgery
Virginia Commonwealth University
Richmond, Virginia

Mark S. Cohen, MD
Department of Surgery
Institute for Minimally Invasive Surgery and Section of
   Endocrine and Oncologic Surgery
Washington University School of Medicine
St. Louis, Missouri

Raul Coimbra, MD, PHD
Division of Trauma
Department of Surgery
University of California San Diego
San Diego California

Daniel G. Coit, MD
Memorial Sloan-Kettering Cancer Center
New York, New York

Gene L. Colburn, PHD
Professor and Chairman
Department of Anatomical Sciences
Ross University School of Medicine
Roseau, Commonwealth of Dominica, West Indies

Anthony J. Comerota, MD
Adjunct Professor of Surgery
Department of Vascular Surgery
University of Michigan
Ann Arbor, Michigan
Director
Jobst Vascular Center
The Toledo Hospital
Toledo, Ohio

Robert E. Condon, MD, MSc, FACS
Emeritus Professor and Chairman
Department of Surgery
Medical College of Wisconsin
Milwaukee, Wisconsin;
Clyde Hill, Washington

Kevin C. Conlon, MCh, MBA, FACS, FRCS, FRCSI
Professor of Surgery
Professorial Surgical Unit
The University of Dublin
Trinity College Dublin
The Adelaide and Meath Hospital
Dublin, Ireland

Willy Coosemans, MD, PHD
Department of Thoracic Surgery
University Hospitals Leuven
Leuven, Belgium

Jeffrey T. Cope, MD
Cardiothoracic Surgeon
Department of Surgery
Lancaster General Hospital
Lancaster, Pennsylvania

Edward E. Cornwell, III, MD
Professor of Surgery
Department of Surgery

Johns Hopkins School of Medicine
Chief, Division of Adult Trauma
Department of Surgery
Johns Hopkins Hospital
Baltimore, Maryland

Jonathan Critchlow, MD
Assistant Professor of Surgery
Beth Israel Deaconess Medical Center
Boston, Massachusetts

Steven A. Curley, MD
Professor
Department of Surgical Oncology
Chief
Department of Gastrointestinal Tumor Surgery
The University of Texas M.D. Anderson Cancer Center
Houston, Texas

Kimberly Moore Dalal, MD
Major, United States Airforce
Chief, Surgical Oncology Department
David Grant U.S.A.F. Medical Center
Travis AFB, California

R. Clement Darling, III, MD
Institute for Vascular Health and Disease
Albany Medical College
Albany, New York

Brian R. Davis, MD
Surgical Endoscopy and ERCP Fellow
Department of Surgery
University of Louisville
Louisville, Kentucky
Minimally Invasive Surgery Fellow
Department of Surgery
Beth Israel Medical Center
New York, New York

James R. DeBord, MD, FACS
Chief, Division of Vascular Surgery
Vice Chairman, Department of Surgery
University of Illinois College of Medicine at Peoria
Peoria, Illinois

Malcolm M. DeCamp Jr., MD
Chief, Division of Cardiothoracic Surgery
Beth Israel Deaconess Hospital
Boston, Massachusetts

Paul De Leyn, MD, PHD
Department of Thoracic Surgery
University Hospitals Leuven
Leuven, Belgium

Luigi De Santis, MD
Dipartimento di Scienze Chirurgiche e
   Gastroenterolgigiche "P. G. Cevese,"
Universita degli Stuid di Padova
Hospedale Civile
Padova Italy

Georges Decker, MD
Department of Thoracic Surgery
University Hospitals Leuven
Leuven, Belgium

Cornelis H.C. Dejong, MD, PHD
Consultant Surgeon
Department of Surgery
University Hospital Maastricht
Maastricht, Netherlands

Eric DeMaria, MD
Chief, Endosurgery
Duke University Medical Center
Durham, North Carolina

Tom R. DeMeester, MD
Department of Surgery
University of Southern California
Los Angeles, California

William C. DeWolf, MD
Professor
Department of Surgery (Urology)
Harvard Medical School;
Chief
Division of Urology, Department of Surgery
Beth Israel Deaconess Medical Center
Boston, Massachusetts

J.C. Meneu Díaz, MD
General and Digestive Surgery Department and
Abdominal Organ Transplant Unit, Hospital
"12 de Octubre"
Madrid, Spain

J. Michael Dixon, MD
Consultant Surgeon and Senior Lecturer
Edinburgh Breast Unit
Western General Hospital
Edinburgh, United Kingdom

Gerard M. Doherty, MD
NW Thompson Professor of Surgery
Department of Surgery
University of Michigan
Ann Arbor, Michigan

Eric J. Dozois, MD
Assistant Professor of Surgery
Colon and Rectal Surgery Department
Mayo Clinic College of Medicine
Consultant Surgeon
Colon and Rectal Surgery Department
Mayo Clinic
Rochester, Minnesota

Roger R. Dozois, MD
Professor of Surgery, Emeritus
Colon and Rectal Surgery Department
Mayo Clinic College of Medicine
Rochester, Minnesota

Richard L. Drake, MD
Director of Anatomy
Cleveland Clinic Lerner College of
Medicine
Cleveland, Ohio

Mark R. Edwards, MD

David T. Efron, MD
Assistant Professor
Department of Surgery
Johns Hopkins Medical Institutions
Baltimore, Maryland

Peter F. Ehrlich, MD, MSc
Associate Professor
Department of Surgery, Section of Pediatric
Surgery
University Of Michigan
CS Mott Childrens Hospital
Ann Arbor, Michigan

John F. Eidt, MD
Professor of Surgery and Radiology
Department of Surgery
University of Arkansas for Medical Sciences
Chief, Vascular and Endovascular Surgery
University Hospital of Arkansas
Little Rock, Arkansas

E. Christopher Ellison, MD
Department of Surgery
Ohio State University
Columbus, Ohio

A. Moreno Elola
General and Digestive Surgery Department and
Abdominal Organ Transplant Unit
Hospital "12 de Octubre"
Madrid, Spain

Scott A Engum, MD
Associate Professor
Department of Surgery
Indiana University
Indianapolis, Indiana

Warren E. Enker, MD
Vice-Chairman and Chief of Colorectal Surgery
Department of Surgery
Beth Israel Medical Center;
Professor of Surgery
Albert Einstein College of Medicine
New York, New York

Sina Ercan, MD
Assistant Professor of Thoracic Surgery
Yeditepe University Hospital
Istanbul, Turkey

Orkan Ergun, MD
Associate Professor of Pediatric Surgery
Department of Pediatric Surgery
Ege University Faculty of Medicine
Izmir, Turkey

Antonio Espinosa-de-los-Monteros, MD
Division of Plastic Surgery
University of Alabama at Birmingham
Birmingham, Alabama

Anthony L. Estreta, MD
Department of Cardiothoracic and Vascular
Surgery
Memorial Hermann Hospital
The University of Texas at Houston
Houston, Texas

W. Steve Eubanks, M.D., FACS
Professor and Chair
Department of Surgery
University of Missouri School of Medicine
Columbia, Missouri

Douglas B. Evans, MD
Professor
Department of Surgical Oncology
University of Texas MD Anderson Cancer
Center
Houston, Texas

Amy R. Evenson, MD
Department of Surgery
Beth Israel Deaconess Medical Center
Boston, Massachusetts

Byron Faler, MD
Research Fellow
Department of Vascular Surgery
Veterans Affairs Medical Center
Washington, District of Columbia

Sheung Tat Fan
Department of Surgery
The University of Hong Kong
Hong Kong, China

Victor W. Fazio, MD
Chairman
Department of Colorectal Surgery
The Cleveland Clinic Foundation
Cleveland, Ohio

Josef E. Fischer, MD
Mallinckrodt Professor of Surgery
Harvard Medical School;
Chairman, Department of Surgery
Beth Israel Deaconess Medical Center
Boston, Massachusetts

Sander S. Florman, MD
Associate Professor of Surgery and
Pediatrics
Chief, Division of Transplant Surgery
Tulane University Hospital
New Orleans, Louisiana

Thomas J. Fogarty, MD
Division of Vascular Surgery
Stanford University School of Medicine
Stanford, California

Yuman Fong, MD
Professor
Department of Surgery
Weill Medical College of Cornell University
Chief, Gastric and Mixed Tumor Service
Murray F Brennan Chair in Surgery
Department of Surgery
Memorial Sloan-Kettering Cancer Center
New York, New York

Henri R. Ford, MD
Vice-President and Surgeon-in-Chief
Childrens Hospital Los Angeles;
Professor and Vice-Chairman, Department of
Surgery
Keck School of Medicine
University of Southern California
Los Angeles, California

Dennis L. Fowler, MD
Department of Surgery
New York Presbyterian Hospital
New York, New York

Glen A. Franklin, MD
Associate Professor of Surgery
Associate Program Director
Department of Surgery
University of Louisville
Louisville, Kentucky

Morris E. Franklin, Jr., MD, FACS
Texas Endosurgery Institute
San Antonio, Texas

Herbert R. Freund, MD
Professor of Surgery
Department of Surgery
Hebrew University
Hadassah Medical School
Chief of Surgery
Department of Surgery
Hadassah University Medical Center-Mount Scopus
Jerusalem, Israel

Julie A. Freischlag, MD
The William Stewart Halsted Professor
Chair of the Department of Surgery
Surgeon-in-Chief
The Johns Hopkins Medical Institutions
Baltimore, Maryland

Nongastrointestinal Transabdominal

Randall S. Friese, MD
Assistant Professor of Surgery
Division of Burn, Trauma, Critical Care
University of Texas Southwestern
*   Medical Center*
Staff Surgeon
Department of Surgery
Parkland Memorial Hospital
Dallas, Texas

Flavio Frigo, MD
Universita degli Studi di Padova
Ospedale Civile
Padova, Italy

Robert D. Fry, MD
Department of Surgery
University of Pennsylvania
Philadelphia, Pennsylvania

Arlan F. Fuller, Jr., MD
Chief, Division of Gynecologic Oncology
Massachusetts General Hospital
Boston, Massachusetts

Stephen C. Gale, MD
Assistant Professor of Surgery
University of Texas Medical School
Houston, Texas

Steven S. Gale, MD, FACS
Jobst Vascular Center
The Toledo Hospital
Toledo, Ohio

James J. Gangemi, MD
Assistant Professor
Department of Cardiac Surgery
University of Rochester Medical Center
Attending Surgeon
Department of Cardiac Surgery
Strong Memorial Hospital
University of Rochester
Rochester, New York

Ian Ganley, MD, PHD, FRCS
Consultant Head and Neck Surgeon
Department of Otolaryngology
Edinburgh Royal Infirmary
Edinburgh, Scotland
United Kingdom

O. James Garden, MD, FRCSED
Regius Professor of Clinical Surgery
Department of Clinical and Surgical Sciences
University of Edinburgh
Head
Department of Surgery
Royal Infirmary
Edinburgh, United Kingdom

Atul A. Gawande, MD, MPH
Assistant Professor of Surgery
Harvard Medical School
Assistant Professor of Health Policy and
*   Management*
Harvard School of Public Health
Surgeon
Department of General and Gastrointestinal Surgery
Brigham and Women's Hospital
Boston, Massachusetts

Keith E. Georgeson, MD
Department of Surgery
University of Alabama at Birmingham School of
*   Medicine, Birmingham, Alabama*

Bruce L. Gewertz, MD
Section of Vascular Surgery
The University of Chicago
Chicago, Illinois

Arthur I. Gilbert, MD
Associate Clinical Professor in Surgery
Hernia Institute of Florida
University of Miami Miller
*   Medical School*
Miami, Florida

Armando E. Giuliano, MD
John Wayne Cancer Institute
Department of Surgery
St. John's Hospital & Health Center
Santa Monica, California

Peter Gloviczki, MD
Professor of Surgery
Mayo Clinic College of Medicine;
Chair, Division of Vascular Surgery;
Director, Gonda Vascular Center
Mayo Clinic
Rochester, Minnesota

Stanley M. Goldberg, MD, FACS
Clinical Professor of Surgery
Division of Colon and Rectal Surgery
University of Minnesota Medical School
Minneapolis, Minnesota

Mitchell H. Goldman, MD
Professor and Chairman
Department of Surgery
University of Tennessee Graduate School of Medicine
University of Tennessee Medical Center
Knoxville, Tennessee

E. Moreno González, MD
Head of the General and Digestive Surgery
*   Department and Abdominal Organ Transplant Unit*
Hospital "12 de Octubre"
Madrid, Spain

Clive S. Grant, MD
Professor
Department of Surgery
Mayo College of Medicine
Rochester, Minnesota

Arin K. Greene, MD
Department of Surgery
Children's Hopsital Boston
Boston, Massachusetts

Jay L. Grosfeld, MD
Riley Hospital for Children
Indianapolis, Indiana

Lorelei Grunwaldt, MD
Beth Israel Deaconess Medical Center
Boston, Massachusetts

Angelita Habr-Gama, MD, PHD
Professor of Surgery,
University of São Paulo School of Medicine
São Paulo, Brazil

Jeffrey A. Hagen, MD
Department of Surgery
University of Southern California
Los Angeles, California

Pegge Alandrees, MD
Department of Surgery

University of Colorado Health Sciences Center
Denver, Colorado

Allen D. Hamdan, MD
Assistant Professor
Department of Surgery
Beth Israel Deaconess Medical Center
Boston, Massachusetts

Kimberley J. Hansen, MD
Professor of Surgery
Head, Section on Vascular and Endovascular Surgery
Division of Surgical Sciences
Wake Forest University School of Medicine
Attending Staff, Vascular and Endovascular Surgery
Department of General Surgery
North Carolina Baptist Hospital
Winston-Salem, North Carolina

Douglas W. Hanto, MD, PHD
Lewis Thomas Professor of Surgery
Department of Surgery
Harvard Medical School
Chief
Division of Transplantation
Beth Israel Deaconess Medical Center
Boston, Massachusetts

Per-Olof Hasselgren, MD, PHD
George H.A. Clowes, Jr. Professor of Surgery
Harvard Medical School
Vice Chair-Research
Director of Endocrine Surgery
Department of Surgery
Beth Israel Deaconess Medical Center
Boston, Massachusetts

Alison R. Hatmaker, MD
Senior Resident
Department of Surgery
Vanderbilt University Medical Center
Nashville, Tennessee

William Hawkins, MD
Hepatobiliary-Pancreatic Surgery
Department of Surgery;
Siteman Cancer Center
Washington University School of Medicine,
St. Louis, Missouri

Michael S. Hayashi, MD
Department of Surgery
University of California-Irvine
Irvine, California

Jeffrey W. Hazey, MD
Department of Surgery
Brody School of Medicine at East Carolina University
Greenville, North Carolina

R. J. Heald, OBE
North Hampshire Hospital
Basingstoke, Hampshire, United Kingdom

Daniel H. Hechtman, MD
Department of Pediatric Surgery
Connecticut Children's Medical Center
Hartford, Connecticut

W. Hardy Hendren, MD, FACS, FAAP, FRCS
Robert Gross Distinguished Professor of
*   Surgery*
Harvard Medical School
Chief of Surgery Emeritus
Children's Hospital Boston
Boston, Massachusetts

B. Todd Heniford, MD, FACS
Chief, Division of Gastrointestinal and Minimally
Invasive Surgery
Department of Surgery
Carolinas Medical Center
Charlotte, North Carolina

Peter K. Henke, MD
Department of Surgery
University of Michigan Health System
Ann Arbor, Michigan

Bradley B. Hill, MD
Assistant Professor
Department of Surgery
Stanford University School of Medicine
Stanford, California

Anil Hingorani, MD
Division of Vascular Surgery
Department of Surgery
Maimonides Medical Center
Brooklyn, New York

Frank Hinman, Jr., MD
Clinical Professor
Department of Urology
University of California, San Francisco
San Francisco, California

Mitchell S. Hoffman, MD
Department of Obstetrics and Gynecology
University of South Florida
Tampa, Florida

George W. Holcomb, III, MD, MBA
Katharine Berry Richardson Professor of
Surgery
Surgeon-in-Chief
Department of Surgery
Children's Mercy Hospital
Kansas City, Missouri

John J. Hong, MD
Assistant Professor
Department of Surgery
UMDNJ-Robert Wood Johnson Medical School
Attending Staff
Department of Surgery
Robert Wood Johnson University Hospital
New Brunswick, New Jersey

Thomas J. Howard, MD
Professor
Department of Surgery
Indiana University
Staff Surgeon
Department of Surgery
Indiana University Medical Center
Indianapolis, Indiana

David B. Hoyt, MD
Department of Surgery
University of California - San Diego Medical
Center
San Diego, California

James C. Hu, MD
Department of Surgery
Brigham and Women's Hospital
Boston, Massachusetts

Jasmine L. Huang, MD
Department of Surgery
Virginia Mason Medical Center
Seattle Washington

William J. Hubbard, MD
Assistant Professor
Department of Surgery
University of Alabama
Birmingham, Alabama

Thomas S. Huber, MD, PHD
Professor
Division of Vascular Surgery and Endovascular Therapy
Department of Surgery
University of Florida College of Medicine
Gainesville, Florida

Kakra Hughes, MD
Section of Vascular Surgery
Medical University of South Carolina
Charleston, South Carolina

Eric S.. Hungness, MD
Assistant Professor
Department of Surgery
Northwestern University
Chicago, Illinois

John G. Hunter, MD
Professor and Chair
Department of Surgery
Oregon Health and Science University
Portland, Oregon

Tam T.T. Huynh, MD
Department of Cardiothoracic and Vascular
Surgery
Memorial Hermann Hospital, The University of Texas at
Houston
Houston, Texas

Thomas H. Inge, MD, PHD
Associate Professor of Surgery and Pediatrics
Cincinnati Children's Hospital Medical Center
Cincinnati, Ohio

George L. Irvin, III, MD, FACS
Professor of Surgery
Chief, Endocrine Surgery
Miller School of Medicine
University of Miami
Miami, Florida

Brian Jacob, MD
Assistant Clinical Professor of Surgery
Department of Surgery
Mount Sinai Medical Center
New York, New York

Carlos Eduardo Jacob, MD, PHD
University of São Paulo School of
Medicine
São Paulo, Brazil

Bernard M. Jaffe, MD
Director of Surgical Research
Tulane Cancer Center
New Orleans, Lousiana

Jerry M. Jesseph, MD
Department of Surgery
Indiana University School of Medicine
Bloomington, Indiana

Blair A. Jobe, MD
Assistant Professor
Department of Surgery
Oregon Health and Science University;
Portland VA Medical Center
Portland, Oregon

Jeffrey L. Johnson, MD
Assistant Professor of Surgery
University of Colorado Health Sciences Center;
Director, Surgical Intensive Care
Denver Health Medical Center
Denver, Colorado

Scott Johnson, MD
Beth Israel Deaconess Medical Center
Boston, Massachusetts

Daniel B. Jones, MD
Associate Professor
Department of Surgery
Harvard Medical School;
Chief, Section for Minimally Invasive Surgery
Beth Israel Deaconess Medical Center
Boston, Massachusetts

Matthew B. Karlovsky, MD
Department of Urology
Banner Desert Medical Center
Mesa, Arizona

Karthikeshwar Kasirajan, MD FACS
Division of Vascular Surgery
Department of Surgery
Emory University School of Medicine
Atlanta, Georgia

Jan Kasperbauer, MD
Professor of Otolaryngology
Mayo Clinic
Rochester, Minnesota

Mukta V. Katdare, MD
Department of Surgery
University of Chicago
Chicago, Illinois

Louis R. Kavoussi, MD
The James Buchanan Brady Urological Institute
Johns Hopkins Medical Institutions
Baltimore, Maryland

Blair A. Keagy, MD
Chief, Vascular Surgery
University of North Carolina
Chapel Hill, North Carolina

Michael R. B. Keighley, MS FRCS
Professor of Surgery
Queen Elizabeth Hospital
Edgbaston, Birmingham, United Kingdom

T. Barry Kelleher, MB, MRCPI
Staff Physician
Division of Gastroenterology
Beth Israel Deaconess Medical Center;
Boston, Massachusetts

Mark C. Kelley, MD
Associate Professor
Department of Surgery
Vanderbilt University Medical Center
Chief
Division of Surgical Oncology
Vanderbilt-Ingram Cancer Center
Nashville, Tennessee

Keith A. Kelly, MD
Professor of Surgery Emeritus
Mayo College of Medicine
Rochester, Minnesota
Consultant in Surgery Emeritus
Mayo Clinic Arizona
Scottsdale, Arizona

Kent W. Kercher, MD
Department of Surgery
Carolinas Medical Center
Charlotte, North Carolina

Lalita Khaodhiar, MD
Instructor in Medicine
Department of Medicine
Harvard Medical School
Staff Physician
Department of Medicine
Beth Israel Deaconess Medical Center
Boston, Massachusetts

Young Bae Kim, MD
Director, Division of Gynecologic Oncology
Beth Israel Deaconess Medical Center;
Assistant Professor of Obstetrics, Gynecology and
* Reproductive Biology*
Harvard Medical School
Boston, Massachusetts

Masaki Kitajima, MD
Department of Surgery
School of Medicine
Keio University
Tokyo, Japan

W. John Kitzmiller, MD
Associate Professor and Chief of Plastic
* Surgery*
Department of Surgery
University of Cincinnati College of
* Medicine*
Chief, Division of Plastic Surgery
Department of Surgery
University Hospital
Cincinnati, Ohio

Mikel V. Knazev
Russia

Ira J. Kodner MD
Professor of Surgery
Washington University
St. Louis, Missouri

Alan J. Koffron, MD
Department of Surgery
Northwestern Memorial Hospital
Chicago, Illinois

Paul B. Kreienberg

Jake E.J. Krige, MD, FACS, FCS (SA),
** FRCS (ED)**
Associate Professor of Surgery
Department of Surgery
University of Cape Town Health Sciences Faculty and
* Surgical Gastroenterology*
Groote Schuur Hospital
Cape Town, South Africa

Irving L. Kron, MD
Professor and Chair
Department of Surgery
University of Virginia Health System
Charlottesville, Virginia

Helen Krontiras, MD
Section of Surgical Oncology
University of Alabama School of Medicine
Birmingham, Alabama

Robert D. Kugel, MD
Hernia Treatment Center Northwest
Olympia, Washington

Alan P. Kypson, MD, FACS
Assistant Professor of Surgery
Division of Cardiothoracic and Vascular Surgery
Brody School of Medicine
East Carolina University
Greenville, North Carolina

Fadi G. Lakkis, MD
Thomas E. Starzl Transplantation Institute
Department of Surgery
University of Pittsburgh Medical Center
Pittsburgh, Pennsylvania

Gregory J. Landry, MD
Division of Vascular Surgery
Oregon Health Sciences University
Portland, Oregon

David W. Larson, MD
Assistant Professor of Surgery
Division of Colorectal Surgery
Mayo Clinic
Rochester, Minnesota

Ian C. Lavery, MB, BS
The Cleveland Clinic Foundation
Cleveland, Ohio

Simon Law, MS, MA (Cantab), MB, BChir,
** FRCSED, FCSHK, FHKAM, FACS**
Professor of Surgery
University of Hong Kong Medical Centre
Queen Mary Hospital
Hong Kong, China

Anna M. Ledgerwood, MD
Professor
Department of Surgery
Wayne State University
Trauma Director
Department of Surgery
Detroit Receiving Hospital
Detroit, Michigan

Bernard Travis Lee, MD
Instructor in Surgery
Harvard Medical School
Division of Plastic Surgery
Department of Surgery
Beth Israel Deaconess Medical Center
Boston, Massachusetts

Jeffrey E. Lee, MD
Professor of Surgery
Department of Surgery
The University of Texas
Professor of Surgery
Department of Surgical Oncology
MD Anderson Cancer Center
Houston, Texas

W. Anthony Lee, MD
Associate Professor
Division of Vascular Surgery and Endovascular Therapy
Department of Surgery
University of Florida College of Medicine
Gainesville, Florida

Luis R. Leon, Jr., MD, RVT
Assistant Professor of Clinical Surgery
Department of Vascular Surgery
University of Arizona Health Sciences Center
Chief
Department of Vascular Surgery
Southern Arizona Veterans Affairs Health Care
* System*
Tucson, Arizona

Antoon E.M.R. Lerut, MD, PHD
Professor
Department of Surgery
Catholic University Chairman
Department of Thoracic Surgery
University Hospitals Leuven
Leuven, Belgium

O. Alex Lesani, MD
University Hospitals of Cleveland
Cleveland, Ohio

Keith D. Lillemoe, MD
Professor and Chairman
Department of Surgery
Indiana University
Chief of Surgery
Department of Surgery
Indiana University Hospital
Indianapolis, Indiana

Timothy K. Liem, MD
Division of Vascular Surgery
Oregon Health Sciences University
Portland, Oregon

Guilherme Lima
The James Buchanan Brady Urological Institute
Johns Hopkins Medical Institutions
Baltimore, Maryland

Philip A. Linden, MD
Harvard Medical School;
Associate Surgeon, Division of Thoracic Surgery
Brigham and Women's Hospital
Boston, Massachusetts

Fred N. Littooy, MD
Emeritus Professor
Department of Surgery
Loyola University Medical Center
Maywood, Illinois

Chi-Leung Liu, MB, BS
Department of Surgery
The University of Hong Kong
Queen Mary Hospital
Hong Kong, China

Chung-Mau Lo, MB, BS
Department of Surgery
The University of Hong Kong
Queen Mary Hospital
Hong Kong, China

Frank W. LoGerfo, MD
Distinguished William V. McDermott Professor of Surgery
Division of Vascular and Endovascular Surgery
Beth Israel Deaconess Medical Center
Boston, Massachusetts

Marios Loukas, MD, PHD
Associate Professor
Department of Anatomical Sciences
St. George's University
Grenada, West Indies
Department of Education and Development
Harvard Medical School
Boston, Massachusetts

Donald E. Low, MD
Head, Section General Thoracic Surgery
Virginia Mason Medical Center
Clinical Instructor
Department of Surgery
University of Washington School of Medicine
Seattle, Washington

Stephen F. Lowry, MD
Professor and Chairman
Department of Surgery
UMDNJ-Robert Wood Johnson Medical School
Attending Staff
Department of Surgery
Robert Wood Johnson University Hospital
New Brunswick, New Jersey

Charles E. Lucas, MD
Professor
Department of Surgery
Wayne State University
Detroit Receiving Hospital
Detroit, Michigan

James D. Luketich, MD
Professor of Surgery
Chief, Heart Lung Esophageal Surgery Institute
Chief, Division of Thoracic Surgery
Co-Director, Minimally Invasive Surgery Center
University of Pittsburgh Medical Center
Pittsburgh, Pennsylvania

Robyn A. Macsata, MD
Chief
Department of Vascular Surgery
Veterans Affairs Medical Center
Washington, District of Columbia

James A. Madura, MD
JS Battersby Professor of Surgery, Emeritus
Indiana University School of Medicine
Indianapolis, Indiana

James W. Maher, MD
Professor of Surgery
Head, Division of General Surgery
Virginia Commonwealth University
Medical College of Virginia Hospitals
Richmond, Virginia

Laurie Maidl, RN
Mayo Clinic
Rochester, Minnesota

Jose M. Martinez, MD
Assistant Professor of Surgery
Division of Laparoendoscopic and Bariatric
Surgery
The DeWitt Daughtry Family Department of
Surgery
University of Miami School of Medicine
Miami, Florida

Joseph Martz, MD
Assistant Professor
Department of Surgery
Attending Surgeon
Colorectal Service
Beth Israel Medical Center
New York, New York

Viraj A. Master, MD, PHD
Assistant Professor
Department of Urology
Emory University School of Medicine
Atlanta, Georgia

Douglas J. Mathisen, MD
Hermes C Grillo Professor of Thoracic
Surgery
Harvard Medical School
Chief, General Thoracic Surgery
Department of Surgery
Massachusetts General Hospital
Boston, Massachusetts

Jack W. McAninch, MD
Chief of Urology
San Francisco General Hospital
Vice Chair, Department of Urology
University of California - San Francisco
San Francisco, California

David A. McClusky, III, MD
Clinical Associate Professor
Department of Surgery
Emory University School of Medicine
Atlanta, Georgia

James F. McKinsey, MD
Site Chief, Division of Vascular Surgery
Columbia University Medical Center
Associate Professor of Clinical Surgery
Columbia University College of Physicians &
Surgeons
Adjunct Associate Professor
Weill Medical College of Cornell University
Assistant Attending Surgeon
New York-Presbyterian Hospital
New York, New York

Jonathan L. Meakins, OC, MD, DSC, FRCS (Hon),
FRCS (C,Glas)
Nuffield Professor of Surgery
Honorary Consultant
Nuffield Department of Surgery
Oxford University
John Radcliffe Hospital
Headington, Oxford
United Kingdom

Manish Mehta, MD, MPH
Institute for Vascular Health and Disease
Albany Medical College
Albany, New York

W. Scott Melvin, MD
Associate Professor of Surgery
Director, Center for Minimally Invasive Surgery
Director, Division of General Surgery
Ohio State University Medical Center
Columbus, Ohio

Robert R. Mendes, MD
Assistant Professor of Surgery
Division of Vascular Surgery
Assistant Professor of Radiology
Division of Interventional Radiology
University of North Carolina- Chapel Hill School of
Medicine
Chapel Hill, North Carolina

Ingrid M. Meszoely, MD
Assistant Professor
Department of Surgery
Vanderbilt University Medical Center
Director, Vanderbilt Breast Center
Division of Surgical Oncology
Vanderbilt-Ingram Cancer Center
Nashville, Tennessee

Fabrizio Michelassi, MD
Lewis Atterbury Stimson Professor
Chairman, Department of Surgery
Weill Medical College of Cornell University
New York, New York

Miroslav N. Milicevic, MD, PHD, FACS
Professor of Surgery
Institute for Digestive Diseases
Belgrade School of Medicine
University of Belgrade
Chief

Department VII–HPB Surgery
The First Surgical Clinic
Clinical Center of Serbia
Belgrade, Serbia

Charles C. Miller, III, PHD
Associate Professor
Chief, Division of Clinical Research and
Outcomes
Department of Cardiothoracic and Vascular Surgery
University of Texas-Houston, Health Science Center
Medical School
Houston, Texas

Matthew Todd Miller, MD
Senior Vascular Resident
Jobst Vascular Center
The Toledo Hospital
Toledo, Ohio

Petros Mirilas, MD, MSurg
Assistant Professor
Department of Anatomy, Neuroanatomy, and
Embryology
University of Crete Medical School
Heraklion, Crete, Greece

Gregory L. Moneta, MD
Professor
Department of Surgery
Chief, Division of Vascular Surgery
Oregon Health & Sciences University
Portland, Oregon

Stephen G. Moon, MD

Ernest E. Moore, MD
Professor and Vice Chair
Department of Surgery
University of Colorado HSC
Chief
Department of Surgery
Denver Health MC
Denver, Colorado

Francis D. Moore, Jr., MD
Professor
Department of Surgery
Harvard Medical School
Chief
Department of General and Gastrointestinal S
urgery
Brigham and Women's Hospital
Boston, Massachusetts

Wesley S. Moore, MD
Professor
Department of Surgery
Division of Vascular Surgery
University of California-Los Angeles
Gonda (Goldschmied) Vascular Center
Los Angeles, California

Christopher R. Morse, MD
Clinical Fellow in Cardiothoracic Surgery
Department of Surgery
Harvard University
Massachusetts General Hospital
Boston, Massachusetts

Mohammed Moursi, MD
Professor of Surgery
Department of Surgery
University of Arkansas for Medical Sciences
Chief, Vascular Surgery
John L. McClellam VAMC
Little Rock, Arkansas

Oliver J. Muensterer, MD
Department of Pediatric Surgery
Dr von Hauner Children's Hospital
University of Munich,
Munich, Germany

John T. Mullen, MD
Instructor of Surgery
Harvard Medical School
Division of Surgical Oncology
Beth Israel Deaconess Medical Center
Boston, Massachusetts

Kenric M. Murayama, MD
Associate Professor of Surgery
Northwestern University Medical School
Director, Minimally Invasive Surgery Program
Northwestern Memorial Hospital
Chicago, Illinois
Professor
Department of Surgery
Vice Chair, Clinical & Hospital Affairs
University of Hawaii
John A. Burns School of Medicine
Honolulu, Hawaii

Sudish C. Murthy, MD, PHD
Department of Thoracic and Cardiovascular
*   Surgery*
Cleveland Clinic Foundation
Cleveland, Ohio

Philippe Nafteux, MD
Department of Thoracic Surgery
University Hospitals Leuven
Leuven, Belgium

Joseph J. Naoum, MD
Clinical Instructor
Department of Surgery
The University of Texas Medical Branch
Galveston, Texas

Mark R. Nehler, MD
Associate Professor
Department of Surgery
University of Colorado Health Sciences Center
Denver, Colorado

Santhat Nivatvongs, MD
Professor of Surgery
Mayo Clinic College of Medicine
Consultant in Colon and Rectal Surgery
Mayo Clinic
Rochester, Minnesota

Mark Nogueira
The James Buchanan Brady Urological Institute
Johns Hopkins Medical Institutions
Baltimore, Maryland

Michael S. Nussbaum, MD, FACS
Professor and Interim Chair
Department of Surgery
University of Cincinnati
Chief of Staff
The University Hospital
Cincinnati, Ohio

Lloyd M. Nyhus, MD
Warren H. Cole Professor of Surgery Emeritus
University of Illinois at Chicago College of
*   Medicine*
Chicago, Illinois

Paul E. O'Brien, MD, FRACS
Director

The Centre for Obesity Research and Education
Monash University
Melbourne, Victoria
Head
The Centre for Bariatric Surgery
Windsor, Victoria
Australia

Shannon P. O'Brien, MD
Resident
Division of Plastic Surgery
University of Cincinnati
Cincinnati, Ohio

Michael P. O'Leary, MD
Associate Professor
Department of Surgery
Division of Urology
Brigham and Women's Hospital
Harvard Medical School
Boston, Massachusetts

Jill Ohland
Mayo Clinic
Rochester, Minnesota

Steven WM Olde Damink, MD, MSC, PHD
Surgeon, Gastrointestinal Surgery
Department of Surgery
University Hospital Maastricht
Maastricht, Netherlands

Keith T. Oldham, MD
Professor and Chief, Division of Pediatric Surgery
Department of Surgery
Medical College of Wisconsin
Marie Z. Uihlein Chair and Surgeon-in-Chief
Children's Hospital of Wisconsin
Milwaukee, Wisconsin

Frank G. Opelka, MD
Associate Dean for Healthcare Quality and
*   Safety*
Louisiana State University School of Medicine
New Orleans, Louisiana

Mark B. Orringer, MD
Professor
Head, Section of Thoracic Surgery
Department of Surgery
University of Michigan
Ann Arbor, Michigan

Kenneth Ouriel, MD
Chairman, Division of Surgery
Department of Vascular Surgery
Cleveland Clinic
Cleveland, Ohio

C. Keith Ozaki, MD
Associate Professor
Department of Surgery
University of Florida College of Medicine
Gainesville, Florida

Soji Ozawa, MD
Department of Surgery
School of Medicine
Keio University
Tokyo, Japan

Kathleen J. Ozsvath, MD
Assistant Professor of Surgery
Institute for Vascular Health and Disease
Albany Medical College
Albany, New York

Juan C. Parodi, MD
Professor of Surgery and Radiology
Washington University School of Medicine
St. Louis, Missouri

Philip S. K. Paty, MD
Associate Professor of Surgery
Institute for Vascular Health and Disease
Albany Medical College
Albany, New York

Benjamin B. Peeler, MD
Assistant Professor of Surgery
Surgical Director for the Virginia Children's Heart
*   Center*
Department of Thoracic Cardiovascular Surgery
University of Virginia Health System
Charlottesville, Virginia

John Pender, MD
Assistant Professor of Surgery
Brody School of Medicine
East Carolina University
Greenville, North Carolina

Rodrigo Oliva Perez, MD
Department of Surgery
University of São Paulo School of Medicine
São Paulo, Brazil

Jane Phillips-Hughes, Mb, Bch, MRCP, FRCR
Honorary Senior Lecturer
Nuffield Department of Surgery
Oxford University
Consultant
Department of Radiology
John Radcliffe Hospital
Headington, Oxford
United Kingdom

Jack R. Pickleman, MD
Maywood, Illinois

Antonio I. Picon, MD
Assistant Professor
Department of Surgery
Attending Surgeon
Gastro-Intestinal Surgery
Beth Israel Medical Center
New York, New York

Kenneth Todd Piercy, MD
Vascular Surgery Fellow
Section on Vascular and Endovascular Surgery
Surgical Sciences Division
Wake Forest University School of Medicine
North Carolina Baptist Hospital
Winston-Salem, North Carolina

C. Wright Pinson, MBA, MD
H. Wm. Scott Professor of Surgery
Hepatobiliary Surgery and Liver Transplantation
Vanderbilt School of Medicine
Associate Vice-Chancellor for Clinical Affairs
Vanderbilt University Medical Center
Nashville, Tennessee

Peter W. T. Pisters, MD
Professor of Surgery
Department of Surgical Oncology
University of Texas MD Anderson Cancer
*   Center*
Houston, Texas

Bertram Poch, MD, PD
Consultant Surgeon
Department of Visceral Surgery

Donauklinikum Neu-Ulm
Neu-Ulm, Germany

Raymond Pollak, MD, FRCS, FACS
Medical Director
Center for Clinical Trials
Edward Hospital
Naperville, Illinois

Alfons Pomp, MD
Associate Professor
Department of Surgery
Weill Medical College of Cornell University
Attending Surgeon
New York Presbyterian Hospital
Cornell Medical Center
New York, New York

Frank B. Pomposelli, Jr., MD
Associate Professor of Surgery
Harvard Medical School
Beth Israel Deaconess Medical Center
Boston, Massachusetts

Jeffrey L. Ponsky, MD
Professor and Chairman
Department of Surgery
Case Western Reserve University School of Medicine
Cleveland, Ohio

Eyal E. Porat, MD
Department of Cardiothoracic and Vascular Surgery
Memorial Hermann Hospital
The University of Texas at Houston
Houston, Texas

Walter J. Pories, MD
Professor of Surgery, Biochemistry, Exercise and Sport
Science
Brody School of Medicine
East Carolina University
Greenville, North Carolina

Richard J. Powell, MD
Department of Surgery
Section of Vascular Surgery
Dartmouth-Hitchcock Medical Center
Lebanon, New Hampshire

Trent Prault, MD
Vascular Surgery Fellow
Department of Vascular Surgery
University of Tennessee Graduate School of Medicine
University of Tennessee Medical Center
Knoxville, Tennessee

Richard A. Prinz, MD
Helen Shedd Keith Professor and Chairman
Department of General Surgery
Program Director - Rush University General Surgery
Residency Program
Rush-Presbyterian-St. Luke's Medical Center
Chicago, Illinois
Voluntary Attending Physician
Department of General Surgery
Cook County Hospital
Chicago, Illinois
Courtesy/Provisional Staff
Department of Surgery
Oak Park Hospital
Oak Park, Illinois

Igor Proscurshim, MS
Department of Surgery
University of São Paulo School of
Medicine
São Paulo, Brazil

Alessandra Puggioni, MD
Fellow, Division of Vascular Surgery
Mayo Clinic
Rochester, Minnesota

Roderick M. Quiros, MD
Department of General Surgery
Rush-Presbyterian-St. Luke's Medical Center
Chicago, Illinois

Faisal G. Qureshi, MD
Pediatric Surgery Fellow
Childrens Hospital of Los Angeles
Los Angeles, California

Hammad N. Qureshi, MB, BS, MD
Research Fellow
Department of Minimally Invasive Surgery
Beth Israel Medical Center
New York, New York
Surgery Resident
Department of Surgery
Metropolitan Group of Hospitals
University of Illinois
Chicago, Illinois

Janice F. Rafferty, MD
Associate Professor
Chief
Division of Colon and Rectal Surgery
University of Cincinnati College of Medicine
Cincinnati, Ohio

Bruce Ramshaw, MD
Associate Professor
Department of Surgery
Chief, Division of General Surgery
University of Missouri- Columbia School of
Medicine
Columbia, Missouri

David Rattner, MD
Professor of Surgery
Harvard Medical School
Department of Surgery
Massachusetts General Hospital
Boston, Massachusetts

Bettina M. Rau, MD, PD **Consultant Surgeon**
Consultant Surgeon
Department of General, Visceral and Vascular Surgeon
University of the Saarland
Homburg, Germany

Feza H. Remzi, MD
Department of Colorectal Surgery
The Cleveland Clinic Foundation
Cleveland, Ohio

Martin I. Resnick, MD
Chairman, Department of Urology
University Hospitals
Lester Persky Professor
Case Western Reserve University
Director, Residency Program
UH Case Medical Center
Cleveland, Ohio

William O. Richards, MD
Professor of Surgery
Vanderbilt University School of Medicine
Director of Laparoendoscopic General Surgery
Vanderbilt University School of Medicine
Staff Surgeon
Chief of Surgical Endoscopy and Laser Surgery
Veterans Administration Medical Center
Nashville, Tennessee

David A. Rigberg, MD
Assistant Professor of Surgery
Division of Vascular Surgery
University of California-Los Angeles Medical
Center
Los Angeles, California

Layton F. Rikkers, MD
Professor and Chair
Department of Surgery
University of Wisconsin—Madison School of Medicine
and Public Health
Madison, Wisconsin

Sean P. Roddy, MD
Associate Professor of Surgery
Albany Medical College
Attending Vascular Surgeon
Albany Medical Center Hospital
Albany, New York

Alexander S. Rosemurgy, II, MD, FACS
Professor of Surgery
Professor of Medicine
Division of General Surgery
University of South Florida
Director
Department of Surgical Digestive Disorders
Tampa General Hospital
Tampa, Florida

Michael J. Rosen, MD
Carolinas Laparoscopic and Advanced Surgery Program
Carolinas Medical Center
Charlotte, North Carolina

James C. Rosser, Jr., MD
Chief, Minimally Invasive Surgery
Director, Advanced Medical Technology Institute
Beth Israel Medical Center
New York, New York

David A. Rothenberger, MD
Program Co-Leader, Translational Research Program
Member, Transplant Biology and Therapy Research
Program
Deputy Chairman and Professor, Department of Surgery
John P. Delaney, M.D. Chair in Clinical Surgical
Oncology
Associate Director for Clinical Research and Programs
University of Minnesota Cancer Center
University of Minnesota Medical School
Minneapolis, Minnesota

Aaron Ruhalter, MD, FACS
Professor of Anatomy
Professor of Surgery
Volunteer Faculty
University of Cincinnati College of Medicine
Cincinnati, Ohio

Robb H. Rutledge, MD
Fort Worth, Texas

Frederick C. Ryckman, MD
Professor of Surgery
Director, Liver Transplant
Surgical Director, Intestinal Transplant Surgery
Department of Pediatric Surgery
Pediatric Liver Care Center
Cincinnati Children's Hospital Medical Center
University of Cincinnati
Cincinnati, Ohio

Hazim J. Safi, MD
Professor and Chairman
Department of Cardiothoracic and Vascular Surgery

The University of Texas at Houston Medical School
Houston, Texas

Atef A. Salam, MD
Professor of Surgery
Emory University School of Medicine
Chief of Vascular Service
Atlanta VA Medical Center
Atlanta, Georgia

Martin G. Sanda, MD
Associate Professor of Surgery
Division of Urology
Department of Surgery
Harvard Medical School
Beth Israel Deaconess Medical Center
Boston, Massachusetts

Lee J. Sanders, DPM
Adjunct Clinical Professor
Department of Podiatric Medicine
Temple University School of Podiatric Medicine
Philadelphia, Pennsylvania
Chief Podiatry Service
Acute Care & Specialty Services
VA Medical Center
Lebanon, Pennsylvania

John L. Sawyers, MD
Foshee Distinguished Professor of Surgery, Emeritus
Vanderbilt University Medical Center
Nashville, Tennessee

Philip R. Schauer, MD
Director, Advanced Laparoscopic and Bariatric Surgery
Department of General Surgery
Cleveland Clinic Foundation
Cleveland, Ohio

Marc Schermerhorn, MD
Assistant Professor
Department of Surgery
Harvard Medical School
Beth Israel Deaconess Medical Center
Boston, Massachusetts

Bruce David Schirmer, MD
Professor of Surgery
Department of Surgery
Division of General Surgery
University of Virginia Health System
Charlottesville, Virginia

Benjamin E. Schneider, MD
Instructor in Surgery
Beth Israel Deaconess Medical Center
Harvard Medical School
Boston, Massachusetts

Richard Schutzer, MD
Division of Vascular Surgery
Department of Surgery
Maimonides Medical Center
Brooklyn, New York

Steven D. Schwaitzberg, MD
Chief of Surgery
Cambridge Health Alliance
Cambridge Hospital
Cambridge, Massachusetts

J. Stephen Scott, MD
Associate Professor of Clinical Surgery
Department of General Surgery
University of Missouri- Columbia School of
*   Medicine*
Columbia, Missouri

Sherry D. Scovell, MD
Instructor in Surgery
Beth Israel Deaconess Medical Center
Boston, Massachusetts

Andrew J. E. Seely, MD, PHD
Divisions of Thoracic Surgery & Critical Care Medicine
Assistant Professor, University of Ottawa
Associate Scientist, Ottawa Hospital Research Institute
The Ottawa Hospital - General Campus
Ottawa, Ontario, Canada

Evelyn G. Serrano, MD
Resident
Department of Obstetrics & Gynecology
University of South Florida
Tampa, Florida

Dhiraj M. Shah, MD
Professor of Surgery
Albany Medical College
Director, The Institute for Vascular Health and Disease
Albany Medical Center Hospital
Albany, New York

Jatin P. Shah, MD
Professor of Surgery
Department of Surgery
Weill Cornell University Medical College
Chief, Head and Neck Service
Elliot w. Strong Chair in Head and Neck Oncology
Department of Surgery
Memorial Sloan-Kettering Cancer Center
New York, New York

David S. Shapiro, MD

Gregorio A. Sicard, MD
Vice Chairman and Professor of Surgery
Chief, Division of General Surgery and Section of
*   Vascular Surgery*
Washington University School of Medicine
St. Louis, Missouri

Anton N. Sidawy, MD
Professor of Surgery
Georgetown University Medical Center
George Washington Medical Center
Chief
Department of Surgery
Veterans Affairs Medical Center
Washington, District of Columbia

J. Rüdiger Siewert, MD
Chirurgische Klinik und Poliklinik
Technical University of Munich
Munich, Germany

Hector Simosa, MD
Department of Surgery
Beth Israel Deaconess Medical Center
Boston, Massachusetts

John E. Skandalakis, MD, PHD
Professor of Surgery
Chris Carlos Distinguished Professor of Surgical
*   Anatomy & Technique*
Director, The Thalia and Michael Carlos Center for
*   Surgical Anatomy & Technique*
Director, The Alfred A. Davis Research Center for
*   Surgical Anatomy & Technique*
Emory University School of Medicine
Clinical Professor of Surgery
The Medical College of Georgia
Senior Attending Surgeon
Piedmont Hospital
Atlanta, Georgia

Lee J. Skandalakis, MD
Clinical Associate Professor of Surgical Anatomy
and Technique
Centers for Surgical Anatomy and Technique
Emory University School of Medicine
Atlanta, Georgia

Panajiotis N. Skandalakis, MD, MS
Clinical Associate Professor
Centers for Surgical Anatomy and Technique
Emory University School of Medicine
Atlanta, Georgia

Donald G. Skinner, MD
Professor and Chair, Department of Urology
Hanson-White Chair in Medical Research
University of Southern California
Keck School of Medicine
Los Angeles, California

Stephen L. Smith, MD
Associate Professor
Department of Surgery
Mayo Clinic
Consultant
Department of Surgery
St. Luke's Hospital
Jacksonville, Florida

Neel R. Sodha, MD
The Department of Surgery and the Division of
*   Cardiothoracic Surgery*
Beth Israel Deaconess Medical Center;
Hrvard Medical School
Boston, Massachusetts

Peter B. Soeters, MD, PHD
Professor Emeritus
Department of Surgery
University of Maastricht
Chief Gastrointestinal Surgery
Department of General Surgery
Academic Hospital Maastricht
Maastricht, The Netherlands

Joseph Solomkin, MD
Professor of Surgery
Surgery-Trauma/Critical Care
University of Cincinnati
Cincinnati, Ohio

Carmen C. Solorzano, MD, FACS
Assistant Professor of Surgery
Section of Endocrine Surgery
Miller School of Medicine
University of Miami
Miami, Florida

Patsy S.H. Soon, MD
Edinburgh Breast Unit
Western General Hospital
Edinburgh, United Kingdom

Nathaniel J. Soper, MD
Professor
Department of Surgery
Northwestern University of Medicine, Feinberg
*   School*
Interim Chair
Department of Surgery
Northwestern Memorial Hospital
Chicago, Illinois

Armando C. Soto, MD
Department of Plastic and Reconstructive Surgery
Mercy Medical Center
Baltimore, Maryland

William Spellacy, MD
University of South Florida
Tampa, Florida

Sasha Stamenkovic, MD
Department of Thoracic Surgery
University Hospitals Leuven
Leuven, Belgium

James C. Stanley, MD
Section of Vascular Surgery
Alfred Taubman Health Care Center
University of Michigan Health System
Ann Arbor Michigan

Thomas E. Starzl, MD, PHD
Thomas E. Starzl Transplantation Institute
Department of Surgery
University of Pittsburgh Medical Center
Pittsburgh, Pennsylvania

John P. Stein, MD
Associate Professor of Urology
University of Southern California;
Norris Comprehensive Cancer Center
Los Angeles, California

René E. Stoppa, MD
Service de Clinique Chirurgicale Universitaire
Amiens, France

Steven M. Strasberg, MD
Head of HPB/GI Surgery
Washington University School of Medicine
St. Louis, Missouri

Li-Ming Su, MD
Associate Professor of Urology
James Buchanan Brady Urological Institute
Johns Hopkins Medical Institutions
Baltimore, Maryland

David J. Sugarbaker, MD
The Richard E. Wilson Professor of Surgical Oncology
Harvard Medical School;
Chief, Division of Thoracic Surgery
Brigham and Women's Hospital;
Philip E. Lowe Senior Surgeon
Dana Farber Cancer Institute
Boston, Massachusetts

Timothy M. Sullivan, MD, FACS
Professor of Surgery
Director, Endovascular Practice of the Division of Vascular
Surgery
Mayo Clinic
Rochester, Minnesota

Tamara Takoudes, MD
Department of Obstetrics, Gynecology and Reproductive
Biology
Beth Israel Deaconess Medical Center
Boston, Massachusetts

Eric P. Tamm, MD
Associate Professor
Department of Diagnostic Radiology
University of Texas MD Anderson Cancer Center
Houston, Texas

Lloyd M. Taylor, Jr., MD
Division of Vascular Surgery
Oregon Health Sciences University
Portland, Oregon

Sumeet S. Teotia, MD
Department of Surgery

Mayo Clinic
Rochester, Minnesota

Oreste Terranova, MD
Professor of Surgery
Department of Surgical and Gastroenterological
*   Sciences*
Univerita degli Studi di Padova
Ospedal Civile
Padova, Italy

Erwin R. Thal, MD
Professor
Department of Surgery
University of Texas Southwestern Medical Center
Staff Surgeon
Department of Surgery
Parkland Memorial Hospital
Dallas, Texas

Sarah K. Thompson, MD
Upper Gastrointestinal Surgery Fellow
Department of Surgery
University of Adelaide
Royal Adelaide Hospital
Adelaide, South Australia

Greg M. Tiao, MD
Assistant Professor of Surgery
Department of Pediatric Surgery
University of Cincinnati
Children's Hospital Medical Center
Cincinnati, Ohio

Adam M. Tobias, MD
Instructor in Surgery
Department of Surgery
Harvard Medical School
Attending Physician
Department of Surgery
Beth Israel Deaconess Medical Center
Boston, Massachusetts

Desmond Toomey, MB, MRCS
Research Fellow
Professorial Surgical Unit
The University of Dublin
Trinity College Dublin
The Adelaide and Meath Hospital
Dublin, Ireland

Jonathan B. Towne, MD
Professor and Chief
Division of Vascular Surgery
Medical College of Wisconsin
Milwaukee, Wisconsin

Courtney M. Townsend, Jr., MD
Department of Surgery
The University of Texas Medical Branch
Galveston, Texas

Tin C. Tran, MD
ERCP Fellow
Department of Surgery
University of Louisville
Louisville, Kentucky

L. William Traverso, MD
Department of General Surgery
Virginia Mason Medical Center
Seattle, Washington

Jorge M. Treviño, MD
Texas Endosurgery Institute
San Antonio, Texas

Donald D. Trunkey, MD
Professor

Department of Surgery
Oregon Health and Science University
Protland, Oregan

Ronald B. Turner, MD
Professor
Department of Pediatrics
University of Virginia
Charlottesville, Virginia

Gilbert R. Upchurch, Jr., MD, FACS
Department of Surgery
Alfred Taubman Health Care Center
University of Michigan Health System
Ann Arbor, Michigan

Joseph Upton, MD
Associate Clinical Professor of Surgery
Department of Surgery
Beth Israel Deaconess Medical Center
Senior Surgeon
Department of Surgery
Children's Hospital Boston
Boston, Massachusetts

Wim G. van Gemert, MD, PHD
Associate Professor
Department of Surgery
University of Maastricht
Staff Surgeon
Department of Surgery
University Hospital Maastricht
Maastricht, The Netherlands

Jonathan A. van Heerden, MD
Department of Surgery
University of Miami School of Medicine
Miami, Florida

Michael van Noord, MD

Dirk Van Raemdonck, MD
Department of Thoracic Surgery
University Hospitals Leuven
Leuven, Belgium

Luis O. Vásconez, MD
Professor and Chief
Division of Plastic Surgery
University of Alabama at Birmingham
Birmingham, Alabama

Dionysios K. Veronikis, MD
St. Johns Mercy Medical Center
St. Louis, Missouri

Eric Vibert, MD
Hospital Paul Brousse
CHB
Villejuif, France

Gary C. Vitale, MD
Professor of Surgery
Department of Surgery
University of Louisville
Director of Centerof Pancreas,
*   Liver and Billary Tract Disease*
Endoscopy Center
Norton Hospital
Louisville, Kentucky

Guy Voeller, MD
Mid-South Center for Minimally Invasive Surgery
Memphis, Tennessee

Charles M. Vollmer, Jr., MD
Department of Surgery
Harvard Medical School;

Attending Surgeon
Beth Israel Deaconess Medical Center
Boston, Massachusetts

Andrew A. Wagner, MD
Instructor of Urology Surgery
Department of Surgery
Harvard Medical School
Director of Minimally Invasive Urologic Surgery
Department of Surgery
Beth Israel Deaconess Medical Center
Boston, Massachusetts

Brad W. Warner, MD
Professor
Department of Surgery
University of Cincinnati College of Medicine
Attending Surgeon
Division of Pediatric General and Thoracic Surgery
Cincinnati Children's Hospital Medical Center
Cincinnati, Ohio

Andrew L. Warshaw, MD
W. Gerald Austen Professor of Surgery
Harvard Medical School;
Head of Department of Surgery
Massachusetts General Hospital
Boston, Massachusetts

David I. Watson, MD, MBBS, FRACS
Professor and Head
Department of Surgery
Flinders University
Head
Gastrointestinal Services
Flinders Medical Center
South Australia
Australia

Jon O. Wee, MD
Department of Surgery
Brigham and Women's Hospital
Boston, Massachusetts

Martin R. Weiser, MD
Assistant Attending
Department of Surgery, Colorectal Division
Memorial Sloan-Kettering Cancer Center
New York, New York

Akuezunkpa O. Welcome, MD
Asst. Professor of Surgery
Columbia University College of Physicians and
Surgeons
New York, New York

Samuel A. Wells, Jr., MD, FACS
Department of Surgery
Duke University School of Medicine
Durham, North Carolina

Lisa A. Whitty, MD
Department of Surgery
University of Illinois College of Medicine
at Peoria
Peoria, Illinois

Samuel E. Wilson, MD
Department of General Surgery
University of California at Irvine Medical
Center
Orange, California

Bruce G. Wolff, MD
Division of Colon and Rectal Surgery
Mayo Clinic
Rochester, Minnesota

John Wong, MB, BS, MD (Hon), PHD, FACS
(Hon.)
Professor and Head
Department of Surgery
University of Hong Kong Medical
Centre
Queen Mary Hospital
Hong Kong, China

Richard A. Yeager, MD
Professor
Department of Surgery
Oregon Health and Science University
Chief
Department of Vascular Surgery
Portland VA Medical Center
Portland, Oregon

Tonia M. Young-Fadok, BM, BCH, MS, FACS,
FASCRS
Associate Professor of Surgery
Mayo Clinic College of Medicine;
Chair, Division of Colon and Rectal Surgery
Mayo Clinic
Scottsdale, Arizona

Jonathan S. Zager, MD
Fellow
Department of Surgical Oncology
University of Texas M.D. Anderson Cancer
Center
Houston, Texas

Christopher K. Zarins, MD
Professor of Surgery
Stanford University School of
Medicine
Stanford, California

Preface: Mastery of Surgery: Fifth Edition

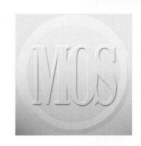

I am delighted to write the preface for the fifth edition of *Mastery of Surgery*. I am indebted to the distinguished predecessors who were kind enough to include me in the third edition many years ago. I learned the craft of being the editor of these volumes at the feet of the masters.

It is interesting to look back at my surgical career beginning in July 1961, when I embarked on my training at the Massachusetts General Hospital while Dr. Churchill was still the chief. Dr. Churchill, of course, is the originator of the rectangular residency program, which is the dominant type of residency program that survives today. It is appropriate to point out that the Halsteadian residency program of graduated responsibility, for which Dr. Halstead appropriately gets credit, was a Germanic, elitist approach in which there was a sharp pyramid. Those who survived it were destined to become professors of surgery and leaders in the surgical field. However, as distinguished as the individuals who graduated from the Hopkins program were, the program did not and had no intention of populating the field of surgery for the needs of the patients of the United States. In addition, although those who failed the sharp pyramid were often placed in excellent programs in which the chiefs were graduates of the Halstead program, depression, anguish, and the stress of being cut from the excellent Hopkins program took its toll on those who did not make the grade. Dr. Churchill, who has many firsts in American surgery, thought that the most important thing he did was to organize the rectangular residency. He had the novel concept that he could choose which fourth year medical students would satisfy the rigid and rigorous criteria that the Massachusetts General Hospital program became.

It is amusing to recall the orientation that I underwent compared to the present. The orientation of our own surgical program is 5 days long; it includes ACLS training, and the residents are also exposed to the head of the laundry, social work, etc. All of this is important but pales in comparison to Dr. Churchill's orientation at noon on July 1, 1961, in which he looked at us, smiled, and said: "Get to work."

I am indebted to those who have been my mentors over the years, including Dr. Claude Welch, the Dean of Boston Surgeons; Dr. Robert Ritchie Linton, whose understanding of liver physiology was intuitive and based on hunches, yet almost always correct because he was such a superb clinician; Dr. William V. McDermott Jr., another mentor who inspired me prior to going to the National Institutes of Health as a research associate for two years, and whose named chair I now hold; Dr. George Nardi, who later became my partner, a delightful and innovative surgeon who made surgery interesting for himself and the residents who assisted him; Dr. Churchill who is among the wisest people I have ever met; later Dr. W. Gerald Austen, under whom I served as his first chief resident; and also my friends and mentors, Dr. Leslie Otinger and Dr. Ashby Moncure, who preceded me as the super-chief.

A critical period of my development was when I went to the National Institute of Mental Health as a research associate (1 of 20). The NIH had put together a fantastic educational program, and I had the privilege of working with Dr. Irwin Kopin, who had just finished a tour in the laboratory with Dr. Julius Axelrod, who later won the Nobel Prize for work that preceded my tenure. Also I was blessed to have a series of excellent technicians, among whom was Dr. Dale Horst, a conscientious objector who became a distinguished pharmacologist in his own right and who was extremely helpful.

Absence makes the heart grow fonder, yes, but it also enhanced my knowledge base. My wife to be, Karen, was still in Boston, so after putting in a 12-hour day at the laboratory, my idea of having a good time was to go to the library and read some of the wonderful classics of surgery; journals, that are not available on the internet, laid the groundwork for my physiologic approach to the practice of surgery.

But enough about me. What is it about this edition that is different? The concept of *Mastery of Surgery,* especially in the first edition was to take advantage of Dr. Nyhus' many contacts abroad and make *Mastery of Surgery* a truly international work. That generation is now no longer on the scene, and what I have tried to do in this edition is restore some of the international flavor from authorities in many countries. Communications being what they are, many of these individuals are well-known to those who will read this book and who see them at meetings such as the Clinical Congress of the American College of Surgeons and at the American Surgical. Thus, the reader will note that the number of international authorities who have contributed to this volume has been increased.

Much has changed in the 5 or 6 years since the fourth edition appeared. Minimally invasive surgery has had a profound effect on general, vascular, cardiac, and thoracic surgery. Minimally invasive technology and approaches have improved. Who is a candidate for the classic big incision open approach? Market forces certainly enter—"smaller is better." For example, witness the limited patient population which is now set for open renal atherectomy for arteriosclerotic disease. Despite the fact that long-term patency is considerably better in the open approach, the mortality of the open approach is not necessarily inferior to that of the endovascular approach. Randomized prospective trials have not yet been done in many areas in which laparoscopic is compared with open surgery. True, the length of stay is usually shorter, days on the respirator in the ICU may be shorter, but it is interesting that the mortality in this group, with many comorbidities, may not be different between open and minimally invasive approach, while the long-term patency seems to be considerably greater. The question of who is a candidate for open and who is a candidate for a minimally invasive approach has not yet been answered. Hopefully by the time the next edition appears, this will have been subjected to rigid randomized clinical trials to produce an evidence based decision. What we have now is bias—a smaller incision is better, even if long-term results are not quite as good.

Evidence based surgery and its emphasis is apparent throughout this volume.

The importance in surgery is outcomes. This is made clear in "pay for performance" accreditation efforts by the American College of Surgeons, and the widespread application of the National Surgical Quality Improvement Program, which not only showed how to improve surgical outcomes in the Veteran's Administration Hospital, but has now been rolled out to more than 200 hospitals,. The emphasis is not only on observed versus expected, which is risk adjusted, but also contains programs for improving outcomes. In internal medicine, pay for performance remains largely process oriented. For example, in internal medicine, pay for performance includes asking a patient to stop smoking. If this were a surgical pay for performance issue, it would likely deal with the outcome: Did the patient stop smoking or did the patient not stop smoking? The administration of perioperative antibiotics is an example of process. We should be concerned about surgical site infection as an outcome, which not only includes perioperative antibiotics but clipping versus shaving, hibiclens scrub for a few days before the operations, and a whole series of other perioperative issues, which will help determine the incidence of surgical site infection.

In a number of other fairly common areas the emphasis has changed based in part on randomized clinical trials in areas such as hernias. If one compares emphasis in the fourth edition between various repairs, the emphasis was on recurrence. While the emphasis on recurrence remains, there is an entirely new area which concerns surgeons: inguinodynia or post herniorhaphy pain. James Madura has written an excellent chapter concerning nerve entrapment, which while not exclusively the province of mesh repairs, nonetheless, has a much lower incidence in open repairs that do not include mesh. In the area of pilonidal sinus and abscess, a very common condition for which surgical attention is sought, there is now accumulating evidence that personal hygiene, removal of hair from the sinus, depilatories, as well as laser treatment in the peripilonidal sinus area may be as or more effective than excision and primary closure of pilonidal sinus.

Another innovation in this book which I think has yielded excellent results is the appointment of an associate editor, Dr. Kirby Bland, who has ably assisted in the identification of authors and in the commentary on surgical oncologic procedures. Assistant Editors Dr. Mark Callery in the hepatobiliary area and Dr. Dan

Jones in the laparoscopic area have helped immensely not only in selecting the authors, but in writing cogent commentaries on the chapters. The explosion of the vascular field, including the proliferation of the endovascular techniques in which the technology is improving and the results are improving with it, has necessitated more in the vascular area including endovascular and open. Dr. Frank LoGerfo helped identify the authors; Drs. Patrick Clagett and James Seeger have been extraordinarily helpful.

The length of the book has necessitated that additional chapters appear on the Web site. Most of these are chapters of historical interest. Additional chapters of interest are those in the gynecological and the urological area, mostly in the area of oncology. The superb approaches utilizing general surgical techniques will be of interest to surgical residents and practicing surgeons alike.

Those of you who have participated in putting together a surgical volume with any number of chapters understand what a tremendous effort and how time consuming it is. I have many individuals to thank. First and foremost, Karen, my wife of 41 years and companion of 46 years, had to endure this time-consuming effort of the past 2 or 3 years, which was also associated with service on the Residency Review Committee, leaving little time for us. Her patience, wisdom, guidance, and love always leave me very grateful for what she has done for my life. My children, Erich and Alexandra, have been squeezed in between these efforts and although they are grown, have their own careers, and are no longer at home, we remain a very close family.

The group at Lippincott headed by Brian Brown has been wonderful to work with; Julia Seto, the Senior Managing Editor, and a group of artists who have translated sometimes crude sketches into excellent artwork. They have all taken my suggestions with patience and good humor and are an extraordinarily talented group of people.

A work such as this does not take place in a vacuum. My office staff has been long suffering, including Iliana Ferguson, Deborah Cruise, Luisa Dello Iacono, and the production/transcription staff, including Anja Duprat, Karen Nehilla, Abigail Smith, and briefly, Stephanie Vrattos.

Time spent on this detracts from my ability to participate and help manage what I consider a superb department of extraordinary surgeons gathered under one roof. I am ably assisted by a series of Senior Faculty members who all pitch in in a "kitchen cabinet" to take some of the pressure off of me, including, in no particular order: Dr. Chip Baker, who serves as Program Director; Dr. Jon Critchlow, who is Associate Program Director; Dr. Scott Johnson and Dr. Alan Hammond as Assistant Program Directors; Dr. Mike Cahalane who is in charge of the surgical clerkship; also a series of talented Senior Vice Chairs including, Dr. Malcolm DeCamp, Dr. Douglas Hanto, Dr. James Hurst, Dr. Callery who serves as chief of General Surgery, and Dr. Donald Moorman, Vice Chair for Safety and Quality. I would be remiss if I did not mention my alter ego, Pat Thurston, the director of the department, business manager, factotum, and person of all work, who takes an enormous amount of pressure off of me. The residents also allow me to do other things as they give superb surgical care.

I have gone on for some time, but a two volume book of 239 chapters does not happen with a sole effort. It is an extraordinarily time-consuming team effort, and I have been privileged to have such an excellent team surround me.

Josef E. Fischer, M.D.

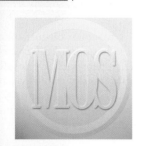

Web-Only Chapters

Chapter 11: Stapling Techniques in Operations on the GI Tract
Iliya M. Buriev and Mikel V. Knazev

The Russians are the originators of the stapling devices. I thought it would be interesting to have an exposition of the current Russian stapling techniques because the instruments are somewhat different than ours, and the techniques are somewhat different than ours because of the instruments that are utilized.

This is an extensive chapter with a number of techniques that are portrayed which should be of interest.

Chapter 21: The Parotid Gland
Kirby I. Bland

The anatomy of the parotid gland is also covered in other areas in the book. However, in many situations, the parotid gland is the province of the plastic surgeon or the general surgeon. The experience of most surgeons in dealing with masses, which could be a tumor of the parotid gland, is not usually current and thus they tend put off dealing with the situation. Hopefully a well-done exposition of the parotid glad as done in this chapter will help.

Chapter 29: Resection of Larynx and Pharynx for Cancer
Jerry R. Castro and Jatin P. Shah

This is a new chapter done kindly by Dr. Jatin Shah, who agreed to do this at the last minute when the original author could not deliver. We are greatly indebted to Dr. Shah who is one of the masters of the field. However, it arrived too late to put in the fabric of the book and thus it is on the website. In the next edition it will appear in the book itself.

Chapter 48: Thoracic Incisions
Sudish C. Murthy and Malcolm M. DeCamp, Jr.

Dr. Malcolm DeCamp and Sudish Murthy have written an excellent chapter, which similarly arrived too late to be included in the book. This is an important chapter and thus it is important to know the various approaches within the thorax, repair of the chest wall as elucidated by one of the masters of thoracic surgery.

Chapter 73: Selective Vagotomy, Antrectomy, and Gastroduodenostomy for the Treatment of Duodenal Ulcer
Lloyd M. Nyhus

Selective vagotomy, antrectomy and gastroduodenostomy for the treatment of duodenal ulcer is an operation that is no longer done. Very frequently parietal cell vagotomy has largely supplanted selective vagotomy, but antrectomy and gastroduodenostomy are useful for carcinoma of the stomach with some slight modifications as pictured elsewhere in the book. This is a classic chapter, and it is included for historical reasons but also because Dr. Nyhus, one of the originators of *Mastery of Surgery* wrote a superb chapter. It can be read with profit.

Chapter 74: Selective Vagotomy and Pyloroplasty
Steven D. Schwaitzberg, John L. Sawyers, and William O. Richards

Dr. Steven Schwaitzberg has written an excellent chapter on selective vagotomy and pyloroplasty. However, as Dr. Schwaitzberg pointed out to me himself, this is an operation that is no longer done very frequently, if at all. However, it is a chapter that elucidates some points concerning surgery of the stomach, unfortunately no longer carried out with any great degree of regularity. It is a chapter that can be read with significant profit.

Chapter 86: Bariatric Surgery
Walter J. Pories and John Pender

This chapter, written by Dr. Walter Pories was intended to be solely concerning the complications of bariatric surgery. It did, however, include a number of other aspects of bariatric surgery, many of which had already been covered in the book. Thus, but owing to the length of the book, it was decided that this would be best seen on the website. It deals with bariatric surgery in general by one of the most experienced bariatric surgeons currently practicing.

Chapter 94A: Echinococcal Cysts: Etiology
E. Moreno González, J. C. Meneu Díaz, and A. Moreno Elola

Dr. Moreno-Gonzalez is one of the foremost liver surgeons in Europe and certainly in the world. He is a vigorous, indefatigable surgeon with a huge practice and tremendous technical abilities (having watched some of his videos myself) and with an enormous following. His approach to echinococcal cysts, which is seen in Chapter 94, led the way to the current thinking of the treatment of echinococcal cysts, that is, not unroofing the cysts and draining it but actual excision.

Although this subject was covered by another chapter by design by another author, Dr. Moreno-Gonzalez' contribution in this area is highly significant and therefore is included in the website as well.

Chapter 124: Intestinal Bypass for Hypercholesterolemia
Henry Buchwald

The Intestinal Bypass for Hypercholesterolemia by Dr. Henry Buchwald is one of the classics of surgical investigation involving basic science, clinical excellence and clinical acumen. In the years prior to the statins, intestinal bypass as practiced by Dr. Buchwald and his group remained one of the efficacious ways to deal with patients with hypercholesterolemia who could not be dealt with in any other way. It is a randomized prospective trial which is extraordinarily well done with long-term follow up and which yields a statistically significant improvement in lifespan.

As Dr. Buchwald himself points out, there still is a place for this operation, rarely in the era of the statins, for example, patients who do not wish to take pills and would prefer an oper-

ation. It is meticulously described and meticulously carried out with excellent surgical results and still can be read with profit.

Chapter 140A: Abdominoperineal Resection (The Miles Operation)
Ira J. Kodner and Janice F. Rafferty

The new colon and rectal surgery, as practiced by some of the advanced colorectal surgeons in many of the major centers around the world, deals with attempts to maintain rectal function under circumstances such as invasion of the sphincter, lesions that go to within three centimeters of the anal verge in an effort to maintain some rectal function and avoid a colostomy. This is where the field is. In other countries surgeons may not want to deal with an increased incidence of recurrence, even in the presence of neoadjuvant therapy, although this reduces the incidence of recurrence to quite a low number. Thus, in their hands, abdominal peritoneal resection, the Miles Operation, which does have a finite incidence of recurrence, is the procedure of choice. This is the identical chapter that appeared in the fourth edition.

Chapter 152A: Calculus Disease: Open Operative Procedures
Martin I. Resnick and O. Alex Lesani

Dr. Resnick is a master urologist. He was kind enough to write a chapter on open procedures, which, as he himself points out, are carried out in a minority of patients with calculous disease. However, it still has a place where necessary. It is a very well done chapter is well argued, meticulously described, and is a model for a procedure which once was the staple of urological training but, alas, has given way to other types of procedures which has led urology to train its people in a much different and innovative fashion.

Chapter 153: Operations on the Ureteropelvic Junction
Frank Hinman, Jr.

"Operations of the Ureteropelvic Junction" is another operation that has given way to minimally invasive and endourological procedures. Dealing with the ureteropelvic junction in open fashion is an art form that will be applied to the minority of patients. Nonetheless, it is important that one know how to do the operation if the occasion demands and the preservation of renal function is at stake.

Chapter 167: Anterior and Posterior Colporrhaphy
Dionysios K. Veronikis

The chapter on anterior and posterior colporrhaphy presented here is a rather detailed chapter and one which can be read with profit. However, the vaginal floor and its repair has become much more complicated and so anterior and posterior colporrhaphy, in and of itself, are used less frequently. They may be used with operations for the prolapse of the rectum and they may be utilized in the more sophisticated approach to cystocele and urethracele.

However, the anatomy which is described in the anatomical repair, is valuable and can shed light in other specialties to the necessity for having pelvic floor repair, for example, or come in useful as stated in my commentary for repair of rectal prolapse.

Chapter 169: Bassini Operation

Oreste Terranova, Luigi De Santis and Flavio Frigo

Drs. Terranova, DeSantis and Frigo, as they have in the past, have contributed to the classic operation which started all repairs of inguinal hernia by Dr. Edoardo Bassini. "The Bassini Operation" probably is the first one that gained credence and has held for approximately 100 years or more. However, as the authors come to the conclusion that "The Bassini Operation" even carried out with repair of the transversalis fascia, as originally described by Bassini and shown here in the original pictures, has a recurrence rate anywhere from 3–22% although it may fall as they say in the text below 1.5–2%. They come to the conclusion that while of historical interest and of interest as far as the anatomy of the inguinal canal, this operation as currently described in and of itself is no longer viable.

The Shouldice operation described elsewhere in this volume may actually disagree with that particular conclusion. But according to the authors, prosthetic material must be used in order to get a reasonable recurrence rate. Thus, despite the importance of Bassini and his operation as it was originally described, this is no longer a contemporary utilization of surgery for inguinal hernia cause of the recurrence.

It is presented on the website for historical interest as it really started everything. One may differ as to whether or not Shouldice repair is useful or whether I use a variant of the Shouldice operation, sometimes with vicryl mesh and seem to have low recurrence rates. However, the reader will decide from all of the repairs which are made available in the hernia section.

Chapter 170: Cooper Ligament Repair of Groin Hernias

Robb H. Rutledge

Dr. Robb Ruttledge is an excellent practitioner who preceded me in the Massachusetts General Hospital residency by a number of years. He is an exemplary gentleman and a superb surgeon who, despite being in private practice is highly academic in his approach. I consider him a friend. The Cooper's ligament repair once was a staple of herniorraphy. Indeed, when I was a resident, the Cooper's ligament repair was the standard procedure we carried out at the Massachusetts General Hospital despite the fact that it is more painful and its primary utility is in the area of femoral hernias. Dr. Ruttledge nicely describes it. The chapter appeared in the fourth edition.

Chapter 172: Iliopubic Tract Repair of Inguinal Hernia: The Anterior (Inguinal Canal) Approach

Robert E. Condon

Chapter 173: Iliopubic Tract Repair of Inguinal and Femoral Hernia: The Posterior (Preperitoneal) Approach

Lloyd M. Nyhus

Chapters 172 and 173 are two classic articles appearing from a golden age in surgery, the collaboration with Dr. Robert Condon and Dr. Lloyd Nyhus. They deal with the anatomy first and foremost of the inguinal canal by two individuals who have made this a major focus of their long and distinguished academic careers. The anatomy is masterfully described and is well argued. Familiarity with this approach is essential because there are times when there is a hernia in the vicinity of the abdomen and anatomical knowledge of this area will enable a repair to be done with less difficulty, thus preventing another operative procedure.

These two classics have appeared in every previous edition and they are included here on the website. At a time when most surgical residents never learn the anatomy of the inguinal canal, which I find unfortunate, these two chapters are superb in how the knowledge of surgical anatomy can lead not only to a concept but also to performance of an excellent clinical operation at that time.

The Pancreas

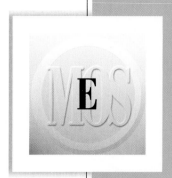

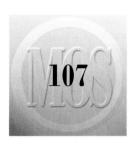

Surgical Anatomy of the Pancreas

107

LEE J. SKANDALAKIS, GENE L. COLBORN,
JOHN E. SKANDALAKIS, MARIOS LOUKAS,
PANAJIOTIS N. SKANDALAKIS, AND
PETROS MIRILAS

The pancreas is neither striking in appearance nor obvious in function. Its early history is hardly more than a list of the names of those who noticed it in their dissections before passing on to more interesting organs. It was only with demonstration of the digestive enzymes by Claude Bernard in 1850 that the pancreas came to be seen as a complete organ with an important function and, thus, an object worthy of study.

In spite of the apparent accessibility of the pancreas, several anatomic relations combine to make its surgical removal difficult. In 1898, Halsted was the first to successfully remove the head of the pancreas and a portion of the duodenum for ampullary cancer. Several surgeons in the United States and abroad subsequently developed two-stage operations for removal of the head of the pancreas. These efforts culminated in 1940 with Whipple's one-stage operation. A major factor in Whipple's success was the use of silk sutures, which tend to resist digestion by enzymes that destroy catgut sutures.

Sir Andrew Watt Kay wrote in 1978, "For me, the tiger country is removal of the pancreas. The anatomy is very complex and one encounters anomalies." The embryogenesis of the pancreas and its deep retroperitoneal anatomy are responsible for the "tiger country." In addition to the normal anatomy of the pancreas, before starting surgery the surgeon should know whether the patient's pancreas has any anomalies such as pancreas divisum or obstruction of the pancreatic duct, or variations in the duct's location or depth, or in the overall vascular structure of the pancreas. No other organ is so closely surrounded by so many anatomic entities (e.g., the duodenum, stomach, spleen, left adrenal, transverse mesocolon and colon, left kidney, right ureter, and jejunum). Figures 1 through 3 show anterior and posterior relations. The proximity of the pancreas to so many organs means that it is prone to invasion by carcinoma. A study by Deziel found that metastases to the pancreas occur most frequently from the lung, followed by the breast, melanoma, stomach, colon or rectum, kidney, and ovary. Similarly, pancreatic cancer is likely to invade other organs. Tables 1 and 2 show two important considerations in pancreatic cancer: organs directly invaded by pancreatic ductal cancer, and areas most likely to be involved by metastatic lesions from pancreatic cancer.

In a study of 7,145 patients, cancer of the pancreas was located in the head in 73.2%, in the body in 19.9%, and in the tail in 6.8%. Partial pancreatectomy and "95 percent" pancreatectomy, first described by Barrett and Bowers and popularized by Frey and Child, are used instead of total pancreatectomy whenever possible because of the high mortality of total pancreatectomy.

The pancreas lies transversely in the retroperitoneal space, between the duodenum on the right and the spleen on the left. It is related anteriorly to the omental bursa above, the greater sac below, and the transverse mesocolon. For all practical purposes, it is a fixed organ.

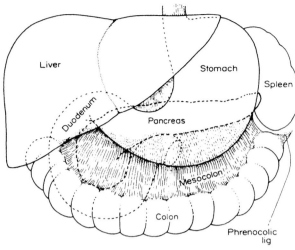

Fig. 1. Anterior relationships. (From JE Skandalakis, Gray SW, Rowe JS Jr, et al. Anatomical complications of pancreatic surgery. *Contemp Surg* 1979;15:17.)

PARTS OF THE PANCREAS

Anatomical Parts

Head

The head of the pancreas is flattened and has an anterior and a posterior surface (Fig. 4). The anterior surface is adjacent to the pylorus and the transverse colon. The anterior pancreaticoduodenal arcade can be seen on the ventral surface of the head of the pancreas, coursing roughly parallel to the duodenal curvature.

The posterior pancreaticoduodenal vascular arcade is a major entity on the posterior surface of the head. This surface of the pancreatic head is close to the hilum and medial border of the right kidney, the right renal vessels and the inferior vena cava, the right crus of the diaphragm, and the right gonadal vein.

The head of the pancreas may be related to the third part of the common bile duct (CBD) in a variety of ways.

Figure 5A and B shows the most frequent conditions: the bile duct is partially covered by a tongue of pancreatic tissue (44%). In Figure 5C, the bile duct is completely covered (30%). The duct is uncovered on the posterior surface of the pancreas in 16.5% of cases (Fig. 5D). In 9% of cases, the third part of the CBD is covered by two tongues of pancreatic tissue (Fig. 5E).

Uncinate Process

An extension of the head of the pancreas (which is variable in size and shape) passes downward and slightly to the left from the principal part of the head. It further continues behind the superior mesenteric vessels and in front of the aorta and inferior vena cava. In sagittal section, the uncinate process lies between the aorta and the superior mesenteric artery (SMA), with the left renal vein above and the duodenum below (Fig. 6). If the junction of the superior mesenteric and portal vein is low, the anterior surface of the uncinate process is related to the su-

perior mesenteric vessels and the portal vein.

The uncinate process may be absent, or it may completely encircle the superior mesenteric vessels (Fig. 7). If the process is well developed, the neck of the pancreas must be sectioned from the front to avoid injury to the vessels. Short vessels from the SMA and vein supply the uncinate process and must be carefully ligated.

Dissection of the head of the pancreas in 20 fresh cadavers resulted in 18 with an uncinate process and 2 without the process. In most cases, the posterior surface of the uncinate process was in contact with the inferior vena cava and aorta and was crossed ventrally by the superior mesenteric vein (SMV) and artery. Efforts to weigh the proximal and distal pancreas with or without the uncinate process did not provide any satisfactory data regarding the weight of the uncinate process.

- The extent of resection of the head or uncinate process is empiric.
- Division at the neck is equivalent to a 60% to 70% resection.
- Division at the proximal body to the left of the portal vein above and to the SMV below is a 50% to 60% resection.
- Even with an 80% pancreatectomy, good exocrine and endocrine activity are present.
- We cannot predict whether the physiology of the in situ remaining pancreas after pancreatectomy will be normal because we do not know how much pancreatic disease is present within the remaining part of the pancreas.

We have seen cases in which the ligament of the uncinate process ends in the vicinity of the SMV. In such cases, the ligament is quite dense, and attaches the process to the SMA. Pancreatitis or cancer makes the fixation even more adherent. An anomalous right hepatic artery may pass through the uncinate process. Because

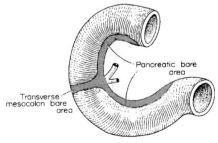

Fig. 2. Bare areas of the duodenum. The pancreas is in intimate contact with the duodenum along the concave surface. The attachment of the transverse mesocolon produces an additional bare area. (From JE Skandalakis, Gray SW, Rowe JS Jr, et al. Anatomical complications of pancreatic surgery. *Contemp Surg* 1979;15:17.)

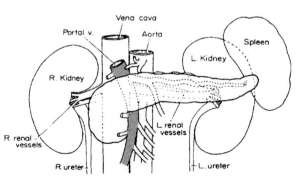

Fig. 3. Posterior relationships. (From JE Skandalakis, Gray SW, Rowe JS Jr, et al. Anatomical complications of pancreatic surgery. *Contemp Surg* 1979;15:17.)

TABLE 1. ORGAN DIRECTLY INVADED (AT AUTOPSY) BY PANCREATIC DUCT CANCER

Anatomic Site Invaded	Total No. Patients	Primary Site		
		Head No. (%)	Body No. (%)	Tail No. (%)
Duodenum	30	24 (67)	6 (24)	0 (0)
Stomach	20	9 (25)	10 (40)	1 (7)
Spleen	8	0 (0)	3 (12)	5 (36)
Left adrenal	5	0 (0)	1 (4)	4 (29)
Transverse colon	6	1 (3)	3 (12)	2 (14)
Left kidney	2	0 (0)	1 (4)	1 (7)
Jejunum	3	1 (3)	1 (4)	1 (7)
Ureter (right)	1	1 (3)	0 (0)	0 (0)
Total (%)	75	36 (48)	25 (33)	14 (19)

From Cubilla AL, Fitzgerald PJ. Metastasis in pancreatic duct adenocarcinoma. In: Day SB, Meyers WPL, Stanley P, et al., eds. *Cancer invasion and metastasis: biologic mechanisms and therapy.* New York: Raven, 1977, with permission.

the aorta is behind the uncinate process, pancreatic carcinoma can be inseparable from the aorta.

Neck

The neck of the pancreas can be defined as the site of passage of the superior mesenteric vessels and the beginning of the portal vein dorsal to the pancreas. This pancreatic segment is 1.5 to 2.0 cm long,

TABLE 2. SITES OF METASTASES FROM CARCINOMA OF THE PANCREAS AS SEEN AT AUTOPSY

Site of Metastasis	Location of Tumor	
	Head (%)	Body and Tail (%)
Regional nodes	75	76
Liver	65	71
Lungs	30	14
Peritoneum	22	38
Duodenum	19	5
Adrenals	13	24
Stomach	11	5
Gallbladder	9	0
Spleen	6	14
Kidney	6	5
Intestines	4	5
Mediastinal nodes	4	5
Other	19	28
No metastasis	13	0

From Howard JM, Jordan JL Jr. Cancer of the pancreas. *Curr Probl Cancer* 1977;2:20, with permission.

and it is partially covered anteriorly by the pylorus. The gastroduodenal artery passes to the right of the neck and provides origin for the anterior superior pancreaticoduodenal (ASPD) artery. Posterior to the neck, the portal vein is formed by the confluence of the superior mesenteric and splenic veins. Near the inferior margin of the pancreatic neck, one can often see the terminations of the inferior pancreaticoduodenal vein and right gastroepiploic vein where they drain into the superior mesenteric or splenic veins or into the portal vein proper. The inferior mesenteric vein drains, with essentially equal frequency, into the splenic vein, the SMV, or the site of formation of the portal vein. Careful elevation of the neck and ligation of any anterior tributaries, if present, are necessary; bleeding makes it difficult

to evaluate the structures lying beneath the neck.

The portal vein receives the posterior superior pancreaticoduodenal, right gastric, left gastric, and pyloric veins. It is fairly common for an anomalous vein to enter the anterior surface.

Body

The anterior surface of the body of the pancreas is covered by the double layer of peritoneum of the omental bursa that separates the stomach from the pancreas. The omental tuberosity (tuber omentale), a blunt upward projection of peritoneum from the body, contacts the lesser curvature of the stomach at the attachment of the lesser omentum. The body is also related to the transverse mesocolon, which divides into two leaves: the superior leaf covers the anterior surface and the inferior leaf passes inferior to the pancreas. The middle colic artery emerges from beneath the pancreas to travel between the leaves of the mesocolon.

Posteriorly, the body is related to the aorta, the origin of the SMA, the left crus of the diaphragm, the left kidney and its vessels, the left adrenal gland, and the splenic vein. Small vessels from the pancreas enter this vein. They must be ligated during pancreatectomy if the splenic vein and the spleen are to be preserved.

Tail

The tail of the pancreas is relatively mobile; its tip reaches the hilum of the spleen in 50% of the cases, lies above the hilum in 8%, and below in 42% (Fig. 8). Together with the splenic artery and the origin of the splenic vein, the tail is contained be-

The Gastrointestinal Tract

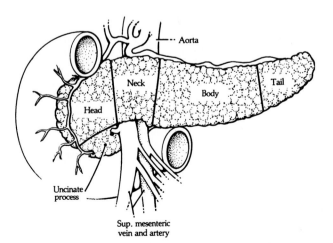

Fig. 4. The five parts of the pancreas. The line dividing the body and tail is entirely arbitrary. (From Skandalakis JE, Gray SW, Rowe JS Jr. *Anatomical complications in general surgery.* New York: McGraw-Hill, 1983, with permission.)

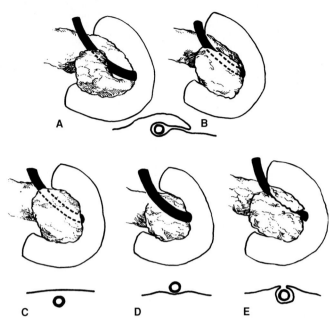

Fig. 5. The relation of the common bile duct to the posterior surface of the pancreas. **A,B:** The most common arrangement (44%); the duct is partially or wholly covered by a tongue of pancreas. **C:** The duct lies within the pancreas (30%). **D:** The duct lies free in the surface of the pancreas (16.5%). **E:** The duct is covered by two small folds of pancreas (9%). (Data from Smanio, 1954; drawing from Skandalakis JE, Gray SW. *Embryology for surgeons*, 2nd ed. Baltimore: Williams & Wilkins, 1994.)

tween two layers of the splenorenal ligament. The outer layer of this ligament is the posterior layer of the gastrosplenic ligament; careless division may injure the short gastric vessels. To avoid bleeding, remember that digital manipulation should stop at the pedicle. Commonly, a caudate branch arises from the left gastroepiploic or an inferior splenic polar branch and passes to the tip of the tail of the pancreas. Anticipate this branch in the pancreaticosplenic ligament.

Segments

Busnardo et al. studied the anatomicosurgical segments of the human pancreas in 30 corrosion casts. Two segments were found, similar to those of the liver. The right (*cephalocervical*) and left (*corporocaudate*) segments of the pancreas are separated by a poorly vascularized area. They are connected by the pancreatic duct and often, according to these authors, by a small artery. Both segments can be used for transplantation.

PANCREATIC DUCTS

The main duct was first described by Wirsung in 1642. The accessory duct and minor duodenal papilla were described by Santorini in 1724, but the findings were not published until 1775. Several researchers studied the pancreas through the years, but the greatest understanding of the anatomy of the pancreatic ducts, their sphincters, and the duodenal wall has

come from studies that Boyden conducted over almost 50 years (1926 to 1971).

Anatomy and Variations

The main pancreatic and accessory ducts lie anterior to the major pancreatic vessels. The main pancreatic duct arises in the tail of the pancreas. Through the tail and body of the pancreas, the duct lies midway between the superior and inferior margins, slightly more posterior than anterior.

The main duct crosses the vertebral column between the twelfth thoracic and second lumbar vertebrae. In more than 50% of persons, the crossing is at the first lumbar vertebra.

In the tail and body of the pancreas, from 15 to 20 short tributaries enter the duct at right angles; superior and inferior tributaries tend to alternate. In addition, the main duct may receive a tributary draining the uncinate process, and, in some individuals, the accessory pancreatic duct empties into the main duct. Small tributary ducts in the head may open directly into the intrapancreatic portion of the CBD.

On reaching neck (depending on its size) or the head of the pancreas, the main duct turns caudad and posterior. At the level of the major papilla, the duct turns horizontally to join the caudal surface of

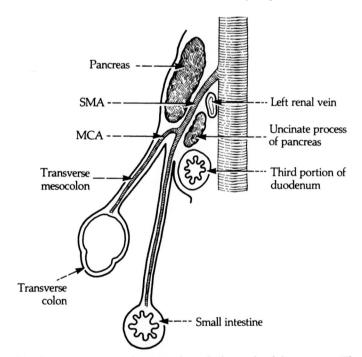

Fig. 6. Highly diagrammatic sagittal section through the neck of the pancreas. The uncinate process and the third portion of the duodenum lie posterior to the superior mesenteric artery (SMA) and anterior to the aorta. The middle colic artery (MCA) leaves the SMA to travel in the transverse mesocolon. (From Akin JT, Gray SW, Skandalakis JE. Vascular compression of the duodenum: presentation of ten cases and review of the literature. *Surgery* 1976;79:515.)

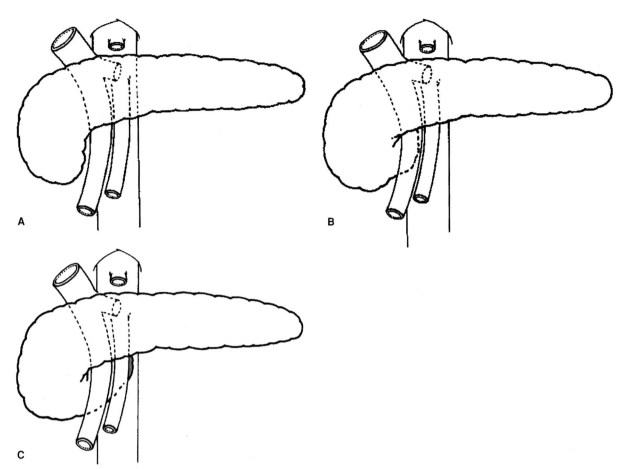

Fig. 7. The uncinate process may or may not extend under the superior mesenteric vessels. **A:** Does not reach the superior mesenteric vessels. **B:** Reaches across the superior mesenteric vein almost to the superior mesenteric artery. **C:** Reaches beyond the superior mesenteric artery. (From JE Skandalakis, Gray SW, Rowe JS Jr, et al. Anatomical complications of pancreatic surgery. *Contemp Surg* 1979; 15:17.)

The Gastrointestinal Tract

the CBD and enters the wall of the duodenum, usually at the level of the second lumbar vertebra.

Frey stated that if the head of the pancreas is 5 cm thick and the distance from the duodenum to the point on the main pancreatic duct at which the duct courses posteriorly and inferiorly is 3 cm, the distance from the junction of the central and dorsal ducts to the hepatopancreatic, or biliaropancreatic, ampulla ("of Vater") is 6 cm. He believes that the major pancreatic duct in the head may not be drained well

by filleting this portion of the surface of the gland.

The accessory pancreatic duct (of Santorini) may drain the anterosuperior portion of the head, either into the duodenum at the minor papilla or into the main pancreatic duct (Fig. 9). Because of the developmental origin of the two pancreatic ducts, several variations are encountered; most can be considered normal. The usual configuration is seen in Figure 10A.

The accessory duct (Santorini) is smaller than the main pancreatic duct (of Wirsung) and opens into the duodenum on the minor papilla. Configurations in Figure 10B through E show examples of progressive diminution in size of the accessory duct. Figure 11 shows examples of prominence of the accessory duct and lessening caliber of the main duct. The configuration shown in Figure 11A is the most common.

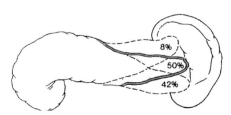

Fig. 8. Relations of the tail of the pancreas to the splenic portas. (From Skandalakis PN, Colborn GL, Skandalakis LJ, et al. The surgical anatomy of the spleen. *Probl Gen Surg* 1990;7:1.)

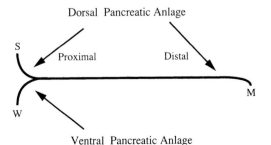

Fig. 9. A highly diagrammatic representation of the embryogenesis of the proximal and distal pancreatic duct. M, main pancreatic duct; S, duct of Santorini; W, duct of Wirsung. (From Skandalakis LJ, Rowe JS, Gray SW, et al. Surgical embryology and anatomy of the pancreas. *Surg Clin North Am* 1993;73:661.)

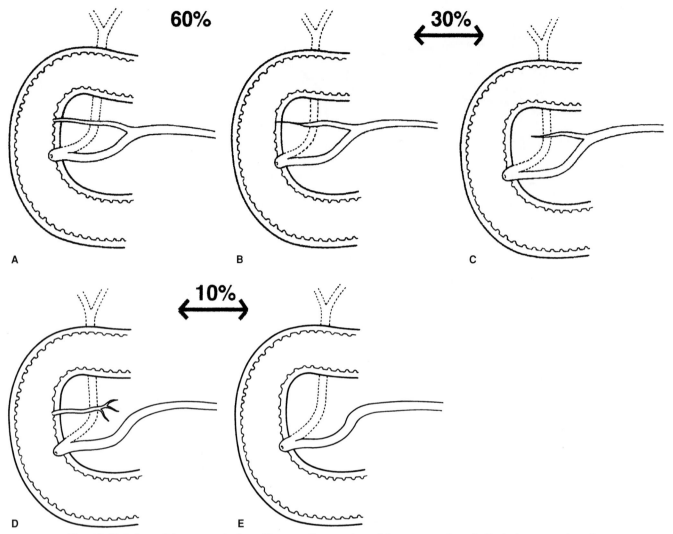

Fig. 10. Variations of the pancreatic ducts. Degrees of suppression of the accessory duct. **A:** Both ducts open into the duodenum (60%). **B,C:** The accessory duct ends blindly (30%). **D:** The accessory duct does not communicate with the main duct (10%). **E:** The accessory duct is absent. (From Skandalakis JE, Gray SW, Rowe JS Jr, et al. Anatomical complications of pancreatic surgery. *Contemp Surg* 1979;15:17.)

In approximately 10% of individuals, there is no connection between the accessory duct and the main duct (Figs. 10D and 11C,D). This fact is important to remember when contrast medium is injected into the main duct. There is no minor papilla in 30% of individuals (Fig. 10B,C, E). In some individuals who have a minor papilla, the terminal portion of the accessory duct is too small to permit the passage of any quantity of fluid. Three papillae have been seen (Fig. 12A,D). A curious loop in the main pancreatic duct (Fig. 12B) was found in 3 of 76 specimens examined by Baldwin; an identical example was reported by Rienhoff and Pickrell.

A 1996 study by Nakamura et al. found that pancreaticobiliary maljunction, an anomaly commonly associated with congenital dilatation of the bile duct, may be a possible cause of recurrent pancreatitis.

Reflux of pancreatic juice into the bile duct is possible through the pancreaticobiliary maljunction. This study suggested involvement of activated phospholipase A_2 in the pathogenesis of choledochal cyst-associated pancreatitis. Sugiyama et al. reported in 1998 that magnetic resonance cholangiopancreatography is an accurate method for the diagnosis of anomalous pancreaticobiliary junction.

Length, Width, and Capacity of the Pancreatic Ducts

Endoscopic retrograde cholangiopancreatography has made the determination of the length, diameter, and capacity of the pancreatic ductal system of considerable importance. Some published values are shown in Figures 13 and 14. The greatest diameter of the main pancreatic duct is in

the head of the pancreas, just before the duct enters the duodenal wall. From this diameter, the duct gradually tapers toward the tail. Like the bile duct, the pancreatic duct is constricted in the wall of the duodenum.

The normal pancreatic ductal system is quite small. Kasugai et al. found that 2 to 3 mL of contrast medium fills the main pancreatic duct in the living patient; and 7 to 10 mL fills the branches and the smaller ducts. In autopsy specimens, Trapnell and Howard found 0.5 to 1.0 mL sufficient to fill the duct system.

Major Duodenal Papilla and Hepatopancreatic Ampulla

There is confusion in the literature about the correct name, definition, and distinguishing points of the major duodenal

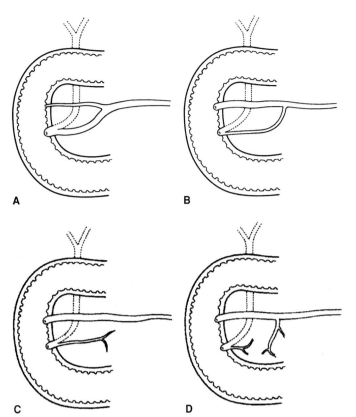

Fig. 11. Variations of the pancreatic ducts. Degrees of suppression of the main duct. **A:** Both ducts open into the duodenum. **B:** The main duct is smaller than the accessory duct. **C,D:** The main duct does not communicate with the accessory duct. (From Skandalakis JE, Gray SW, Rowe JS Jr, et al. Anatomical complications of pancreatic surgery. *Contemp Surg* 1979;15:17.)

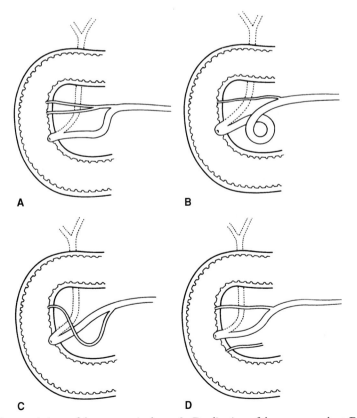

Fig. 12. Rare variations of the pancreatic ducts. **A:** Duplication of the accessory duct. **B:** Loop in main duct. **C:** Anomalous course of accessory duct. **D:** Triple pancreatic ducts. (From Skandalakis JE, Gray SW, Rowe JS Jr, et al. Anatomical complications of pancreatic surgery. *Contemp Surg* 1979;15:17.)

papilla (often referred to as the *papilla of Vater*) and the hepatopancreatic or biliaropancreatic ampulla (often referred to as *ampulla of Vater*). The papilla is a nipple-like projection of duodenal mucosa, located where the main pancreatic duct and the CBD drain into the duodenum. The hepatopancreatic ampulla, which can have several variations, is the union of the pancreaticobiliary ducts.

Major Duodenal Papilla

This papilla often bears the name of Abraham Vater (1684-1751), but the eponym is historically incorrect. The most useful term is *major (or greater) duodenal papilla*.

The papilla is situated on the posteromedial wall of the second portion of the duodenum, 7 to 10 cm from the pylorus. Rarely, the papilla may be in the third portion of the duodenum.

Viewed from the mucosal surface of the duodenum, the papilla is found where a longitudinal mucosal fold or frenulum meets a transverse mucosal fold to form a "T" (Fig. 15). The papilla may not be obvious because too much traction erases the folds, or the papilla may be covered by one of the transverse folds. A study in 1962 by Dowdy et al. found that the papilla was "prominent" and easily found in 60% of their specimens. [EAD10]

At operation, if the T is not apparent and the papilla cannot be palpated, the CBD must be probed from above. A duodenal diverticulum close to the papilla may confuse the surgeon or the endoscopist.

Hepatopancreatic (Biliaropancreatic) Ampulla

Although the ampulla is named after Vater, there is much evidence that it was first described by Santorini. Vater actually described a diverticulum of duodenal mucosa, now referred to as *perivaterian diverticulum*.

The location, or implantation, of the junction of the main pancreatic duct and the CBD is in the descending portion of the duodenum in 75% of cases; in 25% it is primarily in the horizontal portion of the duodenum, to the right of the superior mesenteric vessels, according to Avisse et al.

The ampulla is a dilatation of the common pancreaticobiliary channel adjacent to the papilla and below the junction of the two ducts (Fig. 16A). If a septum is present as far as the duodenal orifice, no ampulla exists (Fig. 16B,C).

The anatomic frequency of an ampulla in several studies ranged from 6% to 90%.

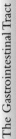

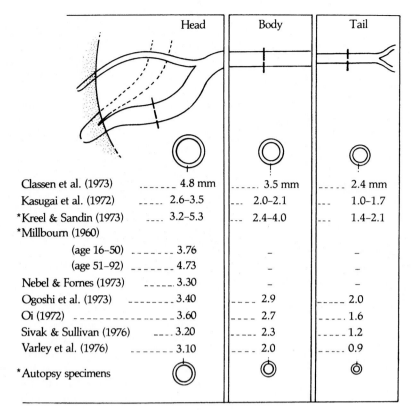

	Head	Body	Tail
Classen et al. (1973)	4.8 mm	3.5 mm	2.4 mm
Kasugai et al. (1972)	2.6–3.5	2.0–2.1	1.0–1.7
*Kreel & Sandin (1973)	3.2–5.3	2.4–4.0	1.4–2.1
*Millbourn (1960)			
(age 16–50)	3.76	–	–
(age 51–92)	4.73	–	–
Nebel & Fornes (1973)	3.30	–	–
Ogoshi et al. (1973)	3.40	2.9	2.0
Oi (1972)	3.60	2.7	1.6
Sivak & Sullivan (1976)	3.20	2.3	1.2
Varley et al. (1976)	3.10	2.0	0.9

*Autopsy specimens

Fig. 13. Diameter of the main pancreatic duct as reported by several authors. Averages and extremes are indicated. (From Skandalakis JE, Gray SW, Rowe JS Jr, et al. Anatomical complications of pancreatic surgery. *Contemp Surg* 1979;15:17.)

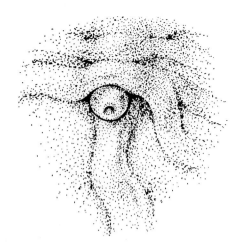

Fig. 15. The "T" arrangement of the duodenal mucosal folds at the site of the major papilla. The papilla is rarely this obvious. This illustration by Santorini was published posthumously in 1775. (From Skandalakis JE, Gray SW, Rowe JS Jr, et al. Anatomical complications of pancreatic surgery. *Contemp Surg* 1979;15:17.)

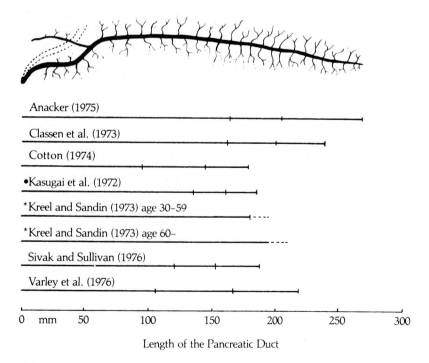

Anacker (1975)

Classen et al. (1973)

Cotton (1974)

•Kasugai et al. (1972)

*Kreel and Sandin (1973) age 30–59

*Kreel and Sandin (1973) age 60–

Sivak and Sullivan (1976)

Varley et al. (1976)

| 0 | mm | 50 | 100 | 150 | 200 | 250 | 300 |

Length of the Pancreatic Duct

*Autopsy specimens
•Standard deviation

Fig. 14. Length of the main pancreatic duct as reported by several authors. (From Skandalakis JE, Gray SW, Rowe JS Jr, et al. Anatomical complications of pancreatic surgery. *Contemp Surg* 1979;15:17.)

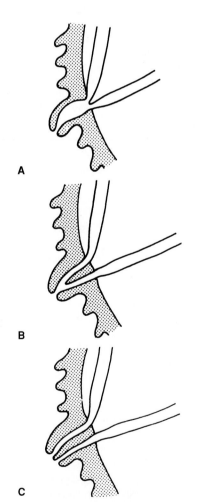

Fig. 16. Variations of the common bile duct and the main pancreatic duct at the duodenal papilla. An ampulla is present in **A;** it is absent in **B** and **C.** (From Skandalakis JE, Gray SW, Rowe JS Jr, et al. Anatomical complications of pancreatic surgery. *Contemp Surg* 1979;15:17.)

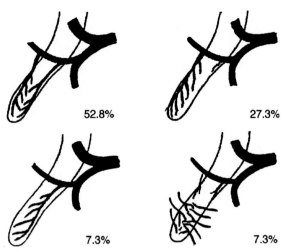

Fig. 17. Frequency distribution of vascular supply of ampulla of Vater. (From Stolte M, Wiessner V, Schaffner O, et al. Vascularization of the Papilla Vateri and bleeding risk of papillotomy. *Leber Magen Darm* 1980;10: 293.)

The Gastrointestinal Tract

Michels collected the findings of 25 investigators in 2,500 specimens and concluded that an ampulla was present in 64% of the specimens. An ampulla was said to be present if the edge of the septum between the two ducts did not reach the tip of the papilla. Actual measurements of the distance between septal edge and papillary tip range from 1 to 14 mm, with 75% being 5 mm or less, according to Rienhoff and Pickrell. The following classification, consisting of three types, was suggested in 1955 by Michels (based on Millbourn and Hjorth's cholangiographic studies [Millbourn (1950), Hjorth (1997)]) and is the most useful.

Type 1. The pancreatic duct opens into the CBD at a variable distance from the opening in the major duodenal papilla (Fig. 16A). Both Hjorth and Millbourn found an ampulla in 85% of the cases they dissected. Where the common channel is less than 5 mm long, there is little or no dilation. When dilation is considered a requirement for the existence of an ampulla, only about 75% of cases would fit the definition.

Type 2. The pancreatic and bile ducts open close to one another, but separately, without an ampulla, on the major duodenal papilla (5%) (Fig. 16C).

Type 3. The pancreatic and bile ducts open into the duodenum at separate points without an ampulla (9%).

The basic embryologic explanation for the above three types is that growth of the duodenum absorbs the proximal bile duct up to its junction with the pancreatic duct. When the resorption is minimal, there is a long ampulla and the junction of the ducts is high in the duodenal wall (type 1, Fig. 16A) or even extramural. With increased—but still partial—resorption of the terminal bile duct, the junction lies closer to the duodenal orifice and, for all practical purposes, does not exist (type 2, Fig. 16B). Maximal resorption results in separate orifices for the main pancreatic duct and the CBD (type 3, Fig. 16C).

Smooth muscle ensheaths the ampulla forming the sphincter of the hepatopancreatic ampulla, which belongs to the broader sphincter complex of Boyden in the hepatopancreatoduodenal area.

There are reports in the literature that mention some of the arteries and veins that participate in the blood supply of the ampulla of Vater, but the topography of the vascular network has not been defined clearly enough to help operators avoid postoperative bleeding. Most of these discussions describe the blood supply of the distal CBD and the pancreatic duct.

What should we surgical anatomists advise the surgeon, laparoscopist, and gastroenterologist about the topography, length, and depth of the incision during sphincterotomy, sphincterostomy, or sphincteroplasty so that bleeding and perforation can be avoided? The incision should be at 10 to 11 o'clock with an approximate length of 5 to 8 mm. The optimal depth to avoid bleeding is not known.

The vessels responsible for bleeding are perhaps the retroduodenal artery and an anomalous right hepatic artery originating from the SMA. These two vessels are located between the distal CBD and the duodenum. We agree with Chassin that during the open method the area behind the ampulla should be palpated to determine whether there is a palpable pulsation. If so, an anomalous artery is present.

The 1980 study by Stolte et al. of the distribution of the vascular supply to the ampulla of Vater is illustrated in Figure 17. The four major types listed below comprised 52 of their 55 cases (94.6%):

■ Equally large ventral and dorsal branches of the posterior duodenal artery (retroduodenal artery) (52.8%) (Fig. 18)

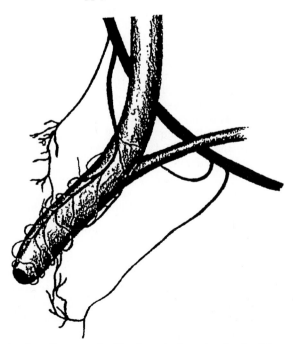

Fig. 18. Schematic of papillary vascular blood supply. Posterior duodenal (retroduodenal) artery crosses bile duct and gives rise to dorsal and ventral branches, which join to form arterial plexus of papillae. (From Stolte M, Wiessner V, Schaffner O, et al. Vascularization of the Papilla Vateri and bleeding risk of papillotomy. *Leber Magen Darm* 1980;10:293.)

- Dominant dorsal branch (27.3%)
- Dominant ventral branch (7.3%)
- No dominant branch (arterial plexus of papilla composed of several vessels entering from sides) (7.3%)
- Rare variations (5.4%)

In 1990 Biazotto reported that three venous networks are associated with the papilla. (i) The deep network resides in the mucous membrane of the intramural bile duct and in the hepatopancreatic ampulla. (ii) The intermediate network is in the deep region of the chorion of the papilla. (iii) The superficial network is in the duodenal submucous membrane covering of the papilla.

Biazotto stated that bleeding during papillotomies is insignificant because the thick veins lie in the body and at the base of the papilla. The location in the apex of the papilla of the many small veins draining into the duodenal submucous membrane also helps to explain the diffuse and low-intensity bleeding.

Sphincter of Boyden/ Sphincter of Oddi

The present concept is that several sphincters of smooth-muscle fibers surround the intramural part of the CBD, the main pancreatic duct, and the ampulla, if present (Fig. 19). The complex has a separate embryonic origin from that of the duodenal musculature and is functionally separate. Although the anatomy has been well described by Boyden and others, the terminology is unsettled. We call the entire sphincter complex the *sphincter of Boyden* in recognition of his contribution to the anatomy of this region, but it was originally described by Oddi in 1887, and some authors refer to it as the sphincter of Oddi.

The total length of the sphincteric complex may be as short as 6 mm or as long as 30 mm, depending on the obliquity of the path taken by the biliary and pancreatic ducts through the duodenal wall. In some instances, the sphincter may extend beyond the duodenal wall into the pancreatic portion of the bile duct. It is important to be aware of this fact when sphincterotomy is performed.

A 1994 study by Flati et al. of the biliopancreatic ducts and sphincteric apparatus of 49 specimens reported the following findings, some of which differ from those of Boyden.

1. On the choledochus duct side, circular muscle fibers were found up to a mean distance of 13.6 mm from the papillary pore, with more rarefied fibers present up to 20.5 mm from the pore.

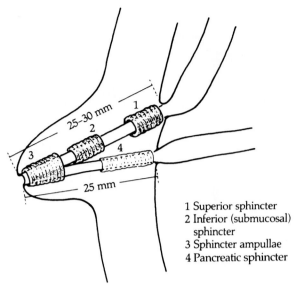

Fig. 19. The four entities composing the sphincter of Boyden. The measurements are from White (1973) . (From Skandalakis JE, Gray SW, Rowe JS Jr, et al. Anatomical complications of pancreatic surgery. *Contemp Surg* 1979;15:17.)

1 Superior sphincter
2 Inferior (submucosal) sphincter
3 Sphincter ampullae
4 Pancreatic sphincter

2. Muscle fibers on the pancreatic duct side stopped 7.3 mm from the papillary pore. The beginning of the sphincter was 2 to 3 mm above the papillary pore.
3. There was no evidence suggesting the presence of upper, middle, and lower biliary sphincters.
4. The shape of the Wirsung-choledochus junction could be categorized as follows:

   Y type (with short or long common channel): 61.2%

   U type (virtually absent common channel): 22.4%

   V type (separate orifices of the Wirsung and choledochus ducts in the same papilla): 14.3%

   II type (one papilla for the choledochus and one for the Wirsung duct): 2.1%
5. The duct of Santorini with a normal papilla was present in 16% of specimens.

Minor Duodenal Papilla

The minor duodenal papilla is situated approximately 2 cm cranial and slightly anterior to the major papilla. It is smaller, and its site does not have the characteristic mucosal folds that mark the site of the major papilla. Baldwin found the minor papilla to be present in all of a series of 100 specimens. However, in a sample of the same size, Dowdy et al. could find no minor papilla in 18 specimens. Some papillae may be difficult to identify, even if they are present.

An excellent landmark is the gastroduodenal artery, situated anterior to the accessory pancreatic duct (Santorini) and the minor papilla. During gastrectomy, duodenal dissection should end proximal to or at this artery. It becomes important in the few patients in whom the accessory duct carries the major drainage of the pancreas.

VASCULAR SYSTEM

The vascular system of the pancreas is complex and nontypical, with several different patterns. In addition to the material presented here, we recommend the publications of Bertelli and Donatini and their colleagues.

Arterial Supply of the Pancreas

Van Damme wrote that the most important pancreatic artery is the splenic artery. The pancreas is supplied with blood from branches arising from both the celiac trunk and the SMA (Figs. 20 and 21). Variations are common, and differing textbook illustrations are all "correct" for at least some patients. For evaluating the topography and anastomosis of pancreatic arteries, Toni et al. reported satisfactory sensitivity of the angiographic approach.

The head of the pancreas and the concave surface of the duodenum are supplied by two pancreaticoduodenal arterial arcades that are always present. These are formed by a pair (anterior and posterior) of superior arteries from the gastroduodenal

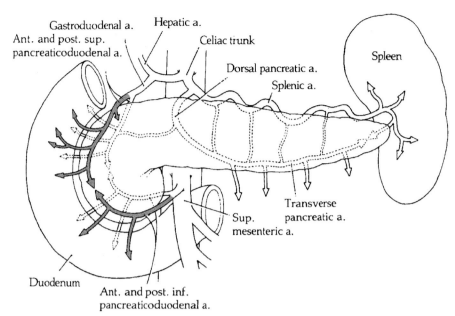

Fig. 20. Anterior view of the major arterial supply to the pancreas (the left and right gastric arteries are omitted). (From Skandalakis JE, Gray SW, Rowe JS Jr, et al. Anatomical complications of pancreatic surgery. *Contemp Surg* 1979;15:17.)

ferior vessels appeared to be absent, but he believed this to be the result of transient spasm.

The anterior inferior pancreaticoduodenal artery arises from the SMA at or above the inferior margin of the pancreatic neck. It may form a common trunk with the posterior inferior pancreaticoduodenal (PIPD) artery. One or both vessels may arise from the first or second jejunal branches of the SMA. Even more striking are instances in which a PIPD artery arises from an aberrant right hepatic artery springing from the SMA. Ligation of the jejunal branch endangers the blood supply to the fourth part of the duodenum.

The supraduodenal artery regularly crosses the bile duct after arising from its gastroduodenal or other source and may supply blood to the bile duct. It and the retroduodenal artery provide arterial supply to the first part of the duodenum. Either or both of these arteries can arise separately or as branches of the PSPD artery.

The PSPD artery arises from the gastroduodenal artery. It then takes a long, spiraling course in a clockwise direction around the CBD to reach the posterior aspect of the head of the pancreas. The terminal part of the course of the PSPD artery is visible only when the pancreas is turned upward to expose its posterior surface (Fig. 21). This also exposes its interconnections with the PIPD artery. Branches may anastomose with other branches of the gastroduodenal artery or with the transverse (inferior pancreatic) artery. Duodenal branches supply the anterior

branch of the celiac trunk that join a second pair of inferior arteries from the SMA. These vascular arcades lie on the surface of the pancreas but also supply the duodenal wall. They are the chief obstacles to complete pancreatectomy without duodenectomy.

At the neck, the dorsal pancreatic artery usually arises from the splenic artery, near its origin from the celiac trunk. A right branch of the dorsal pancreatic artery supplies the head of the pancreas and usually joins the posterior arcade. It may also anastomose with the ASPD artery. One or two left branches pass through the body and tail of the pancreas, often making connections with branches of the splenic artery and, at the tip of the tail, with the splenic or the left gastroepiploic artery. The left and right branches of the dorsal pancreatic artery characteristically lie within a groove on the inferior margin of the pancreas. Here they form the transverse, or inferior, pancreatic artery. All major arteries lie posterior to the ducts.

Pancreatic Arcades

The gastroduodenal artery arises as one of the two terminal branches of the common hepatic artery of the celiac trunk. Shortly after it arises from the common hepatic artery branch, the gastroduodenal artery gives origin to the supraduodenal, retroduodenal, and posterior superior pancreaticoduodenal (PSPD) arteries (Figs. 20 and 21). The supraduodenal and retroduodenal arteries arise, variably, as

branches of the PSPD artery. The gastroduodenal artery ends by dividing into the right gastroepiploic and ASPD arteries.

The ASPD artery lies on the anterior surface of the head of the pancreas, where it contributes 8 to 10 branches to the anterior surface of the pancreas and the duodenum; the main stem ends by anastomosing richly with the anterior inferior pancreaticoduodenal (AIPD) artery at the lower margin of the head of the pancreas. Mellière found four instances in which the anastomosis between superior and in-

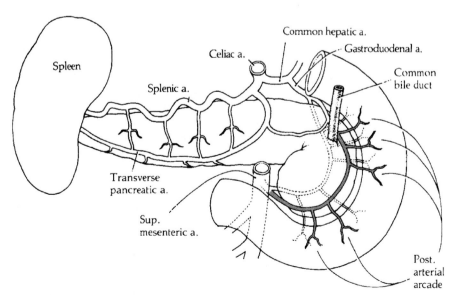

Fig. 21. Posterior view of the major arterial supply to the pancreas (the left and right gastric arteries are omitted). (From Skandalakis JE, Gray SW, Rowe JS Jr, et al. Anatomical complications of pancreatic surgery. *Contemp Surg* 1979;15:17.)

The Gastrointestinal Tract

and posterior surfaces of the second part of the duodenum.

The course of the posterior arcade is farther from the duodenum than is that of the anterior arcade. It passes posterior to the intrapancreatic portion of the CBD.

The posterior arcade, like the anterior, may be doubled or tripled, with the extra arcades joining the PIPD artery or the SMA. The posterior arcade may also anastomose with an aberrant right hepatic artery from the SMA (Fig. 22C), either separately or together with the anterior arcade.

Branches of the Splenic Artery

The splenic artery courses to the left along the posterior surface of the body and tail of the pancreas, looping above and below the superior margin of the organ. This pathway may become more tortuous as the patient ages. If the posterior gastric artery is not present, the first major branch of the splenic artery is the dorsal pancreatic artery, which usually joins one of the posterosuperior arcades after giving off the inferior (transverse) pancreatic artery to the left. The dorsal pancreatic artery arises rather commonly from the celiac trunk or from the common hepatic artery.

The origin of the inferior pancreatic artery varies. It may be doubled or absent. It may or may not freely anastomose with the splenic artery in the body and tail of the pancreas (Fig. 23). The inferior artery often joins the gastroduodenal artery or the ASPD artery to the right. If there are no anastomoses, thrombosis of the inferior pancreatic artery may produce emboli, infarction, and necrosis of the tail and possibly of the distal body of the pancreas.

Great Pancreatic Artery

The great pancreatic (pancreatica magna) artery arises from the splenic artery and reaches the pancreas near the junction of the body and tail. This artery commonly anastomoses with the inferior pancreatic artery.

Caudal Pancreatic Artery

The caudal pancreatic artery arises from the distal segment of the splenic artery, the left gastroepiploic artery, or from a splenic branch at the hilum of the spleen. It anastomoses with branches of the great pancreatic and other pancreatic arteries. The caudal pancreatic artery supplies blood to accessory splenic tissue when it is present at the hilum.

Van Damme studied the pancreatic arteries extensively, paying particular attention to the transverse pancreatic artery

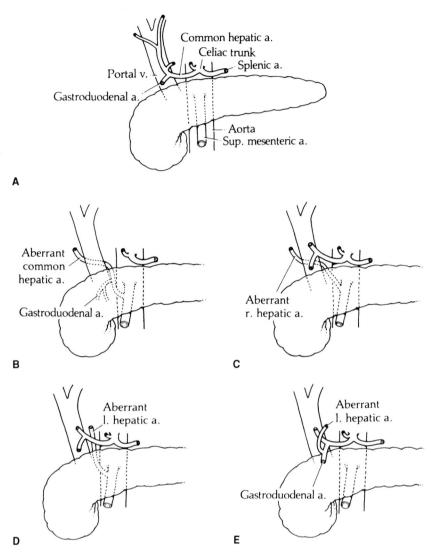

A

B

C

D

E

Fig. 22. Variations of the hepatic arteries. **A:** Normal configuration; the common hepatic artery arises from the celiac trunk. **B:** An aberrant common hepatic artery arises from the superior mesenteric artery. **C:** An aberrant right hepatic artery arises from the superior mesenteric artery. **D:** An aberrant left hepatic artery arises from the superior mesenteric artery. **E:** An aberrant left hepatic artery arises from the gastroduodenal artery. These aberrant arteries may be accessory to, or may replace, normal hepatic arteries. (From Skandalakis JE, Gray SW, Rowe JS Jr, et al. Anatomical complications of pancreatic surgery. *Contemp Surg* 1979;15:17.)

and to some of the important, unnamed arteries that supply the neck, body, and tail of the pancreas.

Anomalous Hepatic Arteries

The common hepatic artery (Fig. 22A) is usually a main branch of the celiac trunk, which arises cranial to the pancreas. The surgeon must always look for a possible anomalous hepatic artery before proceeding with a pancreatic resection. These aberrant arteries may be accessory to, or may replace, normal hepatic arteries.

In 2.0% to 4.5% of persons, an anomalous common hepatic artery arises from the SMA. It is related to the head or neck of the pancreas. Occasionally it passes through the head (Fig. 22B). It subse-

quently passes behind the portal vein. Almost all of the duodenum's blood supply comes from the SMA.

The more frequent anomalous right hepatic artery also arises from the SMA. Its course is unpredictable, but it is related to the head and neck of the pancreas. Such an artery may pass behind the CBD or behind the portal vein (Fig. 22C). An aberrant right hepatic artery was present in 26% of bodies examined by Michels. It may give off the inferior pancreaticoduodenal arteries.

An anomalous left hepatic artery presents a problem in operations on the pancreas only when it arises from the right side of the SMA (Fig. 22D) or from the gastroduodenal artery (Fig. 22E). Michels

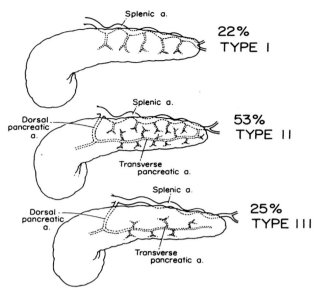

Fig. 23. Diagram of the possible configurations of the blood supply to the distal pancreas. Type I (22%), blood supply from the splenic artery only. Type II (53%), blood supply from splenic and transverse pancreatic arteries with anastomosis in the tail of the pancreas. Type III (25%), blood supply from splenic and transverse pancreatic arteries without distal anastomosis. This type is susceptible to infarction from emboli in the transverse artery. (From Skandalakis JE, Gray SW, Rowe JS Jr, et al. Anatomical complications of pancreatic surgery. *Contemp Surg* 1979;15:17.)

found an anomalous left hepatic artery in 27% of specimens, arising most commonly from the left gastric artery.

Anomalous Middle Colic Artery

A middle colic artery may pass through the head of the pancreas or between the head and the duodenum (Fig. 24). It may arise from the superior mesenteric, the dorsal pancreatic, or the inferior pancreaticoduodenal arteries.

Venous Drainage of the Pancreas

In general, the veins of the pancreas parallel the arteries and lie superficial to them. Both lie posterior to the ducts in the body and tail of the pancreas. The drainage is to the portal vein, the splenic vein, and the superior and inferior mesenteric veins (Figs. 25 and 26).

Veins of the Head of the Pancreas

Four pancreaticoduodenal veins form venous arcades, draining the head of the pancreas and the duodenum. The ASPD vein joins the right gastroepiploic vein. The right gastroepiploic receives a colic vein and forms a short gastrocolic vein. This becomes a tributary to the SMV. According to Helge Baden in a personal communication to John E. Skandalakis (November 23, 1988), this gastrocolic vein— known also as *gastrocolic trunk*—"is a very important structure in pancreatic surgery. It should

be identified and divided before proceeding cephalad on the anterior aspect of the superior mesenteric vein."

The PSPD vein enters the portal vein above the superior margin of the pancreas. The anterior and posterior inferior pancreaticoduodenal veins enter the SMV together or separately. Other small, unnamed veins in the head and neck drain independently into the SMV and the right side of the portal vein.

White wrote that pancreatic tributaries do not enter the anterior surface of the portal or superior mesenteric veins. This reduces the risk of bleeding when incising the neck of the pancreas. Silen, however, warned that in some patients the superior pancreaticoduodenal vein and the gastrocolic vein may enter the portal vein and the SMV anteriorly.

Veins of the Neck, Body, and Tail of the Pancreas

The veins of the left portion of the pancreas form two large venous channels: the splenic vein above and the transverse (inferior) pancreatic vein below. A smaller superior pancreatic vein can sometimes be identified.

The splenic vein, according to Douglass et al., receives from 3 to 13 short pancreatic tributaries. In a few instances, one such tributary enters the left gastroepiploic vein in the tail of the pancreas. The inferior mesenteric vein terminates in the splenic vein in approximately 38% of individuals, and the left gastric vein has a similar ending in 17% of individuals. The inferior pancreatic vein may enter the left side of the SMV, the inferior mesenteric vein, or occasionally the splenic or the gastrocolic veins.

Portal Vein

The portal vein is formed behind the neck of the pancreas by the union of the superior mesenteric and splenic veins (Figs. 25 and 26). The inferior mesenteric vein entered at this junction in approximately one third of specimens examined

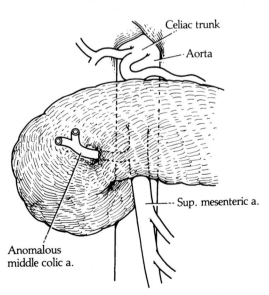

Fig. 24. An anomalous middle colic artery passing through the head of the pancreas. (From Skandalakis JE, Gray SW, Rowe JS Jr, et al. Anatomical complications of pancreatic surgery. *Contemp Surg* 1979;15:17.)

The Gastrointestinal Tract

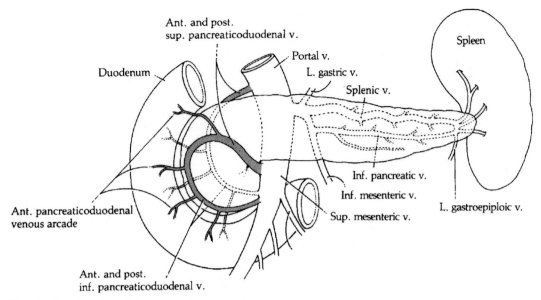

Fig. 25. Anterior view of the venous drainage of the pancreas. (From Skandalakis JE, Gray SW, Rowe JS Jr, et al. Anatomical complications of pancreatic surgery. *Contemp Surg* 1979;15:17.)

by Douglass et al. In another third, the inferior mesenteric joined the splenic vein close to the junction, and, in the remainder, it joined the SMV.

The portal vein lies behind the pancreas and in front of the inferior vena cava, with the CBD on the right and the common hepatic artery on the left. In the absence of disease, the portal vein and the SMV can be separated easily from the posterior surface of the pancreas.

In 23 cadavers dissected by Skandalakis et al., the left gastric (coronary) vein en-

tered the portal vein in 17 and the splenic vein in 6. When drainage flowed to the portal vein, the left gastric vein lay in the hepatogastric ligament.

Rarely the portal vein may lie anterior to the pancreas and the duodenum (Fig. 27), representing persistence of the preduodenal rather than the postduodenal plexus of the embryonic vitelline veins (the normal configuration). Inadvertent section of this vessel could be fatal. It is often associated with anular pancreas, malrotation, and biliary tract anomalies. A

preduodenal portal vein is rare in patients of any age, and extremely rare in adults. Although the 1998 study by Ooshima et al. reported only 20 adult cases of preduodenal portal vein, the surgeon should be aware of this anomaly.

Surgical Considerations

- The right branch of the dorsal pancreatic artery anastomoses with the PSPD artery. This branch does not provide enough

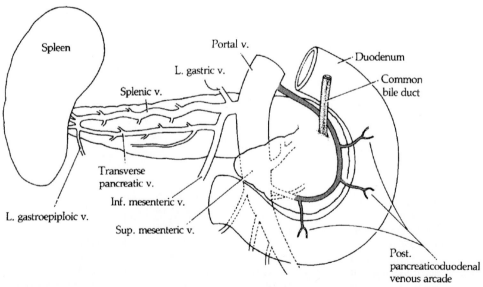

Fig. 26. Posterior view of the venous drainage of the pancreas and the tributaries of the hepatic portal vein. (From Skandalakis JE, Gray SW, Rowe JS Jr, et al. Anatomical complications of pancreatic surgery. *Contemp Surg* 1979;15:17.)

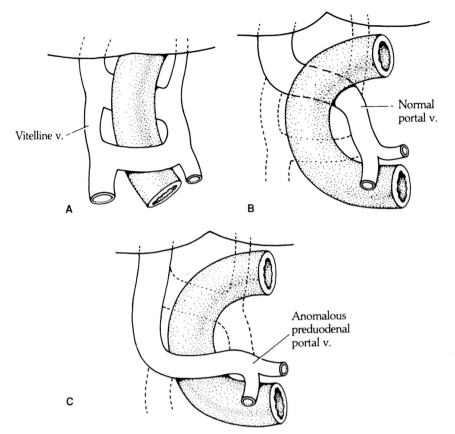

Vitelline v.

A

B

Normal portal v.

C

Anomalous preduodenal portal v.

Fig. 27. Diagram of the embryonic origin of a preduodenal portal vein. **A:** Embryonic, extrahepatic communications between the vitelline veins. **B:** Normal development. The persisting superior communicating vein forms part of the normal, retroduodenal portal vein. **C:** Anomalous persisting inferior communicating vein forms part of an abnormal preduodenal portal vein. (From Skandalakis JE, Gray SW, Rowe JS Jr, et al. Anatomical complications of pancreatic surgery. *Contemp Surg* 1979;15:17.)

- The veins of the pancreatic parenchyma are located between the ducts above and the arteries below.
- Pancreatic veins enter the lateral side of the portal vein or SMV from the pancreas to the right side of the portal vein. Be careful.
- The surgeon must avoid traction on the head of the pancreas and carefully ligate veins in the area.
- There are usually no branches on the anterior surface of the portal vein.
- The four possible vascular anomalies of the portal vein are as follows:
  The portal vein may lie anterior to the pancreas and duodenum.
  The portal vein may empty into the superior vena cava.
  A pulmonary vein may join the portal vein.
  The portal vein may have congenital strictures.
- If there is suspicion of an endocrine tumor of the pancreas that is not seen on computerized tomographic (CT) scan, a pancreatic arteriogram may be helpful in localizing the tumor. CT arteriography is a fairly new technology that also can be useful for localizing subtle tumors of the pancreas.

Lymphatic Drainage of the Pancreas

As might be expected from the position of the pancreas, lymphatic drainage is centrifugal to the surrounding nodes (Fig. 28). None of the efforts to demarcate specific drainage areas of the pancreas have gained wide acceptance, thus no "standard terminology" for the nodes exists. We base our presentation on the studies of Cubilla et al., which has been the basis for most recent works. The lymphatic vessels of the pancreas arise in a rich, perilobular, interanastomosing network. Channels course along the surface of the gland and in the interlobular spaces with the blood vessels. Cubilla et al. divided the peripancreatic lymph nodes into five main groups with subgroups (Fig. 29): (i) *Superior:* superior head, superior body, and gastric; (ii) *Inferior:* inferior head and inferior body; (iii) *Anterior:* anterior pancreaticoduodenal, pyloric, and mesenteric; (iv) *Posterior:* posterior pancreaticoduodenal and CBD; and (v) *Splenic:* lymph nodes at hilum of spleen and at the tail of pancreas.

Superior Nodes

The collecting trunks of this group of nodes arise from the anterior and posterior

blood for survival of the head and duodenum after the arcades are ligated.

- The PSPD artery is the main supply for the ampulla through the epicholedochal plexus.
- Injury may occur to the ASPD artery during the Puestow side-to-side pancreatojejunostomy.
- The superior and inferior pancreaticoduodenal arteries should not be ligated until the neck of the pancreas can be elevated from the underlying vessels. Premature ligation could cause necrosis of the head of the pancreas and duodenum.
- Angiography should be considered before surgery. Lo et al. reported localization rates prior to surgery for pancreatic insulomas using ultrasonography (33%), computed tomography (44%), and angiography (52%). Intraoperative ultrasonography had the highest rate of accurate detection. Huai et al. found that intraoperative ultrasonography also delineated spatial relationships of neighboring anatomic entities such as the splenic and superior mesenteric vessels, portal vein, CBD, and pancreatic

duct, aiding successful resection and avoiding blind pancreatectomy.

- Noncommunication between the splenic and transverse pancreatic arteries is possible. It can result in possible infarction at the area of the tail.
- Ligation of the splenic artery does not require splenectomy; ligation of the splenic vein does.
- Collateral circulation can develop as a result of stenosis of the SMA or celiac artery. Koshi et al. found abnormal blood flow through the pancreaticoduodenal arcade during angiographic examination.
- Ligation of both pancreaticoduodenal arterial arcades results in duodenal ischemia and necrosis.
- Two cadavers used in our first-year dissection laboratory had huge pancreatic carcinomas. We noticed that mesenteric arteries and veins were not obstructed and collateral circulation was not present. This may have been because these unfortunate individuals died at an age before obstruction of the vessels would normally occur.

The Gastrointestinal Tract

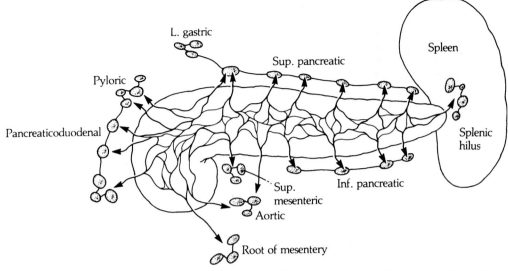

Fig. 28. Lymphatic drainage of the pancreas. Flow is toward the nearest margin of the pancreas. (From Skandalakis JE, Gray SW, Rowe JS Jr, et al. Anatomical complications of pancreatic surgery. *Contemp Surg* 1979;15:17.)

superior half of the pancreas. Most end in the suprapancreatic lymph nodes located along the superior border of the pancreas. The names of the nodes typically reflect the areas drained, such as the superior head and the superior body. Some lymphatics occasionally terminate in the nodes of the gastropancreatic fold or in the lymph nodes of the hepatic chain.

Inferior Nodes

These collecting trunks drain the anterior and posterior lower half of the head and body of the pancreas. They lead into the inferior pancreatic group of lymph nodes, most of which are located along the inferior border of the head and body of the pancreas. Further, they may extend into the superior mesenteric and left lateroaortic lymph nodes. Although infrequent, a collecting trunk may terminate directly in a lumbar trunk.

Anterior Nodes

Two collecting trunks run along the anterior surface of the superior and inferior portions of the head of the pancreas. They extend to the infrapyloric and anterior pancreaticoduodenal lymph nodes. They may also extend to some of the mesenteric lymph nodes located at the root of the mesentery (mesenteric-jejunal nodes).

Posterior Nodes

The posterior nodes follow the posterior surface of the superior and inferior portions of the head of the pancreas. They drain into the posterior pancreaticoduodenal lymph nodes, CBD lymph nodes, right lateroaortic lymph nodes, and some nodes at the origin of the SMA. Most lymphatics of the CBD and ampulla of Vater also end in the posterior pancreaticoduodenal group of lymph nodes.

Splenic Nodes

The splenic lymphatics originate from the tail of the pancreas. They drain into those at the hilum of the spleen, splenophrenic ligament, and inferior and superior lymph nodes of the tail of the pancreas. A few lymphatic channels, however, end in the lymph nodes superior and inferior to the body of the pancreas.

Surgical Considerations

We continue to learn about pancreatic lymphatics. The following paragraphs present some additional information.

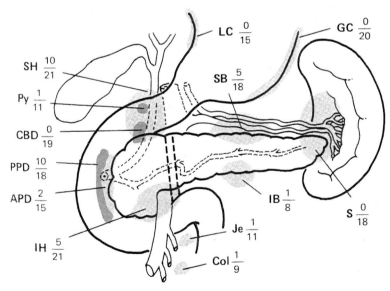

Fig. 29. Metastases of lymph nodes in 21 pancreatectomy resection specimens. Fraction numerators indicate number of patients with metastasis in that lymph node group; denominators indicate number of patients in which lymph nodes in this group were examined. *Stippled line,* Whipple resection; SH, superior head; Py, pylorus; CBD, common bile duct; PPD, posterior pancreaticoduodenal; APD, anterior pancreaticoduodenal; IH, inferior head; LC, lesser curvature; SB, superior body; IB, inferior body; Je, jejunal; Col, midcolic; GC, greater curvature; S, tail of pancreas and splenic. (From Cubilla AL, Fitzgerald PJ. Cancer of the exocrine pancreas: the pathologic aspects. *CA Cancer J Clin* 1985;35:2–18.)

- Deki and Sato wrote that the lymphatics of the anterior surface of the head and neck of the pancreas are associated with the common hepatic group and the superior mesenteric nodal group. All terminate at a lymph node or nodes situated to the right of the origins of the celiac trunk and the SMA. Lymphatics of the posterior surface of the head terminate in a node located behind the previously described node. The lymphatics of the left half of the pancreas terminate in a node to the left of the celiac trunk and SMA. Both the right and left nodes drain into the abdominal aortic nodes.

- The lymphatics of the head and body of the pancreas do not drain toward the tail of the pancreas or the splenic nodes. Rarely, however, the lymph vessels from the tail of the pancreas can terminate in the superior body and inferior body subgroups of nodes.

- By injecting dye into several pancreatic segments and then dissecting, Donatini and Hidden studied the routes of lymphatic drainage from the pancreas. They concluded that dye injected into the body and tail followed the splenic and inferior pancreatic pathways, terminating first to the left interceliacomesenteric node and then to the suprarenal and infrarenal lymph nodes. From the head of the pancreas, dye followed one of three routes:

  The lymphatics of the anterior and posterior aspects of the head followed the superior mesenteric route and reached the right interceliacomesenteric node and then terminated bilaterally in the suprarenal and infrarenal nodes.

  The anterosuperior segment of the head followed two routes. The gastroduodenal joined the right interceliacomesenteric node. An inferior route terminated by flowing backward in direction to the isthmus.

  The drainage of the posterosuperior segment of the head followed the CBD and hepatic artery, reaching the pericholedochal nodes and hepatic pedicular nodes and occasionally the right interceliacomesenteric node.

- Donatini and Hidden consider the right interoceliacomesenteric node the principal relay station for drainage from the head of the pancreas.

- No lymphatic communications exist between the pancreas and the lymph nodes of the greater and lesser curvatures of the stomach.

- Lymph moves from the pancreas to the duodenum, not from the duodenum to the pancreas.

- Based on studies of the lymphatic network of the guinea pig, Bertelli et al. concluded the following: "All lymph vessels in the pancreas are absorbing lymph vessels, characterized by a very thin endothelial wall, anchoring filaments and the absence of a definitive basal membrane."

- Cubilla et al. reported that a total pancreatectomy may include removal of 70 nodes. The Whipple partial pancreatectomy may involve removing 33 nodes. It is the opinion of the authors of this chapter that 15 to 20 is a good harvest.

- The surgeon should be familiar with the anatomic topography of the peripancreatic nodes.

- Delcore et al. reported that 56% of patients undergoing curative resection for pancreatic carcinoma were found to have lymph node metastases.

- It is well known that pancreatic cancer disseminates rapidly because of the retroperitoneal position of the pancreas and its rich lymphatic and venous drainage. Foster wrote that, additionally, pancreatic exocrine adenocarcinomas appear to have an unusually efficient biologic capacity to metastasize.

- Mukaiya et al. wrote that excessive lymph node dissection in advanced cases of ductal adenocarcinoma of the head of the pancreas does not necessarily lead to a favorable prognosis. They found, though, that patients who underwent a radical operation with adequate lymph node dissection had longer survival periods.

- Nakao et al. presented results of histopathologic examination of lymph nodes with metastasis from 139 patients who had cancer of the head of the pancreas. (Fig. 30, Tables 3 and 4). They

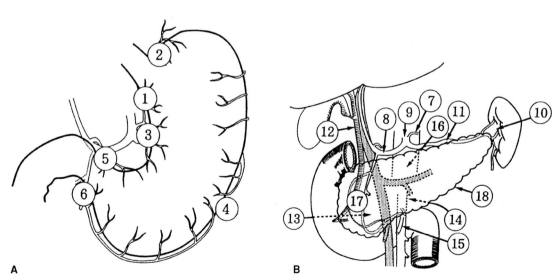

Fig. 30. A: Perigastric lymph nodes in patients who have carcinoma of the head of the pancreas. **B:** Lymph nodes in carcinoma of the head of the pancreas region. 1, right cardiac lymph nodes; 2, left cardiac lymph nodes; 3, lesser curvature lymph nodes; 4, greater curvature lymph nodes; 5, suprapyloric lymph nodes; 6, infrapyloric lymph nodes; 7, lymph nodes around the left gastric artery; 8, lymph nodes around the common hepatic artery; 9, lymph nodes around the celiac trunk; 10, lymph nodes at the hilum of the spleen; 11, lymph nodes along the splenic artery; 12, lymph nodes of the hepatoduodenal ligament; 13, posterior pancreaticoduodenal lymph nodes; 14, lymph nodes around the superior mesenteric artery; 15, lymph nodes along the middle colic artery; 16, para-aortic lymph nodes; 17, anterior pancreaticoduodenal lymph nodes; 18, inferior pancreatic body lymph nodes. (From Nakao A, Harada A, Nonami T, et al. Lymph node metastases in carcinoma of the head of the pancreas region. *Br J Surg* 1995;82:399.)

TABLE 3. OPERATIVE PROCEDURES FOR CARCINOMA OF THE HEAD OF THE PANCREAS REGION[a]

	No. of Total Pancreatectomies	No. of Pancreatoduodenectomies
Carcinoma of the head of the pancreas (n = 90)	48 (48)	42 (41)
Carcinoma of the distal bile duct (n = 22)	1 (1)	21 (2)
Carcinoma of the papilla of Vater (n = 27)	1 (1)	26 (2)

[a]Values in parentheses indicate the number of portal vein resections.
From Nakao A, Harada A, Nonami T, et al. Lymph node metastases in carcinoma of the head of the pancreas region. *Br J Surg* 1995;82:399, with permission.

advised that wide dissection of lymph nodes, including para-aortic nodes, is necessary in patients who have carcinoma of the pancreatic head.

- Vossen et al. reported that pancreatic tumors in children are rare, that the tumor pattern and biologic behavior is not the same as in adults, and that complete surgical excision is the treatment of choice.
- Nakagohri et al. found that intraductal papillary mucinous tumors, a localized malignancy, had a favorable prognosis after surgical treatment. They recommend curative pancreatectomy.
- In contrast, a study by Sho et al. reported that intraductal papillary mucinous tumors have high recurrence at the pancreatic remnant even after curative resection. Their results suggest that intraductal papillary mucinous tumor is a multicentric phenomenon and they advise avoiding incomplete resection.

We quote from Kobari et al.: "Intraductal papillary mucinous tumors may be comprised of 2 clinically distinct subtypes: MDTs [main duct tumors] and BDTs [branch duct tumors]. Initially, although distal pancreatectomy can be recommended for most MDTs, the need for cancer-free margins in this more aggressive type may necessitate total pancreatectomy. Pylorus-preserving pancreatoduodenectomies are recommended for most BDTs, but, because these tumors are more often adenomas, a good prognosis can be expected."

- The enigmatic malignancy of the pancreatic head produces problems for both the patient and the surgeon. The biggest problem for the patient is that quite frequently there is no tissue diagnosis prior to going to the operating room. This means that the patient is accepting on faith (i.e., on the surgeon's very learned opinion) that he or she has a serious problem that may require a very serious operation with a fairly high mortality and morbidity rate. The surgeon, on the other hand, is proceeding with a very serious operation with a high morbidity and mortality rate—comparatively speaking—not because of a tissue diagnosis, but because a distal common duct stricture has a certain look to it that is highly suggestive of pancreatic or distal CBD cancer. Occasionally it happens that a Whipple procedure is done in such a situation, only to find out that there was no malignancy, merely benign disease. That is not to say that an incorrect decision was made; it just confirms that dealing with pancreatic cancer can indeed be enigmatic.

- In regard to diagnosing pancreatic cancer, Warshaw wrote: "If I think there is a mass, I want to be sure I have a high-quality contrast CT scan in hand as my principal imaging modality."
- Yeo and Cameron wrote that "...standard pancreaticoduodenectomy, which in most cases can be performed using the pylorus-preserving technique, should serve as the recommended resectional strategy in patients with adenocarcinoma of the head, neck, or uncinate process of the pancreas." It has been the experience of the authors of this chapter that patients who undergo the pylorus-preserving technique seem to have delayed gastric emptying for a significantly longer period of time. For this reason, the authors have abandoned the pylorus-preserving technique when doing Whipple procedures.

NERVE SUPPLY OF THE PANCREAS

Innervation of the pancreas is by the sympathetic division of the autonomic nervous system through the splanchnic nerves

TABLE 4. LYMPH NODE INVOLVEMENT IN PATIENTS WITH CARCINOMA OF THE HEAD OF THE PANCREAS REGION[a]

Lymph Nodes	Carcinoma of the Head of the Pancreas (n = 90)	Carcinoma of the Distal Bile Duct (n = 22)	Carcinoma of the Papilla of Vater (n = 27)
1	0	0	0
2	0	0	0
3	0	0	0
4	0	0	1 (4)
5	0	0	0
6	13 (14)	0	0
7	0	0	0
8	12 (13)	1 (4)	0
9	2 (2)	1 (4)	0
10	1 (1)	0	0
11	16 (18)	0	0
12	17 (19)	5 (23)	1 (4)
13	46 (51)	3 (14)	11 (41)
14	21 (23)	2 (9)	3 (11)
15	0	0	0
16	23 (26)	2 (9)	0
17	35 (39)	1 (4)	6 (22)
18	3 (3)	1 (4)	0

[a]Values in parentheses represent percentages.
From Nakao A, Harada A, Nonami T, et al. Lymph node metastases in carcinoma of the head of the pancreas region. *Br J Surg* 1995;82:399, with permission.

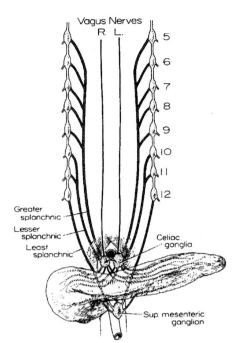

Fig. 31. The nerve supply to the pancreas. (From Skandalakis JE, Gray SW, Rowe JS Jr, et al. Anatomical complications of pancreatic surgery. *Contemp Surg* 1979;15:17.)

and by the parasympathetic division through the vagus nerve (Fig. 31). These nerves generally follow blood vessels to their destinations. The sympathetic and parasympathetic divisions provide efferent (motor) fibers to the wall of the blood vessels, the pancreatic duct, and pancreatic acini. Further, both contain visceral afferent (pain) fibers. The distribution of these in the pancreas, however, is not well understood.

Preganglionic sympathetic innervation is from the greater and lesser thoracic splanchnic nerves. The former is composed of preganglionic efferent fibers from the 5th to the 9th or 10th thoracic segments. The latter is composed of fibers from the 9th and 10th or the 10th and 11th segments. Some fibers may be contributed by the least splanchnic nerve.

The sympathetic nerves pierce the diaphragmatic crura to reach the celiac and superior mesenteric ganglia. Postganglionic fibers arising from neurons in these ganglia accompany branches of the celiac and superior mesenteric arteries to reach the pancreas.

Some afferent fibers cross over the midline in the celiac plexus. The celiac ganglion contains cell bodies of efferent fibers for the pancreas. Cell bodies of afferent fibers are in the dorsal root ganglia at the same spinal nerve levels as those that contribute the preganglionic sympa-

thetic fibers. Interconnections of the afferent fibers from the pancreas with other sensory fibers from the body wall are presumably responsible for referral of pancreatic pain to the surface of the abdominal wall. Pain fibers from the pancreas pass cranially within the greater thoracic splanchnic nerve; they leave it by way of white communicating rami and enter the midthoracic spinal nerves. These neurons have their cell bodies within the dorsal root ganglia of those nerves.

Parasympathetic innervation is by way of the celiac division of the posterior vagal trunk. The efferent fibers are preganglionic axons from cell bodies in the dorsal motor nucleus of the vagus nerve in the brain. The preganglionic vagal fibers synapse with terminal ganglion cells within the pancreas. The postganglionic fibers terminate at pancreatic islet cells. Almost 90% of the fibers carried by the vagus nerve are sensory in function, having to do with stretch, chemoreception, osmoreception, and thermoreception. Grundy states that fewer than 10% of the fibers carried by the vagus are autonomic efferents; the remaining fibers are sensory. These afferent fibers are processes of sensory neurons located in the sensory ganglia of the right vagus nerve at the jugular foramen of the skull. Vagal fibers pass through the esophageal hiatus of the diaphragm, usually as anterior and posterior trunks. The posterior trunk divides into a posterior gastric and celiac division near the lesser curvature of the stomach. The neuronal processes of the celiac division of the posterior vagus traverse the nerve plexuses at the origins of the celiac and superior mesenteric arteries and accompany the branches of these arteries to reach the organs supplied by them. None of the fibers carried by the vagus synapse within the celiac ganglia.

The severe pain of pancreatic disease is not easy to explain anatomically. Bockman et al. wrote that the perineurium is damaged; they, as does Frey, contended that inflammatory cells frequently concentrate around the nerves and ganglia in patients who have chronic pancreatitis. Drapiewski believed the cause in most cases was invasion of the nerves by the tumor. Ductal hypertension is also responsible for the production of pain, and Widdison et al. speculated a compartment syndrome from increased tissue and ductal pressure. Bockman assumes that there are multiple paths for the genesis of pancreatic pain, and that much additional study is needed on its origin and management.

EXPLORATION OF THE PANCREAS

The modern surgeon must understand not only pancreatic anatomy, but how to methodically use diagnostic procedures to evaluate the entire pancreas prior to surgery. A preoperative CT scan should be done, and the surgeon should consider whether a magnetic resonance image of the pancreas and endoscopic retrograde cholangiopancreatography would benefit the patient. Rarely is an arteriogram necessary.

The pancreas can be approached by dividing the gastrocolic ligament (greater omentum) or the hepatogastric ligament (lesser omentum). Under usual circumstances, the gastrocolic ligament is incised widely and provides good exposure of the entire pancreas; this is the approach used by most surgeons. If this exposure proves to be inadequate, the hepatogastric ligament can be divided also, and upward traction can be applied to the stomach. This route is useful in patients with exceptionally ptotic stomachs.

To palpate the head of the pancreas, kocherization of the duodenum is necessary. Mobilization of the duodenum is accomplished by mobilizing the hepatic flexure of the colon and then incising the peritoneum lateral to the second part of the duodenum. Next, the left index and middle fingers are placed posterior to the duodenum and the head of the pancreas, with the left thumb anterior. Palpation of the head of the pancreas and the pancreatic portion of the CBD is then possible. Lymph nodes can sometimes be felt at the distal portion of the CBD, near the upper part of the posterior surface of the head of the pancreas.

The left index finger can continue the exploration posterior to the neck of the pancreas. Occasionally, both index fingers can be used (Fig. 32). The surgeon's left hand approaches the neck from above, with the left index finger posterior to the neck, and the right hand comes from below, with the right index finger also posterior to the neck. The ability to separate the neck from the underlying superior mesenteric and portal veins is considered by many surgeons a criterion for resection for cancer. Silen, however, rejects this maneuver because of possible avulsion of a posterosuperior pancreaticoduodenal vein that may enter the SMV on its anterior surface. It is the opinion of the authors of this chapter, though, that this maneuver is valuable.

The Gastrointestinal Tract

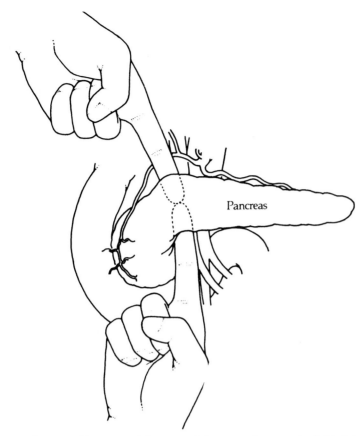

Fig. 32. Exploration of the pancreas. The surgeon's fingers are shown passing behind the neck of the pancreas, which should separate easily from the underlying blood vessels. (From Skandalakis JE, Gray SW, Rowe JS Jr, et al. Anatomical complications of pancreatic surgery. *Contemp Surg* 1979;15:17.)

We believe that the best way to explore the SMV is as follows. After one has done a kocherization of the duodenum, the gastroduodenal artery is identified and, after tying, divided. Further dissection is then done in this area at the superior border of the pancreas. Identify the portal vein. Next, at the inferior border of the pancreas, look for a branch of the middle colic vein that is heading underneath the pancreas, and start your dissection there. As you continue to dissect while staying on top of the vein it will become much larger (it is, in fact, the SMV). Continue very gentle dissection on top of that vein but underneath the pancreas. A very blunt dissecting instrument such as a Kelly clamp is ideal. Once you have proceeded as far as you can comfortably go—alternately using the Kelly clamp, then the finger—switch to the superior border of the pancreas and start dissecting inferiorly, staying on top of the portal vein/SMV. Eventually the superior dissection will connect with the inferior dissection if there is no involvement of the SMV. Even with a successful dissection in this manner the lateral wall of the SMV is frequently

involved with tumor. Thus, successful completion of this maneuver does not necessarily mean that the SMV is not involved.

The uncinate process is the most difficult part of the pancreas to explore and evaluate because of its close relations to the SMA and SMV. The surgeon may find the SMV to be free of cancer anteriorly only to discover cancer in the lateral wall after the pancreas has been divided.

In addition to the routes for abdominal exploration that have already been discussed, there are several others.

- Detach the gastrocolic ligament from the transverse colon. This is time-consuming, but it provides improved visualization of the entire lesser sac.
- Approach through the mesocolon. Disadvantages include limited exposure of the pancreas and risk of injury to the middle colic blood vessels.
- Mobilization of the splenic flexure inferiorly, the spleen, and the tail of the pancreas.

Hermann and Cooperman believe that localized masses in the head of the pan-

creas should be resected, even in the absence of histologic proof of malignancy. They suggest that "the smallest tumors, and perhaps those with the most favorable outcome, may never be resected for lack of histologic proof of the diagnosis." The authors of this chapter fully agree with resection in the absence of histologic proof of malignancy.

Child and Frey have listed several contraindications to pancreaticoduodenectomy: (i) liver metastases or carcinomatous implants on the hepatic serosa; (ii) invasion of the base of the colonic mesentery; (iii) invasion of the hepatoduodenal ligament; (iv) invasion of the gastroduodenal, hepatic, or superior mesenteric arteries; (v) involvement of the porta hepatis; (vi) metastases to the portal vein; (vii) fixation by tumor of duodenum and pancreas to underlying structures; and (viii) metastases to aorta or vena cava.

Positive lymph nodes are not a contraindication for pancreaticoduodenectomy.

SUGGESTED READING

Avisse C, Flament JB, Delattre JF. Ampulla of Vater: anatomic, embryologic, and surgical aspects. *Surg Clin North Am* 2000;80:201.

Deziel DJ. Metastases to the pancreas. In: Howard JM, Idezuki Y, Ihse I, Prinz RA (eds). *Surgical diseases of the pancreas*, 3rd ed. Baltimore: Williams & Wilkins, 1998.

Foster RS Jr. Pancreas [editorial comment]. In: Skandalakis JE, Colborn GL, Weidman TA, et al., eds. *Skandalakis' surgical anatomy: the embryologic and anatomic basis of modern surgery*. Athens, Greece: Paschalidis Medical Publications, 2004:1194.

Huai JC, Zhang W, Niu HO, et al. Localization and surgical treatment of pancreatic insulinomas guided by intraoperative ultrasound. *Am J Surg* 1998;175:18.

Kobari M, Egawa S, Shibuya K, et al. Intraductal papillary mucinous tumors of the pancreas comprise 2 clinical subtypes. *Arch Surg* 1999;134:1131.

Koshi T, Govil S, Koshi R. Problem in diagnostic imaging: pancreaticoduodenal arcade in splanchnic arterial stenosis. *Clin Anat* 1998;11:206.

Mirilas P, Colborn GL, Skandalakis LJ, et al. Benign anatomical mistakes: "Ampulla of Vater" and "Papilla of Vater." *Am Surg* 2005;71:269.

Mukaiya M, Hirata K, Satoh T, et al. Lack of survival benefit of extended lymph node dissection for ductal adenocarcinoma of the head of the pancreas: retrospective multi-institutional analysis in Japan. *World J Surg* 1998; 22:248.

Nakagohri T, Kenmochi T, Kainuma O, et al. Intraductal papillary mucinous tumors of the pancreas. *Am J Surg* 1999;178:344.

Ooshima I, Maruyama T, Ootsuki K, et al. Preduodenal portal vein in the adult. *J Hepatobiliary Pancreat Surg* 1998;5:455.

Sho M, Nakajima Y, Kanehiro H, et al. Pattern of recurrence after resection for intraductal papillary mucinous tumors of the pancreas. *World J Surg* 1998; 22:874.

Sugiyama M, Baba M, Atomi Y, et al. Diagnosis of anomalous pancreaticobiliary junction: value of magnetic resonance cholangiopancreatography. *Surgery* 1998; 123:391.

Vossen S, Goretzki PE, Goebel U, et al. Therapeutic management of rare malignant pancreatic tumors in children. *World J Surg* 1998;22:879.

Warshaw AL, comments in: Lillemoe KD (moderator), Conlon KC, Evans DB, Warshaw AL (panelists). Ductal adenocarcinoma of the pancreas. *Contemp Surg* 2001;57:68.

Yeo CJ, Cameron JL. Pancreatic nodal metastases. *Surg Oncol Clin North Am* 1996;5:145.

The Gastrointestinal Tract

EDITOR'S COMMENT

This is the usual excellent chapter contributed by the Skandalakis group concerning anatomy; they have become and remain the principal surgical anatomists of this generation and the previous one. The anatomy of the hepatobiliary area, including the pancreas, is essential to the development of a relatively new subspecialty of hepatobiliary surgery. The evolution of hepatobiliary surgery is different in the United States and in Europe, depending on whether the hepatobiliary surgeon originates from the field of transplantation, has been specially trained, or because of interest has pursued a career in hepatobiliary surgery. At our own institution we have five individuals who participate in hepatobiliary surgery: Drs. Callery and Vollmer, who principally perform pancreatic surgery, and Drs. Hanto, Johnson, and Karp, who primarily perform hepatic surgery and are liver transplantors as well. The two groups have agreed that they would choose the cystic duct as the dividing line, and that tumors and conditions below the cystic duct would be the province of the pancreatic surgeons and conditions above the cystic duct would fall under the jurisdiction of the liver surgeons. This has worked well and the volume of surgeries has been extraordinary, with more than 120 Whipple procedures carried out in the past year. There is a very low incidence of mortality and an 8.2 days' length of postoperative stay, with an excellent clinical pathway organized by Drs. Callery and Vollmer. The very low mortality indicates that excellent results can be achieved in resection of the pancreas with low mortality and morbidity, a fact that has been confirmed by other groups who have specialized in this area.

When I was a resident in the 1960s, surgeons such as George Crile and Leland McKittrick were of the opinion—given the mortality of pancreaticoduodectomy, which at the time ranged between 15% and 20%, and the low survival advantages as far as long-term cure—that this was not a surgical lesion. Indeed, there were calculations as to the length of life in months that were either gained or lost by operation on carcinoma at the head of the pancreas. The concentration on the hepatobiliary area has borne more fruit, in my humble opinion, as far as survival is concerned, in the hepatic resection area than it has thus far in the area of the pancreas. In the hands of excellent surgeons, most of whom practice in high-volume centers (although individual surgeons in moderate-volume centers have outcomes that approach those of high-volume centers), mortality and complications have decreased remarkably. Survival, although probably slightly increased in carcinoma in the head of the pancreas, has not increased remarkably except with the advent of neoadjuvant chemoradiation therapy, such as practiced by Traverso.

This chapter is very detailed and very practical in that it gives the surgeon the essentials of pancreatic surgery. Early in the chapter, the vagaries of pancreatic resection are enumerated. The authors point out that the extent of resection of the head of the uncinate process is empiric; the division of the neck is not exact, but generally varies between 60% and 70% of the pancreatic bulk; and although with a normal pancreas, even after 80% pancreatectomy, good exocrine and endocrine activity remain, it is difficult to tell its sufficiency, depending on the extent of disease of the pancreas prior to resection.

There are a number of points that have been raised by the authors that one should bear in mind. First, because of the nature of the double-anlage that forms the pancreas and the fact that the dorsal anlage usually develops without any connection to the duodenum, there is no such thing as "normal" or "abnormal" anatomy; all variations are normal. Whether the accessory duct drains into the pancreatic duct is a matter of variation, as to which one is dominant. Whether the accessory duct actually terminates in a single ampulla or a variety of ampullas, and the resorption of the common bile duct, are all variations. When one examines the ampulla, it is important to note whether there is a common channel, not only in biliary tract disease but also in pancreatic disease. For example, with an abnormal or high communication of the pancreatic duct of Wirsung, the result is often the dilatation of the lower end of the common duct of the biliary tree caused by secretion, presumably of activated phospholipase A, into the bile duct, which is thought to be responsible for the choledochal cysts in their various forms. On the other hand, according to the authors, such abnormal arrangements may also result in idiopathic pancreatitis, so when one is confronted with a patient with idiopathic pancreatitis it is wise to look for the dilatation of the lower end of the biliary tree and abnormal communication because this may contribute to what might otherwise be called idiopathic pancreatitis.

Much has been written about finding the ampulla. I usually find this relatively easy. With a wide kocherization of the duodenum and placing one's left hand behind the duodenum, one can usually feel the ampulla at a juncture where the descending portion turns to become the horizontal portion. With the widespread use of endoscopic retrograde cholangiopancreatography and the identification of patients with biliary dyskinesia, one can find someone who does biliary pressures and does them regularly enough so that they are meaningful. The sphincterotomy has become the standard therapy for biliary dyskinesia. However, many patients are not helped by sphincterotomy, which is usually done to a length of 7 or 8 mm, because the procedure does not divide the muscle completely as the muscle ranges in thickness between 13 and 20.5 mm. In

proven biliary dyskinesia patients, sphincteroplasty may be more appropriate provided that they have not had pancreatitis. "Patients with pancreatitis did worse overall, perhaps due to the existence of unappreciated subclinical parenchymal disease not related to sphincter dysfunction" (Nussbaum MS, et al. *Am J Surg* 1989;157:38).

S. Austin Jones has proposed a sphincteroplasty of about 2.5 cm, which is appropriate based on the anatomic data presented in this chapter. The one drawback to these patients, who I have followed for years after performing sphincterotomy, is that after 10 or 15 years most of them develop cholangitis and require either intermittent or constant antibiotics to keep this under control. Thus, it will be interesting to see whether the readily carried out sphincterotomy in which common duct stones are retrieved results in similar cholangitis in these patients.

Another consequence of the complex rotation of the double-anlage of the pancreas is in two anomalies that are both very serious if one is not aware of them and inadvertently divides the structures involved. Of course the SMA may have various paths, including traveling through the pancreas and over the pancreas, but it is rare, occurring in less than 5% of patients; quite honestly, I have never personally seen one. I have, however, seen numerous accessory arteries or replaced right hepatic arteries, and this is dangerous if one is not aware of it and divides it. I have seen patients who have died of acute hepatic necrosis 4 days after division of the large right hepatic artery. I have also seen patients who have died after 1 or 2 months of a steadily inexorable hepatic necrosis. On the basis of these and other experiences, if one divides the right hepatic artery inadvertently it must be repaired. It does seem logical that the right hepatic artery will only provide 50% or less of the blood supply to the right lobe, but apparently in some patients, despite the portal vein increasing its flow in a relatively normal hepatic vasculature, it is not sufficient to prevent these patients from dying. I would also call attention to the right gastroepiploic vein, which sometimes can be troublesome when performing a right hemicolectomy. In the presence of portal hypertension, however, tearing the right gastroepiploic vein from where it comes off the portal vein results in torrential bleeding and can be life-threatening. One must be aware of this vein prior to finishing resection of the hepatic flexure. It usually is found at some point between 3 and 5 cm medial to the hepatic flexure and must be divided early, lest one tear it when taking down the hepatic flexure. The other possibly fatal anomaly is the preduodenal portal vein, which fortunately occurs only rarely.

The nodal structures are given great detail and, as the authors point out, there is no connection between the gastric lymph nodes and the pancreas.

(continued)

There is some sentiment for ever-larger swaths of lymph nodes taken in the pancreatic duodenectomy, and there is some evidence of increased recurrence-free survival, but long-term outcome and long-term survival have not been increased impressively by wider nodal dissection. Indeed, using the analogy of gastric cancer, which has been separately discussed in this volume, one does see increased survival as one gets to a D2 resection for gastric cancer, but the complications and mortality also seem to be increased, at least in some hands. However, the authors believe, and I agree, that given the low mortality and morbidity of a pancreaticoduodenectomy and the horrible painful death of patients who do not have resection, a positive node at the time of surgery may not be a tragedy. Others believe that positive nodes are contraindications to pancreaticoduodenectomy.

Several technical details deserve comment. I agree that a critical maneuver in pancreatico-duodectomy is the passage of one's fingers, a blunt instrument, or in my case a small flexible brain retractor, between the superior mesenteric vein as it becomes the portal vein behind the pancreas. The dissection is achieved by first ligating the gastroduodenal artery and then freeing up the anterior surface of the portal vein and joining the fingers beneath the pancreas; nonetheless, freedom in the anterior plane does not necessarily mean that the tumor has not invaded the superior mesenteric/portal vein somewhere else. In my experience, this is at the most cephalad point laterally, as the pancreas approaches the duodenum. I disagree with Dr. Silen that one will tear vessel branches using this maneuver; and I agree with the authors.

I also agree with the authors that the pylorus-preserving Whipple procedure does have a significant incidence of delayed gastric emptying, so much so that I would suggest that if one is going to do this that one use a gastrostomy and feeding jejunuostomy liberally, so as to enable the patient to get out of the hospital without the prolonged postoperative stay that nasogastric intubation can bring. Finally, as for imaging, the CT angiogram, magnetic resonance imaging, magnetic resonance cholangiopancreatography, and a variety of different types of imaging can also be supplemented if there is a complicated situation revealed by ultrasonography of the pancreas, either perioperatively or intraoperatively. Bertolotto et al. (*Abdom Imaging* 2006;20:1), in an extensive review of ultrasonography of the pancreas and Doppler imaging, have some very nice images as well as a number of suggestions from a group of Italian radiologists based in Trieste and Verona.

Finally, one must congratulate the authors for a fine surgical anatomy chapter that makes a complex operation more accessible and safer.

J.E.F.

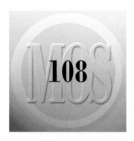

Roux-en-Y Lateral Pancreaticojejunostomy for Chronic Pancreatitis

RICHARD A. PRINZ, MARK R. EDWARDS, AND RODERICK M. QUIROS

Chronic pancreatitis is a disorder with a worldwide distribution. It is an inflammatory disease of the pancreas that is characterized by progressive morphologic and functional damage. If the process is not altered, the parenchyma of the gland becomes fibrotic and displays evidence of acinar cell destruction and lymphocyte infiltration. As the fibrosis continues and the glandular elements are replaced, the microcirculation of the gland is altered. This affects both the exocrine and endocrine functions of the gland and leads to malnourishment, vitamin deficiencies, steatorrhea, and diabetes mellitus.

The hallmark symptom of chronic pancreatitis is intractable abdominal pain. Multiple theories have been used to explain this pain. Some have proposed that the pain is caused, in part, by an inflammatory process that involves pancreatic nerves. Tissue specimens taken from patients suffering from chronic pancreatitis often have multiple foci of inflammatory cells surrounding pancreatic nerves. In a report by Bockman et al., electron microscopy of these nerves showed a damaged perineurium and further invasion of lymphocytes. It is possible that these deleterious alterations may allow inflammatory mediators and pancreatic enzymes access to nerves and lead to the substantial debilitating abdominal pain that is seen.

Di Sebastiano et al., using immunohistochemical staining techniques, have shown a relationship between the extent of perineural inflammation and the severity of clinically apparent abdominal pain.

Glandular hypertension also plays an important role in the disease. This is supported by the findings of pancreatic ductal dilatation, elevated intraductal and intraparenchymal pressures, and pain relief resulting from surgical decompression of the main pancreatic ducts. However, not all patients will have dilated pancreatic ducts and not all patients will be pain-free after surgical decompression. Alternate causes of pain include bile duct stenosis, duodenal stenosis, pseudocyst formation, and parenchymal ischemia.

Excessive ethanol consumption is the leading cause of chronic pancreatitis in the Western world. Alcohol and its metabolites have toxic effects on the acinar and ductal cells, which interferes with intracellular processes and the transport of enzymes. Alcohol not only affects the gland itself but often also the socioeconomic status of the patient. When alcohol is the etiologic factor, a trend toward dependence and addiction to narcotics is not uncommon. Less often seen causes of pancreatitis include pancreatic divisum, traumatic stricture, ductal obstruction by neoplasm, hyperlipidemia, and heredity.

The management of chronic pancreatitis consists of both medical and surgical modalities. Preoperative intervention often includes pancreatic enzyme replacement and cessation of alcohol consumption. Surgical intervention is indicated for management of complications such as pseudocyst formation, pancreatic ascites, symptomatic obstruction of the bile duct and duodenum, or for malignancy, as this occurs in at least 4% of patients with long-standing chronic pancreatitis. The most common indication for operative intervention in chronic pancreatitis is to alleviate intractable abdominal pain. When surgery is indicated for pain relief, the pain is typically refractory to medical therapy and the patient has had multiple hospital admissions for pain control. Social and economic factors such as narcotic dependency and unemployment are also common and have a severe impact on the quality of life.

The goal of surgical intervention for chronic pancreatitis is to safely and reliably relieve pain while preserving the endocrine and exocrine function of the gland. No single operation can accomplish this for all patients, but both ductal drainage and pancreatic resection have proven useful for the relief of pain. These concepts are not mutually exclusive and are often combined, as illustrated by lateral pancreaticojejunostomy with local resection of the pancreatic head.

Lateral pancreaticojejunostomy is the preferred operation for patients with intractable pain from chronic pancreatitis and a dilated pancreatic duct. This operation best approximates the goal of providing pain relief while preserving pancreatic function. With proper patient selection and attention to technical execution, lateral pancreaticojejunostomy can be accomplished with a high likelihood of patient benefit.

HISTORY OF LATERAL PANCREATICOJEJUNOSTOMY

The evolution of the lateral pancreaticojejunostomy began in 1908 when Coffey first performed distal pancreatectomy with pancreaticoenterostomy in dogs. He accurately suggested that this procedure would be beneficial in various clinical situations. Link first performed drainage of the pancreatic duct for chronic pancreatitis in 1911. Several decades later, Duval described distal pancreatectomy, splenectomy, and distal pancreaticojejunostomy for patients with chronic pancreatitis. The distal pancreaticojejunostomy was performed in an end-to-end fashion. His premise for this procedure was that increased pressure in the main pancreatic duct produced pain, which could be alleviated by draining the pancreas by a retrograde route. Criteria for the procedure to proceed included intraoperative documentation of increased pancreatic duct pressure. Duval's procedure addressed the distal pancreatic duct, but it neglected the proximal duct. Puestow and Gillesby addressed the more proximal portions of the duct by longitudinally opening the pancreatic duct in addition to splenectomy and distal pancreatectomy. A pancreaticojejunostomy was formed by the anastomosis of the open end of the jejunum and the proximal pancreas. Although a greater extent of the duct was decompressed, the head of the pancreas remained undrained as the jejunum was not able to be brought to the right of the superior mesenteric vessels.

The Puestow and Gillesby procedure was later modified by Partington and Rochelle, who described a side-to-side anastomosis created from a longitudinal opening in the jejunum as well as the pancreatic duct. Mobilization and resection of the spleen and distal pancreas were not necessary and drainage of the pancreas from the head to the tail was achieved. Most recently, Frey described local resection of the head of the pancreas that has been used in concert with lateral pancreaticojejunostomy. This procedure is important for situations in which the head of the pancreas has become enlarged and contains multiple strictures and retention cysts, which make complete ductal decompression exceedingly difficult.

 PREOPERATIVE PLANNING

Patient selection is the key to a successful outcome with lateral pancreaticojejunostomy. The goals of preoperative assessment are to confirm the diagnosis and rule out other causes of pain, to determine the morphology of the gland, to identify existing exocrine or endocrine insufficiency, and to evaluate the patient's physiologic and psychosocial fitness for surgery.

The diagnosis of chronic pancreatitis should be confirmed first by the presence of characteristic clinical features and review of appropriate imaging studies. A careful history can establish the nature of the patient's pain and the degree of disability. The history usually identifies an etiologic factor for chronic pancreatitis. In most patients, this is excessive alcohol intake. Physical examination may not be revealing in uncomplicated

chronic pancreatitis. The presence of tenderness, an abdominal mass, or jaundice should be assessed, as should signs of nutritional depletion and chronic liver disease. Extrapancreatic causes of abdominal pain, such as calculous biliary tract disease or peptic ulcer disease, must be identified and corrected. In addition, the possibility of pancreatic cancer must be considered, particularly in patients with a pancreatic mass or a history of substantial weight loss in the absence of overt steatorrhea or diminished oral intake. Tumor markers such as CA 19-9 and carcinoembryonic antigen should be obtained preoperatively in patients when malignancy is suspected. However, these tests are not specific for cancer and can be elevated in patients with chronic pancreatitis.

The pancreatic duct must be sufficiently dilated for lateral pancreaticojejunostomy to be technically successful. Multiple studies have demonstrated failure, measured by the persistence of abdominal pain, when lateral pancreaticojejunostomy is performed on a nondilated duct. Recommendations for the minimum caliber of the duct to be satisfactory for decompression vary from 5 to 10 mm. We consider pancreaticojejunostomy for patients with ducts larger than 5 mm.

Computed tomography (CT) and endoscopic retrograde cholangiopancreatography (ERCP) have been the most useful imaging studies for the assessment of chronic pancreatitis. Dynamic CT with 3-mm cuts through the pancreas is obtained in all patients. This study alone often provides sufficient anatomic information for surgical decision-making. CT can demonstrate dilatation of the pancreatic duct and is the most accurate method for detecting ductal and parenchymal calcifications (Fig. 1). CT can also identify associated abnormalities, such as pseudocysts,

The Gastrointestinal Tract

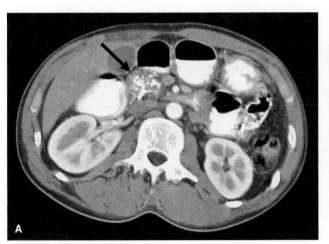
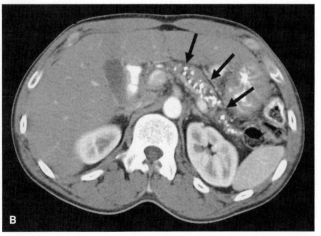

Fig. 1. Computed tomographic scans of a patient with chronic pancreatitis demonstrating enlargement and calcification of the pancreatic head *(arrow)* **(A)** as well as a thickened pancreatic body and tail *(arrows)* **(B)**.

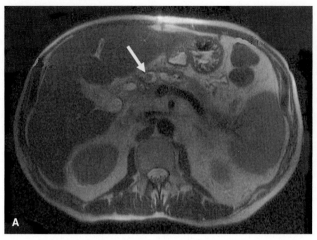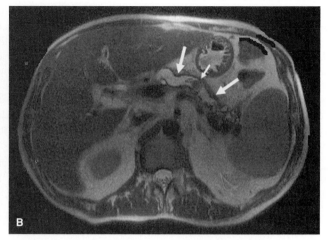

Fig. 2. T2-weighted magnetic resonance images of a patient with chronic pancreatitis demonstrating a large stone *(arrow)* located in the pancreatic duct in the head of the pancreas **(A)** as well as a large stone *(small arrow)* located in the dilated pancreatic duct *(large arrows)* in the body of the pancreas **(B)**.

mass lesions, and dilatation of the bile ducts.

ERCP is now no longer routinely performed before pancreaticojejunostomy. Although ERCP has been considered the most accurate method for determining pancreatic duct size and anatomy, this information is often present on CT scan. ERCP is reserved for patients with suspected chronic pancreatitis when a dilated duct is not seen on CT scan or when associated abnormalities require further evaluation. ERCP can clarify biliary pathology in patients with bile duct stricture or choledocholithiasis. Localized obstruction of the common bile duct and the pancreatic duct, the so-called *double-duct sign*, is best seen by ERCP and suggests pancreatic cancer. ERCP may fail to visualize a dilated pancreatic duct when the duct is obstructed near its entry into the duodenum by a stone or stricture. CT can usually identify the resulting dilatation proximal to this type of obstruction.

Magnetic resonance cholangiopancreatography (MRCP) and endoscopic ultrasound of the pancreas are being used more frequently to evaluate the pancreas and the anatomy of the pancreatic duct. Both are less invasive than ERCP and avoid the risks of inducing pancreatitis or introducing infection into the pancreatic or biliary tract. ERCP still offers unique diagnostic and therapeutic possibilities such as brush biopsy, sphincterotomy, and stent placement. A specific limitation of MRCP is poor visualization of secondary pancreatic ducts. In these situations, ERCP offers enhanced resolution with adequate contrast injection. However, if only a diagnostic study or a determination of the size and course of the pancreatic duct is needed, our practice is to obtain an MRCP (Figs. 2-4) or endoscopic ultrasound of the pancreas after the CT scan.

Preoperative physical evaluation of the patient must include a thorough assessment of their metabolic and nutritional status. Malnutrition and weight loss are common as a result of alcohol use, malabsorption, and pain induced by eating. Hypoalbuminemia is present in approximately one third of patients before pancreaticojejunostomy. Parenteral hyperalimentation for 1 to 3 weeks preoperatively may benefit patients with more pronounced nutritional deficits. Preoperative stabilization of serum glucose is important for the 30% to 40% of patients who are diabetic. The patient's general cardiorespiratory status must, of course, permit a major abdominal operation.

Determination of a patient's suitability for pancreaticojejunostomy also involves evaluation of the psychosocial situation. The extent to which the patient's quality of life has been impaired should be assessed as objectively as possible. Patients who are working, not drinking alcohol, and who have a supportive family structure fare well. A less favorable outcome can be expected in patients who cannot be rehabilitated from alcohol or drug use. In addition, the potential consequences of postoperative diabetes or exocrine insufficiency in the latter group may jeopardize their long-term outcome. Pancreaticojejunostomy preserves function better than resective procedures, but the progressive nature of this disease still adversely affects the metabolic activities of the gland. Patients and surgeons must have realistic expectations as to the anticipated results of operative intervention.

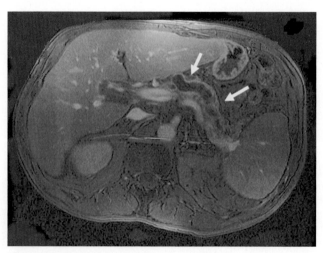

Fig. 3. T1-weighted magnetic resonance image demonstrating a dilated pancreatic duct *(arrows)* with surrounding atrophic parenchyma.

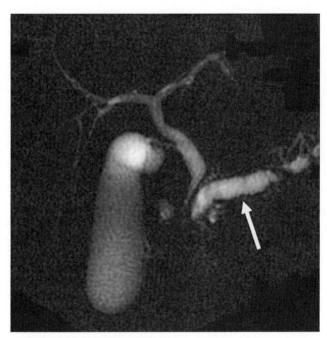

Fig. 4. Magnetic resonance cholangiopancreatography demonstrating a dilated pancreatic duct *(arrow)*.

 SURGICAL TECHNIQUE

The technical performance of lateral pancreaticojejunostomy likely has a substantial impact on the long-term results achieved with pancreatic duct decompression. A broad-spectrum intravenous antibiotic active against Gram-negative enteric organisms is usually administered preoperatively because cultures of pancreatic duct fluid yield organisms in approximately one fourth of patients. A mechanical and antibiotic bowel preparation is advisable, particularly in reoperative cases, because the transverse colon and its vascular supply may be firmly adherent to the retroperitoneal inflammatory process. Sequential compression devices are placed on the legs for the prevention of deep vein thrombosis. Radiographic capability should be available in case intraoperative cholangiography or pancreatography is needed. Digital fluoroscopy is preferred but standard static exposures may suffice.

A bilateral subcostal incision is our preferred method for entering the peritoneal cavity, but a midline incision may be appropriate, depending on the patient's body habitus and the location of previous incisions. A thorough initial exploration should confirm findings of chronic pancreatitis. The pancreas typically has a uniform, firm, and fibrotic consistency. A directed search should be made for evidence of malignancy. Any suspicious liver, peritoneal, or mesen-

teric lesions should be biopsied and sent for frozen section evaluation. If unusually hard areas or a mass is encountered in the pancreas, fine-needle aspiration can be performed with an 18-guage needle, and immediate cytologic analysis of the specimen can be obtained if an experienced cytologist is available. Cancer may also be detected as an area of breakthrough on the surface of the gland or infiltrating along the root of the transverse mesocolon or

small bowel mesentery. Superficial shave biopsies of these areas can be obtained. In any large series of patients undergoing pancreaticojejunostomy for chronic pancreatitis, a few will have cancer diagnosed intraoperatively or within several months.

Complete exposure of the anterior surface of the pancreas is necessary. The lesser sac is entered by sequential ligation and division of the gastrocolic omentum (Fig. 5). The gastroepiploic vessels should be spared. Fibrous adhesions between the pancreas and the posterior wall of the stomach are taken down by cautery or sharp dissection. This can be technically demanding if previous pseudocyst disease has been treated by cystgastrostomy. Care must be exercised to avoid injury to the blood vessels and vagus nerve branches along the gastric lesser curvature because they may be densely adherent. The splenic artery can be palpated at the superior margin of the gland. The firm inferior edge of the pancreas also can be readily identified. At this stage, additional time spent clearing the anterior surface of the pancreas will facilitate suture placement during the subsequent anastomosis. The gastrocolic attachments must be divided all the way to the left, and the transverse colon and splenic flexure must be mobilized downward to provide sufficient access to the more lateral tail of the gland. In chronic pancreatitis, the tail is frequently retracted away from the splenic hilum.

The pancreatic head is mobilized by a wide Kocher maneuver extending from the common bile duct to the superior mesenteric vein. The hepatic flexure of

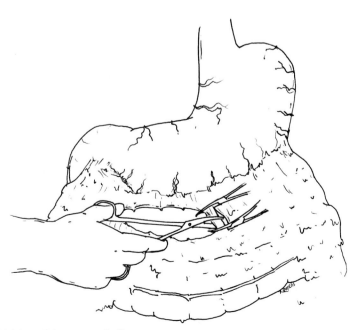

Fig. 5. Division of the gastrocolic ligament.

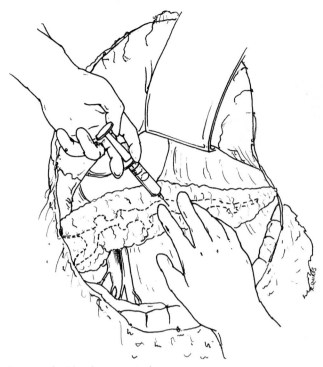

Fig. 6. Identification of a dilated pancreatic duct.

the colon should be mobilized inferiorly to allow complete exposure for this procedure. With normal tissue planes, the duodenum can be delivered bluntly from the retroperitoneum, but in chronic pancreatitis it is best accomplished by sharp dissection to avoid tearing retroperitoneal vessels. The superior mesenteric vein is approached cautiously because it may be obscured by fibrotic reaction and is easily torn or punctured. Tracing the middle colic veins downward helps to identify its location. During this phase of the dissection, the head of the pancreas is exposed, and the adherent mesocolon is mobilized downward. Troublesome bleeding from the mesocolic veins is controlled by fine suture-ligation or venorrhaphy. Division of the gastrocolic ligament and extended kocherization permit complete bimanual palpation of the pancreatic head and evaluation of the uncinate process.

Once the pancreas has been adequately exposed, the pancreatic duct must be identified. The dilated duct usually can be palpated as a soft and compressible depression in the mid-to-distal body of the gland. This is confirmed by needle aspiration that yields water-clear pancreatic fluid (Fig. 6). If a vessel has been punctured during attempted aspiration, the duct fluid may be sanguineous, but it still will be dilute. Cautery is used to cut down directly on the aspirating needle until the duct is entered. If the duct cannot be identified by this method,

intraoperative ultrasonography can be used to determine its location. If intraoperative ultrasonography is not available, a vertical incision perpendicular to the expected course of the duct can be made in the midbody of the gland. The incision should be

to the left of the course of the superior mesenteric vein as this can be injured if the posterior margin of the gland is violated. If the duct is unusually difficult to locate, the preoperative imaging studies should be reviewed again to make certain the duct is suitably dilated for the planned operation.

The ductotomy is extended by incising the overlying parenchyma with cautery (Fig. 7). A dissecting clamp or metal probe is placed in the duct to identify its course. The duct has a more anterior position toward the tail of the gland and dives posteriorly within the head. Thus, the depth of parenchyma that has to be divided is variable. The duct is opened to within approximately 1 cm of the tip of the tail.

The most important and difficult site for decompression is the pancreatic head. The ducts of Wirsung and Santorini are opened as close to the wall of the duodenum as possible. Failure to unroof both the duct of Wirsung and duct of Santorini is a common cause of persistent postoperative pain. Anterior pancreaticoduodenal or gastroepiploic veins that run vertically over the pancreatic head toward the superior mesenteric vein are suture-ligated and divided as the ductotomy is extended to the duodenum (Fig. 7). Because the main pancreatic duct dives posteriorly and inferiorly to the right of the superior mesenteric vein, and because the head of the pancreas is frequently bulky and enlarged in patients

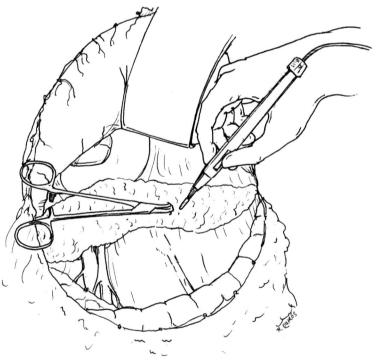

Fig. 7. Extension of the pancreatic ductotomy. In the head of the gland, the anterior-superior and inferior pancreaticoduodenal arteries are often encountered and should be suture-ligated for hemostasis.

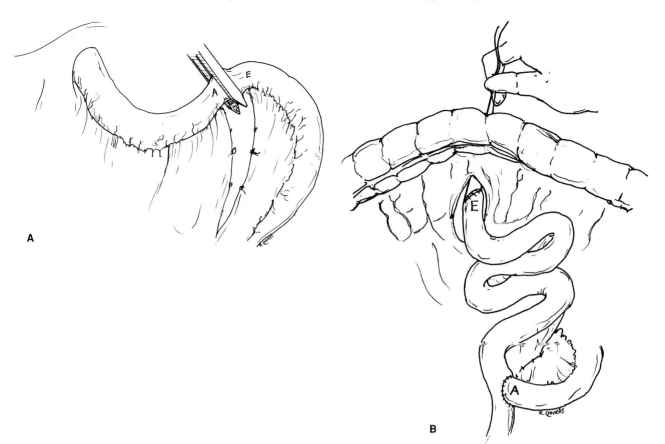

Fig. 8. Construction of a Roux-en-Y limb. **A:** Jejunum is divided distal to the ligament of Treitz. **B:** The jejunal limb is brought up in a retrocolic position for anastomosis to the pancreas. Intestinal continuity is restored by end-to-side jejunojejunostomy. A, afferent; E, efferent.

with chronic pancreatitis, anterior ductotomy alone may not be adequate for drainage of the proximal main pancreatic duct and uncinate process. Local resection (i.e., "coring out") of the pancreatic head described by Frey provides better decompression in this situation. With the fingers of the left hand behind the head of the gland and using cautery, the anterior capsule of the gland and the underlying pancreatic tissue are removed to the level of the duct of Wirsung. Care must be taken to excise sufficient overlying parenchyma to expose the posterior, inferior, and medial extent of the ducts. The posterior wall of the pancreatic duct is within millimeters of the posterior capsule and identifies the posterior extent of the dissection. The superior mesenteric vein and portal vein must be identified during this dissection. A rim of adjacent fibrous tissue of approximately 0.5 cm is preserved for the anastomosis. A probe or balloon catheter can be placed through the cystic duct or a choledochotomy to identify and protect the intrapancreatic common bile duct if there is uncertainty about its location. By palpating the gland with the left fingers posterior and the left thumb anteriorly, the surgeon can

identify residual undrained areas and preserve a posterior rim of pancreatic tissue.

A frozen section is routinely obtained on a portion of the resected head or a slice of parenchyma removed during the ductotomy. This is done not only to confirm the diagnosis but also to rule out a malignancy. Any area in the gland that is suspicious for cancer should be biopsied and evaluated with frozen section. An effort should be made to remove all ductal calculi and debris. This is particularly important in the head of the gland, where they can be the cause of persistent obstruction of tributaries entering the main duct. Concretions of calcium carbonate often extend into the parenchyma and must be firmly extracted. Obviously, not all intraparenchymal calcifications can be removed. Caution is necessary to avoid bleeding. If pancreatic bleeding occurs, it is controlled with cautery, carefully placed suture ligatures, or application of topical hemostatic agents.

A number of authors have emphasized that the pancreaticojejunal anastomosis must be at least 6 to 10 cm to provide optimal results. Focus on a specific length is misplaced because even a long anastomosis is not adequate if portions of the gland

are incompletely decompressed. The surgeon's task is to drain the ductal system as thoroughly as possible, with particular attention to the head of the gland. More complete ductal decompression should be associated with better pain relief.

A 50- to 60-cm Roux-en-Y limb is constructed after dividing the jejunum 20 to 30 cm distal to the ligament of Treitz (Fig. 8). This can be performed quickly with a gastrointestinal stapler. The end staple line closure of the transected distal jejunum is reinforced with sutures. The Roux-en-Y limb is brought up by a conventional route, often in a retrocolic position through a mesenteric window between the right and middle colic vessels (Fig. 8). A longer Roux-en-Y limb may be necessary for concomitant drainage of associated pseudocysts or an obstructed biliary tract. An enterotomy is made along the antimesenteric border of the jejunal loop. The length of the enterotomy should be shorter than that the pancreatic opening because the bowel will stretch. The jejunal opening can easily be extended if necessary.

There have been different recommendations as to the preferred technique for the pancreaticojejunal anastomosis. Alternatives

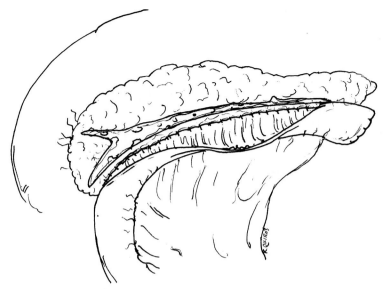

Fig. 9. In the head of the gland, the anterior-superior and inferior pancreaticoduodenal arteries should be avoided or ligated when placing sutures for the anastomosis. We prefer a single-layer continuous absorbable but long-lasting monofilament suture for this anastomosis.

include the use of one or two layers of sutures, the use of continuous or interrupted sutures, and incorporation of the pancreatic capsule, transected edge of parenchyma, or duct mucosa on the pancreatic side. No single method has been proven superior. The technique should be adapted to the size of the duct and thickness of the gland. Interrupted sutures of 3-0 silk have long been used for this anastomosis, but our current preference is for a single-layer continuous anastomosis that uses an absorbable but long-lasting monofilament suture. Bites are taken through the full thickness of the jejunum and pancreatic capsule (Fig. 9). The pancreatic stitch may include a small portion of the transected parenchymal edge. We do not attempt to sew directly to the mucosa of the pancreatic duct, although this may be done toward the tail, where the parenchyma often becomes thin. Sewing the jejunum to the capsule of the pancreas instead of performing a mucosa-to-mucosa anastomosis can allow enhanced decompression of less-dilated ducts. It is thought that sutures placed deep into the gland in an attempt to reach the duct mucosa may occlude side branches and lead to a postoperative leak of pancreatic fluid or limit pancreatic decompression.

The continuous anastomosis is performed by placing two sutures next to each other at the middle of the posterior row. Because access to the tail is more difficult, the left suture is run first. This establishes the left posterior row and a portion of the anterior row after the corner has been reached. Alternatively, the suture line may be started at the tail of the gland. The right suture is then run toward and around the pancreatic head. The anastomosis is completed by tying the two sutures where they meet anteriorly. Care must be taken when performing the anastomosis in the head of the gland to avoid placing sutures through the pancreaticoduodenal vessels, which can cause troublesome bleeding that must be controlled before completing the anastomosis. Rarely, only the head of the pancreas is diseased. In this unusual instance, coring out the head of the pancreas may be all that is required to achieve adequate decompression. The Roux limb is then used as previously described to drain the pancreatic head.

As many as 40% of patients with chronic pancreatitis who undergo lateral pancreaticojejunostomy have associated pancreatic pseudocysts. Concomitant drainage of the pseudocyst and dilated pancreatic duct is the most effective method for treating patients with these coexisting conditions (Fig. 10). Intrapancreatic pseudocysts can be drained by extending the ductal incision into the pseudocyst and incorporating the opening into the jejunal limb. Extrapancreatic pseudocysts can be drained either by using the side or the end of the jejunal limb, depending on their location. When necessary, biliary drainage can be accomplished by choledochoduodenostomy or by anastomosis of the bile duct to the Roux-en-Y limb of jejunum. A gastrojejunostomy can be constructed proximal to the enteroenterostomy for the Roux-en-Y limb if bypass of a fixed duodenal obstruction is required. Pancreaticoduodenectomy is appropriate for management of combined biliary and gastric obstruction in chronic pancreatitis.

Construction of the Roux-en-Y limb is completed by an end-to-side enteroenterostomy (Fig. 8) that is accomplished with either sutures or stapling devices. The opening of the transverse mesocolon is closed around the Roux-en-Y limb to prevent internal small bowel herniation. Likewise, the small bowel mesenteric defect adjacent to the enteroenterostomy is closed. The completed procedure is depicted in Figure 11.

Cholecystectomy is typically performed during lateral pancreaticojejunostomy. A feeding jejunostomy is placed selectively in patients who are extremely malnourished or have had long-standing gastric outlet obstruction. Closed suction drains may be used if there is concern about leakage of bile or pancreatic secretions. The likelihood of this is small, and drains are not usually

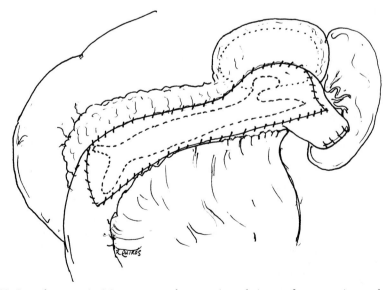

Fig. 10. Lateral pancreaticojejunostomy and concomitant drainage of a pancreatic pseudocyst.

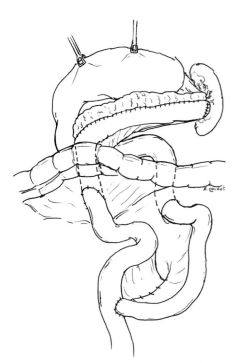

Fig. 11. Completed Roux-en-Y lateral pancreaticojejunostomy.

necessary. Nasogastric decompression is continued postoperatively until bowel function resumes. Oral intake is resumed as after any major abdominal procedure.

RESULTS

A valid assessment of lateral pancreaticojejunostomy for the treatment of chronic pancreatitis cannot be based solely on early operative results. The durability of pain relief, the development of endocrine or exocrine insufficiency, and the patient's eventual functional status must be evaluated. Lateral pancreaticojejunostomy is a reasonably safe procedure, as current operative mortality rates of 0% to 4% affirm. Operative complications develop in 5% to 20% of patients and are typical of the problems that follow any major abdominal procedure. Anastamotic leaks with pancreatic fistulae are uncommon. This is because, in chronic pancreatitis, fibrosis has replaced most of the glandular elements and the parenchyma has a low secretory output. When pancreatic fistulae do occur, they usually close spontaneously within several weeks. Administration of octreotide, a synthetic analogue of somatostatin, may accelerate closure if there is no underlying anatomic abnormality.

The goal of lateral pancreaticojejunostomy is pain relief. Worldwide experience has documented alleviation or elimination

of pain in 65% to 90% of operated patients. In the senior author's evaluation of 100 patients with a mean follow-up of 7.9 years, and a range of 1 to 25 years, pain was improved in 82% of patients. Pain relief was complete in 37% of patients and substantial in 45% of patients. Frey and Amikura reported on 50 patients who underwent lateral pancreaticojejunostomy with local resection of the head to the pancreas to improve decompression. Forty-seven patients were followed for a mean of 37 months. Pain relief was standardized by a verbal scale and quantification of analgesic use was determined to be excellent in 75% of patients and improved in an additional 13% of patients. There has been no standardization of the methods by which most investigators have evaluated postoperative pain. Historic reports also suggest a deterioration of pain relief with time. One major question, however, is whether the extent of ductal decompression achieved in earlier series would be considered adequate on the basis of current understanding.

Exocrine and endocrine insufficiencies are recognized sequelae of untreated chronic pancreatitis. Although lateral pancreaticojejunostomy does not improve established deficits, the operation itself does not impair function. Of 87 patients followed for a mean of 7.9 years by Prinz and Greenlee, almost one-half never became diabetic, only 28% required insulin, and two-thirds did not require enzyme therapy. Only 25% of patients with noninsulin-dependent diabetes required insulin during postoperative follow-up, and only 20% of nondiabetics became diabetic after surgery. Adams et al. reported similar long-term results among 62 patients studied for 1 to 15 years, with a mean follow-up of 6.3 years. Overall, 23% of patients required insulin therapy and 34% required enzyme replacement. These findings were recently collaborated with a study by Maartense et al., who showed that although exocrine function was not improved, endocrine function, using blood glucose levels as an indicator, improved significantly after ductal drainage with lateral pancreaticojejunostomy.

Some data suggest that duct decompression may retard metabolic deterioration in chronic pancreatitis. Nealon et al. observed a slower rate of functional impairment and better weight gain in patients treated with pancreaticojejunostomy as compared with nonoperative therapy. The study groups were not randomized, however, and cannot be considered comparable. Frey and Amikura reported diminished steatorrhea in 20% of patients af-

ter lateral pancreaticojejunostomy and local resection of the head of the pancreas.

Lateral pancreaticojejunostomy has advantages when compared with resective procedures such as pylorus-preserving pancreaticoduodenectomy (PPD) and duodenum-preserving resection of the head of the pancreas (DPRHP). Izbicki and associates have shown in two separate prospective randomized trials that these three procedures are equally as effective in terms of pain relief. Quality of life was improved and endocrine and exocrine functions were preserved with both the lateral pancreaticojejunostomy and DPRHP groups compared with those who underwent PPD. The in-hospital complication rates were increased in both the PPD and DPRHP groups compared with the lateral pancreaticojejunostomy with local pancreatic head excision group. A disadvantage of performing a ductal drainage procedure as opposed to a pancreatic resection is the possibility of missing occult pancreatic carcinoma. A thorough evaluation, including intraoperative biopsies, can minimize this risk. A definitive pancreatic resection should be performed if there is a suspicion of carcinoma and it cannot be ruled out.

Izbicki et al. have reported favorable results when operating on small-duct chronic pancreatitis, defined as Wirsung ductal diameter of 2 mm or less. When draining these small ducts, Izbicki performs a longitudinal V-shaped excision of the ventral pancreas. The pancreatic and jejunal anastomosis is then created using the resulting triangular cavity and a Roux-en-Y loop. Pancreatic drainage occurs via secondary and tertiary pancreatic duct branches into the pancreaticojejunostomy. Thirteen patients who underwent this procedure were followed for a mean of 30 months. A pain-scoring system and quality-of-life questionnaires were used to subjectively evaluate the patients. Exocrine and endocrine function was compared before and after surgery as well. In 92% of the patients, relief of preoperative symptoms was complete. There was an overall decrease in the median pain score by 95%. Quality of life was judged to be improved by 67%. Exocrine and endocrine functions were largely preserved as there were no statistical differences between laboratory measurements taken before and after surgery.

Although lateral pancreaticojejunostomy has been safely and reproducibly effective in relieving the pain of chronic pancreatitis, long-tem results in terms of overall health status and survival have been less satisfactory. Several series have documented late deaths in 25% to 50% of patients, with a mean survival of approximately 5 years. Complications of continued alcohol use, cardiovascular disease, and cancer are leading causes of death. Alcohol and substance abuse and unemployment continue in a substantial number of patients. These results should not dissuade surgeons from offering lateral pancreaticojejunostomy to patients with chronic pancreatitis and dilated pancreatic ducts because it is a well-conceived and usually beneficial treatment. However, recognition of long-term outcomes should reinforce the need for careful preoperative patient selection and long-term rehabilitative care.

SUGGESTED READING

Adams DB, Ford MC, Anderson MC. Outcome after lateral pancreaticojejunostomy for chronic pancreatitis. *Ann Surg* 1994;219:481.

Bockman DE, Buchler M, Malfertheiner P, et al. Analysis of nerves in chronic pancreatitis. *Gastroenterology* 1988;94:1459.

Calvo MM, Bujanda L, Calderon A, et al. Comparison between magnetic resonance cholangiopancreatography and ERCP for evaluation of the pancreatic duct. *Am J Gastroenterol* 2002;97:347.

Di Sebastiano P, Fink T, Weihe E, et al. Immune cell infiltration and growth-associated protein 43 expression correlate with pain in chronic pancreatitis. *Gastroenterology* 1997;112:1648.

Di Sebastiano P, di Mola FF, Bockman DE, et al. Chronic pancreatitis: the perspective of pain generation by neuroimmune interaction. *Gut* 2003;52:907.

Frey CF, Amikura K. Local resection of the head of the pancreas combined with longitudinal pancreaticojejunostomy in the management of patients with chronic pancreatitis. *Ann Surg* 1994;220:492.

Harrison JL, Prinz RA. Surgical management of chronic pancreatitis: pancreatic duct drainage. *Adv Surg* 1999;32:1.

Ho HS, Frey CF. The Frey procedure: local resection of pancreatic head combined with lateral pancreaticojejunostomy. *Arch Surg* 2001;136:1353.

Izbicki JR, Bloechle C, Broering D, et al. Extended drainage versus resection in surgery for chronic pancreatitis: a prospective randomized trial comparing the longitudinal pancreaticojejunostomy combined with local pancreatic head excision with the pylorus-preserving pancreatoduodenectomy. *Ann Surg* 1998;228:771.

Izbicki JR, Bloechle C, Broering D, et al. Longitudinal v-shaped excision of the ventral pancreas for small duct disease in severe chronic pancreatitis: prospective evaluation of a new surgical procedure. *Ann Surg* 1998;227:213.

Izbicki JR, Bloechle C, Knoefel WT. Duodenum-preserving resection of the head of the pancreas in chronic pancreatitis. A prospective, randomized trial. *Ann Surg* 1995;221:350.

Lowenfels AB, Maisonneuve P, Cavallini G. Pancreatitis and the risk of pancreatic cancer. *N Engl J Med* 1993;328:1433.

Maartense S, Ledeboer M, Bemelman WA. Effect of surgery for chronic pancreatitis on pancreatic function: pancreaticojejunostomy and duodenum-preserving resection of the head of the pancreas. *Surgery* 2004;135:125.

Nealon WH, Townsend CN, Thompson JC. Operative drainage of the pancreatic duct delays functional impairment in patients with chronic pancreatitis. *Ann Surg* 1988;208:321.

O'Neil SJ, Aranha GV. Lateral pancreaticojejunostomy for chronic pancreatitis. *World J Surg* 2003;27:1196.

Prinz RA. Surgical options in chronic pancreatitis. *Int J Pancreatol* 1993;14:97.

EDITOR'S COMMENT

Sadly, chronic pancreatitis controls the lives of many patients. As noted, chronic alcohol abuse is to blame in more than 80% of patients, and this has profound implications when surgery becomes necessary. When patients do not abstain from alcohol, the disease inexorably progresses and these patients become more difficult to care for. Pain is the hallmark symptom and it occurs in patients prone to substance abuse, addiction, personality disorders, and noncompliance. Alcoholism leads to nutritional deficiencies, refractory exocrine and endocrine insufficiency, and associated organ dysfunctions that certainly increase risks of perioperative morbidity. Clinicians must carefully consider the psychosocial stigmata associated with chronic pancreatitis before assigning this diagnosis to anyone.

Richard Prinz and colleagues have provided *Mastery* readers a beautifully updated chapter on pancreatic ductal drainage, which is clearly written and quite easy to get through. We learn first of the pathophysiology of disease and next that no single operation can take care of all patients with chronic pancreatitis. This became clear during the evolution of procedures as summarized. Over time, surgeons embraced a complete longitudinal fillet of the pancreatic duct, and abandoned distal pancreatic resection with splenectomy. They learned that full drainage of the pancreatic head was very critical, and for some, such as Charles Frey, this warranted resection (*Arch Surg* 2001;136:1353).

Beyond doubt, the choice of surgical procedures is one of the most active debates among pancreatic surgeons worldwide. Although Dr. Prinz and coauthors cover longitudinal pancreaticojejunostomy, there are salient, intuitive concepts that bridge all chronic pancreatitis operations. Because patients will face an inevitable progressive pancreatic functional loss, the surgeon should work to preserve pancreatic tissue while addressing the anatomic abnormalities found. Longitudinal pancreaticojejunostomy is perfect for "large-duct" disease as it decompresses ductal hypertension (pain) while preserving the pancreas. But remember, there will be no functional exocrine or endocrine gain as the damage has already been done. In experienced hands, operative mortality will be low (less than 1%), morbidity reasonable, pancreatic fistula uncommon, and, if properly selected, 80% of patients will enjoy enduring pain relief (*Ann Surg* 1993;217:458).

Dr. Prinz and colleagues offer excellent detail of the Frey procedure. This couples a coring out of the pancreatic head together with longitudinal pancreaticojejunostomy. Some claim the outcomes are even better. This is a considerably more difficult operation and requires proprioception by the surgeon, and a full understanding of the pancreatic head anatomy to avoid vascular injury and biliary injury. Richard Bell (*J Gastrointest Surg* 2005;9:144) has recently offered a careful description of how he performs this operation, and summarizes his fine results.

My experience also is that preoperative imaging with pancreatic protocol CT scanning is sufficient in large-duct chronic pancreatitis. ERCP in not mandatory, but at times can facilitate a trial of pancreatic duct stenting for patient selection. If the pain goes away, this might predict the success of subsequent surgical duct drainage. I have had variable results with this approach so do not consider it compulsory. MRCP is usually unnecessary. However, ERCP should be performed if a pseudocyst coexists. If the dilated pancreatic duct communicates with the cyst, ductal drainage alone may be sufficient, as recommended by Bill Nealon (*Ann Surg* 2003;237:614).

The finessing of technical elements of longitudinal pancreaticojejunostomy are thoroughly covered in this chapter. That said, there are practical points to emphasize. Full mobilization and anterior exposure of the pancreas is the key. You might expect the distended pancreatic duct to be easily palpable, but be prepared if it is not. For example, it can lie deep within a rock-hard, indurated pancreas and be impossible to palpate. Dr. Prinz and colleagues explain how to localize it using needle puncture that sometimes requires ultrasound guidance. Another option is a vertical incision across the pancreas to expose the dilated pancreatic duct horizontally, which then can be fully opened longitudinally. Yes, this works but it is quite unnerving as you wander into the unforgiving pancreas simply to locate the duct. Although the pancreatic head must be fully drained, it is reasonable to stop before the tail of the pancreas if the duct attenuates. As noted, limit your jejunal enterotomy initially as it will grow. Unlike the authors, I prefer a mucosa-to-mucosa apposition for any pancreatic anastomosis.

Longitudinal pancreaticojejunostomy can certainly be performed laparoscopically in expert hands, although only a few favor this approach. Whatever access method is chosen, the key to surgery remains proper patient selection. Two final points worth emphasizing relate to concerns for malignancy and concomitant biliary obstruction. Our authors nicely detail an approach to ruling out malignancy at the time of longitudinal pancreaticojejunostomy. Occasionally, one must reoperate on a patient on concern for a pancreatic head mass. Pancreaticoduodenectomy can usually be performed properly without sacrificing the original pancreaticojejunostomy anastomosis. With biliary obstruction, I prefer to bring the Roux-en-Y jejunal limb through the gastrohepatic ligament and onto the porta hepatis, where the common hepatic duct can be sewn in. Further down, the pancreaticojejunostomy is created, nicely achieving double duct drainage.

M.P.C.

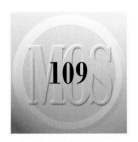

Pancreaticoduodenectomy for Chronic Pancreatitis

L. WILLIAM TRAVERSO

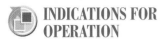 ## INDICATIONS FOR OPERATION

The principles of treating chronic pancreatitis are based on two observations: The "pacemaker" of chronic pancreatitis is in the head of the gland and almost everyone considered for resection has disabling abdominal pain caused by anatomic defects in the pancreas.

Some comments about the "pacemaker" concept would be illustrative here. The phenomenon is so reliable that if the epicenter of the inflammation is not in the head of the pancreas, then some other cause should be considered, such as autoimmune pancreatitis, neoplasm, or continued occult alcohol use. This concept was taught to me during residency in the 1970s, although others have claimed to have described it first in the 1980s.

The following indications for resection have been developed to guide surgeons toward designing surgical resections that will result in pain relief. We have observed, after a long-term follow-up of almost 5 years, the postresection disappearance of *disabling pain* in virtually everyone after applying these indications for resectional surgery. A *pain-free* state was achieved in three quarters of the group. These pain relief outcomes are a tribute to the efficacy of surgical resection because resection was not employed until all other interventional and endoscopic treatments had failed.

To achieve pain relief with head resection, all of the following indications must be met.

Chronic pancreatitis is documented using the 1963 Marseille definition of "residual pancreatic damage, either anatomical or functional, that persists even if the primary cause or factors are eliminated." This irreversible change in the pancreas is usually fibrosis.

The cause of the chronic pancreatitis must have been remedied or eliminated (e.g., gallstones, autoimmune pancreatitis, or current use of alcohol). The latter is usually denied by the patient until pain persists after head resection due to smoldering pancreatitis in the pancreatic remnant.

Imaging studies must show anatomic defects that meet the criteria of "marked" in the Cambridge image severity score, for example, at least a main pancreatic duct stricture with or without stones (Table 1). Resection is designed to address this anatomy, which is almost always in the pancreatic head. As mentioned earlier, the surgeon should use caution if the epicenter of the disease is not in the head. Consider then other causes such as neoplasm, autoimmune, or occult alcohol use. One clue to the presence of continued alcohol abuse is focal upstream "small ductal pancreatitis." Resection is contraindicated as the process is still in evolution.

For those institutions that have an experienced cross-specialty team for chronic pancreatitis, endotherapy before surgical resection can be considered. At least half of our patients have been able to avoid surgery with these new techniques. The same anatomic selection criteria apply.

The Cambridge image severity score has proven very useful. To gain this anatomic information, we depend on several types of modern imaging. In patients with chronic pancreatitis more will be known preoperatively about their pancreatic anatomy than in the patients thought to have cancer. The workup requires computed axial tomography scan of the "pancreas protocol" variety and endoscopic retrograde cholangiopancreatography (ERCP). The latter provides unparalleled fine anatomic details and brush cytology of any stricture potentially malignant. Magnetic resonance cholangiopancreatography (MRCP) has not been helpful as a single source of information. Some patients may require endoscopic ultrasound (EUS). These anatomic criteria will have been correlated with the clinical presentation as well as blood tumor markers such as CA 19-9.

A recent review using "evidence-based medicine" examined a variety of reports that listed pain relief and sequela after all forms of head resection for chronic pancreatitis. Major relief of pain was observed in 70% to 100% of patients from the standard pancreaticoduodenectomy (PD), pylorus-preserving pancreaticoduodenec-

tomy (PPPD), duodenum-preserving head resection (Beger procedure), or the ventral head resection with upstream ductal drainage (Frey procedure). These studies were difficult to compare, although many of them were randomized, controlled trials. The reason for this comparison difficulty was the lack of standard selection criteria for head resection. The criteria listed in the current chapter based on imaging studies would be a great opportunity to standardize. Many head resections in Europe are done just for an inflammatory "pseudotumor" of the head without mention of ductal anatomy. Currently the trend in Europe and North America is to use the less time-consuming and less complex Frey procedure. However, a recent paper from eight German universities that perform pancreatic resections in high-volume centers shows that pancreaticoduodenectomy is still the preferred operation for head resection.

TYPE OF OPERATION

Using the above indications, the patient considered for head resection is highly selected and is in a great position to benefit from modern and safe pancreatic resection. Like the German study, I have preferentially used PD. More specifically, I use PPPD for head resection in an attempt to accrue a 20-year follow-up after the same operation using the Cambridge severity score selection criteria based on anatomy. This effort should prove complementary and supportive of the lesser head resections such as the Beger or Frey procedures and their hybrids. If the premise is correct that the head of the pancreas is the pacemaker of chronic pancreatitis, then removal of the entire head should produce the best pain relief. Since PPPD by itself cannot cause disabling abdominal pain, the incidence of observed *disabling pain* relief after PPPD should be the benchmark that the less extensive head resection procedures should strive to achieve.

To summarize, the indications for head resection are strict and based on anatomic criteria. If these criteria are met, almost all patients should have good (relief of disabling

The Gastrointestinal Tract

TABLE 1. CAMBRIDGE CLASSIFICATION OF "IMAGE SEVERITY" FOR CHRONIC PANCREATITIS

Cambridge Class	Main Pancreatic Duct (MPD)	Abnormal Side Branches
1. Normal	Normal	None
2. Equivocal	Normal	< 3
3. Mild	Normal	> 3
4. Moderate	Abnormal	> 3
5. Marked	Abnormal★	> 3

★Any one of the following anatomic findings will place the case in the "Marked" category:
MPD terminates prematurely (abrupt, tapering, irregular); multiple MPD strictures;
MPD dilated >10 mm; ductal filling defects (stones); intra- or extrapancreatic "cavities" also known as pseudocysts; contiguous organ involvement in or around the pancreas (common bile duct stricture, duodenal stenosis, or arterial venous fistula).
Summarized from Axon ATR, Classen M, Cotton PB, et al. Pancreatography in chronic pancreatitis: international definitions. *Gut* 1984;25:1107.

pain) to excellent (pain-free) outcomes. Beware of the patient with "small ductal" pancreatitis. Another cause should be considered.

PREOPERATIVE EVALUATION

Imaging is acquired that allows the surgeon to view more pancreatic anatomy than was ever possible using older techniques. The result is a picture of the "composite pancreas" through the information gleaned by pancreas protocol computed tomography (CT) and ERCP. EUS may be helpful in some of these patients when enough information cannot be seen from CT. This is particularly true when CT shows a prominent head that is isodense (no low density mass but neoplasm is still suspected). MRCP has not been practical to obtain fine detail of ductal anatomy unless the institution has a dedicated magnetic resonance radiologist willing to spend hours with the image software.

On the day before surgery the patient undergoes mechanical bowel preparation. Antibiotics are administered at induction of anesthesia. A single dose of intravenous cephalosporin and metronidazole is administered. Since almost every patient has or has had biliary or pancreatic duct stents, this method has made abdominal abscess or wound infection an uncommon postoperative occurrence.

TECHNIQUE OF PYLORUS-PRESERVING PANCREATICODUODENECTOMY

Overview

Except for a variety of reconstruction methods, the resective phase of the pylorus-preserving technique is generally performed in the same manner throughout the

world. The most variety is with the reconstruction phase. The procedure removes all of the head of the pancreas and the duodenum (except the duodenal bulb), as shown in Figure 1. Reconstruction in our institution is depicted in Figure 2. Note that the duodenojejunostomy is in an antecolic position, a location we believe minimizes delayed gastric emptying (DGE). The inci-

dence of DGE after the PPPD with this antecolic position should be less than 10% and will be most often associated with an occult or obvious pancreatic anastomotic leak.

Incision and Retractors

An upper midline incision is made from the xiphoid to just above or below the umbilicus. Compared to the bilateral subcostal variety, the midline incision avoids cutting abdominal wall muscle and improves recovery in the postoperative period. When the upper midline incision is combined with epidural anesthesia, the incidence of postoperative pneumonia should be close to zero. Great exposure for better hemostasis can be acquired with this incision if the duodenum is widely mobilized to the midline and the surgeon on the left side of the patient uses his or her left hand for vascular control while disconnecting the head of the pancreas from its dorsal attachments to the superior mesenteric artery (SMA). This technique will be described in more detail below. A retraction system that has proven useful

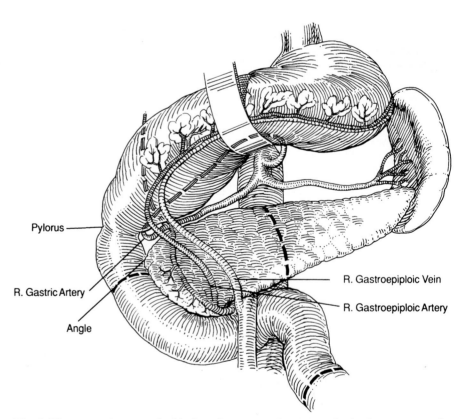

Fig. 1. The areas to be resected with the pylorus-preserving pancreaticoduodenectomy are depicted: Head of pancreas, duodenum (parts 2, 3, and 4), and segment of proximal jejunum. The entire head of the gland is removed. The right gastroepiploic vessels are divided near their origins. The right gastric artery is divided away from the stomach near its origin. This allows the neurovascular supply of the antrum and pylorus to be preserved and may minimize the incidence of delayed gastric emptying. (Reprinted with permission from Traverso LW. The pylorus-preserving Whipple procedure for severe complications of chronic pancreatitis. In: Beger HG, Buchler MW, Malfertheimer P, eds. *Standards of pancreatic surgery,* Heidelberg: Springer-Verlag, 1993:397.)

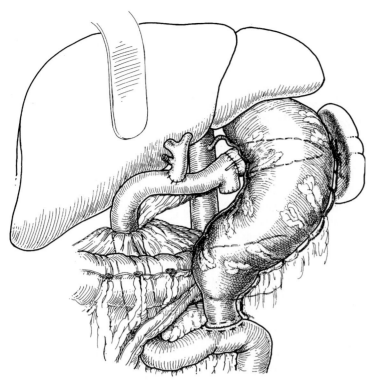

Fig. 2. Reconstruction of the pancreatic duct and bile duct are in a retrocolic fashion. The end-duodenal to side-jejunostomy is in an antecolic position to isolate the duodenal anastomosis from the pancreatic anastomosis and minimize delayed gastric emptying if the latter should leak. (Reprinted with permission from Traverso LW. The surgical management of chronic pancreatitis: the Whipple procedure. In: Cameron JL, ed. *Advances in surgery.* St. Louis: Mosby, Inc., 1999:23.)

with the upper midline incision is the Upper Hand system (Fowler Retractor, Pilling Surgical, Horsham, PA; Fig. 3). With the duodenum mobilized to the midline this retractor system allows superb exposure as it elevates and retracts the costal margins. Also useful is the articulating Martin Arm retractor (Elmed, Addison, IL) to retract the liver off the hepatoduodenal ligament or hold the antrum back while dissecting under the duodenal bulb on the right gastroepiploic vessels and superior mesenteric vein (SMV).

Mobilization of Structures

The round ligament is divided at the liver and the portion between the liver and the umbilicus is excised. A wide Kocher maneuver mobilizes the duodenum to the

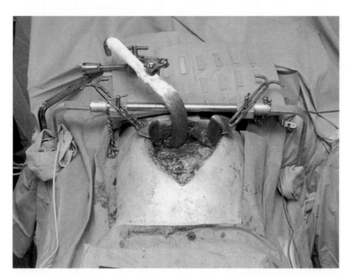

Fig. 3. The retractor setup is depicted with the patient's head at the top. The Upper Hand system's retractor blades hold the costal margin up and out while the multiarticulated Martin arm can hold the liver or stomach back at any angle depending on the dissection task. The system allows sufficient exposure of the pancreatic head through the midline incision.

midline and down to the level of the inferior mesenteric artery. The lesser sac is widely opened by incising the lesser omentum and by removing the entire greater omentum off the transverse colon. Every attempt is made to preserve the greater omentum. The omentum is left attached to the stomach as this "watchdog of the abdomen" may have some ameliorative intra-abdominal properties to promote healing and prevent infection.

The duodenal bulb and pylorus are mobilized for preservation with the stomach. Caution is used here as the neurovascular supply to the pylorus should be preserved where it courses along the cephalad portion of the antrum and pylorus. Wide dissection is required in this location. In order to accomplish wide dissection the following blood vessels are divided at their origins away from the pylorus: The right gastric artery (if present, there usually is not one major vessel) and the supraduodenal vessels of Wilkie. The vessels are more easily dissected by starting at their parent vessels. Ultimately, the superior portion of the duodenal bulb and the pylorus are detached from their neurovascular connections in the hepatoduodenal ligament.

The dorsal inferior surface of the duodenal bulb is next detached from the head of the pancreas, right gastroepiploic artery (RGEA), and the nest of right gastroepiploic vein branches that enter one to three right gastroepiploic veins that then enter the SMV and/or the middle colic vein. The RGEA is divided at the inferior border of the pancreas where it diverges off the pancreas. Experience allows the surgeon to avoid losing blood in this area as each individual vein needs to be divided near the SMV or middle colic vein.

The retropyloric dissection continues along the duodenal bulb until it merges with the pancreas, forming an "angle" (Fig. 1). Here there are several tiny blood vessels shared by the pancreas and duodenum. They are best divided using an ultrasonic dissection instrument. About 3 to 5 cm of duodenum are now free. A stapling device is used to divide the duodenum at the "angle," which, as stated above, is located at the junction of the first and second parts of the duodenum.

Excision of the Pancreatic Head, Remaining Duodenum, and Distal Common Bile Duct

The stomach with the preserved duodenal bulb and omentum are placed in the left upper quadrant and the common bile duct (CBD) is dissected by first dividing the gastroduodenal artery (GDA) near, but

The Gastrointestinal Tract

not at, its origin. To prevent major postoperative bleeding from the stump of the GDA it is triply ligated with nonabsorbable 2/0 silk suture well out onto the head of the pancreas. Once the GDA is divided, the plane behind the GDA provides easy access to the groove between the CBD and the portal vein. The neck of the pancreas is easily isolated from above and below the gland. Now the neck is divided. The electrocautery or ultrasonic scissors are useful in dividing the parenchyma. However, the pancreatic duct should be "cold cut" with a scalpel to avoid devascularizing the duct wall and promoting a pancreatic anastomotic leak.

Then the pancreatic neck is rolled to the right and the CBD encircled with a vascular loop. A bulldog clamp is placed on the upstream side of the CBD and the duct divided. Caution should be exerted here as about a quarter of people will have a large vessel in the retro-CBD area. It is easily palpated before division of the CBD and represents a replaced right, accessory right, or replaced common hepatic artery. Division of a replaced artery will result in a devascularized upstream CBD and subsequent bile anastomotic breakdown.

Next the dorsal pancreatic head attachments to the SMA have to be divided. The lymph nodes do not have to be removed in this noncancer operation, but removing these with the specimen along the SMA sometimes makes the dissection simpler. The dissection to divide these attachments can be bloody because of the variety of veins and arteries that course in this area. Embryologically, the pancreas provides the highest variability for the locations of named arteries (particularly the dorsal pancreatic artery). Every patient is different. The surgeon should know the problem areas and develop a method that works best for them to ensure that no blood is lost during dissection in this SMA area. Blood loss during a Whipple operation should be minimal (< 200 mL) and will usually occur during parenchymal division of the pancreatic neck. Besides the right gastroepiploic vein system, there are two problem areas where major veins can contribute to unacceptable blood loss: The first jejunal vein (posterior and inferior) over the SMA in the retropancreatic head area and the posterior superior pancreaticoduodenal vein. The latter is usually a single large vessel that should be sought as it exits the dorsal superior pancreatic head in a variety of locations. This vein requires suture ligation on the portal vein side. The first jejunal vein does not have to be divided and can be controlled during the dissection, described below.

As the SMA dissection proceeds, much blood can be lost from the specimen side. To decrease blood loss during this retropancreatic head dissection along the SMA, the surgeon on the left side of the patient places his or her left hand over the pancreatic head and uncinate process. Hand compression on the pancreas easily controls hemorrhage from the specimen side where vessels enter and exit from the SMA and portal vein (Fig. 4). The patient side is controlled by clamping and suturing. These attachments carry a variety of veins along with the lymphatics and lymph nodes. As the surgeon moves caudally from above through these attachments, the first jejunal branch entering the back of the SMV is encountered. Just cephalad to this vein is the usual location for the inferior pancreaticoduodenal artery (IPDA).

Usually I begin at the superior head and divide the retro-SMV attachments to the SMA by dissecting slowly toward the uncinate process. Each clamping uses a single long Collar clamp with the tissue divided between the clamp and the specimen. The left hand of the left-sided surgeon nicely controls blood loss from the specimen as the surgeon on the patient's right side ties the sutures behind the clamp. The clamp is re-

moved after a 2-0 silk suture is tied between the clamp and the SMA. Any large bleeders from the specimen are controlled by the surgeon's left compressing hand and can be suture ligated after the pancreatic head is mobilized out of its bed. After several clampings from above, the SMA becomes contiguous with the dissection. This is usually the point where one encounters the IPDA. The IPDA is controlled and ligated in the same manner. The dissection continues along the axis of the SMA while ensuring its location by palpation. As the dissection courses caudad along the SMA and toward the first jejunal vein, the SMA seems to course away from the dissection. The first jejunal branch does not have to be divided; rather, just the branches coming from the uncinate process can be divided before they enter this large vein. The same clamp technique with left-hand vascular control is used to divide the last of the uncinate attachments directly on the surface on the uncinate process while preserving the first jejunal vein. Much blood can be lost in this area. The surgeon should be sure to proceed slowly, with caution, and with profound knowledge of the anatomic variations.

To remove the PPPD specimen, all that remains is to divide the jejunum using the

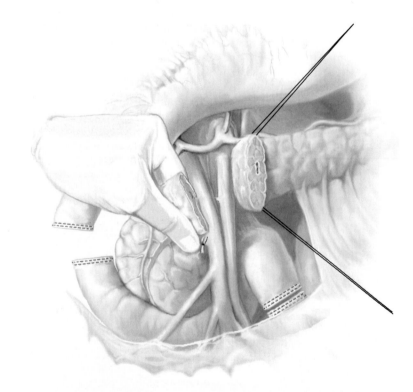

Fig. 4. Hand compression of the specimen is used to control blood loss while the retroperitoneal attachments of the dorsal medial pancreatic head and uncinate process are divided from the superior mesenteric artery. The surgeon on the left side of the patient places his or her left hand on the stout lymph node–laden mesentery attaching the dorsal head and uncinate process to the superior mesenteric artery (SMA) area. As this "mesentery" is sequentially divided from cephalad to caudad along the SMA, the hand pressure controls bleeding from the specimen and the clamps control bleeding from the SMA side.

gastrointestinal stapling device about 6 cm below the ligament of Treitz. The mesenteric vascular attachments of that portion of the jejunum to be removed with the specimen are divided directly on the jejunum. The electrocautery or ultrasonic scissors are very useful here as sutures do not have to be employed.

Prereconstruction Tasks

The avascular window in the transverse mesocolon is located and incised just to the left of the middle colic vein. Then the defect in the ligament of Treitz created by removing the jejunum and fourth part of the duodenum is closed with interrupted sutures to avoid internal hernia. An intraoperative fluoroscopic pancreatogram may be useful to visualize the ductal system in the pancreatic remnant if the duct has not been visualized by ERCP. This ensures that the main cause of persistent pain (smoldering remnant pancreatitis) is minimized by complete main duct decompression. A partial longitudinal incision and lateral pancreaticojejunostomy to the body and tail may be indicated if there are significant chain-of-lake strictures seen on pancreatogram (Fig. 5).

Reconstruction—Pancreatic Anastomosis

The pancreatic and biliary anastomoses will be retrocolic, while the duodenal anastomosis will be antecolic (Fig. 2). The anastomoses are positioned in this way to isolate potential leakage of the bile and pancreatic duct connections from the duodenojejunostomy. This maneuver minimized DGE to 8% in my last 215 cases. The stump of the proximal jejunum is directed toward the pancreatic and bile

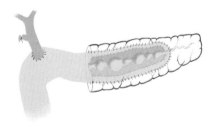

Fig. 5. If multiple strictures from chronic pancreatitis are present in the pancreatic remnant, then the duct must be decompressed using a lateral pancreaticojejunostomy much like with the Puestow lateral drainage procedure. (Reprinted with permission from Traverso LW. Pylorus preserving pancreaticoduodenectomy for chronic pancreatitis. In: Clavien PA, Sarr M, Fong Y, eds. *Atlas of upper abdominal surgery.* Heidelberg: Springer Verlag GmbH & Co., 2006.)

duct remnants through the retrocolic aperture already created in the transverse mesocolon to the left of the middle colic vessels. The stomach, with preserved pylorus and duodenal bulb, is brought antecolic to the left transverse colon, allowing for an easy duodenojejunostomy remote from the other anastomoses.

As stated earlier, if a chain-of-lakes–type ductal dilation is present in the remnant with significant strictures, then a longitudinal side-to-side technique is used, but many patients will have a normal duct in the pancreatic remnant with a diameter of 2 to 3 mm. These small pancreatic ducts are more prone to leak after pancreaticojejunostomy, although chronic pancreatitis and fibrosis make the incidence of leak minimal. After a pancreatic duct to jejunal mucosa anastomosis, an outer layer or "seromuscular envelop" is constructed containing a stented end-to-side, mucosa-to-mucosa pancreaticojejunostomy.

First the back wall of the outer layer is constructed using interrupted 3/0 silk sutures. These knots are tied anteriorly. Then a tiny hole is made in the jejunal mucosa opposite the pancreatic duct. The mucosa-to-mucosa anastomosis is created with interrupted 6/0 Vicryl suture on an RB3 needle (Ethicon, Somerville, NJ). Note that all knots are tied on the outside of the new lumen to avoid sludge and stone formation. If the pancreatic parenchyma is rock hard, then 5/0 polydioxanone suture (PDS) with an RB1 needle will be required as the smaller RB3 needle cannot penetrate a fibrotic pancreas. For small ducts of less than or equal to 3 mm, the task is to place exact mucosal sutures to tack the pancreatic duct wall to the jejunal wall while not crossing these tiny sutures. This four-quadrant apposition is the key to success during pancreaticojejunostomy (Fig. 6). The visual cues available using the surgical microscope at 12.5 to 16.0 power have lowered the leak rate to almost zero when a small duct is present.

A 3 French polytetrafluoroethylene radiodense stent also helps avoid crossing the sutures. The "Geenan" stent is used because it has multiple holes throughout the stent (Wilson-Cook Medical, Winston-Salem, NC). This stent is cut to be about 4 cm long and inserted into the duct just before placement of the last (anterior) mucosa-to-mucosa stitch. The stent is loosely attached in its midportion to just the jejunal mucosa near the last anterior stitch with a single 6/0 Vicryl suture. The stent ensures adequate apposition of the mucosa and decompresses the pancreatic duct upstream from the swollen mucosa due to sutures. It spontaneously passes in about 10 to

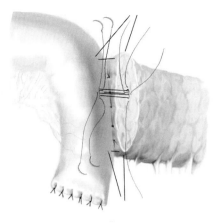

Fig. 6. The back wall of the pancreatic anastomosis has been created with interrupted sutures. These knots have been tied anteriorly. The illustration depicts four-quadrant tacking of the jejunal wall on the left to the pancreatic duct wall on the right. The first suture is the most dorsal and is placed "outside in" through the jejunal wall and then "inside out" through the pancreatic duct wall. This knot will be tied outside the new lumen, but first the superior and inferior sutures are placed. These sutures are also placed so their knots can be tied on the outside of the new lumen. After the second and third sutures are placed, the first suture's knot is tied. The stent is introduced and the fourth and last suture is placed. Then the knots are tied of the second, third, and fourth sutures, respectively. (Modified from Traverso LW. Pylorus preserving pancreaticoduodenectomy for chronic pancreatitis. In: Clavien PA, Sarr M, Fong Y, eds. *Atlas of upper abdominal surgery.* Heidelberg: Springer Verlag GmbH & Co., 2006.

14 days. Its presence can be checked with an abdominal radiograph. The anterior outer layer of interrupted 3/0 silk Lembert sutures is now placed to complete the anastomosis.

Reconstruction—Biliary Anastomosis

The biliary anastomosis begins with placing several sutures "outside-in" on the anterior (ventral) aspect of the bile duct stump. The needles are not removed from the sutures. Clamps hold these sutures and elevate the bile duct into position. Then an opening is cut in the jejunal limb just downstream from the pancreatic anastomosis that is smaller than the bile duct lumen. An end-choledochal–to–side-jejunal anastomosis is created with a single layer of interrupted absorbable 5/0 PDS (Ethicon, Somerville, NJ). Once again all of the knots are placed so they can be tied on the outside (to prevent stone formation on knots of delayed-absorbable suture). A T tube is not used. The jejunal limb is tacked to its exit site through the transverse mesocolon with 3/0 silk sutures.

The Gastrointestinal Tract

Reconstruction—Antecolic Duodenojejunostomy

The stomach, the first part of duodenum, and the omentum are brought over the left side of the transverse colon. Although the duodenal stump may look cyanotic, this is due to venous spasm. I have never had a duodenojejunostomy leak. Vascular supply can be ensured by looking for mucosal integrity inside the lumen of the duodenal bulb when the staple line is excised after the back side of the outer layer has been finished.

The location of the duodenojejunostomy on the jejunal limb is downstream from the biliary and pancreatic anastomoses and about 10 cm below the exit site of the jejunal limb from the transverse mesocolon. The stomach and duodenal bulb are brought over the left transverse colon and an end-duodenal–to–side-jejunal anastomosis is made in two layers. The inner layer is of running 3/0 Vicryl and the outer layer is interrupted 3/0 silk.

Abdominal Wall Closure

A closed suction round 15 French silicone drainage catheter is placed under the biliary and pancreatic anastomoses from a right upper quadrant stab wound. The midline fascia is closed with figure-eight 0 PDS interrupted suture, but nonabsorbable monofilament suture is used if the patient is at risk for nonhealing such as malnutrition, obesity, or preoperative steroids.

RESULTS AFTER HEAD RESECTION WITH PYLORUS-PRESERVING PANCREATICODUODENECTOMY

Over the last decade and a half we have noticed less need for resection due to the improved results of endotherapy. The cases reaching the surgeon are therefore more complicated. In 1997, we reported the short- and long-term outcomes (mean 55 months) from 57 patients that had undergone pancreaticoduodenectomy for chronic pancreatitis. Since then we have extended the experience to over 120 patients. In the original report the indications for head resection were as listed at the beginning of this chapter. All patients had the Cambridge image severity score of "marked," but to be more specific, 96% had main pancreatic duct obstruction and the 4% that did not were patients with intrapancreatic pseudocysts in the head. In addition to main pancreatic duct obstruction or pancreatic head pseudocyst, all patients had multiple other elements of the Cambridge classification to support head resection as listed in the footer of Table 1.

The progressive role of endotherapy was prominent in these patients. Common bile duct obstruction was observed in 65% of patients and therefore 47% of them had undergone prior common bile duct stenting. Pancreatic duct obstruction was seen in 96% of patients, with 39% of them with a documented upstream main pancreatic duct blowout. Pancreatic duct stenting had been used in 35% of patients and these had failed to achieve pain relief. In addition, 19% had required percutaneous drainage of peripancreatic fluid collections. The surgery was safe. There was no hospital or 30-day mortality. PPPD was used in 97% since 3% already had an antrectomy from previous ulcer surgery.

The onset of new diabetes was interesting. We did not see a predisposition for diabetes due to PPPD as has been suggested by others. In those who were not diabetic preoperatively (n = 37), the actual 5-year diabetic occurrence rate was 32%. This diabetes was not a consequence of the resection because no patient became diabetic sooner than 12 months after the resection, indicating that the criteria for surgery had been accurate enough to ensure that only nonfunctional pancreatic tissue had been excised. These data supported the concept that diabetes was a result of continued fibrosis in the pancreatic remnant.

Patients that were at least 1 year after their Whipple operation (n = 43) were then questioned after a mean follow-up period of 55 months. In the 96% of patients that originally had disabling pain as an indication for surgery, every patient indicated that they had a "good" response to surgery and that their pain was no longer disabling. In addition, 76% of the patients indicated that they were pain free. All patients were able to maintain their preoperative weight, and no patients complained of dumping or significant diarrhea. However, 77% of the patients were taking exocrine enzymes and 14% indicated that they had diarrhea if they didn't take exocrine enzymes. Another surprising finding was the incidence of marginal ulceration of 6% in those with PPPD but 44% in those with total pancreatectomy. Since the time of this report we have avoided total pancreatectomy regardless of patients' diabetic status and placed patients on chronic daily proton pump inhibitors.

A cautionary note is provided about those patients thought to have "small ductal pancreatitis." The often discussed need for total pancreatectomy for small ductal pancreatitis has not been necessary in our practice. The vast majority of patients we have seen for "small ductal pancreatitis" were found to be currently drinking alcohol and were therefore not candidates for resective surgery (see the second indication of the introduction).

SUMMARY

After long-term follow-up of almost 5 years after PPPD, the benchmark for relief of disabling pain should approach 100% if patients are selected using strict anatomic selection criteria. It is hoped that this benchmark could be equaled by a variety of promising operations using a more limited head resection, such as the Frey or Beger operations. First the patients should be selected with a standard list of reliable clinical and anatomic imaging criteria such as those used in this chapter. Specific anatomic criteria for limited head resection have not been used in studies for these latter operations. If the premise is correct that the head of the pancreas is the "pacemaker" of chronic pancreatitis in most cases, then limited head resections should approach or equal the pain relief that we have observed after pylorus-preserving pancreaticoduodenectomy.

SUGGESTED READING

Principal References

Axon ATR, Classen M, Cotton PB, et al. Pancreatography in chronic pancreatitis: international definitions. *Gut* 1984;25:1107.

Makowiecz F, Hopt UT, GAST Study Group. Current techniques and complication rates in pancreatic surgery: results of a multi-institutional survey of 6 German centers with 1083 pancreatic head resections (GAST Study Group). *J Gastrointest Surg* 2006.

Schafer M, Mullhaupt B, Clavien PA. Evidence-based pancreatic head resection for pancreatic cancer and chronic pancreatitis. *Ann Surg* 2002;236:137.

Traverso LW, Kozarek RA. Pancreaticoduodenectomy for chronic pancreatitis. Anatomic selection criteria and subsequent long-term outcome analysis. *Ann Surg* 1997;226:429.

ADDITIONAL REFERENCES

Sarles H. Proposal adopted unanimously by the participants of the symposium. In: Sarles H, ed. *Pancreatitis. Symposium Marseilles April 25 and 26, 1963.* Basel: S. Karger, 1963:VII.

Traverso LW. The surgical management of chronic pancreatitis. The Whipple procedure. In: Cameron JL, ed. *Advances in surgery.* Philadelphia: Mosby, Inc., 1999:23.

Traverso LW, Shinchi H, Low DE. Useful benchmarks to evaluate outcomes after esophagectomy and pancreaticoduodenectomy. *Am J Surg* 2004;187:604.

EDITOR'S COMMENT

For chronic pancreatitis, the indications for and techniques of pancreatic head resection are particularly controversial. Head-predominant disease is indeed common, prompting mysterious concepts such as the "pacemaker" of disease and "inflammatory pseudotumor." However described, many argue that some anatomic defect causing pain must exist in the pancreatic head. Collectively, the excellent and enduring results of head resection support their case. Pancreaticoduodenectomy (Whipple procedure) remains the preferred approach (*J Gastrointest Surg* 2005;9:1080) and standard for comparison (*Ann Surg* 1997;226:429). Today, innovative operations that remove the diseased pancreatic head while preserving native anatomy are being scrutinized. In Europe, the duodenum-preserving resection of the pancreatic head (DPPHR, Beger procedure) is quite popular, as detailed elsewhere in *Mastery*.

What really are the inherent controversies? After all, we agree pain control is the goal. When achieved, patients regain their quality of life and personal productivity. Widely cited trials of pancreatic head resection in chronic pancreatitis have yielded pain relief rates of 70% to 100% (*Ann Surg* 2002;236:137). The choice of operation may hinge more on surgeon preference than proven efficacy. As noted by Dr. Traverso, it is difficult to know because we lack standard, agreed-upon selection criteria for pancreatic head resection. This makes comparisons of different procedures confounding. Our author offers his specific indications early in this chapter, and emphasizes an opportunity to standardize. Can we reach consensus for precise selection criteria for pancreatic head resection in chronic pancreatitis? Will they be based on radiographic and anatomic criteria, failure to respond to nonoperative treatments, or clinical criteria such as duration of disease, pain scores, and apparent disability? How will they account for cause? And once established, will consensus selection criteria

reveal one resection technique to be superior to another? Yes, this is an opportunity.

Together with Dr. William Longmire, our author created the pylorus-preserving variant of pancreaticoduodenectomy (PPPD) (*Surg Gynecol Obstet* 1978;156:954). This began a career odyssey in pancreatic surgery well known for both analysis and achievement. The technical details it took him years to refine are now elegantly detailed for *Mastery* readers. While we may not all make the same incision or use the same instruments, the anatomic-based principles for conducting this operation properly really shouldn't change. From nuances like the supraduodenal vessels of Wilkie to precise instruction of how to control bleeding at the superior mesenteric vessels, Dr. Traverso lays everything out clearly, and stresses experience, caution, and a "profound knowledge of anatomic variations." These guidelines cannot be violated, especially when operating for chronic pancreatitis.

The resection should follow a systematic, sequential approach that avoids peril until necessary and reflects the true experience of the pancreatic surgeon. One can avoid blood loss and enhance safety by making the easiest progress first, and not challenging vascular structures too soon. We are learning more about technical elements of the reconstruction, as well. For example, the route by which the afferent limb is delivered up to the pancreas and bile duct does not matter. Some favor behind the mesenteric root; others go through the mesocolon. It does matter how the jejunum is positioned for duodenojejunostomy. As noted by Dr. Traverso, and as recently proven in a randomized, controlled trial by Tani (*Ann Surg* 2006;243:316), antecolic isoperistaltic duodenojejunostomy truly decreases delayed gastric emptying after PPPD, and has been my preference for years. Finally, consider how an operating microscope might help you with a small duct pancreaticojejunostomy. It has helped our author to nearly eliminate postoperative pancreatic anastomotic leakage (*Surgery* 2006;139:735).

The choice of operation is key when the diagnosis of chronic pancreatitis is in question. Autoimmune sclerosing pancreatitis (ASP) often presents in patients older than 50 years of age with upper abdominal pain, variable jaundice, and a fullness in the head of the pancreas. The diagnosis is supported by elevated immunoglobulin G-4 levels or various abnormal autoimmune markers in the serum. Histology shows plasmacytic infiltrates. The differential diagnosis must include a suspected, but unproven, neoplasm. I have often found ASP as the cause in such cases, much as Hardacre et al. at Johns Hopkins would predict (*Ann Surg* 2003;237:853). In years ahead, ASP will factor prominently as patients with presumed idiopathic chronic pancreatitis are evaluated, and the surgeon's role will become better known (*J Gastrointest Surg* 2005;9:11).

Regardless of known chronic pancreatitis, limited pancreatic head resections are inadequate if cancer is suspected. Pancreaticoduodenectomy is necessary based on oncologic principles. Chronic pancreatitis patients develop lethal pancreatic cancer at a rate of 0.2% per year, with a relative risk 15 to 20 times higher than age-matched controls (*N Engl J Med* 1993;328:1433). The morbidity and mortality of pancreaticoduodenectomy is low in experienced hands, even in chronic pancreatitis. Furthermore, patients will often benefit symptomatically even when cancer is not found (*Am J Surg Pathol* 2003;27:110).

Chronic pancreatitis is a difficult disease, usually afflicting patients with complicated medical histories, and with only difficult solutions available. For best results, we promote and adhere to a multidisciplinary team approach to patient evaluation and care. No major decision or invasive intervention should be made without the team's collective agreement. This often requires flexibility and compromise, but patients do benefit.

M.P.C.

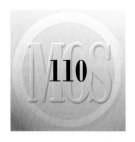

Partial, Subtotal, and Total Duodenum-preserving Resection of the Pancreatic Head in Chronic Pancreatitis and Neoplastic Cystic Lesions

HANS G. BEGER, BETTINA M. RAU, AND BERTRAM POCH

In Western countries, alcohol is the most frequent etiologic factor causing chronic pancreatitis. Approximately 90% of patients with alcoholic chronic pancreatitis suffer a severe abdominal pain syndrome. In alcoholic chronic pancreatitis, as well as in tropical (nutritional) chronic pancreatitis in Asian countries, an inflammatory mass in the head of the pancreas frequently develops in combination with local complications. As a consequence of this chronic inflammatory process, a loss of the endocrine and exocrine parenchyma

occurs, and it is replaced locally by extracellular matrix tissue that results in increased fibrosis. The molecular and pathobiochemical mechanisms causing the inflammation and fibrosis are largely unknown. Pathomorphologically, common features are pancreatic main duct and side branch stenoses and dilations, focal necrosis, and extensive infiltration of leukocytes and immunocytes. Overexpression of epidermal growth factor and transforming growth factor-ß as well as acid and basic fibroblast growth factor is considered to be

crucial for the production of extracellular matrix substances.

Pain in chronic pancreatitis is related to increased duct and tissue pressure in the pancreas. Pathomorphologic changes in the sensory intrapancreatic nerves, which have been identified as being increased in nerve diameter, perineural infiltration of inflammatory cells, and an increased level of neurotransmitter substances, are causally related to the pain syndrome. In long-term follow-up studies, the natural course of chronic pancreatitis after diagnosis reveals persistence of pain in 85% of patients after 5 years and in 55% after 10 years.

The progression of exocrine and endocrine insufficiency, which is frequently observed in chronic pancreatitis, has a limited influence on the pain syndrome and results in only a subgroup of patients in a final burned-out syndrome. Local complications (e.g., pseudocystic lesions, inflammatory mass in the head, common bile duct stenosis, compression or occlusion of the portal, superior mesenteric as well as splenic vein, and narrowing of the periampullary duodenum) are frequently observed. A coexistence of chronic pancreatitis and pancreatic cancer developing years after the diagnosis of chronic pancreatitis is observed, on the basis of epidemiologic studies, in 1.8% to 5.0% of patients and, for extrapancreatic cancers, in 3.9% to 13.0%. The death rate related to chronic pancreatitis is between 12% and 20%. Ten years after diagnosis and treatment of chronic alcoholic pancreatitis, the death rate caused by complications of chronic pancreatitis and continuing alcohol abuse is approximately 30%.

 ## DIAGNOSIS

Diagnosis of chronic pancreatitis is based on contrast-enhanced computed tomography as the "gold standard;" endoscopic retrograde cholangiopancreatography or magnetic resonance cholangiopancreatography provides additional information about the duct changes, including the main pancreatic duct and side branches and the intrapancreatic segment of the common bile duct. In approximately 30% to 50% of the patients suffering from advanced chronic pancreatitis, the intrapancreatic segment of the common bile duct shows a prepapillary stenose. To evaluate the endocrine and exocrine function, an oral glucose tolerance test and a pancreolauryl test, a secretin stimulation test or a fecal chymotrypsin estimation has to be performed.

 ## INDICATIONS

Until now, there has been no preventive therapy for chronic pancreatitis. Except for avoidance of alcohol consumption, medical management has a supportive role in terms of analgesic treatment, supplementation with exogenous enzyme substitutes, and treatment of diabetes mellitus. Medically intractable pain and the development of severe local complications are reasons to change from medical management to surgical treatment (Table 1).

TABLE 1. INDICATIONS FOR DUODENUM-PRESERVING SUBTOTAL/TOTAL PANCREATIC HEAD RESECTION[a]

1. Chronic pancreatitis complicated by
   Inflammatory mass in the pancreatic head
   Stenosis of CBD
   Multiple stenoses and dilatations of PMD
   Severe narrowing of peripapillary duodenum, causing gastric outlet syndrome
   Compression/stenosis of PV/SMV
2. Pancreas divisum, causing CP or recurrent acute pancreatitis
3. Intraductal, papillary mucinous tumor in pancreatic head
4. Mucinous cystic tumor in pancreatic head
5. Large (>2 cm) endocrine neoplasia in pancreatic head

[a]CBD, common bile duct; PMD, pancreatic main duct; PV/SMV, portal vein/superior mesenteric vein; CP, chronic pancreatitis; AP, acute pancreatitis.

 ## SURGICAL TECHNIQUE

The surgical technique of subtotal/total pancreatic head resection includes three principal technical steps (Table 2).

Exposure of the Pancreatic Head

The head of the pancreas is exposed, dividing the gastrocolic and duodenocolic ligaments, which preserves the gastroepiploic vessels. Subsequently, the duodenum is mobilized by a Kocher maneuver. After identification of the superior mesenteric vein at the lower margin of the pancreatic head, preparation of a tunnel between the portal vein and the pancreatic neck has to be performed.

Even in cases of extensive inflammation, the tunneling can be performed without major difficulties. The identification and banding of the common hepatic artery occur on the upper margin of the neck and the head of the pancreas. The common bile duct is identified and banded with a rubber loop in the hepatoduodenal ligament. (Fig. 1).

Resection Phase

Resection of the inflammatory mass in the pancreatic head is initiated with a transverse division of the pancreatic neck at the level of the portal vein (Fig. 1). At the cut surface of the left pancreas, meticulous hemostasis using monofilament 5-0 to 6-0 nonabsorbable sutures is mandatory. The head of the pancreas is rotated forward and to the right (Fig. 2). This can be achieved easily by bluntly freeing the head of the pancreas from the portal vein; small branches entering the portal vein and superior mesenteric vein have to be ligated. The head of the pancreas is removed, using a knife, from the retroperitoneal surface of the pancreas toward the uncinate process without major technical difficulties (Fig. 3A). The subtotal resection of the pancreatic head is completed

TABLE 2. SURGICAL STEPS OF SUBTOTAL/TOTAL, DUODENUM-PRESERVING RESECTION OF THE HEAD OF THE PANCREAS IN CHRONIC PANCREATITIS

Exposure of the pancreatic head
Resection
   Transection of the pancreas between head and body
   Subtotal/total resection of the head
   Decompression of the intrapancreatic segment of the common bile duct

Reconstruction
1. Interposition of a jejunal loop, anastomosis between left pancreas and jejunum (end-to-end) or between jejunal loop and the main pancreatic duct (end-to-side)
2. Anastomosis between jejunal loop and the pancreatic shell-like remainder at the duodenum, including the common bile duct incision as biliary bypass
3. Roux-en-Y anastomosis (jejunojejunostomy)

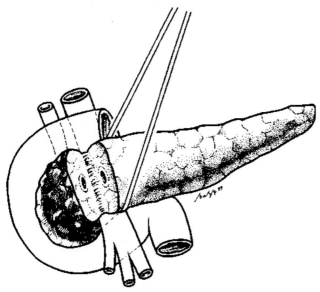

Fig. 1. After exposure of the pancreatic head and formation of a tunnel behind the pancreatic neck ventrally to the portal vein, banding of the pancreas is carried out by passing a tube or drain behind the neck of the pancreas. Transection of the pancreatic head takes place along the duodenal border of the portal vein.

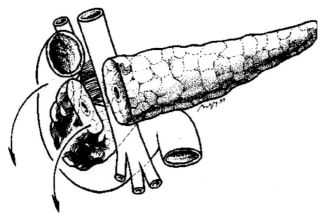

Fig. 2. After completion of the transection of the pancreatic neck, the pancreatic head is rotated into the ventrodorsal axis (upward) for subtotal resection.

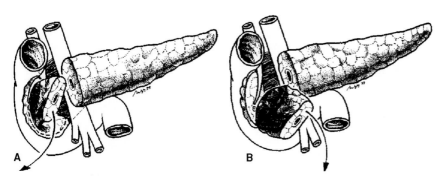

Fig. 3. A: After decompression of the portal vein and dissection of small venous branches between the head of the pancreas and the portal vein, the subtotal resection of the pancreatic head starts at the dorsal part of the pancreatic head toward the uncinate process and along a line 5 mm distant from the ventral duodenal wall. **B:** The intrapancreatic segment of the common bile duct is decompressed by dissecting the pancreatic head along the common bile duct wall. In most patients, this results in a complete decompression of the narrowed common bile duct.

by including the tissue of the uncinate process and excising the pancreatic head tissue at a distance of 5 mm from the duodenal wall. The wet weight of the operative specimen after subtotal pancreatic head resection is 25 to 50 g. It has not proved necessary to preserve the gastroduodenal artery for ensuring an optimal blood supply to the duodenal wall because the supraduodenal vessels, the dorsal pancreaticoduodenal, and the mesoduodenal vessels maintain the blood supply. The dissection of the intrapancreatic segment of the common bile duct is started at the upper margin of the pancreatic head (Fig. 3B). In most cases, decompression of the common bile duct can be achieved by dissecting the pancreatic tissue along the common bile duct wall.

In cases with inflammation in the wall of the common bile duct, the duct is opened by excising a 15- × 5-mm wall segment (Fig. 4). After completion of the subtotal resection of the pancreatic head, a shell-like, 5- to 8-mm wide remnant of the tissue of the pancreatic head is left connected to the duodenal wall (Fig. 5). Meticulous suturing of any bleeding vessels using 5-0 to 6-0 nonabsorbable suture material is recommended.

Reconstruction Phase

Reconstruction is initiated by dissecting the most proximal jejunal loop 20 cm distally to the ligament of Treitz. The aboral jejunal loop is transposed via a retrocolic mesenteric opening to the pancreatic head, and an end-to-end anastomosis using a two-layered technique is fashioned between the pancreatic neck and the jejunal loop (Fig. 6). In patients with a dilated main pancreatic duct and multiple fibrotic duct stenoses, the main pancreatic duct is incised longitudinally at its anterior surface up to the tail of the pancreas. In these patients, the anastomosis is performed as a side-to-side anastomosis, as in a Partington-Rochelle modification drainage of the main pancreatic duct (Fig. 7). A single- or double-layer suture between the jejunum and the residual head of the pancreas along the excision line has to be carried out at a distance of 5 to 8 cm from the anastomosis with the left pancreas.

An additional anastomosis between the common bile duct and the jejunal loop is not mandatory. The opening of the common bile duct is included in the pancreatic anastomosis, which is carried out with the remnant of the pancreatic head on the duodenal wall (Figs. 7 and 8).

For restoration of the food transit, a typical Roux-en-Y anastomosis is carried

The Gastrointestinal Tract

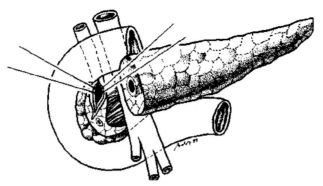

Fig. 4. In case of persistence of common bile duct stenosis caused by an inflammatory process in the wall of the duct, a lateral wall excision of the duct for an internal biliary bypass has to be carried out.

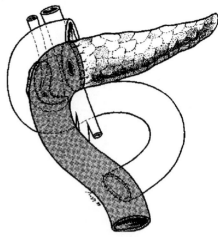

Fig. 6. For restoration of the exocrine pancreatic secretion into the upper jejunum, an end-to-end anastomosis to the distal pancreas and a side-to-side anastomosis between the Roux loop of jejunum and the remnant of the pancreatic head along the duodenal wall have to be performed.

out 20 cm distal to the pancreaticojejunal anastomosis (Fig. 8).

In patients with severe stenosis of the duodenum, dissection of the tissue at the ventral surface of the duodenum, causing an encasement of the duodenum, has to be carried out. The stenosis is caused by fibrous tissue bands at the front wall of the suprapapillary duodenum. Removal of these fibrous layers up to the serosal tissue level results in restoration of a normal food transit through the duodenum. The subtotal resection of the pancreatic head results in decompression of the portal vein and an immediate release of the signs of portal hypertension.

Results after Subtotal Duodenum-reserving Pancreatic Head Resection

Clinical observations and results from immunologic and molecular biologic investigations underline the hypothesis that the pancreatic head is the pacemaker in chronic pancreatitis. The subtotal duodenum-preserving resection of the pancreatic head results in relief of local complications. The coring-out technique of Frey is a modification of the Partington-Rochelle duct drainage procedure resulting in duct decompression, but it conserves the inflammatory mass in the pancreatic head if only 6 g of pancreatic head tissue is excised. In comparison with the Whipple resection and the pylorus-preserving pancreaticoduodenectomy, the subtotal duodenum-preserving pancreatic head resection offers the major advantage of preserving the extrahepatic biliary tree, stomach, and duodenum. In five randomized controlled clinical trials, the superiority of the duodenum-preserving technique in comparison with the Whipple resection or the pylorus-preserving resection has been demonstrated for patients experiencing advanced chronic pancreatitis. In terms of hospital death rates as well as frequency of relaparotomy and complications, the subtotal pancreatic head resection offers the major advantage of low postoperative morbidity (Table 3).

A major advantage of the duodenum-preserving subtotal resection of the pancreatic head in chronic pancreatitis is the preservation of the endocrine function of the pancreas. On the basis of oral glucose tolerance testing after a duodenum-preserving head resection, the glucose tolerance likely undergoes an improvement toward normalization early and late postoperatively; the head resection results in a decrease of the preoperatively increased glucagon and somatostatin levels in the peripheral blood, resulting in a decrease of the anti-insulin effects of these hormones. After a median follow-up of 5.7 years, 39% of the patients had normal findings on the oral glucose tolerance test and 17% had reduced findings on the oral glucose tolerance test, but 44% had insulin-dependent diabetes (Table 4).

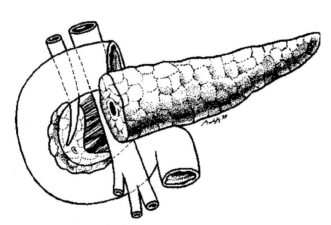

Fig. 5. After subtotal resection, a shell-like remnant of the pancreatic head along the duodenal wall is maintained. Careful surgical hemostasis is important to avoid early postoperative gastrointestinal tract bleeding. The blood supply to the duodenum is maintained by the dorsal pancreaticoduodenal arcades and the supraduodenal and mesoduodenal vessels.

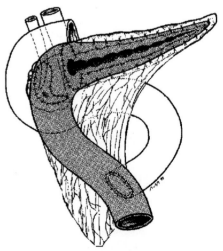

Fig. 7. In cases of multiple pancreatic main duct stenoses, a Partington-Rochelle modification of a drainage procedure between the jejunal loop and the left pancreas is carried out.

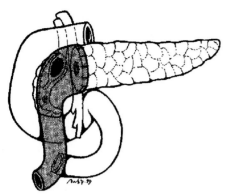

Fig. 8. To maintain the biliary juice flow into the upper jejunum and internal biliary bypass is mandatory in one third of the patients, allowing bile to pass into the duodenum through the ampulla of Vater and also into the Roux limb. The biliary duct incision is included in the side-to-side jejunopancreatic anastomosis.

In terms of the pain status after an observation period of up to 14 years, 79% of the patients were completely pain-free and 9% continued to experience abdominal pain. Regarding further episodes of acute pancreatitis with the need for hospitalization, the late follow-up (median of 6 years and up to 22 years postoperatively) disclosed that only approximately 12% of the patients developed further episodes of acute pancreatitis (Table 5). In terms of quality of life after subtotal duodenum-preserving pancreatic head resection, approximately two thirds of the patients were professionally rehabilitated. Using the Karnofsky index for scoring the quality of life, 72% of the patients scored within the normal range; up to 20% showed a reduced quality of life. After a median observation period of 5–7 years, the late death rate after subtotal pancreatic head resection in chronic pancreatitis was 8.9% and 13.0%. One half of the patients who died in the late postoperative follow-up period died after development of gastrointestinal tract cancer.

Duodenum-preserving Pancreatic Head Resection with Segmental Duodenum and Papilla Resection

Intraductal-papillary mucinous tumor (IPMN) and mucinous cystic neoplasm ([MCN]) have been established as different neoplastic entities of the pancreas. IPMN tumors are located most frequently in the head of the pancreas, followed by the body and tail. The most common subtype is branch duct IPMN; IPMN of the main pancreatic duct is less frequent, but observed equally as often as combined branch duct and pancreatic main duct neoplasia. Communication between the cyst and the pancreatic duct is observed in approximately 60% of the cases; fibrous capsules and mural nodules are found in approximately 15% and 40% of the cases. Additionally, pancreatic diseases (e.g., chronic pancreatitis, acute pancreatitis, and diabetes) are observed in approximately 16% of the patients. Histopathologic examinations of surgical specimens revealed hyperplasia in approximately less than 10% of patients, adenoma in approximately 50%, borderline neoplasia in approximately 2%, and adenocarcinoma in approximately 25% to 40%. Main duct or combined duct IPMN usually leads to surgical resection because of the higher incidence of malignancy. The incidence of malignancy of branch duct-type tumors is lower, compared with main duct type. MCN tumors are observed mostly in women and are more frequently located in the pancreatic body and tail than in the head. Communications between the cysts and the pancreatic duct are observed in approximately 15% of patients; a fibrous capsule in almost two thirds of the patients, and mural nodules in 30%. One third of the patients who had surgical resection for MCN tumor revealed adenocarcinoma. Ovarian-type stroma is the characteristic tissue of the MCN and is composed of densely packed, spindle-shaped cells with round or elongated nuclei and spaced cytoplasm.

The long-term outcome of patients with IPMN and MCN tumors is excellent for patients with adenoma and non-invasive carcinoma. However, the prognosis for patients with invasive carcinoma decreases to less than 50% after 5 years, but it is better than the prognosis for pancreatic ductal adenocarcinoma. The prognosis of MCN tumors after complete resection is excellent in cases of adenoma and noninvasive carcinoma. With an appropriate treatment, both IPMN and MCN tumors, if noninvasive, are completely curable. In patients with IMPN disease in the pancreatic head, incomplete resection leads to recurrence, with the consequence of a reoperation.

TABLE 3. SUBTOTAL, DUODENUM-PRESERVING PANCREATIC HEAD RESECTION IN CHRONIC PANCREATITITS: EARLY POSTOPERATIVE RESULTS

Postoperative hospital stay	14.5 d mean (7–87)
Relaparotomy	5.6% (28 of 504 patients)
Hospital deaths	0.8% (4 of 504 patients)

From Beger HG, Schlosser W, Friess HM, et al. Duodenum-preserving head resection in chronic pancreatitis changes the natural course of the disease. A single-center 26-year experience. *Ann Surg* 1999; 230:512, with permission.

TABLE 4. ENDOCRINE FUNCTION AFTER SUBTOTAL PANCREATIC HEAD RESECTION IN CHRONIC PANCREATITIS[a]

	Preoperative	Late Postoperative		
	1972–1998 504 Patients	1972–1983[b] 56 Patients 2.0 y[d]	1972–1987[c] 109 Patients 3.6 y[d]	1982–1996 303 Patients 5.7 y[d]
	No. (%)	No. (%)	No. (%)	No. (%)
OGTT normal	246 (49)	37 (66)	52 (48)	118 (39)
OGTT reduced	134 (26)	19 (34)	28 (26)	51 (17)
IDDM	124 (25)	—	29 (26)	134 (44)
Glucose-improved	—	3 (15.8)	3 (5.5)	34 (11)
New IDDM	—	2 (5.4)	11 (13.7)	64 (21)

[a]IDDM, insulin-dependent diabetes mellitus; OGTT, oral glucose tolerance test.
[b]From Beger HG, Krautzberger W, Bittner R, et al. Duodenum-preserving resection of the head of the pancreas in patients with severe chronic pancreatitis. *Surgery* 1985;97:467, with permission.
[c]From Beger HG, Schlosser W, Friess HM, et al. Duodenum-preserving head resection in chronic pancreatitis changes the natural course of the disease. A single-center 26-year experience. *Ann Surg* 1999;230:512, with permission.
[d]Median years of follow-up.

The Gastrointestinal Tract

TABLE 5. SUBTOTAL DUODENUM-PRESERVING PANCREATIC HEAD RESECTION IN CHRONIC PANCREATITIS CHANGES THE NATURAL COURSE OF THE DISEASE

	1972–1983 58 Patients[a] 0–11 y 2 y (Median) 57 Patients	1972–1987 128 Patients[b] 0–15 y 3.6 y (Median) 109 Patients	1972–1994 298 Patients[c] 0–22 y 6 y (Median) 258 Patients	1982–1996 388 Patients 0–14 y 5.7 y (Median) 303 Patients
Follow-up rate	100	96	87	94
Pain-free or rare pain	92.8	89	88	91.3[d]
Continuing abdominal pain	7.2	11	12	8.3
Acute episodes/hospitalization from chronic pancreatitis	14	11	10	12.5
Late death	3.6	4.7	8.9	13
Endocrine function improved	15.8	5.5	—	11
Professional rehabilitation	88.7	67	63	69
Quality of life/Kamofsky index 80–100	—	—	—	82

[a]From Beger HG, Krautzberger W, Bittner R, et al. Duodenum-preserving resection of the head of the pancreas in patients with severe chronic pancreatitis. *Surgery* 1985; 97:467, with permission.
[b]From Beger HG, Büchler M, Bittner R, et al. Duodenum-preserving resection of the head of the pancreas in severe chronic pancreatitis. *Ann Surg* 1989;209:273, with permission.
[c]From Büchler MW, Friess H, Bittner R, et al. Duodenum-preserving pancreatic head resection: long-term results. *J Gastrointest Surg* 1997; 1:13, with permission.
[d]Thirty-eight patients (12.5%) are included as pain-free, although they experienced an episode of acute pancreatitis in the period of follow-up observation.

The main goal of preoperative diagnosis in cystic lesions of the pancreatic head is the discrimination between benign and malignant lesion and to objectify the extent of the cystic lesion. In patients with an IPMN tumor in the pancreatic head, larger than 2 cm, a duodenum-preserving complete pancreatic head resection with segmental resection of the duodenal papilla is mandatory (Table 6). For patients with serous cystic lesions, surgical treatment is indicated in cysts more than 2 cm and compressing the pancreatic main duct and, in cases of mass development in the cyst wall, that are suspected to be additional neoplastic lesions.

Indications and Techniques of Duodenum-preserving Total Pancreatic Head Resection in Neoplastic Lesions of the Pancreatic Head

Duodenum-preserving pancreatic head resection with segmental resection of the peripapillary duodenum is indicated in patients suffering from IPMN lesions, located in the pancreatic head up to the duodenal wall (Table 6, Fig. 9A). After transection of the pancreatic head on the duodenal line of the portal vein, the pancreatic head is mobilized up to the wall of the duodenum. One or multiple frozen section controls of the resection margin has to be done to prove the absence of IPMN structures histologically. The common bile duct is identified and transected. The pancreatic head is dissected from the duodenal wall toward the papilla and from the mesoduodenum in the uncinate process toward the papilla.

A segment of the duodenum above and below the papilla is transected to achieve a total pancreatic head resection. Reconstruction is performed in three steps:

1. End-to-end anastomosis between the proximal and distal duodenum (Fig. 9B)
2. Exclusion of the first jejunal loop and interposition between the left pancreas, and the reconstruction of the duodenum using a Cattell anastomosis between the jejunum and the left pancreas (Fig. 9C)
3. End-to-side anastomosis between the common bile duct and the jejunum interponate and a Roux-en-Y anastomosis for reconstruction of the upper intestine. An implantation of the left pancreatic stump into the stomach has been used to avoid an anastomosis with a jejunal loop (Fig. 9D).

A resection of the uncinate process, including a segment of the duodenum, can be performed in patients suffering from a neoplastic lesion that is localized in the uncinate process and is not compressing the pancreatic main duct but is intensively adhesed to the wall of the postpyloric duodenum. Large neuroendocrine tumors localized in the uncinate process and mucinous cystic lesions exclusively including the pancreatic tissue of the uncinate process may have major benefit from this organ-preserving technique (Fig. 10A, B).

A duodenum- and spleen-preserving total pancreatectomy has been performed in patients suffering from IPMN lesions, including those in the pancreatic head, body, and tail. In most patients a dissection of the pancreatic head along the duodenum wall avoids segmental resection of the papilla. However, in the authors' opinion, a segmental duodenum resection and an end-to-side anastomosis between the common bile duct and the postpyloric duodenum are necessary to avoid ischemic lesions of the peripapillary wall of the duodenum (Table 7, Fig. 11A, B).

TABLE 6. INDICATION FOR DUODENUM-PRESERVING TOTAL PANCREATIC HEAD RESECTION[a]

1. IPMN localized in pancreatic head >2 cm main and combined duct type
2. MCN with compression of CBD and PMD
3. Pancreatic endocrine or neuroendocrine neoplastic lesion with adhesion to duodenum

[a]IPMN, intraductal papillary mucinous tumor; MCN, mucinous cystic neoplasm; CBD, common bile duct; PMD, pancreatic main duct.

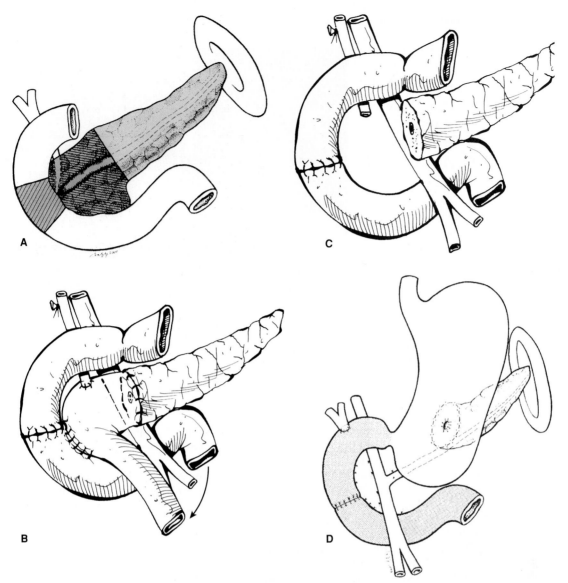

Fig. 9. Duodenum-preserving pancreatic head resection with segmental resection of the peripapillary duodenum is indicated in patients suffering from intraductal-papillary mucinous tumor. A segment of the peripapillary duodenum with close proximity to the intraductal-papillary mucinous tumor of the pancreatic head is transected to achieve a total pancreatic head resection. **A:** An end-to-end anastomosis between proximal and distal duodenum has to be performed. **B,C:** The first jejunal loop is used as an interposition for reconstruction. The pancreaticojejunostomosis is performed as a Catell anastomosis with duct-to-mucosa sutures. **D:** To avoid an anastomosis with jejunal loop, the pancreatic stump is implanted into the wall of the stomach.

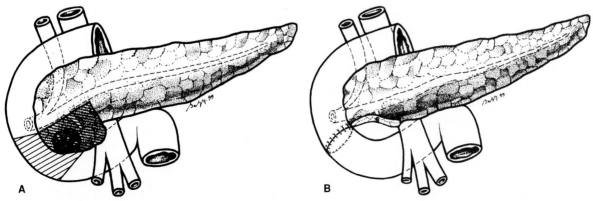

Fig. 10. Neoplastic lesions localized in the uncinate process without compression of the pancreatic main duct are locally resected, including the uncinate process and the postpyloric duodenum segment. **A:** Neuroendocrine tumors localized in the uncinate process are resected with a 4- to 6-cm segment of the postpyloric duodenum. **B:** Reconstruction of the duodenum takes place with an end-to-end anastomosis.

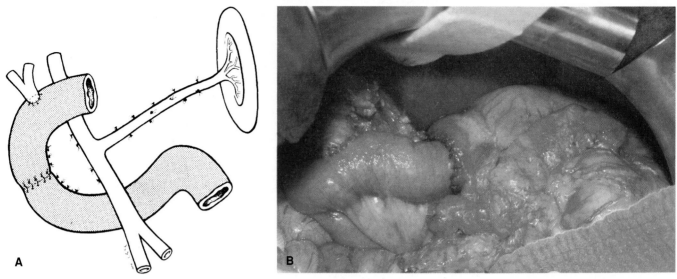

Fig. 11. A: In case of a total pancreatectomy with preservation of the duodenum, a segmental duodenum resection to avoid local recurrence on the duodenum wall has to be performed. **B:** Additionally, an end-to-side anastomosis between the common bile duct and the postpyloric duodenum is necessary.

CONCLUSION

In patients with alcoholic-related chronic pancreatitis who have developed an inflammatory mass in the pancreatic head, a subtotal duodenum-preserving pancreatic head resection results in a change of the natural course of the disease with regard to pain status, frequency of acute episodes of chronic pancreatitis, need for further hospital admissions, late mortality rate, and quality of life. Evaluation of the postoperative outcome of the patients after subtotal head resection confirms observations from other groups that surgical treatment of chronic pancreatitis results in

a delay or even a break in the progressive loss of pancreatic exocrine and endocrine function.

Patients suffering from pancreas divisum that causes chronic pancreatitis or acute recurrent pancreatitis, a duodenum-preserving pancreatic head resection eradicates or alleviates long-lasting pain and further episodes of acute pancreatitis.

Benefits of using duodenum-preserving *total* pancreatic head resection in cystic neoplastic lesions restricted to the head are the preservation of the stomach, duodenum, intestine, and biliary main duct as well as maintenance of the ex-

ocrine and endocrine functions of these mostly young patients. Duodenum and spleen conservation is even recommended in patients suffering from IPMN that is localized in the pancreatic head and body and is treated with total pancreatectomy. However, occasionally, especially in young patients, resection of the uncinate process and a segment of the postpapillary duodenum is performed in cases with mucinous or serous neoplastic lesion and endocrine tumor of the uncinate process.

To avoid the risks of ischemic lesions of periampullary duodenum, total resection of the pancreatic head and a segmental resection of the duodenum, including the papilla, has been introduced in clinical practice. An oncologic pancreatic head resection (e.g., a Whipple-type resection) has to be performed in patients suffering from a cystic neoplastic lesion and an invasive cancer.

SUGGESTED READING

Beger HG, Krautzberger W, Bittner R, et al. Duodenum-preserving resection of the head of the pancreas in patients with severe chronic pancreatitis. *Surgery* 1985;97:467.

Beger HG, Schlosser W, Friess HM, et al. Duodenum-preserving head resection in chronic pancreatitis changes the natural course of the disease. A single-center 26-year experience. *Ann Surg* 1999;230:512.

TABLE 7. MODIFICATIONS OF DUODENUM-PRESERVING PANCREATIC HEAD RESECTION[a]

Duodenum-preserving pancreatic head resection in CP and pancreas divisum.
+ Biliary (CBD) anastomosis (end-to-side)
+ PMD drainage using jejunal loop (side-to-side)
Duodenum-preserving total pancreatic head resection in IPMN and MCN
+ Segmental resection of peripapillary duodenum (end-to-end)
Duodenum-preserving total pancreatectomy in IPMN of pancreatic head and body with conservation of spleen
Duodenum-preserving resection of uncinate process in cases with localized MCN and endocrine tumor with segmental resection of postpapillary duodenum (end-to-end)

[a]CP, chronic pancreatitis; CBD, common bile duct; IPMN, intraductal papillary mucinous tumor; MCN, mucinous cystic neoplasm.

Beger HG, Schlosser W, Poch B, et al. Inflammatory mass in the head of the pancreas. In: Beger HG, Warshaw AL, Büchler MW, et al., eds. *The pancreas.* Oxford: Blackwell Science, 1998:757.

Büchler MW, Weihe E, Friess H, et al. Changes in peptidergic innervation in chronic pancreatitis. *Pancreas* 1992;7:183.

Garcia-Puges AM, Navarro S, Ros E, et al. Reversibility of exocrine pancreatic failure in chronic pancreatitis. *Gastroenterology* 1986;91:17.

Imaizumi T, Hanyu F, et al. Clinical experience with duodenum-preserving total resection of the head of the pancreas with pancreaticocholedochoduodenostomy. *J Hepatobiliary Pancreat Surg* 1995;2:38.

Isaji S, Kawarada Y. Pancreatic head resection with second-portion duodenectomy for benign lesions, low-grade malignancies, and early stage carcinomas involving the pancreatic head region. *Am J Surg* 2001;181:172.

Kimura W. IHPBA in Tokyo, 2002: surgical treatment of IPMT vs MCT: a Japanese experience. *J Hepatobiliary Pancreat Surg* 2003;10:156.

Kimura W, Morikane K, et al. A new method of duodenum-preserving subtotal resection of the head of the pancreas based on surgical anatomy. *Hepatogastroenterology* 1996;43:463.

Lankisch PG, Löhr-Happe A, Otto T, et al. Natural course in chronic pancreatitis. Pain, exocrine and endocrine pancreatic insufficiency and prognosis of the disease. *Digestion* 1993;54:148.

Murakami Y, Uemura K, Yokoyama Y, et al. Pancreatic head resection with segmental duodenectomy for intraductal papillary mucinous tumors of the pancreas. *J Gastrointest Surg* 2004; 8:713.

Nakao A. Pancreatic head resection with segmental duodenectomy and preservation of the gastroduodenal artery. *Hepatogastroenterology* 1998;45:533.

Takada T, Yasuda H, Uchiyama K, et al. Duodenum-preserving pancreatoduodenostomy. A new technique for complete excision of the head of the pancreas with preservation of biliary and alimentary integrity. *Hepatogastroenterology* 1993;40:356.

EDITOR'S COMMENT

The principle role of surgery in chronic pancreatitis is palliative. Patients are typically seen late in the course of their disease and they have irreversible gland destruction that is manifested clinically by pain and exocrine and endocrine insufficiency. Surgeons and patients alike are at early disadvantage. With proper patient selection and care, excellent and durable results can be achieved if the proper operation is performed correctly, and patients remain committed to their successful recovery. Neither of these goals is easy to achieve.

Because surgical drainage of nondilated ducts never helps, resection procedures are used for "small-duct" chronic pancreatitis. The question always is how much of the diseased pancreas to remove. Focal duct strictures and/or cysts in the body and tail causing "segmental" pancreatitis can be nicely managed by distal pancreatectomy. For diffuse small-duct disease, partial to even total pancreatectomy have rendered variable results. Pain does improve, but extended parenchymal resections deepen endocrine/exocrine insufficiency, prompting some to add rescue autologous islet transplantation (*J Gastrointest Surg* 2003;8:978).

Often, it is not about debilitating pain alone. When the fibrosis and inflammation of chronic pancreatitis affects neighboring structures, surgery ultimately becomes necessary. Obstruction of the intrapancreatic common bile duct leads to duct dilation, abnormal liver chemistries, and eventually frank jaundice and episodic cholangitis (*Ann Surg* 1989;210:608). If an isolated symptom, the biliary obstruction can effectively be decompressed through a relatively simple choledochoduodenostomy. More often, however, it is but one symptom of the disease that warrants a larger procedure. Duodenal obstruction occurs next most frequently, and is often associated with biliary obstruction, especially in pancreatic head-predominant disease. Most surgeons employ pancreatic resection procedures in such cases, although a gastrojejunostomy solves isolated duodenal obstruction nicely. Other anatomic consequences of pancreatic fibrosis that can necessitate surgery include colonic obstruction, and occlusions that cause venous hypertension at any segment of the portal/superior mesenteric/splenic venous system (*Surgery* 2004;135:411). For any surgeon, this creates a perilous situation.

Because these anatomic sequelae and pain often relate to an "inflammatory mass" in the pancreatic head, Professor Hans Beger and colleagues have conceived innovative operations that remove most or all of the diseased head, but unlike a Whipple procedure, preserve the native duodenum. Several variants are described and nicely illustrated in this chapter. The authors have extended the indications for these procedures to include intraductal papillary mucinous neoplasms (IPMN), mucinous cystic neoplasms, and larger endocrine neoplasms in the pancreatic head. In Europe, the duodenum-preserving resection of the pancreatic head (Beger procedure) is quite popular for chronic pancreatitis, and compared favorably against the Whipple procedure (*Am J Surg* 1995;169:65; *Surgery* 2003;134:53). This extends the Frey procedure concept that some degree of head resection combined with proper duct drainage is enough (*Ann Surg* 1999;230:512).

Nonetheless, this operation has not attained similar popularity in America and elsewhere. Why not? Some say it relates to different indications for pancreatic head resection, and others point to unique characteristics of respective patient populations. It is also a technically demanding operation, especially for a surgeon without proper training or experience in its intricacies. As a result, the trend worldwide continues to favor either the Frey or Whipple procedures. That said, the clinical results summarized in Tables 4 and 5 are stunning. In follow-up beyond 14 years, 80% of patients remained completely pain-free, two-thirds had been fully rehabilitated professionally, and quality-of-life scores reflected all of this. For some, there was even a mysterious improvement in glucose tolerance. Regardless of lingering doubts or questions, these results long ago earned Professor Beger the international acclaim he rightfully deserves. One must acknowledge these operations push the envelope of pancreatic surgery, and one must admire the results they achieve.

The reader should fully understand, however, that no patient with suspicion of pancreatic cancer in the head of the gland should be treated by duodenum-preserving head resections. These procedures are oncologically inadequate. Pancreaticoduodenectomy is still required. New to *Mastery's* *5th edition* however is Professor Beger's discussion of how these resections can be applied to less-dangerous neoplastic processes, even to the point of including segmental duodenectomy with ampullectomy. With changing landscapes for these diseases, especially IPMN, it seems reasonable to apply innovative surgical techniques with proven track records in patient safety. For actual clinical outcomes, however, time will tell.

M.P.C.

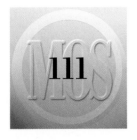

Necrosectomy for Acute Necrotizing Pancreatitis

CHARLES M. VOLLMER JR.

INTRODUCTION

Acute pancreatitis is a significant public health concern that leads to close to a quarter million hospital admissions per year in the United States. This is a disease process historically treated best by surgeons, and today's surgical house officers should continue to embrace the care of these complex patients. Although a benign process, both short- and long-term morbidity can be substantial. There is a full spectrum of affliction ranging from mild, self-limited biochemical enzyme elevation all the way to fulminate systemic illness, and, often, early death. As a consequence of the initial insult to the gland, a significant subset of these patients will have extensive parenchymal necrosis of the pancreas. Management of this condition, both surgical and nonsurgical, is the focus of this chapter, with emphasis on early supportive care and preoperative decision making, followed by description of a preferred surgical approach, when necessary.

FLUID COLLECTIONS AND PANCREATITIS

Perhaps the most vexing aspect of pancreatitis care revolves around the definitions and treatment approaches applied to the findings of peripancreatic fluid collections. Their mismanagement often leads to unnecessary tests and procedures as well as significant morbidity. These collections are common in patients with severe pancreatitis (up to 50%) and are evident very early in the course (within days), not by symptoms per se, but rather through imaging studies used to diagnose or stratify acute pancreatitis.

These collections are the result of the initial inflammation in the pancreatic bed in conjunction with the "quenching" effect of early fluid resuscitation. The overwhelming majority of these will represent *no* disruption of, nor have a communication with, the pancreatic duct. Consequentially, they are not rich in secreted pancreatic enzymes, nor do they develop a defined wall of fibrous granulation tissue—the hallmark of a pseudocyst. It is a common mistake to implicate these complex-appearing, often multiple, peripancreatic collections as the nidus of the patient's overall deterioration (Fig. 1). The vast majority of these will resolve spontaneously and require no specific interventions.

Although they originally appear similar on early imaging, only a small fraction (10%) of these will persist beyond 5 to 6 weeks, and these are then deemed pseudocysts, based on their persistence, prolonged time course, fibrous containment wall, and/or direct communication with the pancreatic ductal system (Fig. 2). The literature is rife with descriptions of drainage interventions (both endoscopically and percutaneously) early in the course for these peripancreatic fluid collections. These should be generally condemned for numerous reasons: (a) they simply often are not necessary (spontaneous resolution is the norm), (b) they can introduce infection to otherwise sterile tissue, (c) they are ineffective at total "clearance" of the bed of necrosis, and finally (d) they can lead to persistent fistulous communications in cases of actual pseudocysts with ductal disruption. More importantly, rarely does this sort of early interventional approach dramatically and immediately "turn around" the course of a sick patient. Obviously there still remain investigational opportunities to elucidate the exact advantages of these approaches, for example, in "temporizing" of poor operative risk patients who are deteriorating.

Pancreatic Necrosis

Necrotizing pancreatitis occurs in approximately a fifth of all cases of acute pancreatitis. Following the parameters delineated in the Atlanta classification scheme (1993), this is defined as a focal, or diffuse, well-marginated zone of nonenhancing, poorly perfused parenchyma on dynamic computed tomography (CT) scan evaluation (Fig. 3), and can be evident even within the first day or 2 of the illness. This should be distinguished from interstitial pancreatitis (indicative of cellular swelling and extracellular edema; Fig. 4) in that necrotizing pancreatitis is the end result of active cellular autolysis leading to nonviable tissue. Organ failure occurs only 10% of the time with interstitial pancreatitis, but rises significantly to around 50% when necrosis is present. Naturally, it follows that once there is any organ failure, there is a substantial risk for mortality. In necrotizing pancreatitis, death rates are 1% or less without evidence of organ failure and 3% with single-system compromise, and they rise exponentially to 50% with multisystem failure. Interestingly, it is not clearly evident that greater amounts of glandular necrosis necessarily lead to higher mortality. Rather, mortality is more closely linked to timing and severity of organ failure rather than degree of necrosis.

There appear to be two distinctly vulnerable timeframes for mortality. Early mortality occurs within the first 1 to 3 days of presentation as a result of an overwhelming systemic inflammatory response syndrome (SIRS) and is *not* necessarily the sequela of infection. A second mortality peak occurs weeks following the initial insult. During this later stage the patient may succumb to lethal infections (pneumonias or line infections) attributed to supportive care measures. Necrotizing pancreatitis is subclassified into sterile and infected (present one third of the time) necrosis, and both conditions may require substantial surgical intervention at some point in the patient's recovery. Less frequently, late demise is the result of this pancreatic necrosis infected with bacterial, and increasingly, fungal species.

Multiple biochemical markers (e.g., C-reactive protein, interleukins) have been proposed to help grade disease severity and predict the patient's course. However, these have not found universal clinical acceptance due to high costs, lack of specificity, and impractical application. Grading scales based on clinical parameters remain the more effective and valid predictive cornerstones for the practitioner caring for these patients. Traditional classifications such as the Ranson and Glasgow criteria have largely been eclipsed by the APACHE-II physiologic score, both in the literature and in daily practice. With greater than 70% predictive value, this has proven to be the most accurate prognostic

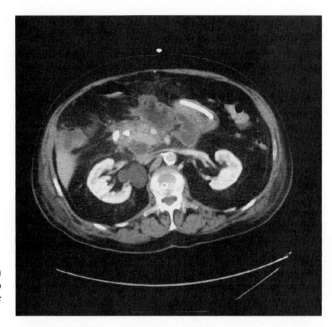

Fig. 1. Peripancreatic fluid collections. In the acute setting (days to weeks) these represent the sequelae of acute pancreatitis and are not exclusive to necrotizing pancreatitis. These are frequently multiple in nature and have characteristic local inflammatory appearances.

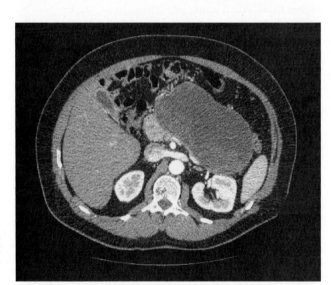

Fig. 2. Pancreatic pseudocyst. This well-delineated fluid collection is the ultimate result of pancreatic necrosis with significant pancreatic ductal disruption. At 8 weeks out, this fluid collection is encapsulated by a fibrous wall contained by the boundaries of the lesser sac. The subtle heterogeneous appearance of its contents reflects a residual necrotic pancreatic tail.

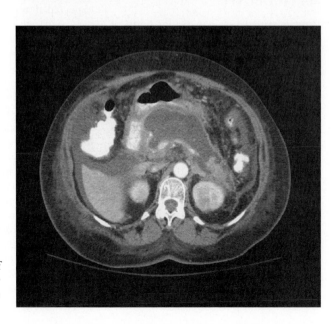

Fig. 3. Necrotizing pancreatitis. A significant portion of the body and tail of the pancreas are nonviable on this computed tomography scan with IV contrast performed 2 days after the inciting event. Note the well-demarcated, enhancing viable pancreatic tissue in the tail.

The Gastrointestinal Tract

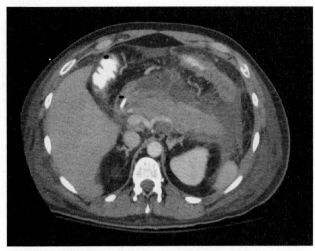

Fig. 4. Interstitial pancreatitis. This well-enhancing, thickened gland appears swollen and wet. Note the peripancreatic edema and fat stranding at its periphery.

system for necrotizing pancreatitis (i.e., higher APACHE-II scores predict escalating morbidity and mortality when necrosis is present).

Lastly, with the ever-improving quality of abdominal cross-sectional imaging, there is recent enthusiasm for the predictive power of helical CT imaging alone. Balthazar has proposed a classification scheme for pancreatic necrosis, based on CT assessment early in the course, which correlates strongly with ultimate morbidity and mortality. However, it must be emphasized that, despite said predictive power, immediate CT imaging is not necessary to make the diagnosis of acute pancreatitis, and lends little to the therapeutic algorithm. It is usually unnecessary in the early stages of disease.

IMMEDIATE PATIENT MANAGEMENT

Patients with severe pancreatitis (with or without a necrotizing component) are best treated in an intensive care setting. Septic hemodynamic patterns (high cardiac output with low vascular resistance) are common and usually require active support. This initial phase is focused on organ-failure prevention and/or support. It is crucial for the practitioner to realize, however, that this "septic" pattern does *not* equate to immediate bacterial infection in this disease. The only exception to this would be if there was overt evidence of obstructive cholangitis from gallstones, which should be relieved endoscopically if present. Surgery during this labile physiologic period is universally morbid, if not even lethal.

The active inflammatory response in the pancreatic bed is analogous to a

retroperitoneal *burn* injury, and therefore the tenets of burn care apply. Fluid resuscitation is mandatory, both to "douse" the peripancreatic inflammation and to support end-tissue perfusion in the setting of cardiovascular compromise. These may be massive requirements—on the order of 10 to 25 L within the first 24-hour period for some. Of all major organs, the pulmonary system is the most frequently, and usually the first, affected. Supplemental oxygenation, at the very least, and more commonly full-fledged ventilator support are required due to the direct effects of pancreatic inflammatory mediators on the pulmonary interstitium, as well as the inevitable volume overload incurred by resuscitation. Inotropic agents or vasopressors are administered with the aim of enhancing tissue oxygen delivery, but should be required less frequently than might be expected if appropriate volume support has been achieved. Renal function is sometimes compromised as these patients often initially present profoundly dehydrated (with elevated hematocrits), a problem that is exacerbated by inadequate volume repletion when pressor support is favored over fluid administration to sustain vascular tone. Significant postresuscitation pharmacologic-assisted diuresis (3 to 4 days after the fact) is the norm, and it is not uncommon to also require volume filtration and/or hemodialysis. Theoretically, biologic and immuno-modulators provide an attractive therapeutic arsenal to combat local inflammatory mediators generated by pancreatic inflammation and cell death, as well as the more advanced systemic responses of SIRS. Disappointingly, to date, none of these has shown singular clinical efficacy in attenuating morbidity and mor-

tality from pancreatitis in humans. This likely reflects the complexity of this biologic cascade with numerous regulatory mechanisms in play.

A common mistake is to apply empiric, broad-spectrum antibiotic coverage to *all* cases of acute pancreatitis from the outset. This is not necessary for the majority of patients, and obviously places the patient in jeopardy of secondary bacterial infections such as *Clostridium difficile* colitis, as well as fungal infections. The current standard of care is to administer antibiotic coverage in *severe* cases (APACHE-II score ≥ 6) of acute pancreatitis *with* necrosis. Antibiotics are applied immediately upon diagnosis and continued, not indefinitely, but for a defined period (usually 10 to 14 days) in a prophylactic fashion with the rationale of *prevention* of pancreatic superinfection, and *not* for generalized therapy for SIRS. The chosen antibiotic should be tailored to provide focal Gram-negative and anaerobic coverage, and should have superior penetration to the pancreatic necrotic tissue. Well-designed prospective studies have identified both the quinolone family and imipenem (more so) as optimal choices in minimizing infectious complications from pancreatic necrosis. Because of the powerful spectrum of coverage with these particular agents, fungal superinfections and fungemia have been on the rise in the last decade. This problem, with its morbid consequences, has prompted most practitioners to concurrently administer antifungal coverage with fluconazole.

Finally, nutritional support is paramount for these patients as they will be in an extended catabolic state from the condition, and will be unable to acquire adequate caloric intake orally—even after they have escaped the initial throes of critical illness. The ideal approach is early feeding via an enteral route and, in the critical care setting, this is almost always achieved through a nasojejunal feeding tube placed beyond the duodenum and into the proximal jejunum. Stimulation of the pancreas is inversely related to tube distance beyond the pylorus. If manual placement of the tube is initially unsuccessful because of failure to pass beyond the pylorus, then efforts should be made with graduated interventional means. The next optimal approach would be fluoroscopic radiology guidance beyond the pylorus. Finally, endoscopic advancement can achieve the goal. These added efforts are preferable to gastric feeding, which poses the risk of aspiration and requires strictly elemental formulas.

Once tube placement has been achieved, a dilute formula should be slowly and gradually advanced as tolerated in that these patients often suffer from a profound ileus initially. Nasogastric drainage is easily achieved in these critically ill patients and can help guide the rate of application of distal feeding, but, in and of itself, does not accelerate the resumption of bowel function. Some advocate the early placement of a percutaneous endoscopic combined gastrojejunal tube (PEG-J) to achieve these goals, citing the improved convenience and patient comfort once the critical care phase has passed. On the contrary, this approach obligates the patient to a potentially risky intervention that almost always can be obviated by simple nasal passage. In fact, many patients will be able to tolerate oral feedings sooner than anticipated, so the risk and expense of such a procedure may be in vain. Furthermore, given that a significant number of these patients will ultimately require operative interventions for their fluid collections (including pseudocyst-gastrostomies), such tubes may hamper subsequent operative approaches.

Reliance on total parenteral nutrition (TPN) is easy and convenient, especially given the fact that these severe patients ubiquitously have central venous access in place. However, it is an inferior approach for three reasons: (a) enteral feedings are more physiologic and prone to fewer metabolic complications. (b) Enteral feedings protect the gut mucosa and reverse the barrier disruption that is the result of hypoperfusion from the initial onset of pancreatitis. The resultant permeability and bacterial translocation theoretically provides a portal of entry for bloodborne pathogens that contribute to endotoxemia and superinfection of pancreatic necrosis. (c) Central catheter–based complications (bacterial infection, fungemia, thrombosis) are real, menacing, and costly. This being said, TPN does have a valuable role to play in select patients after they emerge from the critical care setting (see below).

COURSES OF PROGRESSION

Although generalizations are dangerous, four types of progression are common following the initial onset of severe necrotizing pancreatitis.

Immediate Demise

In a confined group of patients, the initial insult is overwhelming and, despite the measures instituted above, the SIRS response leads to a domino effect of multi-system organ failure. This process can play out early (days) or subacutely (1 to 2 weeks). The urge to intervene operatively at this stage should be resisted in most patients, as outcomes have historically been poor. This is generally due to the fact that the patient is usually too labile physiologically to endure the added surgical stress; the pancreatic bed is actively inflamed with tissues that are not well delineated at this early juncture, resulting in more bleeding complications (sometimes massive); and finally the necrosum is usually *not* infected this early. Thus, the objective of aggressive surgical intervention to relieve presumed local sepsis will be miscalculated.

Obviously there are exceptional patients in any practice, and factors such as extremes in age, presence or absence of comorbidities, and patient/family/cultural preferences must factor into the decision of whether to operate in these dire straits. Sometimes, a fine needle aspiration (FNA) of pancreatic necrosis might determine if infection is present. In the rare case it does, one might offer surgical treatment. In general, however, operative interventions should be very selectively applied in this timeframe.

Rapid Initial Recovery

The vast majority of patients will stabilize and ultimately emerge from critical care support. It is exceedingly rare for this to occur rapidly (in a matter of days from onset) in the setting of pancreatitis with bona fide necrosis. Most will progress, within the next 2 to 3 weeks, to less acute care requirements and will transfer to the floor. Appropriate care for the residual effects of end-organ damage (respiratory, renal, cardiac, etc.) is continued, but many of the initial therapeutic maneuvers can be pared down. Invasive tubes and lines can be selectively removed. Unnecessary, prolonged use of empiric (or directed) antibiotics should be avoided. During this recovery phase, often the most challenging problem is sustaining a suitable nutrition requisite for recovery from the extended catabolic state. Oral intake can be initiated once the patient is neurologically alert enough and can physically swallow, and there is no evidence of paralytic ileus, elevated amylase, or persistent abdominal pain. Physical and occupational rehabilitation is essential for debilitation from extended intensive care unit (ICU) care. This starts in the acute care hospital, but more often than not results in intermediate- or long-care facility placement.

Global Recovery, Inadequate Nutritional Support

In some cases, patients will immediately fail an oral challenge through inadequate caloric intake and/or active pain, nausea, and vomiting. The ability to sustain an adequate caloric intake during this oral trial phase is challenging and unpredictable. CT imaging at this extended time point is helpful as it usually demonstrates either an ongoing active inflammatory process in the lesser sac (made worse by oral stimulation of pancreatic secretions) or the progressive development of a space-filling pseudocyst or an inflammatory mass (pseudotumor) that mechanically distorts the stomach or duodenum. Supplemental means of nutrition will be required during this transition.

In these circumstances it is best to regroup early and put a brake to the process by discontinuing oral intake for a defined period of time. While enteral access is preferred to achieve this support, it is often impractical to rely on the previously placed nasojejunal tubes at this stage once the patient is out of the critical care setting. They become occluded, become dislodged (accidentally or intentionally), or simply are not well tolerated by the patient. A short-term course of parenteral nutrition via a peripherally placed (PIC) central line is a good temporary option. The goal is to sustain the patient for a few weeks only, in which time the inflammatory effects usually subside. Interval CT evaluation will help the practitioner dictate management at this point by demonstrating quelling of inflammation, regression of fluid collections, or maturation of significant pseudocysts that mandate internal enteric drainage. Achieving this objective (nutritional support) will often be the rate-limiting step to the discharge of these patients from the acute care hospital.

Extended, Smoldering Course

Finally, there is a significant cohort of patients that will have neither a severe nor an indolent course, and they are obviously the most challenging for the surgeon. These patients will require prolonged intensive care with relatively stabilized organ failure (ventilatory management, dialysis, pressor support, etc.). Often these patients will have persistent, daily fevers in the 101°F to 103°F degree range during the first 2 to 4 weeks. In lieu of other obvious sources of infection, in an otherwise stable patient this should be attributed to prolonged, active inflammation of the pancreas that contributes to production of poorly regulated cellular mediators. This is

The Gastrointestinal Tract

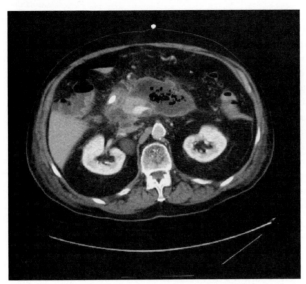

Fig. 5. Pancreatic abscess. Overt gas is evident in a zone of infected pancreatic necrosis 8 weeks following initial presentation of gallstone pancreatitis, and represents an absolute indication for surgical debridement.

referred to as "cytokine storm." This phenomenon is self-limiting, is controlled with antipyretics, and eventually burns out as the pancreatitis subsides.

As these patients linger in the ICU setting for weeks with septic physiology, determination of an infectious nidus is critical, but can be challenging. Pneumonia, line sepsis, and urinary tract infections are the most frequent culprits. Once these are ruled out, pancreatic infection warrants consideration. CT scan evaluation, at this stage, is now advocated to assess for occult infection in the pancreas *only* in the case of a patient with clear deterioration of clinical stability (advancing leukocytosis, newfound pressor support, or advancing ventilator requirements, etc.). At this point, infected pancreatic necrosis must be considered as the source. Gas in the pancreatic bed indicates overt infection (Fig. 5). If the scan shows significant necrosis, without gas, then a fine needle aspirate (with its high sensitivity and specificity) is employed to elucidate firm evidence of pancreatic infection. In some patients with a severe and rapid late deterioration, at this delayed point in time, FNA may be obviated due to the urgency to intervene.

INDICATIONS AND PREPARATION FOR OPERATIVE INTERVENTION

Infected necrosis with clinical deterioration is the prime indication to intervene operatively—observing the surgical principle that any closed-space infection requires

incision and drainage. These procedures often are performed in the setting of physiologic duress. However, a second indication to operate on pancreatic necrosis is failure to progress—otherwise deemed "general unwellness"—in the setting of sterile (or presumed sterile) necrosis. This later concept has been championed by leading pancreatic surgeons to describe those patients who fail to progress to oral diet, have persistent weight loss, or progressively deteriorate 5 weeks or later following the inciting episode of pancreatitis. These procedures are usually performed under more favorable parameters, save for malnutrition and general debilitation.

Once the decision to operate has been secured, a detailed review of the CT scan is imperative as it delineates the anatomic position and extent of the necrosis. Often the necrosis extends beyond the traditional boundaries of the lesser sac (down the paracolic gutters, along the root of the mesentery, superiorly behind the lesser omentum, or within the perinephric space along the Morrison pouch) and therefore requires multiple points of access separate from the lesser sac. This "roadmap" allows the surgeon the ability to focally attack these areas.

Adequate physiologic resuscitation should be achieved, by fluid and/or chemical support, in these deteriorating patients. Arterial, central venous, and even Swan-Ganz monitoring should be secured, and extensive blood loss should be anticipated by cross-matching the patient for 4 to 6 units of blood. Preparations should be made for prolonged intensive care following the operation.

OPERATIVE APPROACHES

Once the decision to intervene on pancreatic necrosis has been made, multiple operative techniques, all a variation of the same theme (incision/debridement/drainage), are available to the surgeon. Three, in particular, have enjoyed widespread use over the last 25 years, yet due to the paucity of cases and the heterogeneity of disease presentation, there is little evidence-based analysis of these approaches to indicate which is more effective. In the end, it comes down to surgeon preference and experience.

The first, more historical, approach relies on operative debridement of the pancreas with subsequent closure of the lesser sac over large-bored sump drains intended to provide continuous irrigation of the necrotic pancreatic bed. The abdomen is usually closed primarily in order to contain the large volumes of fluids that will be utilized. An active lavage process is initiated postoperatively with high-rate saline solution (multiple liters per hour) infused into the excavated pancreas. Infusate is diminished over time and the drains are removed sequentially. Although this is theoretically an attractive means of "diluting" out the local sepsis, management of these patients is cumbersome and prolonged. There is often failure of the drainage system due to clogging of the suction drains from necrotic debris leading to recurrent infections. Furthermore, the large-bored drains are unfortunately not well tolerated by the patient in the recovery phase and their size prevents timely closure of the drain tract leading to persistent pancreaticocutaneous fistulas.

A second approach evolved due to high rates of postoperative intra-abdominal infection and/or incomplete relief of sepsis seen with the aforementioned technique and consists of an open necrosectomy through a "marsupialized" lesser sac, followed with planned interval debridements through the widely opened wound. Most often this is approached through a bilateral subcostal incision for a specific reason. The lesser sac is opened along its entire length and the omental appendages of the stomach and colon are attached to the superior and inferior fascial borders, respectively. This creates a deep open cavity with the pancreatic bed at the base that is packed extensively and deeply with gauze. This then usually consists of extended intubation and critical care support with multiple early reoperations tapering to bedside wound management under sedation in the ICU. Significant, ventral hernia formation is an all too frequent late negative outcome. In order to prevent this unfortunate complication, a variation of this same theme employs a midline incision with re-exploration and open packing performed through an "accessible" incision. This comes in the form of a premade "zipper" device, or a homemade, adjustable temporary mesh applied to the fascial level. Today, this open packing approach has become less popular due to the extended, often unnecessary, use of resources (ICU, operating room, physician's time and effort) and the added costs incurred.

We favor open debridement with primary closure of the lesser sac over small-bored suction drains. When performed in an appropriate interval setting, this can usually be achieved in a single operation with definitive abdominal wall closure. This leads to an expeditious, and lower-cost, recovery period for the patient.

Finally, mention should be made of emerging endoscopic, interventional radiologic, and minimally invasive surgical alternatives to the more traditional open necrosectomy techniques. Percutaneous and/or endoscopic drainage methods may temporize sepsis, but ultimately prove to be inadequate in terms of relieving the bulk of the necrotic tissue that breeds infection. These often result in ultimate open surgical salvage. It should be remembered that in the early time period (1 to 6 weeks), transgastric endoscopic approaches are to be condemned in that there is generally no walling-off process of the lesser sac. Furthermore, this technique (as well as percutaneous drainage), if applied indiscriminately to sterile necrosis, is a set-up for conversion to infected necrosis. However, there is promise that highly selected patients can have an initial percutaneous drainage, followed by a minimally invasive retroperitoneal necrosectomy via drain sites that are upgraded (expanded) to allow for introduction of endoscopic instrumentation for debridement. This approach, however attractive by minimizing incision size and patient satisfaction, is labor- and resource-intensive and is not yet ready for prime-time dissemination. Furthermore, this method should be employed by the few skilled *surgeons* who are trained in the various skill sets required, and who are adept at the overall care of the patient with acute pancreatitis.

Collectively, these less invasive approaches have not yet withstood critical scientific or financial analysis to indicate their validity, nor have they been directly compared to the "gold standard" of open necrosectomy.

PREFERRED TECHNIQUE

When the decision has been made to employ a "closed" transabdominal approach, a midline incision is preferred because it facilitates ultimate placement of exteriorized drains and jejunal, gastrostomy, and cholecystostomy tubes. Initial wound management, whether with primary closure or secondary techniques such as "zippers," meshes, or vacuum devices, is better controlled with a midline incision, and there are more options for long-term hernia management (a frequent occurrence). As is a good principle with any laparotomy, a thorough exploration of the abdomen in all four quadrants should ensue in order to determine other pathologies or additional sources of sepsis, or to prevent postoperative complications. By lifting the transverse colon and greater omentum, the surgeon can get a feel of the inferior extensions of necrosis along the right and left paracolic gutters and along the mesenteric stalk. An important portal of entry to the lesser sac is through the transverse mesocolon on each side of the middle colic vascular arcade (Fig. 2). Unfortunately, it is not uncommon to have direct adherence of the very proximal jejunum (just beyond the ligament of Treitz) to this leaflet, and this can obstruct this entrance point. High-grade proximal bowel obstructions in patients with pancreatitis recovering from the acute event can later occur due to adhesions in this area. Therefore, if it comes easily, these jejunal attachments can be carefully released initially.

The operating surgeon must always remember that, although this operation involves many distinct components, the primary objective is to relieve the contained sepsis in the peripancreatic retroperitoneum. These patients are usually unstable, and operative efficiency is essential. Therefore, the pancreas is the initial target early in the procedure. It is important to be flexible, and not dogmatic, when it comes to avenues to expose the pancreatic necrosis, as no single approach fits all patients. Although I prefer, and describe below, the transomental route to opening the lesser sac, in some instances, an inferior transmesenteric entrance, or a combination of both, is most expeditious.

Using the preoperative CT scan as a guide, a systematic and thorough exposure of the pancreas is required so that necrotic pockets are not neglected. This is best achieved via the gastrocolic ligament. This dissection should start in the safe zone lateral to the left of the midline, closer to the spleen where the gastroepiploic arcade dissipates to the short gastrics, since most necrosis usually occurs in the body/tail region. Although typically foreshortened by local inflammation, there is virtually always enough of a window inferior to the stomach and over the colon to enter the infected space with either a Kelly clamp or through blunt finger penetration (Fig. 6A). I do this in a very controlled fashion in order to minimize bacterial contamination throughout the abdomen. Once a minimal access hole is made, a sump sucker is gently introduced into the cavity in order to achieve a controlled aspiration of the pus. When decompressed, it is mandatory to obtain bacterial and fungal cultures including an immediate Gram

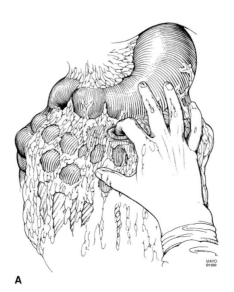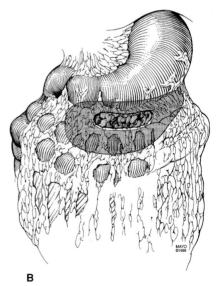

A   **B**

Fig. 6. Entrance into lesser sac area of necrosis. **A:** Bunt probing with finger over area of fluctuance and induration. **B:** Entrance widened carefully to allow complete necrosectomy.

stain from the necrotic tissue bed. This will help to tailor the postoperative antimicrobial needs. Next, the anterior wall of the sac/cavity is unroofed by lateral and medial exposure of the gastrocolic ligament, being careful not to injure the gastroepiploic vascular arcade (Fig. 6B). The necrotic pancreatic tissue is loose and fluffy, resembling stained cottage cheese. This is in contradistinction to viable pancreatic tissue that is firm, hard, white, and fibrotic. Sharp dissection of this tissue is hazardous and unnecessary.

Care should be taken so as not to violate the transverse mesocolon, which is often foreshortened and compromised by extensive local inflammation. With this particular operative approach, it is preferred to contain and drain the infection within the lesser sac so as not to expose the lower abdominal compartment to draining pancreatic juice or sepsis, so integrity of the lower boundary of the lesser sac is useful. In those situations where this region must be transgressed to enter the lesser sac, care should be exercised so as not to compromise the middle colic vascular supply to the transverse colon (Fig. 7). In rare circumstances, the transverse colon is already necrotic upon exploration. If so, a segmental resection with a proximal diverting colostomy is the appropriate move so there is no question regarding potential viability in the recovery period.

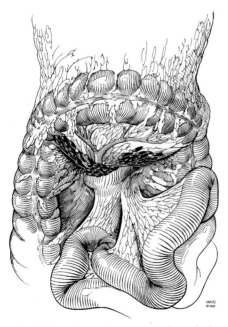

Fig. 7. Necrosis tends to present through the transverse mesocolon to the right of the middle colic vessels if involving the head and uncinate process, and to the left of the middle colic vessels if involving the body and tail regions. Note that necrosis often extends down along superior mesenteric vessels at the base of the mesentery.

The necrosectomy commences with debridement of the tissue that wants to "give" easily to the surgeon. We use a Russian forceps or a sponge-stick instrument (sans sponge) as an effective tool for this. The necrotic tissue is removed in small chunks and some debris should be sent separately for culture. Sometimes a singular, large solid component will lift itself out of the sac with relative ease. Once a working space has been achieved, blunt manual dissection should be gently applied to the cavity—roughing up loose debris only. It is vital to not get overly aggressive with this tactile exploration, yet it helps to understand the boundaries of the necrosis. If a tissue plane does not open up with ease, then it should not be transgressed. Probing the cavity with sharp or blunt instruments is discouraged in order to prevent violation of normal pancreatic tissue, the bile duct, or major vascular structures.

Similarly, it is particularly wise to leave cord-like structures that traverse the cavity alone. These represent the major vascular components of the retroperitoneum (i.e., the splenic and superior mesenteric veins and arteries). Although these firm cords might be thrombosed from the inflammation, the surgeon does not want to find this out the hard way because if they are actually "live," torrential uncontrollable bleeding may ensue. Recovery of such hemorrhage is further complicated by poor exposure, inadequate proximal and distal vascular control, and friable tissues that do not hold sutures well. Should this situation occur, pressure packing using numerous laparotomy pads with a temporary abdominal closure and return to the ICU is most prudent. The temptation to perform a splenectomy, which will be technically formidable, should be avoided; instead, interventional radiographic embolization techniques and planned relaparotomies to salvage the situation should be relied upon. Massive blood loss during necrosectomy, requiring up to 5 to 6 intraoperative units of blood for recovery, should act as an absolute "stop signal" to the surgeon for continuation of the operation in that setting. It is advisable to stabilize the patient and return to fight another day in order to achieve total clearance of the necrosis.

All major necrotic pockets should be explored employing the tenets above. If required, a Kocher maneuver should be employed in order to attack head-based or perinephric disease. The preoperative CT appearance is again useful in determining if the right and/or left pericolic gutters should be explored (not always required). This is best achieved by medially rotating

the colonic attachments off the retroperitoneum. Once all gross necrosis has been removed, Water-Pik irrigation of all involved zones should be performed. This low-pressure, mildly forceful irrigation technique lifts small nonviable debris off the boundaries in a relatively atraumatic fashion and provides a more thorough evacuation while providing concurrent suction.

Wide drainage ensues separately to all involved regions. The principle is to control pancreatic secretions from the remaining, healthy viable tissue through external drainage rather than to allow for intra-abdominal exposure to caustic pancreatic enzymes. Multiple options are available for this step and include the aforementioned large-bored sump suction drains, smaller closed suction Jackson-Pratt drains, and Penrose drains—either de novo or even sometimes modified by stuffing bulky gauze within the lumen in order to tamponade the packed cavity. We prefer to use several closed suction Silastic (19 Blake) drains. A fluted nature allows this drain to retain patency, whereas Jackson-Pratt drains frequently clog with small particulate matter. The Silastic drain's soft consistency is less likely to erode through local structures, thus avoiding hemorrhage or fistula formation. These obviously are carefully placed so as to avoid direct contact with vital structures. Whenever possible, I try to reapproximate the boundaries of the lesser sac over the drain in order to control leakage of the amylase-rich pancreatic secretions. The omentum can also be wrapped around the drain on its course to the abdominal wall, thus ensuring that a good, long drain tract scar will form around the drain as it emerges from the abdomen. When an adequate debridement of the tissue has been performed, this approach can be performed without any fear of retained septic necrosis. Finally, one should place these drain exit sites more medially, rather than laterally as others have advocated, just a 3- to 4-cm distance lateral to the midline incision. This is in anticipation of the potential for a reoperation for internalization of a prolonged pancreaticocutaneous fistula. In this circumstance, it is helpful to have easy access to the fistulous tract in the anterior abdomen, rather than buried in the lateral retroperitoneum.

Whether or not the root cause of pancreatitis is cholelithiasis, a cholecystectomy should be performed. The best time to achieve this is during the index operation and not in the reoperative setting. This being said, there are some instances when this approach is not advisable. One such case is when the porta hepatis is significantly involved with the local effects of the pancreatic inflammation. In some cases, components of true pseudocysts extend into and distort these planes. The porta can be fiercely inflamed with friable bleeding and the cystic duct proper is sometimes not discernible. When this is the case, cholecystostomy tube placement using a small 12 to 14 French rubber tube attached via a purse-string suture at the fundus is appropriate. If the biliary tree has not been imaged heretofore by endoscopic retrograde cholangiopancreatography (ERCP) or interventional transhepatic means, and the patient is stable, an intraoperative cholangiogram using real-time fluoroscopy is advised. This can be achieved through a traditional access route via the cystic duct, or alternatively through the aforementioned cholecystostomy tube. For the factors mentioned above, open common bile duct exploration should be avoided in this setting. If there is any doubt about biliary obstruction that cannot be safely cleared, or even active cholangitis, external drainage via the intact gallbladder or the cystic duct is preferable to T-tube insertion in a normal-caliber bile duct. Furthermore, it is important to achieve this now while one has the chance, and *not* to rely on postoperative ERCP, which can often be thwarted in these patients by the distortion and/or inflammation of the duodenum and ampulla attributed to the pancreatitis.

A final, and crucial, objective of the operation is providing definitive access for enteral feeding and control of gastric secretions. The patient should be expected to make rapid strides to recovery following the definitive debridement, including weaning from the ventilator and release from the intensive care setting. When this occurs, nasojejunal and nasogastric tubes will become impractical. Individual gastric and jejunal feeding tubes can be placed via Stamm and Whitzel techniques, respectively, and these have the ability to be functional for the ensuing weeks to months with improved patient comfort. A combined gastrojejunal (MIC) tube to the anterior fundus of the stomach nicely achieves both purposes. This dual tube has a long jejunal feeding limb that the surgeon can easily navigate around the C-sweep of the duodenum to a position distal to the ligament of Treitz. An intragastric balloon is filled to 10 mL and pulled back in apposition to the gastric mucosa while the stomach is directly applied to the anterior abdominal wall via a traditional Stamm technique.

Some incisions will require secondary closure due to the gross edema of the body wall from the perioperative resusci-tation. However, most incisions can be closed primarily at the fascial level and the skin can be approximated with staples. The abdominal wound should be considered contaminated from the pancreatic infection. I prefer to leave Telfa wicks, placed every inch, for drainage and remove them 3 to 4 days postoperatively.

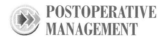

POSTOPERATIVE MANAGEMENT

If an adequate necrosectomy has been achieved, the surgeon can feel confident that a single operation will address the problem. However, although recovery times vary, largely dependent on the patient's preoperative comorbidities, most patients will need continued ICU support (ranging from days to weeks) in the immediate postoperative period. It is not uncommon to actually have a transient hemodynamic deterioration immediately after the case as the process of relieving the closed-space sepsis results in a transient bacteremia. When this occurs, however, it is usually limited to a brief (2- to 3-day) period of instability. The release of these septic mediators can have effects on multiple systems including prolonged ventilatory support, acute renal failure, and cardiovascular collapse. Antibiotics and antifungals should be continued and pared down to directed therapy in short order once the intraoperative cultures have been speciated. Later manifestations (greater than 1 week postoperative) of systemic infection (fever, neutropenia, malaise) come from many sources, with the most prevalent being ventilatory-associated pneumonia and line sepsis. Liberal use of full-torso CT imaging is advocated since intra-abdominal abscess remains a prime culprit as well (15% to 20%). However, currently this complication is most often controlled via percutaneous drainage methods that do not require re-exploration. As stated before, if the initial debridement operation is conducted thoroughly and drained adequately, there should not be any reason to operate in order to redébride, but the surgeon should obviously use clinical judgment and be prepared to re-explore if the patient deteriorates significantly.

Nutrition is best achieved through the newly placed enteral feeding tube. I refrain from removing the nasogastric tube for 2 days so that the operative tube sites can seal to the abdominal wall. The gastric port remains to gravity this whole time. Tube feedings can also be initiated then, but must be started at a trophic level first to ensure tolerance by the jejunum, which is prone to ileus throughout the pre- and postoperative period. Parenteral nutrition can be utilized for a limited period as a nutritional "bridge" until the tube feeds can be safely brought up to goal but should be discontinued as soon as possible to reduce catheter line-based complications.

Once hemodynamically stable and extubated, the patient can be transferred to a floor. Since the patient suffers from weeks of deterioration of strength, conditioning, and weight, the next goal is general rehabilitation, which starts with physical therapy on the ward. A vast majority of these patients, even if relatively healthy before the incident, will require prolonged rehabilitation services in both inpatient and outpatient settings. Cognitive functions and memory decline are commonly experienced and the patient is often frustrated that he or she has no recollection of either the operation or the ICU experience.

Upon discharge, the surgeon must prepare the patient and family for a minimum 3-month overall recovery period. Once converted from the catabolic to the anabolic state nutritionally, rapid strides will be made in wound healing, weight gain, and conditioning. The gastrojejunal tube can be removed 6 weeks after the operation, but only when the oral caloric intake sustains the patient. Intravenous antibiotics will often be required for many weeks postoperatively, as it is common for the pancreatic drains to be infected for an extended period of time. The remaining pancreatic drains can be removed when there is evidence of minimal daily output devoid of infection or high amylase content. A follow-up CT scan at the first postoperative visit (around 1 month) is obtained to confirm resolution of the pancreatic inflammation and resolution of local fluid collections. I prefer to remove these drains slowly over time by removing about 2 in. at a time every 2 weeks in the office.

Persistent pancreaticocutaneous fistulas are infrequent, but are troublesome when they occur (10% to 15% of the time). If the drain has been completely removed, an ostomy-like bag can be attached locally to prevent skin breakdown. Therapeutic approaches to this problem include improving nutritional parameters, extending NPO status, and employing somatostatin analogs. If these fail, consideration should be given to analyzing the pancreatic duct via an ERCP. This is an instance where temporary pancreatic duct stenting can be advocated by the surgeon, with the purpose of relieving upstream obstruction of pancreatic juice effluent into the duodenum. Finally, in some rare and select cases, a significant fistula persists from the phenomenon of a "disconnected pancreatic remnant." In this case, operative intervention is required and this can be achieved through two techniques. Distal pancreatectomy may be considered as a definitive move. However, experience has shown that this is not always practically achievable given the severe fibrotic response of the retroperitoneum following the pancreatitis and the necrosectomy. This fierce scarring incorporates local vascular structures and prevents navigation of the retroperitoneum, making for a dangerous scenario. For this reason, reoperation for formal internal fistula drainage via Roux-en-Y tract-jejunostomy is required. Before embarking on such an operation, the pancreatic fistula should be given at least 3 to 6 months to close spontaneously. During this time, the patient will also improve, and the abdomen will settle, improving the likelihood of an enduring positive outcome.

SUGGESTED READING

Ashley SW, Perez A, Pierce EA, et al. Necrotizing pancreatitis: contemporary analysis of 99 consecutive cases. *Ann Surg* 2001;234:572.

Balthazar EJ. Acute pancreatitis: assessment of severity with clinical and CT evaluation. *Radiology* 2002;223:603.

Banks PA. Practice guidelines in acute pancreatitis. *Am J Gastroenterol* 1997;92:377.

Bradley EL III. A clinically based classification system for acute pancreatitis. Summary of the International Symposium on Acute Pancreatitis, Atlanta, GA, September 11–13, 1992. *Arch Surg* 1993;128:586.

Buchler MW, Gloor B, Muller CA, et al. Acute necrotizing pancreatitis: treatment strategy according to the status of infection. *Ann Surg* 2000;232:619.

Fernandez-Del Castillo C, Rattner DW, Makary MA, et al. Debridement and closed packing for the treatment of necrotizing pancreatitis. *Ann Surg* 1998;228:676.

Howard TJ, Temple MB. Prophylactic antibiotics alter bacteriology of infected necrosis in severe acute pancreatitis. *J Am Coll Surg* 2002;195:759.

Hungness ES, Robb BW, Seeskin C, et al. Early debridement for necrotizing pancreatitis: is it worthwhile? *J Am Coll Surg* 2002;194:740.

Werner J, Feuerbach S, Uhl W, et al. Management of acute pancreatitis: from surgery to interventional intensive care. *Gut* 2005;54:426.

EDITOR'S COMMENT

For training and practicing surgeons alike, severe necrotizing pancreatitis evokes memories of terrible suffering and death. It is a highly lethal and indiscriminate disease that most everyone will encounter during a general surgery career. From the moment it starts until its victim is again safe and healthy, tenacity and very careful decision making are as important as any technical skill. In a community setting, the best first decision may well be prompt transfer to a tertiary hospital. Once there, the decisions shift to how, when, and why to intervene or not. Over time, we have learned more about this disease, often from unorthodox but courageous approaches that have become commonplace. For example, consider the shift over time from open abdominal marsupialization to today's valid nonoperative management of sterile pancreatic necrosis.

I have the pleasure of working each day with Dr. Chuck Vollmer, and can attest to his tenacity, decision making, and technical skills. While he describes our preferred approach to necrotizing pancreatitis, three key points should be stressed. First, our approach is a "hybrid" of many others, some of which are detailed in the references provided. Second, there is always more than one way to do something, especially this complicated. Third, we participate in and adhere to a multidisciplinary team model for treating these complicated patients. And so, *Mastery* readers should remain flexible and refine their own technique with each patient. That said, most of the important foundation knowledge you'll need is presented in this fine chapter.

As detailed, it is the timing and extent of multiple organ failure that determines mortality in this disease, and not the extent of local pancreatic inflammation and eventual necrosis. As such, the key features of patient support during disease escalation are highlighted, including fluid resuscitation, mandatory nutritional support, judicious antibiotic use, and intensive care support. Despite best efforts and care, not all patients will survive early rampant disease, and as correctly noted, early surgery does not change this. Supportive care, and especially resuscitation, helps the patient survive the cytokine and inflammation storm and enter a variable period of watchful waiting during which the need to operate or not becomes apparent.

Surgeons absolutely must be involved during this critical period. If not, decisions get made by others without the surgical skills required to treat the potential consequences. Our author describes somewhat common patterns of disease progression/resolution, but best outcomes require proper decision making. A common scenario is when fevers heighten and persist, almost predictably, 2 and more weeks into disease. Surgeons must participate in decisions for fine needle aspiration (*Ann Surg* 2001;234:572) and antibiotic use. For example, an unnecessary FNA might infect otherwise sterile necrosis that is still evolving. The surgeon is now faced with a pancreatic abscess before necrosectomy should (or not) otherwise have occurred. Mazaki's recent meta-analysis (*Br J Surg* 2006;93:674) shows that prophylactic antibiotics do not prevent infected necrosis or death in this disease. When should they be used? Do they really contribute to later morbidity and mortality from fungal infection? As detailed, it is both safe and best to feed the gut.

Our preferred approach for necrosectomy is described. A midline incision is helpful if access is needed to necrosis dissecting inferiorly along the psoas muscles, colon, and retroperitoneum. One must be precise in both opening and closing it to reduce hernia rates. For necrosectomy, many experts prefer a transmesocolon approach, but our preferred entry via the gastrocolic omentum keeps the approach and exposure anterior. Closed suction pancreatic bed drains are also exteriorized anteriorly and medially for subsequent access to any fistula needing Roux-en-Y internal drainage. They seem to work fine. Lateral and caudal necrosis is accessed and counterdrained inferiorly. Not mentioned is the lateral flank approach to necrosectomy that is at times quite useful. The pulse irrigator does a beautiful job of cleaning up after the manual necrosectomy is completed. I prefer to complete the cholecystectomy before necrosectomy if possible. Finally, these are not late-day add-on cases. The surgeon and anesthesiologist will destabilize an already tenuous patient to achieve the benefit of necrosectomy, and intra- and postoperative courses often reflect this.

Freeny's fine study (*AJR* 1998;170:969) helped show that infected pancreatic necrosis can be treated with catheters (and perseverance) alone. Several, including Horvath (*Surg Endosc* 2001;15:1221), have since shown that pancreatic necrosectomy is indeed possible using laparoscopic and minimally invasive surgical techniques. Those still questioning efficacy might stay tuned for the PANTER trial in Europe (*BMC Surg* 2006;6:6). This randomized, controlled multicenter trial is designed to reveal any reduction in major morbidity by introducing a minimally invasive "step-up approach" instead of traditional necrosectomy by laparotomy in patients with infected necrotizing pancreatitis. Results are expected by 2008.

M.P.C.

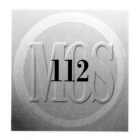

Pancreatic Cystoenterostomy

ANDREW L. WARSHAW AND EMILY R. CHRISTISON-LAGAY

Pancreatic pseudocysts have been recognized as a disease entity for nearly 250 years. Morgagni is credited with the earliest description of a pseudocyst (1761); its surgical management can be traced back to at least 1875 when LeDentu performed a percutaneous drainage of a posttraumatic pseudocyst; and in 1882 Bozeman removed a 10-kg pseudocyst from a 41-year-old patient. The modern surgical history of pseudocysts, marked by the initiation of internal drainage, dates to 1921 when the first cystogastrostomy was performed. Cystoduodenostomy followed in 1928 and cystojejunostomy in 1931. The historic term *pseudocyst* was invoked to differentiate collections of pancreatic juice enclosed by fibrous tissue from "true" cystic pancreatic lesions lined by an epithelium, such as cystic neoplasms or congenital cysts. As noninvasive diagnosis was not possible before the advent of modern radiologic techniques, this histologically based definition was acceptable for the small number of symptomatic surgical encounters on which a pseudocyst was discovered. The development of multiple noninvasive pancreatic imaging modalities such as ultrasound, computed tomography (CT), endoscopic pancreatography (ERCP), and magnetic resonance imaging, have facilitated the identification of incidental (i.e., asymptomatic) pancreatic cystic lesions. The natural history of these lesions has only recently come under scrutiny, and the optimal management of these previously unrecognized diverse cystic lesions remains a topic of debate.

EPIDEMIOLOGY, DEFINITIONS, AND DIAGNOSIS

Although precise figures are not available, it has been estimated that approximately 5,000 new cases of pancreatic pseudocyst arise yearly in the United States. Pseudocysts develop after 5% to 10% of cases of acute pancreatitis and in up to 50% of cases of chronic pancreatitis. Altogether, pancreatic pseudocysts represent more than 75% of cystic lesions of the pancreas.

The behavior (and preferred treatment options) of pseudocysts varies with the cause. Pseudocysts may be broadly divided into acute pseudocysts, which evolve from postpancreatitis acute fluid collections, and chronic pseudocysts, which develop in the setting of chronic pancreatitis. Traumatic pseudocysts arising from pancreatic duct disruption account for 3% to 8% of pseudocyst presentations and behave similarly to acute pseudocysts.

According to the Atlanta classification, which in 1993 sought to delineate a clinically based classification system for acute pancreatitis, an acute pseudocyst is defined as "a collection of pancreatic juice enclosed by a wall of fibrous or granulation tissue, arising as a consequence of acute pancreatitis or pancreatic trauma." The natural history of acute pseudocysts is variable: they may resolve, they may grow, or they may become symptomatic (cause obstruction, pain, or vascular damage). The Atlanta classification further characterized a chronic pseudocyst as "a collection of pancreatic juice enclosed by a wall of fibrous or granulation tissue, arising as a consequence of chronic pancreatitis and lacking an antecedent episode of acute pancreatitis." Chronic pseudocysts rarely resolve, may be associated with other pancreatic duct abnormalities, and are more likely to lead to internal fistulas (causing ascites or pleural effusions) or the rarer complication hemosuccus pancreaticus, an arterial pseudoaneurysm that ruptures into the pancreatic duct system, causing hemorrhage into the gastrointestinal tract. The most operationally and clinically critical aspect of the Atlanta classification system lies in its clear distinction between acute pancreatic fluid collections that often attend a severe episode of pancreatitis and pancreatic pseudocysts. This distinction is made on the basis of time following the instance of pancreatitis (>4 weeks) and the presence of a defined wall. Critics of this broad, binary classification system argue that it does not accommodate more nuanced presentations of pseudocyst such as those arising from cases of acute or chronic pancreatitis. At least two other classification systems have been proposed that attempt to predict the behavior of pseudocysts based on their anatomic relationship with the main pancreatic duct (Nealon) or on a synthesis of clinical presentation and demonstrated ductal anatomy (D'Egidio). Whereas the Atlanta classification seeks to define pseudocysts apart from more acute, unorganized pancreatic fluid collections, these latter classifications strive to segregate pseudocysts into categories that inform clinical management strategies. As such, they may be considered an expansion of the Atlanta classification, which presupposes that the distinction between pseudocyst and acute fluid collection has already been determined. These definitions are more fully delineated in Table 1.

The diagnosis of some type of pancreatic fluid collection should be suspected in every patient with acute pancreatitis who is not significantly better within 1 week of supportive treatment. The diagnosis should also be suspected in patients with chronic pancreatitis and a change in symptoms. CT is the preferred initial diagnostic study as it is able to supply information regarding the common duct, the pancreatic duct, and the presence or absence of pancreatic necrosis. Once a diagnosis has been made by CT, abdominal ultrasound is a suitable radiographic modality for follow-up assessment of interval changes in size, and MRCP is increasingly valuable in demonstrating cyst-duct relationships and communications. The blossoming of advanced radiographic imaging has generated two previously unappreciated clinical dilemmas: (a) the detection of asymptomatic cystic lesions within the pancreas, and (b) the labeling of postpancreatic collections of necrosis as pseudocysts.

The presence of a cystic lesion detected by CT in the absence of any antecedent clinical history of pancreatitis or other abnormalities of pancreatic architecture should be considered a cystic neoplasm until proven otherwise. Cystic neoplasms account for approximately 15% to 20% of all cystic lesions of the pancreas; approximately half of a these neoplasms are either potentially or actually malignant. Clearly, transcutaneous, endoscopic, or internal surgical drainage of a premalignant mucinous cystadenoma or a cystadenocarcinoma under

TABLE 1. CLINICAL DEFINITIONS OF PANCREATIC FLUID LESIONS—ATLANTA INTERNATIONAL SYMPOSIUM

	Acute Pancreatic Fluid Collections	**Acute Pancreatic Pseudocysts**
Definition	Acute fluid collections occur early in the course of acute pancreatitis, are located in or near the pancreas, and always lack a wall of granulation or fibrous tissue.	A pseudocyst is a collection of pancreatic juice that arises as a consequence of acute pancreatitis, pancreatic trauma, or chronic pancreatitis, and is enclosed by a nonepithelialized wall.
Clinical manifestations	Acute fluid collections are common in patients with severe pancreatitis, occurring in 30% to 50% of cases. However, more than half of the lesions regress spontaneously. They are rarely demonstrable by physical findings and are usually discovered by imaging techniques. Often irregular in shape, acute fluid collections do not demonstrate a defined wall.	Pseudocysts in patients with acute pancreatitis are rarly palpable and are most often discovered by imaging techniques. They are usually round or ovoid in shape and have a well-defined wall, as demonstrated by computed tomography or sonography.
Pathology	The precise composition of such collections is not known. Bacteria are variably present. The critical clinical distinction between an acute fluid collection and a pseudocyst (or a pancreatic abscess) is the lack of a defined wall.	The presence of a well-defined wall composed of granulation or fibrous tissue distinguishes a pseudocyst from an acute fluid collection. A pseudocyst is usually rich in pancreatic enzymes and is most often sterile.
Discussion	Acute fluid collections represent an early point in the development of acute pseudocysts or pancreatic abscesses. Why most acute fluid collections regress but others progress to become pseudocysts or abscesses is not known.	Formation of a pseudocyst generally requires 4 or more weeks from the onset of acute pancreatitis. In this regard, an acute pseudocyst is a fluid collection that arises in association with an episode of acute pancreatitis, is of more than 4 weeks' duration, and is surrounded by a defined wall. Fluid collections less than this age that lack a defined wall are more properly termed *acute fluid collections.* In contrast, chronic pseudocysts have a well-defined wall but arise in patients with chronic pancreatitis and lack an antecedent episode of acute pancreatitis. Bacteria may be present in a pseudocyst but often are of no clinical significance because they represent contamination and not clinical infection. When pus is present, the lesion is more correctly termed a *pancreatic abscess.*

Nealon's Classification: Endoscopic Retrograde Cholangiopancreatography

Type	Description	Depiction
I	Normal duct/no communication	Type I
II	Normal duct/with communication	Type II
III	Normal duct with stricture/no communication	Type III
IV	Normal duct with stricture/with communication	Type IV

(continued)

TABLE 1. (continued)

V	Normal duct/complete obstruction	Type V
VI	Chronic pancreatitis/no communication	Type VI
VII	Chronic pancreatitis/communication	Type VII

D'Egidio's Classification of Pancreatic Pseudocysts

Type	Definition
I	Acute "postnecrotic" pseudocysts: occur after an episode of acute pancreatitis and are almost invariably associated with normal duct anatomy and rarely have demonstrable communication with the pancreatic duct. These pseudocysts are often characterized by a shorter disease course, greater size of pseudocyst, and early symptoms.
II	Postnecrotic pseudocysts: occur after an episode of acute or chronic pancreatitis. In type II pseudocysts, the pancreatic duct is diseased but not strictured and there is often a duct-pseudocyst communication (40%).
III	"Retention" pseudocysts: occur in chronic pancreatitis and are uniformly associated with duct stricture and pseudocyst-duct communication.

the mistaken diagnosis of "pseudocyst" may bring with it disastrous consequences. Cystic lesions appearing on CT as multiple small cysts ("the grape sign"), having a "sunburst" appearance, or with multiple loculations are characteristic of neoplasms (typically, serous cystadenomas), with the caveat that most cystic neoplasms are unilocular and, therefore, possibly mistaken for a pseudocyst radiographically (Fig. 1).

Although clinical presentation often informs the diagnosis, it has been suggested that transcutaneous or endoscopic aspiration of the fluid content within the cyst may be of significant assistance in differentiating cystic neoplasms from pseudocysts. In fact, Warshaw et al. were unable to identify any uniformly reliable clinical or radiologic criteria permitting preoperative differentiation of cystic pancreatic lesions. One third of the cystic tumors referred to their group were misdiagnosed as pseudocysts, and many had been treated inappropriately according to this misdiagnosis. Fluid from cystic neoplasms demonstrates positive cytologic evidence of a neoplasm in fewer than 50% of cysts, but markedly increased levels of carbohydrate antigen 19-9 and carcinoembryonic antigen characterize mucinous cystic neoplasms and intraductal papillary mucinous neoplasms, but not

serous cystadenomas or pseudeocysts. Aspiration of mucoid material is pathognomonic for one of the pancreatic mucoid neoplasms. The absence of epithelial cells on aspiration or biopsy, however, should not be used to make a diagnosis of pseudocyst as this may represent a sampling error resulting from a low cell count in the fluid or ulceration of the epithelial lining of a cystic neoplasm.

Another common error is to misread a postpancreatic collection of necrotic tissue mixed with fluid as an "acute pseudocyst." Labeling these sterile collections of necrotic tissue as pseudocysts imposes a 30% to 40% risk of secondary infection and conversion to infected pancreatic necrosis if percutaneous or surgical attempts are made to drain the pseudocyst. All peripancreatic collections in patients with documented necrotizing pancreatitis should be suspected of being neuromas until proven otherwise. Specific recognition requires pancreatic imaging. CT density measurements of the pancreatic collection are usually high in neuromas (>20 Hounsfield units) while remaining low in acute fluid collections and acute pseudocysts (<10 Hounsfield units). Abdominal sonography demonstrates multiple internal echoes within a necuoma but echoless transmission in pure fluid collections. In

rare cases requiring additional differentiation, T2-weighted magnetic resonance imaging shows a variable mixture of fluid and tissue in necuomas in contrast to pure fluid collections, which give off a T2 bright signal.

The Balthazar and Ranson radiographic grading scale of acute pancreatitis correlates with risk of subsequent complication, including pancreatic abscess and pseudocyst (Table 2). None of 51 patients with Grades A–C pancreatitis developed pseudocyst, while 3 of 37 (8%) of those with Grade D or E went on to develop subsequent pseudocysts. Among these 37 patients with Grade D or E pancreatitis, the initial CT examination demonstrated a normally enhancing pancreas in 22 (59%) and pancreatic necrosis in 15 (41%). Pseudocysts developed in two patients without necrosis and in one patient with early evidence of severe necrosis.

PRESENTATION, PATHOGENESIS, AND NATURAL HISTORY OF PANCREATIC PSEUDOCYSTS

Alcohol-related pancreatitis is thought to be the chief cause (59% to 79%) of pseudocysts in countries in which alcohol consumption is relatively high. Alcohol

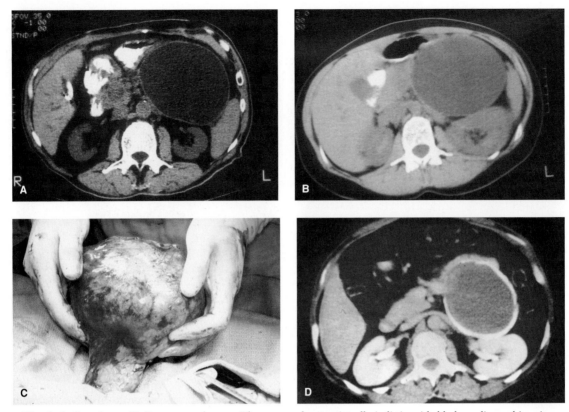

Fig. 1. A: Pseudocyst. **B:** Serous cystadenoma. These examples are virtually indistinguishable by radiographic criteria, emphasizing the importance of a history consistent with pancreatitis and aspiration of "cystic" fluid in making a diagnosis. **C:** The same serous cystadenoma at time of resection. **D:** Serous cystadenocarcinoma. Note the presence of a calcified rim, often indicative of malignant disease.

abuse is the cited cause of pancreatitis in the majority of patients with chronic pancreatic pseudocysts, whereas an acute pseudocyst may develop as a complication of any cause of acute pancreatitis as well as a postsurgical complication when the pancreas is traumatized.

Clinical suspicion for a pseudocyst should arise in the case of persistent abdominal pain despite adequate treatment of acute pancreatitis. Abdominal pain is present in 80% to 90% of patients with pseudocysts; nausea, and obstructive symptoms

TABLE 2. BALTHAZAR AND RANSON GRADING SCALE OF PANCREATITIS	
Grade	**Radiographic Description**
A	Normal pancreas
B	Focal or diffuse enlargement
C	Mild peripancreatic inflammatory changes
D	Single fluid collection
E	Two or more fluid collections or gas within the pancreas or within peripancreatic inflammation

such as jaundice, vomiting, and weight loss can also occur. In approximately 50% of patients, a palpable epigastric mass can be appreciated. Persistently elevated amylase serum amylase levels are present in up to 76% of patients with pseudocysts.

Pancreatic pseudocysts originate in the disruption of the pancreatic ductal system secondary to inflammation. Fluid within the pseudocyst contains pancreatic enzymes susceptible to intracystic zymogen activation. It is the activation of pancreatic protease activity that is likely responsible for such complications as enzymatic erosion into a pancreatic artery with subsequent conversion of the pseudocyst to a pseudoaneurysm or enzyme-induced thinning of the enveloping fibrous membrane and subsequent rupture, resulting in the development of pancreatic ascites or pancreatic hydrothorax. Although the precise mechanism of intracystic activation of pancreatic zymogens remains unknown, circulating plasma protease activators (i.e., plasmin) are suspected candidates.

Active exchange between the enclosed pancreatic juice and the plasma takes place through the enveloping fibrous wall. As the fibrous tissue matures and thickens over time, the ability to exchange with plasma

lessens and it is the reduction in exchange volume that may be responsible for the spontaneous resolution of many pancreatic pseudocysts, although the exact mechanism remains a topic of speculation. Contrast studies or magnetic resonance pancreatography can demonstrate a persistent ductal connection in at least 60% to 80% of pseudocysts; subsequent inflammation and cyst maturation may make this communication inevident by ERCP, although it has been argued that a nondemonstrable connection persists. A persistent ductal communication has therapeutic implications because patients with a demonstrable communication between the pancreatic duct and pseudocyst appear to be at increased risk for a pancreaticocutaneous fistula if treated with percutaneous drainage.

Studies examining the natural history of the untreated pseudocyst have demonstrated that between one quarter and one half of all pancreatic pseudocysts resolve spontaneously (Fig. 2). It is generally agreed that the most influential factors predicting the pseudocyst fate are type of pseudocyst (acute versus chronic) and age (duration of time since formation). Acute pseudocysts resolve spontaneously in 30% to 40% of cases, whereas the ductal scarring and

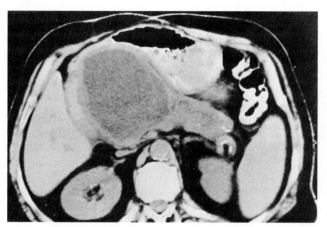 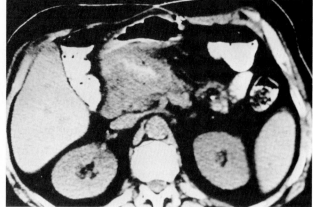

Fig. 2. Spontaneous resolution of a large pseudocyst during several months, probably by acute decompression into the duodenum.

fibrosis that accompanies chronic pancreatitis appear to prevent spontaneous resolution of chronic pseudocysts.

Bradley et al. were the first to follow the natural history of pseudocysts by prospective study in the mid-1970s using abdominal ultrasonography in a population of symptomatic patients. Spontaneous resolution occurred in 42% of patients in whom a pseudocyst was present for less than 6 weeks, but only 8% of patients (1 of 13) with pseudocysts were followed longer than 6 weeks. Moreover, after 6 weeks, prolonged observation was associated with increased risk of severe complications, with mortality rates of 20% to 50%. Warshaw and Rattner corroborated these data, finding that no pseudocyst presenting more than 6 weeks after an episode of acute pancreatitis resolved spontaneously. In their review, the size of the pseudocyst did not affect its likelihood of resolution. Subsequent studies have challenged these findings. Vitas and Sarr expectantly managed 68 patients with pseudocysts; 38% of the pseudocysts resolved more than 6 months after diagnosis. Gouyan et al. re-

ported a pseudocyst resolution rate of 26% with a median time to regression of 29 weeks. In their study, the independent predictive factor of resolution was a size less than 4 cm. Similarly, Aranha et al. reported a mean diameter of 4 ± 1 cm in those cysts that resolved spontaneously and a diameter of 9 ± 1 in cysts that failed to regress. Only 4 of 26 cysts greater than 6 cm at the time of initial evaluation resolved. Yeo et al. expectantly managed 36 patients over a mean period of 1 year. Forty percent of pseudocysts measuring less than 6 cm and 67% of pseudocysts larger than 6 cm required operative management. Twenty-seven percent of large pseudocysts (>10 cm) were managed nonoperatively (Fig. 3).

Based on a collective review of these studies, it is generally accepted to manage most asymptomatic patients expectantly through serial CT scans. The interval development of symptoms, including evidence of biliary or bowel obstruction, recurrent pain with oral intake, persistent nausea, or weight loss, as well at CT evidence of enlargement, bleeding, or rup-

ture, are considered indications for operative intervention. Additionally, intrasplenic pseudocysts have been noted to be associated with a high incidence of hemorrhage (Fig. 4), so the policy at Massachusetts General Hospital is to operate on all such pseudocysts.

ELECTIVE THERAPY

Drainage or excision of a pancreatic pseudocyst is indicated in instances of failed expectant management. Open internal surgical drainage historically has provided the standard of care for symptomatic or complicated pseudocysts; more recently, less-invasive drainage options (percutaneous drainage and endoscopic drainage) have achieved increasing popularity. Additionally, there is an increasing amount of data demonstrating success in laparoscopic drainage, either cystogastrostomy or cystojejunostomy. The choice of treatment typically depends on multiple factors including size, number, and location of the cyst, the presumed presence or absence of infection or residual necrotic tissue, the presence or

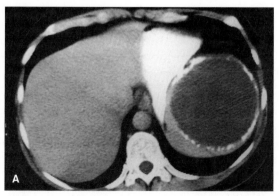 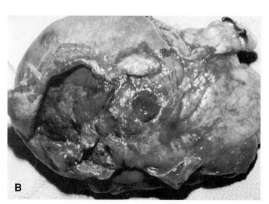

Fig. 3. A: Computed tomographic demonstration of large intrasplenic pseudocyst. **B:** Splenic rupture secondary to large intrasplenic pseudocyst.

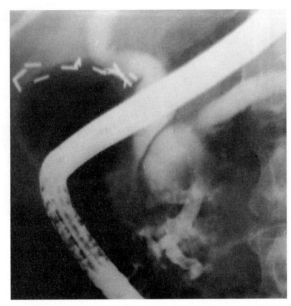

Fig. 4. Pseudocyst causing pancreatic duct and common duct obstruction.

absence of a demonstrable cyst-duct communication, as well as the availability of specialist surgical or interventionalist expertise. In cases in which ductal anatomy is thought to be aberrant or likely to alter the management choice, preprocedural ERCP has been advocated. Instrumentation during ERCP is associated with an increased subsequent risk of biliary tract sepsis, so it is currently recommended that this procedure be performed within 12 to 48 hours of the definitive treatment.

PERCUTANEOUS CATHETER DRAINAGE

CT-guided percutaneous drainage of pancreatic pseudocysts is the least invasive of the treatment options of pancreatic pseudocyst and is the preferred modality for patients unable to tolerate a large operation. Nonetheless, it substitutes small-catheter external drainage for wide internal drainage. These catheters are susceptible to clogging with debris, resulting in failure of drainage with ensuing secondary infection. Simple cyst aspiration results in more than 70% recurrence, whereas the placement of an indwelling No. 10-16 French pigtail catheter has been associated with 42% to 74% success rate during variable drainage periods (2 to 127 days; average, 22 to 79 days). The duration of drainage in Nealon's study correlated highly with type of ductal anatomy, with an average drainage period of 4.4 days in patients with a normal duct (type I and II) by ERCP. In this study, 91% of patients with a ductal cutoff as delineated by ERCP required subsequent oper-

ative drainage of the pseudocyst; the remaining patients requiring conversion from percutaneous to open surgical drainage demonstrated ductal stricture by ERCP. The most common complication related to percutaneous drainage is sepsis, occurring in approximately one third of patients; 75% of these eventually need surgical correction. A recent review comparing percutaneous drainage with surgical drainage across 27,000 pseudocyst admissions to U.S. hospitals found statistically significant adjusted mortality rates, with an inpatient mortality of 5.9% associated with percutaneous drainage and 2.8% associated with surgical drainage.

Percutaneous drainage can be recommended in a selected population of patients with demonstrated normal ductal anatomy following an episode of acute pancreatitis. Patients with chronic pancreatitis and associated pseudocysts are poorly managed by percutaneous drainage as long-term infection of the pancreas results in stricture or even obliteration of the pancreatic duct. Obstruction of the proximal pancreatic duct is associated with the formation of a pancreaticocutaneous fistula along the catheter tract. To lessen the risk of this complication, use of a transgastric drainage approach has been advocated to create a pancreaticogastric fistula. Additionally, it has been speculated that fibrosis of the pancreatic parenchyma in chronic pancreatitis itself prohibits sealing of the cystic cavity. Percutaneous drainage is also not recommended as a therapeutic option in patients with multiple, loculated, or infected pseudocysts,

except as a temporizing measure in the critically ill.

ENDOSCOPIC TRANSPAPILLARY STENTS AND TRANSMURAL DRAINAGE

Two methods of endoscopic drainage exist: creation of a cystoenterostomy (cystogastrostomy or cystoduodenostomy) or transpapillary drainage. In 1989, Cremer et al. reported 33 patients with stable unilocular pancreatic pseudocysts who underwent transmural drainage with a success rate of 73% for cystogastrostomy and 86% for cystoduodenostomy. Although not all studies have replicated these high rates of efficacy, chronic pseudocysts in which the inflammatory reaction contributes to close apposition between cyst and adjacent stomach or duodenum appear to be acceptable candidates for endoscopic drainage. The uncertain degree of adherence and thinner walls associated with acute pseudocysts render them more susceptible to spillage of cystic pancreatic or enteric contents into the peritoneal cavity or retroperitoneum. The use of endoscopic ultrasound has been advocated by some authors to assist in localizing a site for pseudocyst drainage while avoiding vascular structures such as gastric varices or submucosal vessels in the pathway of a possible drainage site.

Complications of transmural endoscopic drainage include bleeding, retroperitoneal perforation, infection, and failure of pseudocyst resolution. The most serious cause of bleeding is endoscopic puncture of previously undiagnosed pseudoaneurysm. Thus, it is crucial that prior to any attempt at transmural puncture, a dynamic bolus contrast CT be performed. When bleeding does occur, infiltration of the bleeding site with a solution of 1:10,000 epinephrine should be performed, followed by endoscopic coagulation or clipping. Perforation into the retroperitoneum can occur with tangential puncture of the cyst or if the pseudocyst is deeply positioned with a distance greater than 1 cm between the gut lumen and the pseudocyst. Finally, infection remains the most common complication of endoscopic transmural pseudocyst drainage through the formation of closed-spaced abscesses, which arise as a consequence of contamination or incomplete evacuation of the pseudocyst cavity. The recognition of residual pancreatic necrosis by preprocedural CT should dissuade attempts at endoscopic drainage as the presence of necrotic debris and devitalized tissue function as a nidus for infection and may be associated

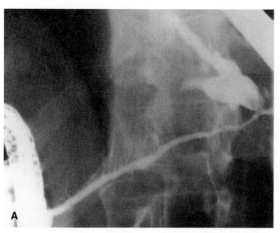
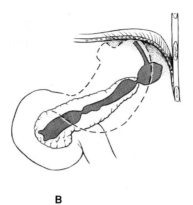
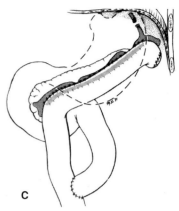

Fig. 9. Complications of pseudocyst. **A:** Endoscopic pancreatography demonstrating pancreatic pseudocyst with pancreaticopleural fistula. **B:** Schematic depicting dilated pancreatic duct with pancreatic tail pseudocyst and pancreaticopleural fistula. **C:** Repair of **B** by Roux-en-Y pancreaticojejunostomy and ligation of fistula.

an expanded pseudoaneurysm. The splenic, pancreaticoduodenal, and gastroduodenal arteries are most frequently involved, although pseudoaneurysms of the hepatic, superior mesenteric, left gastric, and right colic arteries have also been described. Mortality is significantly correlated with type of pancreatitis with a 50% mortality described in association with acute necrotizing pancreatitis versus 11% in chronic pancreatitis. In the past, recognition of this complication was often delayed, and mortality resulted from intraperitoneal rupture of the pseudoaneurysm and exsanguination. In a patient previously known to have a pseudocyst, the development of sudden pain or the development of a pulsatile mass accompanied by a bruit is virtually pathognomonic. Although historically surgical exploration with ligation of the aneurysmal vessel was the mainstay of treatment, during the past decade, advances in percutaneous interventional strategies have al-

lowed an expanding role for mesenteric angiography to improve localization of the aneurysm and transcatheter arterial embolization to treat bleeding pseudoaneurysms either as monotherapy or as a temporizing measure allowing stabilization before surgery. Angiography should be performed only if the patient is stable and if it can be performed quickly (Fig. 10). Approximately one half to two thirds of patients presenting with pseudoaneurysm are candidates for angiography and embolization. The initial success rate in a recent series by Bergert et al. was 88%, with a morality rate of 19% (secondary to rebleeding, pulmonary embolism, and multi-organ system failure following embolization of the hepatic artery). Additionally, their results supported attempt at embolization as the initial therapeutic strategy in patients with acute necrotizing pancreatitis, in whom two of five embolized patients died, whereas two of three died after

surgery. This survival advantage did not exist in patients with chronic pancreatitis.

In the hemodynamically unstable patient, two operative approaches are available: ligation with pseudocyst drainage or partial pancreatectomy. In the former, a direct intracystic approach to the bleeding vessel is most expedient. The pseudocyst should be opened and the culprit artery (most commonly the splenic artery) compressed. Large nonabsorbable sutures are used to oversew the point of bleeding. In some cases, it may be helpful to ligate the feeding vessel directly. When hemostasis has been achieved, the pseudocyst/"pseudoaneurysm" may be internally drained using one of the previously discussed methods. Alternatively, the pseudocyst could be partially closed over a large drainage tube that is externalized for gravity drainage. This last method is likely to be followed by the development of a pancreaticocutaneous fistula, but if hemostasis is adequate, rebleeding is rare. The fistula can be electively rerouted internally at a later time. Alternatively, the pseudoaneurysm may be resected as part of a partial pancreatectomy. This option has a lower attendant risk of rebleeding, but is limited by patient instability and the presence of peripancreatic inflammation (especially associated with acute pancreatitis), which precludes safe anatomic resection.

Figure 11 demonstrates a management algorithm for pancreatic hemorrhage. In the hemodynamically stable patient, the first course of treatment should be attempted embolization. Embolization is associated with a significantly lower rate of rebleeding than initial operative management (12% vs. 37%). Successful embolization requires no further treatment. Embolization failure and hemodynamic

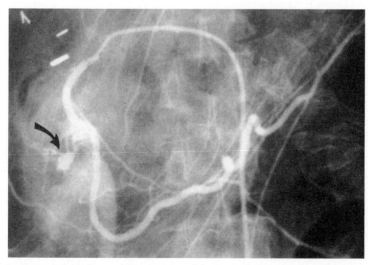

Fig. 10. Angiogram depicting pseudoaneurysm of the gastroduodenal artery (*arrow*).

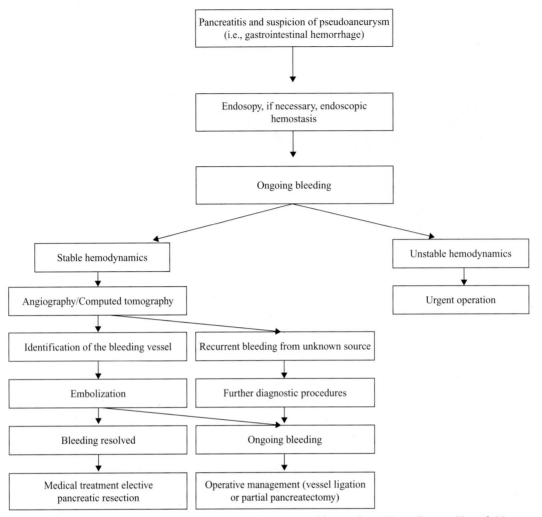

Fig. 11. Management algorithm for suspected pancreatitis-associated hemorrhage. (From Bergert H, et al. Management and outcome of hemorrhage due to arterial pseudoaneurysms in pancreatitis. *Surgery* 2005;137:323.)

instability are indications for operative management.

SUGGESTED READING

Andren-Sandberg A, Dervenis C. Pancreatic pseudocysts in the 21st century. Part I: Classification, pathophysiology, anatomic considerations and treatment. *JOP* 2004;5:8.

Bergert H, et al. Management and outcome of hemorrhage due to arterial pseudoaneurysms in pancreatitis. *Surgery* 2005;137: 323.

Nealon WH, Walser E. Main pancreatic ductal anatomy can direct choice of modality for treating pancreatic pseudocysts (surgery vs percutaneous drainage). *Ann Surg* 2002;235: 751.

Roth JS. Minimally invasive approaches to pancreatic pseudocysts. *Curr Surg* 2003;60:591.

Spivak H, et al. Management of pancreatic pseudocysts. *J Am Coll Surg* 1998; 186:507.

Tsuei BJ, Schwartz RW. Current management of pancreatic pseudocysts. *Curr Surg* 2003; 60:587.

EDITOR'S COMMENT

Drs. Warshaw and Christison-Lagay have provided a precise, detailed, and well-crafted review of the history, natural history, and management of pancreatic pseudocysts. I found their chapter to be especially complete, and a pleasure to read and learn from. Although a relatively uncommon entity in the United States, pseudocysts complicate a fair number of cases of acute pancreatitis, and can be even a more significant problem in chronic pancreatitis. We learn of today's popular classifications for pseudocysts, how and why ductal communication will determine natural history, and why some cystic lesions should not simply be watched. As this knowledge evolved, new treatment modalities emerged, making surgery less common today for this disease.

Pseudocysts are far and away the most common cystic lesions of the pancreas. Mistaking a cystic neoplasm for a pseudocyst can have dire consequences. Even today with our sophisticated imaging and diagnostics, this is not an unusual error. One must carefully consider a patient's antecedent history, radiographic appearance of the lesion, and both serum and cyst fluid laboratory values. At times, the ultrasonographic appearance can help distinguish a cystic neoplasm from a pseudocyst (*Gastrointest Endosc* 2003;57:891). Regardless of imaging modality, however, most agree that radiologic criteria alone are typically inadequate (*Radiographics* 2005;25:671). Dr. Warshaw and his group have been thought-leaders in the diagnostic utility of biochemical cyst fluid analysis. We learn of the pertinent laboratory values, and although a high cyst fluid amylase level could strongly suggest a pseudocyst (*Gastroenterology*

(continued)

1995;108:1230), none of these values should be heavily relied on (*Pancreatology* 2005;5:507) .

Because expectant management fails at times, we must intervene. Our authors provide a thorough and balanced summary of percutaneous, endoscopic, and surgical approaches to pancreatic pseudocysts.

Until the past 10 to 15 years, there was little controversy regarding the management of pancreatic pseudocysts. Observation in the stable patient after a bout of acute pancreatitis would be adequate, as many pancreatic fluid collections would spontaneously resolve. Those that persisted could be treated with an open cystoenterostomy. The advent of minimally invasive techniques has shifted the landscape dramatically. A bevy of options now exist, including percutaneous drainage, endoluminal drainage, and the application of laparoscopy to the classic open procedures. All of the possible approaches are thoroughly outlined by the authors, including common indications for each of them. Nealon and Walser (*Ann Surg* 2005;241:948) re-

cently examined the complications associated with nonoperative pseudocyst management. They concluded that the anatomy of the main pancreatic duct was a strong predictor of treatment failure and future complications. Disruption or stenosis of the duct should lead one away from a percutaneous or endoscopic approach.

There are a few additional technical details about the cystoenterostomy procedures worth highlighting. Whether drainage is to be into the stomach, duodenum, or jejunum, I recommend liberal use of intraoperative ultrasound for cyst localization. Obviously, at times it is unnecessary, but with more practice, it will help you immensely for those times in pancreatic surgery when you do need it. For cystogastrostomy, I favor a limited dissection through the gastrocolic omentum to prove that the cyst and stomach are indeed fused posteriorly, and where. Stapling devices are effective in securing apposition and controlling bleeding as the stomach and pseudocyst walls are brought together. I concur that the duode-

num should not be turned over to accept a cystoduodenostomy. If the cyst cannot be drained easily directly across the medial duodenal wall, then a Roux-en-Y loop of jejunum is the better alternative. Beware of bleeding when draining a cyst across the mesentery. Many pancreatitis patients have at least some degree of venous hypertension at that location. Finally, if you have the skills, and the anatomy is appropriate, consider using laparoscopic approaches to cyst drainage. In my experience, these are most favorable with cystogastrostomy and cystojejunostomy.

Today's newest minimally invasive methods for approaching pseudocysts will require further refinement and randomized clinical studies to evaluate properly their effectiveness in comparison with traditional cystoenterostomy. In addition, improved diagnostic criteria need to be established as the incidence of cystic neoplasms of the pancreas increases.

M.P.C.

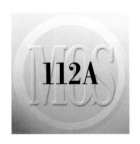

Pancreatic Pseudocyst: Laparoscopic or Endoscopic Versus Conventional Surgery

GARY C. VITALE, TIN C. TRAN, AND BRIAN R. DAVIS

Management of the pancreatic pseudocyst has undergone radical change in the past 10 years with the advent of new laparoscopic and endoscopic methods of drainage. Even the more chronic collections with associated pancreatic necrosis are amenable to these new approaches.

It is important to know the different types of peripancreatic collections in order to select an appropriate treatment strategy. Four pathologic entities of fluid collection are recognized. *Acute fluid collections* occur early as an exudative reaction to pancreatic inflammation, have no fibrous wall, and resolve spontaneously. *Pancreatic necrosis*, diagnosed on dynamic contrast-enhanced computerized tomography, requires early and aggressive cardiorespiratory resuscitation, nutritional support, and possible antibiotic therapy. The development of infection is an indication for operative debridement. *Acute pseudocysts* are collections of enzyme-rich fluid caused by pancreatic ductal disruption that persist 3 to 6 weeks after onset of acute pancreatitis and have a well-defined, nonepithelial fibrous wall. If communication with the ductal system is present, internal enteric drainage is more effective; if communication is not present, the pseudocysts are amenable to percutaneous or endoscopic drainage. *Pancreatic abscesses* are infected, circumscribed

peripancreatic collections that often occur late (4 to 6 weeks) after the onset of severe pancreatitis and may represent infected pseudocysts. Surgical drainage has been the treatment of choice for infected pseudocysts and abscesses, but percutaneous and endoscopic techniques will work particularly when the pseudocyst contents are liquefied and homogenous. If there is a lot of debris or associated pancreatic necrosis with significant infection, open debridement is often still necessary.

CHOICE OF TREATMENT FOR PANCREATIC PSEUDOCYST

Conservative versus Surgical Treatment

Up to 40% of acute pseudocysts will disappear after the pancreatitis resolves. Many patients with pancreatic pseudocysts can be managed conservatively without any procedures if the presenting symptoms can be controlled. However, the success rate is low (approximately 3% to 39%) when a pancreatic pseudocyst is large enough (>5 cm) to cause initial symptoms. Small pseudocysts can resolve without treatment. Asymptomatic patients with a pseudocyst of 6 cm or less in diameter initially can be treated conservatively. If the pseudocyst is larger than 6

cm in diameter and shows no tendency to spontaneous resolution, intervention should be considered. If no complications occur, intervention is postponed until after 6 weeks of observation to allow for maturation of the cyst, which facilitates the cystenteric anastomosis. In pseudocysts related to blunt abdominal trauma, endoscopic retrograde cholangiopancreatography (ERCP) should be performed. If ERCP reveals a major duct disruption, anatomic resection should be considered. In the early stages of cyst development, resolution of the pseudocyst occurs in 20.4% of cases after no intensive therapy with satisfactory clinical follow-up. Cheruvu et al. conservatively treated 36 patients with pancreatic pseudocysts during an 11-year period with a follow-up of 37.3 months. Only 39% of the pancreatic pseudocysts were successfully managed without surgery.

In brief, cysts that are asymptomatic and less than 6 cm in size require no treatment other than follow-up at 3- to 6-month intervals. However, pseudocysts that are caused by chronic pancreatitis are unlikely to resolve spontaneously. Indications for drainage are presence of symptoms, enlargement of the pseudocyst, complications such as infection (14%), hemorrhage (7%), rupture (6%), obstruction, and suspicion of malignancy. The most common indications for invasive intervention are persistent pain (72%), gastric outlet obstruction (18%), jaundice (5%), and dyspepsia with weight loss (5%).

Percutaneous catheter drainage is generally safe and effective in selected patients and should be considered in poor-risk patients, for the treatment of immature cysts, and infected pseudocysts. Percutaneous drainage, however, risks the introduction of secondary infection and the formation of an external pancreatic fistula, and this treatment is associated with high recurrence rates. Contraindications include intracystic hemorrhage and the presence of pancreatic ascites. Andren-Sandberg et al. have reviewed the use of percutaneous catheter drainage in 41 patients. The hospital mortality rate was 2% and postoperative mortality rate was 4%. External drainage was associated with early complications in 40% and recurrent cysts in 33% of patients. Many patients had chronic internal or external pancreatic fistulas. In 1980, Bodurtha et al. reported that the mortality associated with external drainage was 43% and the overall complication rate was 86%. Although treatment has improved in general during the past 25 years, catheter drainage remains complicated. Mortality and morbidity rates are closely related to presence of infection in the pseudocyst.

Internal drainage can be performed by endoscopic transpapillary drainage, endoscopic transmural (transgastric or transduodenal) drainage, laparoscopic pseudocyst-gastrostomy, or pseudocyst-jejunostomy and classic surgeries such as cystogastrostomy or cystojejunostomy.

Pancreatic resection can also be used to remove the pancreatic pseudocyst with the surrounding pancreas, especially when a pseudocyst appears highly suspicious for malignancy.

The choice of procedure depends on a number of factors, including the general condition of the patient; the size, number, and location of the pseudocysts; the presence or absence of communication of the pseudocyst with the pancreatic duct; the presence or absence of infection; and any suspicion of malignancy. For immature pseudocysts, observation is best. If intervention is warranted, percutaneous catheter drainage may be used. For mature cysts in skilled hands, endoscopic drainage should be the first preference. It is less invasive, less expensive, and easier to perform and is associated with a better outcome and less risk of creating an external fistula. Endoscopic expertise is limited, however, and at present, endoscopic drainage cannot be advocated as the procedure of choice in all centers. In the absence of endoscopic expertise, surgical drainage, either laparoscopic or via laparotomy, is the procedure of choice.

ENDOSCOPIC DRAINAGE

Newer endoscopic techniques—a challenge for surgeons—are the major new treatment approach for pancreatic pseudocysts. Given the low complication and mortality rates and the high success rate of endoscopic drainage as compared with surgery, surgical intervention should be reserved only for selected cases. The addition of endoscopic ultrasonography to endoscopic drainage is a new and exciting development and may decrease the risks associated with endoscopic drainage (Table 1).

ERCP has an important role in defining anatomy in the treatment of pancreatic pseudocysts. Evaluation prior to endoscopic drainage of pseudocysts should involve review of a high-quality computed tomography (CT) scan. The endoscopist should attempt to obtain a complete pancreatogram at the index ERCP. Endo-

scopic drainage should be the first preference for the treatment of mature pseudocysts as it is less invasive, less expensive, and easier to perform in many pseudocysts, particularly those involving the pancreatic head. In the absence of endoscopic expertise, percutaneous catheter drainage or surgery is the procedure of choice.

Endoscopic transpapillary drainage is beneficial for pseudocysts that communicate with the pancreatic duct. Endoscopic transmural drainage offers good results in the management of suitably located pseudocysts that complicate chronic pancreatitis. Endoscopic drainage is associated with higher rates of failure in infected pseudocysts and in the presence of pancreatic necrosis (Table 2).

Technically, the endoscopic management of pancreatic pseudocysts is quite effective and safe in experienced hands. ERCP done before the procedure is useful to define anatomy and to evaluate for pancreatic duct disruption. When the cyst does not bulge into gut lumen, an ERCP is necessary for a decision to be made about the feasibility of transpapillary drainage. Most experts agree that endoscopic ultrasonography (EUS) is also useful. It is a valuable supplement to localize the optimal spot for pseudocyst puncture and to avoid hemorrhage from damage to intramural or extramural blood vessels.

Indications

ENDOSCOPIC TECHNIQUES

Transpapillary Drainage

The side-viewing endoscope is passed through the oropharynx to the level of the ampulla. The contours of the gastric wall are briefly studied to evaluate for evidence of an external pseudocyst. The ampulla is

TABLE 1. SOME RESULTS OF ENDOSCOPIC PSEUDOCYST DRAINAGE

Authors	Transpapillary Drainage	Transmural Drainage	Results Success (%)	Results Complication	Long-term Followup
Sharma and Bhargawa 2002 (n = 38)	5	33	100	—	3 (8%) recurrence (44 months)
De Palma et al. 2002 (n = 49)	19	30	84.2 90	—	
Binmoeller et al. 1995 (n = 53)	33	20	94	11% Gallbladder puncture, 1 Bleeding, 2 Abscess, 2	23% (22 months)
Vitale et al. 1999 (n = 36)	9	27	83	1/36 Nonadherent cyst	17% (16 months) recurrent → surgery

TABLE 2. GUIDELINES FOR ENDOSCOPIC DRAINAGE

1. Well-developed cyst wall
2. Nonacute pseudocyst
3. Noninfected pseudocyst
4. Pancreatic ductal disruption or stricture
5. Pseudocyst wall <1 cm
6. Pseudocyst indenting gastrointestinal tract versus endoscopic ultrasonography location of cyst

injected and both biliary and pancreatic ductal systems are opacified if possible. Selective cannulation of the pancreatic duct is essential when endoscopic treatment involving the pancreatic duct is anticipated. Detailed anatomic information is very helpful in determining treatment options in these cases. The first and least-invasive option for patients with a pseudocyst is to access and drain the pseudocyst through the pancreatic duct at the time of the initial ERCP. Injection is accomplished with either a sphincterotome or an injection catheter. In most cases, a sphincterotomy will be performed regardless of whether the pseudocyst is drained through the duct or not. Decompression of the duct with or without stenting is helpful and may be therapeutic in cases when the pseudocyst is connected to the main pancreatic duct.

Sphincterotomy is performed first on the biliary sphincter and then selectively on the pancreatic sphincter. Biliary access is obtained by directing the catheter superiorly and anteriorly in the papilla toward the 11 o'clock direction. In order to accomplish the selective pancreatic sphincterotomy, a guidewire with a hydrophilic tip is usually directed inferiorly, posteriorly, and to the right of where the biliary orifice is found. Pancreatic duct anatomy will determine the next step. The most important information with regard to the pseudocyst is whether it is connected to the pancreatic duct. If the pseudocyst is demonstrated on contrast injection of the pancreatic duct, then transpapillary endoscopic drainage of the cyst is potentially possible. The advantage of the transpapillary approach is that the risk of gastric wall hemorrhage and retrogastric perforation is eliminated, thus reducing the risk of endoscopic pseudocyst drainage.

The anatomy of the pancreatic duct and the presence or absence of a connection to the pseudocyst determines the choice of treatment. If the pseudocyst is opacified, an attempt is made to pass a guidewire through the ampulla and pancreatic duct into the pseudocyst. Usually a straight-tipped hydrophilic guidewire works, but an angled tip wire may be best. A No. 7 French plastic pancreatic stent of an appropriate length is then passed over the guidewire and into the pseudocyst (Fig. 1, A–C). The stent drains the pseudocyst in a transpapillary fashion into the duodenum. If the anatomy demonstrates disruption of the duct with connection to the pseudocyst, but one is not able to access the pseudocyst directly with a guidewire, then placement of the stent in the duct with the tip as close as possible to the origin of the pseudocyst is an acceptable alternative. If the tail of the pancreas is not opacified on injection, one may conclude that there is complete duct disruption and the tail of the pancreas drains into the pseudocyst. If the tail section of the pancreatic duct is visualized beyond the origin of the pseudocyst, drainage of this portion of the duct may allow the pseudocyst to resolve by removing the source of fluid in the cyst. In these cases, passing a pancreatic stent as far into the tail of the pancreas as possible beyond the connection to the pseudocyst may allow the duct disruption to heal and the cyst to resolve spontaneously.

The stent in the pseudocyst is left until the pseudocyst resolves or significantly decreases in size as shown by CT scan. Usually this occurs fairly rapidly during several weeks, but if no improvement occurs, the stent should be removed and the treatment options reviewed in 6 to 8 weeks. If there is no opacification of the tail of the pancreas at the initial ERCP, one can assume the duct is obstructed and may be feeding the pseudocyst. A magnetic resonance image (MRI) with cholangiopancreatography protocol should be helpful in delineating tail ductal anatomy in these cases and may help direct future therapeutic options.

Transmural Drainage

The pseudocyst may be indenting the gastric or duodenal wall. In these cases, direct cyst-gastrostomy or duodenostomy may be possible. The cyst must indent the lumen enough to be recognized and should correspond in location with where the cyst is identified on the CT scan (Table 2). There are several techniques for cyst-enterostomy. A needle knife is used to open into a bulge in the stomach. A small area (2 or 3 mm) is cauterized and then the knife is used to puncture the center of this area. A gush of cyst fluid is encountered when the cyst is entered. A guidewire is then passed through the center of the needle knife after removing the blade, or if a double-lumen knife is used, the wire is passed alongside. The knife is removed and then a

The Gastrointestinal Tract

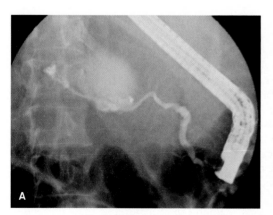
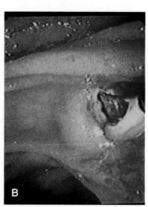
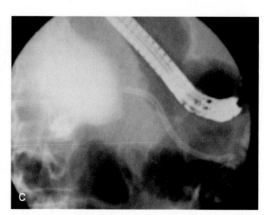

Fig. 1. Techniques of transpapillary drainage of the pancreatic pseudocyst. **A:** The pancreatic duct is injected to prove the connection of the cyst and pancreatic duct. The pancreatic duct anatomy is studied well to make sure that any distal duct strictures are treated. **B:** A selective pancreatic duct orifice sphincterotomy is usually performed to ensure placement of a No. 7 to 10 French pancreatic stent. **C:** A No. 10 French pancreatic stent is placed in the pancreatic duct. Ideally, the end of stent should be placed in the pseudocyst.

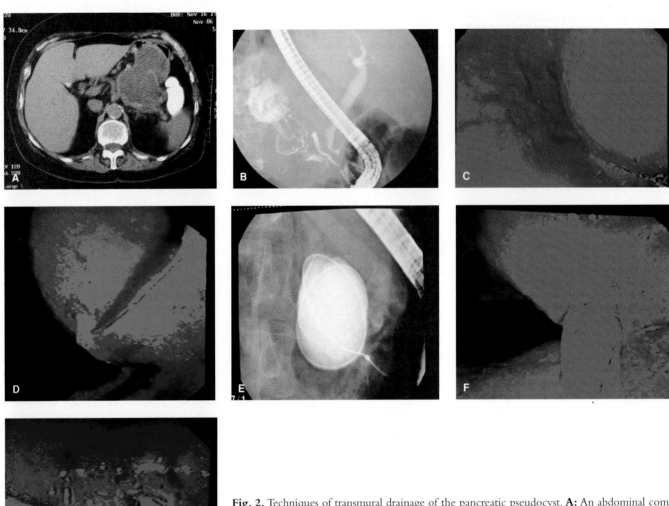

Fig. 2. Techniques of transmural drainage of the pancreatic pseudocyst. **A:** An abdominal computed tomographic (CT) scan is studied carefully before the procedure. An abdominal CT scan with oral and intravenous contrast material is necessary to evaluate the involvement of the cyst with the stomach wall and the visceral vessels. **B:** Pancreatogram should be performed to evaluate the possibility of combined transpapillary drainage. **C:** The lateral-view scope is used to choose the appropriate approach angle. Ideally, the pseudocyst is approached at the right angle. **D:** The precut knife or cystotome is used to make a first cut through the stomach wall. **E:** A guidewire is then passed through the center of the needle knife after removing the blade or, if a double-lumen knife is used, the wire is passed alongside. **F:** A 10- to 15-mm balloon is used to dilate the opening after it is extended by a cannulatome. **G:** One or two No. 10 French single or double pigtail stents are placed.

sphincterotome is passed over the wire to enlarge the opening. A minimum of a 1-cm opening is preferable and is created by orienting the sphincterotome in multiple directions. If the mucosa was prone to bleeding with the initial cut using the needle knife, a balloon can be used to dilate the opening without cutting. In either case, one or two No. 10 French stents are placed into the pseudocyst draining into the stomach (Fig. 2, A–G). Two stents are better than one because they allow the cyst to drain alongside the stents as well as through them. A single stent will drain as long as it is not clogged, but usually the mucosa will grow back right up to the stent, and the pseudocyst will not be able to drain alongside the stent for very long.

Because the stents are left in place a long time, drainage alongside the stent may be more important than the drainage through the stent. Our policy is to leave the stents in for approximately 1 year, and then remove them unless the tail of the pancreas depends on the stent for drainage. This is determined by MRI or ERCP. If there is a tail of the pancreas duct identified by MRI, and it is not connected to the main pancreatic duct, then one can leave the transgastric stent indefinitely to drain the tail.

A relatively new device called the *cystotome* combines a removable electrocautery needle knife with a circumferential electrocautery ring to allow cyst puncture, wire passage, and then cyst-gastrostomy enlarge-

ment without changing catheters (Fig. 3). This makes access to the more difficult cysts easier as no catheter exchange is necessary and the guidewire can be passed through the cutting device, ensuring continuity of the procedure. The size of the cyst-gastrostomy made with this device is similar to that made with the sphincterotome.

Complications and Management

Complications of these procedures include perforation, bleeding, and infection. Endoscopists performing these procedures should have a good understanding of these complications and know how to minimize risks. They should have expert, multidisciplinary backup available at their institution

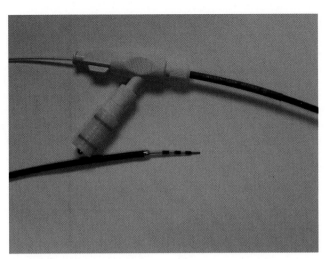

Fig. 3. A cystotome.

in the event of complication or failure. Sharma et al. report experience in 38 patients with endoscopic drainage. Massive bleeding in one patient required surgery, and stent blockage and pseudocyst infection in three patients and perforation in one patient were managed conservatively. ERCP was done before pseudocyst drainage in eight patients because there was no visible bulge into the stomach or duodenum (n = 5), or because obstructive jaundice was present (n = 3). In five patients, ERCP revealed a pseudocyst duct communication. All of these patients were managed by transpapillary drainage, and there was only one asymptomatic recurrence in this group. De Palma et al. also report an experience with 49 patients using an endoscopic approach. Twelve (24.5%) patients had complications: two patients had bleeding, two patients had mild pancreatitis, and eight patients had cyst infections. Five patients with infection had pancreatic necrosis and three patients had a clogged stent.

To reduce bleeding complications, careful electrocautery should be done around the site prior to puncture. Using endoscopic ultrasound, endoscopists can choose the best site for pseudocyst puncture and avoid vessels. With Doppler, endoscopic ultrasound can define the precise location of the pseudocyst and vessels and determine the thinnest point in the gastric wall for puncture. In our experience, a wide opening of the cyst-enterostomy (approximately 1 to 2 cm) is necessary in potentially infected cases to reduce the incidence of infected cyst complications.

Recurrent Pancreatic Pseudocyst

On long-term follow-up, endoscopic drainage has a reported recurrence rate ranging from 8% to 20%. Recurrences are generally seen only with alcoholic pancreatitis. In one study, the biliary pancreatitis group had no recurrences after cholecystectomy and removal of common bile duct stones, if present, and no recurrences in the trauma group. After a 44-month follow-up, Sharma et al. reported the results of endoscopic drainage for 38 pseudocysts. Three patients had symptomatic recurrences, and three had asymptomatic recurrences; all had alcohol-induced pancreatitis. No recurrences were seen in the biliary pancreatitis and trauma group. With a median follow-up of 26 months, De Palma et al. showed a 20.9% recurrence rate.

Causes of recurrent pseudocysts usually involve the obstruction of a cystoenterostomy or stent in the presence of persistent pancreatic disease or ductal stricture. All symptomatic recurrences have been successfully managed either with repeat endoscopic cystogastrostomy and stenting or surgery.

LAPAROSCOPIC DRAINAGE

The evolution of the laparoscopic drainage of pancreatic pseudocysts has followed different strategies, but all have relied on the basic tenets of pancreatic surgery. The first tenet is that the cyst should be drained in a dependent location, and that the choice should be dictated by the best anatomic approach to optimize pseudocyst drainage. The second is to perform biopsy of the cyst wall to rule out a cystic pancreatic neoplasm. The third tenet is to provide adequate exploration and debridement of the cyst cavity. This may be performed by the laparoscope or gastric endoscope. The fourth tenet is to maintain adequate hemostasis on draining the friable pseudocyst wall, whether through the use of an endoscopic stapler or interrupted suture ligation.

Indications for laparoscopic pseudocyst drainage are the same as described previously for other interventions. Symptomatic pseudocysts greater than 6 cm in size that have been present for more than 6 weeks are considered for drainage. Pseudocysts associated with an inflammatory mass in the head of the pancreas or a dilated duct with calculi in the head of the pancreas may be best treated by a pancreatic head resection (Whipple procedure). Patients with pancreatic ductal strictures and a pseudocyst in the tail of the pancreas should be treated with a distal pancreatectomy. Communication with the main pancreatic duct is not a contraindication to laparoscopic drainage, except in patients with multiple pancreatic duct strictures.

Debris evident within the pseudocyst cavity noted on CT indicates the need for a laparoscopic approach for improved pancreatic drainage and direct visualization of pancreatic necrosis for debridement. Some authors have even described the delayed debridement of infected pancreatic necrosis through a cyst-gastrostomy in patients with favorable responses to supportive therapy and systemic antibiotics. This approach should also be considered for patients in whom suspicion of carcinoma requires biopsy and inspection of the pseudocyst wall. Other possible candidates for the laparoscopic approach include patients with portal hypertension or coagulopathy. Because disruption of the other intra-abdominal tissue via dissection is minimal, the laparoscopic treatment of pseudocysts may confer a benefit in patients with chronic pancreatitis and ongoing alcohol abuse as this approach allows for an easier reoperation when attempting more extensive debridement or subtotal pancreatic resection.

Demonstration of the Pseudocyst

Computed tomography of the abdomen and pelvis with thin cuts through the pancreas is the standard of care for localization of pancreatic pseudocysts prior to drainage. Pseudocysts should be drained primarily based on symptoms, and pseudocysts less than 6 cm in size on CT may be managed conservatively. Pseudocysts greater than 10 cm in size should be managed operatively because of the high incidence of complications with conservative management of cysts this size. Endoscopic retrograde pancreatography should also be performed prior to surgery as up to 80% of pseudocysts demonstrate a pancreatic duct stricture or show duct disruption, and this may affect the treatment options. Intraoperatively, the pseudocyst is most commonly localized by needle aspiration. The pseudocysts have also been localized using endoscopic gastric ultrasound and laparoscopic ultrasound.

The Intragastric Cyst-Gastrostomy Approach

The first laparoscopic drainage procedures were performed by Way et al. and Gagner in 1994 via an intragastric approach. Using this technique, a Veress needle is used to gain insufflation of the abdomen and a periumbilical trocar is placed for visualization of the stomach. The stomach is insufflated via a nasogastric tube or a gastric endoscope. Pneumoperitoneum is maintained at 8 to 10 mm Hg while the stomach is inflated and transgastric ports are placed. Multiple techniques have been described for placing these transgastric ports, including specialized trocars with balloons at their tip that can be cinched up to the gastric wall, radially dilating trocars (Inner-Dyne Inc., Sunnyvale, CA) that are placed into the stomach over a Veress needle to create a seal with the

stomach, and standard laparoscopic trocars sutured in place with purse-string sutures. Three intragastric trocars are typically placed through the greater curvature of the stomach under laparoscopic visualization (Fig. 4, A–E). Three ports accommodate an intragastric laparoscope and two operating instruments.

The cyst is localized with either endoscopic ultrasound or needle aspiration. After the cyst has been localized, the cyst cavity is entered either with hook electrocautery or harmonic scalpel dissection. A wedge of cyst wall is sent for pathologic evaluation to rule out cystic neoplasm. A large 4- to 5-cm incision is then made in the cyst wall with either a dissecting instrument or an endoscopic stapler. If the dissecting instrument is used, the cyst-gastrostomy is usually reinforced with interrupted sutures to prevent bleeding complications. After the cyst-gastrostomy has been completed, the trocars are withdrawn and the gastrostomies are closed using figure-of-eight sutures. Park and Heniford have developed a variation of this technique with a minilaparoscopic cyst-gastrostomy in which the stomach is insufflated and the intragastric ports are placed directly

through the skin into the stomach. This technique uses a laparoscopic stapler to complete the cyst gastrostomy. The advantages of this technique are that it avoids the need to establish pneumoperitoneum and obviates the need to close gastrostomies as the ports are only 2 mm in diameter. The main limitations of these approaches are the technical difficulty associated with operating within a limited space and bleeding from the friable cyst-gastrostomy site.

The Anterior Transgastric Cyst-Gastrostomy Approach

The technical challenges of the intragastric approach have led to the development of the anterior approach in which a 5- to 6-cm anterior gastrostomy is performed (Fig. 5). This anterior gastrostomy allows improved access to the posterior wall of the stomach. This access is used for the application of an endoscopic stapler to the cystgastrostomy to create a more hemostatic anastomosis. The anterior gastrostomy is then closed with interrupted sutures or a stapler. The primary disadvantage is the need for two gastrostomies, with the ensuing risk of spillage of gastric contents.

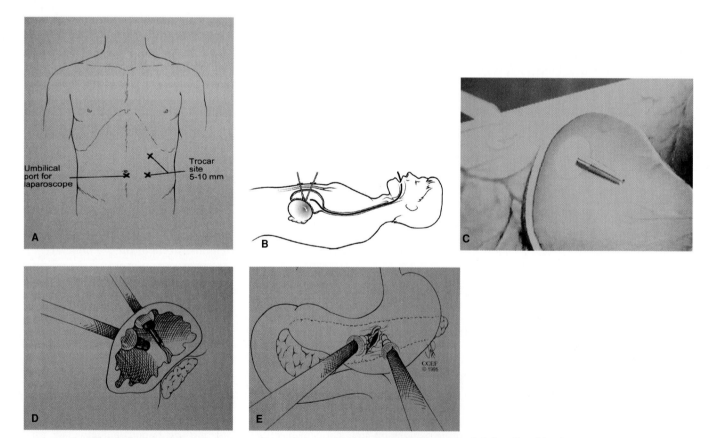

Fig. 4. Intragastric approach to pseudocyst drainage. **A:** Trocar sites. **B:** The stomach is insufflated by the upper gastrointestinal scope to elevate the anterior wall of the stomach closer to the anterior abdominal wall. **C:** Special trocars are used to keep the stomach distended during the procedure. **D:** The operative field in the stomach. **E:** The posterior wall of the stomach and anterior wall of the pseudocyst are cut approximately 2 to 3 cm in length.

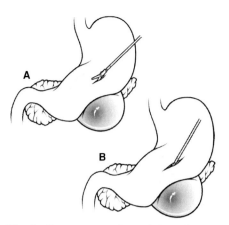

Fig. 5. Cystostomy performed through anterior gastrostomy. **A:** Gastrotomy performed. **B:** Transgastric approach to pseudocyst through gastrotomy.

The Lesser Sac Approach

Park and Heniford describe a technique that addresses the risk of gastric spillage and the technical challenges of this operation by approaching the pseudocyst through the lesser sac and creating a single gastrostomy for effective drainage. The patient is placed in the lithotomy position and pneumoperitoneum is created with a Veress needle. A periumbilical port is placed as well as a left upper quadrant port and a subxiphoid port. The gastrocolic omentum is divided using an ultrasonic dissector, diathermy, or a stapler. The posterior wall of the stomach is then divided from the pancreatic pseudocyst. Localization is performed with needle aspiration. A cystostomy is made with cautery and a cyst wall biopsy is performed. A gastric endoscope is simultaneously introduced into the stomach to determine the optimal position for the posterior gastrostomy. A gastrostomy is then made in the posterior stomach wall in a position that will juxtapose the pancreatic cyst. One arm of the endoscopic stapler is introduced into the gastrostomy and the other into the pancreatic pseudocyst, resulting in a large cystgastrostomy. The laparoscope is then inserted into the pseudocyst and loculations in the cyst cavity are divided. The opening to the cyst-gastrostomy is closed using interrupted sutures (Fig. 6, A–D). After anastomotic completion, the endoscope is introduced into the stomach and insufflated under direct laparoscopic visualization to ensure an airtight anastomosis.

The Cyst-Jejunostomy Approach

This approach was developed to obtain the most dependent and anatomic drainage for pancreatic pseudocysts that are not easily accessed through the stomach. The patient is placed in the lithotomy position and two trocars are placed lateral and superior to the umbilicus on the left. A third trocar is placed in the upper abdomen just lateral to the right rectus muscle. A fourth left lateral, upper abdominal trocar is also placed for the endoscopic stapler. The pseudocyst is localized through the transverse mesocolon by visual inspection, aspiration decompression, or laparoscopic ultrasound. The preferred site of access is just superior and lateral to the ligament of Treitz. The cyst-jejunostomy is performed either with a loop of jejunum or a Roux-en-Y reconstruction. The Roux-en-Y method is the preferred reconstruction according to the literature. The jejunum is transected approximately 30 cm distal to the ligament of Treitz, and the pseudocyst is opened through the transverse mesocolon. The laparoscope is introduced into the cyst under visual control to disrupt loculations and remove necrotic debris. An enterotomy is then performed and a lateral cyst wall-to-jejunal anastomosis is performed with an endoscopic stapler. The cyst-jejunostomy is closed with a running suture layer. The jejunojejunostomy is completed 30 cm distal

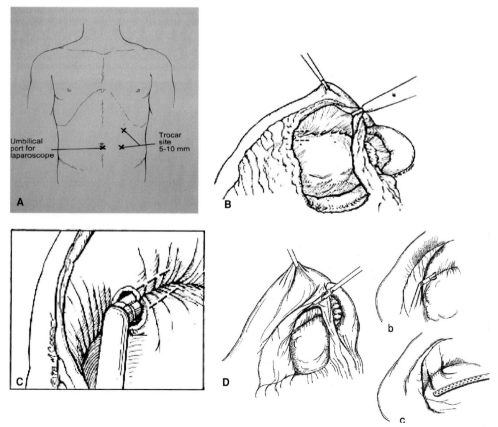

Fig. 6. The lesser sac approach. **A:** Trocar sites. **B:** Dissection of the lesser sac. **C:** Creation of the cystgastrostomy by a laparoscopic stapler. **D:** Completion of the cyst-gastric anastomosis with suture closure of stapler access holes using interrupted sutures.

The Gastrointestinal Tract

to the cyst-jejunostomy. The abdomen must be irrigated thoroughly to remove all pancreatic debris.

Results of Laparoscopic Pancreatic Pseudocyst Drainage

An initial report of intragastric laparoscopic pseudocyst drainage was by Way et al., who later described a series of 18 patients, with successful completion of this laparoscopic procedure in 14 of these patients. Four patients had to be converted to an open approach due to bleeding at the cystgastrostomy. All patients in this series were noted to have resolution of the pseudocyst on long-term follow-up. Trias et al. described a modification of the intragastric technique using a stapler for creation of the anastomosis, which reduced complications of bleeding at the cystgastrostomy. This approach proved technically demanding and led to the development of the anterior transgastric approach described by Obermeyer et al. in a series of five patients with a mean length of hospital stay of 7.5 days with no complications and no recurrences.

Comparing the intragastric and anterior transgastric technique, Hauters et al. studied a series of 12 patients, with 6 patients undergoing each technique. They found comparable results between the two techniques with no differences in the length of hospital stay or cyst recurrence rates. Cysts not adherent to the gastric wall have been addressed by laparoscopic cyst-jejunostomy, which was studied in a series of nine patients by Teixeira et al. This study demonstrated a minor complication rate of 20% with no major complications or mortality, and with total resolution of the pseudocysts and no cyst recurrences. Bhattacharya et al. reviewed the outcomes of laparoscopic pseudocyst drainage in 40 patients, sampled from multiple different series and case reports in the literature, revealing a mean length of hospital stay of 4 days with a success rate of 89%. Complications in this review were seen in two patients, comprising

infection of the pseudocyst contents and recurrence of the pseudocyst. This review also noted that the best results with this procedure were obtained when the cyst-gastric anastomosis was 3 cm or greater in length, with smaller anastomoses potentially leading to inadequate drainage and cyst recurrence. Because this was a review and not a single institution trial, this conclusion may not be accurate.

The largest single series in the literature (28 patients), described by Park and Heniford, uses all four described approaches to pseudocyst drainage and detailed a mean postoperative length of stay from 3 to 4 days, depending on the procedure performed. The most common noted complication was bleeding from the cyst-enteric anastomosis, which was managed with blood transfusions and did not require operative intervention. Long-term follow-up demonstrated cyst resolution with two recurrences. One patient developed necrotizing pancreatitis requiring serial debridements and another required conversion to external pseudocyst drainage with a sump drain.

Postoperative Care

The trend is toward rapid recovery of these patients, most of whom are able to take a clear liquid diet the day after surgery. Most patients can be discharged within 4 days of surgery with no complications and a noted low recurrence rate on follow-up. Patients should be followed at 6-month intervals with serial CT scans until the pseudocyst has resolved.

CONVENTIONAL SURGERY

Newer competing approaches to pseudocyst management such as endoscopic transpapillary or transmural drainage, and laparoscopic internal drainage, laparoscopic pseudocyst-gastrostomy, or pseudocyst-jejunostomy ultimately require objective comparison to the "gold standard" of open surgical drainage. Surgical treatment has

been the traditional approach and is still the preferred treatment in most centers. Multiple pseudocysts, giant pseudocysts, presence of other complications related to chronic pancreatitis in addition to pseudocyst, and suspected malignancy are best managed surgically. Surgery is also the backup management in the event that percutaneous or endoscopic drainage fails. Surgery is chosen for all patients with recurrent pseudocyst, pseudocyst combined with common bile duct or duodenal stenosis, and symptomatic pseudocyst associated with a dilated pancreatic duct. Surgery offers the advantage over endoscopy of obtaining a wedge biopsy specimen of the cyst wall. Any type of endothelium in the wall of the suspected pseudocyst indicates a true cyst or a cystic neoplasm. Surgical procedures for pancreatic pseudocyst include external drainage; internal drainage, which can take the form of cystogastrostomy, cystoduodenostomy, cystojejunostomy, and excision (Table 3).

Owing to advances in pancreatic imaging, cystic lesions of the pancreas are being recognized with increasing frequency. A presumptive diagnosis of pseudocyst, based on CT appearance alone, will prove to be in error in as many as one third of patients. Neoplastic cysts of the pancreas are particularly susceptible to this misdiagnosis, which can result in inappropriate drainage rather than resection. Using a combination of historic features and CT, the differential diagnosis between pseudocyst and cystic neoplasm can usually be made. In borderline patients, transcutaneous aspiration for cytology and analysis of the cyst fluid for neoplastic markers may prove helpful. Final resolution of doubtful cases is achieved by biopsy of the cyst wall.

If the nature of the lesion cannot be determined, it is better to resect a pseudocyst than to drain a cystic neoplasm. Cystic neoplasm should be considered in the differential diagnosis of large pancreatic cystic masses, especially in young female patients. Papillary cystic neoplasm is a rare

TABLE 3. INDICATIONS FOR SURGICAL TREATMENT OPTIONS

External Drainage	Internal Drainage	Pancreatic Resection
1. Free rupture 2. Grossly infected 3. Unstable patients with bleeding 4. Cyst wall not thick enough to allow an anastomosis	1. Mature cysts (>1 cm) 2. Pancreatic duct stricture or leak 3. Benign cyst wall biopsy	1. Cysts in body and tail with possible malignancy 2. Complex cystic diseases of the head 3. Pancreatic pseudoaneurysm
▪ Open drainage ▪ Percutaneous drainage	▪ Cystgastrostomy ▪ Cystoduodenostomy ▪ Roux-en-Y cystojejunostomy	▪ Distal pancreatectomy to include cyst ▪ Pancreatoduodenectomy

malignant tumor of the pancreas that typically occurs in young female patients and has an excellent prognosis. Panieri reported 12 patients with papillary cystic neoplasm. The correct diagnosis was made preoperatively in only five patients. The papillary cystic neoplasm may occur in the head, neck, body, and tail of the pancreas. In those situations, surgical excision such as pancreaticoduodenectomy, central pancreatectomy with pancreaticogastrostomy or distal pancreatectomy should be performed. Panieri has reported on 11 patients treated with this approach who are disease-free and are well at follow-up of 6.6 years (range, 6 months to 15 years).

Surgical management of pancreatic pseudocyst has been eminently successful. Morbidity and mortality rates have been low. Usatoff operated prospectively on 112 consecutive patients for pseudocysts in the setting of chronic pancreatitis. Overall morbidity rate was 28% and the operative mortality rate was 1%. The cyst recurrence rate was 3%. Surgical internal drainage of pancreatic pseudocysts can be performed safely with low morbidity and mortality if patients are carefully selected and their medical management is optimized. Although minimally invasive techniques now offer a variety of treatment options, open surgical drainage is still indicated for a significant number of patients.

The choice of surgical procedure depends on the following factors: size, number, and location of cysts; presence or absence of communication of the cyst with the pancreatic duct; anatomy of proximal pancreatic duct; presence or absence of infection; suspicion of malignancy; and vessel involvement. Endoscopic pancreatography has played a dominant role in the evolution of surgical treatment of pancreatic pseudocysts. Pancreatography helps define operative strategies by identifying associated pancreatic and biliary disease, and predicting outcome of nonoperative treatment.

In the choice of surgical internal drainage, the first concern is the anatomic location of the pseudocysts. If the pseudocyst is bulging against the posterior wall of the stomach, cystogastrostomy is considered. Cystoduodenostomy is considered for the pseudocyst, which closely abuts the duodenal wall (<1 cm) to reduce the risk of bleeding from the amount of pancreatic tissue that must be traversed. For others, the preferred technique for pseudocysts not bulging in the stomach or duodenum is cystojejunostomy. The second concern is the presence or absence of associated lesions, such as

common duct stricture or pancreatic duct stricture. If either common duct stenosis or pancreatic duct dilatation exists in combination with the established pseudocyst, a Roux-en-Y jejunal loop to the common duct and pseudocyst or to the dilated pancreatic duct including the pseudocyst is appropriate.

Timing of Drainage

A better understanding of the natural history of pseudocysts has changed the concepts regarding their management. The old teaching that asymptomatic cysts of more than 6 cm in diameter that have been present for 6 weeks should be drained is open to interpretation. Definite indications for drainage are presence of symptoms, persistent progressive enlargement of the cyst, complications such as infection, hemorrhage, rupture, and obstruction, and suspicion of malignancy (Table 4).

Shantey and Lillehei analyzed 114 patients from the perspective of the timing of operative intervention. In general, the patients undergoing surgical therapy during the first 6 weeks after pseudocyst formation had higher rates postoperatively of morbidity, mortality, and recurrence than did those treated later in the course of the disease. However, further subdivision of the data revealed that the results in patients with uncomplicated pseudocysts were similar, irrespective of the timing of operative treatment. Operative intervention in patients with a pseudocyst who were acutely ill was risky at any time in the course of the disease. Based on these results and on information available in the literature, the optimal timing of the operation in patients with uncomplicated pseudocysts appears to be approximately 4 weeks after formation of the mass.

An accepted approach is as follows. (i) A pseudocyst that occurs after an episode of alcohol-related pancreatitis should be

TABLE 4. GUIDELINES FOR OPEN SURGICAL INTERVENTION

1. Cyst rupture or hemorrhage, or cyst adjacent to vascular structures
2. Cysts with the potential to be cystic neoplasms
3. Patients with multiple or infected pseudocysts
4. Cysts with an associated high-grade pancreatic duct stricture
5. Cyst wall >1 cm
6. Pancreatic pseudoaneurysm

observed for 4 to 6 weeks with regular follow-up ultrasound examinations of the abdomen. (ii) After 6 weeks, observation should continue if the size of the cyst is less than 6 cm and the patient is asymptomatic or if there is decrease in size of the cyst. (iii) Therapy is indicated if the patient is symptomatic or if the cyst size is more than 6 cm, the cyst is increasing in size, the cyst is infected, or there is a suspicion of malignancy. (iv) Immediate drainage is safe in cysts that have a mature wall or in those arising in chronic pancreatitis. Similarly, presence in the serum of an isoamylase is a reliable indicator for safety of internal drainage, regardless of the apparent age of the pseudocyst. Warshaw and Rattner observed that, in the presence of old amylase, 14 of 14 pseudocysts were suitable for internal drainage, but that in its absence, 4 of 5 pseudocysts required external drainage.

The current literature suggests that the old 6 cm/6 week criteria for intervention should be a relative rather than an absolute indicator. Asymptomatic pseudocysts, regardless of size and duration, can be safely observed if they are carefully monitored and are not rapidly increasing in size. Intervention is mandatory only in the presence of symptoms, complications, or if there is any suspicion of malignancy.

Elective versus Urgent Surgery

Most surgical treatments, approximately 87%, for pancreatic pseudocyst are elective. Urgent operation for pancreatic pseudocyst is approximately 13% and involves higher postoperative morbidity, 67% versus 10%. Internal drainage operations and pancreatic resection are usually scheduled.

Erosion of a major pancreatic or peripancreatic vessel leads to free rupture or formation of pseudoaneurysm that subsequently may rupture. The splenic artery is the most commonly involved vessel, followed by the pancreaticoduodenal, left gastric, hepatic, and small intrapancreatic arteries. Pseudoaneurysm should be suspected in the event of repeated episodes of gastrointestinal bleeding, presence of an enlarging pulsatile abdominal mass, or an abdominal bruit, and in patients with increasing abdominal pain. Bolus dynamic CT scan is the most useful initial diagnostic test; it detects the presence of hemorrhage (attenuation >30 HU) and pseudoaneurysms.

Angiography is the procedure of choice for both identification of the source of bleeding and therapeutic embolization. Embolization facilitates surgical control of bleeding and eliminates unnecessary harmful extra dissection. Angiography should be attempted preoperatively in stable patients. A postoperative superior mesenteric artery pseudoaneurysm that communicates with a pancreatic pseudocyst after aortic surgery is a difficult management problem. Untreated, this condition can lead to exsanguination. Traditional surgical treatment has many potential complications. Endovascular repair has the potential for avoidance of surgical complications. Cowan reported the first superior mesenteric artery pseudoaneurysm successfully treated with a polytetrafluoroethylene covered stent.

Surgical intervention is indicated in patients with pseudoaneurysm involving pseudocysts who are hemodynamically unstable, or when embolization is technically not possible or when it fails to stop the bleeding. Surgical options consist of (i) proximal and distal ligation of bleeding vessels with drainage of pseudocyst or necrotic tissue, and (ii) distal pancreatectomy when bleeding arises from the body or tail of the pancreas.

Massive hemorrhage occurs in approximately 5% to 10% of patients with pseudocysts, and this is the most feared complication. Most commonly, there is massive bleeding into the gastrointestinal tract, followed by intra-abdominal bleeding, and rarely there is bleeding into the pancreatic duct (hemosuccus pancreaticus).

The high mortality associated with pancreatic hemorrhage makes prompt and aggressive management essential. Balthazar reported that in 1,910 patients diagnosed as having pancreatitis in the last 10 years, 26 developed hemorrhagic complications (1.3%). These complications were detected from 2 months to 8 years (mean, 2.3 years) after one or several episodes of pancreatitis. The cause of hemorrhage was bleeding pseudoaneurysm in 16 patients (61%); diffuse bleeding with pancreatic necrosis in 5 patients (19.5%) and hemorrhagic pseudocysts in 5 patients (19.5%). Intra-abdominal hemorrhage developed in 21 patients and gastrointestinal bleeding in 5 patients. Early detection followed by angiography, embolization, and/or surgery has decreased mortality rates.

In a study by Carr et al., 16 patients had pancreatic pseudoaneurysms. Ten of 16 patients initially underwent operative therapy, 4 elective and 6 emergency surgeries, whereas 6 stable patients were initially treated with percutaneous arteriography embolization. The surgical morbidity rate was 62% (8 of 13) and that of embolization was 50% (5 of 10). Three deaths occurred after emergency operations, two of which procedures failed to stop the bleeding. There were no deaths following embolization. A trend was noted toward increased death with necrotizing pancreatitis ($P = 0.07$) and emergency surgery ($P = 0.06$). The mean size of pseudoaneurysms that required operative intervention for secondary complications was 13.9 cm, compared with 7.7 cm for all others in the series ($P = .046$). Long-term follow-up was available in all 13 survivors at a mean of 44 months (range, 1 to 108 months).

SUMMARY

In summary, new minimally invasive surgical options along with nonoperative endoscopic approaches appear to decrease the morbidity of treatment without a significant reduction in effectiveness. Surgeons should embrace these new techniques, including endoscopic options, or risk becoming peripheral in the treatment schema of pancreatic pseudocyst disease.

SUGGESTED READING

Adkisson KW, Baron TH, Morgan DE. Pancreatic fluid collections: diagnosis and endoscopic management. *Semin Gastrointest Dis* 1998;9:61.

Amorri BJ. Laparoscopic transgastric pancreatic necrosectomy for infected pancreatic necrosis. *Surg Endosc* 2002;16:1362.

Beckingham IJ, Krige JE, Bornman PC, et al. Endoscopic management of pancreatic pseudocysts. *Br J Surg* 1997;84:1638.

Bhattacharya D, Ammori BJ. Minimally invasive approaches to the management of pancreatic pseudocysts: review of the literature. *Surg Laparosc Endosc Percut Tech* 2003;13:141.

Binmoeller KF, Siefert H, Walter A, et al. Transpapillary and transmural drainage of pancreatic pseudocysts. *Gastrointest Endosc* 1995;42:219.

Bodurtha AJ, Dajee H, You CK. Analysis of 29 cases of pancreatic pseudocyst treated surgically. *Can J Surg* 1980;23:432.

Cheruvu CV, Clarke MG, Prentice M, et al. Conservative treatment as an option in the management of pancreatic pseudocyst. *Ann R Coll Surg Engl* 2003;85:313.

Cooperman AM. An overview of pancreatic pseudocysts: the emperor's new clothes revisited. *Surg Clin North Am* 2001;81:391.

De Palma GD, Galloro G, Puzziello A, et al. Personal experience with the endoscopic treatment of pancreatic pseudocysts. Long-term results and analysis of prognostic factors [in Italian]. *Minerva Chir* 2001;56:475.

Gagner M. Laparoscopic pancreatic cystgastrostomy for pancreatic pseudocyst. *Surg Endosc* 1994;8:239.

Hauters P, Weerts J, Peillon C, et al. Treatment of pancreatic pseudocysts by laparoscopic cystogastrostomy [in French]. *Ann Chir* 2004;129:347.

Norton ID, Peterrsen BT. Interventional treatment of acute and chronic pancreatitis. Endoscopic procedures. *Surg Clin North Am* 1999;79:895.

Park AE, Heniford BT. Therapeutic laparoscopy of the pancreas. *Ann Surg* 2002;236:149.

Sharma SS, Bhargawa N, Govil A. Endoscopic management of pancreatic pseudocyst: a long-term follow-up. *Endoscopy* 2002;34:203.

Way LW, Legha P, Mori T. Laparoscopic pancreatic cystgastrostomy: the first operation in the new field of intraluminal laparoscopic surgery. *Surg Endosc* 1994;8:235.

EDITOR'S COMMENT

Pancreatic pseudocysts result from acute or chronic pancreatitis, and often involve some disruption of the pancreatic ductal system. Traditionally, these have been managed by open surgical drainage or resection techniques, as described herein and elsewhere in *Mastery*. In the past decade, minimally invasive techniques have emerged to treat pancreatic pseudocysts with sound efficacy and acceptable complication rates. As both a surgeon and expert endoscopist, Dr. Gary Vitale is highly qualified to update our readers on these options. Although techniques have changed, our basic principles of pseudocyst management have not.

Not all who intervene on pseudocysts are hybrid endoscopist-surgeons, however. For the techniques Dr. Vitale and coauthors describe to be safest and most effective, all camps should work together: multidisciplinary management decisions are best. Complications arising from misguided unilateral decisions can and should be avoided. A surgeon embarks on open internal drainage for something that easily could be managed endoscopically and the patient suffers postoperative sepsis. An endoscopist underestimates hypertensive portal gastropathy and cannot control hemorrhage during pseudocyst drainage. Which is worse? Neither is, because both are terrible but potentially avoidable when careful multidisciplinary evaluation and management is the rule.

Once the team ascends the learning curve together, many decisions can be made safely independently. Ours is a high-volume pancreatic

(continued)

surgery and endoscopy center where decisions are still most often made together. Other centers agree, and offer compelling clinical results. Hookey (*Gastrointest Endosc* 2006;63:635) has recently demonstrated the efficacy of endoscopic drainage techniques in 116 patients presenting with a variety of acute fluid collections and acute and chronic pseudocysts. The endoscopic drainage technique was transpapillary in 15 patients, transmural in 60, and both in 41 patients; 88% of patients were treated successfully. One might safely assume the majority avoided surgery. Complications did occur in 11%, and six patients died within 30 days. Only one death (0.8%) was directly related to the procedure. Such fine outcomes reflect a requisite expertise that is not available everywhere.

Several key principles of endoscopic drainage are worth highlighting. As with open surgical drainage, pancreatic ductal communication should be determined first by ERCP. Transpapillary stent drainage may be all that is necessary. If the cyst is bulging through the posterior wall of the stomach, transluminal drainage is ideal and, as noted by our authors, most effective when multiple pigtail stents are placed. Endoscopic ultrasound is compulsory, not as much for cyst localization but to avoid large gastric wall varices that can occur following severe

pancreatitis. Thankfully, today's endoscopic techniques have replaced most percutaneous drainage techniques, which rarely worked well, especially when pancreatic ductal communication existed. Recurrences are more typical in alcoholic pancreatitis and not biliary pancreatitis.

Like most minimally invasive surgical procedures, the laparoscopic techniques for pancreatic pseudocysts replicate open surgical procedures. It is not surprising, therefore, that they are effective. They do require advanced laparoscopic skills, also not available everywhere. Unlike endoscopic procedures, they require general anesthesia and a major operating room setting. They are facilitated by laparoscopic ultrasound for localization and safety, and also by today's advanced endoscopic stapling devices. The surgeon needs to be capable in laparoscopic suturing, and experienced in open pseudocyst surgery. I prefer a transgastric anterior laparoscopic approach for pseudocyst drainage. This is useful and familiar, should conversion to open operation be necessary. The same tenets hold for transmesocolon Roux-en-Y cyst-jejunostomy. An added feature of laparoscopic cyst-enterostomy is the debridement and removal of necrotic cyst content (*Ann Surg* 2002;236:149), something not usually possible with endoscopic techniques. Laparoscopic visualization of the cyst-

visceral anatomy allows for accurate determination of fused "mature" surfaces. This is not foolproof with endoscopic approaches, and after transluminal endoscopic cyst entry, free peritonitis will occur without suitable cyst fusion.

These minimally invasive techniques can have fine long-term outcomes in experienced hands Sharma SS, et al. (*Endoscopy* 2002;34:203), and patient morbidity will be less. Again, I stress multidisciplinary decision-making. Conclusions about reduced costs often neglect the many follow-up radiographic procedures required, but nonetheless, these techniques are probably less expensive. Unusual complications can occur such as stent migration and loss into the cyst, peritonitis, and severe gastric wall bleeding.

Finally, open surgical intervention is still preferred when any question of neoplasia exists. Just as internal drainage of a pancreatic cystic neoplasm is wrong, an attempt to do the same using the endoscope or laparoscope is equally misguided. Recurrence rates will be high and, worse, the potential for malignant transformation might be overlooked. Going forward, however, all of today's less-invasive procedures will still be compared with a successful history of open surgical management for pancreatic pseudocysts.

M.P.C.

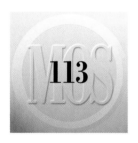

Pancreaticoduodenectomy (Whipple Operation) and Total Pancreatectomy for Cancer

DOUGLAS B. EVANS, JEFFREY E. LEE, ERIC P. TAMM, AND PETER W. T. PISTERS

The standard surgical treatment for adenocarcinoma of the pancreatic head remains the pancreaticoduodenectomy, first described by Whipple et al. in 1935. Their two-stage pancreaticoduodenectomy consisted of biliary diversion and gastrojejunostomy during a first operation and, after the patient recovered (usually about 3 weeks later), resection of the duodenum and pancreatic head. The world experience by 1941 totaled 41 cases, with a perioperative mortality rate of 30%. The original technique did not include reanastomosis of the pancreatic remnant to the small bowel, and the high mortality rate was largely the result of pancreatic fistula from the oversewn pancreatic remnant. Whipple modified his reconstruction in 1941 to include a pancreaticojejunostomy, with the entire procedure done in one operation. In 1946, Waugh and Clagett modified the one-stage procedure to its current form. The goals of surgical therapy outlined by Waugh and Clagett have not changed in the past 50 years: (i) there should be a reasonable opportunity for cure, (ii) the risk of death should not outweigh the prospects for

cure, and (iii) the patient should be left in as normal a condition as possible.

Recent advances in surgical technique, anesthesia, and critical care have resulted in a 30-day in-hospital mortality rate of less than 2% for pancreaticoduodenectomies performed at major referral centers by experienced surgeons. Achieving such a low surgery-related mortality rate appears to be a function of the level of experience of the individual surgeon and institution. Patient selection, preoperative medical evaluation, surgical technique, and postoperative care are all critically important in minimizing patient morbidity and mortality and optimizing long-term oncologic outcome. A reasonable level of experience with major pancreatic resection is thus necessary to achieve good results.

Current treatment strategies for patients with localized pancreatic cancer are based on knowledge of the disease's natural history and patterns of treatment failure. Patients who undergo multimodality therapy that includes pancreaticoduodenectomy for adenocarcinoma of the pancreatic head have a long-term survival

rate of 10% to 20% and a median survival of approximately 24 months. This relatively low cure rate and modest median survival following pancreaticoduodenectomy mandate that treatment-related morbidity be low and treatment-related death is rare. Following pancreaticoduodenectomy for localized pancreatic cancer, local recurrence occurs much too often. Accurate preoperative imaging and proper surgical technique will minimize local recurrence, and the routine use of multimodality therapy (chemotherapy with or without chemoradiation) will maximize survival duration by treating microscopic metastatic disease, which is present in most patients at the time of surgery. Because the goal of therapies directed at the primary tumor is to maximize local-regional tumor control and thereby enhance the quality and duration of patient survival, pancreaticoduodenectomy should be performed only when there is a reasonable expectation that all gross disease can be encompassed within the resection. Operations resulting in grossly positive margins offer no survival benefit to the patient compared with palliative chemotherapy and irradiation. With currently available endoscopic, percutaneous, and laparoscopic methods of biliary decompression, laparotomies in patients with unresectable, locally advanced disease can often be avoided.

This chapter focuses on the proper use of preoperative diagnostic studies and the technical maneuvers involved in the performance of pancreaticoduodenectomy and total pancreatectomy. Investigational techniques for early diagnosis and details on multimodality therapy are beyond the scope of this chapter but have been reviewed in recent publications listed in the Suggested Reading list.

PRETREATMENT DIAGNOSTIC EVALUATION

Current technology allows accurate preoperative radiologic staging and assessment of resectability. There is rarely a need for "exploratory" surgery in the management of patients with biopsy-proven or suspected pancreatic or periampullary cancer.

Our preoperative evaluation includes a careful physical examination, chest radiography, and computed tomography (CT) of the abdomen. The development of multislice or multidetector CT (MDCT) allows imaging of the entire pancreas during peak contrast enhancement. In addition, scan data can be processed to display images in three-dimensional and multiplanar formats. Helical CT performed with contrast enhancement and a thin-section technique can accurately assess the relationship of the low-density tumor to the celiac axis, superior mesenteric artery (SMA), and superior mesenteric–portal vein (SMPV) confluence. For MDCT scanning at our institution, patients receive 1,000 mL of water or a 2% barium sulfate suspension (Readi-CAT; E-Z-EM, Inc., Westbury, NY) to opacify the stomach and small bowel. Noncontrast-enhanced CT scans are then obtained through the liver and pancreas at a slice thickness of 5 mm, contiguous, to localize the pancreas. Intravenous (IV) contrast enhancement is achieved with nonionic contrast material (300 to 320 mg iodine per milliliter) administered by an automatic injector at a rate of 3 to 5 mL/sec for a total of 150 mL.

At least two phases of contrast-enhanced helical scanning are performed. The first (arterial) phase begins 25 seconds after contrast injection and is performed during a 20-second breathhold, with imaging done from the diaphragm through the horizontal portion of the duodenum at a slice thickness of 2.5 mm contiguous, reconstructed to 1.25-mm slice thickness for multiplanar reconstructions. Imaging during this first phase includes the pancreas at 35 to 45 seconds after contrast injection, which, at this rate of contrast injection, optimizes the difference in density between the pancreas and tumor (pancreatic parenchymal phase). The second (venous) phase, which is done to look for metastases in the liver and abdomen, begins 55 seconds after the start of IV contrast injection and covers the entire liver and upper abdomen at a 2.5-mm slice thickness, which is then reconstructed to a 1.25-mm slice thickness.

Our current algorithm for the diagnosis and treatment of patients with presumed or biopsy-proven adenocarcinoma of the pancreatic head or periampullary region is illustrated in Figure 1. Patients with a low-density mass in the pancreatic head on contrast-enhanced CT scans are eligible for preoperative chemoradiation if a tissue diagnosis of malignancy has been obtained. The more widespread use of endoscopic ultrasonography (EUS)-guided fine-needle aspiration (FNA) biopsy will allow the frequent use of preoperative

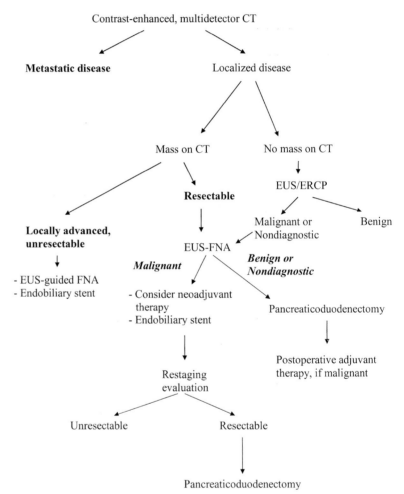

Fig. 1. Management algorithm for patients with suspected or biopsy-proven adenocarcinoma of the pancreatic head or periampullary region. Patients without a histologic or cytologic diagnosis of adenocarcinoma who have a low-attenuation, resectable mass in the pancreatic head on contrast-enhanced computed tomography (CT) undergo endoscopic ultrasonography (EUS)-guided fine-needle aspiration (FNA) biopsy. This management philosophy is based on the ongoing use of protocol-based preoperative chemotherapy with or without chemoradiation at our institution. If preoperative therapy is not considered, biopsy confirmation of adenocarcinoma may be less important. In the absence of a mass on CT, diagnostic EUS is usually performed. When there is no obvious mass to biopsy, or if pretreatment biopsies are nondiagnostic, patients who have clinical and radiologic findings suggestive of a pancreatic or periampullary neoplasm undergo pancreaticoduodenectomy. Endoscopic retrograde cholangiopancreatography (ERCP) is performed in patients with biliary obstruction as both a diagnostic study (when the cause of the biliary obstruction is not apparent), or as a therapeutic modality to place an endobiliary stent when surgery is to be delayed (for the delivery of preoperative therapy).

colic vein is divided proximal to its junction with the SMV. Division of the middle colic vein allows greater exposure of the infrapancreatic SMV and prevents iatrogenic traction injury to the SMV during dissection of the middle colic vein-SMV junction, especially when dealing with large tumors or tumors extending inferiorly from the uncinate process. In fact, the base of the transverse mesocolon and the anterior leaf of the small bowel mesentery can be left attached to the tumor and resected en bloc with the pancreatic head. Such caudal or inferior tumor extension is not a contraindication to pancreaticoduodenectomy but does add complexity to the operation during this step when the infrapancreatic SMV is identified.

Mobilization of the retroperitoneal attachments of the small bowel and right colon mesentery is performed in patients with uncinate tumors extending into the small bowel mesentery and in those patients who require venous resection and reconstruction. This maneuver was first described by Cattell and Braasch for exposure of the duodenum. The visceral peritoneum of the small bowel mesentery is incised to the ligament of Treitz, thereby mobilizing the small bowel mesentery. When complete, this maneuver allows cephalad retraction of the right colon and small bowel, exposing the third and fourth portions of the duodenum.

Occasionally, when there is extensive inflammatory change or scarring at the root of mesentery, usually the result of a prior attempt at resection, we may not identify the SMV early in the operation. In such a case, the SMV will be exposed during step 6 when the pancreas is divided in a caudal direction from the level of the portal vein. This can be a dangerous maneuver because of the lack of vascular control; however, it is a valuable technique for the experienced surgeon who deals with more complicated pancreatic resections, often in the reoperative setting.

2. The Kocher maneuver is begun at the transverse portion (third portion) of the duodenum by identifying the inferior vena cava. All fibrofatty and lymphatic tissue medial to the right ureter and anterior to the inferior vena cava is elevated, along with the pancreatic head and duodenum (Fig. 9). The Kocher maneuver is continued to the left lateral edge of the aorta, with care taken to identify the left renal vein. The right gonadal vein is usually preserved as it courses anterior to the right ureter and serves as a good landmark to help prevent inadvertent injury to the ureter. A complete Kocher maneuver is necessary for the subsequent dissection of the pancreatic head from the SMA (step 6). Particularly important is the division of the leaf of peritoneum that is posterior to the mesenteric vessels; incision of this portion of peritoneum is necessary prior to performing the SMA dissection. Traditionally, the relationship of the tumor to the SMA would be assessed by manual palpation following a completed Kocher maneuver. As previously stated, preoperative MDCT more accurately predicts resectability and obviates this maneuver.

3. The portal dissection is initiated by exposing the common hepatic artery (CHA) proximal and distal to the right gastric artery and the gastroduodenal artery (GDA) (Fig. 10). The CHA is exposed by removing the large lymph node that lies directly anterior to this vessel. The right gastric artery and then the GDA are ligated and divided. The GDA often has a small proximal branch, which may originate anteriorly or just along its lateral border. It is often helpful to ligate and divide this branch separately to obtain adequate length on the proximal GDA to perform a safe ligation and division. If there is tumor extension to within a few millimeters of the GDA origin, one should obtain proximal and distal control of the hepatic artery and divide the GDA flush at its origin. The resulting arteriotomy can be closed with interrupted 6-0 Prolene (Ethicon, Inc., Somerville, NJ) sutures. Overly aggressive dissection at the GDA origin can result in intimal dissection of the hepatic artery; this is usually the result of blunt dissection and inadequate vascular control of the proximal and distal hepatic artery. Dissection of the hepatic artery should be performed with gentle, sharp dissection, especially in patients who have received prior external-beam radiation therapy and in those with extensive scar formation from prior surgery. Division of the GDA allows mobilization of the hepatic (common, proper) artery off of the underlying PV, which can be found within the triangle formed by the CHA, GDA, and superior border of the pancreas. The PV should always be exposed prior to dividing the common hepatic duct. Cholecystectomy is then performed and the common hepatic duct is transected at its junction with the cystic duct.

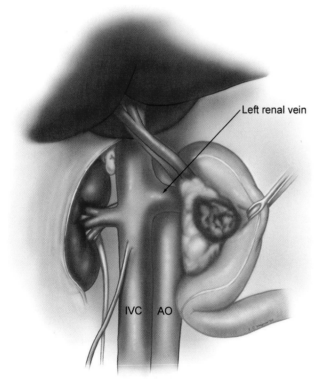

Left renal vein

IVC   AO

Fig. 9. Illustration of step 2. A Kocher maneuver has been performed by first identifying the inferior vena cava (IVC) at the level of the proximal portion of the transverse segment of the duodenum (D3). One can then mobilize the duodenum and pancreatic head off of the IVC in a cephalad direction, thereby removing all soft tissue anterior to the IVC. The right gonadal vein is usually preserved, if possible, as it serves as a good landmark to help prevent inadvertent injury to the underlying ureter (which is usually posterior and slightly lateral to the gonadal vein). Note that the Kocher maneuver is continued to the left lateral border of the aorta (AO). An accessory right renal artery (which is an end artery) may travel anterior to the IVC and should be seen and preserved; rarely, the main right renal artery may be anterior to the IVC.

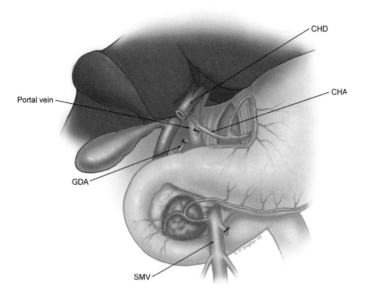

Fig. 10. Illustration of step 3. Dissection of the porta hepatis begins with identification of the common hepatic artery (CHA) by removal of the large lymph node that commonly sits anterior to this vessel. The CHA is then followed distally to allow identification and ligation and division of the right gastric artery (not shown) and the gastroduodenal artery (GDA). This allows the CHA-proper hepatic artery to be mobilized cephalad and medial off of the underlying anterior surface of the portal vein. The portal vein is always identified prior to division of the common hepatic duct (CHD). Careful palpation of the porta hepatis prior to division of the bile duct should alert one to the possibility of an accessory or replaced right hepatic artery traveling posterior to the bile duct and lateral to the portal vein. The CHD is divided at the level of the cystic duct. SMV, superior mesenteric vein.

Review of the preoperative CT scan and careful palpation of the porta hepatis prior to division of the bile duct should alert one to the possibility of anomalous hepatic arterial circulation. A replaced or accessory right hepatic artery arising from the proximal SMA may course posterolaterally to the PV. Rarely, the entire CHA may arise from the SMA (type IX hepatic arterial anatomy). If the foramen of Winslow was initially closed because of adhesions, it should have been re-established at the time of the Kocher maneuver (step 2). Access to the foramen of Winslow is necessary to palpate the porta hepatis and appreciate anomalous hepatic arterial circulation. Rarely, the right hepatic artery arising from the proper hepatic artery courses posterior to the PV. In addition, a low-lying right hepatic artery may be injured when the bile duct is divided in an inflamed porta hepatis. Following transection of the bile duct, bile fluid cultures are sent for evaluation and the indwelling biliary stent, when present, is removed. Intraoperative bile cultures are used to guide therapeutic antibiotic treatment postoperatively in the event of an intra-abdominal or superficial wound infection. When possible, we place a gentle bulldog clamp on

the transected bile duct to prevent bile spillage until the time of bile duct reconstruction.

The anterior wall of the PV is further exposed following division of the common hepatic duct and medial retraction of the CHA. The PV itself should be identified but not extensively mobilized until step 6, at which time the stomach and pancreas have been divided. The superior pancreaticoduodenal vein is a constant venous tributary of the PV, which drains the cephalad aspect of the pancreatic head and is located at the superolateral aspect of the PV. Bleeding caused by traction injury to this venous tributary may be difficult to control at this time in the operation.

4. The stomach is transected with a linear gastrointestinal stapler (Ethicon, Inc.) at the level of the third or fourth transverse vein on the lesser curvature and at the confluence of the gastroepiploic veins on the greater curvature so as to perform a standard antrectomy (Fig. 11). Care should be taken to ligate and divide the terminal branches of the left gastric artery along the lesser curvature of the stomach prior to gastric transection. However, when opening the lesser omentum and one should specifically look for an accessory or replaced left hepatic artery arising from the left gastric artery. Overly aggressive division of the filmy lesser omentum (with the cautery) in a caudal direction

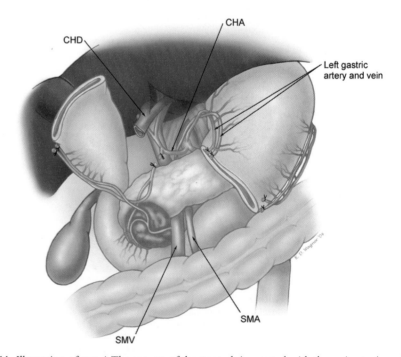

Fig. 11. Illustration of step 4. The antrum of the stomach is resected with the main specimen by dividing the stomach at the level of the third or fourth transverse vein on the lesser curvature. CHD, common hepatic duct; CHA, common hepatic artery; SMV, superior mesenteric vein; SMA, superior mesenteric artery.

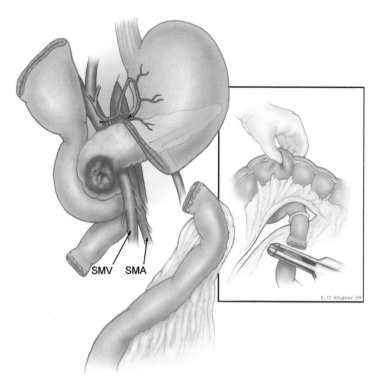

Fig. 12. Illustration of step 5. Transection of the jejunum is followed by ligation and division of its mesentery. The loose attachments of the ligament of Treitz are taken down, and the fourth and third portions of the duodenum are mobilized by dividing their short mesenteric vessels. The duodenum and jejunum are then reflected underneath the mesenteric vessels in preparation for the final and most important part of pancreaticoduodenectomy. SMV, superior mesenteric vein; SMA, superior mesenteric artery.

aorta, allowing the devascularized segment of duodenum and jejunum to be reflected beneath the mesenteric vessels.

6. The most oncologically important and difficult part of the operation is step 6. After traction sutures are placed on the superior and inferior borders of the pancreas, the pancreas is transected with electrocautery at the level of the PV. If there is evidence of tumor adherence to the PV or SMV, the pancreas can be divided at a more distal location in preparation for segmental venous resection. The specimen is separated from the SMV by ligation and division of the small venous tributaries to the uncinate process and pancreatic head (Fig. 13). Complete removal of the uncinate process from the SMV is required for full mobilization of the SMPV confluence and subsequent identification of the SMA. Failure to fully mobilize the SMPV confluence risks injury to the SMA and usually results in a positive margin of resection caused by the incomplete removal of the uncinate process and the mesenteric soft tissue adjacent to the SMA (Fig. 14). In addition, without complete mobilization of the SMV, it is difficult to expose the SMA—a maneuver necessary for direct ligation of the inferior pancreaticoduodenal

can easily injure a replaced left hepatic artery. The omentum is then divided at the level of the greater curvature transection with the harmonic scalpel (Ethicon Inc.). Pylorus preservation may be considered in patients with small periampullary neoplasms, but should not be performed in patients with bulky pancreatic head tumors, duodenal tumors involving the first or second portions of the duodenum, or lesions associated with grossly positive pyloric or peripyloric lymph nodes. To ensure adequate blood supply to the duodenojejunostomy (if pylorus preservation is performed), the anastomosis is created 1.0 to 1.5 cm from the pylorus.

5. The loose attachments of the ligament of Treitz are taken down with care to avoid injury to the inferior mesenteric vein. The jejunum is then transected with a linear gastrointestinal stapler approximately 10 cm distal to the ligament of Treitz, and its mesentery is sequentially ligated and divided (Fig. 12). We prefer to tie the mesenteric (staying) side and use the harmonic scalpel on the serosal (bowel) side. This dissection is continued proximally to involve the fourth and third portions of the duodenum. The duodenal mesentery is divided to the level of the

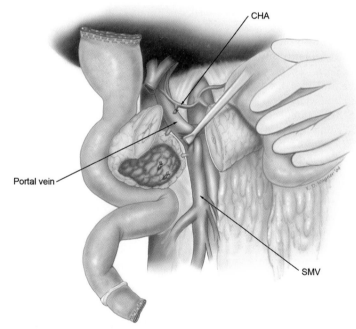

Fig. 13. Illustration of step 6. The pancreatic head and uncinate process are separated from the superior mesenteric-portal vein confluence. The pancreas has been transected at the level of the portal vein and the pancreatic head is reflected laterally, allowing identification of small venous tributaries from the portal vein and superior mesenteric vein (SMV). These tributaries are ligated and divided. There is one fairly constant venous tributary of the portal vein to the most cephalad pancreatic head, often referred to as the superior pancreaticoduodenal vein. Some surgeons prefer to leave this venous branch intact until they have divided at least one of the more caudal inferior pancreaticoduodenal arteries (off of the superior mesenteric artery), thereby minimizing venous hypertension in the specimen, which contributes to increased blood loss during this portion of the dissection. CHA, common hepatic artery.

The Gastrointestinal Tract

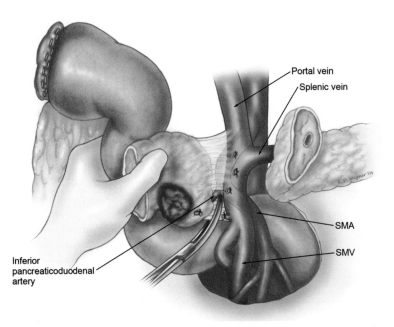

Fig. 14. Illustration of attempted removal of the pancreaticoduodenectomy specimen from the mesenteric vessels without mobilization of the superior mesenteric vein (SMV) and direct identification of the superior mesenteric artery (SMA). This maneuver should not be performed, as it risks injury to the SMA and inadequate control of the inferior pancreaticoduodenal arteries because of their mass ligation with adjacent soft tissue. Failure to directly identify and individually ligate the inferior pancreaticoduodenal arteries is the major cause of postoperative hemorrhage. SMA injury and postoperative hemorrhage are avoidable complications if the SMA is routinely exposed for identification (rather than the surgeon relying on palpation). This technique also facilitates a complete retroperitoneal/mesenteric dissection, minimizing the potential for a margin-positive resection.

SMA, a situation that greatly facilitates this dissection. The jejunal branch usually gives off one or two venous tributaries to the uncinate process; these tributaries should be divided. If tumor involvement of the SMV (at the level of the jejunal branch) prevents dissection of the uncinate process from the SMV, the jejunal branch should be divided. Injury to the distal SMV at this level, or a tangential laceration in its jejunal branch (as it courses posterior to the SMA), is difficult to control and probably represents the most frequent cause of iatrogenic SMA injury as one attempts to suture a venous injury prior to full exposure of the SMA. Once the uncinate process is separated from the distal SMV, medial retraction of the SMPV confluence allows one to expose the SMA. The specimen is then separated from the right lateral wall of the SMA, which is dissected to its origin at the aorta (Fig. 16). Direct exposure of the SMA avoids iatrogenic injury and ensures direct ligation of the inferior pancreaticoduodenal artery or arteries.

Most patients have one or two pancreaticoduodenal arteries that are identified and ligated in continuity at their origins

artery or arteries. Mass ligation of this vessel (or vessels) with mesenteric soft tissue is the major cause of postoperative hemorrhage as this vessel retracts from its poorly placed tie or ligature.

Once the pancreatic head and uncinate process are completely separated from the SMV and SMPV confluence, one may experience bleeding from the specimen because of the resulting venous hypertension (the inferior pancreaticoduodenal arteries from the SMA are still intact). One option we occasionally employ is to leave the superior pancreaticoduodenal vein (located at the superolateral aspect of the PV) intact until the more caudal inferior pancreaticoduodenal artery is ligated. This usually does not limit the mobilization of the SMV at the level of the uncinate process and therefore still allows exposure of the SMA.

Proper mobilization of the SMV involves identification of the jejunal branch of the SMV (referred to by some as the first jejunal branch). This branch originates from the right posterolateral aspect of the SMV (at the level of the uncinate process), travels posterior to the SMA, and enters the medial (proximal) aspect of the jejunal mesentery (Fig. 15). Very rarely, the jejunal branch may course anterior to the

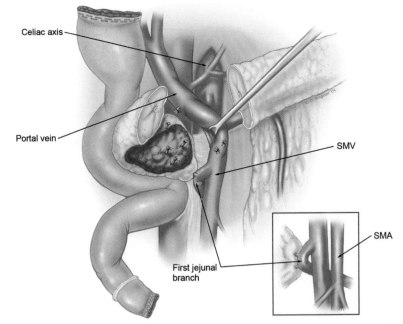

Fig. 15. Illustration of the important surgical anatomy of the superior mesenteric vein (SMV) at the level of the uncinate process. The SMV usually bifurcates into two main branches, one to the ileum and one to the jejunum. Adequate venous return from the small bowel requires that one or the other of these two main SMV tributaries is intact. The jejunal branch of the SMV (often referred to as the first jejunal branch) drains the proximal jejunum, travels posterior to the superior mesenteric artery (SMA), and enters the SMV along its posterolateral wall. The jejunal branch usually has a few venous tributaries that drain the uncinate process *(inset)*. If necessary, the jejunal branch can be divided. The most feared complication during this part of the operation is a tangential laceration of the jejunal branch extending posterior to the SMA. In an attempt to control such an injury, poorly placed sutures may result in an injury to the SMA. Rarely the jejunal branch will travel anterior to the SMA, which simplifies this part of the operation.

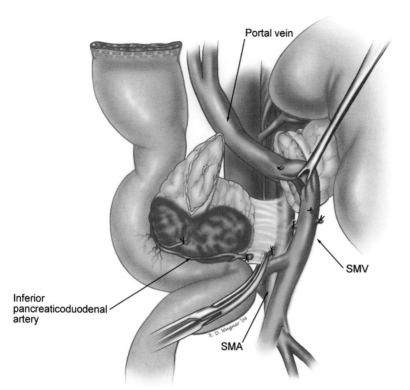

Fig. 16. Illustration of the continuation of step 6, and the final step in resection of the specimen. Medial retraction of the superior mesenteric-portal vein confluence facilitates dissection of the soft tissues adjacent to the lateral wall of the proximal superior mesenteric artery (SMA); this site represents the SMA margin. The inferior pancreaticoduodenal artery (or arteries) is identified at its origin from the SMA, ligated, and divided. SMV, superior mesenteric vein.

from the SMA. Failure to accurately identify and ligate these vessels may be a common cause of early postoperative bleeding. As mentioned previously, the soft tissue adjacent to the proximal SMA represents the SMA (or retroperitoneal) margin. A grossly positive SMA margin should not occur if high-quality preoperative imaging is performed. A microscopically positive SMA margin will occur in 10% to 20% of cases; margin positivity can result from tumor spread along perineural sheaths and does not always result from direct extension of the primary tumor.

Frozen-section evaluation of the pancreaticoduodenectomy specimen is limited to analysis of the pancreatic and common hepatic duct transection margins. Positive resection margins on the bile or pancreatic duct mandate further resection until clear margins are achieved. However, changes caused by pancreatitis should not be confused with margin positivity. Pancreatitis usually involves the entire body and tail of the pancreas distal to the tumor within the pancreatic head. This may result in dysplastic cells at the pancreatic transection margin on frozen-section evaluation. Further resection of the pancreas should be performed only if there is

histologic evidence of invasive carcinoma (on frozen-section analysis) at the margin; dysplasia in the absence of carcinoma is not an indication for further pancreatic resection. Invasive carcinoma extending along the main pancreatic duct is uncommon.

Complete permanent-section analysis of the pancreaticoduodenectomy specimen requires that it be oriented for the pathologist to enable accurate assessment of the SMA margin of excision and other standard pathologic variables. Because we remove all tissue to the right of the SMA, further resection at this margin is not possible. However, the SMA margin must be identified and inked with the pathologist; it cannot be assessed retrospectively.

The operation as described here emphasizes full mobilization of the SMPV confluence, exposure of the SMA, and removal of all mesenteric soft tissue and perineural tissue to the right of this vessel. The high incidence of local recurrence following pancreaticoduodenectomy mandates that greater attention be paid to the SMA margin (the soft tissue margin along the right lateral border of the proximal 3 to 4 cm of the SMA). During step

6 of pancreaticoduodenectomy, full mobilization of the SMPV confluence is necessary to allow complete exposure of the SMA. Dissection of the specimen from the proximal SMA is necessary to obtain a negative SMA margin; therefore, this is the most important technical aspect of this operation. Direct exposure of the SMA should be a routine part of pancreaticoduodenectomy, will minimize the risk for iatrogenic injury of this vessel, and will ensure direct ligation of the inferior pancreaticoduodenal artery(s), thereby minimizing the risk for postoperative intra-abdominal hemorrhage.

Vascular Resection

It is important to emphasize the distinction between regional pancreatectomy and pancreaticoduodenectomy with segmental resection of the SMV or SMPV confluence. We do not consider venous resection as an attempt to improve en bloc lymphatic and soft tissue clearance, as is performed in regional pancreatectomy. It is unlikely that larger local-regional resections (to the left of the SMA and celiac axis) in poorly selected patients with advanced disease will have an impact on survival. Venous resection should be performed only in carefully selected patients who have tumor adherence to the SMV or SMPV confluence but no evidence of tumor extension to the SMA or celiac axis. Because the need for venous resection is unexpected in many patients and is discovered only after gastric and pancreatic transection, when nonresectional procedures are no longer an option, surgeons who perform pancreaticoduodenectomies should be familiar with standard vascular techniques for resection and reconstruction of the SMPV confluence.

Steps 1 through 5 of pancreaticoduodenectomy are completed as described. Before segmental resection of the SMPV confluence and tumor removal, the right colon is returned to its normal anatomic position, removing the clockwise twist in the mesentery that often occurs during the retroperitoneal/mesenteric dissection. Tumor adherence to the lateral wall of the SMPV confluence prevents dissection of the SMV and PV off of the pancreatic head and uncinate process, thereby inhibiting medial retraction of the SMPV confluence (and lateral retraction of the specimen). The standard technique for segmental venous resection involves transection of the splenic vein. Division of the splenic vein allows complete exposure of the SMA medial to

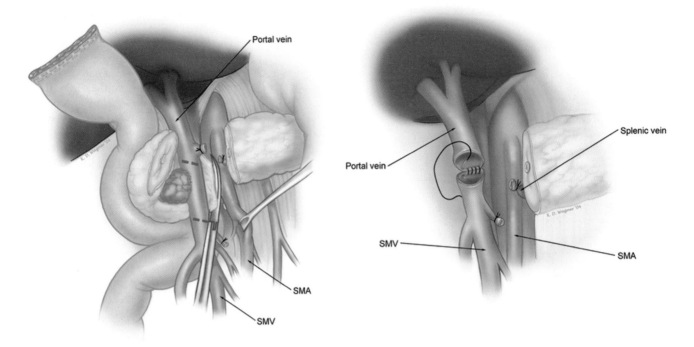

Fig. 17. Illustration of the final step in pancreaticoduodenectomy when segmental venous resection is required and the decision is made to divide the splenic vein. In the early experience with resection and reconstruction of the superior mesenteric-portal vein confluence, splenic vein ligation was routine. Currently, we ligate the splenic vein only when the tumor involves the splenic vein confluence. By dividing the splenic vein, the superior mesenteric artery (SMA), which is identified medial to the superior mesenteric vein (SMV), can be exposed to its origin from the aorta and the pancreatic head removed from the right lateral border of the SMA. This dissection is considerably more difficult when the splenic vein-SMV-portal vein confluence is intact. The tumor is then attached only by the superior mesenteric-portal vein confluence, which can be divided proximally and distally to the involved segment. Reconstruction is performed (during inflow occlusion) by an end-to-end anastomosis of the portal vein and the SMV with interrupted 6-0 Prolene sutures. The anastomosis can be run (as shown) or interrupted. The authors frequently interrupt the anastomosis, especially when there is a size discrepancy between the portal vein and the SMV.

the SMV and provides increased SMV and PV length (as they are no longer tethered by the splenic vein) for a primary venous anastomosis following segmental resection (Fig. 17).

The retroperitoneal dissection is completed by sharply dividing the soft tissues anterior to the aorta and to the right of the exposed SMA; the specimen is then attached only by the SMPV confluence. Vascular clamps are placed 2 to 3 cm proximal (on the PV) and distal (on the SMV) to the involved venous segment, and the vein is transected, allowing tumor removal. A generous 2- to 3-cm segment of SMPV confluence can be resected without the need for interposition grafting if the splenic vein is divided. Venous resection is always performed with inflow occlusion of the SMA to prevent small bowel edema (which makes pancreatic and biliary reconstruction more difficult). Systemic heparinization is employed prior to occluding the SMA if coagulation function is normal at this point in the operation. The free ends of the vein are reapproximated using interrupted sutures of 6-0 Prolene.

Contrary to previously published reports, we have seen upper gastrointestinal hemorrhage caused by sinistral portal hypertension following splenic vein ligation. This usually results when both the splenic and the inferior mesenteric veins are ligated because the inferior mesenteric vein enters the portion of SMV to be resected. When the inferior mesenteric vein enters the splenic vein, it provides a route for collateral venous flow out of the splenic vein in a retrograde fashion. Therefore, in contrast to the standard technique of venous resection previously described, we currently preserve the splenic vein-PV junction whenever possible, especially if the inferior mesenteric vein needs to be ligated and divided. Splenic vein preservation is possible only when tumor invasion of the SMV or PV does not involve the splenic vein confluence (Fig. 18). Preservation of the splenic vein-SMV-PV confluence significantly limits the mobilization of the PV and prevents primary anastomosis of the SMV (following segmental SMV resection) unless segmental resection is limited to 2 cm or less. There-

fore, in most patients who undergo SMV resection with splenic vein preservation, an interposition graft is required. Our preferred conduit for interposition grafting is the internal jugular vein. Preservation of the splenic vein adds significant complexity to venous resection because it prevents direct access to the most proximal 4 to 5 cm of the SMA (medial to the SMV). Venous resection and reconstruction can be performed either before the specimen has been separated from the right lateral wall of the SMA or after complete mesenteric dissection by separating the specimen first from the SMA. Both techniques require significant experience with pancreaticoduodenectomy and are described in detail in previous publications (see "Suggested Reading"). The different forms of venous resection and reconstruction that we have used are illustrated in Figure 19.

An aberrant right hepatic artery may arise from the SMA as an accessory right hepatic artery (type VI, VII, or VIIIb hepatic arterial anatomy), in which case a normal right hepatic artery also arises

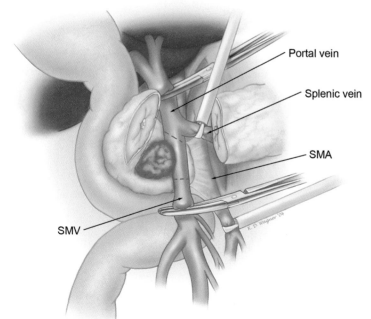

Fig. 18. An illustration of resection of the superior mesenteric vein (SMV) with splenic vein preservation. The intact splenic vein tethers the portal vein, making a primary anastomosis impossible in most cases. With the splenic vein intact, one cannot complete the dissection of the specimen from the right lateral border of the superior mesenteric artery (SMA) to the origin of this vessel in standard fashion. Therefore, options include either placing the graft prior to specimen removal or separation of the pancreatic head from the SMA by medial rotation of the specimen, as described by Leach et al. Segmental resection of the SMV with splenic vein preservation adds significant complexity to this operation but prevents the potential complications of hypersplenism (which may result in mild-to-significant thrombocytopenia, thereby possibly complicating the delivery of cytotoxic chemotherapy) and sinistral portal hypertension (with the risk for gastroesophageal varices and hemorrhage).

from the celiac axis; ligation of the accessory artery in such a case would not affect hepatic or bile duct arterial flow. A replaced right hepatic artery arising from the SMA (type III or VIIIa), unlike an accessory right hepatic artery, represents the only direct arterial inflow to the right hepatic lobe. Because the right and left hepatic arteries communicate within the liver, ligation of the right hepatic artery should be tolerated, assuming a normal level of serum bilirubin and normal flow in the PV. However, because the proximal bile duct receives virtually all of its arterial supply from the right hepatic artery following interruption of cephalad flow from the GDA, it has been our practice to revascularize this vessel when possible. Although an aberrant hepatic artery arising from the SMA is prone to tumor encasement at the posterosuperior border of the pancreatic head, it has been our experience that pancreaticoduodenectomy in this situation rarely requires removal of

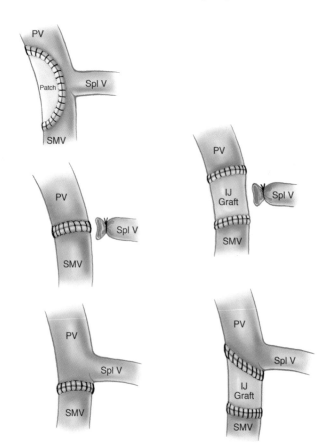

Fig. 19. Illustration of the different types of venous reconstruction used at the time of pancreaticoduodenectomy. When a patch is needed, we use the saphenous vein; when an interposition graft is needed, we use the left internal jugular (IJ) vein. PV, portal vein; Spl V, splenic vein; SMV, superior mesenteric vein. (Modified from Tseng JF, Raut CP, Lee JE, et al. Pancreaticoduodenectomy with vascular resection: margin status and survival duration. *J Gastrointest Surg* 2004;8:935.)

this vessel because the majority of resectable tumors are located more anteriorly in the pancreatic head or uncinate process. Rarely, the entire CHA may arise from the SMA (type IX). Failure to recognize this anatomic variant and inadvertent ligation of the hepatic artery may result in fatal hepatic necrosis.

Celiac axis stenosis with compensatory retrograde flow in the GDA from the SMA may result from atherosclerotic disease, median arcuate ligament syndrome, or inflammatory entrapment. We always assess the hepatic artery pulse at the time of surgery; if the pulse is noted to significantly decrease in intensity or disappear on ligation of the GDA, the CHA is then dissected to its origin at the celiac axis in an attempt to differentiate extrinsic compression from atherosclerotic disease. If flow is not improved, we proceed with a reversed saphenous vein interposition graft between the aorta and the hepatic artery at the site of the GDA origin (Fig. 20). This event is infrequent; however, a clearly defined strategy for intraoperative management is required.

Pancreatic, Biliary, and Gastrointestinal Reconstruction

Reconstruction after pancreaticoduodenectomy proceeds first with the pancreatic anastomosis.

1. The pancreatic remnant is mobilized from the retroperitoneum and splenic vein for a distance of 2 to 3 cm. Failure to adequately mobilize the pancreatic remnant results in poor suture placement at the pancreaticojejunal anastomosis. Injury to the proximal splenic artery can occur when mobilizing the pancreatic remnant if one does not appreciate the location of this vessel. The transected jejunum is brought through a generous incision in the transverse mesocolon to the left of the middle colic vessels. We prefer to bring the jejunum retrocolic rather than retroperitoneal (posterior to the mesenteric vessels in the bed of the resected duodenum). A two-layer, end-to-side, duct-to-mucosa panceaticojejunostomy is performed over a small Silastic stent (Dow Corning, Midland, MI) (Fig. 21). If the pancreatic duct is dilated, a stent is not employed. Following completion of the posterior row of interrupted 4-0 seromuscular monofilament sutures, a small full-thickness opening is made in the bowel. The anastomosis between the pancreatic duct and the small bowel mucosa is completed with 4-0 or 5-0 monofilament sutures. Each stitch incorporates a generous bite of the pancreatic

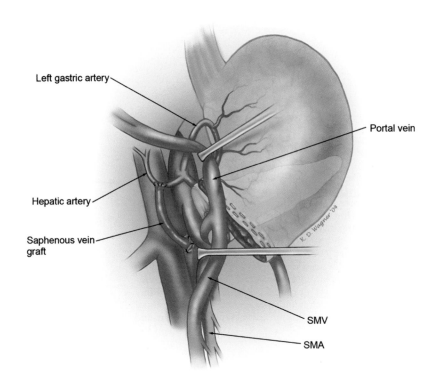

Fig. 20. Illustration of our preferred method of celiac revascularization using a reversed saphenous vein graft between the aorta and the origin of the gastroduodenal artery. SMV, superior mesenteric vein; SMA, superior mesenteric artery. (Modified from Evans DB, Lee JE, Leach SD, et al. Vascular resection and intraoperative radiation therapy during pancreaticoduodenectomy: rationale and technique. *Adv Surg* 1996;29:253.)

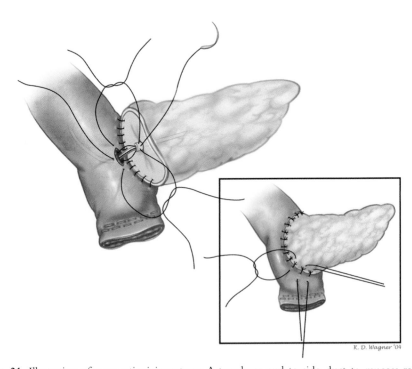

Fig. 21. Illustration of pancreaticojejunostomy. A two-layer, end-to-side, duct-to-mucosa retrocolic pancreaticojejunostomy is performed with (when the pancreatic duct is not dilated) or without a small stent. When used, the stent (4 to 5 cm long) is sewn to the jejunum with a single absorbable monofilament suture. Inset shows the completed anastomosis with an anterior layer of interrupted sutures.

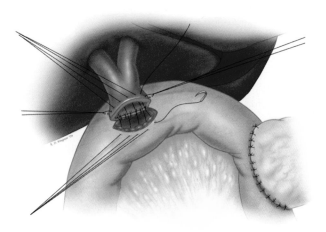

Fig. 22. Illustration of hepaticojejunostomy. A one-layer, end-to-side hepaticojejunostomy is performed with 4-0 or 5-0 absorbable monofilament sutures distal to the pancreaticojejunostomy. A stent is rarely placed in this anastomosis. Care is taken to allow enough distance between the pancreatic and biliary anastomoses so the falciform ligament can be placed between the anastomoses anterior to the hepatic artery and posterior to the jejunal limb.

duct and a full-thickness bite of the jejunum. The posterior knots are tied on the inside, and the lateral and anterior knots are tied on the outside. Prior to the anterior sutures being tied, the stent is placed across the anastomosis so that it extends into the pancreatic duct and small bowel for a distance of approximately 2 to 3 cm. The anastomosis is completed with placement of an anterior row of 4-0 seromuscular monofilament sutures. When the pancreatic parenchyma is soft, we often use vascular pledgets for the anterior row of sutures to prevent them from causing a tear in the pancreatic tissue.

When the pancreatic duct is not dilated and/or the pancreatic substance is soft (not fibrotic), one can perform a two-layer anastomosis that invaginates the cut end of the pancreas into the jejunum. The outer posterior row of 4-0 sutures is placed as outlined previously. The bowel is then opened for a length equal to the transverse diameter of the pancreatic remnant. Using a running, double-armed, 4-0 nonabsorbable monofilament suture, the pancreatic remnant is sewn to the jejunum. The anastomosis is completed with placement of an anterior row of 4-0 seromuscular sutures. However, we rarely use this technique because even a nondilated pancreatic duct can usually be anastomosed using the duct-to-mucosa technique.

2. A single-layer biliary anastomosis is performed using interrupted 4-0 absorbable monofilament sutures (Fig. 22). It is important to align the jejunum with the bile duct to avoid tension on the pancreatic and biliary anastomoses. A stent is rarely used in the construction of the hepaticojejunostomy.

3. An antecolic, end-to-side gastrojejunostomy is constructed in two layers. Starting from the greater curvature, 6 to 8 cm of the gastric staple line is removed. A posterior row of 3-0 silk sutures is followed by a full-thickness inner layer of running monofilament sutures; the anterior row of silk sutures completes the anastomosis. The distance between the biliary and gastric anastomoses should be at least 50 cm, thereby allowing the jejunum to assume its antecolic position (for the gastrojejunostomy) without tension, and also preventing bile reflux cholangitis. We prefer an antecolic gastrojejunostomy to prevent possible outlet obstruction caused by the colonic mesentery. Lastly, the jejunal limb should be aligned so that the efferent limb is adjacent to the greater curvature of the stomach. A No. 10 French feeding jejunostomy tube may be placed distal to the gastrojejunostomy. We rarely use a gastrostomy tube for postoperative gastric decompression.

Prior to abdominal closure, the abdomen is carefully irrigated in all four quadrants. In patients with a previous indwelling endobiliary stent, the bile is contaminated and often has had free access to at least the right upper quadrant of the abdomen; careful irrigation may prevent postoperative infectious complications. In addition, in patients who have contaminated bile from an endobiliary stent or a previous biliary bypass, we often place one drain in the right upper quadrant; we no longer place a drain near the pancreatic anastomosis. The use of drains remains an active area of controversy in the field of pancreatic surgery, and many surgeons still drain the pancreaticojejunostomy. Finally, we place the mobilized falciform ligament (carefully preserved when the abdomen was opened) between the hepatic artery, at the level of the GDA stump, and the afferent jejunal limb to cover the GDA stump (Fig. 23). This is one simple strategy to

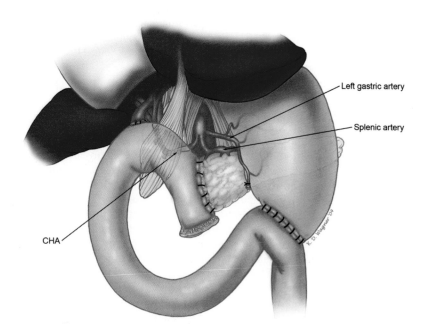

Fig. 23. Illustration of the completed reconstruction after pancreaticoduodenectomy. The falciform ligament, mobilized on opening the abdomen, is placed over the hepatic artery to cover the stump of the gastroduodenal artery, thereby separating the hepatic artery from the afferent jejunal limb. We are careful to leave at least 50 cm between the biliary and the gastric anastomoses to prevent the possible complication of reflux cholangitis. CHA, common hepatic artery.

The Gastrointestinal Tract

minimize the risk for pseudoaneurysm formation at the site of the GDA stump in the event of a pancreatic anastomotic leak and resultant abscess formation.

Pylorus Preservation

Preservation of the antropyloroduodenal segment in combination with pancreatico-duodenectomy was first described by Traverso and Longmire in 1978. Since then, increasing numbers of pancreatic surgeons have employed this modification of the procedure, particularly for patients with benign disease or small periampullary neoplasms. Proponents of this technique argue that preservation of the antropyloric pump mechanism results in improved long-term upper gastrointestinal tract function with enhanced weight gain and few nutritional sequelae. Detractors of pylorus preservation counter that the reported improvements in gastrointestinal and nutritional functions are small, if any, and that they come at the expense of an increased incidence of early postoperative delayed gastric emptying. Further, leaving the distal stomach and duodenum may compromise margins of excision and prevent adequate peripyloric lymphadenectomy. Published data to date involve retrospective comparisons that have yielded mixed results. Despite the controversy, most pancreatic surgeons would agree that pylorus preservation should not be performed for patients with bulky tumors of the pancreatic head, duodenal tumors involving the first or second portions of the duodenum, or lesions associated with grossly positive pyloric or peripyloric lymph nodes.

The steps in pylorus-preserving pancreaticoduodenectomy are identical to those in standard pancreaticoduodenectomy except in the approach to the antrum, pylorus, and duodenum (steps 3 and 4). Pylorus preservation involves not only simple proximal division of the gastrointestinal tract beyond the pylorus but, more critically, preservation of sufficient blood supply to the proximal duodenum and preservation of vagal innervation to the antrum and pylorus. Therefore, appropriate caution must be exercised during the portal dissection to avoid unnecessary injury to the nerves of Latarjet. This is the fundamental technical difference in the pylorus-preserving procedure and is essential to avoid postoperative gastroparesis.

The duodenum is divided approximately 2 to 3 cm beyond the pylorus with the linear gastrointestinal stapler and the gastroepiploic arcade divided at that level. The staple line is removed prior to performance of the

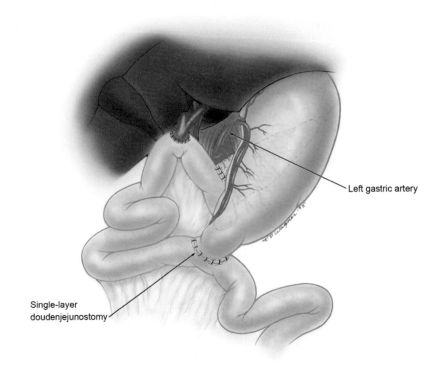

Fig. 24. Illustration of the completed reconstruction following pylorus-preserving pancreaticoduodenectomy. The duodenojejunostomy can be placed either retrocolic or antecolic (colon not shown in this illustration); we prefer an antecolic anastomosis so that there is no potential for obstruction of the jejunum as it exits the transverse mesocolon. When pylorus preservation is performed, we often place a jejunostomy tube distal to the duodenojejunostomy because of the concern for poor gastric emptying in the first few weeks following surgery.

duodenojejunostomy so as to leave approximately 2 cm of duodenum distal to the pylorus. A short segment of duodenum ensures adequate vascularity of the remaining duodenum. The duodenojejunostomy is performed in an end-to-side fashion using a single-layer technique with monofilament absorbable sutures (Fig. 24).

TOTAL PANCREATECTOMY

Total pancreatectomy is rarely required for adenocarcinoma of the pancreas. Adenocarcinomas arising in the neck, body, and tail of the pancreas are usually locally advanced at the time of diagnosis and not amenable to complete surgical resection. Adenocarcinoma of the body and tail of the pancreas is diagnosed late in the disease course of patients with this cancer because of the absence of biliary obstruction. The presenting complaints of most patients with pancreatic body and tail tumors are pain and gastrointestinal dysfunction resulting from tumor invasion of the neural plexus surrounding the celiac axis and SMA, symptoms that should alert the surgeon to the potential for celiac or SMA encasement.

Total pancreatectomy is accomplished by performing dissection of the proximal

splenic artery and dissection of the left upper quadrant of the abdomen, following step 3 of our six-step pancreaticoduodenectomy. After identification of the infrapancreatic SMV and completion of the portal dissection, the proximal splenic artery is exposed and, if possible, ligated (but often not divided). The greater omentum is separated from the left side of the transverse colon, and the splenic flexure is mobilized. The peritoneum lateral to the spleen is then incised in a cephalad direction to the gastroesophageal junction. The short gastric vessels are ligated and divided, allowing medial and cephalad retraction of the stomach (Fig. 25). Mobilization of the spleen and pancreas from their retroperitoneal attachments to the kidney and adrenal gland is then completed. The inferior mesenteric vein is divided if it enters the splenic vein, and the mesenteric root divided from the left lateral border of the SMV to the left lateral border of the aorta, staying anterior to the SMA. Exposure of the SMA inferior to the neck of the pancreas will allow the dissection to proceed directly anterior to this vessel under direct vision. Division of the splenic vein is often delayed until the completion of steps 4 (gastric or duodenal transection) and 5 (ligament of Treitz,

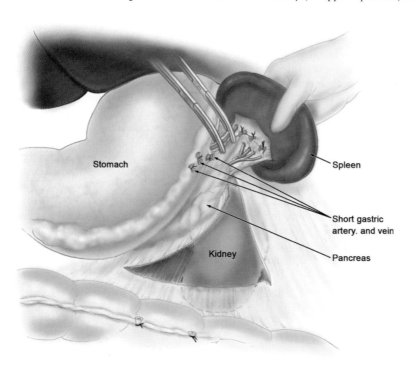

Fig. 25. Illustration demonstrating mobilization of the spleen and distal pancreas followed by ligation and division of the short gastric vessels as performed in total pancreatectomy. This allows the stomach to be separated from the spleen, which facilitates completion of the dissection of the spleen and pancreas from their retroperitoneal attachments.

proximal jejunum and duodenum). Then, in preparation for completion of the retroperitoneal dissection, the spleen and distal pancreas are again reflected medially, exposing the origin of the splenic vein-SMV junction; the splenic vein is then ligated and divided (Fig. 26). The splenic artery origin may not be adequately exposed until this time; if so, we always try

to divide the splenic artery before the splenic vein to minimize blood loss.

When dealing with tumors in the pancreatic neck, there are two technical points worthy of note.

1. Preservation of islet cell function is particularly important in younger patients with cystic or solid pseudopapillary neoplasms and islet cell tumors. When a tumor arises in the pancreatic neck or proximal body of the pancreas, a complete distal pancreatectomy may leave only a small portion of pancreatic head and uncinate process; the patient may not have adequate islet cell mass for normal glucose metabolism and therefore may require insulin injections. Accordingly, in patients with relatively small tumors of the pancreatic neck of favorable histology (i.e., neuroendocrine carcinoma, solid pseudopapillary neoplasm, mucinous cystic neoplasm), segmental resection of the pancreatic neck and proximal body with preservation of the splenic artery and vein (when possible) is preferred to ensure adequate islet cell reserve. Reconstruction requires Roux-en-Y pancreaticojejunostomy to the remaining segment of distal pancreas.

2. When anticipating the need for distal pancreatectomy in the rare patient with potentially resectable adenocarcinoma of the pancreatic neck, the surgeon should avoid having to perform unnecessary total pancreatectomy because of an unexpected positive proximal transection margin in the pancreatic head. In such a situation, it may be unclear both on preoperative CT scans and at the time of surgery whether the patient should undergo extended right (pancreaticoduodenectomy) or left (distal pancreatectomy) pancreatectomy. Because of the appropriate desire to perform the less-complicated (and potentially less-morbid) procedure, one might elect to perform distal pancreatectomy, only to discover on frozen-section analysis that the pancreatic transection margin is positive and, thus, that completion pancreaticoduodenectomy is needed. This situation can be avoided by completing the proximal pancreatic transection prior to committing to distal pancreatectomy. Frozen-section analysis of the proximal transection margin, if negative, enables one to perform a negative-margin distal pancreatectomy. A positive proximal transection margin indicates the need for extended pancreaticoduodenectomy. In either situation, total pancreatectomy is not necessary.

When distal pancreatectomy is performed, it is important that the site of pancreatic transection be closed with a technique—either suture or staple—that will

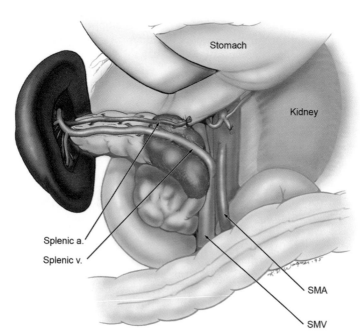

Fig. 26. Illustration demonstrating medial rotation of the spleen and distal pancreas as performed when completing total pancreatectomy. The splenic artery has been divided in preparation for division of the splenic vein at its junction with the superior mesenteric vein (SMV). It is important not to narrow the SMV during ligation of the splenic vein. The authors prefer to close the SMV-splenic vein junction with a running 6-0 Prolene suture or the vascular linear stapling device. SMA, superior mesenteric artery.

minimize the potential for pancreatic leak. The most important factor is identification and suture ligation of the pancreatic duct. For those who prefer to staple the pancreas, note that the staple line secures the pancreatic duct, prevents its retraction into the pancreatic substance, and allows its identification; a 5-0 monofilament suture can then be used to close the pancreatic duct. The staple line is then reinforced with 5-0 monofilament sutures on pledgets. However, when the pancreas is divided just medial to the intrapancreatic portion of the common bile duct, the pancreatic transection line is too thick for a stapling devise. Again, identification of the pancreatic duct is critical to prevent pancreatic leak. When performing distal pancreatectomy, we routinely bring the mobilized falciform ligament through the lesser omentum and allow it to cover the stump of the splenic artery and the pancreatic transaction site, which is analogous to the use of the falciform ligament following pancreaticoduodenectomy, discussed previously.

PERIOPERATIVE MANAGEMENT AND COMPLICATIONS

As with all complex surgery, a good outcome after pancreatectomy depends on meticulous perioperative care. We routinely use combined epidural-general anesthesia, we monitor hemodynamics with an arterial line, and most patients receive a central venous catheter. Pulmonary artery catheters are rarely used. All postoperative pancreatectomy patients are managed overnight in the recovery room and transferred to the floor on postoperative day 1. A short course of perioperative antibiotic coverage is used, but prolonged postoperative IV antibiotic use in the absence of documented or suspected infection is discouraged.

The pancreatic anastomosis is not routinely drained. A lateral subhepatic drain is often placed, especially in patients with indwelling endobiliary stents or in those who had a previous biliary bypass because of the presence of contaminated bile. The right upper quadrant drain is removed on postoperative day 2 if the output is less than 200 mL per 24 hours. Sips of clear liquids are allowed on postoperative day 1; solid food is provided after the nasogastric tube is removed. In those patients who undergo a pylorus-preserving pancreaticoduodenectomy, jejunostomy tubes are often used because of the known difficulty with early gastric emptying. In such patients, jejunostomy feeding provides adequate nutritional support; there is no urgency to rapidly advance oral intake. Jejunostomy feeding is initiated at a rate of 10 mL per hour on postoperative day 2 or 3 and then increased daily if gastrointestinal function has returned. With the institution of an oral diet, jejunostomy feeding is converted from continuous to nighttime administration. Patients are routinely discharged while receiving supplemental continuous or nighttime jejunostomy feedings.

Postoperative fevers occurring after postoperative days 3 to 4 demand careful evaluation. Potential sources of fever include those that are common to all major abdominal surgery: pneumonia, deep venous thrombosis, central line sepsis, urinary tract infection, and wound infection. Patients who undergo pancreaticojejunostomy are at risk for the development of intra-abdominal abscess as a result of leakage from the pancreatic anastomosis. Because leaks from either the biliary or gastric anastomoses are very uncommon, intra-abdominal sepsis is considered to be caused by a pancreatic anastomotic leak, until proven otherwise. The study of choice for evaluation of presumed intra-abdominal sepsis is CT of the abdomen and pelvis with oral and IV administration of contrast material. The finding of a localized fluid collection in the region of the pancreaticojejunostomy should be considered for CT-guided aspiration.

We are selective in our use of CT-guided aspiration based on the general condition of the patient, standard laboratory evaluation (especially the degree of leukocytosis), and the presence or absence of an air-fluid level in the fluid collection. Percutaneous catheter drainage is indicated if the aspirated fluid appears infected grossly or on Gram stain. It is common to identify nonloculated ascitic fluid on postoperative CT scans in patients who have undergone pancreatectomy; this finding rarely represents infection or anastomotic leak and does not demand aspiration or drainage unless clinical signs of sepsis persist and another source of infection has not been identified. Pancreaticojejunostomy-related anastomotic leaks generally close once adequate drainage is established. We commonly use octreotide and antibiotics when treating established pancreatic anastomotic leaks that have required percutaneous drainage.

Postoperative gastrointestinal or drain tract bleeding should prompt immediate evaluation with arteriography. Although uncommon, an arterial-enteric fistula occasionally occurs in the postoperative setting (rarely before postoperative day 10). The most common cause is a pancreatic anastomotic leak with surrounding inflammation and infection, resulting in blowout of the ligated GDA stump. Gastrointestinal or drain tract bleeding represents a true emergency; the only patients likely to survive are those in whom the diagnosis is made immediately. Experience with this complication is anecdotal, but we would proceed with embolization of the hepatic artery at the time of diagnostic arteriography; endovascular stent placement may be an alternative. Surgical control of hemorrhage from the stump of the GDA is exceedingly difficult in a postoperative pancreaticoduodenectomy patient and, in our opinion, carries a higher mortality rate than that associated with hepatic artery embolization.

Patients are ready for discharge when they are afebrile, independent with the majority of self-care activities, and have adequate caloric intake from a combination of oral and jejunostomy feedings. Patients are discharged with a regimen of pancreatic enzyme replacement and a proton-pump inhibitor.

SUMMARY

A detailed preoperative assessment of resectability prevents needless laparotomy in patients with advanced pancreatic cancer, and a standardized technique of tumor resection minimizes perioperative complications. We recommend dividing pancreaticoduodenectomy into six well-defined maneuvers. Attention to detail and a standardized approach to postoperative care minimize patient morbidity and hospital stay.

Future progress in the treatment of pancreatic cancer will involve techniques for early diagnosis and effective systemic therapy. For now, the best results can be achieved by careful attention to patient selection, preoperative assessment of resectability, surgical technique, and postoperative care.

ACKNOWLEDGMENT

The authors thank Kathleen Wagner, senior medical illustrator at The University of Texas M. D. Anderson Cancer Center, Houston, who has created all of the illustrations used in the publications of the Pancreatic Cancer Working Group during the past 15 years.

SUGGESTED READING

Bilimoria MM, Cormier JN, Mun Y, et al. Pancreatic leak after left pancreatectomy is reduced following main pancreatic duct ligation. *Br J Surg* 2003;90:190.

Cattell RB, Braasch JW. A technique for the exposure of the third and fourth portions of the duodenum. *Surg Gynecol Obstet* 1960; 111:378.

Greene FL, Page DL, Fleming ID, et al. *AJCC cancer staging manual,* 6th ed. New York: Springer-Verlag, 2002.

Leach SD, Davidson BS, Ames FC, et al. Alternative method for exposure of the retropancreatic mesenteric vasculature during total pancreatectomy. *J Surg Oncol* 1996; 61:163.

Lowy AM, Lee JE, Pisters PWT, et al. Prospective, randomized trial of octreotide to prevent pancreatic fistula after pancreaticoduodenectomy for malignant disease. *Ann Surg* 1997;226:632.

Mullen JT, Lee JH, Gomez HF, et al. Pancreaticoduodenectomy after placement of endobiliary metal stents. *J Gastrointest Surg* 2005;9:1094. Pisters PWT, Lee JE, Vauthey JN, et al. Laparoscopy in the staging of pancreatic cancer. *Brit J Surg* 2001;88:325-337.

Pisters PWT, Wolff RA, Crane CH, Evans DB. Combined-modality treatment for operable pancreatic adenocarcinoma. *Oncology* 2005; 19:393.

Porter GA, Pisters PWT, Mansyur C, et al. Cost and utilization impact of a clinical pathway for patients undergoing pancreaticoduodenectomy. *Ann Surg Oncol* 2000;7: 484.

Raut CP, Grau AM, Staerkel GA, et al. Diagnostic accuracy of endoscopic ultrasound-guided fine-needle aspiration in patients with presumed pancreatic cancer. *J Gastrointest Surg* 2003;7:118.

Tseng JF, Raut CP, Lee JE, et al. Pancreaticoduodenectomy with vascular resection: margin status and survival duration. *J Gastrointest Surg* 2004;8:935.

Tyler DS, Evans DB. Reoperative pancreaticoduodenectomy. *Ann Surg* 1994;219:211.

Varadhachary GR, Tamm EP, Crane C, et al. Borderline resectable pancreatic cancer. *Curr Treat Options Gastroenterol* 2005;8:377.

Whipple AO, Parsons WW, Mullin CR. Treatment of carcinoma of the ampulla of Vater. *Ann Surg* 1935;102:763.

Wolff RA, Crane CH, Li D, et al. Neoplasms of the exocrine pancreas. In: Kufe DW, Bast RC, Hait WN, et al., eds. *Holland-Frei cancer medicine,* 6th ed. Ontario: BC Decker, Inc., 2006:1331.

EDITOR'S COMMENT

More than 30,000 Americans will succumb to pancreatic cancer this year. Survival rates are abysmal and have not changed during 3 decades (Sener SF, et al., *J Am Coll Surg* 1999;189:1). For certain early subgroups, new advances in surgical and medical care may be helping (Shaib YH, et al., *Aliment Pharmacol Ther* 2006; 24:87), but certainly not enough. Only 10% to 15% of tumors are resectable at diagnosis, and even then, resection confers at most a 20% 5-year survival. Death for patients with unresectable or metastatic disease comes quickly, and reflects how profoundly resistant is the tumor to today's chemotherapy and radiation. Although a patient's best hope, surgery alone is not enough (Traverso LW, *Surg Endosc* 2006;20:S446), and even postoperative chemoradiation has recently fallen into question (Neoptolemos JP, et al., *N Engl J Med* 2004;350:1200). Despite these tragic statistics, pancreatic cancer sadly remains underrepresented in both clinical and basic research compared with other cancer sites. Anyone dealing with pancreatic cancer is justifiably desperate.

Dr. Doug Evans leads a program in pancreatic cancer care at M. D. Anderson Cancer Center that is recognized worldwide for its superb ongoing contributions. From landmark studies of neoadjuvant therapy to analyses of the technical elements of vascular resection, Dr. Evans and his colleagues set a pace few can match. It is no surprise that this *Mastery* chapter is second to none that is currently available elsewhere. It is complete, beautifully written and illustrated, and based on tested, rational thought processes about why, when, and how to remove this disease. Experience is stressed as being required for best outcomes. In his recent report of 1,000 consecutive pancreaticoduodenectomies that he performed individually, Dr. John Cameron (*Ann Surg* 2006;244:10) reveals impact of experience, and the oncologic efficacy of this operation for pancreatic cancer. Indeed, during our recent

"golden era" (Lillemoe KD, et al., *Ann Surg* 2006;244:16), this operation has been taken to near-optimal results. If only more patients could survive the disease. The answers to pancreatic cancer must lie in the biology of the disease, and not whether it can be safely removed.

Futile, unnecessary laparotomy should be avoided whenever and however possible so that we can maintain quality and comfort in the final stages of a patient's life. As such, preoperative staging and evaluation is critical, and this is properly detailed by the authors. Today, the highest resolution MDCT angiography may be as much as we need, but even this will fall short in predicting resectable disease, despite its strengths in unresectable disease. If you embrace laparoscopy, you'll use it selectively in pancreatic cancer (Callery MP, et al., *J Am Coll Surg* 1997;185:33), as recommended by the authors. If you favor preoperative chemoradiotherapy, as do they, you will need endoscopic ultrasound for diagnosis and staging, otherwise it is unnecessary and cannot replace CT angiography based on today's available evidence (Dewitt J, et al., *Clin Gastroenterol Hepatol* 2006;4:717). Plastic biliary stents, if necessary, are inexpensive and effective if operation is planned soon, but for extended neoadjuvant therapy, metal biliary stents do better in controlling jaundice and cholangitis, and contrary to earlier myth, do not complicate eventual pancreaticoduodenectomy (Mullen JT, et al., *J Gastrointest Surg* 2005;9:1094).

I find the step-by-step instruction of how and why to perform this operation very logical and helpful. It is great for training residents. The critical oncologic feature is achieving a negative posterior margin along the uncinate process. There are many ways to achieve this and other key margins, but we all must specify in our operative notes whether we have achieved an R0, R1, or R2 resection. The authors' expose on expanding indications, options, and techniques for vascular resection/reconstruction is superb. These procedures require an even higher level

of experience and technical ability, however. Randomized trials have indicated that extended lymphadenectomy is not necessary. Finally, the literature swells with options as how best to re-establish pancreatic, biliary, and gastrointestinal continuity. The techniques described in this chapter are certainly sound. Find what technique you are best at, and stick with it. Concerns about the oncologic efficacy of pylorus preservation are fading, and delayed gastric emptying is infrequent if an isoperistaltic antecolic duodenojejunostomy if performed (*Tani M, et al., Ann Surg* 2006;243:316). Feeding jejunostomy is not compulsory, except perhaps in elderly patients.

As noted, total pancreatectomy should be required infrequently for pancreatic cancer. Left-sided resections, however, are not uncommon, but the survival results have consistently been discouraging. Dr. Steve Strasberg et al. (*Surgery* 2003;133:521) have promoted the radical antegrade modular pancreatosplenectomy (RAMPS) procedure as a solution. The rationale is to provide an anatomically based resection of left-sided cancers that achieves comparable primary tumor clearance, negative margins, and N1 nodal clearance that pancreaticoduodenectomy does for head lesions. Its true oncologic impact should become clear with broader use over time.

Better operations have naturally facilitated postoperative care and recovery. Ours is one of many centers now benefiting from defined clinical pathway care of patients who have undergone a Whipple procedure. With minimal blood loss and restricted intraoperative fluid administration, blood transfusion is infrequent, as is postoperative need for intensive care unit stay. Durations of stay, when all goes well, are 7 to 8 days. Properly designed clinical pathways allow a high-volume center to mitigate higher patient acuity, and to control costs without sacrificing quality.

M.P.C.

The Gastrointestinal Tract

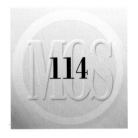

Operative Management of Pancreatic Trauma

EDWARD E. CORNWELL AND DAVID EFRON

A surgeon managing any patient who has abdominal trauma must consider the possibility of pancreatic injury. The effects of pancreatic disruption can be devastating, but the sometimes subtle findings associated with pancreatic injury make diagnosis difficult in patients who do not have obvious indications for laparotomy. The mortality rates of patients with pancreatic injury vary from 9% to 25%, and death is mainly due to associated injuries. Of those surviving initial hemorrhage, as many as 50% of patients have a complication of their pancreatic wound, such as fistula, abscess, pseudocyst, and hemorrhage from false aneurysms, as well as anastomotic leak. The surgical management of these injuries is complicated by the gland's complex anatomic relationship with the duodenum, biliary tract, splanchnic vessels, liver, spleen, vena cava, and aorta. Operative decisions are challenging because of the unforgiving nature of the gland, relative unfamiliarity with the techniques, controversy regarding the technical details, and judgment required to decide on the extent of surgery.

CAUSES

The rising frequency of pancreatic trauma can be traced to the fast-paced and increasingly violent nature of the American lifestyle. Patients with penetrating injuries to the pancreas experience trauma in equal frequency along the head, body, and tail of the organ. On the other hand, the deceleration and direct compression mechanism of injury involved in victims of blunt trauma explain why the neck of the pancreas, in the prevertebral area of the gland, is the most commonly injured region.

Associated injuries occur in as many as 90% of cases of pancreatic trauma and account for most fatalities. Specifically, hemorrhagic shock from associated major vascular injuries (e.g., inferior vena cava, portal vein, and superior mesenteric vessels) is the single most common cause of early mortality in patients sustaining pancreatic trauma. Solid organs (e.g., liver and spleen), as well as the stomach and diaphragm, are also frequently injured in patients with pancreatic trauma. It should be

clear, therefore, that as with all cases of intra-abdominal injury, control of hemorrhage has the highest priority in the management of pancreatic trauma.

 ## DIAGNOSIS

Patients with torso trauma who manifest early indications of intra-abdominal bleeding or peritonitis require operative intervention, at which time direct evaluation of the pancreas should be carried out. The only penetrating injury with a significant likelihood of causing an isolated pancreatic injury is a posterior abdominal stab wound, and even this is quite unusual. The stable patient with blunt abdominal trauma is the person in whom timely diagnosis of pancreatic injury is most challenging.

Serum amylase should be obtained routinely. Eighty percent of patients with blunt pancreatic injury have elevation of serum amylase. This figure is much lower for penetrating wounds, but, in either case, an elevated amylase mandates a focused evaluation of the pancreas. An elevated amylase can be the result of bowel perforation, salivary gland trauma, and nondisruptive pancreatic injury, and as such is not a very specific test. Serum lipase may be used if there is confusion; it is not elevated when hyperamylasemia is of salivary origin. Pancreatic isoenzyme fractionation can identify salivary amylase but is often not available. It is often useful to repeat the serum amylase in patients being observed for abdominal trauma, because the first blood specimens may be drawn so close to the time of wounding that a misleading normal value may result.

Additional diagnostic studies are indicated if there is suspicion of pancreatic injury. Such patients are those with amylase elevation and mild abdominal tenderness and distention. Plain or contrast radiographs and peritoneal lavage offer little assistance. The dynamic rapid sequence computed tomography (CT) scan has been helpful in identifying major parenchymal (and therefore potential ductal) disruption (Fig. 1). Although this examination is helpful, there are some important pancreatic in-

juries that it may miss. The study should be performed with oral contrast, because occasionally a retroperitoneal rupture of the duodenum is responsible for elevation of the serum amylase without obvious signs of peritonitis.

In cases in which the clinical findings leading to the CT scan are persistent, and the CT scan is equivocal, or even negative, we use endoscopic retrograde cholangiopancreatography (ERCP) to delineate the pancreatic ductal anatomy (Fig. 2). Although this situation occurs infrequently, ERCP can identify major ductal disruption well before clinical signs lead to laparotomy. Early identification and treatment of pancreatic injury reduces morbidity. The most important elements in the diagnostic search are a strong suspicion of and healthy respect for pancreatic injury.

INTRAOPERATIVE EVALUATION

In most cases of traumatic pancreatic injuries, the diagnosis is confirmed intraoperatively. Evaluation of pancreatic trauma requires several surgical maneuvers. A Kocher maneuver entails incising the lateral peritoneal attachments to the second and third portion of the duodenum and mobilizing the duodenum and the head of the pancreas to the patient's left (Fig. 3). This proceeds along the avascular plane to the superior mesenteric artery. Occasionally a replaced right hepatic artery is encountered as a branch of the superior mesenteric artery and care must be taken as it can be injured during this dissection. This facilitates inspection of the posterior aspect of the head of the gland as well as the posterior wall of the duodenum and provides a view of the suprarenal inferior vena cava.

The anterior aspect of the entire gland may be evaluated by entering the lesser sac through the gastrocolic omentum. With a wide incision through that omentum and retraction of the stomach superiorly and the transverse colon inferiorly, thorough evaluation of the gland becomes possible. Any hematomas overlying the gland must be evacuated and thoroughly explored, because they commonly mask underlying severe pancreatic parenchymal or ductal injury

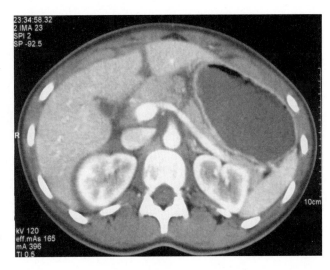

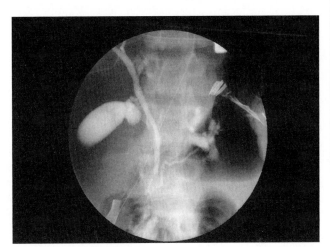

Fig. 1. Abdominal computed tomography scan demonstrating disruption of the pancreas anterior to the spine.

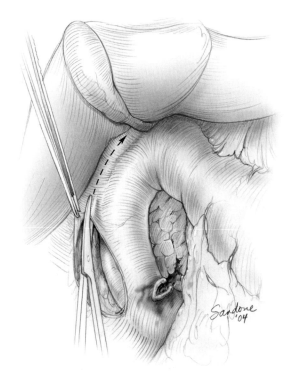

Fig. 2. Endoscopic retrograde cholangiopancreatography demonstrating a pancreatic duct disruption with extravasation of dye.

Fig. 3. The Kocher maneuver showing incision of the peritoneum overlying the lateral aspect of the second portion of the duodenum.

The Gastrointestinal Tract

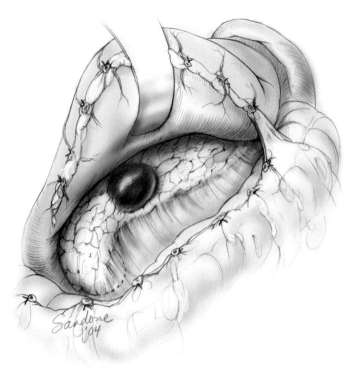

Fig. 4. Exposure of the pancreas in the lesser sac through the gastrocolic ligament. A contained hematoma is shown in the proximal body of the gland.

(Fig. 4). Occasionally, a patient may present with severe injury to the posterior aspect of the pancreas, with the anterior capsule intact. This is seen most commonly in patients with blunt mechanisms of injury. When hematoma or contusion raises an index of suspicion for injuries that may involve the posterior aspect of the gland, an incision should be made in the peritoneum and areolar tissue along the inferior aspect of the pancreas. This most commonly applies in the prevertebral region of the pancreas. After division of the peritoneum along the inferior border of the pancreas, the surgeon's finger is slipped behind the gland to evaluate for palpable parenchymal defects by palpation and direct visualization (Fig. 5).

Full evaluation of the tail of the pancreas can be facilitated by the Aird maneuver. Originally described in 1955 to facilitate adrenalectomy, this procedure entails division of the avascular splenic ligaments (i.e., splenorenal, splenocolic, and splenophrenic) and mobilization of the spleen and the tail of the pancreas from the patient's left to right (Fig. 6).

TREATMENT OF INJURIES TO THE TAIL AND BODY OF THE PANCREAS

Minor contusions and lacerations that do not transect major ducts (Wirsung or

Santorini) require drainage only, usually of the closed suction type (Fig. 7). Closure of the pancreatic capsule with sutures is of no proven value. Major disruption of the pancreatic tissue requires a decision regarding

the likelihood of major ductal injury. Even in many major trauma centers, the "gold standard" ERCP is not available intraoperatively in the middle of the night. Suspicion of ductal involvement is raised by the anatomic location of the injury and the amount of local pancreatic tissue disruption. Occasionally, pancreatic juice can be seen leaking at the open ends of a duct. When major ductal injury is suspected, it should, in most instances, prompt definitive therapy. Under some circumstances, such as cardiovascular instability, drainage alone should be performed, after which the patient almost always has a pancreatic fistula, the management of which is covered later in this chapter.

Definitive treatment of major ductal injury due to blunt trauma is required commonly for injuries over the vertebral column through the neck of the pancreas. When ductal injury has occurred at that location, the body and tail of the pancreas should be resected. Additionally, any penetrating injury to the left of the pancreatic head with major ductal injury should be managed in the same way. The physiologic consequences, endocrine or exocrine, are usually minimal and well tolerated. Some have suggested preservation of the tail of the pancreas by Roux-en-Y pancreaticojejunostomy or end-to-end suture of the pancreas. These do preserve more pancreatic function, but they add considerable

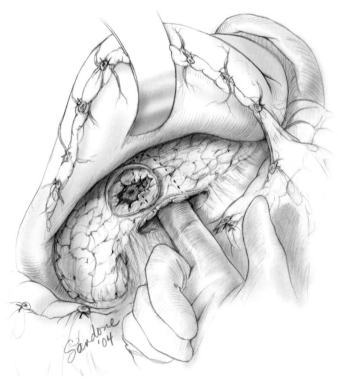

Fig. 5. With the hematoma unroofed, the posterior aspect of the gland is palpated, and may be visualized after incision of the peritoneum along the inferior aspect of the body and tail.

placed over the cut end as horizontal mattress sutures. Some have used gastrointestinal stapling devices (5-mm staples) to close the proximal end. Because occasional pancreatic fistulae occur no matter how closure is performed, the transected end should be drained with two closed suction drains (Jackson-Pratt).

Preservation of the spleen is possible if the splenic vein is treated with care. This is a much more tedious operation, because the short veins draining the pancreas are easily torn. As shown in Figure 8, the operation can proceed from right to left after division of the pancreas. The distal pancreas is lifted anteriorly, slightly cephalad, and, as dissection proceeds, rolled to the left and separated from the splenic artery and vein. A fine right-angle clamp may be used to dissect the small branches of the splenic vein and artery. These branches are tied in continuity with 4-0 silk suture and cut with Potts scissors. The cut end of the retained pancreas is managed as mentioned previously, including drainage. If, during the procedure, the splenic vein is torn or narrowed, splenic preservation should be abandoned.

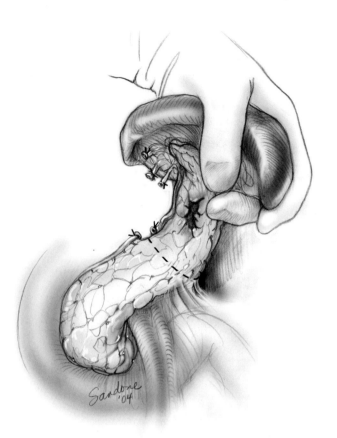

Fig. 6. The Aird maneuver to elevate the spleen, tail, and distal body of the pancreas. After freeing the spleen from its attachments, the pancreas is elevated out of the retroperitoneum and rotated medially.

complexity to the operation and increase the chance of serious complications.

In most cases, the distal pancreas is resected with the spleen, but this leaves the patient, especially children, vulnerable to the postsplenectomy sepsis syndrome. Distal pancreatectomy and splenectomy should be performed when the patient is hemodynamically unstable, has multiple organ injuries, or has a major splenic injury. Mobilization of the spleen and tail of the pancreas should proceed from left to right by first dividing the ligamentous attachments of the spleen and lifting the spleen and tail of the pancreas anterior and to the right (the previously described Aird maneuver, Fig. 6). The splenic artery and vein are identified from behind and individually suture-ligated at a point 1 cm to the right of the proposed pancreatic transection. Any residual intact pancreatic tissue at the area of trauma is transected, and a search is made for the pancreatic duct. Magnification may be helpful. If identified, the proximal end of the duct should be suture-ligated with a fine nonabsorbable suture such a 4-0 Prolene. Mattress sutures of silk or Prolene are also

COMBINED PANCREATICODUODENAL INJURIES

Once hemorrhage is controlled in the management of pancreatic trauma, delayed complications such as pancreatic fistulae

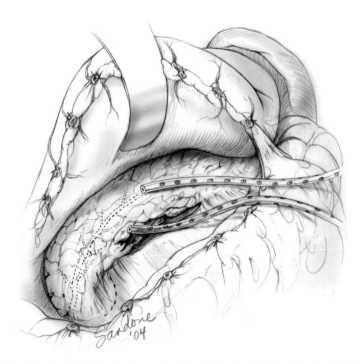

Fig. 7. Injury is not felt to involve the major duct drained with closed suction Jackson-Pratt drains. The pancreatic duct is seen within the gland as the dotted lines.

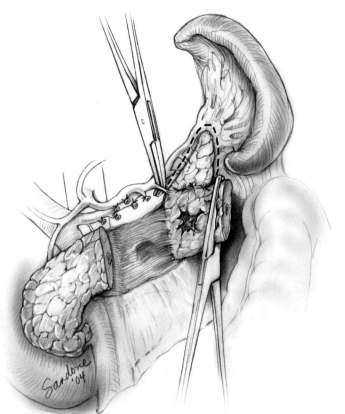

Fig. 8. Careful dissection with a fine right-angle clamp to ligate the small branches of the splenic artery and vein is required for splenic preservation with distal pancreatectomy. This is appropriate only in the stable patient. As with any distal pancreatectomy, the main duct is identified at the edge of the remaining gland and specifically ligated in addition to oversewing the edge of the gland. The dotted line demonstrates the extent of the dissection.

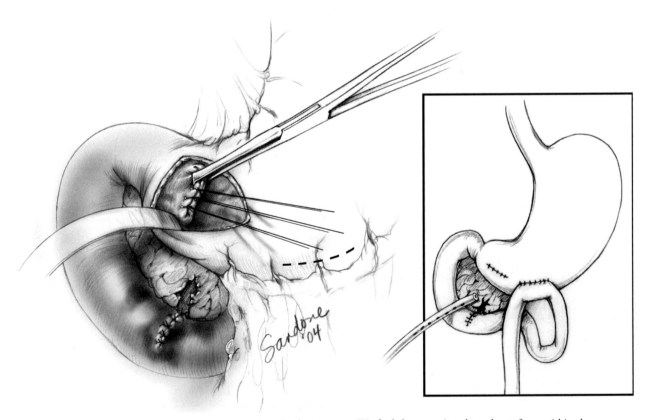

Fig. 9. The pyloric exclusion is achieved via a distal gastrotomy. We find that grasping the pylorus from within the stomach with an Allis clamp allows better visualization and facilitates ease of suturing. The pylorus may be closed with interrupted, running, or, as is our preference, a purse-string suture. Additionally, the pylorus may be closed with a TA stapler device applied externally. A gastrojejunostomy is then performed to maintain gastroenteric flow. The gastrojejunostomy may be performed at a site separate from the initial gastrotomy (*dotted line*) or, if appropriate, at the gastrotomy used for the pyloric exclusion. The inset shows the final positioning.

viously described, in the unstable patient, the resection is performed and the re-establishment of enteric continuity is delayed until the patient has been stabilized.

CONSIDERATIONS IN POSTOPERATIVE MANAGEMENT

When drainage is performed for major pancreatic injuries, our guideline for removing the drain is tolerance of regular oral feedings and the absence of high volume or high amylase content in the drainage fluid. A feeding jejunostomy is an important adjunct to complex pancreatic injury, pyloric exclusion, and the Whipple procedure because of the accumulated evidence showing the importance of early enteric feeding in maintaining the immune function of the gut in critically injured patients.

Rarely, late management of the pancreatic fistula that shows no sign of closure after many weeks of nonoperative management or the patient who forms a pseudocyst after drain removal requires internal drainage via a Roux-en-Y jejunal limb. Postoperative pancreatic bed infection usually demands open debridement and wide drainage. However, single, uniloculated collections in the absence of much pancreatic necrosis (as determined by dynamic CT scanning) may respond to percutaneous CT-guided drainage with large catheters.

SUGGESTED READING

Aird I, Helman P. Bilateral anterior transabdominal adrenalectomy. *BJM* 1955;2:708.

Bradley EL III, Young PR Jr, Chang MC, et al. Diagnosis and initial management of blunt pancreatic trauma. *Ann Surg* 1998;227:861.

Frey C, Araida T. Trauma to the pancreas and duodenum. In: Blaisdell FW, Trunkey D, eds. Abdominal trauma, New York: Thieme Medical, 1993:1881.

Jones RC, Foreman ML. Pancreas: In: Ivatury RR, Cayten CG, eds. *Penetrating trauma.* Baltimore: Williams & Williams, 1996:631.

Kao LS, Bulger EM, Parks DL, et al. Predictors of morbidity after traumatic pancreatic injury. *J Trauma* 2003;55:898.

Patton JH Jr, Lyden SP, Croce MA, et al. Pancreatic trauma: a simplified management guideline. *J Trauma* 1997;43:234.

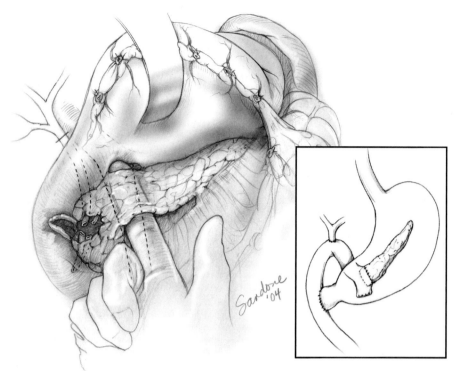

Fig. 10. The avascular plane between the neck of the pancreas and the superior mesenteric vein allows for safe and expedient mobilization of the gland for resection as is performed during the Whipple procedure. The inset demonstrates re-established enteric connections.

and pseudocysts, intra-abdominal abscesses, and multisystem organ dysfunction correlate in frequency with the severity of the pancreatic injury. Therefore, the most extensive surgical procedures in the management of pancreatic trauma are reserved for patients with combined pancreaticoduodenal injuries. The overall goals of these surgical procedures are to (a) maintain pancreatic-enteric and biliary-enteric flow, (b) provide wide drainage for all pancreatic and duodenal injuries and anastomoses, and (c) divert the gastrointestinal stream so as to minimize stimulation of pancreaticobiliary secretions.

When pancreatic injuries are associated with major duodenal injuries, drainage or resection of the pancreas can be combined with suturing or stapling of the pylorus ("pyloric exclusion procedure") to divert gastric flow from the duodenum. Gastrointestinal continuity is then accomplished by gastrojejunostomy (Fig. 9). It is quite remarkable that gastroduodenal continuity is

re-established 4 to 6 weeks after pyloric exclusion even when heavy nonabsorbable sutures or staples are used. The pyloric exclusion procedure has largely replaced the duodenal diverticularization procedure, which entails antrectomy and gastrojejunostomy, as well as drainage and decompression of the duodenal injury and drainage of the pancreatic injury.

When pancreaticoduodenal trauma is so severe that hemorrhage control or extensive destruction of tissue necessitates resection of the second portion of the duodenum or the head of the pancreas, a pancreaticoduodenectomy (Whipple procedure) is indicated. An important step in this maneuver is the establishment of the avascular plane between the anterior wall of the portal vein and the posterior wall of the pancreas, which is achieved by digital exploration (Fig. 10). Care is taken to stay directly anterior to the portal vein to avoid transverse venous tributaries into the side wall of the vein from the head of the pancreas. As pre-

The Gastrointestinal Tract

Thankfully, pancreatic trauma is relatively rare. When it does occur, it must be recognized promptly or else severe morbidity and even death will occur. Drs. Cornwell and Efron provide a great overview of pancreatic trauma, and many of its key points warrant emphasis. First and foremost is the "unforgiving nature" of the pancreas. Missed injuries become huge problems. Second, the astute clinician must be alert to the mechanism of injury, remain suspicious, and persevere through sometimes subtle clinical findings to discover and treat a pancreatic injury. Typically, associated hemorrhage will determine early deaths, but the missed pancreatic injury itself will determine longer-term sequelae such as pancreatic fistula, abscess, and sepsis. These too can ultimately be fatal.

There are additional considerations as related to the causes of pancreatic injury. Penetrating injuries will be the most lethal when associated with major vascular injury. When not, missed associated injuries, which occur commonly, will determine the outcome whether or not the pancreas has been treated properly. Blunt injuries are often caused by steering shaft or seatbelt impact during motor vehicle accidents. The body and neck of the gland are suddenly compressed back against the vertebral column and fractures. In children, a latent pseudocyst or pancreatic fistula in the absence of a defined trauma event should raise concerns for abuse. Not mentioned are iatrogenic pancreatic injuries that still occur and are often missed. Typical scenarios include urgent or elective splenectomy, colectomy, and some laparoscopic procedures (*Urology* 2004;64:1089) when the pancreatic tail is unknowingly injured.

Diagnosis can be difficult in a stable blunt trauma patient. There may not be evidence of other injury on physical examination or axial imaging. The value of serially rising amylase levels is stressed. Serial CT scans may be necessary to reveal progressive evidence of parenchymal disruption. Pancreatic duct injury may be diagnosed using endoscopic and less commonly magnetic resonance pancreatography. Ultimately, however, the prudent approach to haziness or fluid in the lesser sac will be laparotomy. This usually indicates a careful surgeon's suspicion based on injury mechanism, and proper fear of pancreatic disruption. Olah (*Dig Surg* 2003;20:408) demonstrated the higher pancreas-specific morbidity and mortality of delayed surgical intervention after unsuccessful nonoperative management of pancreatic trauma.

Once in the operating room, the key to proper evaluation is the deliberate and complete mobilization of the pancreas. Our authors detail how to accomplish this using a regional approach that allows both an anterior and posterior assessment of the gland and surrounding structures: Mobilize the head and uncinate process by a Kocher maneuver, visualize the neck and body by traversing the gastrocolic omentum, and rotate the tail and spleen using the Aird maneuver. If suspicion of pancreatic injury is low during trauma laparotomy, such extensive mobilization is not necessary. At a minimum, though, the pancreas should be visualized. Because of its retroperitoneal location, proper evaluation of pancreatic injury is difficult to achieve laparoscopically (*Surg Endosc* 2002;16:217), so this is not recommended.

Major injuries to the left of the portal confluence are best managed by resection with or without splenectomy in stable patients. There is uncertain value, only risk, to preserving left-sided pancreatic parenchyma by constructing an unnecessary pancreatic-enteric anastomosis. Lin et al. (*J Trauma* 2004; 56:774) reviewed 48 major blunt pancreatic trauma patients who required operation. Distal pancreatectomy with or without splenectomy had the lowest complication rates (22%). Debridement, wide drainage, and control of hemorrhage are advisable in unstable patients, and also in stable patients where no main ductal injury is found. Pancreatic head disruptions requiring pancreaticoduodenectomy are exceedingly rare, probably because the penetrating injury also disrupted the portal vein, inferior vena cava, or aortic vessels, causing death. It is difficult to find published series of Whipple procedures for trauma. In general, the overall mortality for it would appear to be at least 50%. As noted, it may safely be performed as a two-stage operation. Duodenal injury rarely requires complete resection as summarized. Of course, there will be many variations to all these approaches to injury.

These patients can have stormy postoperative courses. Most agree that feeding tubes are essential for enteral nutritional support. The occurrence of a late pancreatic fistula should be managed expectantly with ERCP pancreatic duct stenting and operative or radiologically placed drains. At least 2 months of observation, support, and recovery should pass before any attempt at surgical repair of pancreatic fistula is undertaken.

Finally, if you need help, get help. Pancreatic regional anatomy is complex and perilous. The principal operations detailed elsewhere in *Mastery* are challenging enough when elective, much less in a trauma victim. If available, summon an experienced trauma or pancreatic surgeon to help you save the life. If not available, consider stabilizing, controlling associated injuries, draining the pancreas widely, and transferring to a trauma facility for definitive care.

M.P.C.

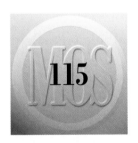

115

Splanchnic Denervation of the Pancreas for Intractable Pain

KEITH D. LILLEMOE AND THOMAS J. HOWARD

INTRODUCTION

The treatment of intractable pain in patients with either chronic pancreatitis or pancreatic cancers is one of the most challenging clinical situations faced by the surgeon. The pancreas is a highly innervated visceral organ incorporating both exocrine and endocrine tissue into an integrated functional unit. The autonomic nerves orchestrating this function, in addition to providing neurohumoral regulation, are sensitive to both chemical and mechanical stimuli that can be transmitted back to the central nervous system as pain. The precise molecular pathophysiology of pancreatic pain remains incompletely understood, and most data seeking to clarify this issue come from studies in patients with chronic pancreatitis. Based on these investigations, two general theories for the genesis of pain have been proposed: (a) Increased pancreatic duct pressure with tissue hypertension and poor microvascular perfusion and (b) pancreatitis-associated neuritis with alterations in the perineural sheath. Both theories have their advocates; however, neither is sufficiently comprehensive to explain pain generation in all clinical circumstances. It remains entirely possible, as with most complex, neural-mediated pain syndromes, that potential overlap and considerable synergism exists between these two competing theories. For the purpose of our discussion in this chapter, regardless of the exact pathophysiologic mechanism responsible for the genesis of pain, sensory autonomic nerve endings located in the pancreatic parenchyma transmit neural afferent information to the celiac ganglion. The celiac ganglion plexus of nerves then serves as a way station for pain impulses traveling toward the central nervous system where they are processed, localized, and interpreted. The greater (T5 to T10) and lesser (T10 to T11) splanchnic nerves are composed of postganglionic sympathetic nerve fibers that carry visceral sensory impulses to the spinal cord, which are then transmitted on to the thalamus and subsequently to the cerebral cortex.

Pain referable to the pancreas is commonly described by the patient as either a sharp stabbing pain or a dull boring pain, localized in the midepigastrium or left upper quadrant. This pain frequently radiates to the back between the T12 and L2 dermatomes. Occasionally, the pain becomes so severe that it doubles the patient over, causing him or her to bend forward at the waist in a knee-to-chest configuration, the so called "pancreatitis position." The pain occurs predominately postprandial, at least early in its course, and is associated with nausea. Colicky pain is unusual in this setting and should arouse suspicion of a biliary tract rather than pancreatic cause. Pain severity differs markedly from patient to patient, and severity can also vary considerably from day to day in the same patient. In both chronic pancreatitis and pancreatic cancer, as the disease advances the pain becomes progressively more severe and unrelenting.

The treatment of pain in patients with chronic pancreatitis has been recently addressed in a position statement by the American Gastroenterologic Association (AGA) (Table 1). In this algorithm, total abstinence from alcohol and initial pain management with nonsteroidal anti-inflammatory drugs (NSAIDs), antidepressants, and a low-fat diet are recommended. Imaging studies should be carried out to look for treatable causes of pain (i.e., pancreatic pseudocyst, biliary stricture, duodenal stenosis, or peptic ulcer disease). If the initial treatments rendered prove ineffective, an 8-week course of oral pancreatic enzyme supplementation and acid suppression is insti-

tuted. Failure of these treatments leads to the use of opioid analgesics and consideration should then be given to either endoscopic or surgical management. Imaging studies should also be used to categorize patients with chronic pancreatitis into anatomic (large duct, small duct, minimal change) and morphologic (enlarged hypertrophic pancreatic head, small pancreatic head, obstructive pancreatitis) variants. Once categorized, patients can be treated rationally with the most appropriate type of endoscopic or surgical intervention.

For patients with pancreatic cancer, use of transdermal or long-acting narcotic analgesics that provide a steady-state basal plasma level, supplemented with the intermittent use of short-acting narcotic analgesics for breakthrough pain, is the preferred initial treatment method. Antidepressant medication also facilitates pain management in patients with both chronic pancreatitis and pancreatic cancer. Percutaneous or endoscopic ultrasound–directed celiac plexus blocks are useful, minimally invasive adjuncts to achieve pain control in patients with either chronic pancreatitis or pancreatic carcinoma.

Failure of the above-mentioned treatment regimen makes a patient a potential candidate for bilateral thoracoscopic splanchnicectomy (BTS). Patients with pancreatic cancer with more than 3 months to live, with significant pain recalcitrant to narcotic analgesics, and who are candidates for a general anesthetic should be considered for BTS to improve their pain management. In our experience, patients with

small duct pancreatitis without an endoscopic or surgical target (i.e., pancreatic duct stricture, dilated pancreatic duct) or patients who have failed first-line endoscopic or surgical treatment are also candidates for BTS. We would advocate that all patients with chronic pancreatitis considered for BTS have a differential epidural anesthetic done to document the transmission of pain through the splanchnic nervous system. By recording the subjective sensation of pain after injections of either normal saline (placebo control) or local anesthetics, pain perceived by the patient can be characterized as visceral, nonvisceral, or central in origin. Use of a validated quality-of-life (QOL) instrument and/or a visual analog scale (VAS) helps to objectively quantify the severity of pain and an individual patient's response to treatment.

The differential epidural anesthetic involves access to the epidural space followed by a placebo injection, a complete epidural block, and dissipation of the complete epidural block to only a sympathetic, small-fiber epidural block. After each of these stages of the anesthetic, patients are queried on their level of pain. When significant improvement in pain occurs after placebo injection alone, patients are considered placebo responders. Patients experiencing a reduction in pain after complete epidural block that returns early after the return of lower extremity motor function are felt to have somatic nonpancreatic pain. Patients who have pain relief after complete epidural block that maintain their pain control even after return of lower extremity motor function during continued sympathetic blockade (i.e., temperature differences remain between upper and lower extremities) are felt to have visceral pancreatic pain. Patients with no pain relief after complete epidural blockade have high centralization of their pain (including psychogenic pain). Only patients with chronic pancreatitis who have visceral, sympathetic-mediated afferent pain pathways should be considered candidates for BTS.

ANATOMY

The celiac ganglion innervates the upper abdominal viscera and is the largest plexus of nerves in the abdominal aortic sympathetic plexus. It contains both preganglionic and postganglionic sympathetic fibers, preganglionic parasympathetic fibers, and visceral afferent (pain) fibers. The celiac plexus is composed of bilateral celiac ganglia, located in front of and on both sides of the abdominal aorta at the level of the celiac

TABLE 1. AMERICAN GASTROENTEROLOGICAL ASSOCIATION (AGA) MEDICAL POSITION STATEMENT ON THE TREATMENT OF PAIN IN CHRONIC PANCREATITIS

Initial Therapy			
Abstain from alcohol	Nonnarcotic analgesics	Low-fat diet	Quality of life questionnaire
No Response			
	Gastric acid suppression	8-week trial of high-dose pancreatic enzymes	
No Response			
	Consider endoscopic therapy		
No Response			
Watchful waiting vs. narcotic analgesics vs. surgery Surgery decided			
Small Ducts		**Large Ducts**	
Nerve ablation Pancreatic resection		Surgical drainage	

The Gastrointestinal Tract

artery. Plexus fibers cross in front of the aorta both above and below the celiac axis. Organs innervated by the celiac ganglia include the stomach, liver, gallbladder, pancreas, adrenal glands, kidneys, and intestines to the level of the transverse colon. The sympathetic plexus ganglia vary in number from one to five on each side of the aorta, and range from an aggregate size of 0.5 to 4.5 cm. Without extensive dissection, the origin of the celiac artery can be identified intraoperatively by palpation of the common hepatic and splenic arteries, the two most consistent arterial branches off the celiac artery. Radiographically, the plexus can be found by identification of both the celiac and superior mesenteric arteries.

The splanchnic nerves, usually three (greater, lesser, and least), consist primarily of preganglionic sympathetic and accompanying visceral afferent fibers. These nerves vary much in their origin; however, the greater splanchnic nerves usually arise from the 5th through 9th thoracic ganglia (Fig. 1). The unison of these roots forms a nerve of considerable size (larger than the continuation of the sympathetic trunk into the abdomen) that descends on the front of the vertebral column and pierces the muscular part of the diaphragm to end in the celiac ganglion. The lesser splanchnic nerve usually arises from the 9th and 10th or last two thoracic sympathetic ganglia. It runs parallel and medial to the greater splanchnic nerve but lateral to the sympathetic trunk. This nerve trunk is constituted at or above the

level of the 10th thoracic vertebra, and descends along the spine where it is bound by the parietal pleura. The lesser splanchnic nerve generally supplies the submesenteric organs and forms from the trunks of the 10th and 11th thoracic ganglia and runs parallel to the greater splanchnic nerve in the chest. Both nerves penetrate the crus of the diaphragm and enter the abdomen. The greater splanchnic nerve ends in the celiac ganglia, and the lesser splanchnic nerve ends in the aorticorenal ganglion. The vagus nerves run in the lower thoracic cavity along the esophagus below the parietal pleura. The role of the vagal fibers in the transmission of pain sensation from the pancreas is unclear. Bilateral vagotomy has been advocated in early series as a method of increasing the completeness of splanchnic denervation. Currently, most surgeons limit their operation to the splanchnic nerves as the postvagotomy sequelae of delayed gastric emptying and diarrhea can often be formidable.

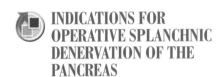

INDICATIONS FOR OPERATIVE SPLANCHNIC DENERVATION OF THE PANCREAS

Pancreatic Cancer

Survival of patients with locally advanced, unresectable pancreatic cancer is 6 to 12 months, while patients with metastatic dis-

ease to the liver or peritoneal cavity survive approximately 3 to 6 months. The majority of patients in both groups will have pain requiring increasing doses of narcotic analgesics during the course of their illness. In cases in which pancreatic cancer is found to be inoperable based on preoperative studies, nonsurgical techniques for pain control are indicated. However, in those patients where the tumor is found to be unresectable at the time of laparotomy, intraoperative chemical celiac plexus block should be done in conjunction with appropriate surgical palliative procedures such as biliary bypass and/or gastrojejunostomy. This procedure is indicated whether or not the patient has significant pain at the time of surgery, as the natural course of the disease is pain that becomes progressively more severe and unrelenting. The technique is applicable whether the tumor arises in the head, body, or tail of the gland. There are currently no good data to support prophylactic celiac plexus block in patients who have undergone a complete R0 surgical resection, despite the fact that almost 50% of such patients will eventually develop retroperitoneal tumor recurrence as a component of disease relapse.

There is little indication for open laparotomy for the sole purpose of performing celiac plexus block in patients who otherwise are not candidates for surgical resection or palliation based on the extent of their disease, age, or medical disability. The availability of percutaneous celiac plexus block using fluoroscopic or computed tomography (CT) guidance or using endoscopic ultrasound to visualize the celiac axis has eliminated the need for laparotomy solely for this purpose. In patients with pancreatic cancer and unmanageable pain who are unable to be adequately palliated by percutaneous or endoscopic celiac plexus block, bilateral thoracoscopic splanchnicectomy should be considered, as complete transaction of the afferent nerves above the level of the celiac axis can often be beneficial.

Chronic Pancreatitis

Currently, there is a paucity of data regarding the concomitant use of celiac plexus block as an adjunct for postoperative pain control during an operation where either a resection (Whipple, duodenal-sparing pancreatic head resection) or drainage procedure (Puestow) is being done for patients with chronic pancreatitis and recurrent abdominal pain. In the usual circumstances, the resection or drainage procedure is done without denervation. If the

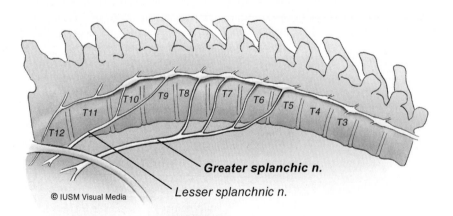

Fig. 1. Diagram showing the standard location of the greater splanchnic nerve as viewed through the right chest in the prone position. It is composed of the rami communicans of the 5th through the 8th thoracic sympathetic ganglia, funneling down toward the diaphragm. The lesser splanchnic nerve is derived from fibers arising from the 9th and 10th thoracic sympathetic ganglia and courses parallel to the greater splanchnic nerve.

patient is carefully selected and the operation is appropriately matched to the ductal anatomy and pancreatic morphology, a 70% to 80% long-term success rate in achieving postoperative pain control can be anticipated. In those patients who fail to achieve pain relief or in patients who develop recurrent pain during the postoperative follow-up period, radiographic and endoscopic investigation of postoperative anatomy should be carried out. If there is no anatomic explanation for their recurrent symptoms (biliary stricture, fluid collection, pancreatic duct stricture, disease progression), percutaneous or endoscopic ultrasound (EUS)–guided celiac plexus block should be considered to assist in pain management. If further denervation is required, bilateral thoracoscopic splanchnicectomy can be considered if the patient shows an appropriate response to a differential epidural anesthetic.

 ## SURGICAL TECHNIQUE

Open Celiac Plexus Block

Open celiac plexus block has become a standard approach to pain management in patients undergoing laparotomy for unresectable pancreatic cancer. The procedure was first described by Copping et al. in 1969. In an update of their series in 1978, including 41 patients with pain due to pancreatic cancer, 88% of patients experienced relief of pain postoperatively. Most patients underwent palliative biliary and gastrojejunal bypass at the same operation. These results were compared with a group of historic controls in which only 21% of patients had pain control after similar palliative procedures. Since that time, this procedure has been advocated by a number of authors in anecdotal reports describing successful control of pain in the majority of patients. In 1993, a prospective, randomized, placebo-controlled study of this treatment was completed, with results demonstrating that open chemical neurolysis with a 50% alcohol solution significantly reduces or prevents pain in patients with unresectable pancreatic cancer when compared to a placebo injection with saline. This beneficial effect was observed in all randomized patients, including both subgroups of patients, those with and without preoperative pain. Interestingly, this study also showed a significant improvement in survival in patients with significant preoperative pain who received the alcohol neurolysis when compared with placebo, implying that better pain control and a reduced requirement for

narcotic analgesics may prolong, as well as improve, the quality of life in patients with end-stage pancreatic cancer.

Through an upper midline or bilateral subcostal incision the abdomen is entered, and careful assessment of the tumor for resectability is done. After determining that the cancer is unresectable, the operating surgeon's focus should switch from aggressive tumor extirpation to palliation. After completion of the appropriate operative bypasses of the biliary system and/or gastric outlet, chemical neurolysis should be considered. Forty milliliters of a 50% alcohol solution is prepared in a sterile fashion by diluting 20 mL of absolute ethanol with 20 mL of sterile injectable saline solution (1:1). A 20-mL syringe with a 22-gauge spinal needle is used for delivery of this solution to the para-aortic tissues. The lesser omentum is incised over the bare area and the celiac axis can be palpated through the retroperitoneum as it arises from the aorta, behind the stomach, near the diaphragmatic crura. A palpable thrill due to the high blood flow through the celiac axis is usually apparent. The operating surgeon, using his or her left hand, then straddles the celiac axis, putting the

index finger on the splenic artery and the middle finger on the common hepatic artery while stabilizing this orientation with the thumb on the left side of the abdominal aorta (Fig. 2). The 22-gauge spinal needle is then advanced into the soft tissue on both sides of the aorta, both below and above the level of the celiac artery (10 mL of 50% alcohol solution is injected into all four quadrants). Both before and episodically during the injection, the syringe should be aspirated to ensure that the inferior vena cava, coronary vein, aorta, or adjacent lumbar vessels have not been inadvertently cannulated. If blood flow is obtained with this maneuver, the surgeon simply withdraws the needle, repositions, aspirates again, and resumes infiltration of the ethanol solution into the para-aortic soft tissue. Instillation of at least 40 mL of 50% ethanol solution is considered necessary to achieve an adequate celiac block.

After completing the injection in all four quadrants, the sites are inspected for hemostasis. If minor bleeding is observed, the area is packed and compressed for a short period of time. At the time of injection, the anesthesiologist should be notified of the procedure. Occasionally, with an ad-

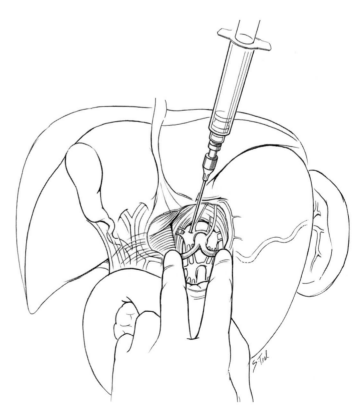

Fig. 2. Intraoperative celiac plexus block (CPB). After incising the avascular area of the hepatogastric ligament, the celiac trunk is palpated by placing the surgeon's left index finger on the splenic artery and left third finger on the common hepatic artery while steadying his or her hand by abutting the thumb to the left lateral aspect of the aorta. The surgeon's right hand uses the 10-mL syringe to inject 50% ethanol into four quadrants around the celiac axis.

The Gastrointestinal Tract

equate sympathetic blockade, some degree of hypotension may be observed. This situation can generally be managed easily by the anesthesiologist giving additional intravenous fluids or the judicious use of pharmacologic blood pressure support. As a general rule, celiac plexus block is quite well tolerated with few complications, and it requires no alteration in the postoperative management of patients undergoing laparotomy and palliative bypass procedures for unresectable pancreatic cancer. Mild complications include bleeding and postural hypotension; both are generally self-limiting and easily managed. Bleeding can generally be controlled by direct pressure intraoperatively. During the first attempts at postoperative ambulation, the patient should be observed for any evidence of orthostatic hypotension. However, this effect, if noted at all, is seldom long-lasting. In patients who have only had exploration and biopsy for tissue diagnosis in which a celiac plexus block is also done, oral intake can be resumed as tolerated, and the patient can be discharged as soon as possible after the procedure. Serious complications are rare but include diarrhea, gastroparesis, chylothorax, retroperitoneal abscess, superior mesenteric vein thrombosis, extradural abscess, and reversible paraparesis. There has been a single case report of paraplegia after celiac plexus block.

The predominant reasons for failure of an adequate celiac plexus block are either poor localization of the injection to the celiac plexus or use of an inadequate volume of neurolytic agent. With large tumors involving the pancreatic neck/proximal body or with tumors with extensive associated celiac lymphadenopathy, identification of the appropriate intraoperative anatomy is often problematic and these patients are often better approached percutaneously using CT guidance as a separate procedure after recovery from the operation. Pain relief even with a successful celiac plexus block will often be poor when the tumor is extensive enough to involve somatically innervated sites in the abdominal wall, Glisson capsule, or diaphragm.

Bilateral Thoracoscopic Splanchnicectomy

The transthoracic approach for pancreatic splanchnic denervation has gained increasing popularity, particularly in patients with intractable pain who have undergone previous abdominal procedures. Pancreatic denervation to interrupt the flow of painful stimuli from the pancreas through the central nervous system has conceptually intrigued surgeons since its first report by Mallet-Guy in 1943. The ability to relieve pain from chronic pancreatitis with a single therapeutic intervention without disrupting the pancreas or digestive tract or reoperating through a scarred abdomen remains an extremely attractive option for a large segment of patients with chronic pancreatitis. In 1993, two groups combined the theories of Mallet-Guy with the burgeoning technology of video thoracoscopy to report on the use of thoracoscopic splanchnicectomy to treat the pain from pancreatic cancer. This marriage, combining the mystique of neuronal ablation with minimally invasive surgery, re-energized the surgical community in search of a simple, straightforward procedure to address the vexing problem of pain from chronic pancreatitis. The operation was extended to patients with chronic pancreatitis and modified to include bilateral nerve ablation through a posterior approach, and patients were screened by the use of a differential epidural anesthetic to identify those individuals who would have a high likelihood of success with the procedure.

The operative technique we use is similar to that originally described by Cuschieri et al. with minor modifications. Briefly, the procedure is done under a general endotracheal anesthetic with double-lumen intubation to provide for sequential single-lung ventilation. The patient is then placed in the full prone jackknife position with a Foley and orogastric tube, TED hose, and SCDs. Operative access is established using a three-port technique: A 10-mm port (camera port) is positioned in the sixth intercostal space at the posterior axillary line, and two 5-mm ports (working ports) are placed in the fourth and eighth intercostal spaces approximately half the distance between the posterior axillary line and the spine (Fig. 3). Local anesthetic (0.5% Marcaine) is used liberally in the thoracic access sites, the lung on the operative side is deflated, and single-lung ventilation is continued on the contralateral side. Once access to the chest has been gained, the sympathetic chain is often easily identified through the parietal pleura running along the posterior chest wall above the vertebral bodies. Occasionally, due to prior pleural disease (effusions, inflammation), the parietal pleura is thickened and opaque and the neural anatomy cannot be identified without opening the mediastinal pleura. Once the mediastinal pleura is opened in a cephalad-to-caudad direction perpendicular to the vertebral bodies, the greater splanchnic nerve is identified by following small ramus fibers from the fifth to eighth sympathetic ganglia, which coalesce into the main greater splanchnic trunk. Dissection continues along its entire course in the mediastinum to the diaphragm, clipping and dividing all rami communicans from the sympathetic ganglia and then clipping and dividing the proximal and distal segments to completely remove the entire nerve (Fig. 4). Rami communicans from the 8th to 11th intercostal space (lesser splanchnic nerves) can occasionally

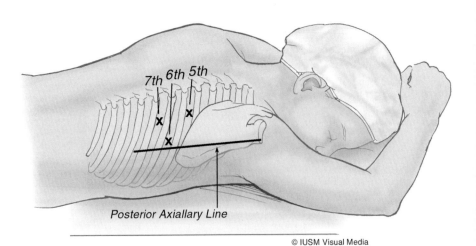

© IUSM Visual Media

Fig. 3. This image shows the trocar positioning for bilateral thoracoscopic splanchnicectomy. In our setup, we use the posterior axillary line in the sixth intercostal space where we place a 10-mm trocar for camera placement. We then use a triangular positioning of the two 5-mm working ports in the fifth and seventh intercostal spaces, halfway between the posterior axillary line and the vertebral column.

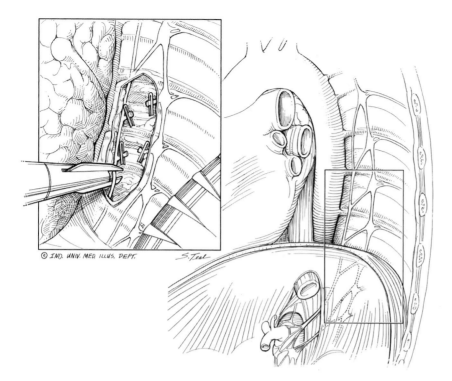

© IND. UNIV. MED. ILLUS. DEPT.   S. Teat

Fig. 4. Intraoperative diagram in which the boxed image illustrates a magnified view of the operation from the surgeon's perspective. In this image, through an opening in the mediastinal pleura, the surgeon is dissecting and dividing the small rami communicans from the thoracic sympathetic ganglia to the greater splanchnic nerve while isolating the nerve throughout its length in the chest.

be found and are easily disrupted using the hook electrocautery when identified. It is important to completely remove the entire greater splanchnic nerve as regrowth of sympathetic nerves is possible. Diaphragmatic elevation, particularly in the left chest, can occur from gastric dilation caused by air trapped in the stomach as a result of vigorous bag masking during the induction phase of a general endotracheal anesthetic. This elevated diaphragm obscures the full course of the greater splanchnic nerve, particularly the lower rami communicans (T7 and T8), resulting in an incomplete splanchnicectomy. Gastric decompression with an orogastric tube can often reduce the diaphragm elevation and improve visualization inferiorly in the chest, allowing a more complete nerve dissection.

After nerve resection, hemostasis is obtained and the lungs are reinflated under direct vision. The chest is then closed in layers using subcutaneous 3-0 Vicryl and a subcuticular stitch using 4-0 Vicryl; during

closure the lung is completely expanded using a gentle Valsalva maneuver. Steristrips and a sterile dressing are placed and the surgeons go to the other side of the patient and repeat the procedure on the contralateral side. At the end of the procedure, the patient remains intubated and is moved to an adjacent gurney and is positioned sitting upright while a chest radiograph is done in the operating room. This film is read prior to the reversal of the anesthetic. If a significant pneumothorax is identified, a small-bore chest tube is inserted through a prior trochar site in the appropriate chest and secured in place while the patient remains anesthetized. If no pneumothorax is seen, the anesthetic is reversed and the patient is extubated and taken to the recovery room.

Perioperative morbidity rate in our series was 11% (three chylothoraces, two wound infections, one pneumonia), and the average postoperative hospital stay was 3.6 days (range 2 to 27 days). Two patients required reoperation for persistent

chylothoraces recalcitrant to closure by use of standard medical treatment. Six patients (11%) had postoperative intercostal neuralgia persisting for longer than 30 days postoperatively. Five of the six had eventual pain relief, on average 3 months from the operation. One patient had continued neuralgia requiring re-referral to our pain clinic for evaluation and intercostal nerve blocks. There were no deaths related to the operative procedure. The most common causes of failure from this operation are either misidentification of the greater splanchnic nerve or incomplete mobilization of the nerve (particularly T7 and T8 in the inferior part of the dissection) to ensure that all rami communicans through the splanchnic nerve to the abdomen are ablated.

CONCLUSION

Splanchnic denervation to manage intractable pancreatic pain is a rarely indicated procedure. However, when used in the proper situation, in a carefully selected patient, it can be an extremely effective therapeutic option.

SUGGESTED READING

Buscher HCJL, Jansen JBMJ, van Dongen R, et al. Long-term results of bilateral thoracoscopic splanchnicectomy in patients with chronic pancreatitis. *Br J Surg* 2002;89:158.

Copping J, Williz R, Draft R. Palliative chemical splanchnicectomy. *Arch Surg* 1969;98:418.

Cuschieri A, Shimi SM, Crothwaite G, et al. Bilateral endoscopic splanchnicectomy through a posterior thoracoscopic approach. *J R Coll Surg Edinb* 1994;39:44.

Howard TJ, Swofford JB, Wagner DL, et al. Quality of life after bilateral thoracoscopic splanchnicectomy: long-term evaluation in patients with chronic pancreatitis. *J Gastrointest Surg* 2002;6:845.

Lillemoe KD, Cameron JC, Kaufman HS, et al. Chemical splanchnicectomy in patients with unresectable pancreatic cancer: a prospective randomized trial. *Ann Surg* 1993;217:447.

Mallet-Guy PA. Late and very late results of resections of the nervous system in the treatment of chronic relapsing pancreatitis. *Am J Surg* 1983;145:234.

Warshaw AL, Banks PA, Fernndez-del Castillo C. AGA technical review on treatment of pain in chronic pancreatitis. *Gastroenterology* 1998;115:765.

Woodham MJ, Hanna MH. Paraplegia after celiac plexus block. *Anaesthesia* 1989;44(6):487.

The Gastrointestinal Tract

EDITOR'S COMMENT

Intractable pancreatic pain is awful and debilitating. For pancreatic cancer patients, it ruins their quality of remaining life. For chronic pancreatitis patients, it makes their lives unmanageable as recurrent hospitalizations and narcotic addictions become the norm for some. The psychosocial stigmata that can result are terrible. We have every desire to solve intractable pancreatic pain and stop such needless suffering. However, it seems we cannot.

Keith Lillemoe and Tom Howard speak from experience for *Mastery* and beautifully lay out the anatomy, pathophysiology, and clinical realities of pancreatic pain. There are so many collateral anatomic elements of pancreatic pain that it is no wonder we have failed. In this comprehensive chapter, our authors summarize the treatment algorithm endorsed by the AGA (Table 1), which brings patients from lifestyle changes through pancreatic enzymes to nerve blocks and ultimately endoscopic or surgical treatments. The description of the differential epidural anesthetic to discriminate true pancreatic pain is quite interesting. Finally, we are provided sensible indications for the splanchnic denervation procedures, and clear technical instruction for how these procedures should be performed.

One understands why intractable pancreatic pain occurs and can be so severe, and why its refractory nature is determined by the redundant neural anatomy pathways described. All of our current strategies to control this pain are detailed, but all of them target peripheral pathways. As noted, the purposeful interruption of visceral pain afferents to the pancreas took hold many years ago, and today, is accomplished via the minimally invasive and open techniques described. All these techniques carry risks, and despite how well applied and performed, have variable efficacy and durability. Do not lose hope, however. As I will describe, new emerging data suggest that our best solutions may lie centrally, not peripherally.

Some very practical technical points regarding celiac plexus block warrant mention. First, does your operating room actually have sterile absolute alcohol available? You will need to be sure of this and otherwise properly prepared to avoid annoying delays. I have always followed the precise technique illustrated herein for open celiac plexus block since it is not difficult and is safe (*Ann Surg* 1993;217:447). Despite the useful straddle maneuver illustrated in Figure 2, this still is to some degree a deep blind stick into the para-aortic soft tissues. Also, my routine is to instill four-quadrant 5-mL injections initially, and move on to performing the palliative biliary and gastrointestinal bypasses as indicated. I return before closing and repeat four-quadrant 5-mL injections, reaching the total recommended 40-mL volume. Though I have no proof that this matters, conceptually it could render a more complete neurolysis.

As noted, a resurgence of interest in BTS for the treatment of intractable pancreatic pain has been fueled by video thoracoscopy technology. Ihse et al. (*Ann Surg* 1999;230:785) evaluated BTS prospectively in 23 pancreatic cancer patients and 21 chronic pancreatitis patients with follow-up of 3 and 43 months, respectively. Both pain scores and indicators of pancreatic function were evaluated. All patients had decreased narcotic use and at least a 50% reduction in pain scores. Howard (*J Gastrointest Surg* 2002;6:845) and Hammond (*Am Surg* 2004;70:546) have each subsequently evaluated BTS for chronic pancreatitis with solid results. While critics will point to limited responses of short duration, our authors correctly emphasize that patients qualify for BTS once other pain-control measures have failed. As such, BTS is a salvage therapy, and any positive response is valuable. Although minimally invasive, BTS is not an innocuous procedure, with significant complications such as chylothorax noted in all available series. One could question exposing end-stage pancreatic cancer patients to such risks of BTS and the anesthetic and operation required.

Lastly, the question has arisen whether central mechanisms of intractable pancreatic pain should be targeted. After all, up to 40% of chronic pancreatitis patients have persistent same pain even after total pancreatectomy. This refractory nature of pancreatic pain prompted Freedman et al. to hypothesize that a central, not peripheral, mechanism was to blame. They have implicated abnormal brain cortical regulation of visceral sensation, suggesting that symptoms are sustained by a pancreas-independent, neural-based mechanism. To test their hypothesis, they performed a double-blind, sham controlled pilot trial of repetitive transcranial magnetic stimulation (rTMS) to suppress cortical excitation (*Ann Neurol* 2005;58: 971; *Pain* 2006;122:197). They have convincingly shown that low-frequency rTMS applied to the right secondary somatosensory area can decrease pain and narcotic use in patients with idiopathic chronic pancreatitis. A larger study with longer duration rTMS is under way, and hopefully will reveal a better treatment for intractable pancreatic pain.

M.P.C.

Portal Hypertension and Its Treatment

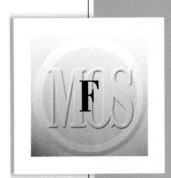

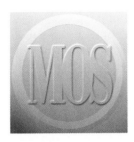

Introduction to the Treatment of Portal Hypertension

JOSEF E. FISCHER

The treatment of portal hypertension has become a critical issue in preserving lives of cirrhotic patients. Whereas previously in this country alcoholism was the principle reason for bleeding esophageal varices, the increased incidence of hepatitis B and hepatitis C have resulted in a reservoir of patients that may bleed from esophageal varices and ultimately are candidates for hepatic transplantation. In considering hepatic transplantation, it is important to carry out whatever therapy for portal hypertension one can and at least try to preserve the opportunity to carry out a liver transplant later. The principal anatomic necessity means that whatever mechanism one uses to carry out the control of bleeding esophageal varices, it should, whenever possible, leave the porta hepatis free of previous surgery.

For the most part, many centers of liver transplantation will also deal with patients with bleeding esophageal varices. This is done either by endoscopy, as detailed elsewhere in this section, either by injection or by rubber band obliteration of bleeding esophageal and gastric varices. When these techniques fail, a transjugular intrahepatic portosystemic shunt (TIPS) procedure is done, in which one provides an egress of high-pressure portal flow from the portal system into the systemic system by means of a shunt traversing the hepatic parenchyma. For the most part, in the present state of knowledge, TIPS cannot be used as definitive therapy for bleeding esophageal varices, but are used as a bridge in patients who must by necessity undergo liver transplantation in the finite future. The

stenosis rate of the TIPS conduit is high, ranging between 30% and 50% or even higher at the end of 1 year. Thus, there are many techniques for actually dilating stenoses so that the patient can undergo subsequent hepatic transplant.

However, there remains a group of patients in whom cessation and arrest of bleeding esophageal varices and gastric varices cannot be accomplished with TIPS and other means of controlling the often-torrential hemorrhage. In these patients, shunt surgery then becomes a necessity.

In addition, there are a group of patients, mostly class A patients, in whom the state of hepatic function is such that it is thought they can survive for a long period of time without liver transplant. In these patients, some type of shunt surgery, which is described in the subsequent chapters, then becomes a necessity. The hypothetical equation in carrying out shunt surgery is to do enough to decrease portal pressure to a reasonable level so that bleeding from esophageal varices stops in this instance and can be prevented from happening again. The obverse of this equation is to provide enough forward portal pressure to allow hepatic perfusion so that hepatic failure is not the result of shunt surgery. In order to understand the complexities of this pressure equation, it is necessary to understand the basics.

The liver is supplied by two perfusion systems, the hepatic artery, a splanchnic artery that is usually responsible from between 20% and 25% of hepatic flow under normal circumstances. The portal vein is not generally oxygen-deprived; thus, the hepatic artery, rather than most organs supplying all of the essential oxygenation, supplies only 50% of the oxygen requirement of the liver. The portal vein, which normally supplies between 75% and 80% of the flow, also supplies 50% of the oxygen requirement of the liver, as well as the lion's share of nutrients derived from the gut and its absorption of nutrients. The liver, sitting astride the portal vein, absorbs and processes and, in some cases, stores for release into the general circulation the nutrients, which appear in the portal vein. The liver probably processes nearly 100% of the carbohydrate presented to it. It also processes the majority of the amino acids presented to it, notably the aromatic amino acids, of which two in particular, phenylalanine and its hydroxylated product tyrosine, are principal components of hepatic protein synthesis, but also form the substrate for the sympathetic nervous system as well as many of the amines, which perform vital functions within the brain. Lipids are separately absorbed, and are usually absorbed in their triglyceride form in the lymphatics, which then enter the venous system through the thoracic duct and thus do not pass through the liver.

The age-old question that has persisted for a century is, does the liver require all of the nutrients that pass through it for its own structural integrity, including structural protein synthesis, or does it only require a portion of it, and the rest can be distributed to the periphery? The evidence that is slowly building up seems to indicate that the liver does in fact require all of these nutrients in order to maintain its integrity. This is surprising, because some of the older, classic data from the 1950s and 1960s indicate that, of a protein load that is given enterally in dogs, only approximately 21% ends up as amino acids, which are available in the general circulation. More than half finally end up as urea, after going through gluconeogenesis. The question this raises is, if there is something special about the glucose which is produced from protein, is it required at a certain place at a certain time? With the advent of knowledge of the cytoskeleton, in which the location of various nutrients as close to the various enzyme systems that do not float free in the cell as a bag but are firmly fixed to the cell membrane, or other aspects of the cytoskeleton, there appears to be an answer to this important question. The answer is that glucose, which is created through gluconeogenesis, does end up as glycogen immediately adjacent to certain enzyme systems, which then use the substrate for specific functions such as aerobic glycolysis, as our laboratory showed in the 1990s and in the first years of this century.

Aerobic glycolysis produces considerably less adenosine triphosphate than glucose that goes through the Krebs cycle—considerably less. However, it is important because of its location in the cytoskeleton to a series of membrane-bound enzymes that make the glucose, which ends in glycogen, a very valuable commodity for essential cellular functions. It has also created the controversy as to whether lactate, which remains elevated in response to epinephrine (James JH, et al. *Lancet* 1999; 354:505; James Fischer. *Crit Care Med* 2001;29:454; James JH, et al. *Am J Physiol* 1999;277:E176)—and thus overresuscitating a patient simply on the basis of elevated blood lactate, when in fact every other parameter indicates complete resuscitation—may be injurious to the entire organism.

In addition to the nutrients that course in the portal vein, there are trophic factors that seem to be essential for the integrity and normal functioning of the liver. Beginning in the late 1950s and in the early 1960s, there was a great deal of interest in insulin and glucagon and other putative peptides that appear to originate in the pancreas. In addition, the needs of regeneration of the liver appear to involve a substance known as *ileal factor*, which results from grinding up ileum and giving it in experiments of hepatic regeneration. This probably consisted of the vascular endothelial and epidermal growth factors and also some putative peptides present in the liver, which were essential, and not only permissive, for hepatic regeneration.

As bridging necrosis and replacing the reticulum elastic framework with fibrosis occurred in a liver that was progressively being destroyed by whatever disease was operant, the resistance to portal flow, either presinusoidal, sinusoidal, or postsinusoidal, depending on the pattern of the disease, elevated the resistance to portal flow. Under normal circumstances, flow would drop. Here, however, a feature of portal hypertension enters, and that is the presence of pumps, as it were, in which arterial admixture with portal flow provided increased positive pressure to the portal vein perfusion, thus maintaining portal flow to the liver. To the surgeon, portal flow is a nuisance. It results in variceal bleeding, collaterals around the rectum, gastric varices, the caput medusae at times, and large variceal collaterals in adhesions in the abdominal wall, varices around such structures as ileostomies, which, of course, are deleterious to the entire organism. To the liver, however, portal hypertension is probably a good thing, an attempt to maintain flow despite increased resistance. Thus, in all of the chapters that follow, there is always the question of balance: balance between forward perfusion of portal flow to the liver, and decompressing the portal system sufficiently so that the patient did not exsanguinate from variceal bleeding.

Early studies from Rousselot in the 1950s revealed that following end-to-side portacaval shunt and using flow meters around the hepatic artery so that those patients that did well following end-to-side hepatic portacaval shunt were those who had the ability to increase hepatic artery flow to take the place of portal flow and perfuse the liver. I prefer to look at this phenomenon as indicating the stage of liver disease. Those patients who could increase their portal flow had an earlier stage of cirrhosis, and for those who could not, that inability to increase hepatic artery flow indicated a late stage of the disease. Unfortunately, the advent of transplantation decreased research in this area, so that for many of the mystical concepts concerning hepatic regeneration, trophic factors necessary for the integrity of the liver now became irrelevant if one was going to replace a diseased liver that was fibrotic with a newly transplanted liver in which the portal flow was delivered, and normal hepatic function might result.

Finally, as one reads these various chapters and reads the claims of various individuals concerning specific shunts: For example, as one will read in the subsequent chapter, there were claims made that a distal splenorenal shunt was somehow magical and could prevent the inexorable desire, as it were, of blood at high pressure to seek a lower pressure. Indeed, Maillard et al. (*Surgery* 1979;86:663), among others, demonstrated by primitive angiography that within 24 hours of the distal splenorenal shunt, collaterals between the portal system and the systemic system arose rather quickly, thus robbing the liver of forward flow. The answer was the portal azygos disconnection—an operation that is beyond the technical abilities of most surgeons—to prevent this phenomenon from occurring. However, I believe this is futile, and our own studies have shown that in time, comparing distal splenorenal shunts with central splenorenal shunts, forward flow decreases progressively and the rates of encephalopathy, as a good mark for diminished hepatic function, proceeded at the same pace (Fischer JE, et al. *Ann Surg* 1981;194:531).

These are the choices one has to make in portal hypertension. The idea that somehow one can magically lower the pressure, leaving some portal hypertension to perfuse the liver, is superior to one shunt or another may be a goal that cannot be reached. However, what is clear is that there are certain operations that do preserve some portal flow; these are either small interposition shunts, distal splenorenal shunts, and/or central splenorenal shunts whose diameter is controlled, as Dr. Robert Linton taught me when I was his resident and a young staff person, so that forward perfusion of the liver occurs.

This whole area remains a fascinating area of physiology in which surgeons have always been interested because it applies directly to the welfare of their patients.

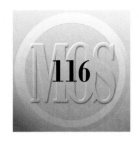

Anatomy of the Portal System

RICHARD H. BELL, JR., AND ALAN J. KOFFRON

The word *portal* is derived from the Latin *porta,* meaning "gate" or "passage." In Babylon, the livers of sacrificed animals were interpreted to predict the future. The Babylonians considered the liver the seat of the soul; the port of entry to this structure was therefore accorded special significance. Similarly, for modern surgery of the pancreas, liver, and portal hypertension, the portal vein has special importance. Knowledge of its anatomy and variants is crucial to ensure surgical success in performing such procedures.

DESCRIPTIVE ANATOMY

The portal vein arises from the postduodenal plexus of the embryonic vitelline veins. Rarely, the preduodenal plexus persists, giving rise to a portal vein that lies anterior to the duodenum. This anomaly, which is potentially lethal if it is not recognized and the portal vein is transected during surgery in this area, is associated with annular pancreas, malrotation, and biliary tract anomalies.

In the adult, the portal vein and its tributaries have no valves, those that existed during fetal circulation having been resorbed. The vein delivers blood from the spleen, the pancreas, and the digestive tube to the liver. It provides approximately 75% of hepatic blood flow and 50% of the oxygen delivery to this organ.

The portal vein can be thought of as the trunk of a tree, with the visceral veins (superior mesenteric, inferior mesenteric, and splenic) forming the roots, and the intrahepatic portions of the right and left portal veins forming the branches (Fig. 1). The vascular delta formed by the mixing of portal venous and hepatic arterial blood in the sinusoids of the liver then drains into the inferior vena cava through the three hepatic veins.

The portal vein trunk is 4.8 to 8.8 cm long, with an average length of 6.4 cm, and 0.6 to 1.2 cm wide, with an average width of 0.9 cm. It is formed behind the neck of the pancreas, at the level of the second lumbar vertebra, by the confluence of the superior mesenteric vein (SMV) and the splenic vein (Fig. 2). In approximately one third of the population, the inferior mesenteric vein joins the portal vein directly at

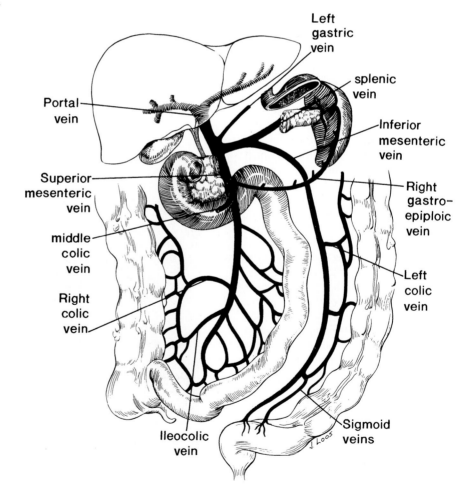

Fig. 1. Overview of the entire portal venous system within the abdominal cavity. (Modified from Monsen H. Anatomy of the portal system. In: Nyhus LM, Baker RJ, eds. *Mastery of surgery,* 2nd ed. Boston: Little, Brown and Company, 1992; and from Williams PL, Warwick R, eds. *Gray's anatomy,* 36th ed. New York: Churchill Livingstone, 1980.)

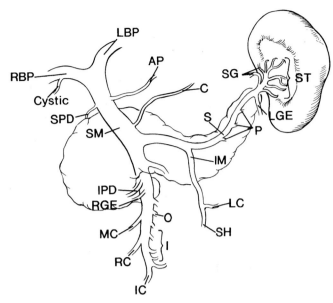

Fig. 2. Anatomy of the extrahepatic portal venous system. AP, accessory pancreatic vein; C, coronary vein; I, ileal veins; IC, ileocolic vein; IM, inferior mesenteric vein; IPD, inferior pancreaticoduodenal vein; LBP, left branch of portal vein; LC, left colic vein; LGE, left gastroepiploic vein; MC, middle colic vein; O, omental vein; P, pancreatic veins; RBP, right branch of portal vein; RC, right colic vein; RGE, right gastroepiploic vein; S, splenic vein; SG, short gastric veins; SH, superior hemorrhoidal vein; SM, superior mesenteric vein; SPD, superior pancreaticoduodenal vein; ST, splenic trunks. (Modified from Douglass B, Baggenstoss A, Hollinshead WH. The anatomy of the portal vein and its tributaries. *Surg Gynecol Obstet* 1960;91:564. By permission of *Surgery, Gynecology, & Obstetrics,* now known as the *Journal of the American College of Surgeons.*)

this point, forming a trifurcation; in the remaining cases, it drains into the splenic vein (38%) or the SMV (29%). The portal vein then passes to the right and cephalad behind the first portion of the duodenum and into the hepatoduodenal ligament, which forms the ventral boundary of the foramen of Winslow. Within the hepatoduodenal ligament, the portal vein lies posterior to the hepatic artery and common bile duct, usually slightly to the left of the duct. It bifurcates in the porta hepatis at the right aspect of the hilar plate—a thickening of the liver's fibrous capsule at the hilum (Fig. 3). The right branch, which supplies the right hepatic lobe, is shorter (0.5 to 1.0 cm long), wider, and more variable than its sinistral counterpart. It often divides into anterior and posterior branches at its point of entry into the liver parenchyma. The more constant and longer left portal vein, with a 4-cm average length, supplies the left hepatic lobe and runs left in the hilar plate as the pars transversa until it enters the fissure for the ligamentum venosum (Fig. 4). At this point, the vein receives the attachment of the ligamentum venosum and then curves anteriorly, becoming the pars umbilicus, which ends by attaching to the ligamentum teres hepaticus in the umbilical fissure. The caudate lobe is supplied by two to three branches arising from the

bifurcation of the portal vein or from its right or left branches.

Of great importance to the surgeon are the sundry side branches that feed into the portal vein as it forms behind the pancreas and runs cephalad in the hepatoduodenal ligament (Fig. 2). The portal vein usually receives the pancreaticoduodenal vein(s) and the pyloric vein, which is also known as the *right gastric vein*. More variable in their point of insertion are the coronary vein, which is also known as the *left gastric vein*, and the accessory pancreatic vein. The superior pancreaticoduodenal vein usually enters the right aspect of the portal vein at or just above the superior margin of the pancreas. The inferior pancreaticoduodenal vein usually enters the right aspect of the SMV just before it joins the splenic vein to form the portal vein proper. In approximately 38% of cases, there is only a single pancreaticoduodenal vein, which joins the portal vein at the same juncture as the superior pancreaticoduodenal vein. The pyloric vein is present in 80% of the population and, in 75% of the population, terminates in the anterior aspect of the portal vein (inside the hepatoduodenal ligament), within 3.0 cm of the portal vein bifurcation. The coronary vein inserts at the superior aspect of the junction of the splenic and SMVs in 60% of the population, in the portal vein proper in 25% of the population, and in the splenic vein (just

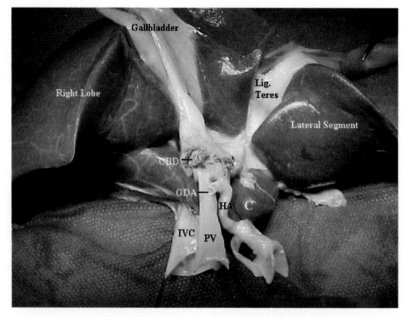

Fig. 3. The portal vein entering the visceral surface of the liver as viewed from below. The portal vein (PV) reaches the liver hilum posterior to the common bile duct (CBD) and hepatic artery (HA). The right branch of the PV enters quickly into the liver, whereas the left branch of the PV courses to the ligamentum teres (Lig. teres) within the umbilical fissure (medial to the left lateral segment). Note the relationship of the PV and inferior vena cava (IVC). GDA, gastroduodenal artery; C, caudate lobe.

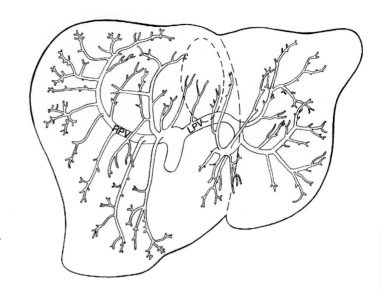

Fig. 4. The intrahepatic branching of the portal vein. Note that the caudate lobe often receives branches from both the right portal vein (RPV) and left portal vein (LPV) branches. In addition, note that the LPV enters the umbilical fissure before giving off branches that traverse back to the left medial segment. (Modified from Healey JE. Clinical anatomic aspects of radical hepatic surgery. *J Intern Coll Surg* 1954;22:542.)

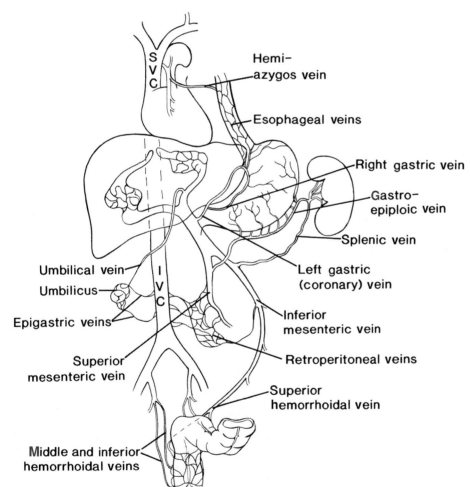

Fig. 5. Sites of formation of portosystemic collaterals in patients with portal hypertension. Connections between the portal and systemic venous system are normally present, but they carry increased flow when there is a block to portal venous flow through the liver. The sites of portosystemic collateral connections shown in this figure are (a) from the portal vein through the right and left gastric veins to the esophageal veins and the hemiazygos vein to the superior vena cava (SVC); (b) from the superior mesenteric vein through retroperitoneal veins to the inferior vena cava (IVC); (c) from the left portal vein through the (recanalized) umbilical vein to epigastric veins to the vena cava; and (d) from the inferior mesenteric vein through the superior hemorrhoidal vein to the middle and inferior hemorrhoidal veins to the iliac veins. (Modified from Orloff MJ. The biliary system. In: Sabiston DC, ed. *Textbook of surgery*, 10th ed. Philadelphia: WB Saunders, 1972.)

before its junction with the SMV) in 15% of the population. In a series of 92 dissections, 29 specimens had an accessory pancreatic vein terminating in the superior aspect of the midportal vein.

Another anatomic aspect of the portal system that is of importance to the surgeon are the points of communication between the portal and systemic (caval, azygous, and hemiazygous) venous systems (Fig. 5). Normally, these anastomotic channels are small, but the combination of portal hypertension and the lack of valves in the adult portal system leads to reversal of flow, with consequent dilatation and tortuosity. Clinically, the most important portosystemic anastomoses are the veins of the proximal stomach and distal esophagus, which receive flow from the coronary and short gastric veins and drain into the superior vena cava via the azygous system. Dilatation and tortuosity in this plexus of relatively unsupported veins results in varices that can rupture, causing exsanguinating hemorrhage. Other significant anastomotic areas include:

1. The submucosal venous plexus in the rectum between the superior hemorrhoidal veins (the portal system) and the middle and inferior hemorrhoidal veins (the caval system). Large bleeding rectal varices, although rare, can arise here in patients with portal hypertension.
2. The paraumbilical veins, which connect the left portal vein via a recannulated umbilical vein to the epigastric venous network of the abdominal wall, which drains into the caval system. This plexus can become the variceal "caput Medusae" in patients with portal hypertension. Accidental transection of one of these varices during surgery that

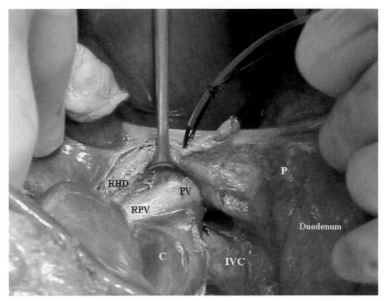

Fig. 6. Relationship of the portal vein (PV) to the inferior vena cava (IVC) before reconstruction of a portacaval shunt. View from the patient's right of exposure of the portal vein through an incision in the right posterolateral aspect of the hepatoduodenal ligament. The common bile duct is retracted anteriorly. RHD, right hepatic duct; RPV, right branch of the portal vein; C, caudate lobe of the liver; P, pancreas.

involves the anterior abdominal wall can result in significant blood loss.

3. Retzius veins, a group of small but numerous retroperitoneal veins that connect abdominal viscera, both tubular and solid, with the caval system via intercostal, phrenic, lumbar, and renal veins. In the patient with portal hypertension, bleeding from these veins can make any upper abdominal operation, from a cholecystectomy to a splenorenal shunt, extremely dangerous according to the amount and location of retroperitoneal dissection required.

4. Finally, significant venous collaterals can form in surgical adhesions, making reoperative surgery and stomal takedowns more dangerous in patients with portal hypertension.

 APPLIED ANATOMY

Portosystemic Shunts

One of the more common categories of surgical operations in which a detailed knowledge of portal anatomy is necessary is that of portosystemic shunts. A detailed review of the multiple causes of portal hypertension and the advantages and disadvantages of the various kinds of shunts is beyond the scope of this chapter; rather, the anatomic points of portal vein anatomy relevant to the performance of three frequently performed shunts are discussed.

The creation of a side-to-side portacaval shunt necessitates mobilizing a portion of the suprarenal inferior vena cava, as well as exposing the portal vein where it lies posteriorly in the hepatoduodenal ligament, which is best performed through a longitudinal incision over the right posterolateral aspect of the palpable vein (Fig. 6). Not infrequently, to

obtain good apposition of the two vessels, it is necessary to dissect out the portal vein circumferentially (Fig. 7). Great care should be taken during this maneuver because a pyloric, accessory pancreatic, or coronary vein can arise from the anteromedial aspect of the vein in the area of dissection. It is sometimes necessary to excise some of the peripancreatic tissue that covers the lateral aspect of the portal vein (where it emerges from the pancreas) to expose enough vein for the anastomosis. The superior pancreaticoduodenal vein usually joins the portal vein precisely in this area and should be ligated and divided (Fig. 7). Another anatomic point to keep in mind during the performance of this shunt is the aberrant or replaced right hepatic artery. In this variant, which is present in 15% to 20% of the population, the right hepatic artery arises from the superior mesenteric artery (SMA) and runs posterolateral to the common bile duct on top of the portal vein and, occasionally, behind the portal vein itself. A pulse in this area should alert the surgeon; the artery must be preserved because, in 60% to 80% of patients, it is truly a replacement vessel, supplying the entire right hepatic lobe. The portal vein usually crosses this aberrant vessel anteriorly as the artery originates from the SMA. The vein may become kinked at this point and partially obstructed when pulled posteriorly to appose the vena cava. This may cause shunt occlusion and persistent portal hypertension postoperatively.

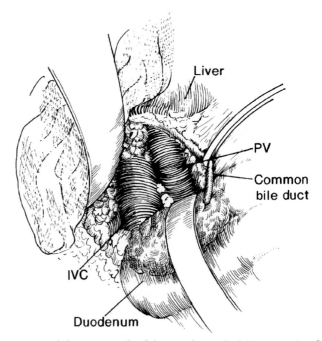

Fig. 7. Dissection around the main trunk of the portal vein (PV) in preparation for a portacaval shunt. The accessory pancreatic (AP) and superior pancreaticoduodenal (SPD) veins have been identified in preparation for ligation and division. IVC, inferior vena cava. (Modified from Zollinger RM Jr, Zollinger RM. *Atlas of surgical operations*, 6th ed. New York: Macmillan, 1988.).

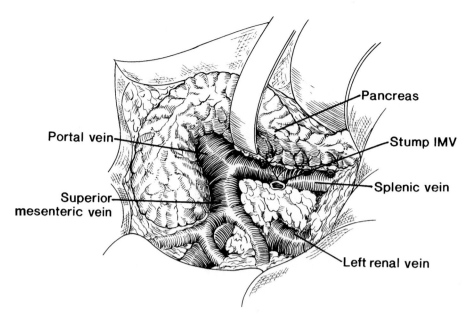

Fig. 8. Anatomy of splenorenal shunt as viewed from below. The splenic vein has been freed from the pancreas by ligation of small side branches from the pancreatic parenchyma. IMV, inferior mesenteric vein. (Modified from Zollinger Jr RM, Zollinger RM. *Atlas of surgical operations,* 6th ed. New York: Macmillan, 1988.)

The mesocaval shunt, in which the SMV is joined to the inferior vena cava with an interposition graft, necessitates exposure of the SMV at the root of the small bowel mesentery. This exposure is obtained by retracting the transverse colon cephalad and the small bowel caudad, and incising the peritoneum over the SMV, where it lies in the base of the mesointestine just to the right of the pulsatile SMA. Some texts make mention of the phenomenon of an absence of the SMV trunk, with, in its stead, several small mesenteric veins joining the splenic vein to form the origin of the portal vein. Such a configuration would make construction of an adequate mesocaval shunt impossible. However, in cadaveric dissection studies in which the vein was followed up to the level of the uncinate process of the pancreas, the SMV was always identified without difficulty and was a single large trunk.

The construction of a splenorenal shunt involves dissecting a portion of the splenic vein free of the posterior aspect of the pancreatic body and tail and anastomosing it to the immediately adjacent left renal vein (Fig. 8). This process requires ligation and the division of numerous small side branches from the pancreas that feed into the splenic vein. In some cases (up to 25% in cadaveric dissections), the groove that the splenic vein runs in is obscured by overhanging pancreatic tissue, necessitating division of pancreatic tissue to expose the vein. In the setting of portal hypertension,

the retroperitoneal Retzius veins are often dilatated and tortuous, making the dissection for splenorenal shunt quite difficult.

Pancreaticoduodenectomy

Another category of surgical procedure that requires a working knowledge of the portal vein is pancreaticoduodenectomy. When this operation is performed for a neoplasm of the pancreatic head, it is crucial to determine whether the portal and SMVs are free from tumor invasion as they course posterior to the neck of the pancreas. Exposure of the neck of the pancreas can be considerably improved by division of the right gastroepiploic vein as it courses across the anterior surface of the neck of the gland to insert into the SMV. Portal and SMV involvement by tumor can then be determined before resection, by establishing a "tunnel" underneath the neck of the pancreas, anterior to the portal vein. First, the anterior surface of the portal vein within the hepatoduodenal ligament is identified. Then, with a Kuttner dissector or other blunt-tipped instrument, the anterior surface of the portal vein is gently separated from the posterior aspect of the pancreas. Once a few centimeters have been cleared, the tunnel should be completed from below. This step involves entering the lesser sac, incising the peritoneum over the inferior margin of the pancreas, and identifying the SMV where it runs underneath the pancreas by

following the middle colic vein down the cephalad aspect of the transverse mesocolon to the junction of the two veins (Fig. 9A). The vein (initially the SMV, then the portal vein proper) is gently separated from the posterior aspect of the pancreas. In the absence of neoplastic invasion, the vein should separate easily from the pancreas. The patency of the tunnel can be confirmed with a finger or a long, blunt clamp (Fig. 9B). It is stated in some texts that venous tributaries do not enter the anterior surface of the portal or SMVs. Others have disputed this observation, however, and cadaveric dissections have documented the frequent insertion of the pyloric vein and the right gastroepiploic vein into the anterior surface of the portal and SMV, respectively. Therefore, this dissection must be performed with care.

Once resectability has been established, pancreatic neck is transected, allowing full exposure of the portal outflow system including the portal vein, SMV, and splenic vein (Fig. 9C). The head of the pancreas must now be separated from the portal vein. This necessitates the careful identification, ligation, and division of the branches running from the pancreatic head and uncinate process into the right lateral aspect of the portal vein and SMV. These include, with some variability, the superior and inferior pancreaticoduodenal veins (Fig. 9C), the right gastroepiploic vein, and other, anomalous branches arising as a result of the nearby neoplastic process. These venous branches must be managed carefully to control hemorrhage, preserve hepatic arterial inflow in the presence of a replaced right hepatic artery (Fig. 9C), and preserve the enteric venous outflow (Fig. 10).

Hepatic Resection

Knowledge of portal vein anatomy is also useful in performing hepatic resections. As mentioned in "Descriptive Anatomy," the portal vein usually bifurcates in the fibrous tissue at the right lateral aspect of the hilar plate. It is therefore possible to ligate and divide either branch at this point before resecting hepatic parenchyma when undertaking a formal right or left hepatic lobectomy. Exposure of the right portal vein can be improved by mobilizing the liver (i.e., incising the coronary, triangular, and falciform ligaments) and retracting the right lobe to the left and anteriorly. In 12% of patients, the anterior and posterior branches to the right lobe arise directly from the portal trunk (as opposed to the branching off of a proper right portal vein trunk as it enters the

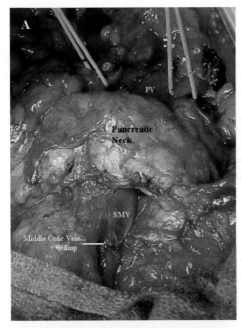

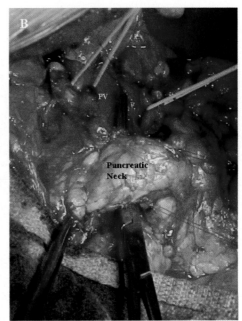

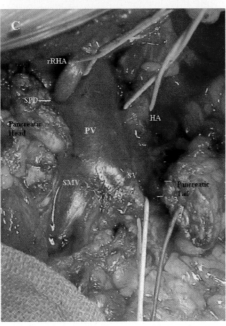

Fig. 9. A: Identification and dissection of the superior mesenteric vein (SMV) as it passes beneath the inferior border of the neck of the pancreas. Note the SMV may be initially located by following the middle colic vein to its entrance into the SMV. **B:** Demonstrating the patency of the tunnel between the anterior surface of the portal vein (PV) and the posterior surface of the neck of the pancreas. **C:** The pancreatic neck has been divided. Note the confluence of the SMV and splenic vein (SV) becomes the PV directly posterior to the pancreatic neck. Other pancreatic veins (e.g., superior pancreaticoduodenal vein, SPD) contribute to the portovenous system in this area. rRHA, replaced right hepatic artery; HA, hepatic artery.

hepatic parenchyma), giving the appearance of a trifurcation in the porta hepatis. The left portal vein can usually be exposed with minimal dissection where it runs as the pars transversa in the left lateral aspect of the hilar plate. When performing a right trisegmentectomy (right lobe plus left medial segment) or a left lateral segmentectomy, the surgeon must be cognizant of the portal blood supply to the left medial and lateral segments and thus avoid resection through the umbilical fissure. The previously described pars umbilicus of the left portal vein runs in the umbilical fissure, heading anteriorly until it fuses with the ligamentum teres hepaticus. The portal branches to the left medial segment run from the pars umbilicus

in the fissure back toward the right. The branches to the left lateral segment feed from the pars umbilicus in the fissure toward the left (Fig. 11). Therefore, in the case of right trisegmentectomy, hepatic parenchymal dissection should be performed to the right of the umbilical fissure to avoid devascularizing the remaining left lateral segment. Conversely, in the case of left lateral segmentectomy, dissection should be performed to the left of the fissure to avoid devascularizing the left medial segment.

 IMAGING PORTAL ANATOMY

The modern practitioner of pancreatic, hepatic, and portal hypertensive surgery

must not only recognize portal anatomy intraoperatively, but must know the methods to image it preoperatively and postoperatively. Principal reasons for performing such assessments include checking for thrombosis in the portal vein or its tributaries before attempting a portosystemic shunt or hepatic transplant, postoperative documentation of shunt or portal vein patency, and determining proximity to or invasion of the portal vein by neoplasms.

Portography used to be the "gold standard" for imaging the portal vein. However, helical computed tomography (CT) has become the diagnostic tool of choice for imaging the portal vein. Portography

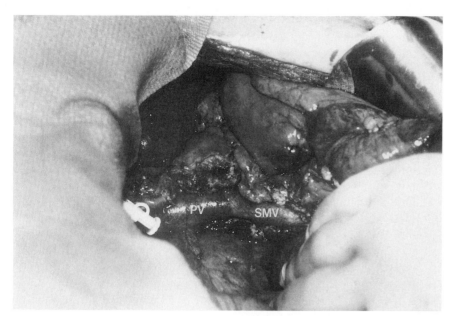

Fig. 10. View from the patient's right of the portal vein (PV) and superior mesenteric vein (SMV) after the head of the pancreas and the duodenum have been resected. A clamp has been placed on the transected common bile duct.

than regular ultrasonography, CT, and portography for diagnosing portal venous invasion by pancreaticobiliary carcinomas. Intraportal endovascular ultrasonography is a new diagnostic procedure that may prove even more sensitive in evaluating tumor involvement of the portal vein. These advances in ultrasonic diagnostics may prove particularly useful for preoperative planning in light of recent evidence that tumor invasion of the portal vein is not a contraindication for pancreatic resection.

Magnetic resonance (MR) imaging has become a valuable diagnostic tool in portal venous evaluation. Although surgical shunts are being performed less frequently, the increasing numbers of both cadaveric and live-donor liver transplants has led to advances in MR imaging. This modality is noninvasive and without significant complications. With improved technology, particularly the combination of nonnephrotoxic intravenous contrast and novel computer software, the spatial resolution is approaching that of CT, further augmented by the ability to perform MR three-dimensional reconstruction. MR angiography and MR venography is superior to DU in imaging the splenic vein and SMV, as well as in detecting either thrombus and deep portosystemic collaterals.

and CT are expensive and can result in hemorrhage, nephrotoxicity, and contrast reactions in an already ill patient population. Duplex ultrasonography (DU) costs much less than CT and has no known complications.

Despite the usual limitations of ultrasonography (e.g., level of operator experience with the technique or poor visibility in patients with abundant bowel gas or obesity), DU is highly sensitive (it approaches 100% when compared with invasive contrast studies in some series) for demonstrating postoperative patency of surgically placed portacaval shunts. It is also useful preoperatively to screen for thrombosis in the portal system. With DU, however, thrombosis of the SMV and splenic veins can be more difficult to identify than portal vein thrombosis. Therefore, if a complete evaluation of the SMV and splenic vein is desired (i.e., when planning a mesocaval or splenorenal shunt, respectively) but not obtainable by DU, CT should be performed. If DU demonstrates an apparently normal portal vein and an incompletely visualized splenic vein in a patient with an enlarged spleen and bleeding gastric varices (suggesting splenic vein thrombosis), helical CT should be carried out to clarify the diagnosis before a surgical procedure is performed. Additional uses of DU are determining portal flow direction (i.e., hepatofugal versus hepatopetal) if the surgeon deems this important in deciding what kind of shunt to perform, and intraoperative location of the

portal vein and its branches (i.e., finding the pars transversa of the left portal vein in the hepatic hilum before dissection).

Intraoperative ultrasonography has also proved to be more sensitive and specific

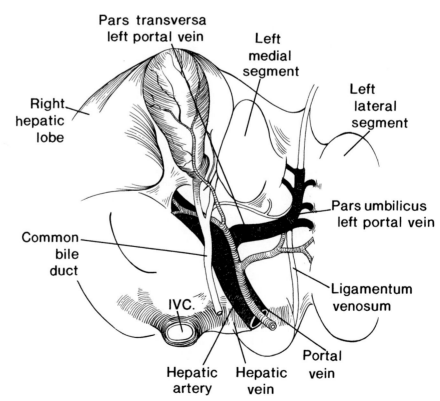

Fig. 11. Anatomy of the left portal vein in the umbilical fissure. IVC, inferior vena cava. (Modified from Yamaoka Y, Ozawa K, Shimahara Y, et al. A simple and direct approach to the portal triad structures for a left lobectomy or a left lateral segmentectomy. *Surg Gynecol Obstet* 1988;166:78.)

The Gastrointestinal Tract

More recently, the development of MR cholangiopancreatography has added the ability to accurately define extrahepatic biliary and intrapancreatic ductal anatomy and pathology that may influence operative conduct. MR angiography and MR venography should be considered when DU is inadequate and CT is contraindicated or inadequate. Additional uses of MR angiography and MR venography include (a) determining the anatomic relationship between the splenic vein and the left renal vein when considering a splenorenal shunt, (b) planning major hepatic resection in which portal vein resection and reconstruction is a possibility, (c) planning the surgical approach in hepatic transplantation to avoid large collateral vessels in the porta hepatis or manage the removal of the increasing numbers of transjugular intrahepatic portosystemic shunts, (d) evaluation and surgical management of the portal vein during live-donor liver transplantation, and (e) the ability to simultaneously evaluate arterial, venous, and ductal anatomy using a single imaging modality in efforts to reduce patient inconvenience and medical cost.

SUGGESTED READING

Bach AM, Hann LE, Brown KT. Portal vein evaluation with US: comparison to angiography combined with CT arterial portography. *Radiology* 1996;201:149.

Douglass BE, Baggenstoss AH, Hollinshead WH. The anatomy of the portal vein and its tributaries. *Surg Gynecol Obstet* 1950;92:562.

Furukawa H, Kosuge T, Mukai K. Helical computed tomography in the diagnosis of portal vein invasion by pancreatic head carcinoma: usefulness for selecting surgical procedures and predicting the outcome. *Arch Surg* 1998;133:61.

Ger R. Surgical anatomy of hepatic venous system. *Clin Anat* 1988;1:15.

Kaneko T, Nakao A, Takagi H. Intraportal endovascular ultrasonography for pancreatic cancer. *Semin Surg Oncol* 1998;15:47.

Koslin BD, Mulligan SA, Berland LL. Duplex assessment of the portal venous system. *Semin Ultrasound CT MRI* 1992;13:22.

Lomas DJ, Britton PD, Alexander GJM, et al. A comparison of MR and duplex Doppler ultrasound for vascular assessment prior to orthotopic liver transplantation. *Clin Radiol* 1994;49:307.

Meyers W, Jones RS. *Textbook of liver and biliary surgery.* Philadelphia: JB Lippincott Co, 1990.

Nghiem HV, Winter TC, Schmiedl UP. MR angiography of the portal venous system. *Semin Ultrasound CT MRI* 1996;17:360.

Schwartz SI. Pancreas. In: Schwartz SI, ed. *Principles of surgery,* 5th ed. New York: McGraw-Hill, 1989.

Skandalakis U, Rowe JS Jr, Gray SW, et al. Surgical anatomy and embryology of the pancreas. In: Skandalakis JE, ed. *Surgical anatomy and embryology.* Philadelphia: WB Saunders, 1993.

Sugiyama M, Hagi H, Atomi Y. Reappraisal of intraoperative ultrasonography for pancreaticobiliary carcinomas: assessment of malignant portal venous invasion. *Surgery* 1999;125:160.

VanDamme J-P J. Behavioral anatomy of the abdominal arteries. In: Skandalakis JE, ed. *Surgical anatomy and embryology.* Philadelphia: WB Saunders, 1993.

Yamaoka Y, Ozawa K, Shimahara Y, et al. A simple and direct approach to the portal triad structures for a left lobectomy or a left lateral segmentectomy. *Surg Gynecol Obstet* 1988;166:78.

Zollinger RM Jr, Zollinger RM. *Atlas of surgical operations,* 6th ed. New York: Macmillan, 1988.

EDITOR'S COMMENT

"Anatomy of the Portal System" is written by Drs. Richard Bell and Alan Koffron. Dr. Bell's credentials for writing this chapter are beyond reproach, as he trained with two of the giants in the area of portal hypertension and the portal venous system, Dr. Marshall Orloff and Dr. Tom Starzl. This is a succinct chapter that indicates the anatomic variance in the portal system and what one must be careful about when encountering them. Violating the anatomic relationships that Dr. Bell has so clearly delineated may result in either torrential hemorrhage, as if one were to inadvertently transect or damage a collateral, or a basic anatomical venous draining structure as it approaches either the superior mesenteric vein or the portal vein. In addition, given the adage that there is no normal portal anatomy, there are only variations, more often than not, Dr. Bell gives many of them. A disastrous complication of working within the porta is the replaced right hepatic artery, which usually supplies the entire right lobe of the liver. Inadvertent transection of the right hepatic artery almost invariably results in the death of a patient from right lobular necrosis, either acutely, in which case death occurs early, or a chronic loss of right lobe function, resulting in the death of a patient after 1 or 2 months. At autopsy, central lobular necrosis is usually present. Thus, one must be especially vigilant to anticipate these different anatomic arrangements in order to be on guard when performing the operation within or near the portal triad, as in a side-to-side portacaval shunt. For many of these reasons, end-to-side portacaval shunts or side-to-side portacaval shunt is no longer performed as often as it was, for example, when I was a resident and young staff person, when we did not have the expertise in rubber banding or injection of esophageal or gastric varices such as we do now, and TIPS did not exist.

One of the things that aids the surgeon is the incredible progress that has been made in vascular imaging, be it a helical CT, MR image, or ultrasound. As the authors correctly point out, with the progress in ultrasound for which there are no known complications, one may be able to get a detail of anatomy that is sufficient to allow the operating surgeon to proceed with confidence that he or she knows the anatomy of the portal system in the patient about to be encountered.

Others have attempted to use more advanced computer-generated enhancements of ultrasound in order to make the diagnosis of cirrhotic liver disease by getting a better view of peripheral hepatic vasculature. Zheng et al. (*World J Gastroenterol* 2005;11:6348) have used contrast-enhanced, code-phase inversion harmonic ultrasonography to get a better view of the peripheral vasculature in cirrhosis. In 20 patients, including 5 normal volunteers and 16 patients (10 with established liver cirrhosis and 6 with chronic hepatitis), using a 6- to 8-MHz convex-arrayed wide-band transducer. The time when microbubble appeared in the peripheral vessel was also recorded. These authors found that the microbubble arrival time at peripheral artery, portal, and hepatic vein was shorter in cirrhotic patients than in the patients with chronic hepatitis and normal subjects. They also rated their findings on the basis of marked, slight, and no morphologic changes in peripheral hepatic vasculature. They proposed this methodology as an improved diagnostic method for ascertaining patients with hepatic cirrhosis.

Finally, the anatomic approach to the hepatic plate is critical for liver resections, and is undertaken with great regularity at many of our academic centers. If one is lowering the hepatic plate, the variations in the right portal vein, especially, are necessary to get an accurate delineation of the vasculature in performing resection.

The final issue is whether there are any branches anterior to the portal vein when one is attempting portacaval shunt in the rare instances when this is necessary. I have rarely seen one, but as the authors make the point, some of the coronary vein insertions, pyloric vein insertions, as well as other veins from the pancreas, if torn or transected in the anterior aspect of the portal vein, may result in torrential hemorrhage and, at times, death of the patient. Also, Kubo (*Clin Anat* 2000;13:134) described the extremely rare situation of aberrant left gastric veins or the coronary vein draining into the liver. Thus, one can actually decompress the varices by an end-to-side portacaval shunt and hemorrhage would still persist because the left gastric vein draining into the liver would not be decompressed. This is an extremely rare variant, but one needs to be aware of it. Failure to recognize it may result in a situation in which a successful shunt is carried out but the variceal bleeding persists.

J.E.F.

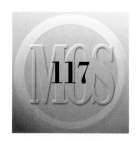

End-to-Side and Side-to-Side Portacaval Shunts

LAYTON F. RIKKERS AND KENRIC M. MURAYAMA

Portal hypertension is usually caused by increased vascular resistance in the portal venous system or liver. The most common cause of portal hypertension worldwide is schistosomiasis; in the United States, however, cirrhosis is the cause of more than 90% of cases. The most lethal complication of portal hypertension is gastrointestinal hemorrhage, with mortality rates for the first episode of bleeding ranging from 15% to more than 50%.

Surgical treatment of portal hypertension dates back to 1877, when Nikolai Eck created a portacaval anastomosis in dogs to treat ascites. In 1893, Pavlov described the physiologic consequences of complete diversion of portal flow by an Eck fistula in dogs. He clearly defined a *meat intoxication* syndrome in these animals, which is the equivalent of what is known today as *portosystemic encephalopathy*. He astutely attributed this "intoxication" to nitrogenous compounds diverted away from the liver into the systemic circulation. In 1903, Vidal performed the first end-to-side portacaval shunt in a patient. Unfortunately, this patient, in whom encephalopathy developed, died 4 months later of septic complications. Because of the devastating consequences of early attempts at total portal decompression, interest turned to partial diversion of portal flow. The first successful side-to-side portacaval shunt was performed by Rosenstein in 1912, but, in general, early attempts at partial portal decompression were also not successful.

In 1945, Whipple et al. reported their experience with portacaval and splenorenal shunts in patients with portal hypertension. Their success in ten consecutive patients heralded the beginning of the modern era of surgery for portal hypertension. Their reintroduction of portosystemic shunting for treatment of portal hypertension was based on a lack of any other effective therapy and on their recently developed improvements for vascular anastomoses. This impressive series of cases from Columbia Presbyterian Hospital stimulated others to adopt this new strategy for management of variceal bleeding. Worldwide, several hundred end-to-side and side-to-side portacaval

shunts were performed; the consensus was that these procedures were the most effective means for prevention of recurrent variceal hemorrhage.

This anecdotal experience was subjected to randomized trials in the 1960s. The results of these studies were discouraging. There was no survival advantage, and the incidence of encephalopathy was increased in patients who underwent shunting as compared with medically treated controls. Because of the results of these trials, new procedures have been developed that can prevent variceal hemorrhage and maintain portal perfusion of the liver. Although these newer operations may be preferable in most patients, the portacaval shunt is still indicated in certain clinical situations.

Portosystemic shunts can be classified as selective or nonselective. Selective shunts, such as the distal splenorenal shunt, often preserve portal blood flow to the liver, and nonselective shunts do not. Preservation of hepatic portal blood flow results in continued delivery of hepatotrophic hormones, such as insulin, to the liver, and continued extraction of intestinally absorbed cerebral toxins, which are metabolized by the liver before entering the systemic circulation. Because of this feature, several trials have demonstrated a lower frequency of encephalopathy after selective shunts than after nonselective shunts.

Nonselective shunts include the end-to-side portacaval shunt and several types of side-to-side portosystemic shunts. All nonselective shunts completely decompress the splanchnic venous circulation, but the intrahepatic hemodynamic effects differ. After an end-to-side portacaval shunt, the liver is completely dependent on the hepatic artery for its blood supply, and the hepatic sinusoidal pressure varies depending on the intrahepatic vascular resistance.

The initial proposed benefit of the side-to-side portacaval shunt and other side-to-side shunts was partial preservation of portal blood flow, but subsequent studies have shown that a side-to-side shunt of sufficient caliber to remain patent completely diverts portal blood away from the liver. Because

the hepatic end of the portal vein remains in communication with the vena cava, side-to-side portacaval shunts have the added feature of reliably relieving hepatic sinusoidal hypertension. Because the liver is a major site of ascites formation, side-to-side portosystemic shunts are the most effective shunts for treating intractable ascites as well as variceal hemorrhage.

Portacaval shunts, whether end-to-side or side-to-side, provide excellent control of variceal hemorrhage; the incidence of recurrent variceal bleeding after either procedure is less than 5%. Because it is a vein-to-vein anastomosis and receives flow from the liver and the splanchnic organs, the side-to-side portacaval shunt has the highest patency rate of all shunts. The major disadvantage of portacaval shunts is that they completely divert portal flow and thereby predispose patients to portosystemic encephalopathy and, possibly, earlier onset of hepatic failure. In addition, these operations, especially the side-to-side portacaval shunt, require an extensive hilar dissection, which makes future liver transplantation more difficult.

INDICATIONS

Because it reliably controls bleeding and can be performed rapidly, the portacaval shunt is often preferred over other shunts in the emergency setting. However, the rate of mortality from liver failure after an emergency portacaval shunt is extremely high in most series. Therefore, nonsurgical attempts to control hemorrhage should be undertaken first. If the patient is a potential candidate for transplantation, an interposition mesocaval shunt or a transjugular intrahepatic portosystemic shunt may be a better alternative in the emergency situation. When the setting is urgent rather than emergent (e.g., bleeding has been temporarily controlled by balloon tamponade), a selective shunt may also be a reasonable option.

A surgeon who is inexperienced in shunt surgery and who is confronted with an acutely bleeding patient in whom nonoperative therapies have failed to control hemorrhage should

The Gastrointestinal Tract

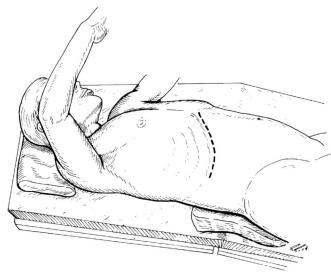

Fig. 1. The patient is placed in the left lateral oblique position, and a bean bag posterior to the right flank or elevation of the kidney rest is used to improve exposure. A right subcostal incision *(dashed line)* extends from the midline to the midaxillary line.

not attempt to perform an emergency shunt procedure. Although less effective in the long-term prevention of rebleeding, transabdominal esophageal transection and reanastomosis using the EEA stapling device combined with coronary vein ligation would have a higher likelihood of success in this setting.

The location of variceal bleeding is also an important determinant of shunt type. Selective shunts are effective only when portal hypertensive bleeding is from the esophagus or stomach. A nonselective shunt, such as the portacaval shunt, is indicated when bleeding is from stomal varices (e.g., colostomy or ileostomy), portal hypertensive colopathy, or, more rarely, from uncontrolled hemorrhoidal bleeding or small bowel varices.

Two other indications for a nonselective side-to-side shunt, such as the side-to-side portacaval shunt, are (a) variceal bleeding in a patient with ascites that has been intractable to medical management, and (b) the Budd-Chiari syndrome in its early stages, before cirrhosis has developed. Once cirrhosis has developed, liver transplantation is a preferable option.

All patients being considered for portacaval shunt surgery should undergo either visceral angiography, with specific interest in the venous-phase views, or duplex ultrasonography. Information regarding the anatomy and patency of the portal vein and its tributaries is essential. Thrombosis of the portal vein or inferior vena cava is an obvious contraindication to a portacaval shunt. Partial thrombosis of the portal vein or a recanalized portal

vein is a strong relative contraindication because the risk of shunt thrombosis is high.

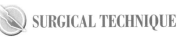

SURGICAL TECHNIQUE

The initial steps in performance of an end-to-side and a side-to-side portacaval shunt are similar. The patient is placed in the left lateral oblique position, with his or her right side elevated 15 to 20 degrees. Placement of a bean bag posterior to the right flank or elevation of the kidney rest may improve exposure. A right subcostal (Kocher) incision is used and is extended laterally to the midaxillary line (Fig. 1). If an end-to-side portacaval shunt is planned, special care is taken to preserve the umbilical vein in the falciform ligament because it provides the only route for retrograde flow of portal blood and hepatic sinusoidal decompression postoperatively. If a patient has reversal of portal flow before the operation, suggesting that the portal vein is a major outflow pathway for the liver, medically intractable ascites may develop after an end-to-side portacaval shunt if the umbilical vein is interrupted. Gentle abdominal exploration is performed, with care taken to avoid injury to fragile portosystemic collaterals within the retroperitoneum and surgical adhesions. Special care should be taken to suture-ligate all vessels and lymphatics and to avoid cauterization to minimize postoperative bleeding and lymphocele formation. The liver should be assessed for the potential presence of a hepatoma.

Extensive duodenal mobilization is usually not necessary and risks injury to retroperitoneal collaterals. The lateral, anterior, and medial surfaces of the inferior vena cava are cleared along its length from the caudate lobe of the liver to the right renal vein (Fig. 2). Careful and complete dissection of the infrahepatic vena cava is crucial to facilitate the anastomosis to be performed between this vessel and the portal vein. Although there are no lumbar veins superior to the renal vein, the right adrenal vein can be located anywhere from the retrohepatic vena cava to the renal vein and may be injured during the lateral dissection of the inferior vena cava. Hepatic venous branches from the caudate lobe to the inferior vena cava may also bleed profusely if injured.

The portal vein is next identified and dissected. The duodenum and transverse colon are gently retracted inferiorly and medially. The surgeon places a finger into the foramen of Winslow to identify the portal vein and hepatic artery by palpation. An aberrant right hepatic artery, which is present in approximately 20% of patients, is usually located just lateral to the portal vein and must be carefully preserved. The peritoneum over the lateral aspect of the hepatoduodenal ligament is dissected, and the common bile duct is identified (Fig. 3). This may be difficult to do in some patients with edematous and thickened overlying tissue. In such cases, the dissection should be initiated as far inferior and posterior as possible to avoid injury to the common bile duct. The common bile duct is dissected off the portal vein and is retracted medially and superiorly with vein retractors (Fig. 4). The

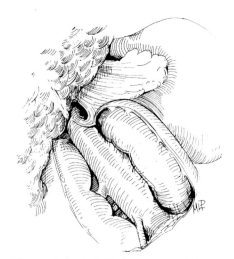

Fig. 2. A limited Kocher maneuver is performed to expose the inferior vena cava adequately. The lateral, anterior, and medial aspects of the inferior vena cava are cleared from the caudate lobe of the liver, superiorly, to the right renal vein, inferiorly.

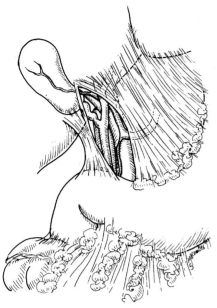

Fig. 3. The hepatoduodenal ligament is incised, and the structures within the portal triad are identified. The lateral aspect of the ligament is cleared to facilitate identification of the portal vein posterolaterally.

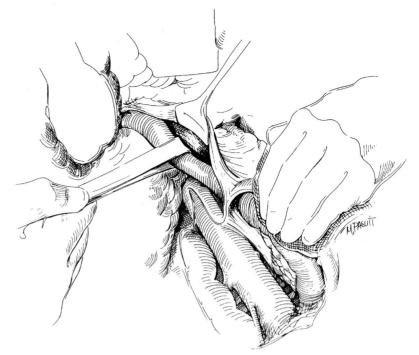

Fig. 5. The portal vein must be circumferentially dissected from its bifurcation at the liver hilum to the level at which it becomes retropancreatic inferiorly.

portal vein is circumferentially dissected from its bifurcation in the hilum of the liver to the level at which it becomes retropancreatic inferiorly (Fig. 5). The portal vein is then encircled with a vessel loop, which can be used to retract it inferiorly. Special caution must be taken in dissecting the medial aspect of the portal vein to avoid avulsion of the left or right gastric veins. These veins most often enter the portal vein near the confluence of splenic and superior mesenteric veins beneath the pancreas and are

usually out of the field of dissection. Any branches of the portal vein that are encountered are doubly ligated in continuity and divided.

END-TO-SIDE PORTACAVAL SHUNT

Once the dissection of the portal vein and inferior vena cava is complete, the hepatic end of the portal vein is ligated in continuity with a 2-0 monofilament vascular

suture and then suture-ligated (Fig. 6). After occlusion of the portal vein with vascular clamps at the level where it becomes retropancreatic, the portal vein is divided near the suture-ligated hepatic end (Fig. 7). Alternatively, when the portal vein is large in diameter, a vascular clamp is placed across it at the bifurcation; the vein is divided and then oversewn with a running 4-0 monofilament vascular suture. A side-biting vascular clamp (e.g., a Satinsky clamp) is placed on the anteromedial surface of the inferior vena cava (Fig. 8). Selection of the proper clamp is important. The jaws should be deep enough to allow

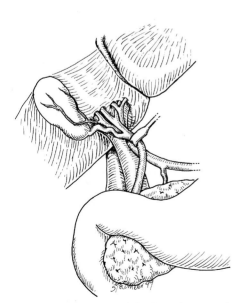

Fig. 4. The common bile duct is retracted with a vein retractor to facilitate dissection of the portal vein.

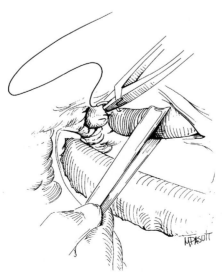

Fig. 6. The hepatic end of the portal vein is ligated in continuity with a 2-0 monofilament vascular suture and is subsequently suture-ligated.

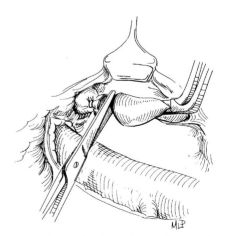

Fig. 7. A vascular clamp is placed across the portal vein inferiorly, and the portal vein is divided just inferior to the suture-ligated hepatic end.

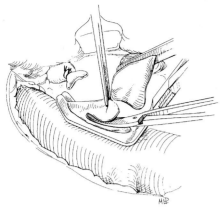

Fig. 8. A side-biting vascular clamp is placed across the anteromedial surface of the vena cava, and a button of the vena cava wall is excised. The button should approximate the size of the cut end of the portal vein.

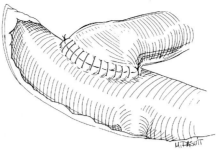

Fig. 10. Once the vascular anastomosis is completed between the portal vein and the inferior vena cava, the vena caval clamp is released first, followed by release of the portal vein clamp to establish portacaval flow.

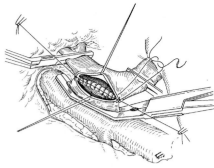

Fig. 12. A continuous vascular anastomosis is performed between the side of the portal vein and the side of the inferior vena cava. Special care should be taken to evert the portal vein and inferior vena cava edges if possible.

incorporation of half the diameter of the vena cava, and the handle should angle inferiorly away from the area of the anastomosis. A button of vena cava wall, approximately the size of the portal vein in cross section, is excised. The lengthwise diameter of the cavotomy should be approximately three-fourths of the diameter of the compressed end of the portal vein to avoid a discrepancy in size. The portal vein is brought down to the inferior vena cava in a gentle arc, with care taken to avoid torsion. If the portal vein kinks, it is trimmed to an appropriate length.

A continuous vascular anastomosis is subsequently performed between the portal vein and the inferior vena cava with 4-0 or 5-0 monofilament vascular suture (Fig. 9). Two corner sutures are first placed with the knots on the outside, and then one is brought to the inside through the inferior vena cava. The posterior suture line is then run, everting the edges of the portal vein and inferior vena cava if possible. The anterior anastomosis is performed by running each corner suture to the mid-

dle and then tying it. Before completion of the anastomosis, the portal vein clamp is released and immediately reclamped to flush the portal vein, which is irrigated with heparinized saline. Once the anastomosis is complete, the vena cava clamp is released, followed by the portal vein clamp, thus establishing portacaval flow (Fig. 10).

SIDE-TO-SIDE PORTACAVAL SHUNT

The side-to-side portacaval shunt is more difficult than the end-to-side portacaval shunt because more extensive dissection of the portal vein and inferior vena cava is necessary and because a prominent caudate lobe of the liver can occasionally prevent tension-free approximation of the two vessels. In this situation, part of the caudate lobe can be resected, or an interposition portacaval shunt that uses either knitted Dacron or a ribbed polytetrafluoroethylene (Teflon) graft can be constructed.

Once dissection is complete, vascular clamps are placed across the portal vein at

the liver hilum and at the superior border of the pancreas. Alternatively, Rumel tourniquets may be used. A side-biting vascular clamp (e.g., a Satinsky clamp) is placed on the anteromedial surface of the inferior vena cava in a direction parallel to the portal vein (Fig. 11). Subsequently, a similar-size elliptical button of vein wall that is approximately 2.0 to 2.5 cm long is removed from the opposing surfaces of the inferior vena cava and the portal vein. The two vessels are brought into approximation, and a continuous vascular anastomosis is performed with 4-0 or 5-0 monofilament vascular suture, as described for the end-to-side portacaval shunt (Fig. 12). Before completion of the portacaval anastomosis, the portal vein clamps are opened in sequence to flush debris out of the portal vein, which is irrigated with heparinized saline. The portacaval anastomosis is completed, and the vena cava clamp is removed first, followed by the portal vein clamps, establishing portacaval flow (Fig. 13).

After completion of either type of portacaval shunt, the adequacy of portal

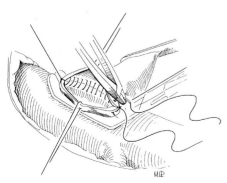

Fig. 9. A continuous vascular anastomosis is performed between the portal vein and the inferior vena cava.

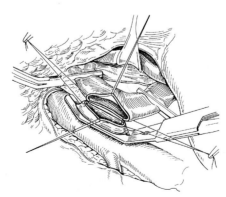

Fig. 11. A side-biting vascular clamp is placed on the anteromedial surface of the inferior vena cava. Corner sutures are placed between the side of the portal vein and the side of the vena cava to facilitate a symmetric anastomosis between the portal vein and the inferior vena cava.

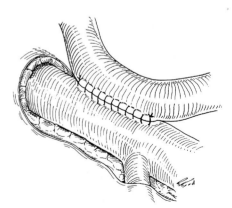

Fig. 13. Once the portacaval anastomosis is complete, the vena caval clamp is removed first, followed by the portal vein clamps, to establish portacaval flow.

decompression should be evaluated by measuring the pressure gradient across the anastomosis. This is achieved by direct puncture of both vessels with a 20-gauge needle attached by sterile tubing to either a handheld manometer or a pressure transducer. After a successful portacaval shunt, the gradient should be less than 5 cm of saline. After hemostasis is ensured, the abdomen is irrigated, and the incision is closed in a standard two-layer fashion without drains. Care should be taken to make the closure watertight so that an ascites leak does not develop. If indicated, a needle liver biopsy should be carried out before closing.

SUGGESTED READING

Johansen K, Helton WS. Portal hypertension and bleeding esophageal varices. *Ann Vasc Surg* 1992;6:553.

Levine BA, Sirinek KR. The portacaval shunt: is it still indicated? *Surg Clin North Am* 1990;70:361.

Nussbaum MS, Schoettker PJ, Fischer JE. Comparison of distal and proximal splenorenal shunts: a ten-year experience. *Surgery* 1993;114:659.

Orloff MJ, Orloff MS, Orloff SL, et al. Three decades of experience with emergency portacaval shunt for acutely bleeding esophageal varices in 400 unselected patients with cirrhosis of the liver. *J Am Coll Surg* 1995;180:257.

Rikkers LF. Emergency shunt for variceal bleeding. *J Am Coll Surg* 1995;180:337.

Rikkers LF, Jin G. Surgical management of acute variceal hemorrhage. *World J Surg* 1994;18:193.

Rikkers LF, Sorrell WT, Jin G. Which portosystemic shunt is best? *Gastroenterol Clin North Am* 1992;21:179.

Spina GP, Santambrogio R, Opocher E, et al. Emergency portosystemic shunt in patients with variceal bleeding. *Surg Gynecol Obstet* 1990;171:456.

Suc B, Vinel JP, Rousseau H, et al. Intrahepatic portocaval shunt in patients waiting for transplantation. *Transplant Proc* 1995;27:1715.

EDITOR'S COMMENT

As Drs. Rikkers and Murayama indicate in this direct chapter, end-to-side portacaval shunts are now rarely performed except in emergency situations where control of variceal bleeding cannot be achieved by any other means. The end-to-side portacaval shunt is the classic nonselective shunt because all of the portal blood is diverted away from the liver. There is ample evidence that this shunt results in decrease in hepatic function and increasing incidence of hepatic encephalopathy and perhaps early liver failure. In the studies carried out by the Boston Intrahospital Liver Group in the 1960s, there was a slight advantage to patients who received end-to-side portacaval shunt, but the expense in the postoperative period was considerably greater than the medical therapy because of repeat hospitalization for hepatic encephalopathy. Also the mode of death was different. The patients who died following portacaval shunt died of hepatic failure and hepatic encephalopathy, while patients with medical therapy often died of repeat variceal bleeding.

With the exception of the end-to-side and side-to-side portacaval shunts, the other shunts tend to be more selective than I believe the authors indicate. The size of the shunt generally is a balance between an attempt on the part of the surgeon to maintain some aspect of hepatic perfusion. If an increase in portal pressure continues, new collaterals develop, as I have previously stated in the introduction to these chapters. The side-to-side shunt, like the central splenorenal shunt, is useful in treating patients with ascites. Dr. Linton, who had popularized the central splenorenal shunt, always taught that, when needed, a central splenorenal shunt should be no larger than 1 cm or at the very most 1.2 cm in order to decompress the portal hypertension, but at the same time provide some low-grade perfusion of the liver. Indications for side-to-side shunts are generally in patients with intractable ascites, very much as the central splenorenal shunt. When performing a side to side shunt, one should measure venous pressures both above and below the portal vein clamp. If clamping the portal vein increases the pressure within the liver in the hepatic side, a side-to-side shunt is indicated. This will both prevent the ascites but unfortunately decompress the liver, which may contribute to hepatic encephalopathy by robbing the

liver of its portal perfusion. However, the alternative is not attractive: intractable ascites, which is difficult to control with medical therapy.

As far as the emergency shunt is concerned, the mortality is considerable. Orloff continues to advocate emergency shunts, but what is often forgotten is that the emergency shunt is part of the system that Orloff has proposed so that patients are operated on quickly and are not allowed to bleed with repeated episodes of hypotension, aspiration, pneumonitis, and depletion of coagulation factors. If a patient comes into an institution on the medical service and there are repeated attempts with sclerotherapy, the Sengstaken-Blakemore tube, aspiration pneumonia, 12 units of blood given, the depletion of clotting factors, and then subjected to emergency shunt, the mortality is sky high. The emergency shunt, as advocated by Orloff, should take place within 8 hours. No one has tried this approach; it makes sense to try to get patients so that the bleeding is stopped first and foremost, before all of these other negative prognostic factors occur.

The technique described by Drs. Rikkers and Murayama is the usual technique. It is important to preserve the umbilical vein, as the authors propose, as it is the only egress from the liver if one performs end-to-side portacaval shunt and the liver needs to be decompressed. I have occasionally taken both saphenous veins from the distal side from the leg, turned them up subcutaneously, dilated the umbilical vein, and decompressed the liver through that mechanism, with diuresis of the ascites. This is a tour de force that should be carried out only under circumstances under which the patient is viable except for the horrendous ascites, which may occur once an end-to-side portacaval shunt is carried out when the side-to-side shunt should have been used. My technique in carrying out an end-to-side portacaval shunt is similar except that I identify the portal vein first, dissect it out, and put a vessel loop around it so that one can identify it easily once it has been completely dissected free of the porta. I then go directly posterior to the vena cava. This avoids unnecessary clearing of vena cava, which is usually surrounded by engorged lymphatic tissue, and which, as Drs. Rikkers and Murayama point out, must be suture-ligated to prevent the accumulation of lymphatic ascites following the operation. As far as the back wall is concerned, I use a running everting mattress suture, such as I describe in Chapter 120. If prop-

erly done, there will be no suture exposed to the blood on the back wall, which tends to give a shunt with less turbulence. I also tend to do an interrupted mattress suture on the front wall of the portal vein, again minimizing the amount of monofilament that is exposed to blood in the portal vein. Drs. Rikkers and Murayama do make a very good point as far as indications for end-to-side portacaval shunt, and that is that massive bleeding from varices that occur (not from esophageal or gastric varices) may be controlled by either rubber band ligation or sclerotherapy, but there is massive hemorrhage from collaterals around adhesions to small bowel areas or around ileostomies that cannot be controlled by suture.

As stated in this chapter, the transjugular intrahepatic portosystemic shunting is most often performed as a bridge to hepatic transplant. Klempnauer and Schrem (*Metab Brain Dis* 2001;16:21) prefer transjugular intrahepatic portosystemic shunting as do many centers in which the end game in these patients is hepatic transplantation. They do stenose, as pointed out in the chapter, but if the transplant can be done expeditiously, the porta is not disturbed and transplantation, of course, does away with portal hypertension.

Others, such as Yan and Yan (*Hepatobiliary Pancreat Dis Int* 2003;2:202), have experimented with portacaval hemitransposition, especially in the areas of portal vein thrombosis. These authors have performed a total of 23 cases. Mortality was high: 8 of the 23 patients died. Fifteen patients are alive and have normal liver and kinase function and no dietary restrictions. They and others, such as Molmenti et al. (*Pediatr Transplant* 2001;5:381), have used a modified, temporary end-to-side portacaval shunt and liver and small bowel transplantation in which a temporary portacaval shunt and small-for-size livers enable the decompression of the liver so that the liver does not become swollen and does not function well. A similar technique has been described by Takada et al. (*Liver Transplant* 2004;10:807) in which there were disparities in size and in living donors in which the graft was small for size. They state that the advantages of avoiding portal hypertension as well as sufficient portal flow to the graft enabled success in these patients that might have otherwise occurred had they not diverted portal flow.

J.E.F.

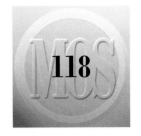

Small-Diameter Interposition Shunt

ALEXANDER S. ROSEMURGY, II

Partial portal decompression gained popularity after its reintroduction by Sarfeh et al. in the early 1980s. Numerous publications and works since then have shown that the concept is safe and efficacious. Sarfeh et al. have also studied patients undergoing various degrees of partial portal decompression and have found that smaller (8-mm) H-graft portacaval shunts lead to superior results when compared with larger (12- to 16-mm) prosthetic shunts. My experience with partial portal decompression at the University of South Florida has confirmed some of their work.

In the late 1980s, after reading about Dr. Sarfeh's technique with small-diameter prosthetic portacaval shunting, I began to use this shunt technique as my preferred method of portal decompression. I have modified his technique to achieve an approach with which I am pleased. My basic approach differs from his in that the graft I use is shorter, I remove a portion of the caudate lobe to accommodate the placement of the shorter graft, and I do not aggressively attempt to ligate collaterals from the portal vein. This operative approach has been undertaken in more than 170 patients, with results that have strongly encouraged its continued use.

SURGICAL TECHNIQUE

After the patient is positioned supine on the operating table, an endotracheal tube is placed, and then a Foley catheter and a nasogastric tube are placed. Neither vasopressin nor octreotide is given perioperatively, unless active bleeding is occurring. Although such agents may decrease operative blood loss, I generally have not found blood loss to be significant. The operation can be undertaken without significant blood loss and almost always without blood transfusions; therefore, I find the intraoperative use of vasopressin or octreotide to be superfluous. Prophylactic antibiotic therapy is always used.

The patient is rolled into a 30-degree left lateral decubitus position by means of a bed sheet rolled tightly and placed just to the right of the spine. After being pre-

pared and draped in the usual manner, the patient is operated on through a rather transverse incision. The exact placement of this incision depends on the size of the liver, which is often palpable below the costal margin. I try to place the incision over the liver edge, making the incision more transverse than oblique. I generally do not cross the midline in making this incision, and I usually incise only a small portion of the musculature lateral to the rectus muscle. As is my preference, I use wound protectors and Clorpactin solution for irrigation. Once the peritoneal cavity is entered, I irrigate the wound liberally with this solution and place the wound protector so that the wound is bathed by Clorpactin solution throughout the remainder of the operation.

If the falciform ligament is divided during the incision, it is divided carefully because large collaterals may reside in this ligament. Suture ligation of the falciform ligament at the time of division is usually undertaken.

A table-mounted Omni bariatric retractor is used during these operations. All retractor blades are well padded, and the sternal blade of the Omni bariatric retractor is then placed to move the incision cephalad. The foramen of Winslow is a key landmark. A Kocher maneuver is undertaken, always maintaining orientation with the foramen of Winslow. High-energy electrocautery is liberally used, although visible venous collaterals are ligated before division, as are lymphatic channels. A common mistake in the early part of this operation is that, with the patient in a 30-degree left lateral decubitus position, the dissection is undertaken in a much too lateral direction, deviating from the vena cava. With this error in dissection, the renal capsule or hilum is often exposed needlessly. The Kocher maneuver does not need to be extensive but just enough to expose approximately 5 cm of inferior vena cava and to allow for placement of a side-biting vascular clamp. The exposed segment of the inferior vena cava should include the portion of the inferior vena cava that forms the posterior boundary of the foramen of Winslow. The cephalad portion of this seg-

ment of cava may lie dorsal to the inferior tip of the caudate lobe. If necessary, this portion of the caudate lobe is excised to expose the vena cava, so that the portal vein can be bridged to the vena cava easily with a short segment of polytetrafluoroethylene (PTFE) graft.

If necessary, the caudate lobe is easily resected. The tip of the caudate lobe is grasped using a ringed forceps. Electrocautery is used to separate the caudate lobe from the rest of the liver. Then pressure is placed on the cut edge of the liver to control bleeding. Bleeding veins can generally be controlled with electrocautery, but suture ligation occasionally may be necessary.

Exposure of the inferior vena cava is completed as the dissection is carried cephalad and caudad to expose the 4 to 5 cm of inferior vena cava necessary to undertake the shunt. It is very important that the inferior vena cava be well exposed medially and laterally so that a vascular clamp can be placed on the inferior vena cava easily. I generally try to expose at least half the circumference of the 4- to 5-cm segment of the inferior vena cava to facilitate clamp placement and anastomosis. After the inferior vena cava is exposed, a traction suture is placed into the loose tissue adjacent to the right side of the inferior vena cava. This suture is further placed into the lateral abdominal wall and then tied to retract this tissue laterally and to optimize exposure.

Once the inferior vena cava has been adequately exposed, attention is turned toward the hepatoduodenal ligament. With the splanchnic blade of the Omni retractor placed carefully over a well-padded gallbladder, the gallbladder is retracted toward the patient's left shoulder. This lifts and rolls the gallbladder and the common bile duct ventrally and medially. The hepatoduodenal ligament is opened posteriorly and laterally. This area is rich with lymph vessels, and liberal ligation of lymphatic structures is important in minimizing ascites. The dissection in the hepatoduodenal ligament is undertaken along the length of the ligament, parallel and posterior (dorsal) to the common bile duct to minimize chances of ductal injury.

A segment of 8-mm, externally reinforced PTFE graft is used for the portacaval shunt. This graft is no longer than 3 cm from toe to toe and 1.5 cm from heel to heel, with the bevels of the graft at 90 degrees to each other. Orienting the bevels in this way allows the graft to be oriented to the portal vein and to the vena cava. The portal vein is not parallel to the vena cava but oriented approximately 60 degrees to the vena cava.

Once the graft is cut, it is placed in a syringe full of heparinized saline. With the tip of the syringe occluded by a fingertip, suction is placed on the syringe and air bubbles can be seen to emanate from the graft. With a rather firm tapping on the side of the syringe, the air bubbles are dislodged and, with removal of the suction, the PTFE graft should no longer float. Through this action, air has been removed from the graft and replaced by heparinized saline. This makes it much easier to scan the graft with color-flow Doppler ultrasound postoperatively.

The graft is then placed on the inferior vena cava to determine whether a portion of the caudate lobe needs to be excised, as discussed previously. If the graft lies so that a portion of the caudate lobe needs to be excised, it is excised without difficulty. A ringed forceps is used to grab the most caudad portion of the caudate lobe. A vein retractor is placed on the portal vein to ensure that it is not injured. Electrocautery at a high energy level is used to score and remove the designated portion of the caudate lobe. Traction is placed along the ringed forceps as the cautery is applied to facilitate this excision. This traction pulls the piece of the caudate lobe up and off the vena cava so as to protect it. Blood loss during excision of a portion of the caudate lobe is much less than would be imagined. Once the portion of caudate lobe is excised, a small cotton gauge sponge is placed over the cut edge of caudate lobe and pressure applied. After 1 or 2 minutes, most bleeding stops. Bleeding that does not stop can be controlled by electrocautery, again using high-energy levels or suture ligatures.

Once bleeding from the cut edge of caudate lobe has stopped, a side-biting Satinsky clamp is placed on the anterior vena cava. A ringed forceps is used to pull the anterior wall of the inferior vena cava ventrally to facilitate placement of the side-biting clamp. This clamp should be closed completely so that the vena cava does not slip out of the clamp (Fig. 2). Volume loading before application of the clamp is generally not necessary. Hypotension is virtually never a problem because the vena cava

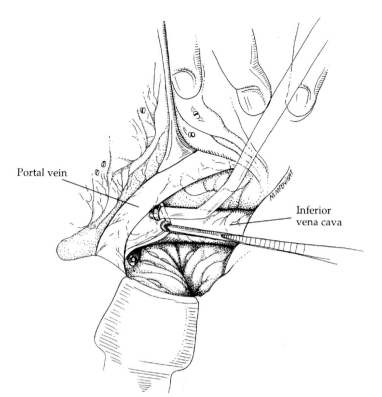

Fig. 1. The Yankauer sucker is used to raise the portal vein off the tissue of the posterior hepatoduodenal ligament. A Russian forceps is used to minimize chances of tearing tissue. A vein retractor is helpful in the dissection. Here, it is retracting tissue containing the common bile duct medially. The vena cava is seen at the base of this view. A portion of the caudate lobe has already been excised. The line of excision of the caudate lobe lies posterior to the cephalad aspect of the portal vein. The patient's head is to the left. This view is from the patient's right side, where the surgeon is standing.

Often, the portal vein is not readily identified because of thick lymphatic tissue in this area. Once the portal vein is identified, further dissection should be undertaken only to better define the portal vein. The common bile duct should be retracted ventrally and medially with a vein retractor to facilitate exposure of the portal vein. Palpation of this area is important to detect and locate an accessory or aberrant right hepatic artery. An accessory right hepatic artery should not be injured because an injury can greatly interfere with necessary blood flow to the liver. If present, an aberrant or accessory right hepatic artery should be retracted with the common bile duct and thereby retracted ventrally and medially. As the portal vein comes into view, a Russian forceps is used to grasp the portal vein. A substantial portion of vein should always be grasped to minimize chances of tearing it. Dissection of the portal vein is greatly facilitated with use of a plastic Yankauer sucker (Fig. 1).

I have found this to be a very superior technique to dissect the portal vein. This technique does not injure any side branches off the vein and greatly speeds circumferential dissection of the portal vein. With Russian forceps holding the enveloping tissue of the posterior hepatoduodenal ligament, a vein retractor is placed on the portal vein, retracting it ventrally and medially. The Yankauer sucker is then used to separate the portal vein from the posterior enveloping tissue. Once this dissection is carried quite medially, the portal vein is released from the vein retractor, and the vein retractor is placed on the accessory right hepatic artery, if one is present, or on the common bile duct. With these structures drawn ventrally and medially, the portal vein is grasped with the Russian forceps; the ventral surface of the portal vein is freed from overlying structures with the Yankauer sucker. At this point, a right angle is passed over the ventral surface of the portal vein and then around the vein. Circumferentially, the portal vein is controlled by a vessel loop. This vessel loop is useful in subsequent placement of the side-biting Satinsky clamp on the portal vein; it is also helpful if bleeding problems develop because it can provide secure control of the portal vein in the proximal hepatoduodenal ligament. If circumferential control of the portal vein is excessively difficult, lateral exposure of the vein can suffice.

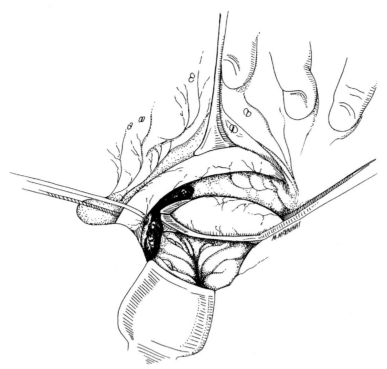

Fig. 2. A Satinsky clamp has been placed across the anterior surface of the inferior vena cava. A vessel loop is around the cephalad portion of the portal vein. The cauterized edge of the caudate lobe is the black area at the tip of the Satinsky clamp. A generous portion of inferior vena cava is controlled by the Satinsky clamp. The patient is positioned so that the head is to the left in this drawing. This view is from the patient's right, where the surgeon stands.

is not completely occluded with this clamping. Once the side-biting Satinsky clamp is placed on the anterior surface of the vena cava, a small window must be cut from the vena cava so that outflow from the graft is adequate; merely opening the vena cava is not sufficient. The window is cut in a downward, or ventral-to-dorsal, direction, rather than in a caudad-to-cephalad direction (Fig. 3). The primary orientation of the cut must be downward; otherwise, the window is much longer than necessary. When the vena cava is opened, the vein excised should be approximately 4 mm long and 1 to 2 mm wide ex vivo. This will provide an adequate hole in the vena cava (Fig. 4).

The graft is placed on the vena cava so that the bevel in the graft allows the graft to lean cephalad (Fig. 4). Suturing with 5-0 polypropylene is undertaken in a running fashion to construct the anastomosis. The suture is initially placed as a horizontal mattress stitch at the most cephalad aspect of the anastomosis (Fig. 5). This anastomosis is initiated in this manner so that sewing along the length of the anastomosis is always from inside-out on the vein and outside-in on the graft, allowing easy placement of the sutures in the vein. The back wall in the anastomosis is constructed first, until the midline (or toe of the graft)

is crossed. At that point, the suturing returns to the most cephalad aspect of the anastomosis, using the other limb of the 5-0 polypropylene suture. The front wall of the anastomosis is then completed.

Before the knot is tied, a suture is reversed so that the knot is tied across the anastomosis. When the graft is being anastomosed to the vena cava, the initial sutures are placed so that the graft is parachuted down on the anastomosis (Fig. 5). This facilitates placement of the first few sutures, which otherwise can be quite difficult. Once the

graft has been parachuted down on the vena cava, tension is maintained on the suture line as the anastomosis is sewn so that the anastomosis is not loose and so that the sutures need not be tightened with a nerve hook on completion of the anastomosis. Certainly, the sutures and the anastomosis should be visually inspected for defects and gaps before the suture is tied. As well, a nerve hook may be used to test for tautness of the sutures before the knot is tied.

Once the anastomosis has been completed and the knot tied, a right-angled clamp is placed across the graft, and the side-biting Satinsky clamp is removed from the inferior vena cava (Fig. 6). This tests the anastomosis; it should not leak, and it should bleed only at needle holes and then only minimally. The side-biting Satinsky clamp is then replaced on the vena cava, and the right-angled clamp is removed from the graft. The graft is then vigorously irrigated with heparinized saline delivered through an 18-gauge angiocatheter attached to a 30-mL syringe.

The portal vein–graft anastomosis is now constructed. The common bile duct and accessory right hepatic artery, if present, are retracted ventrally and medially, exposing the portal vein well. With the vessel loop around the portal vein, a Russian forceps is used to grab the lateral wall of the portal vein and retract it laterally. A right-angled side-biting clamp is then placed on the portal vein. This clamp does not have to occlude all flow in the portal vein, but it must be securely placed to prevent bleeding once the portal vein is open. Once the Satinsky clamp has been placed, the posterior lateral aspect of the portal vein is opened with a No. 11 knife blade. Once the vein is entered, Potts scissors are used to lengthen the opening to accommodate placement of the graft. A window does not

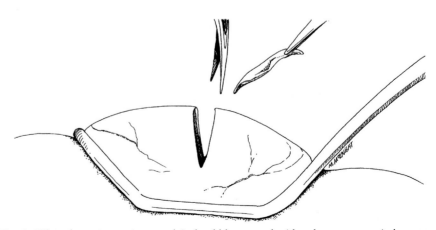

Fig. 3. When the vena cava is opened, it should be opened with a deep narrow window cut, as shown in this drawing. The window is cut to improve graft outflow. This window elongates considerably and easily accommodates the graft anastomosis.

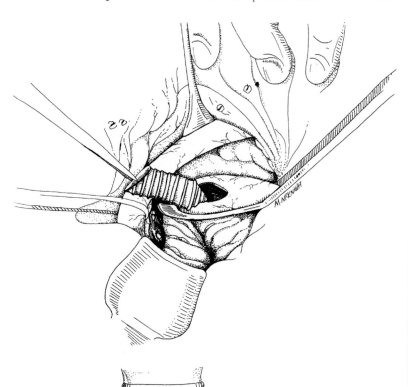

Fig. 4. A window has been cut in the inferior vena cava. The graft is being placed into position for completion of the anastomosis. Note the orientation of the beveled ends of the graft. The patient's head is to the left. This view is from the patient's right side.

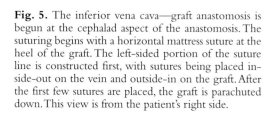

Fig. 5. The inferior vena cava—graft anastomosis is begun at the cephalad aspect of the anastomosis. The suturing begins with a horizontal mattress suture at the heel of the graft. The left-sided portion of the suture line is constructed first, with sutures being placed inside-out on the vein and outside-in on the graft. After the first few sutures are placed, the graft is parachuted down. This view is from the patient's right side.

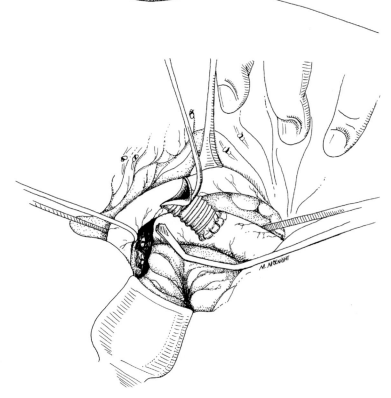

Fig. 6. After the inferior vena cava-graft anastomosis has been completed, a right-angled clamp is placed to occlude the graft. The Satinsky clamp is then opened, and the anastomosis is tested.

The Gastrointestinal Tract

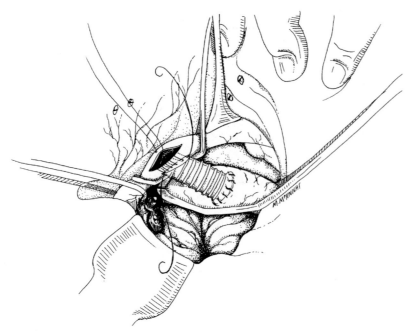

Fig. 7. With the vena cava again occluded, the lateral wall of the portal vein is controlled with a small Satinsky clamp. The portal vein is opened posterolaterally. A traction suture of 5-0 Prolene is placed to retract the anterior lip of the venotomy, thereby facilitating placement of sutures along the posterior anastomosis. The graft—portal vein anastomosis is begun in the midportion posteriorly. The anastomosis is begun with a horizontal mattress suture placed inside-out on the vein and outside-in on the graft. This view is from the patient's right side.

need to be cut in the portal vein. A 5-0 polypropylene suture is placed in the ventral edge of the hole in the portal vein to act as a retraction suture, so as to "open up" the hole in the portal vein (Fig. 7). With this exposure, the posterior wall of the portal vein is then sewn to the graft with a double-armed 5-0 polypropylene suture. The anastomosis is initiated by placing a horizontal mattress suture of polypropylene in the midportion of the posterior wall of the portal vein. This suture is passed inside-out on the portal vein and outside-in on the graft with each end of the polypropylene suture. Once this horizontal mattress suture has been placed, all sewing of this anastomosis is inside-out on the portal vein and outside-in on the graft. When one of the corners is reached, a rubber-shod clamp is placed on that end of the polypropylene suture, and sewing is initiated with the other end of the suture. As sewing is carried around both the cephalad and caudad corners of the anastomosis, the sutures along the back wall are drawn taut with a nerve hook. This is the last time that this back wall of the anastomosis will be visible, and it is important that the sutures be drawn taut at this time. As the sewing continues toward the middle of the anterior portion of the anastomosis, the clamp on the portal vein is momentarily opened so that clot and debris within the portal

vein will be blown out of the portal vein before completion of the anastomosis. After this result is achieved, heparinized saline again is applied liberally to dislodge debris from the graft. A small bore intravenous

catheter on the tip of a 20-30 cc syringe that contains heparinized saline is placed through the anterior defect in the anastomosis and heparinized saline is injected forcefully down the graft. The anastomosis is then completed, with one of the sutures being reversed so that the knot is tied across the anastomosis. The clamp on the vena cava is removed first, and then the clamp on the portal vein is removed (Fig. 8). The clamp on the portal vein can sometimes be difficult to remove.

There should be a thrill in the vena cava just cephalad to the anastomosis. This thrill should be easily detected by means of exquisitely light palpation to the vena cava. If no thrill is felt, it is unlikely that the shunt will prove to be patent.

Pressures within the portal vein and inferior vena cava are measured early in the operation, before the portal vein or vena cava is clamped. I record these pressures with a 25-gauge needle and a pressure-transducing setup identical to that used for an arterial line. A gradient of 20 mm Hg usually is present before shunting, with a pressure of approximately 30 mm Hg in the portal vein and approximately 10 mm Hg in the vena cava. On completion of the shunt, pressures in the portal vein and inferior vena cava are measured again. Caval pressures generally rise a bit with construction of the shunt, and portal pressures fall significantly. Accordingly, the portal vein–inferior vena cava pressure gradient should

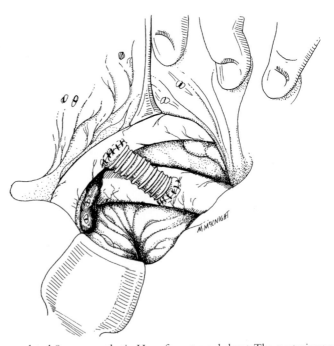

Fig. 8. The completed 8-mm prosthetic H-graft portacaval shunt. The posterior portion of the portal vein–graft anastomosis must be drawn taut before completing the anterior part of anastomosis. One limb of Prolene suture is reversed before the knot is tied. There should be a thrill in the inferior vena cava once both Satinsky clamps are removed.

fall considerably with shunting. The gradient should be less than 10 mm Hg on completion of the shunt, with gradients of 6 to 8 mm Hg being common. If pressures within the portal vein fall by 10 mm Hg with shunting and the gradient is less than 10 mm Hg, postoperative graft patency is virtually certain. Appropriate pressures after shunting, combined with a palpable thrill in the vena cava, uniformly predict graft patency in the immediate and late postoperative periods.

The vena cava-graft anastomosis is marked by large hemoclips placed on tissue adherent to the vena cava and cephalad and caudad to the anastomosis, which allow the radiologist easily to identify and cannulate the anastomosis when undertaking routine postoperative transfemoral cannulation of the shunt. The shunt is evaluated to document patency and to measure pressures 3 to 6 days after shunting and during late postdischarge follow-up, generally at 1, 3, 5, and 10 years after shunting.

The operative field is copiously irrigated, the retractors are removed, and the wound is closed along anatomic layers using 0- polypropylene suture. Sutures must be placed with good purchase of fascia and in close proximity to each other so that the chances of postoperative ascitic leak are minimized. The fascia is closed in two layers. The polypropylene sutures are generally started on each corner of the incision and then run to the middle, where they are tied, for the anterior and posterior layers of rectus fascia. The subcutaneous tissues are copiously irrigated, and the skin is closed with a running nylon suture. The skin sutures are not removed in the immediate postoperative period, but generally after several weeks. They are removed once they are loose, which signals wound contraction. Nylon sutures are used to minimize problems with wound failure or leakage of ascitic fluid. Wound morbidity can be a problem in patients with liver disease, but I have been pleased with this method of wound closure.

A diligent second assistant, often a scrub nurse, is important to the operation. Such an assistant is necessary to suction accumulating ascitic fluid while the graft-caval anastomosis is undertaken and to keep the graft full of heparinized saline during portal vein-graft anastomosis. I generally stand to the patient's right side while undertaking this operation, and the first assistant stands to the patient's left.

COMMENT

I was initially attracted by this shunt because of perceived operative simplicity. Although I have been very pleased with its results, I find the operation to be somewhat tedious and demanding because it requires extreme attention to detail. If the guidelines within this chapter are followed, I believe this shunt can be undertaken by any surgeon familiar with hepatobiliary or vascular surgery. I do not believe that the technique is inordinately difficult, although, as mentioned, there are several points that are important.

SUGGESTED READING

Rosemurgy AS, Bloomston M, Clark WC, et al. H-graft portacaval shunts versus TIPS: ten-year follow-up of a randomized trial with comparison to predicted survivals. *Ann Surg* 2005;241:238.

Rosemurgy AS, McAllister EW, Kurto HZ, et al. Postprandial augmentation of portal hepatic inflow after 8 mm H-graft portacaval shunt. *Am J Surg* 1992;163:213.

Rosemurgy A, Serafini F, Zervos E, et al. Small diameter prosthetic H-graft portacaval shunt: definitive therapy for variceal bleeding. *J Gastrointest Surg* 1998;2:585.

Rosemurgy AS, Zervos EE. Management of variceal hemorrhage. *Curr Prob Surg* 2003; 40:253.

Sarfeh IJ, Rypins EB, Conroy RM, et al. Portacaval H-graft: relationships of shunt diameter, portal flow patterns, and encephalopathy. *Ann Surg* 1983;197:422.

Sarfeh IJ, Rypins EB, Mason GR. A systematic appraisal of portacaval H-graft diameters: clinical and hemodynamic perspectives. *Ann Surg* 1986;204:356.

EDITOR'S COMMENT

Dr. Rosemurgy has given us a very nice chapter on an interposition shunt, which is intentionally small (8 mm) and short (1.5 to 3.0 cm) with a bevel and a direct anastomosis between the portal vein and the inferior vena cava. The technique is clearly described. The purpose of this shunt—as with many other shunts in this section—is to preserve hepatic perfusion while decreasing portal pressure sufficiently to arrest variceal hemorrhage.

There have been a number of studies involving transjugular intrahepatic portosystemic shunting, distal splenorenal shunts, and these small interposition shunts. A recent study from Italy by Capussotti et al. (*Surgery* 2000;127:614) compared a randomized trial for 46 good-risk patients with cirrhosis and documented variceal hemorrhage. A partial shunt procedure—in this case, a 10-mm diameter interposition portacaval H-graft—was compared with direct, small, side-to-side portacaval anastomosis with which the authors had significant prior experience and had decided that this, in fact, despite their attempts to make a small anastomosis, finally became a total shunt. There was no mortality in this relatively good-risk category. The authors found that the 10-mm interposition shunt had a significantly longer encephalopathy-free survival in the interposition group ($P = 0.025$) and that the encephalopathy in the two groups was statistically significant, with three patients in the interposition partial shunt group and nine in the direct shunt group. The combination of a 13% to 39% difference in encephalopathy, and a 70% survival rate in the interposition group versus 45% in the total shunt group, is impressive and indicates that the 10-mm graft, which does not dilate, does apparently preserve some flow to the liver. This is the advantage of this shunt, and one presumes it is because the PTFE graft is rigid, and does not apparently enlarge to rob the liver of its flow.

A similar attitude was expressed by Batignani et al. (*Hepatobiliary Pancreat Dis Int* 2004;3:516), who reported 29 cirrhotic patients with a ringed PTFE interposition prosthesis of 8 or 10 mm. The 8-mm grafts apparently result in a lower mortality and morbidity, presumably because hepatofugal flow was preserved better in the 8-mm prosthesis. The Class C prosthesis resulted in an extraordinarily high mortality and morbidity. Shunt thrombosis was greater in the 8-mm group than in the 10-mm group (16% vs. 8%, respectively). Variceal rebleeding occurred in four patients. The individuals who performed this study are quite satisfied that small interposition shunts seem to be reasonable for Italian patients, most of whom do not have cirrhosis from alcoholism.

Taken together, there is now a large body of literature indicating that either the 8-mm or the 10-mm shunt provides long-term patency, an acceptable rate of encephalopathy, and an acceptable rate of rebleeding from varices. The hypothesis that a rigid PTFE graft, which does not dilate, will allow hepatofugal flow, thus preventing encephalopathy and later death of liver failure, seems to be borne out.

J.E.F.

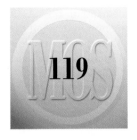

Distal Splenorenal Shunts: Hemodynamics of Total versus Selective Shunting

ATEF A. SALAM

The goal of any portosystemic shunt is effective decompression of the gastroesophageal veins. There are two distinct types of portosystemic shunts: those that are associated with total diversion of portal blood away from the liver (i.e., total shunts), and those that maintain portal blood supply to the liver (i.e., selective shunts). Examples of total shunts include portacaval, mesocaval, and central splenorenal shunts (CSRSs). An example of a selective shunt is the distal splenorenal shunt (DSRS), for which the terms *selective* and *DSRS* are often used interchangeably. The only other truly selective shunt, the coronocaval shunt, is rarely used today.

The concept of selective shunting was first introduced by Warren and his associates in 1967. These authors emphasized the increased morbidity and mortality associated with liver failure and hepatic encephalopathy after total shunting procedures. They attributed these problems to loss of liver portal perfusion. Their goal for the ideal operation for the treatment of patients with variceal bleeding was to achieve effective variceal decompression while preserving portal blood flow to the liver. The operation they devised to achieve these objectives was the DSRS.

The DSRS is created by anastomosing the splenic end of the divided splenic vein to the side of the left renal vein. The portal end of the splenic vein is oversewn. A functioning DSRS achieves variceal decompression by establishing a route for gastric venous drainage that offers less vascular resistance than the anastomotic channels between the gastric and esophageal veins. This route is sequentially made of the short gastric and splenic veins, splenorenal shunt, and left renal vein.

The second important goal of the selective shunt is to maintain portal blood flow to the liver. Because the splenorenal anastomosis is not in direct communication with the superior mesenteric or portal veins, the pressure in these vessels remains elevated. Such pressure elevation is crucial in maintaining portal blood flow to the cirrhotic liver in the face of increased vascular resist-

ance. Portal blood flow to the liver, however, can be maintained only if the high-pressure portomesenteric venous compartment is anatomically disconnected from the low-pressure splenic venous zone. This is the rationale for combining the selective shunt with interruption of the coronary gastroepiploic and inferior mesenteric veins. Any overlooked communicating channels between these two pressure zones are likely to develop into a major conduit for diversion of portal blood away from the liver to the decompressed splenic vein.

INDICATIONS

In the early years after the introduction of the DSRS, it was the practice with my group to recommend the procedure for nearly all patients who presented with or had a documented history of variceal bleeding. The only exceptions were patients with intractable ascites or signs and symptoms of hepatic decompensation. Increased popularity of sclerotherapy in the 1970s prompted us to conduct a prospective trial in which we compared sclerotherapy with the DSRS operation. We concluded that patients who received sclerotherapy with the DSRS as a safety net for sclerotherapy failure had better overall survival than those who received DSRS as their first line of treatment. Meanwhile, reports began to appear in the literature showing improved survival of patients with advanced liver disease treated by liver transplantation. In view of these developments, our current policy is to treat all patients initially with sclerotherapy. Patients with rebleeding after obliteration of the variceal bed are stratified according to their degree of liver function. Patients with adequate liver reserve (Child class A or B) receive DSRS. Patients with severe liver dysfunction are evaluated for liver transplantation. Patients with intractable ascites are unsuitable for DSRS. Patients with bleeding gastric varices who are good operative candidates are considered for DSRS as initial treatment because these varices are difficult to sclerose.

PREOPERATIVE PLANNING

Preoperative evaluation for DSRS should include liver function tests, liver serologic evaluation, splenoportography, and left renal venography. Hepatic wedge venography and pressure measurement are useful in differentiating between presinusoidal and postsinusoidal portal hypertension. An angiographic evaluation of the inferior vena cava and hepatic veins is indicated in patients with Budd-Chiari syndrome. Liver ultrasonography or computed tomographic scanning is used to determine the liver volume and to uncover nodules that may suggest hepatoma formation. Such nodules should be subjected to biopsy preoperatively for histologic verification. Liver biopsy is also indicated to determine the nature of the underlying liver disease in atypical cases and in patients with clinical evidence of active viral or alcohol-related liver disease.

It is our policy to postpone the operation until the liver function and nutritional status of the patient are maximally improved. Patients who are actively drinking alcohol are referred to appropriate centers, and the operation is deferred until there is a reasonable chance that they will abstain. Patients with ascites are treated medically until the problem is resolved. Intractable ascites is a contraindication to DSRS operation.

SURGICAL TECHNIQUE

The patient is placed in the supine position. Slight hyperextension of the lumbar spine helps to improve surgical exposure. The procedure is most commonly performed from a subcostal incision. The incision begins in the left midaxillary line and extends one fingerbreadth below the costal margin, across the midline, to the lateral border of the right rectus muscle. This incision provides excellent exposure, particularly to the region of the tail of the pancreas and hilum of the spleen. It may, however, weaken the abdominal wall. The midline incision (Fig. 1) is also adequate

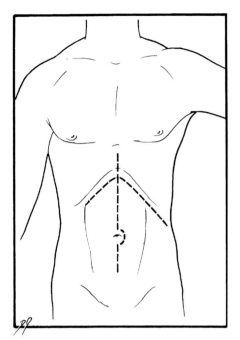

Fig. 1. Bilateral subcostal and midline incisions, both suitable for the distal splenorenal shunt operation.

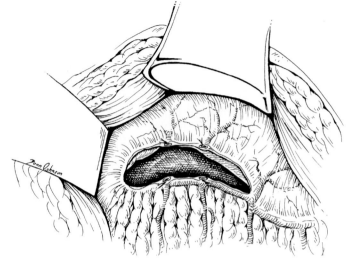

Fig. 2. The lesser sac is entered by dividing the gastrocolic ligament. The gastroepiploic vessels are disconnected from the stomach. Both right and left gastroepiploic veins are ligated to prevent maldiversion of portal blood to the decompressed splenic vein.

for this procedure and has, in fact, become my preference in recent years. In patients who have previously undergone midline abdominal operations, fewer adhesions may be encountered if the subcostal incision is used. Abnormal bleeding from the skin edges and abdominal muscles is common in patients with portal hypertension. Well-developed venous collaterals are often encountered around the umbilicus and in the falciform ligament. All bleeding should be securely controlled before proceeding with the operation. Persistent incisional bleeding can cause considerable perioperative blood loss in patients with portal hypertension. Another potential source of bleeding in these patients is the portosystemic collateral veins, which form in the adhesions between the abdominal contents and the abdominal wall. These adhesions should be meticulously divided by appropriate hemostatic techniques.

After all the adhesions crossing the surgical field are lysed, the abdomen is explored. Any suspicious nodule in the liver is sampled and examined for malignancy. The gallbladder is palpated for stones. In patients with cirrhosis, one should avoid cholecystectomy if at all possible. The morbidity and mortality from this procedure are quite high in such patients. Enlargement of the gallbladder is common among these patients, and this finding should not be mistaken for acute obstructive cholecystitis unless there are obvious signs of acute inflammation.

Adequate exposure is of crucial importance in the DSRS operation because of the depth of the operative field. In our experience, the Omni retractor is extremely useful for this purpose, particularly during dissection of the splenic and left renal veins. It should be remembered, however, that the tissues of patients with portal hypertension are congested and, if injured, can cause troublesome bleeding. This fact is especially true of the mesentery and spleen. Thus, it is important to use gentle retraction and to use proper padding under the retractor blades. The next step is to proceed with devascularization along the greater curvature of the stomach (Fig. 2). The gastric vessels are isolated individually, then divided between clamps and ligated according to proper surgical techniques. Devascularization is carried close to the wall of the stomach in a stretch extending from the pylorus to the first short gastric vein. The right and

left gastroepiploic veins are suture-ligated for the aforementioned reasons. Next, the splenic flexure is carefully mobilized by dividing its peritoneal attachment to the lower pole of the spleen. The stomach is then retracted superiorly, and the transverse colon is retracted inferiorly, using appropriate retractor blades. This procedure brings the pancreas into view. The stage is now ready for exposure of the splenic vein.

We routinely use headlight and magnifying loupes for mobilization of the splenic vein. First, the pancreas is mobilized by dividing the peritoneum along its inferior border (Fig. 3). Mobilization of this border is completed before dissection is carried deeper in the retropancreatic space. With the pancreas carefully retracted, the surgeon starts looking for the splenic vein. In most instances, it loops inferiorly as it approaches the superior mesenteric vein. It is, therefore, easier to identify the splenic vein

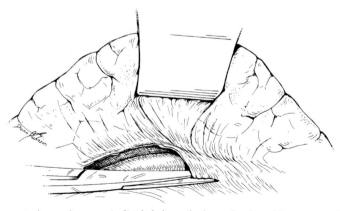

Fig. 3. The posterior peritoneum is divided along the lower border of the pancreas. The latter is retracted gently to visualize the splenic vein.

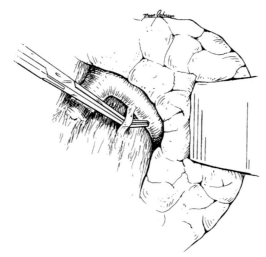

Fig. 4. The inferior mesenteric vein is identified in preparation for its division. In some cases, the inferior mesenteric vein is used as a guide for the splenic vein.

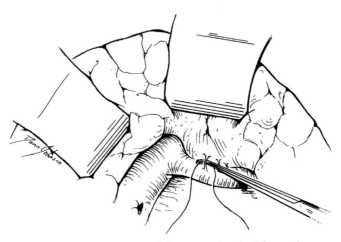

Fig. 5. Technique for isolation and division of the pancreatic veins. These veins are encircled, ligated, and then divided using meticulous surgical technique. Laceration of these fragile veins causes troublesome bleeding.

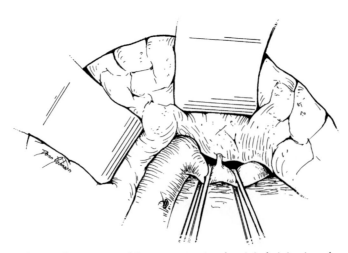

Fig. 6. The technique for exposure of the coronary vein when it is draining into the splenic vein instead of the portal vein. The splenic vein is encircled on either side of the coronary vein. Traction on the tape encircling the splenic vein facilitates exposure of the coronary vein.

first medially, then to proceed with its mobilization in the direction of the hilum of the spleen. The inferior mesenteric veins may be used as a guide to find the splenic vein unless it is joining the superior mesenteric vein (Fig. 4).

The splenic vein should be mobilized first inferiorly, then anteriorly, and posteriorly, leaving dissection of its superior border until adequate length of the vein has been exposed. The pancreatic veins along this border of the pancreas require special handling because they are friable and, if torn, can cause troublesome bleeding. Our technique for isolation of these veins starts with careful dissection until a sufficient length of the vein is exposed. A fine silk suture is then applied around the mobilized vein and ligated flush with the splenic vein. A fine-tip clamp is applied to the other side, and the vein is transected between the clamps. The pancreatic end of the divided vessel is then ligated using meticulous surgical technique (Fig. 5). These veins are sometimes too short to be safely controlled with simple ligatures, in which case it is safer to use 5-0 Prolene to suture the divided veins. Dissection of the pancreatic veins is the most challenging part of the DSRS operation. In my experience, the tearing of these vessels is most often caused by excessive pancreatic retraction, a premature attempt to encircle the splenic vein, or a premature attempt to encircle the pancreatic veins. Another complicating factor in this dissection is the coronary vein, which joins the upper border of the splenic vein in approximately one-fifth of patients. In some cases, the coronary vein may be as large as the splenic vein. Tearing of the coronary vein can cause severe bleeding and may lead to irreversible damage to the splenic vein. The safest way to deal with this situation is to free the upper border of the splenic vein and encircle it on both sides of the coronosplenic venous junction. Gentle traction on the splenic vein facilitates further mobilization of the coronary vein (Fig. 6). The mobilization is continued until there is sufficient room for safe clamping and division of the coronary vein.

Once an adequate segment of the splenic vein is mobilized, attention is shifted to the left renal vein. This vessel can be approached either above or below the transverse mesocolon. In the superior approach, the colon is retracted inferiorly, and the duodenojejunal junction is exposed. The posterior peritoneum and the underlying tissue are divided along an imaginary line that stretches from the lateral border of the fourth part of the duodenum to the hilum of the left kidney. Once the left renal vein is identified, it is mobilized by dividing as many tributaries as necessary, including the adrenal and gonadal veins (Fig. 7).

In the infracolonic approach to the left renal vein, the colon is retracted superiorly, and the third part of the duodenum is exposed. The duodenum is mobilized by dividing the peritoneum along its inferior border, and the dissection is advanced superiorly until the left renal vein is exposed. Once the left renal vein is identified, the colon is retracted inferiorly, and mobilization of the left renal vein is completed as described previously. The advantage of this approach is the ability to locate the left renal vein with minimal untargeted dissection in the retroperitoneal space. This advantage is important because the retroperitoneal tissue of patients with portal hypertension is often dense and loaded with distended lymph vessels and collateral veins. Any transected tissue in this dissection should be securely ligated to minimize perioperative blood loss and postoperative lymphatic leakage. Uncontrolled lymphatic leakage causes postoperative ascites and, if the intestinal lymphatics are involved, chylous ascites may develop, a condition that is often difficult to treat.

With the left renal vein fully exposed, the surgeon turns back to the splenic vein, dividing it between vascular clamps near its junction with the portal vein. We use a Cooley clamp on the portal end of the splenic vein flush with the portal vein (Figs. 8, 9). It is important to leave a sufficient rim exposed to ensure secure closure of the stump of the splenic vein. A 5-0 Prolene stitch is used for the closure (Fig. 10). The splenic end of the splenic vein is now less anchored in place; hence, more of the deeply located pancreatic veins can be readily brought into view (Figs. 11 and 12). Mobilization of the splenic vein is advanced laterally until an adequate length of the vessel is exposed.

The stage is now set for shunt construction. A Satinsky clamp is applied to the left renal vein (Fig. 13). The splenic end of the splenic vein is then approximated to the clamped segment of the left renal vein. Any apparent tension should be corrected by further mobilization of either of the two veins. It is also important to trim any excess in the splenic vein; otherwise, it will become acutely angulated when circulation is restored. Optimal orientation of the two vessels can usually be achieved by rotating the splenic vein in a clockwise direction for 45 degrees. The shunt is placed as medially as possible in relation to the left renal vein to prevent sharp bending of the splenic vein.

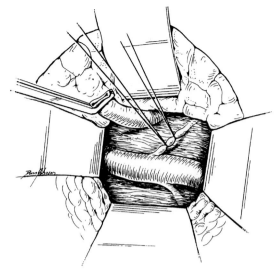

Fig. 7. The left renal vein is exposed by dividing the overlying peritoneum. The vein is mobilized by dividing its tributaries, including the gonadal and adrenal veins.

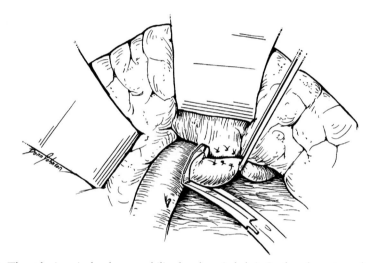

Fig. 8. The splenic vein has been mobilized and encircled. A Cooley clamp is applied to the splenic vein at its junction with the superior mesenteric vein.

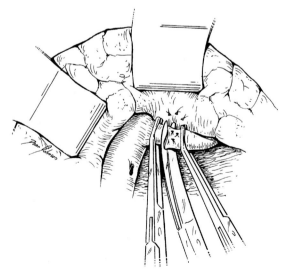

Fig. 9. The splenic vein is divided between clamps, leaving sufficient rim medially to allow safe control of the stump of the splenic vein. Accidental slippage of the clamp or faulty stump closure may cause bleeding and tearing of the splenomesenteric-portal vein junction.

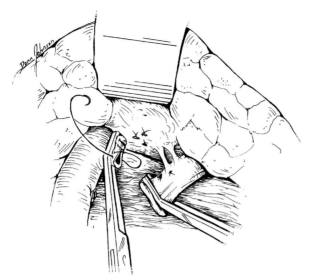

Fig. 10. Oversewing of the stump of the splenic vein using 5-0 running Prolene.

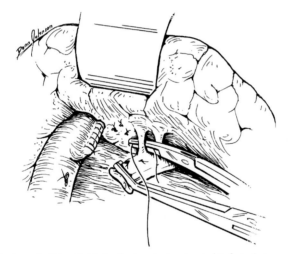

Fig. 11. The splenic end of the divided splenic vein is retracted inferiorly to expose more of the pancreatic veins laterally.

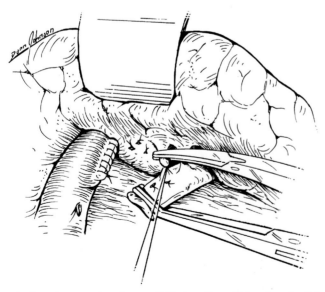

Fig. 12. The splenic and pancreatic veins are divided until a sufficient length of the splenic vein is disconnected from the pancreas.

With the two veins properly approximated, shunt construction is begun by removing a disk 10 × 15 mm from the superior wall of the left renal vein (Fig. 14). A stay stitch is used to keep the opening in the vein well exposed. The anastomosis is started at the most medial end (or toe) using double-armed 5-0 Prolene. One needle is passed from the outside to the inside of the left renal vein. This needle is used as a running stitch to close the posterior wall. A new 5-0 Prolene corner stitch is then applied at the lateral corner (or heel) of the anastomosis and ligated. One end of this suture is tied to the one used for the posterior row. At this stage, there is one stitch at each corner of the anastomosis. These two stitches are advanced so that the anastomosis is finished in the middle of the anterior row (Figs. 15–19). Both veins are adequately flushed before the anastomosis is completed. The potential purse-string effect of the running suture is minimized by interrupting the suture line at the toe and heel of the anastomosis. In children, we routinely interrupt the entire anterior row to allow for growth.

The final step in the DSRS procedure is coronary vein ligation. The stomach is retracted anteriorly and superiorly, and the peritoneal fold stretching between the highest point of the lesser curvature and the posterior wall of the lesser sac is exposed. The coronary vein is identified and ligated in this location. Any accessory coronary veins in the region should also be ligated. It is important to protect the nerve of Latarjet while exposing the coronary vein.

The operative field is then thoroughly examined, and any remaining bleeding points or lymphatic leaks are controlled. The abdomen is closed without any drains. Draining the abdominal cavity in the presence of ascites leads to massive postoperative fluid loss and profound electrolyte disturbances. Abdominal drains also enhance the risk of secondary bacterial invasion.

MODIFICATION OF THE DSRS OPERATION

Temporary Clamping of the Splenic Artery

In patients with hyperdynamic splenic circulation and massive splenomegaly, I routinely clamp the splenic artery until the shunt construction is completed. In patients with schistosomiasis, for example, the spleen, which is usually quite large, grows even larger with clamping of the splenic vein. The difficult exposure is compounded by the extreme engorgement of the pancreatic and splenic veins. The decongestive

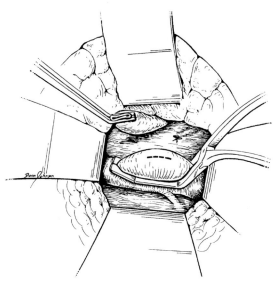

Fig. 13. A Satinsky clamp is applied to the left renal vein. The more medial the segment of the vein selected for the shunt, the better the angle of the meeting of the splenic and left renal veins.

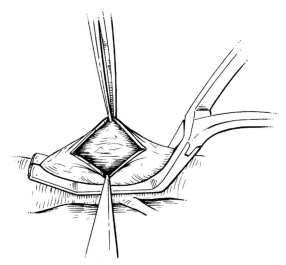

Fig. 14. A disk is removed from the wall of the left renal vein. Stay stitches may be used to retract on the anterior rim of the vein.

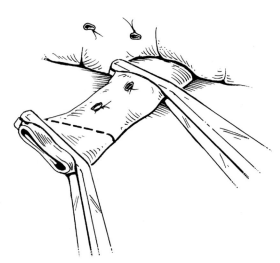

Fig. 15. The splenic vein is being prepared for the shunt. The vessel is rotated one fourth of a circle clockwise. The splenic vein is shortened to avoid any redundancy that might lead to kinking of the vessel when the flow is restored.

effect of splenic arterial clamping helps to reduce the size of the spleen and congestion in the operative field.

Renosplenic End-to-Side Shunt

In a renosplenic end-to-side shunt (Fig. 20), the left renal vein is divided near the hilum of the kidney, and its central (or caval) end is swung upward to be anastomosed to the side of the left renal vein. The total shunt thus created is then converted into a selective shunt by ligating the splenic vein at some point between the renosplenic anastomosis and the portal vein. Patients with portal hypertension tolerate well the interruption of the renal vein because of pre-existing collateral venous circulation. Normally, a longer segment of a free vessel can be procured by mobilizing the left renal vein as compared with the splenic vein. The renosplenic technique is therefore advantageous when a long conduit is needed to cross the gap between these two veins. Compression of the left renal vein by the superior mesenteric artery is a potential problem with this technique and is usually caused by excessive traction on the left renal vein.

Splenocaval Shunt

For patients in whom left renal veins are absent or unsuitable, a selective shunt can be created by anastomosing the splenic end of the divided splenic vein to the side of the inferior vena cava (Fig. 21). The splenocaval shunt is also useful when one is dealing with an unusually tortuous splenic vein. The tortuosity of the vessel is partly corrected as it is stretched in a straight line to meet the inferior vena cava. Conversely, these angulations may be accentuated as the direction of the splenic vein is changed, first inferiorly and then posteriorly, to reach the left renal vein.

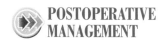

POSTOPERATIVE MANAGEMENT

Fluid and electrolyte balance should be monitored carefully because patients with cirrhosis have an increased tendency to retain fluid and salt. The aim is to slow down the rate of postoperative ascitic accumulation. Approximately half of the daily fluid requirement is given as 5% albumin in the first 24 to 48 hours. Ranitidine is administered to reduce gastric acidity. Cephalosporin is used for antibiotic prophylaxis, with the first dose given

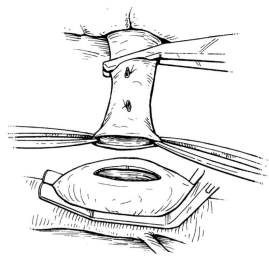

Fig. 16. The splenic vein is approximated to the left renal vein.

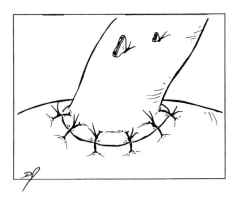

Fig. 18. Shunt construction. In children, the anterior row of sutures is interrupted.

1 hour before operation and the coverage extended during the procedure and for 24 to 48 hours after the operation. Diuretic therapy is started on the 3rd postoperative day in the form of spironolactone. Furosemide (Lasix) may be added in the management of problematic ascites.

QUESTIONS FREQUENTLY ASKED ABOUT THE SELECTIVE SHUNT

How Effective Is the Shunt in Preventing Rebleeding?

Rebleeding after a selective shunt occurs in 5% to 7% of cases; this compares favorably with the incidence for total shunts. In an emergency situation, a selective shunt may not be as effective as a total shunt in controlling the bleeding. In most instances, however, recurrent bleeding in the presence of a patent DSRS can be controlled with variceal injection.

What Is the Incidence of Shunt Occlusion?

Shunt failure is usually caused by faulty technique. The incidence of this complication should not exceed 5%. Excessive tension, kinking, twisting, and renal venous hypertension secondary to tenting of the left renal vein are among the main causes of early shunt failure. Poor selection of patients may be another reason for this complication. The risk of shunt thrombosis is high in patients with alcohol-related pancreatitis and a small splenic vein. Late shunt occlusion is rare, but late stenosis has been seen infrequently.

Is There a Role for the Selective Shunt in Patients with Ascites?

Existing preoperative ascites is likely to get worse after DSRS. First, cirrhotic patients with ascites have an increased tendency to retain fluid after major operations. Second, the selective shunt does not correct the major cause of ascites in such patients—the high pressure in the portal and superior mesenteric veins. Third, lymphatic leakage is known to occur after the selective shunt because several retroperitoneal lymph vessels are likely to be transected during mobilization of the left renal vein. Therefore, the selective shunt is not suitable for the treatment of patients who present with intractable ascites. On the other hand, ascites precipitated by the selective shunt is usually easily controlled with medical treatment. Chylous ascites, however, is more difficult to treat and may require prolonged periods of hospitalization. Intravenous hyperalimentation and repeated paracentesis is the recommended treatment for this condition.

What Is the Incidence of Encephalopathy after the Selective Shunt?

Early encephalopathy after DSRS occurs in 5% of patients. This percentage compares favorably with the reported incidence of 30% to 40% after total shunts. Assessment of the available data suggests that encephalopathy seen in patients with total shunts is more likely to be severe and incapacitating.

Long-term studies of patients with selective shunts have shown that the incidence of encephalopathy increases from

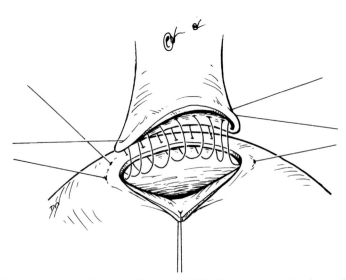

Fig. 17. Shunt construction: First, double-armed 5-0 Prolene suture is placed at each corner of the anastomosis. The medial corner suture is ligated. One end of this suture is used for the posterior wall.

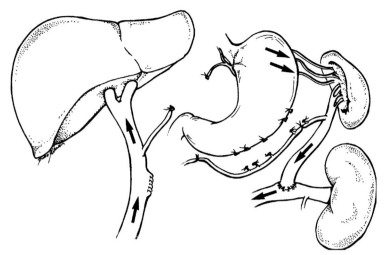

Fig. 19. A diagrammatic illustration of the distal splenorenal shunt.

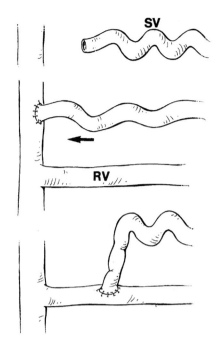

Fig. 21. A splenocaval shunt is desirable in patients with tortuous splenic vein (SV) because a standard distal splenorenal shunt may be difficult to construct without the risk of kinking the SV. RV, renal vein.

5% to a range of 10% to 15% in 3 to 5 years. Deterioration of liver function from worsening of underlying liver disease, together with progressive reduction in the level of liver portal venous perfusion, accounts for delayed-onset encephalopathy in these patients.

How Durable Is Selectivity of the Selective Shunt?

Early postshunt angiography has shown continuing portal perfusion in most cases. Late follow-up studies, however, have shown progressive formation of collaterals, reduction of portal vein diameter, and decreasing prograde portal flow after DSRS. Three main routes for mesoportal to splenic venous collaterals have been described: (a) the transpancreatic (pancreatic syphon) pathway, (b) the transgastric pathway, and (c) the colosplenic pathway. It has been proposed that, to minimize transpancreatic collateralization, the operation be modified so that the splenic vein is disconnected from the pancreas as far as the hilum of the spleen. Splenopancreatic disconnection, however, adds to the technical difficulty of the operation, and there is some evidence that it may compromise the decompressive effect of the procedure.

Is There a Difference in Survival after Selective as Opposed to Total Shunt Operation?

Studies have shown a trend in favor of the selective shunt in patients who have adequate liver reserve (Child classes A and B). This trend, however, did not reach statistical significance. Survival advantage of one type of shunt as compared with another is difficult to demonstrate in alcoholic patients. As the majority of these patients continue to drink postoperatively, death from hepatic failure remains high irrespective of the type of shunt operation. Conversely, patients with schistosomiasis tend to live longer because of the relative stability of their underlying liver disease. It is of interest to note that reports from Egypt and Brazil have shown that DSRS does improve survival of these patients.

Operative Technique for CSRS

In the CSRS procedure (Fig. 22), the spleen is removed and the central end of the splenic vein is anastomosed to the side of the left renal vein. The CSRS diverts all the portal blood away from the liver; hence, it has no physiologic advantage over the portacaval shunt. Further-

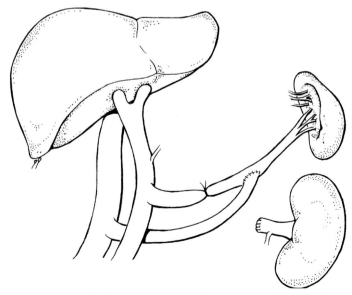

Fig. 20. Renosplenic shunt. The left renal vein is divided near the hilum of the kidney. The central end of the divided vein is anastomosed end-to-side to the splenic vein. The splenic vein is ligated between the shunt and the portal vein.

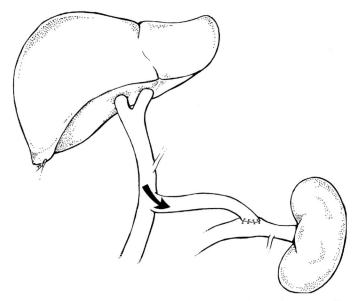

Fig. 22. A diagrammatic illustration of the central splenorenal shunt. The *arrow* indicates total diversion of portal blood away from the liver across the shunt to the left renal vein.

more, it may be technically more difficult because of the problems associated with removing the spleen in patients with portal hypertension. In addition, the patency rate of the CSRS may not be as good as the portacaval shunt. Hypercoagulability after splenectomy and a slower flow rate across the shunt may adversely affect shunt patency.

CSRS procedures are performed from an extended subcostal incision. The first step in the operation is to remove the spleen according to standard operative techniques. Because of the hypervascularity of the field, it is advisable to ligate the splenic artery before attempting to mobilize the spleen.

The splenic vein is divided near the hilum of the spleen. After removal of the spleen, the splenic vein is mobilized by dividing the pancreatic veins. These veins are easier to deal with in CSRS than in DSRS because they become less congested after the spleen has been removed.

The central end of the mobilized splenic vein is then anastomosed to the side of the left renal vein. The technical aspects of CSRS are similar to those described for DSRS.

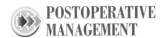 **POSTOPERATIVE MANAGEMENT**

The outline for postoperative care after DSRS also applies to CSRS. Ascites is less of a problem after CSRS. Rebleeding is usually secondary to shunt occlusion. This complication can generally be successfully treated with sclerotherapy because the varices are partially decompressed after removal of the spleen. In contrast, rebleeding associated with DSRS usually requires reoperation. Finally, encephalopathy occurs in 30% to 40% of patients after CSRS, although the incidence may be falsely reduced if patients with silent shunt occlusion are not excluded.

SUGGESTED READING

Abdel-Wahab M, el-Ebidy G, Gad el-Hak N, et al. Fundal varices: problem and management. *Hepatogastroenterology* 1999;46:849.

Ezzat FA, Abu-Elmagd KM, Sultan AA, et al. Schistosomal versus nonschistosomal variceal bleeders: do they respond differently to selective shunt (DSRS)? *Ann Surg* 1989;209:489.

Hasegawa I, Tamada H, Fukui Y, et al. Distal splenorenal shunt with splenopancreatic disconnection for portal hypertension in biliary atresia. *Pediatr Surg Int* 1999;15:92.

Henderson JM, Millikan WJ, Galloway JR. The Emory perspective of the distal splenorenal shunt in 1990. *Am J Surg* 1990;160:54.

Inokuchi K, Sugimachi K. The selective shunt for variceal bleeding: a personal perspective. *Am J Surg* 1990;160:48.

Jenkins RL, Gedaly R, Pomposelli JJ, et al. Distal splenorenal shunt: role, indications, and utility in the era of liver transplantation. *Arch Surg* 1999;134:416.

Langer B, Taylor BR, Greig PD. Selective or total shunts for variceal bleeding. *Am J Surg* 1990;160:75.

Lopes Filho G de J, Haddad CM. Late clinical, biochemical, endoscopic, and electroencephalographic evaluation of patients with schistosomal portal hypertension treated with distal splenorenal shunt. *Int Surg* 1998;83:42.

Maffei-Faccioli A, Gerunda GE, Neri D, et al. Selective variceal decompression and its role relative to other therapies. *Am J Surg* 1990; 160:60.

Richards WO, Pearson TC, Henderson JM, et al. Evaluation and treatment of early hemorrhage of the alimentary tract after selective shunt procedures. *Surg Gynecol Obstet* 1987;164:530.

Rikkers LF. The changing spectrum of treatment for variceal bleeding. *Ann Surg* 1998;228:536.

Salam AA, Ezzat FA, Abu-Elmagd KM. Selective shunt in schistosomiasis in Egypt. *Am J Surg* 1990;160:90.

Selim N, Fendley MJ, Boyer TD, et al. Conversion of failed transjugular intrahepatic portosystemic shunt to distal splenorenal shunt in patients with Child A or B cirrhosis. *Ann Surg* 1998;227:600.

Spina G, Santambrogio R, Opocher E, et al. Improved quality of life after distal splenorenal shunt. *Ann Surg* 1988;208:104.

Zacks SL, Sandler RS, Biddle AK, et al. Decision-analysis of transjugular intrahepatic portosystemic shunt versus distal splenorenal shunt for portal hypertension. *Hepatology* 1999;29:1399.

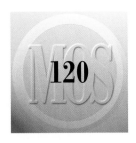

Central Splenorenal Shunts

JOSEF E. FISCHER

The nature of therapy for bleeding varices and cirrhosis has changed dramatically since the introduction and popularization of hepatic transplantation. However, it remains largely believed that unless the patient has demonstrated abstinence from alcohol for a period, it is inappropriate to consider hepatic transplantation. Therefore, arrest of variceal bleeding and the use of shunting procedures remain appropriate.

In considering shunting procedures, it is best that such procedures not involve the porta hepatis so that future transplantation is not compromised. Thus, the central and distal splenorenal shunts have gained increasing acceptance by those who previously carried out portacaval shunts because they do not interfere technically with the opportunity to do an expeditious liver transplant at some future time. One should not lose sight of the fact that, in a patient with bleeding esophageal varices who shows no signs of stopping despite aggressive therapy, one should move early to emergency portacaval shunt to stop the bleeding before the patient becomes coagulopathic and unsalvageable. Although this would make future liver transplantation difficult, it does not render it impossible.

Central and distal splenorenal shunts are generally not emergency procedures, as the decrease in portal pressure is not usually sufficient to arrest bleeding acutely. One should rely on Pitressin, somatostatin, iced saline lavage, Sengstaken-Blakemore tubes, and sclerotherapy to provide immediate cessation of bleeding. The patient should be prepared for operation carefully at an interval, in the hospital, if possible, or at home, with abstinence from alcohol, good nutrition, vitamins, and modest exercise. If the patient is protein-intolerant, a high branched-chain amino acid diet should be used to minimize encephalopathy, in addition to lactulose or neomycin, or both. The patient should be admitted to the hospital the evening before operation, and a central venous pressure or Swan-Ganz catheter placed if there is doubt about the cardiovascular status. The prevalence of left-right dissociation makes a Swan-Ganz cathether particularly useful. Antibacterial washes to the abdomen and chest should have been carried out several days before to minimize the skin bacterial count, and vitamin K administered to get a maximum prothrombin time. Because the Child class is directly related to mortality (Table 1), one should seek to obtain maximum improvement in nutrition, albumin, and overall nutritional and functional status before undertaking operation. I use a standard Nichols-type bowel preparation, generally with erythromycin and neomycin, in case the colon is entered inadvertently during the procedure, and it is also probably useful in preventing encephalopathy. The patient should be hydrated overnight; 10% glucose or a branched-chain-enriched amino acid parenteral nutrition solution may be used. Perioperative antibiotics are given as a single dose, usually of a first-generation cephalosporin, at the induction of anesthesia, and repeated every 3.5 hours of the operative procedure.

CENTRAL SPLENORENAL SHUNT

The central splenorenal shunt (Fig. 1) is carried out through a 10th rib thoracoabdominal incision, as popularized by Linton. The patient should be carefully positioned to be in the right lateral decubitus position, with the left side turned up at 45 degrees (Fig. 2). The entire abdomen and chest are prepared. The incision is carried out from the area of the umbilicus through the 10th rib proximally to the posterior axillary line. The 10th rib is removed (Fig. 3). I find it easier to enter the abdomen through the peritoneum anterior to the 10th rib and then work posteriorly to resect the rib. If the break in the table is properly placed under the opposite 10th rib, the operator is positioned right over the splenic vein and where the renal vein is ultimately located centrally in the operative field (Fig. 4).

The key to the operative procedure is not to lose control of the splenic vein or the spleen with respect to hemorrhage and blood loss during the splenectomy. I have found it helpful to ligate the splenic artery before attacking the spleen. This generally can be carried out by identifying the splenic artery at a convenient point at the superior border of the pancreas, passing a 0 silk tie around it, and ligating it (Fig. 5). This decreases the blood loss if there is an inadvertent tear in the spleen. The splenic vein may be encircled with a vessel loop, but need not be tied at this point.

The splenectomy is carried out by taking down the attachments to the colon between Kelly clamps and tying with 0 cotton, if available, or silk if it is not. The retroperitoneum is then entered between Schnidt or Reinhoff clamps and suture-ligated on both sides with 2–0 silk. This is the most tedious part of the procedure, but it is essential if one is to dissect the splenic vein free in controlled fashion. One then proceeds laterally along the entire border of the spleen. It is best to take down the spleen 2 cm lateral to its peritoneal attachment (Fig. 6) because one can get a good purchase on the retroperitoneum, and suture ligation is

TABLE 1. CHILD'S CLASSIFICATION OF LIVER CIRRHOSIS

Finding	Class		
	A	**B**	**C**
Ascites	None	Controlled	Uncontrolled
Bilirubin	<2.0	2.0–2.5	>3.0
Encephalopathy	None	Minimal	Advanced
Nutritional status	Excellent	Good	Poor
Albumin	>3.5	3.0–3.5	<3.0
Operative mortality (%)	2	10	50

The Gastrointestinal Tract

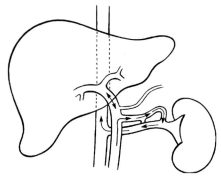

Fig. 1. The path of flow *(arrows)* after central splenorenal shunt. Intestinal flow and some proximal portal flow tend to be diverted into the shunt. Flow from the short pancreatic branches and the proximal portal vein probably continues to perfuse the liver at a pressure of 10 to 15 mm Hg.

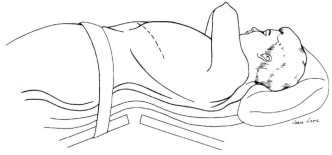

Fig. 2. Positioning of the patient. The thoracoabdominal incision centered over the 10th rib *(dotted line)* is carried from the midaxillary line toward, but not to, the umbilicus.

relatively easy; it is also less bloody in that plane. Remember that the basic idea of carrying out a central splenorenal shunt is to get behind the spleen and the pancreas and bring the pancreas anterior so that the splenic vein, which is a retroperitoneal structure, can be easily identified and managed.

The short gastric vessels are then ligated in continuity with 2–0 silk. The highest short gastric vessel may be especially difficult because it is very short and the stomach may be inadvertently entered. The greater curvature should be closed with 4–0 silk sutures where the short gastric vessels have been ligated to prevent the uncommon complication of perforation of the greater curvature.

After the spleen has been mobilized medially, the hilum is then addressed. The splenic vein is then dissected free and its branches are ligated, as are the branches of the splenic artery. If the splenic artery has not been previously ligated, it should be ligated so that postoperative hemorrhage can be avoided. The spleen is then delivered. One must take care not to involve the pancreas in the resection or dissection of the splenic hilum.

After the splenic vein has been isolated and the tail of the pancreas elevated in the wound, the next step is to identify the renal vein (Fig. 7). The purpose of this is to make certain that one does not mobilize too much of the splenic vein, making it redundant. One identifies the renal vein by palpating the upper and lower borders of the kidney and then feeling the renal artery. Between clamps, and with suture ligation of the divided retroperitoneum, the renal vein is identified. It is necessary to clamp the fatty areolar tissue in this

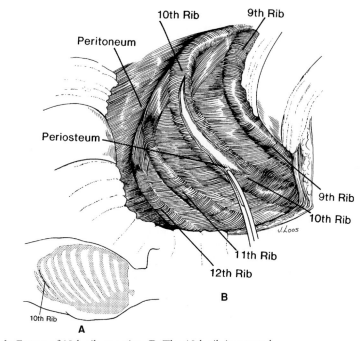

Fig. 3. A: Extent of 10th rib resection. **B:** The 10th rib is resected.

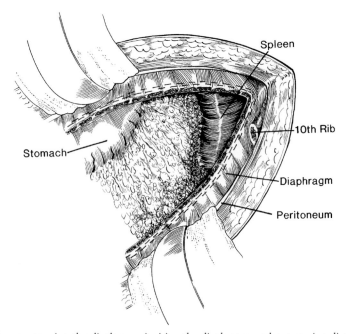

Fig. 4. View on opening the diaphragm, incising the diaphragm, and oversewing diaphragm cut edges with mattress sutures.

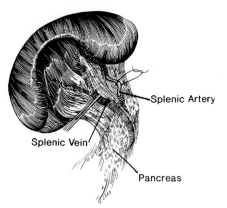

Fig. 5. Ligating the splenic artery.

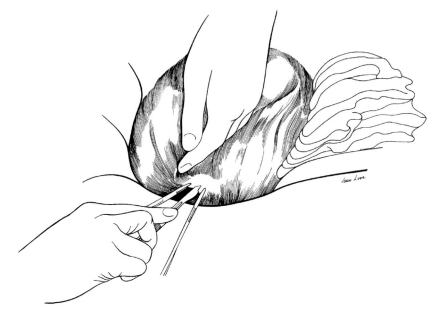

Fig. 6. The critical maneuver of removing the spleen. Clamps are placed approximately 2 cm lateral to the splenic edge in the areolar tissue of the retroperitoneum, which contains large collaterals. These are subsequently suture-ligated with nonabsorbable sutures of 2-0 silk.

area, not only because of bleeding, but also because of the lymph vessels that abound here and the proximity to the cisterna chyli. The renal vein is identified and vessel loops are then passed around the renal vein. It may be necessary to ligate the adrenal vein later in the procedure to obtain a reasonable spot for the anastomosis.

After the renal vein is identified, an appropriate portion of the splenic vein is dissected out. There are no branches of the splenic vein on the posterior aspect of the splenic vein, and the overlying peritoneum may be sharply divided; the branches of the splenic vein to the pancreas occur laterally at approximately 1-cm intervals. They are fine, but do not be fooled: ripping one of the tributaries may result in torrential hemorrhage if portal pressure is too high, which it usually is. I use the technique of insinuating a right-angle Jacobson clamp, grasping 4–0 silk on either side (Fig. 8) and tying it proximal and distal, and then cutting between these silk sutures with a knife. Others may use different techniques, but the

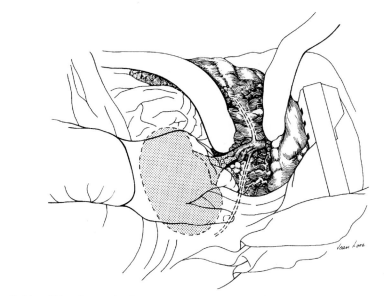

Fig. 7. Identifying the renal vein.

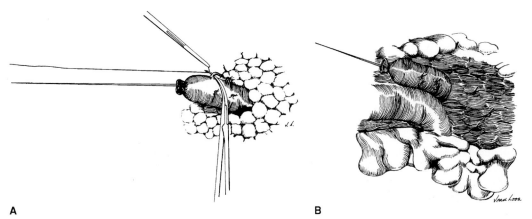

A   **B**

Fig. 8. A: Dissecting the splenic vein. There are short branches, which are paired approximately 1 cm apart. These must be taken carefully. **B:** A length of splenic vein is now available.

The Gastrointestinal Tract

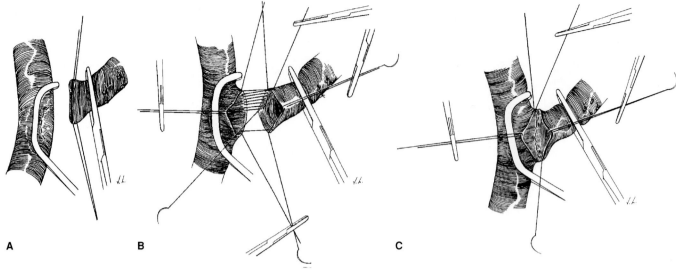

A   **B**   **C**

Fig. 9. A: Stay sutures at corners of splenic vein. A specially fashioned Satinsky clamp is placed on the splenic vein and an ellipse is excised. **B:** Stay sutures placed between the corners of the renal vein incision and the splenic vein. A horizontal everting mattress of 5-0 sutures is then used to bring the two veins together posteriorly. **C:** The horizontal everting mattress is then snugged up posteriorly. Properly performed, there should be little or no suture material showing on the posterior wall.

purpose is to elevate a portion of the splenic vein from the pancreatic bed.

Once an appropriate portion of splenic vein is elevated, one must then judge what will happen to the anastomosis when the pancreas is replaced back in its natural position. Vascular clamps are then applied to the splenic vein, and a miniature Satinsky clamp is applied to the renal vein. A small ellipse of renal vein is then excised (Fig. 9A). The back wall of the splenic vein is then anastomosed in running everting mattress fashion to the renal vein, as illustrated in Figure 9B, C. The front wall is then sutured with interrupted horizontal mattress sutures of 5-0 Prolene (Fig. 10A). The renal vein clamp is released just before completion of the anastomosis to vent the anastomosis and get rid of clots (Fig. 10A, B). The splenic vein clamp is then released. Any leaks are sutured with doubly armed 6-0 Prolene. Dr. Linton frequently liked to resect the tail of the pancreas so that the splenic vein would lie better, whereas I have not found it necessary to do this.

After irrigation, one should oversew the lateral border where the spleen has been removed with a running suture to secure hemostasis (Fig. 11). The abdominal closure is carried out carefully in multiple layers, making certain that if the patient accumulates ascites, there is no ascitic leak. The diaphragm, which has been taken down to provide access to the spleen, is then closed with mattress sutures of 0 silk and any running nonabsorbable suture over the cut edge to secure hemostasis. It can be expected that ascites will

be well controlled. An open shunt can frequently be estimated clinically by measuring serial urinary sodium concentrations. If the concentration is higher than 10 mg/dL, the shunt is almost certainly open.

Postoperatively, sodium-containing fluids are minimized, and the urinary sodium is measured frequently. Abdominal girths are measured to make certain that ascites is not accumulating. The nasogastric

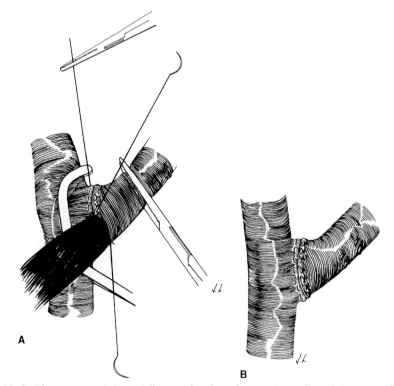

A

B

Fig. 10. A: The anastomosis is partially completed on the anterior wall, with interrupted horizontal mattresses of 5-0 Prolene. The vein is flushed. The remainder of the sutures are then held before being finally tied. **B:** The completed anastomosis. The anastomosis should be between 1.0 and 1.2 cm. The splenic vein is rarely larger than this. A thrill may be felt by placing a finger along the renal vein. It is customary to place a needle through the renal vein and pull back the needle, measuring pressures across the splenic vein. A gradient of more than 3 or 4 mm suggests that the anastomosis should be redone.

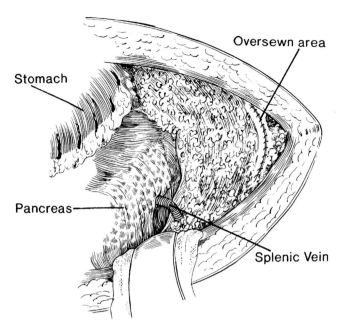

Fig. 11. Oversewing the cut edge of the splenic bed with a running chromic suture.

tube may be removed on the 2nd or 3rd postoperative day, as gastric ileus usually occurs after this procedure. A chest tube that has been placed in the event of a diaphragmatic leak or bleeding is removed 48 hours postoperatively.

If the patient experiences hepatic failure, it is treated with fluid restriction and total parenteral nutrition with a branched-chain-enriched amino acid solution. Encephalopathy is similarly treated, with the addition of neomycin or lactulose, or both.

The critical aspect of central splenorenal shunt is meticulous hemostasis at the time of operation. Some have used a hypotensive spinal anesthesia, and that is perfectly appropriate. However, one must make certain that the normal blood pressure has been restored before closing. If not, bleeding may supervene postoperatively when normal pressure is restored.

In a time when distal splenorenal shunts have become most popular as a bridge to transplantation, or in relatively good-risk patients who are not thought to require transplantation, the central splenorenal shunt should be performed in patients with tight ascites. The experience of my group and that of others have shown that these patients are not likely to do well after distal splenorenal shunt. Others have argued that the central splenorenal shunt turns into a total shunt before long. This is not true in our experience when we have measured portal flow. The reason is that one must limit the size of the anastomosis to between 1.0 and 1.5 cm. When pressures are measured under these circumstances, the splenic vein pressure should remain between 10 and 15 cm of water so that some flow to the liver persists. The central splenorenal shunt is a side-to-side shunt. However, it should be a small side-to-side shunt, not a total

shunt. In this, we differ with the late Dean Warren, Dr. Salam in Chapter 119, and others who are the devotees of the distal splenorenal shunt, as we have had excellent results with the central splenorenal shunt.

The other group that may benefit from a central splenorenal shunt, as opposed to a distal splenorenal shunt, are patients with hypersplenism. After end-to-side portacaval shunt in McDermott's early series published in the *New England Journal of Medicine* in 1962, there were a number of patients who responded, with amelioration of their hypersplenism, but some did not. Similarly, in our experience, an occasional patient with hypersplenism has not done well from the standpoint of thrombocytopenia. Those patients probably would have done better with a central splenorenal shunt.

This remains a good operation that can be performed with low mortality and morbidity, provided it is carefully done. It requires the utmost in surgical technique and gentleness in handling of tissues and, because the splenic vein tends to be a thin vein, one must use a maximum of care in its anastomosis. However, if one does so, the results are gratifying and many patients continue to do well years after surgery, with a minimum of encephalopathy.

SUGGESTED READING

Fischer JE. The technique for central splenorenal shunt. In: Schwarz S, ed. *Modern techniques in surgery.* Vol. 13: *Abdominal surgery.* New York: Futura Publishing, 1982:1.

Fischer JE, Bower RH, Atamian S, et al. Comparison of distal and proximal splenorenal shunts: a randomized prospective trial. *Ann Surg* 1981;194:531.

Linton RR. The definitive treatment of bleeding esophageal varices. In: Linton RR. *Atlas of vascular surgery.* Philadelphia: WB Saunders, 1973:168.

Nussbaum MS, Schoettker PJ, Fischer JE. Comparison of distal and proximal splenorenal shunts: a ten-year experience. *Surgery* 1993;114:659.

The Gastrointestinal Tract

EDITOR'S COMMENT

The principal indication for both of the shunts described in Chapters 119 and 120 is a Child class A or B cirrhotic patient who is expected to be reasonably stable over the next several years, has proven bleeding esophageal varices, with the unlikelihood of transplantation in the future and, in the Middle East, the presence of schistosomiasis. Occasionally, a patient will present with massive splenomegaly and thrombocytopenia, necessitating a splenectomy. Data have accumulated that suggest

that these patients would probably do better if, in fact, they have a central splenorenal shunt at the time of splenectomy. The workup of these patients with both these conditions is similar. I tend to use a less elaborate workup than Dr. Salam does. A helical computed tomographic scan will show the vessels reasonably well, and will usually show the suitability of both the renal vein, its distance from the splenic vein, and the diameter of the splenic vein. It is useful to know in both of these operations that the patient

has not had chronic pancreatitis with fibrosis. This situation makes the operation quite difficult.

As in the portacaval shunt, I believe it is essential that one does not do a lot of needless dissecting of the retroperitoneum in both of these operations. In the first place, it is bloody; in the second place, there are lots of lymphatic vessels, and the cisterna chyli is not far from the site. Thus, excellent exposure, good help, good lighting, and mechanical retractors are essential if the operation is

(continued)

to be carried out well. To me, there is no difference in outcome between the distal splenorenal and central splenorenal shunts. A randomized prospective trial (Fischer JE, et al., *Ann Surg* 1981;194:531) revealed almost identical survival and identical incidence of hepatic encephalopathy and liver failure. The reason for these identical results is, I believe, something that Dr. Robert Ritchie Linton, who basically originated and popularized the operation as it is currently done, emphasized to me as he was teaching me how to do it: that is, that one does not want a huge shunt, that one wants a controlled shunt with a 1.0- to 1.2-cm diameter opening in order for the portal pressure to remain between 10 and 15 mm Hg so that there is some prograde flow to the liver. If one forgets that and makes a large shunt, then, in fact, Dr. Salam is right: this is a total shunt. However, if the shunt is intentionally kept on the small side, one can expect protection from bleeding esophageal varices and, when appropriately selected, the patient should be free of ascites. Dr. Salam makes clear that a patient with unmanageable or tight ascites is not a candidate for distal splenorenal shunt. What concerns me is his seeming refusal to consider the central splenorenal shunt under these circumstances. I disagree on this violently because of my own personal experience in which patients with tight ascites who undergo a proper central splenorenal shunt with a controlled size of anastomosis have prolonged survival and minimal encephalopathy. In my own randomized prospective trial, the incidence of encephalopathy was quite low, and was identical in each procedure.

The approaches are the same, and one can do a central splenorenal shunt through the subcostal incision. However, I think it is more difficult. Although removing the 10th rib and dividing the diaphragm has a slightly higher morbidity as well as the opportunity for an ascitic leak into the chest, if the central splenorenal shunt is patent there will be no ascites to leak into the chest, and the diaphragm can be closed well, in two layers.

The difficulty with both operations is isolating the splenic vein. The pancreatic branches usually occur at 1-cm intervals. My own technique is to insinuate a Jacobson right-angle clamp under the vein, and then pass a 4–0 silk on either side, tying them far enough away from each other so that one can cut the vein between the sutures with either Potts scissors or a No. 15 blade. Remember that the fascia overlying the splenic vein at the dorsal side of the pancreas is usually avascular, and one can divide that relatively easily with the scissors, thus allowing the splenic vein to bulge. When the patient has chronic pancreatitis, the operation can become quite difficult.

In dissecting out the renal vein, it is best not to go too far medially because that is where the cisterna chyli or those lymph vessels that help make up the cisterna chyli are located. Despite the fact that one can suture-ligate the lymphatics in the retroperitoneum, and one should, and not depend

on cautery for either hemostasis or sealing lymphatics one can still get into difficulty with chylous ascites, which is a very significant complication.

As Dr. Salam says, occasionally it is necessary to divide the renal vein and turn it up to the splenic vein, that is, a renosplenic shunt. The reason that this is able to be performed under these and most circumstances is that adequate drainage can be obtained through the gonadal vein, provided one preserves it. The adrenal vein is less important, and it may be necessary sometimes to divide the adrenal vein in order to get a suitable site for anastomosis.

I will use perioperative antibiotics, usually in two doses, using a first-generation cephalosporin, and repeating after 3.5 hours.

The patients undergoing this procedure may benefit from a parenteral nutrition in the perioperative period with a branched-chain amino acid-enriched aromatic amino acid-deficient solution, given as parenteral nutrition, such as HepatAmine. In addition, if volume shifts are large, these patients have a remarkable difference between their left atrial pressure and their wedged pulmonary artery pressure, often as much as 8 or 9 mm Hg. This may be because of the arterial venous shunts that open up, particularly in the bronchial circulation, with the amount of circulating estrogen, which is not well metabolized by the damaged liver. It may be necessary in the postoperative period in both groups, as the duration following the successful shunt increases, to use an oral branched-chain amino acid supplement in order to prevent encephalopathy and to maintain nutrition.

Others, such as Wong et al. (*Arch Surg* 2002; 137:1125), claim that the splenic shunt, appropriately distal and central, the latter with tight ascites, is an excellent operation for patients who come to the medical centers in Hawaii, often from Pacific Island hospitals as far away as 3,800 miles, because transjugular intrahepatic portasystemic shunt may stenose, and these patients are sufficiently from far away that they will not get medical attention in time. Of the 34 patients who underwent splenorenal shunt in the Wong et al. report, both distal and central, 24 were either homeless, actively involved in substance abuse, or were being treated for psychiatric problems—not the patient population that one would choose to undergo liver transplantation.

As stated previously, schistosomiasis is a reasonable indication for either central or distal splenorenal shunt. Melo et al. (*J Surg Res* 2004;121:108) reported on a series of 30 patients who were randomized for either distal splenorenal shunt or distal splenorenal shunt plus splenic artery ligation. They reported no mortality or encephalopathy in both groups, a result similar to the experience of most other individuals. Although they thought that the splenic artery ligation associated with distal splenorenal shunt was associated with a substantial increase in postoperative pain and fever, nonetheless it did not contribute to an increased incidence of shunt thrombosis, and did improve white cell and platelet count as well as reduce the spleen size.

Rocko et al. (*Am Surg* 1986;52:81) reported on a series of 80 patients in a randomized prospective trial, as well as an additional 30 patients in whom a mesocaval shunt was carried out. The mortality in mesocaval shunts, including emergency shunts, was 9%. Incidence of encephalopathy was 10%, although it is not clear exactly how long was the follow-up.

Much of the world's literature seems to revolve around reporting large or small numbers of cases in the treatment of portal hypertension and the enumeration of simple outcomes such as mortality, morbidity, and encephalopathy. An exception to this is a report by Orloff et al. (*J Am Coll Surg* 2002;194:717), who reported the largest and longest experience, they claim, of the use of portal-systemic shunts to treat esophageal varices from extrahepatic portal hypertension associated with portal vein thrombosis. The three types of splenorenal shunts used were a central side-to-side shunt without splenectomy, a central end-to-side shunt with splenectomy, and a mesocaval end-to-side cavomesenteric shunt. All patients survived the operation, and 15-year survival rates were 95%. Five patients (2.5%), all with central end-to-side splenorenal shunts (which I find quite difficult), rebled because of thrombosis of the shunt. There was no encephalopathy.

Xin-Bao Xu et al. (*World J Gastroenterol* 2005;11:4552) did a 10-year study in China of 508 patients with portal hypertension who were treated with a mélange of different approaches, including porta-azygous devascularization, porta-systemic shunt, distal splenorenal shunt, combined portasystemic shunt and porta-azygous devascularization, and liver transplantation. The operative mortality was 5.91%. The remainder of the article looked at outcomes in smaller and smaller numbers of different operations.

Distal splenorenal shunt with splenopancreatic and gastric disconnection in patients with idiopathic portal hypertension was reported by Hase et al. (*World J Surg* 2005;29:1034). Fifteen patients had idiopathic portal hypertension, which is an interesting disease. One patient died within 3 years of surgery, yielding a 3-year survival rate of 93%. The 10-year survival rate was 64%. The cause of this condition is not known. Several article many years ago suggested that catecholamines originating from somewhere in the portal circulation was responsible for this condition, but this has never been proven.

Finally, Shah and Robbani (*Tex Heart Inst J* 2005;32:549) proposed a simplified technique of performing splenorenal shunt. In reading this article, the technique looks exactly like the one I used and that Dr. Linton used, and may be found in his excellent atlas. It does involve getting around the back of the pancreas and lifting it up in order to make it accessible. I agree entirely with this technique, and believe it is a standard technique that people have always used.

                                                                    J.E.F.

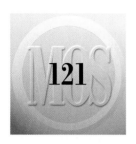

Endoscopic Therapy in the Management of Esophageal Varices: Injection Sclerotherapy and Variceal Ligation

JAKE E.J. KRIGE AND PHILIPPUS C. BORNMAN

PORTAL HYPERTENSION

An increase in portal vein pressure over 12 mm Hg (normal 5–10 mm Hg) causes portal hypertension with resultant compensatory portosystemic venous collateral formation, increased splanchnic blood flow, and disturbed intrahepatic circulation. These factors cause the important complications of chronic liver disease, which include variceal bleeding, hepatic encephalopathy, ascites, hepatorenal syndrome, recurrent infection, and coagulopathy. Esophagogastric varices are part of the collateral venous system that diverts high-pressure portal blood via the coronary, short gastric, and esophageal perforator veins to the azygous system. These varices are the major source of hemorrhage and mortality, although bleeding from congestive gastropathy and anorectal varices also occurs. Epigastric and abdominal wall collateral vessels may enlarge with recanalization of the umbilical vein, and multiple retroperitoneal collaterals may form, which complicate surgical intervention. Splenomegaly and hypersplenism develop with impeded splenic vein outflow.

Cause

Two mechanisms lead to portal hypertension: (a) increased portal resistance and (b) increased portal flow. Increased resistance to flow is classified as presinusoidal, sinusoidal, and postsinusoidal (Table 1). Increased flow is caused by either an arteriovenous fistula or increased splenic arterial flow. Portal hypertension has a wide variety of causes and geographic prevalences; while cirrhosis dominates in the Western world, schistosomiasis is most common overall.

Natural History

Rational management of esophageal varices depends on a clear understanding of the risks of bleeding and rebleeding and the response to therapy. One third of compensated cirrhotics have varices on diagnosis. Bleeding risk can be predicted by (a) large varices, (b) portal pressures over 12 mm Hg, and (c) advanced liver disease. Thirty percent of patients with varices will bleed, and of these, one quarter die as a consequence of the bleeding. There is a 70% chance of subsequent rebleeding with a similar mortality.

Careful assessment of hepatic functional reserve is necessary before selecting the appropriate treatment. Dynamic tests of hepatocellular function (aminopyrine breath test, galactose elimination capacity, or hepatic amino acid clearance) have been used, but the Child classification is the most useful and practical predictor of survival

(Table 2). The operative mortality for Child grade A patients is less than 5%, while for Child grade C mortality is over 25%.

In Western countries, variceal bleeding accounts for 7% of all upper gastrointestinal bleeding, although this varies geographically (11% in the United States, 5% in the United Kingdom), depending on the prevalence of alcoholic liver disease.

MANAGEMENT OF ACUTE VARICEAL BLEEDING

Choice of Therapy

The possibility of variceal bleeding should be considered in all patients who present with upper gastrointestinal bleeding and have known risk factors for chronic liver disease or clinical evidence of portal hypertension. The modern management of acute variceal bleeding requires a variety of therapeutic options to be available that may have to be used either sequentially or combined in an individual patient (Table 3). Several important considerations influence the choice of therapy as well as the prognosis in individual patients. These include the natural history of the disease causing the portal hypertension, the location of the bleeding varices, residual hepatic function, the presence of associated systemic disease, continuing drug or alcohol abuse, patency of major splanchnic veins, and the response to each specific treatment.

TABLE 1. CAUSES OF PORTAL HYPERTENSION

1. Increased resistance to blood flow
   a. Presinusoidal
      (i) Extrahepatic
         Portal vein thrombosis
         Splenic vein thrombosis
      (ii) Intrahepatic
         Schistosomiasis
         Sarcoidosis
   b. Sinusoidal
      Cirrhosis
      Hemochromatosis
      Wilson's disease
      Congenital hepatic fibrosis
   c. Postsinusoidal
      Budd-Chiari syndrome
      Congestive heart failure
      Veno-occlusive disease
2. Increased portal blood flow
   Increased splenic blood flow
   Arterial-portal venous fistula

TABLE 2. THE CHILD CLASSIFICATION OF FUNCTIONAL LIVER STATUS

	Number of Points		
	1	**2**	**3**
Bilirubin (μmol/L)	<34	34–51	>51
Albumin (g/L)	>35	28–35	<28
Prothrombin time	<3	3–10	>10
Ascites	None	Mild	Moderate to severe
Encephalopathy	None	Mild	Moderate to severe

Grade A: 5–6 points
Grade B: 7–9 points
Grade C: 10–15 points

The Gastrointestinal Tract

TABLE 3. MANAGEMENT OF ACUTE VARICEAL BLEEDING

Treatment Options
1. Pharmacologic agents
   a. Somatostatin
   b. Glypressin
   c. Octreotide
   d. Vasopressin and nitroglycerine
2. Endoscopic therapy
   a. Band ligation
   b. Injection sclerotherapy
      i. Sclerosants
      ii. Cyanoacrylate ("superglue")
      iii. Thrombin
3. Balloon tamponade
4. TIPS
5. Surgery
   a. Shunt procedures
   b. Esophageal transection

TIPS, transjugular intrahepatic portosystemic shunt.

General Strategy

All patients with suspected acute variceal bleeding require hospitalization. The immediate aims of emergency treatment involve hemodynamic stabilization, blood-volume replacement, control of bleeding, support of vital organ function, and prevention of complications due to hypovolemic shock and impending liver failure. Patients should be nursed in an intensive or high care unit whenever possible, and standard resuscitation for major hemorrhage instituted. Although variceal bleeding stops spontaneously in 60% of patients, it is not possible to predict which patients will continue to bleed and require further specific emergency therapy. Patients should preferably be transferred to a center with appropriate facilities and expertise as soon as they have been adequately resuscitated and are stable, because subsequent management is difficult if bleeding continues or recurs and may require advanced multidisciplinary investigations and therapy. A suggested management algorithm is shown in Figure 1.

Initial Measures

Many patients with acute variceal hemorrhage have liver decompensation with encephalopathy, ascites, coagulopathy, bacteremia, and malnutrition. The extent and urgency of initial therapy depend on the severity of bleeding. Stable patients with intermittent bleeding are candidates for endoscopic therapy, whereas the occasional patient with exsanguinating bleeding may require balloon tamponade to control bleeding before endoscopy is performed.

Maintenance of a secure airway and prompt resuscitation with restoration of circulating blood volume are vital and precede any diagnostic studies. Intravenous access is obtained via a central venous cannula. While blood is being cross-matched, crystalloid solution is rapidly infused until the blood pressure is restored and the urine output, measured with a Foley catheter, is adequate. Infusions of saline may aggravate ascites and must be avoided. Overzealous expansion of circulating blood volume may precipitate further bleeding. Central venous pressure should be maintained at no greater than 2 to 5 cm H_2O, measured from the sternal angle. Patients who are hemodynamically unstable, who are elderly, or who have concomitant cardiac or pulmonary disease should be monitored using a pulmonary artery catheter because injudicious administration of crystalloids, combined with vasoactive drugs, may lead to the rapid onset of edema, ascites, and hyponatremia. Clotting factors are often deficient and fresh blood, fresh frozen plasma, and vitamin K_1 are frequently required. Platelet transfusions may be necessary. Sedatives should be avoided.

Pharmacologic Therapy

Although vasoactive drugs aimed at controlling variceal bleeding have been used for decades, their efficacy remains controversial. Previously, a continuous intravenous infusion of vasopressin at 0.4 units per minute, combined with glyceryl trinitrate given as a sublingual tablet or applied as a skin patch, was used. Vasopressin is seldom used today because newer agents are superior. Glypressin (terlipressin), the synthetic analog of vasopressin, has the advantage of being effective in 2-mg intravenous bolus doses administered every 4 to 6 hours and is simpler to administer. Early administration of Glypressin in a French study showed improved survival.

The most widely used agent is somatostatin, which does not cause systemic vasoconstriction like vasopressin, but reduces splanchnic and hepatic blood flow. Somatostatin is administered as a continuous intravenous infusion of 250 μg/hr. An initial bolus dose of 250 μg is administered and additional bolus doses are given if bleeding continues. Somatostatin appears to be more effective than its synthetic analog, octreotide.

Most endoscopy units recommend that pharmacologic therapy be commenced when a diagnosis of variceal bleeding is suspected and before emergency endoscopy is performed. This policy has the theoretical advantage of controlling bleeding before the initial endoscopy, which should make both diagnosis and immediate endoscopic therapy easier.

Emergency Endoscopy and Immediate Endoscopic Therapy

Emergency diagnostic endoscopy is mandatory to confirm that a patient is bleeding from esophageal varices. Patients with varices can usually be separated into three groups: those with active variceal bleeding, those with variceal bleeding that has stopped, and those who have varices but are bleeding from another lesion. These other lesions should be treated appropriately.

Emergency endoscopy should be performed in the endoscopy unit where all the necessary equipment is available. Many units have a fully equipped emergency endoscopy trolley that, if necessary, can be taken into the operating room or the intensive care unit. It is imperative that full resuscitative facilities are available together with skilled staff experienced in dealing with emergencies. Two endoscopy assistants should be present throughout, and adequate monitoring is necessary during the procedure. Emergency endoscopy should not commence until satisfactory venous access and central venous pressure measurement are established and volume replacement and resuscitation procedures with blood transfusions are initiated to correct hypovolemia. If bleeding is profuse or if the patient is stuporous, endotracheal intubation is essential before endoscopy to protect the airway and avoid aspiration.

Patients who have endoscopically proven active variceal bleeding or in whom variceal bleeding has stopped should have immediate endoscopic sclerotherapy or variceal ligation (Fig. 1). If sclerotherapy or variceal ligation is deferred until the next elective endoscopy list in patients who have stopped bleeding, there is a distinct danger of further major acute variceal bleeding during the interval period, with substantial morbidity and mortality. If acute or recurrent major variceal bleeding continues despite endoscopic and pharmacologic therapy, mechanical control by balloon tamponade is required.

Failure of Emergency Endoscopic Therapy

Endoscopic therapy is successful in controlling acute variceal bleeding in over

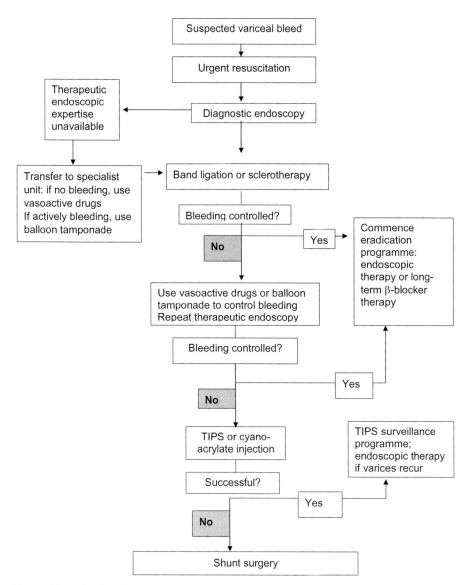

Fig. 1. Algorithm for the management of acute variceal bleeding. TIPS, transjugular intrahepatic portosystemic shunt.

90% of patients after one or two treatment sessions. Current evidence suggests that variceal ligation is as effective as sclerotherapy. Any patient who rebleeds after two successive emergency endoscopy treatments during a single hospital admission has a prohibitively high mortality if endoscopic therapy is pursued. Such patients should have a balloon tube inserted, be resuscitated, and then be treated by an alternative technique. A transjugular intrahepatic portosystemic shunt (TIPS) stent is recommended for patients who continue to bleed despite two endoscopic band or sclerotherapy sessions. In patients being considered for liver transplantation, a TIPS stent is the preferred treatment to provide a bridge to transplantation.

Balloon Tube Tamponade

Acute variceal bleeding can be temporarily controlled by a correctly placed balloon tube (Fig. 2). If the patient continues to bleed after a balloon tube has been inserted and the balloon is correctly positioned, a further emergency endoscopy is required. This endoscopy usually reveals another bleeding lesion that was overlooked or obscured by blood during the first diagnostic endoscopy.

The balloon tube should always be inserted by an expert. The technical details are presented later. The tube should be left in situ for as short a time as possible while the patient is being resuscitated and preparations are made for endoscopic treatment by an experienced endoscopist.

A balloon tube is used when emergency endoscopic therapy cannot be successfully performed because visibility is obscured by major variceal bleeding, or when patients have continued active variceal bleeding despite attempted control by emergency endoscopic therapy. Balloon tube tamponade is also used to control a subsequent massive variceal bleed or tide a patient over while preparing for alternative therapy when endoscopic therapy is considered to have failed (i.e., a further major acute variceal bleed occurs after two apparently successful emergency endoscopic treatments during a single hospital admission).

Alternative Emergency Management Options

The main secondary alternatives to primary pharmacologic and endoscopic therapy for acute variceal bleeding are TIPS stenting, portosystemic shunts, esophageal transection operations, and hepatic transplantation. In patients with recurrent bleeding it is crucial to identify the cause and site of bleeding, because the management of injection-induced esophageal ulceration, recurrent variceal bleeding, gastric varices, and portal hypertensive gastropathy differs.

A TIPS shunt is the emergency procedure of choice in patients with failed endoscopic therapy. Recent data confirm the utility and efficacy of TIPS shunts as a salvage procedure for refractory variceal bleeding unresponsive to endoscopic and pharmacologic treatment. Immediate control of variceal bleeding is achieved in over 90% of patients. However, TIPS in uncontrolled variceal bleeding still has a high mortality. Prognosis is poor if patients have developed sepsis or require inotropic support and ventilation and have deteriorating liver and renal function. Established renal failure in a decompensated cirrhotic patient with uncontrolled bleeding is a contraindication to TIPS placement in most units.

The need for emergency surgical shunts to control acute variceal bleeding has diminished dramatically in the past decade because of the improved efficacy of pharmacologic, endoscopic, and radiologic treatment. While a successful surgical shunt effectively stops acute variceal bleeding and prevents recurrent bleeds, the role of emergency shunting procedures is currently restricted to patients who have failed endoscopic therapy and cannot be salvaged by a TIPS stent for technical reasons. Emergency shunt surgery has an operative mortality of 25%, which is largely determined by the degree of liver decompensation.

The Gastrointestinal Tract

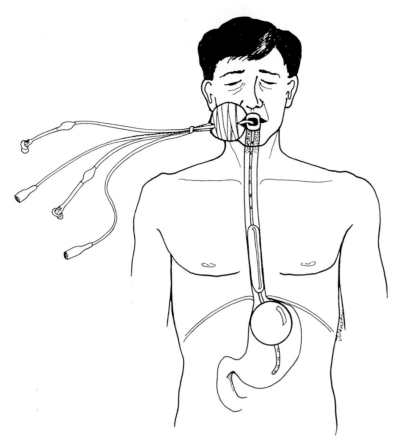

Fig. 2. Four-lumen balloon tube. The gastric balloon, which is filled with air, is held firmly against the esophagogastric junction by fixing a split tennis ball to the tube at the patient's mouth.

A variety of devascularization and transection operations that disconnect the high-pressure portal system from the esophageal varices have been devised. As a basic principle, the most simple procedure should be used. Simple esophageal transection using a staple gun is the preferred procedure for patients in whom endoscopic therapy has failed and TIPS or an operative shunt is not feasible. Previous sclerotherapy may increase the difficulty and risk of performing the operation due to sclerosant-induced ulceration and periesophageal fibrosis. Esophageal transection combined with an extensive esophageal and gastric devascularization procedure is not justified in the emergency setting. Four trials have compared sclerotherapy with esophageal transection and one with portacaval shunt after failure of medical treatment. Failure to control bleeding was higher with sclerotherapy, and rebleeding, assessed in three trials, was significantly higher with injection sclerotherapy. No significant differences in mortality were found.

Emergency liver transplantation has been advocated but, in our view, is best performed after initial control of the variceal hemorrhage, preferably using an endoscopic technique, as this will interfere least with a subsequent transplant. For the failures of endoscopic therapy in potential transplant recipients, TIPS is used as a bridge to transplantation.

Patients with end-stage liver disease who are not candidates for liver transplantation and who do not respond to initial standard emergency therapy should be seriously considered for expectant treatment only. This poses difficult moral and ethical issues but must be a realistic option today.

LONG-TERM MANAGEMENT AFTER VARICEAL BLEEDING

Once the acute bleeding episode has been controlled and the patient is stabilized, a detailed evaluation is undertaken to identify the cause of the portal hypertension, the severity of any underlying liver disease, and the likely natural history and the location and extent of bleeding varices.

Although the chances of a recurrent variceal bleed diminish with time, up to 70% of patients will have further variceal bleeding. For this reason, all patients who have had a variceal bleed should be con-

sidered for long-term management aimed at preventing further variceal bleeds. Endoscopic therapy is the primary treatment of choice. The options and second-line alternatives are summarized in Table 4 and are detailed below.

Injection Sclerotherapy

In the past, injection sclerotherapy was the most widely used endoscopic treatment. Sclerotherapy has now been replaced by endoscopic variceal ligation as first-line endoscopic therapy. Sclerotherapy, when used, is performed using a video endoscope and a freehand injection technique without an oversheath. Unlike most other forms of therapy used in the management of esophageal varices, sclerotherapy techniques are not standardized. The injections may be placed directly into the varices ("intravariceal") with the objective of thrombosing the varices, or into the submucosa adjacent to the varices ("paravariceal") to produce submucosal edema to stop acute variceal bleeding and to cause thickening of the mucosa, which prevents later bleeding. Many endoscopists use a combination of these two techniques (Fig. 3).

Sclerotherapy Technique

Sclerotherapy is performed with different levels of skill and in protocols using variable frequencies of injections and endoscopic review. It is, therefore, not surprising

---

TABLE 4. LONG-TERM MANAGEMENT TO PREVENT VARICEAL REBLEEDING

Treatment Options
1. Endoscopic therapy
   a. Variceal band ligation
   b. Injection sclerotherapy
2. Pharmacotherapy
   a. Beta-blockers
   b. Other drugs
3. Surgery
   a. Shunt
      i. DSRS
      ii. Portocaval
   b. Nonshunt
      i. Esophageal transection and esophagogastric devascularization
      ii. Splenectomy for gastric varices due to splenic vein thrombosis
4. TIPS
5. Liver transplantation

DSRS, distal splenorenal shunt; TIPS, transjugular intrahepatic portosystemic shunt.

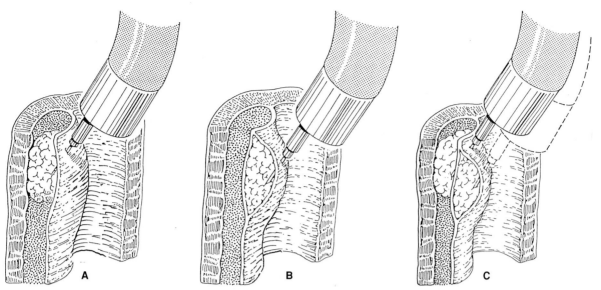

Fig. 3. Technical variants of injection sclerotherapy. **A:** Intravariceal injection. **B:** Paravariceal or submucosal injection. **C:** Combined intravariceal and paravariceal injections.

that controlled trials comparing sclerotherapy with other specific therapies, including variceal ligation, have yielded conflicting results. We prefer a combined para- and intravariceal technique for the management of acute variceal bleeding and utilize a predominantly intravariceal technique for long-term management when varices are smaller. Our sclerosant of choice is ethanolamine oleate 5%. Injection treatments are continued at weekly intervals until the varices have been eradicated. Thereafter, the patient is first assessed at 3 months and then at 6 month and subsequently at yearly intervals. Whenever recurrent varices are diagnosed, a repeat course of weekly sclerotherapy is undertaken until re-eradication is achieved.

Esophageal Variceal Ligation

The concept of endoscopic variceal ligation or banding is similar to the technique used for treating hemorrhoids, and was devised by Stiegmann of Denver. The use of endoscopic band ligation represents a seminal development in the endoscopic treatment of varices. Hemostasis is achieved by physical constriction of the varix by the rubber band. Ischemic necrosis of the strangulated mucosa and submucosa trapped within the band occurs, followed by sloughing of the banded varix. The resulting shallow mucosal ulcer re-epithelializes over the next 14 to 21 days, with replacement of the varix by maturing scar tissue. Two different types of ligating devices are used. The original Stiegmann apparatus allows the placement of one band at a time and requires the use

of an overtube to allow multiple withdrawals and reinsertions of the endoscope. The newer multiband apparatus allows the placement of eight to ten bands during a single insertion of the endoscope, obviating the need for an overtube. The band ligation procedure is repeated at weekly intervals until all the varices are obliterated.

Endoscopic variceal ligation has been shown to be as effective as injection sclerotherapy in the emergency management of bleeding esophageal varices. Variceal eradication using ligation requires fewer endoscopic treatment sessions, and causes substantially less local esophageal complications. Current data demonstrate a clear advantage for ligation in preference to sclerotherapy. Ligation should therefore be regarded as the endoscopic treatment of choice in the management of esophageal varices.

ALTERNATIVE LONG-TERM MANAGEMENT OPTIONS

Although we prefer endoscopic therapy as the primary therapy for most patients, pharmacologic therapy with propranolol alone or combined with nitrates is an acceptable alternative primary long-term therapy in selected patients. Operative shunts, particularly the distal splenorenal shunt, also have a role in good-risk Child A or B patients.

Pharmacologic Therapy

The use of beta-blockers as primary long-term therapy has considerable support in the current literature. Several meta-analy-

ses have concluded that beta-blockers, principally propanolol, significantly reduce the incidence of recurrent bleeding and improve long-term survival when compared with placebo. Unfortunately, beta-blockade is not without its drawbacks. There are a large number of relative contraindications to beta-blockade, including bronchial asthma, chronic obstructive pulmonary disease, peripheral vascular disease, congestive cardiac failure, and unstable insulin-dependent diabetes mellitus. Once treatment is initiated, beta-blocker–induced side effects may be a problem. The most common side effects are loss of energy, depression, impotence, and headaches. In a minority of patients, these side effects may be sufficiently severe to cause discontinuation of treatment. Thus, a significant proportion of the population at risk may not be suitable for treatment with beta-blockers or stop taking the drug as a result of side effects. In addition, one third of patients treated with standard doses of beta-blockers do not have a significant reduction in portal venous pressure.

Where patient compliance is reliable, long-term propranolol therapy is an alternative option to endoscopic management of varices. If patients have a recurrent bleed while on adequate propranolol therapy, alternative treatment, particularly endoscopic therapy, should be instituted. The risk of side effects has led to the evaluation of other drugs to reduce portal hypertension. The other main group of drugs is nitrates, with isosorbide-5-mononitrate being increasingly used in clinical practice. Other oral medications such as α_2-agonists (e.g., clonidine), calcium channel antagonists (e.g., verapamil), and serotonin antagonists (e.g., ketanserin) have been evaluated in studies but have not gained wide clinical acceptance.

Surgical Shunts

Portosystemic shunts are classified as (a) nonselective, (b) selective, or (c) partial. Successful nonselective end-to-side or side-to-side portacaval shunts effectively control acute variceal bleeding and prevent recurrent bleeding and were the "gold standard" with which other forms of therapy were compared in the past. Portacaval shunts are, however, a major operation in poor-risk patients and are associated with severe and unpredictable side effects—particularly encephalopathy and deteriorating liver function.

The most popular selective shunt for long-term management is the distal splenorenal shunt (DSRS). A DSRS should be considered for patients who do not have readily available tertiary care, including repeated endoscopic therapy, or who are unlikely to be compliant with follow-up. This shunt has the theoretical advantage of selectively shunting left upper quadrant portal venous blood away from the esophagogastric varices, while preserving superior mesenteric blood flow to the liver. Although prograde flow tends to diminish with time, this shunt has a lower encephalopathy rate than standard portacaval shunts. The DSRS remains the shunt of choice for patients who have recurrent variceal bleeding despite pharmacologic and endoscopic treatment and are good surgical candidates with preservation of liver function. The narrow-diameter polytetrafluoroethylene (PTFE) H-graft partial shunt is an effective alternative to the distal splenorenal shunt.

Devascularization and Transection Operations

Although simple esophageal transection was previously used in the management of acute variceal bleeding, a more extensive gastric and esophageal devascularization with transection of the lower esophagus has been used in some centers for long-term management. These major procedures are particularly popular in Japan. Controlled trials have shown that although this procedure is as effective as repeated endoscopic therapy, long-term endoscopic therapy is simpler and much less costly. Devascularization and transection proce-

dures are generally reserved for patients with recurrent variceal bleeding despite endoscopic and pharmacologic treatment who are not candidates for TIPS and have vasculature unsuitable for shunt operations.

Transjugular Intrahepatic Portosystemic Shunt

Until recently, major surgery was the only method of creating a portosystemic shunt. TIPS is a nonoperative interventional radiologic stent that can be inserted under local anesthesia. In principle, a catheter is inserted into a hepatic vein via the jugular vein. A rigid needle is inserted through the catheter and passed from the hepatic vein through a bridge of liver tissue into a major portal vein branch. This is followed by placement of a guidewire and withdrawal of the needle. The tract within the liver tissue is dilated using a 10-mm angioplasty balloon catheter and the communication between the hepatic vein and the portal vein is held open with an expandable metal stent, usually a Palmaz or Wallstent (Fig. 4).

The major advantage of TIPS stenting is its use in treating the failures of endoscopic therapy in patients with acute variceal bleeding. The procedure can be performed with low morbidity by an expert interventional radiologist, even in poor-risk patients. TIPS is also an ideal bridge to liver transplantation in patients with acute variceal bleeding.

Disadvantages of the TIPS procedure include the cost (each Wallstent costs

more than $1,000), particularly when more than one procedure is required. Another disadvantage is that with time, the encephalopathy rate increases to a level similar to the rate that occurs after standard portacaval shunts. The most significant problem has been narrowing and occlusion of these shunts within 1 to 2 years. The incidence of occlusion at 1 year is approximately 50%.

Liver Transplantation

Liver transplantation is the only treatment that both cures the underlying liver disease and eradicates the portal hypertension. All patients presenting with variceal bleeding and significant liver decompensation should be considered for hepatic transplantation, even though only a small percentage of patients will ultimately become transplant candidates.

In potential transplant candidates with acute variceal bleeding, emergency endoscopic therapy is considered the treatment of choice. If endoscopic therapy fails to control active variceal bleeding and if a donor liver is not immediately available, an emergency TIPS procedure should be performed as a salvage procedure to control bleeding before transplantation. Once the patient has recovered from the acute variceal bleed, early transplantation should be performed if further evaluation confirms that the patient is a suitable liver transplant candidate. Patients with good liver function should be considered for a distal splenorenal shunt and not a transplant.

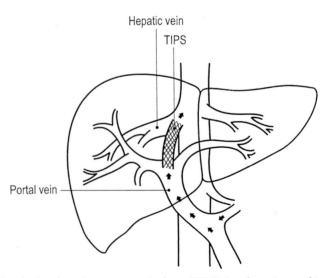

Fig. 4. Transjugular intrahepatic portosystemic shunt (TIPS). A catheter is passed into the hepatic vein via the jugular vein. A needle, inserted through the catheter, is passed from the hepatic vein through liver tissue into a major portal vein branch. This is followed by the placement of a guidewire and withdrawal of the needle. The liver tract is dilated with an angioplasty balloon catheter and the tract is kept open after deployment of an expandable metal stent.

No Therapy: Observation Only

Patients with end-stage liver disease who present with major esophageal variceal bleeding complicated by multiorgan failure and who are not candidates for liver transplantation should not be subjected to major emergency procedures without careful evaluation. Withholding treatment in these circumstances is a difficult clinical and ethical decision but one that must be considered in today's cost-conscious medical environment.

TECHNIQUE OF BALLOON TUBE INSERTION

Acute esophageal variceal bleeding can be temporarily controlled in most patients by a correctly placed balloon tube (Fig. 2). The four-lumen Minnesota tube is the most widely used balloon tube; control of bleeding allows time for resuscitation and planning for management. Although the initial bleeding episode is effectively controlled, if no additional measures are used, 60% of patients will rebleed after removal of the tube with a high associated mortality rate. Either variceal ligation or injection sclerotherapy is performed when the tube is removed.

Before a balloon tube is inserted in a stuporous or comatose patient, the airway should be protected by placing an endotracheal tube to prevent aspiration. A new tube should always be used, and the balloons should be tested by inflating them under water to confirm a complete air seal. The deflated lubricated balloon tube is passed through a bite-guard via the mouth, after adequate topical pharyngeal anesthesia. Awake patients are instructed to swallow while the tube is being passed. In a stuporous patient, placing the index finger within the mouth assists in guiding the tip of the tube over the posterior tongue and through the cricopharyngeus, thereby preventing coiling of the tube in the pharynx. At times it may be difficult to negotiate the tube through the cricopharyngeus, particularly in patients with an endotracheal tube in place. Under these circumstances, a McGill forceps and laryngoscope are used, and the tube is passed under direct vision. The tube is inserted as far as possible.

The position of the balloon in the stomach is confirmed by injecting air into the aspirating lumen of the gastric tube using a 50-mL syringe and auscultating over the epigastrium, while instilling air. Thereafter, the gastric balloon is cautiously inflated with 50-mL increments of air until a total of 250 mL has been inserted. The air should be easy to inject; if the tube is curled in the esophagus, resistance is felt and inflation must be stopped immediately and the balloon deflated, or the esophagus may be ruptured. Water and oily contrast media are contraindicated because they are difficult to inject via the narrow lumen of the tube and, even more important, are difficult to aspirate before the tube is removed. The tube is then pulled up until the inflated gastric balloon is positioned firmly against the esophagogastric junction.

The tube is held in place by a split tennis ball that is strapped to the tube adjacent to the mouthguard. The central portion of the tube is therefore made taut between the gastric balloon below and the tennis ball at the mouth above. This has proven to be the most effective method of maintaining tamponade at the esophagogastric junction. Adequate tension on the gastric balloon can be checked regularly at the mouth. The mouthguard helps to protect the patient's lips from the pressure of the tennis ball. Inflation of the esophageal balloon is not usually necessary as traction on the gastric balloon is generally sufficient. If esophageal balloon inflation is used, this is achieved by a three-way tap and a blood pressure manometer. The esophageal balloon is inflated to 40 mm Hg and the tube clamped. This pressure should be checked regularly. The third lumen, which opens in the esophagus, is placed on constant suction to keep the esophagus clear of saliva. The gastric lumen is used for either suction or administering medication, such as lactulose.

Patients with a balloon tube in place should be monitored carefully in an intensive care unit to avoid complications. The position of the gastric balloon must be checked by a flat roentgenogram of the abdomen, which will confirm the siting of the air-filled gastric balloon in the stomach. Once the balloon tube has been inserted and fixed and bleeding has been arrested, resuscitation is continued, clotting defects are corrected, and the patient is made as fit as possible for the necessary subsequent management. The balloon tube should be removed after 6 to 12 hours, with a maximum time of 24 hours and either variceal ligation or injection sclerotherapy performed.

If bleeding persists after insertion of the tube, the tube should be checked by a senior staff member, and if found to be correctly sited, a further diagnostic endoscopy is required. A nonvariceal bleeding source, missed during the initial endoscopy, is usually found.

INJECTION SCLEROTHERAPY TECHNIQUES

Trained assistants are essential and adequate resuscitative facilities must be available. A flexible video endoscope is used without general anesthesia.

Technical Variants

Three basic techniques are used (Fig. 3). The aim of direct intravariceal injection (Fig. 3A) is to thrombose the varices, thereby preventing recurrent hemorrhage. Paravariceal or submucosal injection (Fig. 3B) produces submucosal edema, which stops acute bleeding by compression and later causes mucosal thickening, thereby preventing recurrent bleeding. Combined paravariceal and intravariceal techniques have been proposed in the hope of combining the advantages of both techniques. The combined technique is depicted in Figure 3C. A double-channel endoscope is preferred and either an end-viewing or side-viewing instrument can be used. The end-viewing endoscope is more versatile for both diagnosis and therapy, although the oblique-viewing endoscope has the advantage of the built-in forceps elevator, which helps in aiming the injector, particularly for small varices during subsequent elective sclerotherapy.

In obtunded patients, the airway must be protected by prior endotracheal intubation. If the patient has a balloon tube in place, the balloons should only be deflated and the tube either removed or pushed further inward when the team is ready to begin endoscopy and sclerotherapy. Once the varix that was bleeding has been controlled, the remaining varices are injected and the diagnostic endoscopy completed.

Several sclerotherapy injectors with retractable needles are commercially available and are preferable to the flexible, reusable, metal injectors. Injectors have either a 23- or 25-gauge needle attached. The larger needle is preferred because it facilitates injection of the viscous sclerosant solution.

Sclerosants

There is a wide variety of sclerosant agents available with different mechanisms of action and varying complication rates. The most common sclerosants are ethanolamine oleate 5%, sodium morrhuate 2% to 5%, and sodium tetradecyl sulfate in varying concentrations. These agents have been mainly used for intravariceal injections, although ethanolamine oleate is also used in the combined technique. Polidocanol (1%

The Gastrointestinal Tract

to 3% concentration) has mainly been used by endoscopists in Europe for a predominantly paravariceal or a combination technique. The best sclerosant and the best route of administration have yet to be defined, although the few controlled trials available tend to favor ethanolamine oleate for intravariceal or combined injection therapy.

Tissue Adhesives

Two types of cyanoacrylate tissue adhesives, Histoacryl and bucrylate, have been used to treat variceal bleeding. These have proved effective in the control of acute bleeding with a success rate of more than 90% with a single injection. The cyanoacrylate hardens within 20 seconds when activated by water and more rapidly on contact with blood. Thus, the tissue adhesives potentially offer immediate control of bleeding. Their administration, via an endoscope, utilizes a similar technique to traditional sclerosant injection but with slight modifications. There are serious risks of equipment damage by tissue adhesives in inexperienced hands. Care must be taken to ensure that the adhesive does not come into contact with the endoscope and block the channels of the instrument. This can be minimized by the application of silicone oil to the tip of the instrument and by mixing the adhesive with lipiodol to delay premature hardening. A further precaution is to ensure that the endoscope needle is correctly placed within the varix before injection. When the needle is in position, the tissue adhesive is injected in 0.5- to 1-mL aliquots; if the adhesive leaks, the endoscope should be immediately withdrawn and cleaned before the polymer can set.

Thrombin

In initial studies, control of variceal bleeding has also been achieved using either human or bovine thrombin (as components of a thrombogenic cocktail) to thrombose the bleeding varices. Thrombin injection is technically easy to perform, utilizing the same freehand injection technique as for sclerotherapy, without the technical difficulties associated with the use of tissue adhesives. Uncontrolled trials have shown that thrombin is equally effective in controlling bleeding from either esophageal or gastric varices.

Elective Sclerotherapy Technique

Elective sclerotherapy is performed in an outpatient clinic with two assistants trained in endoscopy techniques. One assistant

reassures the patient, provides suction of the patient's mouth to avoid aspiration, and ensures that the bite-guard is not dislodged. The other assistant, usually a trained nurse, advances and retracts the injector needle and administers the sclerosant under the direction of the endoscopist.

The patient is placed in the left lateral decubitus position at the top of the endoscopy bed, with the head on a pillow and the neck slightly flexed. The pharynx and posterior tongue are anesthetized with 10% Xylocaine spray. A small butterfly needle is inserted into a superficial hand vein for administration of sedation. We usually administer small incremental doses of midazolam (2.5 mg). All the instruments, including the endoscope, are checked before use, and commands such as "advance needle" and "retract needle" are rehearsed, if an inexperienced assistant is present. Each time an injection is required, this is called for by the endoscopist and acknowledged by the assistant. The assistant is instructed to comment if resistance is encountered during injection, because resistance may indicate that the varix is thrombosed or that the needle is not correctly positioned.

The endoscope is inserted through the mouthguard, and the moderately flexed tip is passed over the tongue. The tip is extended in the upper pharynx. The opening of the cricopharynx is identified and negotiated, with gentle pressure coinciding with a swallow. The endoscope is then passed under direct vision, keeping the lumen of the esophagus in view while controlling the position of the endoscope tip. Small amounts of air are insufflated intermittently to maintain sufficient distension of the lumen for visibility. Mucus and fluid are removed through the suction channel, and the lens cleared with a water jet whenever necessary. The complete esophagus is examined and the presence of esophageal varices noted and documented, including their number, size, and extent. In the elective setting, bleeding will usually not be present and a full diagnostic panendoscopy is performed first to exclude other lesions, before commencing injection of varices. Once the stomach is reached, the tip of the endoscope is passed distally under vision, insufflating enough air to display the lumen ahead. Once the pylorus is in view, air is insufflated to distend the distal stomach and relax the pylorus. As this occurs, the tip is gently advanced into the duodenum, which is carefully evaluated. The endoscope is then withdrawn into the stomach and the cardia, gastric fundus, and upper portion of the lesser curve are viewed by retroflexion

of the tip of the endoscope within a moderately gas-distended stomach. The presence, extent, and size of gastric varices and the degree of portal hypertensive gastropathy are noted and documented.

Once the full panendoscopy has been completed, the endoscope is withdrawn into the esophagus and positioned above the esophagogastric junction so that the varices in the lower 5 cm of the esophagus can be injected. The endoscope is maneuvered into position, and the target varix is identified. The endoscopist then passes the injector through the biopsy channel into the field of view and the tip is positioned 2 cm beyond the end of the endoscope. To prevent the needle damaging the injector sheath, the injector should only be passed when the endoscope tip is in a nonflexed position. The needle must remain in the retracted position until the tip of the injector has passed through the endoscope and is visible to the endoscopist. All movements and manipulation of the injector must be performed only by the endoscopist. A practice-aiming pass of the injector, with the needle retracted within the sheath, is useful to determine the direction that the advancing needle will take. The assistant advances the needle on instruction, and a small volume of sclerosant solution is discarded into the lumen of the esophagus to ensure that the injector is filled. The endoscopist inserts the needle directly into the center of the most prominent part of the varix, near the esophagogastric junction, by advancing the injector a further 5 to 10 mm. Once the needle has been satisfactorily placed within the lumen of the varix, the assistant is instructed to inject 1 mL of sclerosant (Fig. 5). If this is achieved without resistance, further sclerosant is injected under instruction. The varix should be seen to distend above and below the injection site and become a paler color. At this time the injection should be stopped. A total of no more than 5 mL of ethanolamine oleate is usually required for a large varix. Smaller varices usually require less sclerosant. Thereafter, any additional varices are injected at the same level. A second injection is placed 2 to 3 cm higher in large varices. Usually, only 2 to 3 mL of sclerosant are injected into the upper site. Smaller varices are only injected at the lower site.

The injection needle must be placed accurately into the varix. Only the needle should enter the varix. If the angle is too acute, the injection may penetrate the back wall of the varix and pass into the esophageal wall, which potentially gives rise to serious complications, rather than

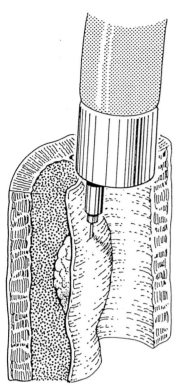

Fig. 5. Intravariceal injection technique. After an initial test injection of 1 mL of sclerosant, up to 5 mL of ethanolamine oleate is injected directly into the varix immediately above the esophagogastric junction.

life. If recurrent varices are noted at any time, repeat endoscopy and injections are performed at weekly intervals until the varices have again been eradicated.

Emergency Sclerotherapy

The initial resuscitative measures required have been presented earlier. The patient should be in as stable a condition as possible before commencing sclerotherapy. The procedure is performed in a fully equipped endoscopy suite. If the patient is stuporous or comatose, an endotracheal tube will have been inserted. Severely ill patients should have the injection treatment performed in the intensive care unit or, when active bleeding is present, the patient should be taken to the operating room and placed on a tilting operating table.

The patient is placed in the left lateral decubitus position, as for elective sclerotherapy. However, if active bleeding is present, the patient is placed on his or her back on an operating table and the table head is elevated to between 30 and 45 degrees to improve visualization. The lower esophagus is vigorously flushed with saline and active suction is used, which usually permits adequate visualization to perform the first injection.

Intravariceal Injection

An intravariceal injection technique similar to that described for elective sclerotherapy can be used (Fig. 6). However, some endoscopists prefer the combined paravariceal and intravariceal injection technique described below for patients with active variceal bleeding.

Combined Paravariceal and Intravariceal Injection

The needle is inserted in a paravariceal position immediately proximal to the bleeding point and 1 mL of 5% ethanolamine oleate solution is injected. The aim is to raise a submucosal wheal (Fig. 7A) and thereby to control the active bleeding by compression (Fig. 7B). If this does not completely control the acute bleeding, a further paravariceal injection is performed alongside the bleeding point. Once the bleeding has been controlled, the procedure for that varix is completed by an intravariceal injection of 3 to 5 mL of ethanolamine oleate (Fig. 7C). The same technique is used, even if the active bleeding has ceased at the time of the emergency endoscopy. All additional

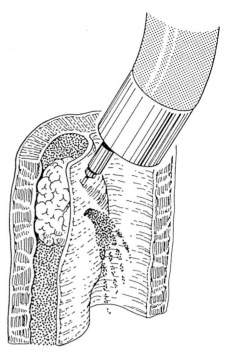

Fig. 6. Emergency sclerotherapy. An intravariceal injection technique is used to treat an actively bleeding varix.

The Gastrointestinal Tract

variceal channels are injected either with a combined or an intravariceal technique. Large varices are injected with a further intravariceal injection 2 to 3 cm above the initial injection site. Although most bleeding varices occur near the esophagogastric junction, occasionally the bleeding site is at a higher level, and the initial injections are performed at this site. The remaining varices are then injected near the esophagogastric junction.

When bleeding is profuse, vigorous lavage via the endoscope channels and elevation of the head of the operating table to 30 or 45 degrees will improve visibility and will usually allow identification and treatment of the bleeding site. Blind attempts at injection should never be performed as this may injure the esophagus. If the bleeding is so profuse that injection treatment cannot be safely completed, a balloon tube is inserted, as described previously.

After an emergency injection treatment, the patient is returned to the intensive care unit. The patient is allowed oral fluids for the first 24 hours and thereafter a regular diet is recommended. In stuporous or comatose patients, intravenous feeding is continued until they regain consciousness and can manage fluids by mouth.

Retrosternal discomfort and a low-grade pyrexia may develop in some patients after injection sclerotherapy, which usually

into the variceal lumen. Care must be taken to ensure that only the needle and not the injector catheter above the needle enters the variceal wall because the latter may cause a large defect in the variceal wall, which may give rise to troublesome bleeding. No attempt should be made to inject the varices while the patient is restless or heaving. Such uncontrolled injections may result in laceration of the varix wall by the needle with resultant major bleeding.

After the procedure, the patient is observed in the outpatient endoscopy suite recovery room for an hour and then discharged home. It is unusual for bleeding to complicate an elective sclerotherapy session.

Subsequent sclerotherapy injections are performed at weekly intervals until all the varices have been eradicated. Severe local esophageal mucosal ulceration or slough may delay injection of the underlying varix, but the other variceal channels should be injected. Once eradication of the varices has been achieved, a further endoscopic assessment is performed at 3 months to confirm continued eradication. Further surveillance evaluations are performed every 6 months for 2 years and then annually for

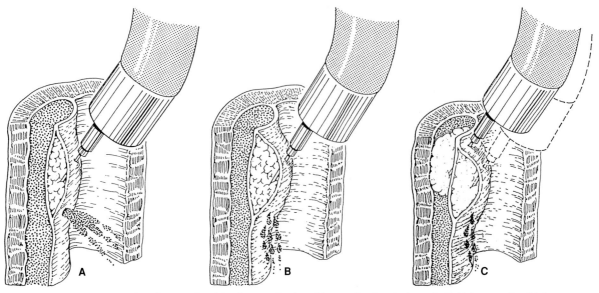

Fig. 7. Emergency sclerotherapy: Combined paravariceal and intravariceal technique. **A:** Initial paravariceal injection immediately proximal to the bleeding point. **B:** Bleeding controlled by the paravariceal injection. **C:** An intravariceal injection completes the procedure.

resolves within 24 hours. If pain is excessive or if dysphagia develops, a contrast swallow examination (using Gastrografin) is indicated to exclude a local injection site leak.

Most patients (70%) respond to a single injection treatment and have no further bleeds. If bleeding does recur, the patient must be re-endoscoped urgently. Pharmacologic therapy (somatostatin or Glypressin) can be commenced, or reintroduced, if previously used. Bleeding varices are injected as before. If the bleeding is from an esophageal ulcer, somatostatin infusion is used and oral sucralfate administered. Noting that the success rate of a single injection treatment is 70%, some 30% of patients will have a further bleed and require additional injection treatment. Two injection treatments usually control variceal bleeding in more than 95% of patients. Subsequently, repeated elective sclerotherapy sessions are undertaken at weekly intervals until all varices have been eradicated.

When a further bleeding episode occurs after two injection treatments during a single hospital admission, this is defined as failure of emergency endoscopic therapy. The patient should have a balloon tube inserted to control the bleeding. After resuscitation, he or she should have an alternative procedure, which is usually a TIPS procedure, or occasionally, when appropriate, injection of the varices with cyanoacrylate.

Complications

The major complication after sclerotherapy is esophageal perforation caused by inadvertent intramuscular esophageal wall injection of sclerosant. This is uncommon. Less severe complications include a minor injection site leak. This is diagnosed on Gastrografin swallow and is usually treated with parenteral nutrition or nasogastric feeding through a fine Silastic tube and antibiotics. The minor leaks usually resolve on conservative therapy. The main danger is recurrent bleeding during the treatment phase but long-term sequelae are unusual. The most common local esophageal complication is esophageal mucosal ulceration, which is a frequent occurrence but usually of no consequence and heals without further problem. Pneumonia may occur in patients with acute variceal bleeding, irrespective of the management used, and may be aggravated by aspiration of blood. With repeated sclerotherapy, complications are cumulative, but with increasing experience, are of relatively minor importance.

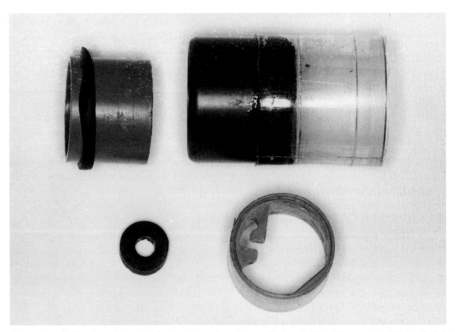

Fig. 8. Single band endoscopic device. Inner banding cylinder (left) is illustrated with loaded O ring ready for application and unstretched band for comparison.

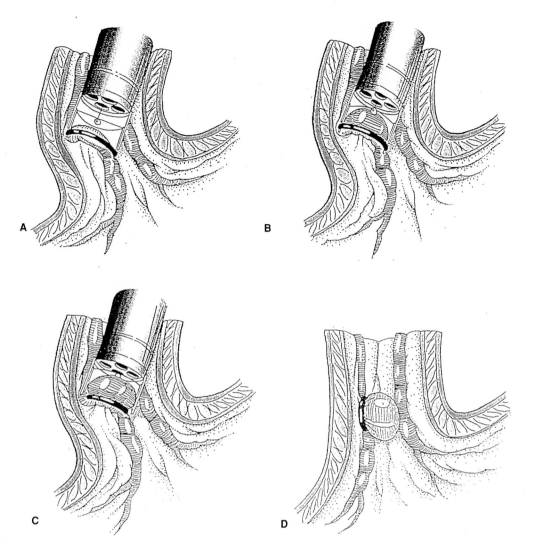

Fig. 9. Endoscopic ligation of esophageal varices using the flexible endoscope. **A:** Varix is approached under direct vision by the endoscopist. Full contact is made between the end of the ligating device and the tissue to be ligated. **B:** Endoscopist activates the endoscopic suction, which results in aspiration of esophageal mucosa, submucosa, and the varix into the ligating device. **C:** Trip wire (which runs through the biopsy channel of the endoscope) is pulled, which moves the inner cylinder (over which the elastic O ring is stretched) toward the endoscope, displacing the small elastic band. **D:** Elastic band encircles the neck of the now ligated tissue, resulting in strangulation and thrombosis.

ENDOSCOPIC VARICEAL BAND LIGATION

Single Band Application

The original endoscopic variceal banding device (C.R. Bard, Tewksbury, MA) has a housing, or outer, cylinder and a banding, or inner, cylinder, and is completed with a trip wire and a single latex O ring (Fig. 8). The outer housing cylinder is attached to the end of the endoscope via a silastic friction mount. The banding cylinder is a smaller cylinder fitted with a clasp that allows insertion of the trip wire. It is constructed to fit snugly yet slide smoothly inside the housing cylinder. The trip wire consists of a monofilament strand, to which a flange

has been attached at the distal end. The small latex O rings are mounted on the banding cylinder (Fig. 8).

The banding technique is the same whether performed for an acute variceal bleed or for an elective banding procedure. A diagnostic panendoscopy is performed first, when possible. After confirming the need for variceal banding, the endoscope is removed and reinserted after backloading an overtube. After reinserting the endoscope into the stomach, the overtube is carefully advanced and passed through the cricopharyngeus and into the upper esophagus. The endoscope is removed again and the banding device is attached to the end of the endoscope. A trip wire is passed through the vacuum lock of the biopsy channel entry port and exits via

the distal biopsy channel opening. The trip wire is secured to the clasp in the banding cylinder and the banding cylinder is "backed" into the housing cylinder. The banding cylinder is positioned so that approximately 1 mm of the cylinder protrudes beyond the O ring, which is seated against the end of the housing cylinder. The endoscope is reinserted into the patient's esophagus via the overtube. The endoscope has to be passed repeatedly for each banding procedure and then removed to disconnect the used inner cylinder, which is replaced with a fresh cylinder with an O ring.

The varix that is to be banded must be clearly identified. The endoscope is advanced under direct vision until the banding cylinder is in full 360-degree contact with the varix (Fig. 9A). Once full contact is made, suction is applied. This draws the varix and the surrounding mucosa into the banding chamber (Fig. 9B). Once the chamber is completely filled with the varix, this gives rise to a "red-out" view down the endoscope. The trip wire is pulled and the latex O ring is dislodged from the inner cylinder and becomes securely fixed around the base of the target varix (Fig. 9C,D). A disadvantage is that multiple variceal ligations are required, which necessitates removal and reinsertion of the endoscope for each separate variceal ligation.

The treatment begins with ligation of the bleeding varix or the most distal part of the target variceal column. Each column has a single band placed at its lower end. Large varices have additional bands placed more proximally, 2 to 5 cm higher up the esophagus. On average, a total of six to nine bands are applied during the initial session, and progressively fewer bands are required at subsequent sessions as the varices decrease in size. If small volume injection sclerotherapy is performed in addition, intravariceal injections are placed in visible veins, usually above the upper band.

After banding, it is necessary for patients to chew food well, but they do not require any specific dietary restrictions. The postoperative care is the same as for patients who have received injection sclerotherapy. Repeated banding treatments are performed at 1-week intervals until all varices have been eradicated.

Multiband Application

The multiband ligator carries five, six, eight, or ten bands (Fig. 10). The bands are singly activated by a drawstring, which passes from the ligator through the biopsy channel and is attached to a trigger unit mounted on the biopsy channel port of the endoscope, which allows repeated individual firings of the bands. The multiband system obviates the need for an overtube. The multiband variceal ligator is a significant technical advance over the single-shot device, but because the unit is disposable and cannot be reused, the current retail cost of $200 per unit may limit the widespread use of the multiband device.

Complications

Complications can be divided into two categories. The first relates to the overtube and the second to the elastic bands. The esophagus can be injured by inadvertently pinching the esophageal wall in the gap between the overtube and the endoscope while advancing the overtube. This has led to mucosal tears and rarely esophageal perforation. Overtubes with a new improved design should eliminate this problem. The second problem has been engorgement of the varices in the distal esophagus, which may lead to rupture and bleeding before banding, which may be life threatening. If this occurs, the overtube should be withdrawn until the distal end just protrudes through the cricopharyngeus into the esophagus. The engorgement should then

resolve. Complications related to the banding itself are uncommon. Bleeding at an ulcer site, after the band has fallen off, has been a less frequent complication than that occurring with sclerotherapy ulcers.

CONCLUSION

The range of treatment options for bleeding esophageal varices has expanded markedly during the past two decades. Increasingly sophisticated methods of management have developed in response to the evolving understanding of the pathophysiologic processes underlying portal hypertension. Endoscopic treatment has become the principal first-line intervention in patients with bleeding esophageal varices, both during the acute event and for long-term prevention of recurrent bleeding. The treatment of both acute and persistent recurrent variceal bleeding is best accomplished by a skilled, knowledgeable, and well-equipped team using a multidisciplinary integrated approach. Optimal management should provide the full spectrum of treatment options including pharmacologic therapy, endoscopic treatment, interventional radiologic procedures, surgical shunts, and liver transplantation.

SELECTED READING

Bosch J, Abraldes JG, Groszmann R. Current management of portal hypertension. *J Hepatol.* 2003;38:S54.

Ferguson JW, Tripathi D, Hayes PC. Review article: the management of acute variceal bleeding. *Aliment Pharmacol Ther* 2003;18:253.

Garcia-Tsao G. Current management of the complications of cirrhosis and portal hypertension: variceal hemorrhage, ascites, and spontaneous bacterial peritonitis. *Gastroenterology* 2001;120:726.

Gow PJ, Chapman RW. Modern management of oesophageal varices. *Postgrad Med J* 2001; 77:75.

Grace ND, Groszmann RJ, Garcia-Tsao G, et al. Portal hypertension and variceal bleeding: an AASLD single topic symposium. *Hepatology* 1998;28:868.

Krige JEJ, Botha JF, Bornman PC. Endoscopic variceal ligation for bleeding esophageal varices. *Dig Endosc* 1999;11:315.

Krige JEJ, Terblanche J. Injection sclerotherapy of oesophageal varices. In: Carter D, Russell RCG, Pitt HA, Bismuth H, eds. *Rob and Smith's operative surgery. Hepatobiliary and pancreatic surgery,* 5th ed. London: Chapman and Hall Medical, 1996:163.

Mihas AA, Sanyal AJ. Recurrent variceal bleeding despite endoscopic and medical therapy. *Gastroenterology* 2004;127:621.

Sharara AI, Rockey DC. Gastroesophageal variceal hemorrhage. *N Engl J Med* 2001; 345:669.

Tait IS, Krige JEJ, Terblanche J. Endoscopic band ligation of oesophageal varices. *Br J Surg* 1999;86:437.

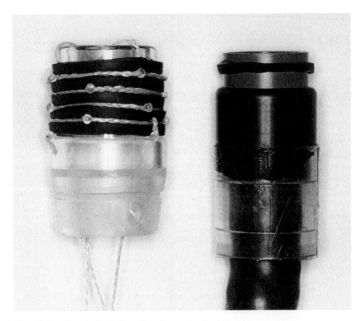

Fig. 10. Loaded multiband and single band endoscopic devices.

EDITOR'S COMMENT

This is a very nice chapter and comes from the hospital that once again popularized endoscopic therapy and sclerotherapy for bleeding esophageal varices. The history is well known; Crafoord, a Swedish otorhinolaryngologic surgeon, first proposed sclerotherapy in approximately 1939 for the treatment of esophageal varices. It was forgotten for a while, but then reintroduced by John Terblanche using a rigid Negus esophagoscope, which required general anesthesia. A necessary general anesthetic contributed to the mortality of endoscopic sclerotherapy, and it wasn't until the flexible endoscope was then utilized, which did not require general anesthesia, that the mortality dropped to where it is today, approximately 20% or 30%, depending on the Child class of the patient.

Esophageal varices are much more damaging to the liver than, for example, a bleeding duodenal ulcer, because in addition to the hypotension, there is the decreased portal flow as the bleeding varix acts as a vent, decreasing portal pressure and flow. The authors are correct in that portal hypertension is a complex set of hemodynamics. Normally, if flow is constant and pressure is constant, then the presence of an obstruction, either presinusoidal, sinusoidal, or postsinusoidal, results in a decrease in flow. In the case of portal hypertension, the flow continues, and that is because of the presence of arterial shunts, which many have attributed to the presence of increased amounts of estrogen that are not metabolized, thus opening, for example, arteriovenous shunts between the bronchial and the gastrointestinal circulation.

In resuscitating these patients, in addition to a central venous pressure, which the authors advocate, this is the one situation where the Swan-Ganz wedge pulmonary artery pressure may result in a better appreciation of where the patient actually is. This is because of the left–right association that occurs in portal hypertension between the right side and the left side of the heart, probably due in major part to the bronchial circulation and the effects of estrogen.

The authors stress speed, and nowhere in the treatment of any patient is speed as to the definitive therapy important. Marshall Orloff pioneered this concept years ago in which he proposed that the workup and definitive therapy, in his case portocaval shunt either end to side or side to side, were carried out within 8 hours. There were a number of skeptics as to this approach, but Orloff's results have been verified by any number of individuals and in fact has one simple hypothesis: When the patient comes in they are relatively intact, and it is repeated episodes of bleeding, repeated episodes of hypotension, aspiration, hypovolemia, pneumonitis, and repeated episodes of hypoxia that converts a class B cirrhotic, for example, after 48 hours into a class C, at which point surgery is consulted.

In this case, the sclerotherapy needs to be carried out quickly and efficiently in a well-equipped endoscopy suite, operating room, and intensive care unit to prevent complications. If one episode of sclerotherapy or variceal ligation is not sufficient, then depending on the skill of the endoscopist, a second attempt should be made. If this is not successful and there are no other lesions seen, a Sengstaken-Blakemore tube or Minnesota tube is placed, which is well described, and TIPS or some sort of shunt is carried out. If the patient is a candidate for transplant, then TIPS is the better alternative. If the bleeding does not stop with a TIPS procedure, one should stay out of the portal area, and a distal splenorenal or central splenorenal shunt if the patient has ascites carried out. The authors point out that there is a place for expectant therapy, in patients that are critically ill and have very little chance of survival. Expectant therapy is a difficult ethical and moral choice. However, if one does adopt expectant therapy, then blood transfusion and transfusion of blood products, intensive care, etc., should cease. This is extraordinarily difficult for most physicians, but if there is little chance for survival, this is essential, rather than allowing the blood bank to be depleted.

As the authors state, Rikker's data have shown that if patients live a distance from a medical center so that repeat sclerotherapy or variceal ligation cannot easily be carried out, then some form of shunt is appropriate. I would like to disabuse people of the notion of selective and nonselective shunts. All shunts are nonselective, since they go from areas of high portal pressure to low. The French, especially Henri Maillol, showed that within 24 hours of a distal splenorenal shunt, collaterals opened within the pancreas to the systemic circulation, thus diminishing portal flow. The concept that somehow magically blood does not go from a high pressure to a low pressure is contraintuitive. It may not be as much. In response to this finding, Dean Warren and his group (Chapter 119) proposed an azygoportal disconnection. This is beyond the skill of most surgeons, and it is not clear that additional collaterals do not open up.

The central splenorenal shunt is useful for patients with ascites, which the distal splenorenal does not decompress. Dr. Linton was clear that the shunt should not be any larger than 1 cm in diameter to maintain some portal perfusion. Indeed, our own randomized prospective trial (Fischer JE, et al. *Ann Surg* 1981;194:531) showed no difference in hepatic failure and portosystemic encephalopathy in follow-up.

In brief, these are terribly fragile patients who can go sour very quickly. It takes a well-trained team to make certain that these patients are well cared for. Meticulous technique, very careful attention to detail, and support of a patient with respect to hemodynamics, prevention of aspiration, treatment of encephalopathy, appropriate transfusion, and appropriate transfusion of coagulation factors may lead to a live patient at the end of the day. I know of no other condition compared with bleeding esophageal varices where timing, meticulous patient care, and meticulous intensive care will more likely than not result in a live patient and that any digression from these principles will result in mortality.

J.E.F.

The Gastrointestinal Tract

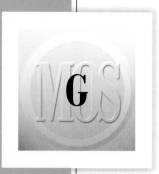

Surgery of the Small Intestine

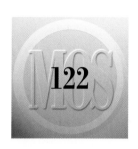

122 | Small and Large Bowel Obstruction

JACK R. PICKLEMAN AND JOSEF E. FISCHER

SMALL BOWEL OBSTRUCTION

Small bowel obstruction is defined as a partial or complete interference with the passage of stool distally in the small intestine. It is one of the more common acute abdominal emergencies and is associated with significant morbidity and mortality, especially if it has progressed to bowel ischemia. Obstruction is to be differentiated from paralytic ileus, which is associated with a wide variety of intraperitoneal and extraperitoneal processes that interfere with the normal motility of the intestine and that resolve spontaneously once the inciting cause has been eliminated.

In as many as 70% of all patients in the United States with small bowel obstruction, adhesions are the cause, usually secondary to previous abdominal operations. Other less common causes of adhesions are congenital disorders, blunt trauma to the abdomen, inflammatory processes within the abdomen, and an indirect inguinal hernia with adhesion formation at the internal ring. Adhesion formation appears to be especially frequent after gynecologic surgery, total abdominal colectomy, abdominoperineal resection, and laparotomy for blunt or penetrating abdominal trauma.

The second most common cause of bowel obstruction is incarceration of the intestine in an inguinal, femoral, or ventral hernia. Although these are generally obvious on physical examination, the diagnosis of a femoral hernia may be obscure, particularly in obese individuals. Malignant tumors of the colon are frequently seen with large bowel obstruction, but obstructing tumors in the right colon may lead to a clinical and radiologic picture indistinguishable from that of small bowel obstruction. Metastases from any primary tumor can likewise cause small bowel obstruction, as can primary small intestinal lesions such as carcinoma, carcinoid, lymphoma, and benign and malignant soft tissue tumors, which are often seen with obstruction secondary to intussusception.

Most patients with small bowel obstruction manifest abdominal pain, nausea and vomiting, obstipation, and abdominal distention. Distention may be mild or massive but is often absent with proximal bowel obstructions. Bowel sounds are classically high-pitched and active, coming on in rushes coincident with crampy pain. Thin people may manifest visible peristalsis. Abdominal tenderness tends to be diffuse and mild in simple small bowel obstruction but may be localized to a single quadrant in strangulation obstruction. The stool is generally negative for occult blood, unless bowel ischemia has supervened. Evidence of dehydration is frequent, with tachycardia, postural hypotension, and decreased urinary output.

The presence of small bowel obstruction should be suspected in any patient presenting with abdominal pain, vomiting, distention, and obstipation. Most patients have either a visible hernia or a laparotomy scar, and the diagnosis becomes far more unlikely if neither of these is present. The essential diagnostic test in all such patients is four radiographic views of the abdomen: an upright chest, an upright abdomen, a supine abdomen, and a left lateral decubitus view.

The presence of significant amounts of colonic gas should raise the suspicion of the presence of obstruction of the large bowel rather than the small bowel. The relationship between the onset of pain and the first episode of vomiting is a clue to how high the obstruction is. The frequency of the cramps is also somewhat indicative of how high the obstruction is.

The utility of upper gastrointestinal contrast studies is controversial, and their use should be discouraged. Although these films can document the presence of an obstruction, this is information that is generally already appreciated. Likewise, such studies may fail to distinguish complete from incomplete obstruction. As such, they are of limited use to the clinician. Computed tomographic (CT) scans, on the other hand, may provide valuable additional information to conventional abdominal radiography in selected situations. Sometimes, the diagnosis of small bowel obstruction will be obscure and a CT scan with oral contrast may prove diagnostic. Also, CT scans with intravenous contrast can determine the presence of edematous bowel or provide evidence of bowel gangrene through the demonstration of pneumatosis of the bowel wall or free intraperitoneal air. This should not be construed as a blanket recommendation for CT scanning in all cases of suspected bowel obstruction; such testing would be both superfluous and expensive in most situations, in which a carefully performed history and physical examination, coupled with four views of the abdomen, is sufficient.

No discussion of bowel obstruction would be complete without reference to the syndrome of strangulation obstruction of the small intestine. This may be one of the most difficult acute abdominal conditions to recognize, but it is clearly one of the most important, because it is life-threatening if the diagnosis is delayed. In contrast to patients with simple mechanical small bowel obstruction, patients with strangulation obstruction may have little vomiting or distention. In addition, watery stools are seen frequently. One characteristic of this syndrome is a severe constant abdominal pain that appears out of proportion to the physical findings on abdominal examination. The strangulated loop of intestine rapidly fills up with fluid, and therefore the usual radiographic signs of dilated bowel with air–fluid levels are often absent. Any patient with a scar on the abdomen and such a clinical picture should be promptly operated on after volume replacement.

Once the diagnosis of small bowel obstruction has been made, the most important initial step is to rehydrate the patient.

Volume losses can be profound, and large quantities of lactated Ringer's solution may be required. An indwelling Foley catheter is mandatory, as the production of an adequate volume of urine is the most useful sign of successful volume resuscitation, and urine output must commence prior to induction of general anesthesia. If this does not occur there is a significant chance of acute tubular necrosis, as renal blood flow drops precipitously with the induction of general anesthesia. Depending on the clinical circumstances, a central venous pressure line or a Swan-Ganz pulmonary artery catheter may be required. The use of antibiotics, as in many areas in surgery, is controversial. Surely, any patient who is being prepared for operation should receive perioperative antibiotics, and any drug regimen effective against the more common Gram-positive and Gram-negative aerobic and anaerobic bacteria is sufficient. More controversial is the recommendation to use antibiotics in simple small bowel obstruction during the brief period of nonoperative management, while the decision to operate is still pending. Whereas the normal gut mucosa is relatively impermeable to bacteria, distended or ischemic bowel may allow the passage of toxins and bacteria into the portal circulation and peritoneal cavity. Accordingly, I favor the use of prophylactic antibiotics during the brief observation period before deciding about operation. This practice is supported by the early laboratory results of Dr. Isidor Cohn, Jr.

With regard to the timing of surgery, all patients should be operated on promptly after volume resuscitation if any evidence or suspicion arises that bowel is ischemic. Most but not all of these patients have some of the following signs: tachycardia, localized tenderness, fever, leukocytosis, or an abdominal mass. In order to understand the progression of symptoms in nonischemic intestinal obstruction to the symptoms of ischemic bowel, one must review the innervation of the abdomen and abdominal wall. The intestine and its visceral peritoneum do not have alpha fibers; that is, the myelinated pain fibers that can localize abdominal pain. Only delta fibers, which are nonmyelinated, tend to localize the midline and respond only to distention and spasm. One feels the pain of intestinal obstruction caused by spasm and cramping as well as distention of the small bowel loops. However, the pain is rarely localized. Once the bowel becomes ischemic, the irritation of the small bowel against the parietal peritoneum then enables the alpha fibers to become irritated and the pain to become localized. Thus, the development

of point tenderness tends to be associated with ischemic bowel with the transudation of bowel fluid and/or the irritation of the serosa.

Not all of the visceral peritoneum has access to alpha fibers. These are notably absent in the pelvic peritoneum. Thus, when I have seen dead bowel in the true pelvis and I have seen patients with dead bowel for several days without any abdominal tenderness and, interestingly enough, without any signs of ischemic bowel. Occasional patients, however, may harbor ischemic bowel in the absence of these signs. The clinician must therefore differentiate between complete and incomplete small bowel obstruction. In complete small bowel obstruction, no significant flatus or stool has been passed in the previous 12 hours and no significant colonic gas is apparent on abdominal radiographic films. The percentage of patients with ischemic bowel is higher in such a circumstance than in incomplete obstruction, and in up to 80% of such patients the condition will not resolve with intestinal suction alone. Therefore, I favor immediate operation for all patients with a complete small bowel obstruction. On the other hand, patients with an incomplete small bowel obstruction and no evidence of ischemic bowel may be safely treated for some time because resolution may be expected in up to 80% of this group. Most of the patients who are successfully treated nonoperatively show definite signs of clinical improvement within 24 hours, and nearly all by 48 hours. Accordingly, this should be the maximum period of observation; after 48 hours, laparotomy is indicated.

The choice of intestinal decompression tube remains more emotional than it probably should be, with most authorities advocating a standard Levin tube and others a long intestinal tube with a weighted balloon to promote passage through the loops of small intestine. The theory behind the use of a long intestinal tube is that providing suction closer to the point of obstruction decreases the luminal pressure and bowel edema, and therefore increases venous and arterial circulation adjacent to the obstructed loop, which hastens resolution. Although this is an appealing concept, the difficulties involved in placing and passing these tubes seem to far outweigh their theoretical advantages. Frequent positioning of the patient and advancement of the tube into the nares is required, and serial radiographic films must be made to gauge the progression of the tube. Also, some patients require a concomitant nasogastric tube because the intestinal tube will not decompress a distended stomach. Furthermore, prolonged nonoperative treatment of some patients may allow progression to ischemic bowel. Accordingly, I see no advantage to such tubes over a standard nasogastric tube.

The anesthesiologist plays a critical role in the operative management of these patients. Many anesthesiologists choose to perform endotracheal intubation with the patient awake but lightly sedated in an attempt to minimize the possibility of aspiration during induction of anesthesia. After this, excellent muscle relaxation is required not only to aid in exploration but also to facilitate closure of the abdomen in the presence of markedly distended bowel. The anesthesiologist should be cautioned against using nitrous oxide in this clinical situation; this agent leads to severe bowel distention.

The choice of the operative incision is critical. Because adhesions are likely to form on the undersurface of previous incisions, in many instances, making a new incision is wise. If the prior laparotomy incision is midline, a transverse incision just above or below the umbilicus will satisfy all the requirements for exposure within the abdomen and pelvis, and provide a structurally sound incision. Alternatively, the incision can be extended cephalad and the abdomen entered above the old incision. The other advantage of placing a new incision away from a scar is that the abdomen can be entered in a virgin area, which hopefully minimizes the potential for bowel injury during the initial dissection. The character of the peritoneal fluid should be observed, and whether this is serous, turbid, or bloody should be noted; the latter two types would tend to indicate the presence of ischemic bowel. Aerobic and anaerobic cultures of this fluid should be carried out. If possible, the exploration should begin at the ileocecal valve and should continue proximally. In certain instances, a single obstructing band will be noted, with dilated bowel proximally and decompressed bowel distally. After lysis of such a band, the surgeon is assured that the cause of the obstruction has been eliminated, and lysis of remaining adhesions is unnecessary.

In other instances, however, to ascertain the exact point of obstruction is far more difficult because multiple segments of dilated and partially decompressed bowel are present. In such a circumstance, lysing all adhesions from the ileocecal valve to the ligament of Treitz is essential. Often, it may be advantageous for the more experienced surgeon to act as the first assistant because exposing difficult tissue planes is probably harder than dissecting them once they are exposed. Also, instances are seen in which use of sharp, even scalpel, dissection is far safer than blunt dissection, as the latter may tend to deserose bowel. When bowel is damaged by dissection, it should be repaired only if mucosa is visible, preferably with a 5-0 monofilament suture, which is nonreactive. If merely a serosal tear is involved, the defect need not be repaired, and indeed, repair of such a defect may predispose to increased adhesion formation, especially if silk isused.

The determination of bowel viability may be extremely difficult in certain circumstances. Although color, the presence of motility, and arterial pulsations are reassuring, these are not definite indicators of viable bowel. The use of several intraoperative aids has been advocated to determine bowel viability, including intestinal Doppler studies, fluorescein staining, and bowel wall oxygen tension measurement. Although these will probably indicate the state of bowel viability in the majority of patients, some will be found in whom this determination cannot be made accurately. In such a situation, placing the suspect loop of intestine in warm packs for approximately 15 minutes and observing it later may provide the answer. If the loop is still questionable, it should be resected and a primary anastomosis carried out. If the suspect loop is a long one, however, and concern exists about creation of short-gut syndrome, the bowel can be replaced in the peritoneal cavity, the abdomen closed, and a second-look operation carried out the following day.

At the end of the lysis of adhesions, if it is technically possible, the distended bowel should be emptied of its luminal contents. This not only improves the blood supply of the bowel but also facilitates abdominal closure. The two most practical ways to accomplish this are to milk the intestinal contents in a proximal direction with aspiration by either a nasogastric tube or an intestinal tube placed in the jejunum. Alternatively, milking of the intestinal contents distally into the right colon may be accomplished. Probably no circumstances exist in which an enterotomy or colotomy should be made to evacuate bowel contents, as this may unnecessarily contaminate the peritoneal cavity. Whether a viable segment of intestine that is densely adherent in the pelvis should be resected or bypassed remains a matter of judgment. Surely, in some circumstances, it will be obvious that attempts to dissect free such a loop will result in damage to the loop and surrounding structures, and lead to the need for resection and anastomosis. In such a circumstance, the preferable course may be to perform an enteroenterostomy or enterocolostomy to bypass a segment, provided the area bypassed is a short length of intestine. Bypass of long segments of small intestine tend to yield poor long-term results, with problems of stasis and bacterial overgrowth in the long segment and chronic intestinal symptoms.

Fascial closure of the abdomen should be accomplished in every situation. Whether the skin should be closed depends on whether gangrenous bowel is present. If so, the skin and subcutaneous tissues should be left open and a delayed primary closure accomplished. However, a delayed primary closure has a wound infection rate of 5%; a useful alternative is primary closure with prolonged closed suction drainage.

In certain situations, extremely dense adhesion formation may be encountered, termed an *obliterated abdomen*. Arduous dissection may result in multiple bowel resections and anastomoses, along with many areas of deserosed and edematous remaining bowel. This often results in postoperative obstruction, abscess, and fistula formation. In such a circumstance, if real concern exists regarding the integrity of the remaining intestine, a proximal jejunostomy and distal mucous fistula can be constructed, with subsequent barium studies through the distal segment to rule out leaks and obstruction. Reanastomosis can then be accomplished when deemed appropriate (Fig. 1). This technique is applicable in any situation including gastrointestinal cutaneous fistulas, whether or not bowel has been resected, when the ability of the remaining distal small bowel to heal without breakdown is a concern.

When suturing bowel, I prefer a single-layer open anastomosis with 4-0 Tevdek sutures. A hemostat is passed through the mesentery adjacent to the bowel, and small bites of mesentery are taken between hemostats and then ligated (Fig. 2). After the mesentery is ligated, the bowel is defatted for approximately 1 cm so that Block-Potts bowel clamps can be cleanly applied, always by grasping from the antimesenteric-to-mesenteric borders to prevent twisting of the bowel (Fig. 3). A 9-inch Kocher clamp is applied on the specimen side, and the bowel is transected between the clamps with a scalpel. The clamps are removed, and hemostasis is accomplished with cautery. The bowel ends are aligned, and the posterior row of seromuscular sutures are placed. Each suture is grasped with a hemostat, and all hemostats are maintained over a ring forceps (Figs. 4 and 5). When all posterior row

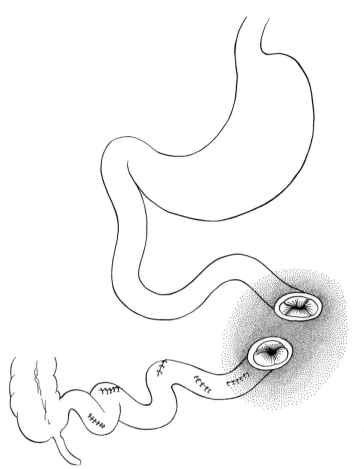

Fig. 1. The jejunum exits the abdominal wall as a jejunostomy. The proximal end of the distal limb is brought out as a mucous fistula.

sutures have been placed, the knots are then tied. The end sutures are kept separate, and all others cut. Next, the anterior row of sutures is tied as they are placed (Fig. 6). If the mesenteric defect lends itself easily to closure, this is accomplished. If the tissues are too fragile, however, or if tension is present, this step can be omitted.

LARGE BOWEL OBSTRUCTION

Large bowel obstruction generally results from either an advanced colon carcinoma or sigmoid diverticulitis; less commonly, a sigmoid volvulus is present. The presence of a large bowel obstruction may be suggested by a long history of symptoms, rather than their abrupt onset, the presence of positive occult blood in the stool, or the presence of significant amounts of colonic gas on a supine abdominal radiographic views. In all patients with these features, an unprepared thin barium enema should be carried out. Likewise, a patient who presents with signs and symptoms of obstruction and a radiologic picture of small bowel obstruction on conventional abdominal views but who has

no external hernia or abdominal scar should undergo a barium enema because no apparent cause is present.

Oftentimes, a patient who appears to have a complete large bowel obstruction on barium enema examination, with no passage of barium proximal to the obstructing lesion, continues to have liquid bowel movements. Sometimes, however, this ex-

amination may show contrast agent proximal to the lesion, and yet the patient is clinically obstructed with no passage of stool or flatus. Therefore, the clinician should be guided by the patient's symptoms rather than the radiographic views in determining which patients require urgent operation as opposed to an elective operation after mechanical bowel preparation. A patient whose bowel cannot be adequately prepared preoperatively has several treatment options, depending on the location of the lesion, the amount of gas and stool proximal to the lesion, and the patient's general status.

Lesions of the right colon can generally be resected with a primary anastomosis. In an ileocolic resection and ileotransverse colostomy, once again the mesentery to be resected is delineated and ligated between hemostats (Fig. 7). A stapler is fired across the terminal ileum, and the staple line is then oversewn with 4-0 Tevdek sutures (Figs. 8, 9). A Block-Potts bowel clamp is applied to the transverse colon, which is then transected. A one-layer side-to-end anastomosis is carried out, which eliminates the problem of suturing bowel of differing sizes (Fig. 10). Once again, all posterior-row sutures are placed before tying, with the anterior row tied as they are placed. In a patient with a left-sided obstruction, however, a local resection and anastomosis is often contraindicated because of excessive proximal stool. In such an instance, rectal enemas are given preoperatively, and a subtotal colectomy is carried out (Fig. 11). This permits anastomosis to the terminal ileum, which generally contains only liquid contents; these can be milked proximally before applying an occluding bowel clamp. A side-to-end anastomosis can be easily fashioned, which eliminates the difficulties involved in suturing together the ends of bowel of differing diameters (Fig. 12).

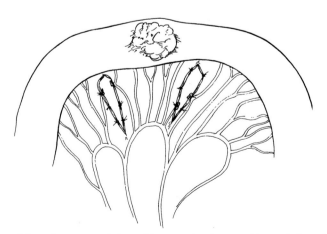

Fig. 2. The small bowel mesentery is ligated between hemostats, with care being taken to maintain the blood supply of each end.

The Gastrointestinal Tract

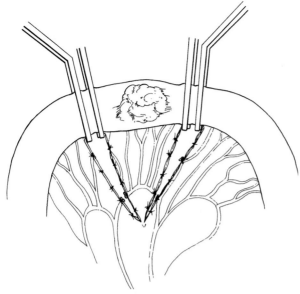

Fig. 3. Block-Potts bowel clamps are applied from the antimesenteric to mesenteric border to avoid twisting. A Kocher clamp is applied on the specimen side, and the bowel is transected with a scalpel.

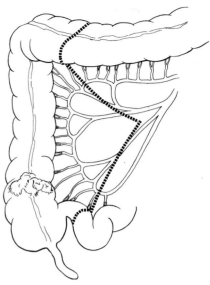

Fig. 7. Schematic representation of the mesenteric dissection required for an ileocolic resection.

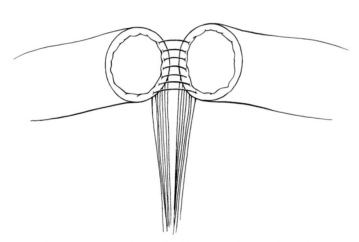

Fig. 4. The posterior row of sutures is placed, with each stitch grasped by a hemostat and kept in order over a ring forceps.

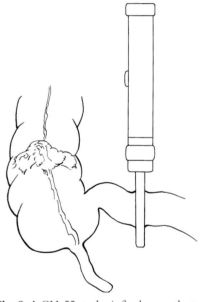

Fig. 8. A GIA 55 stapler is fired across the terminal ileum.

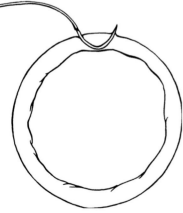

Fig. 5. Cross-sectional view of the intestine showing the depth of each suture. Deep seromuscular bites are taken that do not enter the lumen.

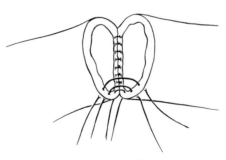

Fig. 6. The posterior row of sutures has been tied, and all but the end sutures cut. The knots on the posterior row are within the lumen. Next, the anterior row sutures are tied as they are placed.

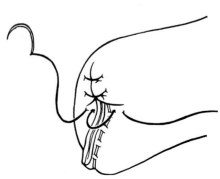

Fig. 9. Inverting Lembert sutures additionally cover the staple line.

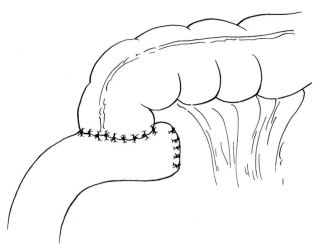

Fig. 10. A side-to-end ileotransverse colostomy, which eliminates the problem of suturing bowel of different diameters. Note the very short stump of small intestine beyond the anastomosis.

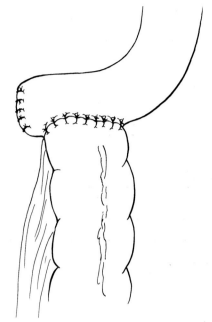

Fig. 12. A side-to-end ileoproctostomy; once again the short stump of small bowel distal to the anastomosis is demonstrated.

In the case of left-sided colon obstruction, cancer and stricture are the usual causes. In the past, this has created quite a quandary for the surgeon as far as having to operate on an unprepared bowel, especially when there is a carcinoma at the splenic flexure. Because of questions of blood supply and the lack of preparedness of the bowel, one of the alternatives is perform a subtotal colectomy and ileorectostomy. More recently, stenting associated with dilatation of a neoplastic stricture and other strictures may be carried out acutely in the presence of large bowel obstruction. This enables evacuation of the bowel and a decrease in the diameter of the distended colon. Some preparation then can be taken before the patient is operated on semielectively. Because the colorectal community has recently done several studies showing that the preparation of the large bowel is or may be deleterious, the preparation is relatively minor, but the bowel is in much better shape and is suitable to undergo an elective operation when it is neither distended nor thinned and with good blood supply.

In other instances of left-sided obstruction, performing an initial transverse loop colostomy, with subsequent resection of the obstructing lesion and colostomy closure carried out as second and third stages at a later time, may be judged safer. In recent years, I have come to favor performing an ileostomy rather than a right transverse colostomy in such a situation, as an ileostomy tends to be easier for the patient to manage than a colostomy. A loop ileostomy is constructed sufficiently proximal to the ileocecal valve so that subsequent ileostomy takedown is simplified. A standard two-stage Hartmann's resection is usually contraindicated by the large diameter of the proximal remaining left colon and the potential for fecal spillage.

The third area, concerning post-operative ileus which will undoubtedly alter the way the patients are treated postoperatively and which will minimize their postoperative stay, is twofold. The first is the advent of the mu-opioid receptor antagonist for decreasing the duration of postoperative ileus, and the other is the use of what has been described by Henrik Kehlet as a series of maneuvers to minimize postoperative stay by so-called fast-track surgery.

New Opioid Receptor Antagonists

Four well-done randomized prospective trials have indicated a shortening of several end points following gastrointestinal track surgery, most of all colectomies. The drug, which has not been released as yet, alvimopan, shortens the postoperative ileus as indicated by the passage of flatus, first bowel

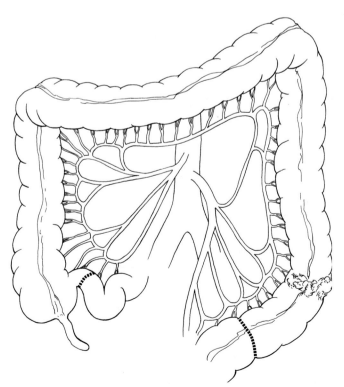

Fig. 11. Schematic representation of the mesenteric dissection required for a subtotal colectomy.

movement, and/or solid diet with either 6 or 12 mg given 2 hours preoperatively and twice a day thereafter. Unfortunately, the four trials themselves have not given a clear indication of a dose-response curve as the trials actually differ on whether 6 mg or 12 mg is more effective. However, the data itself are internally consistent and do seem to indicate that even in the presence of a clinical pathway in which at least one of the institutions in which the trial took place had instituted four colonic resections, the results are effective. Unfortunately, the trials were marred by the presence of hysterectomy, which has a very short length of stay. Apparently this was intended to increase the usefulness of alvimopan when and if it ever reached the market. The utility of this drug, and whether it will be on hospital formularies, will likely be decided on the basis of length of stay. In one of the studies, the difference in postoperative ileus was 22 hours and in another it was 15 hours, both probably long enough to result in earlier discharge of the patient, which in the United States at least will result lower expenditure of Diagnosis Related Group (DRG) which is the basis on which most hospitals get paid. Thus, there will be pressure to get it on the hospital formulary.

The successful submission to the Food and Drug Administration has been marred by a rather poorly done European study comprising nine different studies in which the data are all over the place and in which the discharge order was as long as 36 or 54 hours after end points, indicating the discharge in those countries, many of which had little to do with when the patient was ready for discharge, but more on social issues. This, unfortunately, is holding up the submission to the Food and Drug Administration and the successful release on the market. Whether or not these issues can ever be resolved is unclear.

Fast-Track Surgery

Henrik Kehlet is generally credited with the fast-track way in which patients are managed postoperatively. Kehlet, who works in Denmark and is a professor of both anesthesiology and surgery, has created an entirely different way in which patients are treated postoperatively. First, patients are in the hospital prior to operation, unlike in the United States. The key to the way in which Kehlet treats patients is first to avoid postoperative opioids, and second to minimize the amount of crystalloid that is given, thus decreasing postoperative swelling of the anastomosis and delay in the first bowel action. A successful epidural is an important part of the postoperative management because an effective epidural prevents the use of opiates, which, together with the excessive use of crystalloids during the operative and postoperative period, contributes to an increase in postoperative ileus and length of postoperative stay.

At our own institution we are currently completing some pilot studies in the use of the Kehlet fast-track type of regimen in an effort to reduce postoperative stay following colectomy. The components of this particular pathway are an effective epidural, thereby decreasing the need for postoperative opiates. In the first 24 hours, epidurals very frequently result in hypotension, so one usually adds some type of opiate to the epidural, but this comes out of the epidural after the first 24 hours postoperatively. In addition, brief periods of Neo-Synephrine may be necessary for maintenance of renal perfusion and hemodynamic stability intraoperatively and, at times, for a short time postoperatively.

The regimen for intraoperative fluids includes 250 or 500 mL of 5% albumisol (the manufacturing process for albumisol has been changed, so the price is now sharply reduced), 800 to 900 mL of crystalloid, a decrease from the usual 2,500 to 3,000 mL for a colectomy, and/or the use of 500 mL of Hespan, which is less frequently used. The regimen has also been impressive regarding the first flatus time between 48 and 60 hours postoperatively, early feeding, and readiness for discharge at 4.5 to 5 days postoperatively, even in 70- and 80-year-old patients. This regimen is not quite as good as Kehlet's data

reports, but it is certainly much faster than our previous 6 to 7 days to discharge. In addition, hospitals are dangerous places nowadays, and getting the patient out of the hospital protects them.

SUGGESTED READING

Beck DE, Opelka FG, Bailey R, et al. Incidence of small bowel obstruction after adhesiolysis after open colorectal and general surgery. *Dis Colon Rectum* 1999;42:241.

Brolin RE, Krasna MJ, Mast BA. Use of tubes and radiographs in the management of small bowel obstruction. *Ann Surg* 1987;206:126.

Cheadle WG, Garr EE, Richardson JD. The importance of early diagnosis of small bowel obstruction. *Am Surg* 1988;54:565.

Deitsch EA. Simple intestinal obstruction causes bacterial translocation in man. *Arch Surg* 1989;124:699.

Deitsch EA, Bridges SM, Ma JW. Obstructed intestine as a reservoir for systemic infection. *Am J Surg* 1990;159:394.

Frager DH, Baer JW, Rothpearl A, et al. Distinction between postoperative ileus and mechanical small-bowel obstruction: value of CT compared with clinical and other radiographic findings. *AJR Am J Roentgenol* 1995;164:891.

Landercasper J, Cogbill T, Merry W, et al. Long-term outcome after hospitalization for small bowel obstruction. *Arch Surg* 1993;128:765.

Lau PW, Lo CY, Law WL. The role of one-stage surgery in acute left-sided colonic obstruction. *Am J Surg* 1995;169:406.

Luque DE, Leon E, Metzger A, et al. Laparoscopic management of small bowel obstruction: indications and outcome. *J Gastrointest Surg* 1998;2:132.

Phillips RK, Hittinger R, Fry JS, et al. Malignant large bowel obstruction. *Br J Surg* 1985;72:296.

Pickleman J, Lee RM. The management of patients with suspected early postoperative small bowel obstruction. *Ann Surg* 1989;210:216.

Sarr MG, Bulkley GB, Zuidema GD. Preoperative recognition of intestinal strangulation obstruction. *Am J Surg* 1983;145:176.

Selby RR, Mertz GH, Gilsdorf RB. Spontaneous resolution of intestinal obstruction while receiving home parenteral nutrition. *Am J Surg* 1983;146:742.

Stewardson RH, Bombeck CT, Nyhus LM. Critical operative management of small bowel obstruction. *Ann Surg* 1978;187:189.

EDITOR'S COMMENT

The management of small bowel obstruction has not changed a great deal during the past two decades. As the author points out, there is still controversy over the use of long tubes as opposed to short nasogastric tubes in the management, but as yet there has not been a reasonable series of prospective randomized trials that indicate that in the nonpostoperative period long tubes are more effective than nasogastric tubes. I have always been taught to believe that the only time one really should use a long tube is in the immediate postoperative period when adhesions are not necessarily firm, and decompressing the bowel may enable it to recover from a kink or twist that is not fixed. The difficulty of passing a long tube and the time that is lost in decompression of the bowel stand as negatives in the routine use of long tubes for intestinal obstruction.

(continued)

In the diagnosis of intestinal obstruction, volvulus and the tendency toward gangrene might conceivably be aided by the routine use of C-reactive protein elevations. As yet there is not a great deal of data on whether ischemic and gangrenous bowel has an increase in C-reactive protein as compared with normal intestinal obstruction. Many institutions use serum lactate as a marker for decreased peripheral perfusion, presumably the result of compromise in bowel perfusion. However, it should be pointed out that serum lactate may also be the result of aerobic glycolysis from stored adjacent glycogen, which is a series of membrane-bound enzymes stimulated by epinephrine. Thus, the use of serum lactate solely as an indicator of ischemic bowel is probably not accurate.

One must also think of small bowel volvulus as a cause of intestinal obstruction that leads rapidly to gangrene. An excellent clinical marker, I have found, is back pain, almost always an indicator of small bowel volvulus as it occurs in very few other conditions other than those associated with aortic occlusions in patients with small bowel obstruction. Very often, this is the result of incomplete rotation of the small bowel and incomplete fixation of the small bowel mesentery against the retroperitoneum. One must be very sensitive to this because if one does not move quickly to manage these patients, they may result in complete loss of small bowel viability. Huang et al. (*J Gastroenterol Hepatol* 2005;20:1906) reported 19 adults whose mean age was 61 years and who suffered from small bowel volvulus. The authors claim that this finding, at least in their practice in Taiwan, is rare. Primary volvulus was present in nine patients; that is, no predisposing factors were found in the patients. In my experience, if one looks at patients with small bowel

volvulus with an eye toward looking to the degree of fixation of the small bowel mesentery, one will find that it is relatively narrow.

Other rare causes of small bowel obstruction include endometriosis, in which, at least in our society, there usually is some indication that it exists prior because of the investigation of abdominal pain and the use of laparoscopy. Paksoy et al. (*Mt Sinai J Med* 2005;72:405) reported on a premenopausal woman in Turkey who did not have this diagnosis and underwent both hysterectomy and colonic resection because of failure to diagnose what was really the issue, which was endometriosis, rather than a neoplasm. Paraduodenal hernias and other rare hernias must also be considered (Huang YM et al., *World J Gastroenterol* 2005;11:6557). Small bowel tumors are not often encountered in the normal diagnoses of small bowel obstruction, but should at least be thought of when someone presents with a small bowel obstruction without previous scars on the abdomen or with hernias. Catena et al. (*Aust New Zealand J Surg* 2005; 75:997) presented an interesting series of 34 consecutive cases of small bowel tumors treated in Bologna. Intestinal obstruction was the most common clinical presentation, although perforation and gastrointestinal bleeding were also common (15 cases, 11 cases, and 8 cases, respectively). Lymphoma was the most common type of tumor seen, and five of the nine patients presented with perforation secondary to chemotherapeutic treatment. The next most common type of tumor was stromal tumor; eight patients had this lesion and all of presented with gastrointestinal bleeding. Seven carcinoid patients presented with bowel obstruction because of the bulk of the tumor and because of the desmoplastic reaction causing constriction and small bowel occlusion. Two patients with melanoma metastasis had intussusception. This finding

is apparently reported in the literature but is not currently emphasized. It is of note that none of the carcinoid patients had the carcinoid syndrome, but all had increases in the level of 5-hydroxyindoleacetic acid. This is a nice series that indicates that each type of small bowel tumor does different things. It is also of note that of the four gastric stromal tumors in which radiological embolization was attempted, embolization was only successful in two cases.

In the United Kingdom, 15% of all colorectal cases are initially seen as large bowel obstruction (Hughes E, *Nurs Stand* 2005;19:56). In a study from Corfu, 45% of those patients presenting with large bowel obstruction turned out to have colonic cancer, and this was the first indication that the patients had of this finding (Gatsoulis et al., *Technological Coloproctology* 2004;8:S82). Colonic cancer in their series represents 25% of all intestinal obstructions. It is notable that the mortality of this group was 14%. Small bowel obstruction in the series represented 39% of those patients presenting with intestinal obstruction. It is probably far better if an endoscopic stent can be placed, enabling the patient to be treated nonemergently.

In summary, the world of intestinal obstruction has changed significantly, as stated at the introduction to the chapter. With computed tomography playing a major role, endoscopic stenting of rectal and sigmoid lesions enable a major alteration in how these patients are treated, and, in large measure, obviate the difficulties of emergency surgery in this group. Fast-track surgery decreases postoperative ileus, not only in rectosigmoid colectomies but also in ileocolonic resections for Crohn disease (Andersen et al., *Colorectal Dis* 2005;7:394).

J.E.F.

The Gastrointestinal Tract

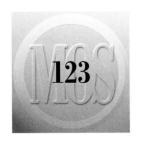

Adjunctive Procedures in Intestinal Surgery

RAYMOND POLLAK

Although parenteral nutrition has changed our ability to support patients, most surgeons performing tertiary-quaternary abdominal operations also prefer access to the gastrointestinal tract. In addition, access is particularly useful in older patients, especially after prolonged intubation when swallowing problems may exist, making feeding jejunostomy desirable. In this chapter, some of the more useful techniques applied to gain access to the small intestine are described. Intubation of the small intestine and its usefulness in preventing recurrent intestinal obstruction are discussed. Finally, excision of Meckel diverticulum is described.

ENTEROSTOMY

Enterostomy is defined as an opening made in the wall of the small intestine that com-

municates with the exterior through the anterior abdominal wall. It may be proximal (in the jejunum) or, less commonly, distal (in the ileum). Current indications for enterostomy include the need for a temporary (or permanent) route of access to the gastrointestinal tract for alimentation. Enterostomy might be done before or after major procedures in which the stomach could not be successfully intubated, when parenteral alimentation is thought inadvisable, or in addition to parenteral nutrition access. Enterostomy is also indicated as a vent for decompression in instances of adynamic ileus in which conventional nasogastric intubation is inadequate or the cause cannot be removed. Similarly, it may be used to decompress fragile areas of resection and anastomoses, especially following duodenal and gastric operations.

Preoperative preparation is determined by the disease involved. Enterostomy may be done as an isolated procedure or together with a major resection of the gastrointestinal tract. When enterostomy is an isolated procedure for feeding purposes or a temporary decompression measure for obstruction of the small intestine, laparoscope-guided or laparoscope-assisted techniques may be utilized.

In the open operative technique, the skin incision is usually placed in the left upper quadrant in the area of the ligament of Treitz. If the enterostomy is part of a major abdominal operation, the site is usually a separate abdominal stab wound, well away from the primary incision. Currently, the Witzel or Stamm technique of enterostomy is used, the former being preferred when long-term intubation is thought likely.

In both the Witzel and Stamm techniques, a loop of proximal jejunum 15 to 20 cm from the ligament of Treitz is delivered into the wound. The proximal and distal ends are identified by the direction of the mesentery, and noncrushing (such as Glassman) or linen-shod clamps are applied after the loop has been emptied of its contents. In the Witzel technique, a catheter is placed through an incision in the antimesenteric surface of the intestinal wall. A simple purse-string suture of 000 chromic catgut is placed in the desired area, and an incision is made in the intestinal wall in the center of the suture (Fig. 1). The catheter is threaded into the lumen the desired distance, and the purse-string suture is tied. A serosal tunnel is made using the same suture in a running manner for a distance of 5 to 6 cm and anchored finally around the proximal tube with another purse-string suture (Fig. 2). The tube is delivered through the abdominal wall through the separate stab incision. The adjacent loop of intestine is anchored to the parietal peritoneum using two 000 silk sutures. A skin suture is placed around the tube as a further anchor. In both techniques the attachments of the intestinal loop to the parietal peritoneum should be broad-based to avoid a volvulus about a small fixed point.

In the Stamm technique, after the intestine has been prepared as described, two concentric purse-string sutures of 000 silk are placed in the submucosa on the antimesenteric border of the jejunal loop. An incision is made in the center of the concentric sutures, using a knife or diathermy (Fig. 3). The catheter is then passed into the intestinal lumen, and the inner suture is tied. After the clamps are released, the outer suture is tied, which anchors the tube to the intestinal wall. The catheter is delivered through the abdominal wall through a stab incision and fixed to the parietal peritoneum and skin as described for the Witzel technique (Fig. 4). Use of a button jejunostomy device rather than a catheter, inserted in a similar fashion, may lead to fewer complications of catheterization, such as leakage, obstruction, and inadvertent removal, but the tube is more difficult to change.

The catheter can now be used as a drainage device or for alimentation. It can be removed at the desired time by simple traction, and the resulting fistula should close within 3 to 4 days without complications. However, in order to make certain the bowel does not leak, it is best to wait for 2 weeks before tube removal, to ensure that a good seal has been established.

Needle catheter jejunostomy, as described by Delaney et al., is a modification of the Witzel technique that can be used without an enterostomy. A large-bore needle (14 or 16 gauge) is tunneled subserosally for its entire length; its tip is then introduced into the intestinal lumen. A catheter is threaded through the needle the desired distance into the lumen, and the needle is withdrawn. The intestinal loop is anchored to the parietal peritoneum as previously described, and the catheter is sewn to the skin (Fig. 5). The catheter, which is too small to be an adequate route for decompression of the gastrointestinal tract, has been used largely for enteral nutrition. However, its use has been largely abandoned because of the limited choice of nutritional solutions, as most enteral feeds will obstruct the tube. Complications have been few. On withdrawal of the catheter, the serosal tunnel should seal any potential leak or resultant fistula. Conversion to a larger jejunostomy tube can be achieved with a J-wire and the Seldinger dilator-sheath technique.

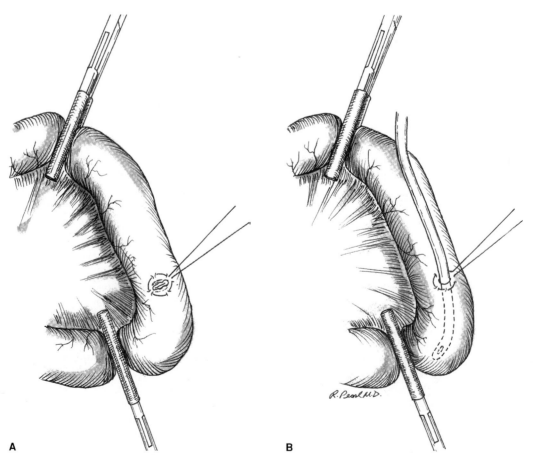

A   **B**

Fig. 1. Enterostomy, Witzel technique. **A:** Incision made in center of purse-string suture. **B:** Catheter threaded into intestinal lumen.

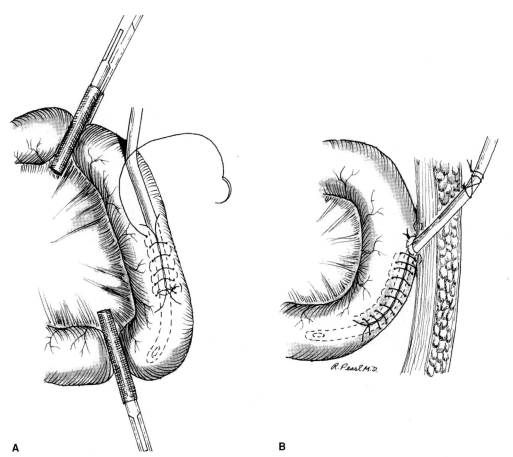

Fig. 2. Enterostomy, Witzel technique. **A:** Formation of serosal tunnel. **B:** Catheter anchored with purse-string suture and delivered through abdominal wall.

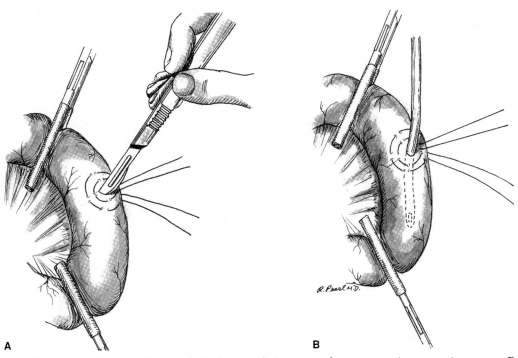

Fig. 3. Enterostomy, Stamm technique. **A:** Incision made in center of two concentric purse-string sutures. **B:** Catheter passed into intestinal lumen and inner of two concentric purse-string sutures tied.

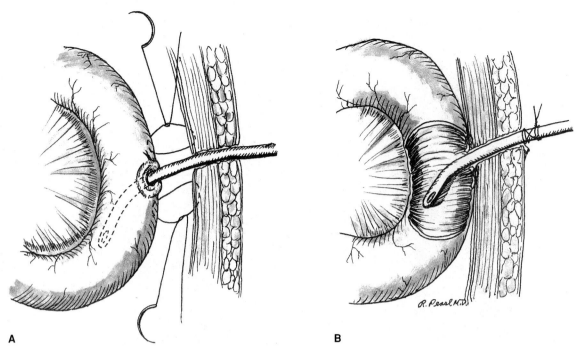

A   **B**

Fig. 4. Enterostomy, Stamm technique. **A:** Catheter delivered through abdominal wall. Loop of intestine anchored to parietal peritoneum. **B:** Skin suture around tube acts as further anchor.

Laparoscopic surgery has also been successfully applied to the creation of enterostomies. After the induction of general anesthesia and the pneumoperitoneum, a laparoscope port (10 to 12 mm) is placed at the umbilicus. Two accessory ports are placed (one in the upper midline, the other in the left or right lower quadrant), and the ligament of Treitz is identified. At a point 30 to 45 cm (12 to 18 in.) distal to the ligament, an enterotomy can be made for a 12 French catheter, and thereafter a Witzel or Stamm technique is used to secure the catheter. Alternatively, the Seldinger introducer-sheath technique can also be used. In all instances, the jejunal segment is sutured to the underside of the peritoneum from within. Under visual guidance, saline can be injected through the newly placed tube to confirm absence of leakage and aboral positioning. The tube is anchored to the skin, and the incisions closed after release of the pneumoperitoneum. Feedings can begin early—often within 24 hours of tube place-ment. Finally, laparoscope-assisted placement of jejunostomy tubes via an enteroscope is also being developed as a further refinement of this technique.

INTUBATION OF THE SMALL INTESTINE

The prevention of recurrent obstruction through plication of the small intestine was first suggested by Noble in 1937. Although some good results have been

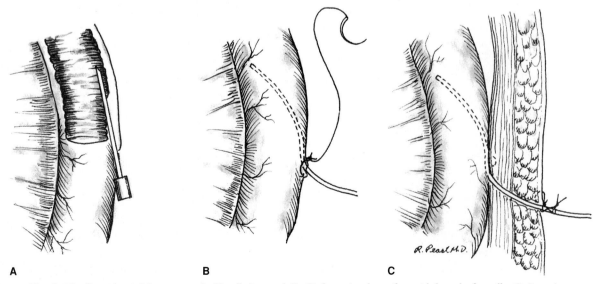

A   **B**   **C**

Fig. 5. Needle catheter jejunostomy. **A:** Needle inserted. **B:** Catheter in place after withdrawal of needle. **C:** Intestinal loop anchored to parietal peritoneum.

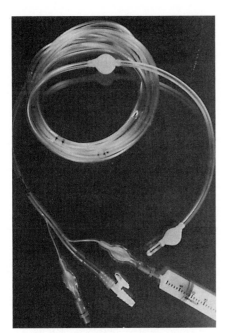

Fig. 6. Modified Baker tube. Note second inflatable balloon proximal to first.

reported, suturing dilated, edematous intestine carries the risk of causing an abscess or fistula. Childs and Phillips therefore modified the technique by applying transmesenteric sutures, although this also is a needlessly traumatic procedure. The one instance in which the external plication technique would seem to be useful is in Peutz-Jeghers syndrome or other rare forms of diffuse polyposis of the small intestine in which recurrent episodes of intussusception occur.

Baker described a long jejunostomy tube to be used for intraoperative decompression of the obstructed intestine. Left in for a time postoperatively, this catheter also internally plicated the small intestine in gentle loops to prevent recurrent obstruction. Performing an enterotomy on obstructed intestine is hazardous, however, as the concentration of bacteria in the obstructed intestine is enormously increased, and jejunal enterocutaneous fistulas have the worst spontaneous rate of closure of fistulas at any point in the gastrointestinal tract. Stewardson et al. reported a significant increase in wound infection rate in patients who had an enterotomy during operations for small-intestinal obstruction. In Chilimindris and Stoneseifer's hospital experience with the Baker tube, two thirds of the patients had complications believed to be directly attributable to the jejunostomy. Stewardson therefore suggested that the Baker tube be inserted by the nasogastric route. Although this route is much safer, passing the tip of the catheter from the pylorus to the ligament of Treitz is

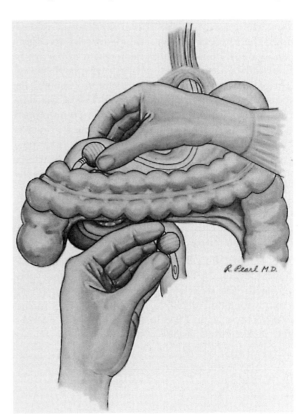

Fig. 7. Insertion of modified Baker tube. (With permission from *Surgery, Gynecology & Obstetrics.*)

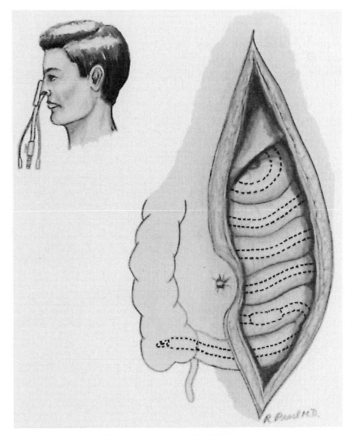

Fig. 8. Internal plication of small intestine by modified Baker tube.

The Gastrointestinal Tract

difficult. To facilitate the passage of the Baker tube through the retroperitoneal portion of the duodenum, Nelson and Nyhus added a second balloon to the Baker tube 25 cm proximal to the first (Fig. 6). This modification permits easy insertion of the long intestinal tube either by the nasogastric route or through a gastrostomy (Fig. 7). Adequate intraoperative decompression and internal plication of the small intestine are thus achieved, and the risks of jejunostomy in dilated intestine are avoided (Fig. 8).

MECKEL DIVERTICULUM

Meckel diverticulum was first described in 1598 by Fabricius Hildanus. Meckel is credited, however, with the first gross anatomic analysis of this condition in 1809. It is a "disease of twos": It occurs in 2% of the population, is twice as common in men

as in women, and is usually found 2 ft from the ileocecal valve. Embryologically, it is the remnant of the primitive vitellointestinal duct that has failed to close, and thus it occurs on the antimesenteric border of the intestine 95% of the time and may have a fairly wide communication with the lumen. It is usually lined with ileal mucosa, but in up to 20% of instances, it may contain heterotopic gastric, colonic, or pancreatic mucosa, either singly or in combination. A flimsy mesentery carrying an independent blood supply from an ileal arcade may be present. The lifetime risk of symptom development is estimated to be 4% to 6% and decreases with age.

The diagnosis is made only when a complication supervenes or incidentally during laparotomy for other reasons.

Complications include inflammation, often simulating appendicitis; hemorrhage, with heterotopic acid-producing gastric

mucosa causing ulceration in normal ileal mucosa; obstruction, by bands or intussusception; and fistula to the abdominal wall or elsewhere in the intestine. Radioisotopic techniques using technetium may locate ectopic gastric mucosa in the diverticulum with gastrointestinal hemorrhage.

Treatment is surgical; indications for excision are the complications. Presence of a diverticulum found incidentally at laparotomy for other reasons is generally not advised.

If an elective excision is thought necessary, as in hemorrhage, a right lower transverse incision is made. The cecum and ileocecal valve are identified. One follows the ileum proximally. The diverticulum usually is found within 2 ft (40 to 50 cm) of the ileocecal valve. The diverticulum and adjacent intestine are delivered into the wound. If a mesodiverticulum is present, it is divided and ligated between clamps. The

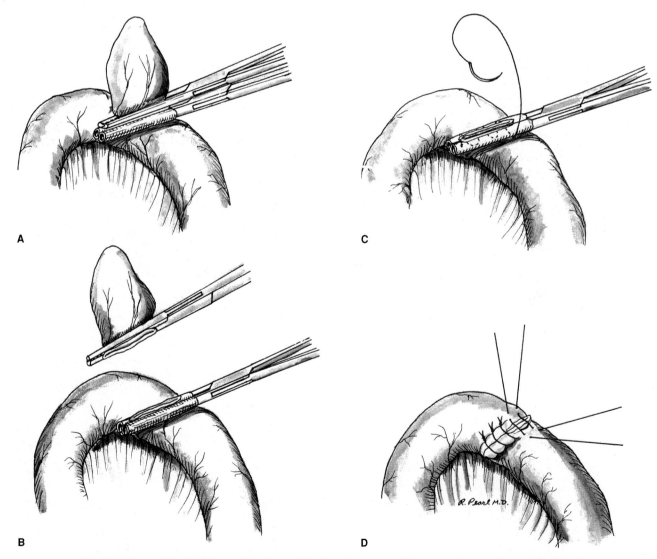

Fig. 9. A: Base of Meckel diverticulum clamped. **B:** Specimen excised between clamps with cautery. **C:** Full-thickness sutures placed beneath clamp. **D:** Inverting interrupted Lembert sutures placed in seromuscular layer.

lumen of the diverticulum is emptied of its contents, and the base is clamped with two linen-shod or noncrushing clamps. The specimen is then excised between the clamps with cautery. Two traction sutures of 000 silk are placed beyond the margins of the line of excision to approximate the serosa. An inner layer of continuous full-thickness 000 Vicryl (polyglactin 910) sutures is placed beneath the clamp, and when this layer is complete the clamp is removed. Inverting interrupted Lembert sutures of 000 silk are placed in the seromuscular layer as a second and final closure (Fig. 9). A surgical stapling device may also be used if the neck of the diverticulum is narrow and the staple line is oversewn similarly with Lembert sutures. Most times, however, the anatomy of the diverticulum does not permit a simple excision; a sleeve resection that encompasses the diverticulum and 2 to 3 cm of the adjacent intestine is performed. A single-layer end-to-end anastomosis of the intestinal defect can then be effected using seromuscular sutures of 3-0 silk. The lumen is then tested for patency between thumb and index finger, and the intestine is returned to the peritoneal cavity. The abdominal wall is closed routinely in layers.

Laparoscopic surgery allows for the resection of these diverticula as well. The techniques utilized in the open procedures can be readily applied to laparoscopic resections (see Suggested Reading).

Morbidity is minimal, and rapid return of intestinal function can be anticipated. When the resection is being done for a complication (inflammation, hemorrhage, obstruction, intussusception, or fistula), a segmental resection of the uninvolved ileum is recommended, with a standard end-to-end anastomosis in one or two layers. This would be especially appropriate for ulceration of the adjacent ileal mucosa because of ectopic gastric epithelium. Postoperative morbidity, ileus, and wound infections are more likely when the operation is performed for a complication. Much debate still continues over the management of these diverticula when found incidentally at laparotomy or laparoscopy, although fewer surgeons favor resection for uncomplicated Meckel diverticula ("don't poke a skunk"). The reader is referred to the list of suggested readings for further discussion of this issue.

SUGGESTED READING

Baker JW. A long jejunostomy tube for decomprising intestinal obstruction. Surg Gynecol obstet 1959;109;519.

Childs WA, Phillips RB. Experience with intestinal plication and a proposed modification. Ann Surg 1969;152:258–265.

Chilimindris CP, Stoneseifer GL. Complications associated with the Baker tube jejunostomy. Am Surg 1978;44:707.

Delaney HM, Carnevale NJ, Garvey JW. Jejunostomy by needle catheter technique. Surgery 1973;73:786.

Di Giacomo JC, Cottone FJ. Surgical treatment of Meckel's diverticulum. South Med J 1993;86:671.

Grassi CJ. Modified gastrojejunostomy tube: percutaneous placement for gastric decompression and jejunal feeding. Radiology 1989; 173:875.

Jönsson HJ, Zederfeldt B. Breaking strength of small intestinal anastomoses. Am J Surg 1983;145:800.

Lee KH, Yeung CK, Tam YH, et al. Laparoscopy for definitive diagnosis and treatment of gastrointestinal bleeding of obscure origin in children. J Pediatr Surg 2000;35:1291.

Matsagas IM, Fatouros M, Koulouras B, et al. Incidence, complications and management of Meckel's diverticulum. Arch Surg 1995; 130:143.

Nelson RL, Nyhus LM. A new long intestinal tube. Surg Gynecol Obstet 1979;149:581.

Noble, Jr TB. Plication of the small intestine: second report. Am J Surg 1939; 45:574–80.

Sangster W, Swanstrom L. Laparoscopic guided feeding jejunostomy. Surg Endosc 1993;7:308.

Schmid SW, Schafer M, Krahenbuhl L, et al. The role of laparoscopy in symptomatic Meckel's diverticulum. Surg Endosc 1999;13:1047.

Stewardson RH, Bombeck CT, Nyhus LM. Critical operative management of small bowel obstruction. Ann Surg 1978;187:189.

St. Vil D, Brandt ML, Panic S, et al. Meckel's diverticulum in children: a 20-year review. J Pediatr Surg 1991;26:1289.

Weigelt JA, Snyder WH III, Norman JL. Complications and results of 160 Baker tube plications. Am J Surg 1980;140:810.

EDITOR'S COMMENT

Adjunctive procedures in dealing with the gastrointestinal tract are extremely important, as they often may spell the difference between a smooth postoperative course and one that is troublesome. As with any surgical procedure, attention to detail and meticulous technique are essential, but in some of these procedures, such as a jejunostomy or a feeding jejunostomy, avoidance of intestinal obstruction with small sutures not narrowing the lumen and fastening to the abdominal wall are critical if one is to have a smooth postoperative course.

In a previous edition, I might have argued for the inclusion of gastrostomy in this chapter. However, it is not included, and I will not include it. The reason for this is the fact that evidence that nasogastric tubes do not change postoperative course and outcome has accumulated. While previously I would use gastrostomies routinely in left-sided colonic resections and even, fearing duodenal ileus, in a right hemicolectomy, I, like many other surgeons, am barely using nasogastric tubes, and if I do use one, for example, in a patient in whom I've carried out a left or right hemicolectomy, the nasogastric tube usually comes out the next day. The only situation in which I use a nasogastric tube for a more prolonged period of time is following, for example, a 6- or 8-hour fistula resection and reconstruction, in which the lysis of adhesion is generally carried out from the ligament of Treitz down to the ileocecal valve. There I may leave a nasogastric tube in for 48 hours, or possibly 60 or 72 hours on occasion. But that is the exception rather than the rule. Thus, in my practice nowadays, which includes many reoperative procedures and repair of enterocutaneous fistulas, inclusion of a gastrostomy done at a time of another procedure is a rarity rather than commonplace, as it once was. Inclusion of feeding jejunostomy, however, is common. I will use a feeding jejunostomy in any patient who has been hospitalized for a long time, and has had malnutrition, kwashiorkor, or marasmus as a diagnosis in a previously septic illness from which the patient has recovered, or is still septic when urgent operation is required. In a patient who has had what I call an "upper abdominal rearrangement," for example, in a gastrectomy that is not done well or in a Roux-en-Y that has become obstructed. Patients with preoperative weight loss, such as carcinoma of the esophagus in whom an Ivor Lewis procedure will be carried out, always get a feeding jejunostomy at the time of operation, and patients who are candidates for perioperative total parenteral nutrition (TPN) always get a feeding jejunostomy. My goal in the latter situation is to switch over from parenteral nutrition to enteral nutrition. There are times when this is not possible, and one must continue both parenteral and enteral nutrition. However, good evidence has accumulated that shows that even in the event one cannot meet all of the caloric and protein goals by enteral nutrition, giving as little as 20% of the total calories and protein is enough to result in the beneficial effects of enteral nutrition, which, to me, include stimulation of hepatic protein synthesis, stimulation of acute-phase protein from the liver, and perhaps a better outcome for multiple anastomoses due to early enteral feeding. Notice I have not said anything about maintaining the integrity of the tight junctions of the gut or preventing translocation. Happily, I have not heard those phrases in some time, and since the idea that the tight junctions are somehow disrupted by TPN have happily faded from the scene. Translocation is a normal phenomenon in which the macrophages and lymph nodes on the opposite side of the barrier sample those potential invaders that might be lurking and invade a weakened barrier, perhaps because of ischemia or a major burn. My technique for feeding jejunostomy differs from that described by Dr. Pollak. The reason is that I think a continuous suture in producing a Witzel tunnel may, in fact, prevent the placement of sutures that are particularly meticulous in narrowing as much of the small bowel as one can. Like Dr. Pollak, I use a 000 chromic purse-string on the antimesenteric border. I then make a hole and use a 14 Robinson nephrostomy catheter, with an extra hole cut, and pass the catheter distally, until only

(continued)

approximately one third of the catheter is showing. I then tie the purse-string, and place the suture through the serosa of the tube, not into the lumen, but enough to catch the rubber and tie it in place. Then the difference: to create the Witzel tunnel, I will place five or six interrupted 0000 silk sutures, and hold them until I believe that I adequately cover the tube but do not narrow the small bowel to too great an extent. These are then tied. The tube is passed through a stab wound in the abdominal wall retrograde, and I then place 0000 silk sutures on either side of the tube hole to fixate it on a broad base, similar to what Dr. Pollak describes, to make certain that a volvulus around the feeding jejunostomy does not occur. One also should be meticulous at not narrowing the jejunostomy. There is a phenomenon of hold-up of the jejunostomy at 5 to 7 days, similar to that of stomal dysfunction, which one used to see in the old gastrectomy days. Usually it is associated with vomiting a bilious material while the tube feedings continue unobstructed. If one wishes put Gastrografin down, one sees a hold-up at the tube jejunostomy. In my experience, placing a nasogastric tube at this point, and placing it in suction for 2 days, generally results in the obstruction subsiding, without any need to do anything except nasogastric suction.

Noble plications and Baker tubes are mentioned only as a matter of historic interest. Dr. Pollak is right that doing a Noble plication to a distended edematous gut has no place in the armamentarium, and it does result in many postoperative fistulas. Data are beginning to emerge that there may be a place for long Miller-Abbot tube decompression early in the postoperative period, following postoperative obstruction. Again, the data are very soft, and nasogastric tube suction may be as good, but there are glimmers of data suggesting that this may be the case. However, one cannot say this with certainty.

If one is inclined to pass a Miller-Abbot tube, this is a skill that has long been lost. I believe that the Miller-Abbot tube is superior to most of the other substitute tubes. The following is the way I place the tube:

1. Measure where the tip is with respect to where you think the pylorus lies. Mark the tube where it comes out of the nares.
2. Then insert the tube. The patient is placed on the right side. The tube is not placed to suction.
3. Allow the patient to stay on his or her right side for 2 hours, and then send the patient down to radiography for a KUB (kidneys, ureters, and bladder), judging whether or not the tube is in the first or second portion of the duodenum. If it is not, ask the radiologist to pass it.
4. If difficulty is encountered in the tube's passage, perform endoscopy and pass the tube through the pylorus.
5. Initially, the tube is placed to gravity with a 4- to 6-in. loop taped to the side of the face. Once the tube passes the pylorus and heads downstream, it is advanced 3 in. every 4 hours, again taking it off suction while advancing and leaving it taped to the side of the face with the loop.

Meckel diverticula are frequently encountered in laparotomies, as they occur in 2% of the population. In my dealing with the Meckel diverticulum that is asymptomatic and uncomplicated, I make certain there is no mass, for occasionally an adenocarcinoma occurs in the Meckel diverticulum. If there is no mass, it is left alone. I think the number of times that one can place a stapler across the base of a rather broad Meckel diverticulum is few and far between, but if the occasion occurs, then one oversews that with a running suture line of 000 chromic and then 000 Lembert on the way back, followed by some 0000 silks. But as I say, this is few and far between. I think it is easier and far better to do a formal small bowel resection, with two layers of interrupted 0000 silk. As expected, one sometimes has difficulty in determining whether or not the Meckel diverticulum is symptomatic. This is a diagnosis of exclusion.

Of course, laparoscopy has also entered into the field of deciding when to do feeding jejunostomies. To my way of thinking, a short left upper quadrant incision under local sedation, determining the oral and abdominal–oral path of jejunum between 15 and 20 cm from the ligament of Treitz at the very shortest, and doing the usual feeding jejunostomy are described. Laparoscopic feeding jejunostomy is, of course, carried out. However, if feeding jejunostomy needs to be carried out as part of a more major procedure such as, for example, colectomy or a resection for Crohn disease, the reader can learn more about this in Chapter 127 in this book.

J.E.F.

Chapter 124, see www.masteryofsurgery.com

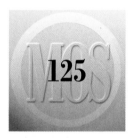

125

The Continent Ileostomy

ERIC J. DOZOIS AND ROGER R. DOZOIS

The continent reservoir ileostomy, commonly referred to as the *Kock pouch*, comprises an internal ileal reservoir that stores stool and gas between intubations, a stoma and outflow tract needed to intubate and evacuate the contents of the reservoir, and a surgically created biologic valve interposed between the other two components to act as a pressure barrier and provide continence. The major advantages of this operation over the conventional spout ileostomy are the elimination of the necessity for the patient to continually wear an external appliance and a much less conspicuous stoma.

HISTORICAL BACKGROUND AND RATIONALE

Although patients and their caregivers recognize the benefits of proctocolectomy and Brooke ileostomy, a curative operation that restores the patient's health, it has become evident that for many ileostomates, the need to constantly wear an external appliance to collect the effluent of an incontinent stoma can interfere with some of their daily activities and their social life, and be detrimental to their overall quality of life. Also, the material necessary to pouch the stoma is expensive. Although an incontinent Brooke-type stoma is acceptable to most ostomy patients, primarily because they regain their general health, as many as 40% of these patients long for a better alternative. By surgically devising an internal reservoir capable of collecting the bowel contents and by rendering it continent by adding a valve mechanism so that patients no longer have to wear an external appliance, Nils Kock of Göteborg, Sweden, revolutionized the concept of surgically created continence and unknowingly paved the way for the ileal pouch anal anastomosis.

The construction of an intestinal reservoir to substitute for the loss of rectal capacity evolved rapidly when a U-shaped, double-folded reservoir was designed by Kock and his colleagues. The means to achieve continence, however, were slower to evolve. At first, Kock hoped that continence could be achieved by external compression of the outflow tract brought through the rectus abdominis muscle, but this proved unreliable. Interposition of an antiperistaltic segment of ileum between the reservoir and the stoma also proved inefficient. In 1972, Kock ingeniously devised the intussusception ileal valve, the so-called nipple valve, using an isoperistaltic portion of the outflow tract, which resulted in a far more reliable continence mechanism.

A number of technical refinements were later added to compensate for the weaker mesenteric side of the intussuscepted ileal segment, including stripping off the peritoneum and defatting the mesentery of the valve, placement of "rotation" sutures, reinforcement by a mesenteric sling of synthetic mesh encompassing the outflow tract, and stapling the antimesenteric side of the valve to the side wall of the reservoir.

At the Mayo Clinic, the efforts to construct and perfect the continent ileostomy were spearheaded by Oliver H. Beahrs in the early 1970s. Initially, the valve was made 3 cm in length and anchored in place with through-and-through nonabsorbable silk sutures. Subsequently, and with the hope of reducing valve slippage and valve fistula, the nipple was made longer (5 cm), was anchored in place with both absorbable sutures and staples, and interrupted sutures were added between the base of the reservoir and the outflow tract to further anchor the intussusceptum. We have been reluctant to use Marlex mesh, which may result in fistula formation across the nipple valve.

CURRENT INDICATIONS AND CONTRAINDICATIONS

Although the ileal pouch anal anastomosis is now preferred by most patients requiring proctocolectomy, the continent ileostomy remains a viable alternative to the Brooke ileostomy for certain categories of patients, which include (a) patients with an existing conventional Brooke ileostomy with no possibility of an ileal pouch anal anastomosis (no anal sphincter) who want to improve their quality of life, (b) patients requiring a proctocolectomy who wish to preserve continence but are not suitable candidates for an ileoanal anastomosis, most often because of poor anal sphincter function, (c) the rare patients whose daily work takes them away from toilet facilities for long periods of time and who prefer a continent ileostomy to an ileoanal anastomosis, and (d) patients with a failed ileoanal anastomosis who desire to preserve continence and avoid an external appliance if the failure is unrelated to Crohn disease or severe pouchitis.

Use of the Kock pouch should be discouraged in (a) older patients who may be more prone to postoperative complications, including valve dysfunction, and may not tolerate reoperation, (b) patients with Crohn disease, (c) obese patients, (d) critically ill patients such as those with toxic megacolon, (e) psychologically unfit patients who may not be able to intubate properly or tolerate complications and reoperations, and (f) patients in whom a significant amount of small intestine has already been removed.

THE OPERATION

The distal 45 cm of the ileum is used to construct the reservoir, the valve, and the

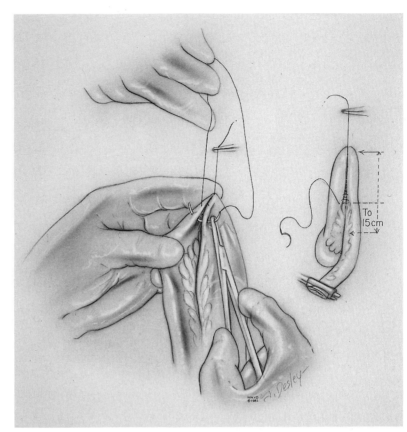

Fig. 1. The two 15-cm limbs of the folded 30-cm loop are approximated with continuous 2-0 chromic catgut placed near the mesenteric border of the bowel. (Modified from Beahrs OH. Continent ileostomy. In: *Surgical techniques illustrated,* vol 3. Boston: Little, Brown and Company, 1978.)

outflow tract (efferent limb). Beginning 15 cm from the cut end of the distal ileum, a 30-cm segment of ileum is measured and fashioned into a U (Fig. 1). The antimesenteric borders of the two 15-cm limbs of the U are approximated with continuous suture of 2-0 chromic catgut. The two limbs are then incised on their antimesenteric borders, with the incision extending 4 to 5 cm longer on the afferent limb than on the efferent limb so that the two limbs separate as the pouch is constructed. A second layer of continuous chromic catgut is used to approximate the mucosa and complete the posterior wall of the reservoir (Fig. 2).

The valve is then fashioned. The serosal surface of the efferent limb of the ileum is scarified, with the electrocautery beginning at the pouch and extending for a distance of 10 cm toward the cut end. The peritoneum of that same segment is also stripped from the adjacent mesentery, which is also defatted. These maneuvers are designed to promote adherence of the ileum and its mesentery when the efferent limb is intussuscepted into the pouch to fashion the valve.

The 10-cm efferent limb is intussuscepted into the pouch to form a nipple valve of approximately 5 cm in length. The intussusceptum is fixed in place with through-and-through sutures of 2-0 Vicryl (polyglactin 910) and three cartridges of stainless steel staples along both sides of the mesentery, care being taken to avoid injury to the vascular supply, and immediately opposite the mesentery using the GIA (U.S. Surgical Corp., Norwalk, CT) autosuture apparatus (Fig. 3). The placement of the staples and sutures is facilitated by "stenting" the lumen of the intussusceptum with a No. 28 French catheter.

The bottom of the U is then folded over to construct the anterior wall of the reservoir, using two layers of continuous 2-0 chromic catgut (Fig. 2). The outflow tract is sutured to the base of the pouch with interrupted 3-0 nonabsorbable sutures at the exit of the limb from the pouch to further anchor the intussusceptum in place (Fig. 3).

A circumferential defect is created through the abdominal wall just above the pubic hairline in the right lower quadrant, and the outflow tract is brought through the defect and amputated flush with the skin and matured into a stoma with interrupted 3-0 chromic catgut. The length of ileum between the pouch and the stoma

The Gastrointestinal Tract

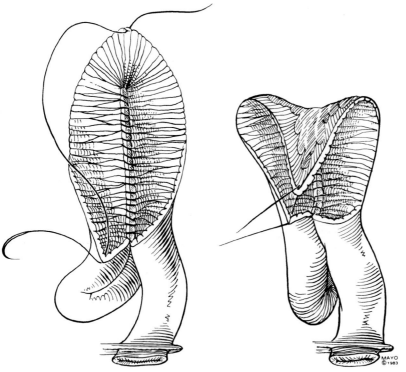

Fig. 2. The two approximated limbs are incised and a second row of continuous 2-0 chromic catgut sutures is used to approximate the mucosa before the apex of the opened loop is folded over. (From Dozois RR, Kelly KA, Beart RW, et al. Continent ileostomy: the Mayo Clinic experience. In: Dozois RR. *Alternatives to conventional ileostomy.* Chicago: Year Book Medical Publishers, 1985.)

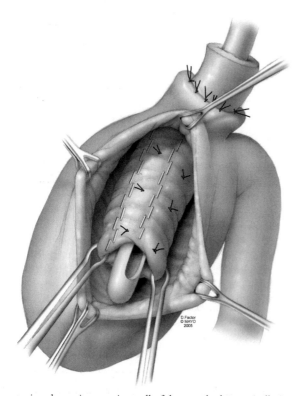

Fig. 3. Prior to suturing the entire anterior wall of the pouch, the surgically intussuscepted efferent limb is held in place with interrupted sutures of 2-0 polyglycolic acid and three rows of stainless steel staples to form the nipple valve. This is facilitated if done over a catheter. Interrupted sutures of 2-0 polyglycolic acid placed between the base of the reservoir and efferent ileal limb help anchor further the intussuscepted segment within the pouch. Suturing of the anterior wall of the pouch is then completed in two rows. For revisions caused by valve slippage, the same procedure can be performed after the anterior wall of the pouch is reopened and the valve pulled back into the reservoir with Babcock clamps.

should be kept short to avoid tortuosity and facilitate later intubation of the reservoir. This is aided by suturing the pouch to the undersurface of the anterior abdominal wall so that the nipple valve is perfectly aligned with the stoma (Fig. 4).

A No. 28 French catheter is passed through the stoma, efferent limb, and nipple valve, and its tip is positioned within the lumen of the pouch before the incision is closed. A suture of heavy silk is tied around the catheter at the level of the stoma so that the exact position of the catheter can easily be ascertained in the postoperative period. These precautions help prevent pouch perforation or tube slippage during postoperative recovery.

POSTOPERATIVE AND POSTHOSPITALIZATION CARE

In the immediate postoperatiave days, the ileal pouch is irrigated with 25 mL of physiologic saline twice a day to maintain the patency of the catheter, which is connected to a drainage bag. When spontaneous bowel function returns, oral alimentation can be resumed. Before dismissal from the hospital, approximately 8 to 10 days postoperatively, patients are taught self-catheterization by the stoma therapist.

On leaving the hospital, patients are given a catheter designed to drain the pouch (either an ileostomy catheter, M8730 [Atlantic Surgical Co., Inc., Merrick, NY], or an ileal pouch catheter [Dow-Corning Co., Midland, MI]). The Atlantic ileostomy catheter has a diameter of approximately 9 mm (No. 28 French) and a length of 30 cm, whereas the Dow-Corning ileal pouch catheter has a diameter of approximately 1 cm (No. 30 French) and a length of approximately 64 cm. Each catheter has a thin wall and large holes at the insertion end just proximal to its bullet-shaped blunt tip. The patient keeps the catheter in a small plastic case, which is carried at all times.

When the patient experiences a sensation of fullness, the pouch requires emptying. To empty the pouch, the patient passes the catheter through the stoma into the pouch, usually in the sitting position. The ileal contents spontaneously drain by gravity through the catheter directly into the toilet or another suitable receptacle. The Valsalva maneuver and direct manual compression of the abdomen over the pouch area may at times facilitate drainage, but routine irrigations are not required. The catheter then is removed from the pouch, rinsed clean, and replaced in its case for later use. A soft gauze pad with a waterproof surface is taped over the stoma to absorb

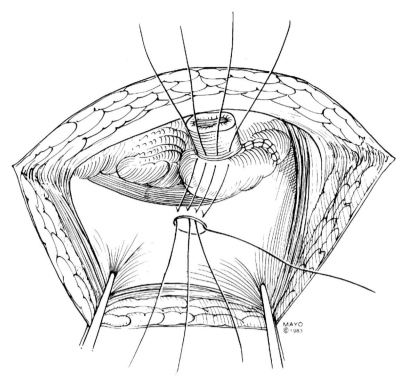

Fig. 4. The reservoir and outflow tract are anchored to the undersurface of the abdominal wall immediately underneath the stoma site to facilitate future intubation. (From Dozois RR, Kelly KA, Beart RW, et al. Continent ileostomy: the Mayo Clinic experience. In: Dozois RR. *Alternatives to conventional ileostomy.* Chicago: Year Book Medical Publishers, 1985.)

any mucus secreted by the stoma. Patients rapidly become proficient at this procedure, which requires 5 to 10 minutes to complete. None of our patients has ever perforated the pouch with the catheter.

Some patients have found that partially digestible substances, such as seeds, apple skins, celery, and mushrooms, may plug the catheter, so they have avoided these foods. Others, however, have found that all foods can be eaten, provided they are thoroughly masticated before being swallowed.

Four to 6 weeks after operation, restrictions on physical activities are removed. Pregnancy is not contraindicated. Many patients who have undergone this procedure have become pregnant and have delivered healthy babies, either vaginally or by cesarean section.

RESULTS

Between November 1971 and December 1981, 460 patients had a continent ileostomy constructed at the Mayo Medical Center in Rochester, Minnesota. Since 1982 and with the advent of the ileal pouch anal anastomosis, approximately 12 continent ileostomies are either constructed or revised each year.

In our series of patients, no pouch-related deaths occurred intraoperatively or postoperatively. The mean postoperative

hospital stay was 10 days. Because of careful patient selection, greater experience, avoidance of a Kock pouch in patients with Crohn disease, and favoring of valve revision over pouch excision when serious complications occur, we have had to excise the reservoir in fewer than 3% of cases.

REVISIONAL SURGERY

Persistent difficulties with pouch intubation and/or incontinence related to nipple valve malfunction has necessitated reoperation in 10% to 20% of patients. In most patients, valve dysfunction occurs within 6 months after construction of the pouch (Fig. 5), after which the need for revision decreases dramatically. Malfunction is most often caused by extrusion of the valve and its mesentery, which results in elongation and tortuosity of the efferent limb. As a consequence, the pouch is difficult to intubate as the tip of the catheter may not be maneuvered easily into the pouch lumen, and the pouch leaks. A pouchogram can confirm the clinical suspicion of valve deintussusception. If intubation by the patient or the treating physician is impossible, bowel obstruction will ensue, and a rigid endoscope must be inserted into the pouch lumen to aspirate its contents and place a catheter.

Factors that influence the need for valve revision include age, gender, type of operation, and body habitus (Table 1).

Pouch Malfunction from Valve Failure

When valve malfunction occurs, most often reoperation is necessary. The nature of valve revision needed depends on the type of complication and the anatomic configuration of the valve at the time of surgical exploration. After the stoma, the efferent limb, and the reservoir are dissected free from the abdominal wall and fully mobilized, the

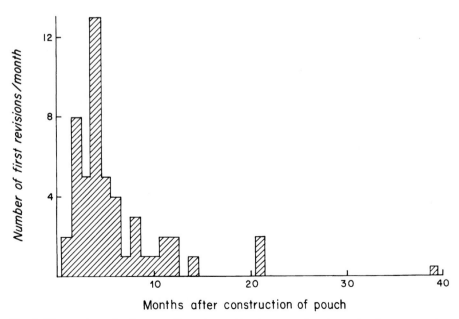

Fig. 5. The number of patients needing valve revision is greatest 2 to 6 months after construction of the pouch (From Dozois RR, Kelly KA. The surgical management of ulcerative colitis. In: Kirsner JB, ed. *Inflammatory bowel disease*, 5th ed. Philadelphia: WB Saunders, 2000:626.)

The Gastrointestinal Tract

TABLE 1. FACTORS INFLUENCING VALVE REVISION IN PATIENTS UNDERGOING THE KOCK POUCH PROCEDURE

Factor	Revisions (%)	P value[a]
Age[b]		
<40 y	20	<.05
≥40 y	35	
Gender[b]		
Women	17	<.05
Men	28	
Operation[b]		
Colectomy and pouch	16	<.05
Conversion of ileostomy	30	
Obesity[c]		
Yes	75	<.05
No	23	

[a]Estimates of cumulative probability were based on multivariate analysis.
[b]Data from Dozois RR, Kelly KA, Ilstrup E, et al. Factors affecting revision rate after continent ileostomy. *Arch Surg* 1981;116:610.
[c]Data from Schrock TR. Complications of continent ileostomy. *Am J Surg* 1979;138:162.

pouch lumen is entered through an incision in its anterior wall. If the valve has become deintussuscepted into the mesenteric side of the reservoir and outflow tract, the existing nipple valve is pulled back into the reservoir with Babcock clamps and the valve is reanchored with a combination of sutures and stainless steel staples. The pouch incision is closed in two layers, the pouch is again fixed to the undersurface of the abdominal wall, and the stoma is rematured in the same location. If the existing valve cannot be used because of extensive fibrosis, stenosis, or a fistula through the valve, then the stoma, the efferent limb (outflow tract), and the valve are excised and a new valve is created from the afferent limb (inflow tract), which is transected approximately 15 cm proximally (Fig. 6A). The proximal cut edge is then anastomosed to the ileal pouch at the site of the excised valve (Fig. 6B) after the pouch has been rotated clockwise.

Failed Ileoanal Anastomosis Converted to Kock Pouch

On rare occasions, a poorly functioning ileal pouch-anal anastomosis can be converted to a continent ileostomy using the existing ileal reservoir. In order to qualify for this type of revisional surgery, failure of the ileoanal anastomosis must NOT be attributable to either Crohn disease or severe, recalcitrant pouchitis. Indeed, in our institution, patients who have had their ileoanal converted to a Kock pouch were patients with poor functional results primarily to the result of inadequate anal sphincters, and who had a strong desire to preserve continence.

If the patient still elects to have the failed ileal pouch-anal anastomosis converted to a

Kock pouch after detailed and frank discussions about the limitations and risks of such an attempt, the existing ileal reservoir may be used, as long as the pouch can be fully mobilized from the pelvis intact after disconnection it from the anal canal (Fig. 7A). The ileum immediately above the reservoir is then transected 15 cm proximally and serves to construct the valve, the efferent limb, and stoma (Fig. 7A,B). The proximal cut end is then anastomosed to the defect in the reservoir, resulting from disconnecting the ileal reservoir from the anal canal area (Fig. 7B).

POUCHITIS SYNDROME

Some patients develop a nonspecific inflammation of the reservoir characterized clinically by the sudden onset of diarrhea, cramping, low-grade fever, and, at times, bleeding. Endoscopic findings include mucosal erythema, friability, and easy bleeding. In the majority of patients, symptoms and signs of pouchitis abate readily with administration of oral antibiotics such as metronidazole or ciprofloxacin, which suggests that overgrowth of anaerobic bacteria in the pouch or the more proximal jejunoileum may be responsible for the diarrhea syndrome. In some cases, however (<5%), the pouchitis recurs soon after discontinuation of therapy or may be recalcitrant to treatment and lead to failure.

QUALITY OF LIFE

The crucial consideration in assessing the value of the continent ileostomy is whether it is sufficiently continent for the

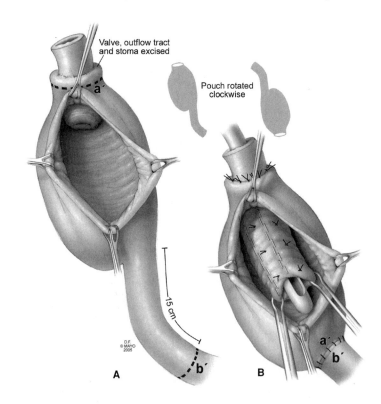

Fig. 6. If the existing valve cannot be used because of extensive valvular fibrosis, ischemia, or a fistula, the existing outflow tract and valve need to be excised (dotted line, a')**(A)**, the pouch is rotated clockwise after transecting the inflow tract, and a new valve, outflow tract, and stoma are reconstructed from the "old" inflow tract **(A)**. The operation is completed by suturing the proximal cut end of the inflow tract (b') to the defect created by removing the dysfunctional valve (a')**(B)**.

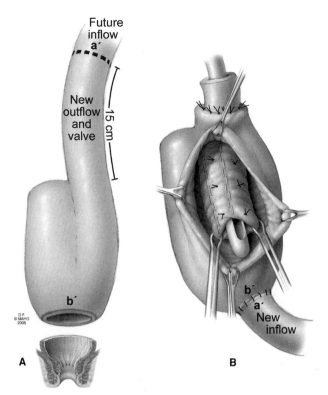

Fig. 7. Conversion of failed ileoanal anastomosis to Kock pouch. After mobilization of the entire ileal reservoir through an abdominal incision, the ileal reservoir is transected proximal to the anal anastomosis **(A)**. The ileum is then transected 15 cm proximal to the pouch. The latter segment of ileum is then used to create the valve mechanism and outflow tract **(B)**. The operation is completed by anastomosing the cut end of the proximal ileum (a') to the transected ileal reservoir (b'), thus creating a new inflow tract.

concerns about the social, psychological, and sexual disadvantages of the Brooke ileostomy. The long-term effects of the continent ileostomy are unknown. As yet, metabolic, nutritional, hepatic, renal, and oncologic complications have not appeared after continent ileostomy. The Kock pouch procedure should be done primarily in centers at which the operation is performed in sufficient numbers to enable the surgical team to become proficient, and at which careful follow-up is available.

ACKNOWLEDGMENTS

The senior author is deeply indebted to Oliver H. Beahrs for his invaluable teaching of this operation, and to Kathleen Polikowsky and Rosemary Armstrong for their expert assistance in the conduct of several of these operations during a period of more than 20 years.

SUGGESTED READING

Beahrs OH, Kelly KA, Adson MA, et al. Ileostomy with ileal reservoir rather than ileostomy alone. *Ann Surg* 1974;179:634.

Cohen Z. Evolution of the Kock continent ileostomy. *Can J Surg* 1982;25:509.

Dozois RR, Kelly KA, Beart RW. Improved results with continent ileostomy. *Ann Surg* 1980;192:319.

Dozois RR, Kelly KA, Ilstrup D, et al. Factors affecting revision rate after continent ileostomy. *Arch Surg* 1981;116:610.

Fazio VW, Church JM. Complications and function of the continent ileostomy at the Cleveland Clinic. *World J Surg* 1988;12:148.

Kelly DG, Phillips SF, Kelly KA, et al. Dysfunction of the continent ileostomy: clinical features and bacteriology. *Gut* 1983;24:193.

Kock NG. Continent ileostomy: historical perspectives. In: Dozois RR, ed. *Alternatives to conventional ileostomy*. Chicago: Year Book Medical Publishers, 1985:133.

Kock NG, Darle N, Kewenter J, et al. Quality of life after proctocolectomy and ileostomy: a study of patients with conventional ileostomies converted to continent ileostomies. *Dis Colon Rectum* 1974;17:287.

Mullen P, Behrens D, Chalmers T, et al. Barnett continent intestinal reservoir: multicenter experience with an alternative to the Brooke ileostomy. *Dis Colon Rectum* 1995; 38:573.

Pemberton JH, Dozois RR. The continent ileostomy. In: Farnell MB, McIlrath DC, eds. *Problems in general surgery*. Philadelphia: JB Lippincott, 1984:1:27.

Pemberton JH, Phillips SF, Ready RR, et al. Quality of life after Brooke ileostomy and ileal pouch-anal anastomosis: comparison of performance status. *Ann Surg* 1989;209:620.

Schjonsby H, Halvorsen JF, Hofstad T, et al. Stagnant loop syndrome in patients with continent ileostomy (intra-abdominal ileal reservoir). *Gut* 1977;18:795.

patient to avoid the need to wear an external appliance. In our experience, as well as that of others, more than 90% of patients eventually are continent enough that they never have to wear an appliance (Table 2). Also, when quality of life after continent ileostomy was compared with that after a Brooke ileostomy, satisfaction was found to be greater, and the desire to change to a different alternative was found to be less in patients with a Kock pouch than in those with a Brooke ileostomy. Finally, in each performance category, more patients with a Kock pouch than patients with an incontinent Brooke ileostomy improved in their daily activities. Although the role of continent ileostomy is more limited since the advent of the ileoanal anastomosis, our experience as well as that of many others confirm the favorable results of Kock himself, and encourage its continued use in specific circumstances.

Because of its substantial physical and psychological benefits over the conventional ileostomy, the appliance-free continent ileostomy continues to have an important place in the overall armamentarium for dealing with ulcerative colitis or familial polyposis.

The current refined operative approach offers a high probability of complete continence. Careful selection of patients further increases the chances of success and reduces the need for reoperation. The operation is most attractive to young people, especially the unmarried, who have great

TABLE 2. QUALITY OF LIFE AFTER CONTINENT ILEOSTOMY

Reference	Never Wear Appliance (%)
Kock (1985)	98
Cohen (1982)	97
Fazio and Church (1988)	91
Ecker (1999)	98
Mullen et al. (1995)[a]	92
Schrock (1979)	90
Dozois and Kelly (2000)	95

[a]Used Barnett continent intestinal reservoir, a modification of the Kock pouch that includes a "living collar" of small bowel wrapped around the outflow tract to help improve continence.

EDITOR'S COMMENT

It is clear from writings and the literature that, except for a few centers, namely, University of Goteborg and the Barnett Clinics, that most patients who end up with a continent ileostomy fall into two categories, the first being a failed ileal pouch-anal anastomosis and the second being conversion from a standard ileostomy. As the authors state, many of their patients, in whom they have performed almost 500 procedures, are patients who would like to have converted a standard ileostomy to a continent ileostomy. The reasons for the standard ileostomy are not difficult to understand. Many patients are quite ill when undergoing proctocolectomy and their focus is on getting better. It is only when they do get better and they review their situation that they would like a better quality of life, which, one suspects, is the principal reason why most patients receive a continent ileostomy.

One should make the point that a continent ileostomy only restores quality of life when, in fact, it is continent, which is of course its Achilles heel. Reoperations are common, and not infrequently—perhaps up to 30% or 40%—one has to deal with a slipped valve. Nor is it necessarily true, as the authors state, that some patients undergo continent ileostomy because they are somewhat tired of having to worry about finding a bathroom when they go outside. Indeed, Berndtsson et al. (*J Wound Ostomy Continence Nurs* 2005;32(5):321) described long-term adjustment for patients with a continent ileostomy. There were 68 patients (25 male and 43 female) who apparently underwent continent ileostomy and proctocolectomy as their initial operation for ulcerative colitis. The mean time of follow-up was 31 years (range, 29 to 36) and the median subject age at this point was 60, which makes sense as ulcerative colitis tends to be a young person's disease. A 36-item questionnaire was used to assess adjustment to the continent ileostomy, and subjects used a 6-point Likert scale for grading. If they did not like the question, they could avoid it. High median adjustment ratings were found for all 36 statements, but the maximum median rating of 6 appeared on 28 items. Eight items had low median ratings which included embarrassing situations, activity, body image, sexuality, and good care. Despite the analysis, which indicated that the patients, for the most part, were self-reliant, impediments to bowel evacuation outside the home were common in their responses to the questionnaire, indicating that they had limited outside-the-home activity. Specifically, they mentioned the quality and availability of public restrooms, which reduced their daily activities away from home. Apparently, this finding is for patients with continent ileostomies and not incontinent ileostomies, which, if it occurs, tends to really interfere with activity and requires revision.

The authors state that Kock probably was the person who ultimately was responsible for the concept of the pouch. This subsequently evolved with the aid of Sir Alan Parks, who proposed the S pouch initially, but with a long spout, which necessitated

that these patients catheterized themselves. Lester Martin, a pediatric surgeon in Cincinnati with whom I had the pleasure of working, probably is responsible for taking the concept of the Soave procedure in Hirschsprung disease and, with the mucosal stripping, applying it to the ileal pouch-anal anastomosis with a short spout, thus obviating the need for self-catheterization. Dr. Ollie Beahrs at the Mayo Clinic was among the first to apply the Kock pouch to the American population. The main problem with a Kock pouch is the nipple. There have been innumerable ways of trying to stabilize the nipple so that it does not slip. These methods include through-and-through nonabsorbable sutures, through-and-through absorbable sutures, scarification of the serosa, stripping of the mesentery, Marlex mesh, and stapling. The authors have stated that they have not used Marlex mesh for fear of fistula, which I suppose is a possibility. In patients that I have operated on for continent ileostomies, I have tended to use mesenteric stripping, almost to the point of rendering the nipple ischemic (my response to residents who point out that the nipple is blue, is that at least it's not black). I then use Marlex mesh and four rows of staples. The problem is, however, on the side that is close to the ileal wall, generally the side of the mesentery. And here one must use through-and-through sutures because stapling is too difficult to carry out with the ileostomy adjacent to the wall. This probably provides the most secure form. In addition, a flat abdominal film can always be obtained if one is concerned about slippage, and whether or not the staples form a line then becomes easily known to the surgeon.

Castillo et al. (*Dis Colon Rectum* 2005;48(6):1263) reviewed 24 patients: 13 were operated on for a Brooke ileostomy, which they wanted continent; 7 for a failed ileal pouch; 3 for colonic inertia and incontinence; and 1 patient with multiple failed operations for Hirschsprung disease. Twenty-eight revisions were performed in 14 patients (58%), with 6 patients requiring multiple procedures. This is not unusual. Of these revisions, 11 operations were for valve repairs and 12 were for skin level revision for stenosis. Two patients lost their pouches, one because of Crohn disease and the other because of inability to manage the pouch. In a report on a conference in Israel headed by Rachmelewich, Kock reported on a group of patients; 92% were continent, but some required six revisions. In this chapter the need for revision in 12 months was 29%, but the average time period before the first revision was 24 months. Total failure rate was 8.3%. Ninety percent of the patients still have their pouches and are satisfied with pouch function, although this was not formally evaluated. The unhappiness with the pouch has led some, including the group headed by Dr. Robert Beart Jr. at the Keck School of Medicine, University of Southern California (Kaiser AM, et al. *Dis Colon Rectum* 2002;45(3):411), to try to adapt a T-pouch valve concept, which has been used for urinary reservoirs by Dr. Skinner and his group in the creation of an ileostomy. The valve is apparently created by embed-

ding a segment of bowel with blood supply intact in a serosa-lined tunnel of two apposed limbs of bowel that will form the pouch reservoir. They reported six patients with complete continence of the pouch. This is an interesting, but sounds like a very complicated, solution to a difficult problem. I have been unable to locate any article written in follow-up of the report.

Another problem that has not received a great deal of publicity is neoplasia in patients with familial adenomatous polyposis who undergo pouch surgery (Church J. *Dis Colon Rectum* 2005;48 (9):1708). We are all familiar with the ileal pouch-anal anastomosis and anastomotic cancers, and this is variously blamed on rectal mucosa, which is not completely stripped or is covered by the pouch. However, the risk factors with adenomas or adenomatous epithelium in contact with rectal epithelium are not known. Therefore, it comes as some surprise that, in this review of the literature, the median time from pouch construction to pouch adenomas was 4.7 years. Eight patients with cancer at the ileal pouch-anal anastomosis site were diagnosed a median of 8 years after pouch construction. What was of interest was that there were eight case reports of cancer described in ileostomy in patients with familial adenomatous polyposis, in which the problem of a rectal segment interacting with the ileostomy presumably was not present. Here, the median time from construction of the ileostomy to the discovery of the cancers was 25 years, with a range of 9 to 40 years. The author blames fecal stasis, adenomatous epithelium, a germline APC mutation, with the emphasis on fecal stasis, as a recipe for epithelial neoplasia. Although it does happen in ileostomy, it seems to happen much faster in an ileal pouch. One assumes that this is the same possibility that one must be on guard for with a continent ileostomy, in which stasis is a continuing issue.

Pouchitis is a continual problem in these patients, as it is in patients with ileal pouch-anal anastomosis. My technique differs slightly, not only with the nipple, but in the use of a Malecot or perhaps the Pezar catheter, which does not run the risk of dislodgement, although it is a little more difficult to get the catheter out, especially if it's large (No. 28 or 30), without damaging the bowel.

All in all, the continent ileostomy remains a reasonable alternative to patients who would like to be continent, particularly if sexual difficulties are paramount in their minds. It is true that these patients have second thoughts about the ileostomy, which they may have accepted the first time but not as time went on. After 400 ileal pouch-anal anastomoses, with quite a low complication rate, except for pouchitis (chronic pouchitis in 6%), which I attribute to too long a spout, to my mind this is a useful alternative under circumstances in which the sphincter has been removed, and one does not get a wink and total removal of the anal and rectal mucosa.

J.E.F.

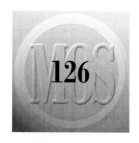

Gastrointestinal-Cutaneous Fistulae

JOSEF E. FISCHER AND AMY R. EVENSON

Enterocutaneous fistulae (ECF) represent catastrophic complications from abdominal diseases and surgical procedures. Although rare, the physiologic challenges to patients, the resources used, and the morbidity and mortality resulting from their occurrence are substantial. Modern management strategies have resulted in an improved overall mortality from nearly 50% in the 1940s to between 10% and 20% in recent series, with complications of sepsis responsible for the majority of deaths.

Gastrointestinal fistulae may be categorized as internal or external. Abnormal connections between hollow viscera that do not communicate with the skin are classified as internal fistulae. Examples of internal fistulae include ileoileal fistulae, ileocolic fistulae, enterovesical or colovesical fistulae, gastrocolic fistulae, enterovaginal or colovaginal fistulae, and fistulae to the thoracic cavity. Intervention for internal fistulae is indicated when the communication is dangerous or symptomatic. Appropriate therapy for internal fistulae requiring treatment consists of resection and reanastomosis. The focus of the current discussion is external fistulae, or communications between the gastrointestinal system and the skin.

Enterocutaneous fistulae may complicate nearly any abdominal surgical procedure during which the bowel integrity is compromised either intentionally or inadvertently. Given the substantial impact of ECFs, an understanding of their cause and prevention as well as their identification and management is important for all surgeons of the peritoneal cavity.

ETIOLOGY AND PREVENTION

Enterocutaneous fistulae result from one of several conditions: (a) extension of bowel abnormalities to surrounding structures, (b) extension of adjacent disease to normal bowel, (c) inadvertent or unrecognized trauma to the bowel, or (d) anastomotic disruption (Table 1). Seventy to ninety percent of ECFs occur in the postoperative period. Operations for complications of inflammatory bowel disease, resection of malignancy, or adhesiolysis for intestinal obstruction are common antecedent procedures. Preoperative factors may increase the likelihood of development of an ECF. These factors include malnutrition, infection, and emergency procedures with concomitant hypotension, anemia, hypothermia, or poor oxygen delivery. In the elective procedure, these aggravating factors should be corrected prior to operation with nutritional support, bowel preparation, and control of physiologic parameters such as cardiac output, blood glucose, and anemia. Ideally, the serum albumin level should be greater than 3 g/dL and the patient will not have lost more than 10% to 15% of body weight in the preceding months. Diabetes should be controlled, and the patient should not be anemic. Mechanical and antibiotic bowel preparation as well as intravenous antibiotics just prior to incision will further decrease the incidence of intra-abdominal and wound infections and abscesses, thus further reducing the likelihood of developing an ECF.

For patients undergoing emergency procedures, however, optimization of resuscitation and performance of a technically meticulous procedure may be the only steps the surgeon can take to prevent ECF. Sound surgical technique including adequate mobilization, use of healthy bowel with good blood supply for anastomosis, avoidance of tension, and prevention of hematoma will minimize the risks of formation of an ECF. Additionally, prior to abdominal closure, the bowel should be inspected for inadvertent bowel injury, and all enterotomies or serosal injuries should be appropriately repaired.

Spontaneous ECFs most commonly occur in settings of inflammation, malignancy, or irradiation. Inflammatory causes of ECFs include Crohn disease, ulcerative colitis, peptic ulcer disease, appendicitis, diverticulitis, pancreatitis, and ischemic bowel. Of these inflammatory conditions, ECFs in patients with inflammatory bowel disease represent a special concern for the surgeon. Often, fistulae in these patients will resolve with nonoperative management with parenteral nutrition, only to reopen on resumption of enteral feedings. These ECFs are best resected once closed, to prevent recurrence. A second important distinction that is specific to patients with Crohn disease involves whether the fistula arises in healthy bowel (following resection of a diseased segment) or in diseased bowel (not necessarily following bowel resection). The former type responds to nonoperative therapy and has a significant likelihood of spontaneous closure, and the latter type has a low rate of nonoperative closure. Patients with this type of ECF may benefit from early resection. ECFs in patients with malignancy or following radiation therapy are another special case because many of these fistulae will not close without resection. An understanding of the etiology of an ECF may provide information about the likelihood of successful closure, with or without intervention.

It must be remembered that more than one of these predisposing conditions may exist in any patient and the risks are compounded when multiple factors are present.

 CLINICAL PRESENTATION

The recognition of a postoperative ECF typically occurs 7 to 10 days following the procedure. The patient has typically suffered a slow course, with fevers and a prolonged ileus, culminating in the development of wound erythema and, finally, drainage of

TABLE 1. CAUSES OF ENTEROCUTANEOUS FISTULAE

Cause	Frequency (%)
Postoperative	85
Spontaneous	15
Crohn disease	39
Ulcerative colitis	13
Malignancy	9
Radiation	6
Diverticular disease	5
Other[a]	27

[a]Other includes rare conditions such as enteric vasculitis or myopathy or no associated condition.
From Hollington P, Mawdsley J, Lim W, et al. An 11 year experience of enterocutaneous fistula. *Br J Surg* 2004;91:1646.

The Gastrointestinal Tract

enteric contents through the wound spontaneously or following opening of the skin over the wound. At this point, the patient likely is suffering from at least one of the three major causes of morbidity and mortality among ECF patients: fluid and electrolyte imbalances, malnutrition, and sepsis.

With the diagnosis of postoperative ECFs, patients are typically intravascularly dry with multiple electrolyte deficiencies, especially sodium, potassium, phosphate, and magnesium. Patients have taken minimal oral fluid or nutrition, and often have significant "third-spaced" fluids. Further loss of fluid and electrolytes from the fistula combined with movement of fluid into the bowel wall and lumen contribute to fluid losses. Given the sophisticated electrolyte monitoring capacities available, it may seem surprising that these deficiencies persist, but recent series and our own experience demonstrate this to be a real problem. Frequently, monitoring of serum electrolyte values, careful measurement of the patient's fluid status, and aggressive repletion of electrolytes can aid in overcoming this problem. Additionally, in complicated cases, analysis of the electrolyte composition of the fistula fluid may aid in tailoring repletion (Table 2). For high-output fistulae, measures to decrease fistulae output (which will be discussed later) may also facilitate maintenance of normal serum electrolyte values. Once nutritional support commences, refeeding syndrome presents a new set of challenges in maintaining normal serum electrolytes. Aggressive monitoring and supplementation of magnesium, phosphate, and potassium is required in this setting to prevent further complications.

Malnutrition that complicates ECFs is multifactorial. Postoperative patients have often endured 1 to 2 weeks of poor enteral intake prior to recognition of their fistulae. Patients with spontaneous fistulae often have inflammatory bowel disease or malignancies and concomitant poor nutrition. All patients have ongoing protein losses from their fistulae and may have a limited surface area for enteral absorption of nutrients, depending on the level of the fistula. Further, ECFs are often accompanied by varying degrees of sepsis and inflammation, which increase metabolic needs.

Nutritional status is associated with complications and mortality from ECFs. In one large series, patients with serum albumin levels less than 2.5 g/dL had an increased mortality, and those with normal levels (>3.5 g/dL) suffered no mortality. Hypoalbuminemia may also limit wound healing and may lead to bowel dysfunction. Other serum markers of nutrition, including transferring, retinol-binding protein, and thyroxin-binding prealbumin, are also useful in predicting morbidity and mortality in patients with ECFs. Enteral nutrition appears to provide an advantage over parenteral nutrition in promoting intestinal and respiratory integrity. However, parenteral support may be initially necessary until a transition to total enteral nutrition is possible.

The ability to optimize nutritional status in patients with ECFs depends on the successful control and elimination of sepsis. Modern series all report sepsis or multisystem organ failure from sepsis as the leading cause of mortality among patients with ECFs. Fistula formation is one of several potential outcomes of bowel perforation or anastomotic breakdown. Enteric contents escaping the bowel lumen may be contained in a local abscess, may spill freely throughout the peritoneal or thoracic cavities, or may track through the abdominal wall and form an enterocutaneous fistula. Closed-space sepsis, such as an abscess, must be drained before the patient will be able to achieve positive nitrogen balance. The liberal use of computed tomography, ultrasound, or magnetic resonance imaging in making the diagnosis of an ECF will allow early identification of and potential percutaneous management of abscesses in these patients. Peritonitis resulting from free spillage of enteric contents requires an urgent laparotomy to contain the spillage and prevent further soilage. A proximal diverting enterostomy may be required at this stage. Local wound sepsis from an ECF can be treated with antibiotics and wound-care techniques to protect the surrounding abdominal wall (this will be discussed later).

Finally, blood, urine, and sputum cultures should be obtained to evaluate for concomitant infections. In considering antibiotic use in patients with ECFs, in order to avoid selection of multiagent resistant organisms, antibiotics should only be used to treat identified infections using the narrowest spectrum agent available for the shortest duration possible. Of note, it is important to remember that central venous access catheter should not be placed for 24 hours after the drainage of any septic focus to avoid contamination of the catheter.

MANAGEMENT

The goal of treating enterocutaneous fistulae is to restore bowel continuity, to achieve oral nutrition, and to close the fistulae. Whether achieved with or without surgical intervention, management of these complex patients is best conceptualized in stages with specific goals for each phase (Table 3). Stabilization of the patient with identification of the fistula, initial resuscitation, and steps to contain fistula drainage occur in the first 24 to 48 hours. Investigation into the origin, course, and anatomic characteristics of the fistula occur during the first 7 to 10 days. Whether the fistula will close spontaneously or will require operative intervention is decided during the next several weeks. Should operative intervention be required, definitive surgical therapy requires a well-prepared patient and team; the best timing for this procedure is usually after at least 4 to 6 weeks from the initial procedure. Finally, the patient must be sustained via nutritional support and have physical and emotional rehabilitation during the healing phase to help prevent recurrence of the fistula and return the patient to his or her original level of function.

Phase 1: Stabilization

Resuscitation

By the time a postoperative ECF has become clinically apparent, the patient typically has significant deficits in lean body mass, intravascular volume, red blood cell

TABLE 2. ELECTROLYTE COMPOSITION OF BODY FLUIDS[a]					
Source	**Volume (mL/d)**	**Na**	**K**	**HCO₃**	**C1**
Gastric	2,000–2,500	60	10		90
Pancreatic	1,000	140	5	90–110	30–45
Bile	1,500	140	5	35	100
Small bowel	3,500	100–130	15	25–35	100–140
Diarrhea	1,000–4,000	60	10–20	10	45–65
Urine	1,500	20–40	20–40		20
Urine + Lasix		40–60	20–40		60–100
Sweat		50	5		55

[a]All electrolyte values are mEq/L.
From Grant JP. *Handbook of total parenteral nutrition*, 2nd ed. Philadelphia: WE Saunders, 1992:174.

TABLE 3. PHASES OF MANAGEMENT FOR ENTEROCUTANEOUS FISTULAE

Phase	Description	Timing
Stabilization	■ Rehydration ■ Correction of anemia ■ Electrolyte repletion ■ Drainage of sepsis ■ Control of fistula drainage ■ Local skin care measures ■ Commencement of nutritional support	■ 24–48 h
Investigation	■ Fistulogram to define anatomy ■ CT/US/MRI[a] to localize collections and guide drainage	■ 7–10 d
Decision	■ Assess likelihood of nonoperative closure ■ Plan therapeutic course ■ Decide optimal surgical timing	■ 7–10 d to 4–6 wk
Definitive therapy	■ Plan operative approach ■ Bowel resection with end-to-end anastomosis ■ Secure abdominal closure (+/− flap) ■ Gastrostomy ■ Jejunostomy	■ 4–6 wk or if spontaneous closure unlikely
Healing	■ Continue nutrition support ■ Transition to total oral/enteral feedings ■ Physical and emotional rehabilitation	■ 5–10 d after closure

[a]CT, computed tomography; US, ultrasound; MRI, magnetic resonance imaging.

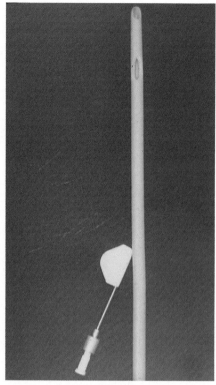

Fig. 1. Sump system for management of fistulae.

mass, and serum proteins. Resuscitation commences with crystalloid to restore intravascular volume lost in fistula drainage and "third spacing." Electrolytes should be replaced with frequent monitoring of serum levels until stable values are obtained. Red blood cells should be transfused to optimize oxygen delivery; although a target hematocrit is controversial, our practice is to maintain a value of 30%. Similarly, albumin has be suggested to aid in wound healing and intestinal function as well as transporting certain nutrients and medications; we administer albumin to a serum level of 3 g/dL to support these functions unless sepsis-induced capillary leak is present. Invasive monitoring with central venous or pulmonary artery catheters may be necessary to guide therapy in patients with poor cardiopulmonary reserve.

Drainage of Sepsis

Should the patient demonstrate any evidence of ongoing sepsis (such as fever, hypotension, low systemic vascular resistance, elevated white blood cell count, and positive blood cultures), an exhaustive search for septic foci should commence.

Computed tomography or ultrasound examination of the abdomen and pelvis will reveal abscesses and may guide percutaneous aspiration and drainage. Aspirated material should be sent for microbiologic culture along with blood, urine, and sputum samples. Patients with peritonitis should be explored expeditiously to prevent further peritoneal contamination and allow for copious irrigation of the peritoneum. Proximal diversion may be necessary to control ongoing leakage. In the case of abscesses, consideration should be given to performing a fistulogram by injecting water-soluble contrast into the abscess cavity to provide information on the course and character of the fistula.

Control of Fistula Drainage and Skin Care

To prevent continued irritation and destruction of the abdominal wall and to guide resuscitation, fistula drainage must be contained and quantified. Low-output fistulae may be adequately managed with a dry dressing; however, should the external opening of the fistula close, an abscess will result. Higher-output fistulae would require multiple dressing changes that be-

come cumbersome to maintain. Thus, we manage our fistulae with a sump system to keep the wounds clean and provide an accurate measurement of output. A Robinson nephrostomy tube is placed in the wound, vented with a 14-gauge catheter, and attached to suction (Fig. 1) This type of catheter is soft at body temperature and will not erode into the bowel or abdominal wall structure. DuoDerm, stoma glue, ion exchange resins, or karaya powder can be placed around the wound to prevent the surrounding skin from drainage and tape from dressing changes. A skilled enterostomal therapist can be useful in constructing an appropriate dressing system. Recently, several groups have reported the use of vacuum-assisted closure devices to aid in the management and closure of these complicated wounds, especially in cases of low-to moderate-output fistulae (Fig. 2). The largest series published to date involved 74 patients with good results. It must be kept in mind, however, that this device is not currently approved for use in ECFs. Additionally, some groups advocate use of split-thickness skin grafting to the bowel around a fistulous opening as a biologic dressing that reduces protein and fluid loss, and their effects on patient nutritional status.

Reduction of Fistula Output

Several measures may be used to reduce fistula output. Gastric acid suppression

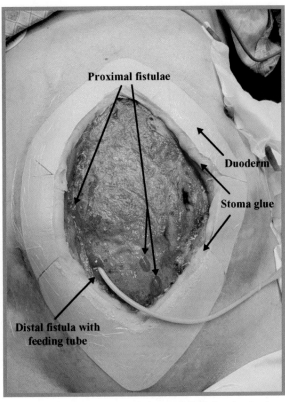
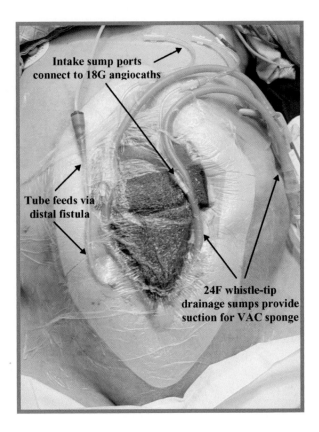

Fig. 2. Vacuum-assisted closure (VAC) dressing in situ.

with histamine blockers or proton pump inhibitors reduces the production of gastric fluid. Sucralfate, a gastric mucosal protective agent, may also contribute to constipation and reduce fistulae output. Nasogastric drainage is useful only in cases of distal obstruction or severe ileus; the long-term use of nasogastric drainage may result in alar necrosis, sinusitis, distal esophageal stricture, and aspiration pneumonia. Somatostatin and its analog, octreotide, have also been evaluated in the management of ECFs. Data have mixed reports as to their overall effectiveness in reducing fistulae output and increasing rates of spontaneous closure; however, some authors suggest that a 48-hour trial of these agents should be attempted. If a reduction in fistula output occurs, then the agent is continued. Octreotide is not a standard agent used in the management of our patients. Risks associated with the use of these agents include cholecystitis, hyperglycemia, mucosal atrophy, and interruption of intestinal adaptation.

Infliximab, a monoclonal antibody to tumor necrosis factor-α, has been extensively evaluated in the setting of fistulae from Crohn disease. A recent, large, randomized controlled trial suggests that maintenance of patients with fistulizing Crohn disease with infliximab reduces hospitalizations and surgeries in this popula-

tion. A new approach to patients with Crohn disease and with fistulae refractory to infliximab involves the use of long-term oral tacrolimus. Several small series suggest that this agent may aid in both closing persistent fistulae and allowing patients to be weaned from steroid and other immunosuppressive therapy. Additionally, there are several case reports of patients with chronic, non-Crohn fistulae that achieved permanent closures of their fistulae following single infusions of infliximab. Further studies will be required before general recommendations to use either of these agents in the routine management of ECFs can be made, especially in settings of clinically important acute infection, in which use of these agents is not recommended.

Nutritional Support

Once sepsis has been controlled, optimization of nutrition must be commenced. Provision of nutritional support in combination with control of sepsis may be sufficient to allow for spontaneous closure of ECFs. Should operative intervention ultimately be necessary, restoration of nutritional parameters will allow for the best opportunity for successful fistulae closure. Metabolic needs can be estimated using the Harris-Benedict equation and appropriate stress factors. Frequent use of metabolic cart analysis (indirect calorimetry)

can provide more accurate assessment of the macronutrient balance. As general guidelines, we provide 25 to 32 kcal/kg/d with a calorie-to-nitrogen ratio of 150:1 to 100:1, and at least 1.5 g/kg/d of protein. Constant reassessments of the clinical progress of the patient and laboratory indicators of nutritional status are required to fine-tune the nutritional management of these patients.

The original large series of ECFs reported the success of total parenteral nutrition (TPN) in promoting fistulae closure, but the paradigm has shifted to prefer enteral nutrition whenever possible. Even so, TPN may represent the only means of providing nutrition in some critically ill patients. If enteral support is ultimately an option, full nutritional support via the enteral route may take several days to accomplish, or may never be fully achieved. For these reasons, most patients with ECFs begin parenteral nutrition once sepsis has been controlled. Enteral support requires the presence of approximately 4 feet of small intestine for absorption. This length of small bowel may be proximal to or distal to the fistula. Enteral feeds may be taken by mouth, infused via nasoenteric tube, or may be fed into the fistula (fistuloclysis) if sufficient bowel distal to the fistula is present. Enteral feeding has the advantages of preserving the gastrointestinal mucosa as well as supporting the immunologic and hormonal functions of the gut and liver. Authors from an intestinal failure unit have also reported that, at operation, the bowel of patients fed via fistuloclysis had improved bowel caliber, thickness, and ability to hold sutures than bowel from patients maintained on parenteral nutrition alone.

Phase 2: Investigation

During the initial stabilization of the patients with an ECF, computed tomography may be used to look for undrained abscesses as a source of sepsis. Within 1 to 2 weeks of adequate nutritional support in the absence of sepsis, most ECFs will have matured enough to allow for intubation with soft catheters for the purpose of obtaining fistulograms. This form of imaging can provide information that is not otherwise obtainable, and may be valuable in planning the ultimate management of the patient. Ideally, the most senior surgeon involved in the patient's care and a senior radiologist will jointly perform the fistulogram using water-soluble contrast. Information from early images may be most revealing and provide information on the length and diameter of the tract, site of bowel wall defect, health of the adjacent bowel, and the presence of strictures, abscess cavities, distal obstruction, or anastomotic dehiscence. The details specific to each fistula will provide information that will help determine whether the fistula is likely to close spontaneously with continued nutritional support and local wound care or whether operative intervention will likely be necessary for ultimate closure (see following discussion).

Traditional contrast examinations (upper gastrointestinal series, barium enema) rarely demonstrate fistula tracts and do not provide information not seen on a well-executed fistulogram. Similarly, fistula tracts are not often seen using computed tomography, although computed tomographic scans are useful in identifying abscesses and other, extraluminal pathologic findings. When the use of multiple imaging techniques is considered, the order of the examinations is important to avoid the effects of residual contrast on subsequent studies.

Phase 3: Decision

The goal of this phase of management of patients with ECFs is to determine the likelihood that a fistula will close with continued nonoperative management or will require definitive surgical therapy. If surgical intervention is required, a decision must be made as to the optimal time to perform the definitive operation. Several factors must be considered in arriving at these decisions: (a) fistula location and characteristics, (b) pattern of fistula output, (c) status of the surrounding bowel, and (d) response to nonoperative management (Table 4).

Certain characteristics of the fistula may provide information about its ultimate likelihood of closure. Fistulae arising from the oropharynx, esophagus, duodenal stump or lateral duodenum, pancreaticobiliary tree, or jejunum are more likely to resolve without operative intervention than are fistulae originating from the stomach, ligament of Treitz, or ileum. Longer fistula tract length also suggests a greater likelihood of closure, and very short tracts are unlikely to spontaneously resolve. Larger defects are similarly less likely to resolve without intervention.

Fistulae may be classified according to the amount of fluid drained daily. High-output fistulae drain more than 500 mL/day and are often of small bowel origin. Low-output fistulae drain less than 200 mL/day and pose less of a challenge in the management of metabolic and nutritional complications than high-output fistulae. The output does not clearly predict the likelihood of closure, but most fistulae that will undergo spontaneous resolution demonstrate a decrease in output prior to closure. Thus, close monitoring of fistulae output can provide evidence of whether closure is likely.

The status of the bowel surrounding the fistula also affects whether nonoperative management will be successful. Those fistulae likely to close arise in otherwise healthy bowel. The presence of distal obstruction or stricture, adjacent abscess, active inflammation or inflammatory bowel disease, or bowel discontinuity diminishes the likelihood of spontaneous closure. Fistulae arising in the setting of malignancy, radiated tissue, or the presence of foreign bodies are also unlikely to close. The presence of nonabsorbable mesh used in the management of ventral hernia defects represents a growing cause of ECFs. Although mesh may be required for successful treatment of large herniae, adhesions between the bowel and the mesh should be expected unless measures are taken to keep these surfaces separate during the healing phase. Interposition of omentum or the development of nonadhesive surfaces for mesh will help minimize the development of adhesions and subsequent ECFs resulting from the use of mesh. Once an ECF has developed in association with mesh, the mesh must usually be removed to allow for successful healing of the fistula.

If fistulae closure has not occurred after 4 to 5 weeks of adequate nutrition and in the absence of sepsis, it is unlikely that the fistulae will spontaneously close. In most series, 80% to 90% of those fistulae that eventually close spontaneously will have done so by this time. Provided that nutritional support is adequate and the patient can tolerate the fistula and its attendant care (such as sumps, vacuum-assisted closure, TPN, and tube feedings), it is actually

TABLE 4. PREDICTORS OF SPONTANEOUS CLOSURE

Factor	Likely to Close	Unlikely to Close
Anatomical location	Oropharyngeal	Gastric
	Esophageal	Ligament of Treitz
	Duodenal stump	Ileal
	Lateral duodenal	
	Pancreaticobiliary	
	Jejunal	
Tract length	>2 cm	<2 cm
Defect size	<1 cm^2	>1 cm^2
Fistula output	Decreasing	Stable or increasing
Surrounding bowel	Healthy	Distal obstruction or stricture
		Abscess
		Active inflammation
		Bowel discontinuity
		Crohn disease
Etiology	Appendicitis	Malignancy
	Diverticulitis	Radiation
	Postoperative	Foreign body (mesh)
Nutritional status	Well-nourished	Malnourished
Sepsis	Absent	Present

The Gastrointestinal Tract

of significant benefit to delay surgery for a total of 4 to 6 months from the date of the original procedure. This delay allows for softening of the adhesions created at the original operation and allows one to avoid operating in the setting of "obliterative peritonitis," which is described by Fazio et al. as existing from 10 days to 6 weeks following laparotomy complicated by peritonitis or fistula formation. Retrospective series have shown that mortality is doubled in the group of patients who require operation during this time frame. Waiting 4 to 6 months also allows for adequate healing of any abdominal wall sepsis, which will permit a secure closure.

Phase 4: Definitive Therapy

Definitive operative reconstruction of an ECF requires the investment of significant time and resources. Optimal nutritional parameters and complete freedom from any form of infection are important patient prerequisites. Tube feedings should be tapered in the days preceding the operation to allow for mechanical and antibiotic preparation. Intravenous antibiotics should be chosen based on a review of the patient's microbiologic data and the pattern of known hospital pathogens. The patient and his or her family should be mentally and emotionally prepared to participate in the difficult recovery and rehabilitation that often follows procedures of such magnitude.

The surgical team should anticipate a long procedure and, in complicated cases, should involve a plastics and reconstructive surgery (PRS) team to perform a musculocutaneous flap closure of the abdominal wall. The plastics and reconstructive surgery team should be involved early in the patient's course to allow adequate planning for the reconstructive procedure.

Entrance to the peritoneum should commence through a new incision to avoid potential sources of inflammation or adhesions. Often, use of a transverse incision will allow the best opportunity to enter the abdomen without danger of damaging adherent bowel. Thoroughly wrung, antibiotic-soaked wound towels may be sutured to the fascia to prevent contamination of the subcutaneous tissues during the dissection. The goal of the initial phase of the operation is to free all bowel from adhesions, drain all abscess, and correct all areas of obstruction; this process has been termed "refunctionalization." Dissection may not proceed from one end of the bowel to the other as it is often easier to tackle areas of least-dense

adhesions first. Our practice is to use the scalpel and scissors to sharply dissect adhesions to avoid inadvertent injuries from tension on the bowel. Approaching adhesions from the side, rather than head-on, also minimizes injury. Allowing particularly troublesome loops of bowel to rest in antibiotic-soaked laparotomy pads often creates edema that facilitates further dissection. Closure of all enterotomies and serosal tears will minimize further fistula formation.

All authors recommend resection of fistulized bowel with reanastomosis over bypass, Roux-en-Y drainage, or simple closure or wedge resection. In a recent large series, the only predictors for fistula recurrence were use of wedge repair or oversewing of the fistulae tracts. The authors note that these suboptimal options were used only when it was technically impossible to perform a resection.

The new anastomosis should be performed using an end-to-end, two-layer, interrupted nonabsorbable suture technique. Avoidance of tension and assurance of good blood supply will maximize the chances of a successful repair. Consideration should be given to the creation of a proximal protecting stoma until healing is assured. Given the magnitude of the laparotomy performed, many patients suffer from a prolonged postoperative ileus. In order to avoid prolonged nasogastric tube drainage, a gastrostomy tube may be placed at the time of surgery. Similarly, a catheter jejunostomy tube may be placed to facilitate enteral nutrition early in the postoperative period.

Prior to abdominal closure, the entire bowel surface should be inspected to ensure that no unrecognized injuries exist. Irrigation with copious amounts of saline and antibiotic solution should be performed. Closed suction drains may be left in abscess cavities, or in the case of complicated dissections. Optimally, the omentum should be placed between the anastomosis and the abdominal incision to prevent formation of adhesions to the anterior abdominal wall. A secure abdominal closure is then performed by the primary team or with the assistance of a special reconstructive team.

Several groups have recently reported experience with laparoscopic approaches to the operative management of ECFs with minimal complications or conversions to open procedures. Laparoscopic operations for fistulous disease may provide advantages over laparotomy that include decreased pain, faster resumption of bowel function, and shorter length of stay.

As expertise with laparoscopic approaches to complex abdominal problems increases, one can expect to see more procedures performed with these techniques. It must be remembered, however, that these procedures require advanced laparoscopic skills and require a steep learning curve. Given the significant preoperative investment of time and resources in patients with ECFs, the choice of operative technique must ensure patients' best possible outcomes.

Phase 5: Healing

Whether fistula closure occurs by operative or nonoperative management, continued nutritional support is required to promote wound healing and avoid recurrence. Oral feedings are commenced once the postoperative ileus has resolved. The traditional diet advancement protocol (sips to clears to fulls to regular diet) may not be tolerated by these patients. Instead, we typically start patients on a soft diet 1 week postoperatively and advance quickly to a regular diet. The patient should be encouraged to eat his or her favorite foods, and the patient's family should be encouraged to bring in any special requests. Tube feedings may be cycled during the nighttime hours to supplement oral nutrition until the patient is able to consume at least 1,500 kcal/d. Zinc supplementation has proven useful to improve taste and increase oral intake.

After a 4-to 6-month medical ordeal, patients are often physically and emotionally fatigued. The limitations imposed by a cumbersome wound dressing as well as the metabolic and septic challenges endured by these patients often leads to limited ambulation and deconditioning. Use of inpatient physical and occupation therapy resources can limit some of these losses, and continued rehabilitation may be required on discharge from the hospital. Similarly, the emotional, mental, and financial ordeals brought about by an ECF may require additional support in the form of involvement of case managers, social workers, and psychiatric consult-liaison services. A coordinated effort may be necessary to allow for a patient's successful reintroduction to an active lifestyle. The consistent and continued involvement of the senior surgeon involved in the patient's care must be emphasized as a mechanism to ensure that the multiple services required by the patient are coordinated, and to avoid confusion and fear on the part of the patient and his or her family.

DUODENAL FISTULAE

The dictum that fistulae are best resolved by resection and end-to-end anastamoses is not true in duodenal fistulae. Whether lateral duodenal fistulae from sphincterotomies, for example, or perforated duodenal ulcers, which have not been completely repaired, or an end-duodenal fistula following a gastrectomy, the fact that resection usually requires a pancreaticoduodenectomy makes this option an unreasonable choice for this type of fistula. Instead, we have had excellent results with bypass, such as a gastrojejunostomy, thus excluding the fistula. This is, of course, in deviance to the technique that has been espoused for other fistulae, which is resection and end-to-end anastamoses, but in this situation, it seems it works well.

The overwhelming majority of biliary and pancreatic and duodenal fistulae will close spontaneously or nonoperatively. Octreotide, 50 to 100 μg three times a day is useful in this fistula, a group that has not been useful in others. In the event that spontaneous closure does not occur, it is important to stay out of the area, which is extraordinarily difficult, and one may do a lot of damage. In the case of a duodenal fistula, bypass with a gastrojejunostomy is most useful. A feeding jejunostomy should be included so that nutrition in the postoperative area can be administered through the feeding jejunostomy. I have not usually used the vagotomy in these patients in whom gastrojejunostomy is performed. This is because most of these patients do not have an ulcer diathesis, and therefore an acid and motility reducing operation is probably meddlesome.

THE INFLUENCE OF TPN ON MORTALITY IN GASTROINTESTINAL-CUTANEOUS FISTULAE

One would expect the drop in mortality with fistulae occurred with the introduction of TPN. This is not the case, and the reasons may be several. First, some forms of nutrition took place in the 1960s, whether these were tube feedings, 10% dextrose, albumin, Lipomul (an early and somewhat imperfect form of fat), 5% amino acids in dextrose, or various forms of oral supplementation. Dr. Claude Welch, one of my brilliant teachers who dealt with a lot of ECFs, always liked his patients to take a lot of peanut butter. He jokingly said it was sticky and it might bring the wounds together. Obviously, peanut butter is a great source of protein and fat calories. Given these various primitive forms of nutritional supplementation, the mortality actually dropped between 1960 and 1970, probably because of intensive care, more intelligent use of antibiotics, and greater expertise in respiratory and other forms of support.

The introduction of TPN did not result in any decrease in mortality in two centers that were accustomed to dealing with gastrointestinal cutaneous fistulae (Table 5). Thus, from the standpoint of parenteral nutrition, it is a useful adjunct and enables one to make certain that the patient is in the most optimum shape for a long and tedious operation, but in itself does not appear, at least in selected centers, to have resulted in improved outcome in patients with gastrointestinal-cutaneous fistulae. This may be somewhat contraintuitive, but that is what the data appear to show.

TABLE 5. MORTALITY

1946–1959	45% (138 patients - MGH)
1960–1970	15% (119 patients - MGH)
1970–1975	19% (145 patients - MGH)
1982–1991	20% (79 patients - UH)

SUGGESTED READING

Berry SM, Fischer JE. Enterocutaneous fistulae. In: Wells SA Jr, ed. *Current problems in surgery.* St. Louis: Mosby-Year Book, 1994:469.

Edmunds LH, Williams GH, Welch CE. External fistulas arising from the gastrointestinal tract. *Ann Surg* 1960;152:445.

Haffejee AA. Surgical management of high output enterocutaneous fistulae: a 24-year experience. *Curr Opin Clin Nutr Metab Care* 2004;7:309.

Hollington P, Mawdsley J, Lim W, et al. An 11-year experience of enterocutaneous fistula. *Br J Surg* 2004;91:1646.

Kuvshinoff BW, Brodish RJ, McFadden DW, et al. Serum transferring as a prognostic indicator of spontaneous closure and mortality in gastrointestinal cutaneous fistulas. *Ann Surg* 1993;217:615.

Lichtenstein GR, Yan S, Bala M, et al. Infliximab maintenance treatment reduces hospitalization, surgeries, and procedures in fistulizing Crohn's disease. *Gastroenterology* 2005;128:862.

Lynch AC, Delaney CP, Senagore AJ, et al. Clinical outcome and factors predictive of recurrence after enterocutaneous fistula surgery. *Ann Surg* 2004;240:825.

Regan JP, Salky BA. Laparoscopic treatment of enteric fistulas. *Surg Endosc* 2004;18:252.

Soeters PB, Ebeid AM, Fischer JE. Review of 404 patients with gastrointestinal fistulas: impact of parenteral nutrition. *Ann Surg* 1979;190:189.

Teubner A, Morrison K, Ravishankar HR, et al. Fistuloclysis can successfully replace parenteral feeding in the nutritional support of patients with enterocutaneous fistula. *Br J Surg* 2004;91:625.

The Gastrointestinal Tract

EDITOR'S COMMENT

Drs. Fischer and Evenson provide a masterful review of enterocutaneous fistulae (ECF), which follow major complications arising from intrinsic intestinal disease, trauma, and/or surgical procedures. The remarkable changes in management strategies, including the use of electrolyte replacement solutions, total parenteral nutrition (TPN), advances in anesthesia, blood coagulation therapy, and antibiotics, have all contributed to a reduction in mortality of ECF, which exceeded half of patients in the 1930s to 1940s, to less than one in five patients with recent series of advanced ECFs related to the complications listed.

As indicated by the authors, gastrointestinal fistulae are best categorized as internal or external, with categorization of origin: intestinal (gut-to-gut), extraintestinal (genitourinary, biliary, vascular, respiratory), or external (cutaneous high or low output). ECF may result as a circumstance in which there is breach of bowel integrity with establishment of an inflammatory, and thereafter, functional continuity between bowel, abdominal viscera, or cutaneous sites (Pickhardt PJ, Bhalla S, Balfe DM. *Radiology* 2002;224:9). As indicated by the authors, fistulae formation represents a long-standing expectant event in Crohn disease, with occurrence in 20% to 40% of such patients described in various surgical series (Delaney CP, Fazio VW. *Surg Clin North Am* 2001;81:137). Consistent are the development of sinus tracts in fistulae. These tracts involve distal small bowel, peritoneal abscess, and produce phlegmon associated with these presentations (Rubesin SE, et al. *Surg Clin Am North Am* 2001;81:39). Because of the wide clinical presentations, radiographic manifesta-

tions vary as well; internal fistulae can involve virtually any organ site, although enterovesical and ileocolic fistulae are the most common variants (Glass RE. *Br J Surg* 1985;72(suppl):93). External fistulae, as indicated by McClane and Rombeau (*Surg Clin North Am* 2001;81:169), are common presentations, especially in perianal Crohn presentations. Although fistulae formation, and specifically ECF, is less common in chronic ulcerative colitis, such fistulous events are possible despite the fact that ulcerative colitis is only a mucosal disease and is differentiated from the transmural pathology of Crohn disease (Gore RM, et al. *AJR Am J Roentgenol* 1996;167:3).

Chronic diverticulitis represents the most common cause of colonic fistulae formation; fistulae communication with the urinary bladder is

(continued)

commonly seen (Woods RJ, et al. *Dis Colon Rectum* 1988;31:591). Following hysterectomy, colovaginal fistulae may occur in women who present with antecedent sigmoid colon diverticulitis. Fistulae may be evident in as many as one fifth of such patients who are treated surgically for diverticular disease (Stollman NH, Raskin JB. *J Clin Gastroenterol* 1999;29:241).

Drs. Fischer and Evenson document the historical chronology for use of TPN. Table 5 in their presentation documents the lack of reduction in mortality in academic medical centers that are accustomed to management of ECF. Even though mortality has plateaued in ECG management, TPN represents a highly useful and appropriate adjunct for preoperative nutritional and electrolyte replenishment of the patient who has planned major resectional surgery, as a method to support these individuals postoperatively.

The recent article by Truong et al. of Germany (*Surg Endosc* 2004;18:1105) notes that periodic success can be achieved with very simple measures following anastomotic leaks or fistulae following surgery for upper gastrointestinal cancer. Under sedation, endoscopic lavage of the sinus cavity at the site of anastomotic leakage was identified and completed. The entrance to this cavity was obstructed/closed with Vicryl mesh, and thereafter sealed with fibrin glue. Endoscopy repeated in a water-soluble contrast study indicated that seven of nine treated patients had complete healing of the anastomotic leak. However, such techniques can only be considered a temporary support and "bridging" technique to manage what almost certainly will become a recurrent ECF.

The recent analysis by Parsi et al. (*Am J Gastroenterol* 2004:445) from the Cleveland Clinic Foundation determines the association between type of fistulae and complete response to infliximab therapy for patients with fistulous Crohn disease. The highest rates of closure in response to infliximab were external fistulae and perianal fistulae associated with Crohn disease. Rates of closure with this drug for patients with rectovaginal fistulae were only 14%, compared with those with perianal fistulae of Crohn disease (78%; *P* = 0.0007). For mixed fistulae group patients, a modest achievement of only 11% was evident for complete response within infliximab. Moreover, relapse was higher for smokers than nonsmokers. These results have also been confirmed by Sands et al. (*N Engl J Med* 2004;350:876) in the multicenter study of infliximab maintenance therapy for fistulizing Crohn disease. In this double-blind, randomized, placebo-controlled trial of 306 adult patients with Crohn disease, 5 mg of infliximab per kilogram of body weight indicates the time to loss of response was significantly longer for patients who received infliximab maintenance therapy than for those receiving placebo maintenance. At 54 weeks, there was 19% closure for the placebo group versus 36% in the infliximab maintenance group (*P* = 0.009).

More recently, the publication by Mahadevan et al. (*Aliment Pharmacol Ther* 2003;18:1003) determined that the efficacy of methotrexate allowed induction and maintenance of remission in luminal Crohn disease. These authors confirmed that in 33 patients with luminal and/or fistulizing Crohn disease, there was an overall response to methotrexate in 62%, and 6% had significant adverse events. Thus, 56% of patients treated with methotrexate had a complete or partial response. Clearly, prolonged detailed analyses are necessary to confirm the role of methotrexate alone in fistulizing Crohn disease and/or its combination with other therapies.

Bell et al. (*Aliment Pharmacol Ther* 2003;17:387) of the St. Mark's Hospital, United Kingdom, advocate the use of magnetic resonance imaging to identify clinical sepsis, to assess fistulae tract healing following infliximab therapy. As iterated by the authors, fistulae may persist despite clinical remission. Magnetic resonance imaging may represent a useful, noninvasive method of assessing such patients before and after therapy. However, magnetic resonance imaging was unable to reliably identify fistulae tract infections with abdominal ECF or significant surgical scarring.

The authors have made a most salient point with admonition of a key management principle: "If fistulae closure has not occurred after 4 to 5 weeks of adequate nutrition and in the absence of sepsis, it is unlikely that the fistulae will spontaneously close." This admonition must be acknowledged as 80% to 90% of such ECFs will have eventually closed by this time interval. The authors prefer to delay surgery for a total of 4 to 6 months when proper nutritional support can be achieved and tolerated by the patient with dysfunctional gut. Such intervals of delay allow "softening of the adhesions" initiated with the original operation, and allows the operating surgeon to avoid remarkable inflammatory responses of obliterative peritonitis previously described by Fazio et al. We agree with this principle to delay 4 to 6 months to provide optimal nutritional support and subsequent management.

An attitude of temperance and patience is essential in the management of patients with ECF. A surgeon should plan to have many hours available for the disposal of patient care when initiating such a major procedure of re-exploration following surgically initiated ECF. Nutritional optimization of the patient, electrolyte management, and blood availability, are standard principles of care, as have been iterated by the authors.

K.I.B.

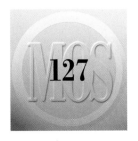

127 Surgical Treatment of Crohn Disease

FABRIZIO MICHELASSI, MUKTA V. KATDARE, ALESSANDRO FICHERA, AND ROGER D. HURST

INTRODUCTION

Crohn disease is a chronic inflammatory disorder of the gastrointestinal tract that can result in strictures, inflammatory masses, fistulas, abscesses, hemorrhage, and cancer. Crohn disease may affect any region of the gastrointestinal tract from the mouth to the anus, and often involves multiple areas simultaneously. Crohn, Ginsberg, and Oppenheimer first identified the disorder as a unique clinical entity in 1932. Although the cause of Crohn disease remains unknown, the prevailing theory is that, in patients with a genetic predisposition, exposure to particular environmental stimuli triggers an altered immune response, resulting in inflammation and ulceration of intestinal tissues.

The histopathology of Crohn disease is characterized by transmural inflammation with multiple lymphoid aggregates in a thickened submucosa. The earliest gross manifestation of Crohn disease is the development of small mucosal ulcerations, called *aphthous ulcers,* that eventually progress to larger ulcerations. These mucosal ulcerations can penetrate through the submucosa to form intramural channels that have the potential to bore deeply into the bowel wall and create sinuses, abscesses, or fistulas.

It is estimated that the incidence of Crohn disease in the United States is approximately 4 new cases per year for every 100,000 persons, and the prevalence is between 80 and 150 cases per 100,000 persons. Crohn disease can affect patients of all ages, but the peak incidence occurs between the 2nd and the 3rd decades. In the United States, the incidence of Crohn disease is highest among whites, low among African Americans, and lowest among Hispanics and Asians. Crohn disease is three to four times more common in the ethnic Jewish population, and it appears slightly more predominant in women than in men.

Curative treatment for Crohn disease does not exist. Current medical therapy is often effective abating the progression of the disease, but even with the newer medical treatment, complications often occur that require surgical intervention. Modern principles of surgical management dictate that intestinal resections be limited, without wide margins of normal tissue. This is supported by the evidence that recurrence of Crohn disease is unaffected by the presence of macroscopically involved bowel at the anastomotic line, as demonstrated by the long-term results obtained with stricturoplasty or when microscopic involvement is present at the resection margin. Greater understanding of the clinical course of Crohn disease has led to a more conservative strategy, with surgery reserved for the treatment of complications of the disease, and bowel-sparing approaches advocated.

GENERAL CLINICAL ASPECTS

Crohn disease is commonly categorized according to the affected intestinal site. Approximately 40% of patients have distal ileal disease with or without involvement of the right colon. Proximal small bowel disease without colonic involvement is observed in 30% of patients, whereas isolated colonic involvement without small bowel disease occurs in approximately 25% of patients. Involvement of the anorectal region, the perianal region, or both, without proximal small or large bowel is found in only 5% of patients.

Crohn disease may also be categorized by its clinical manifestations and grouped into one of three general entities: stricturing, perforating, or inflammatory disease. These are not truly distinct forms of the disease, but rather are terms that are used to describe the predominant gross pathologic manifestation. Stricturing Crohn disease results in the development of fibrotic scar tissue that constricts the intestinal lumen and may result in a partial or complete obstruction. These fibrostenotic scars are not reversible with medical therapy; therefore, once they become symptomatic, surgical intervention is required. Perforating Crohn disease is caused by deep mucosal ulcerations that can develop into sinus tracts, fistulas, and abscesses. The inflammatory pattern of Crohn disease is characterized by mucosal ulceration and bowel wall thickening that may lead to an adynamic segment of intestine and luminal narrowing, causing obstructive symptoms in the small intestine and diarrhea in the colon.

The onset of symptoms is often insidious, with most patients presenting with complaints of intermittent abdominal pain, bloating, diarrhea, nausea, vomiting, weight loss, and fever. Patients may also experience symptoms related to complications of the disease, including abdominal masses, pneumaturia, or perianal pain and swelling. The particular signs, symptoms, and complications of Crohn disease exhibited by a patient depend greatly on the affected sites.

There is no specific laboratory test that is diagnostic for Crohn disease, and although computed tomographic (CT) scans or magnetic resonance imaging may be useful for diagnosing complications of the disease, there is little role for these advanced imaging studies in the initial diagnosis. Upper intestinal contrast studies, colonoscopy with biopsies, and capsule endoscopy can all be useful in the differential diagnosis. However, the diagnosis of Crohn disease still relies heavily on the history and physical examination.

INDICATIONS

Although medical therapy can only palliate the symptoms of Crohn disease, it may afford long periods of remission and delay surgical treatment. However, approximately 80% of patients will still require surgical intervention during their lifetime. The main goal of surgery is to treat complications and to palliate symptoms while minimizing complications and side effects.

FISTULAS

Although one-third of patients with Crohn disease will develop an intestinal fistula, these are rarely the primary indication for surgery. Surgical treatment is generally reserved for intestinal fistulas that connect with the genitourinary tract and result in repeated urinary tract infections or renal impairment; for enterocutaneous and enterovaginal fistulas that cause the patient personal embarrassment or discomfort; and for fistulas that result in the functional bypass of a major intestinal segment, causing malabsorption and diarrhea.

INFLAMMATORY MASSES AND ABSCESSES

Abscesses that occur in the setting of Crohn disease are often the result of sealed perforations of the bowel. They are most frequently located in the right lower quadrant of the abdomen or along the descending colon. Most abscesses can be treated initially with percutaneous CT-guided drainage and antibiotics. However, an abscess usually originates from a severely diseased segment of bowel and thus, without a resection of the involved segment, is likely to recur or result in an enterocutaneous fistula. Therefore, after successful interventional drainage, elective surgical resection is recommended. The presence of abscesses not amenable to percutaneous drainage, such as multilocular abscesses,

multiple interloop abscesses, or inflammatory masses that are refractory to antibiotic therapy is an indication for surgical intervention.

PERFORATION

Free perforation of the small or large bowel only occurs in approximately 1% of patients with Crohn disease. The clinical signs of peritonitis or the identification of free intraperitoneal air on a plain radiograph or CT scan are diagnostic of free perforation. Once diagnosed, urgent surgery is required, with resection of the perforated bowel and any associated involved segments. A stoma may be necessary in the presence of significant intra-abdominal contamination.

OBSTRUCTION

A partial or complete intestinal obstruction may require surgical intervention. A partial intestinal obstruction that is caused by acute inflammation and bowel wall thickening can often be treated with medical therapy. However, obstructions that are caused by high-grade fibrostenotic lesions will not respond to medical management and are an indication for surgery. In an effort to limit the length of bowel to be resected, attempts initially should be made to treat partial or complete intestinal obstructions conservatively with nasogastric decompression, intravenous hydration, and intravenous steroids, allowing for a definitive procedure to be conducted electively when decompression is achieved.

CARCINOMA

Crohn disease is a risk factor for adenocarcinoma of the small bowel and the colon. The incidence of cancer occurrence correlates with the duration and extension of disease. The risk of malignancy also increases in defunctionalized segments of bowel. Therefore, bypass surgery of the small intestine should be avoided, and defunctionalized rectal stumps should either be restored to their function or excised.

HEMORRHAGE

Severe hemorrhage in the setting of Crohn disease is extremely rare and often requires definitive surgical treatment. Massive gastrointestinal hemorrhage occurs most frequently from Crohn colitis. Hemorrhage from Crohn disease of the small bowel tends to be indolent with episodic or chronic bleeding that may require intermittent blood transfusions, but rarely requires emergent surgical intervention. However, the risk of a recurrence is high with spontaneous cessation of a small bowel hemorrhage; therefore, elective surgery of the actively diseased segment should be considered after the first episode of hemorrhage.

TOXIC MEGACOLON

Toxic megacolon is a rare but potentially fatal complication of Crohn disease. Unstable patients or patients who do not readily respond to supportive measures, including adequate fluid resuscitation, antibiotics, and medical therapy, require surgery. A subtotal colectomy with creation of an ileostomy is the preferred surgical option. The decision between creating a mucous fistula and closing the distal rectosigmoid stump is based on the degree of inflammation and disease of the distal bowel.

GROWTH RETARDATION

Twenty-six percent of children with Crohn disease experience growth retardation as a result of either steroid treatment or the malnutrition associated with active intestinal disease. Persistent growth retardation in the face of adequate medical and nutritional therapy is an indication for surgical intervention.

FAILURE OF MEDICAL TREATMENT

Failure of medical treatment, the most common indication for surgery, occurs when (a) maximal medical treatment proves inadequate; (b) patients who are asymptomatic on maximal induction medical therapy develop recurrence of symptoms with tapering of these medications that do not have an acceptable safety profile for use as maintenance therapy; (c) the disease progresses with worsening symptoms or a complication arises despite maximal medical treatment; or (d) the patient experiences significant treatment-related complications.

PREOPERATIVE PLANNING

A complete assessment of the gastrointestinal tract is required prior to surgery to evaluate the full extent of disease and any associated complications that may require management before surgical intervention. Small bowel follow-through or enteroclysis adequately assesses the entire small intestine.

Crohn disease is a relative contraindication for capsule endoscopy because of the high incidence of strictures. However, if a contrast study has ruled out lesions that could prevent capsule passage and clinical questions are still unanswered, capsule endoscopy can be safely and effectively used. A colonoscopy provides the best evaluation of the colon and rectum and, with the intubation of the terminal ileum, biopsies can be obtained to confirm the diagnosis of Crohn disease. If colonic strictures prevent the passage of a colonoscope, a barium enema may be helpful. If the patient presents with a fever or an abdominal mass, a CT scan should be obtained to assess for the presence of an intra-abdominal abscess and enable percutaneous drainage.

The use of mechanical bowel preparation is controversial in patients with Crohn disease during an acute attack and in the presence of severe diarrhea, and is clearly contraindicated when a perforation or a complete obstruction is present. All patients should be administered prophylactic broad-spectrum antibiotics and patients on long-term steroid therapy should receive stress-dose steroids. In the event that the patient cannot undergo primary restoration of the gastrointestinal continuity, a potential stoma site should be marked preoperatively.

SITE-SPECIFIC PLANNING

Esophagus, Stomach, and Duodenum

Gastroduodenal involvement in Crohn disease is reported in only 2% to 4% of cases and is rarely confined to only the gastroduodenal segment. In a study conducted by Yamamoto et al., 96% of patients with gastroduodenal Crohn disease had disease elsewhere. In general, more than 50% of patients have known distal involvement before the diagnosis of gastroduodenal disease, and approximately 30% of patients present with duodenal and distal Crohn disease simultaneously. The most common distribution of gastroduodenal Crohn disease is contiguous involvement of the gastric antrum, pylorus, and the duodenal bulb. However, in a series of 89 patients from the Lahey clinic, isolated duodenal disease with gastric sparing was reported in 40% of patients.

Crohn disease of the upper gastrointestinal tract may produce symptoms of nausea, vomiting, dysphagia, or odynophagia and is often misdiagnosed as peptic ulcer disease. The failure of antiulcer medications to resolve symptoms often leads to further investigation, including endoscopy and upper

gastrointestinal imaging. Based on radiologic, endoscopic, and pathologic studies, the earliest findings in gastroduodenal Crohn disease are edema, aphthous ulceration, nodularity, cobblestoning, and irregular mucosal thickening, which often progresses to stricture formation and stenosis.

The use of medications to suppress gastric acid secretion and corticosteroid therapy is effective for patients with mild or moderate gastrointestinal Crohn disease. However, approximately one third of patients affected by gastroduodenal Crohn disease will require surgical intervention in their lifetime, most commonly for obstruction resulting from stenotic disease. Intractable pain, bleeding, and fistulas are also indications for surgical treatment. Options for surgical management of complicated gastroduodenal Crohn disease include bypass, stricturoplasty, and, less frequently, resection.

Traditionally, the "gold standard" for treating obstruction of the first and second portion of the duodenum has been to bypass the duodenum via a gastrojejunostomy. This procedure effectively relieves duodenal obstructive symptoms caused by Crohn strictures, but it carries a high risk for stomal ulcerations. Therefore, it is suggested that a vagotomy be performed along with the gastrojejunostomy. A highly selective vagotomy is preferred over a truncal vagotomy to reduce the incidence of vagotomy-related diarrhea. If the stricturing disease is limited to the third or fourth portions of the duodenum, a Roux-en-Y duodenojejunostomy to the proximal duodenum is preferred over a gastrojejunostomy because it eliminates the concern of developing acid-induced marginal ulceration.

Because of the frequency of morbidity and risk for recurrence with gastrojejunostomy, alternatives to bypass procedures have been sought. Ross et al. published a series of patients who had undergone bypass procedures for obstructing duodenal Crohn disease and reported a 70% reoperation rate for complications including marginal ulceration, recurrent obstruction, and duodenal fistula formation with a follow-up of 17 years. Given the focal nature of stricturing disease of the duodenum, stricturoplasty has become a viable option. The type of stricturoplasty depends on the location, the length, and the number of strictures present. Strictures in the first, second, and proximal third portion of the duodenum can effectively be managed with a Heineke-Mikulicz stricturoplasty. In order to safely accomplish a Heineke-Mikulicz stricturoplasty, the duodenum must be fully mobilized with a generous

Kocher maneuver. Strictures of the first and fourth portion of the duodenum are best handled with a Jaboulay and a Finney stricturoplasty, respectively, constructed by creating an enteroenterostomy between the greater curvature of the stomach and the first portion of the duodenum, or the fourth portion of the duodenum and the first loop of the jejunum.

The safety and efficacy of stricturoplasty in the management of obstructive gastroduodenal Crohn disease has been studied in a number of recent series. In a retrospective study conducted by Yamamoto et al., 13 patients underwent stricturoplasty for obstructive duodenal Crohn disease. Eleven of 13 patients had follow-up for more than 8 years. Three of 13 patients (23.1%) required further surgery because of early postoperative complications, and 6 of the 13 patients (46.2%) developed recurrent strictures at the previous stricturoplasty site. When compared with bypass surgery, the authors found that, after a median follow-up of 143 months, 9 of 13 patients (69.2%) who underwent stricturoplasty required reoperation, compared with 6 of 13 patients (46.2%) treated with bypass after a median follow-up of 192 months. Worsey et al. reported a more favorable experience with duodenal stricturoplasty when they compared this procedure with bypass surgery for the treatment of duodenal Crohn disease in a retrospectively study. They found that after a mean follow-up of 8 years, 1 of 21 patients (4.8%) who underwent a bypass procedure required reoperation for recurrent disease, and after a mean follow-up of 3.6 years, one of 13 patients (7.7%) treated by stricturoplasty required reoperation for recurrence, a difference that was not significant. They concluded that although the follow-up was shorter for stricturoplasty, it afforded the same rates of symptom relief and reoperation, but had fewer complications than traditional bypass surgery.

In recent years stricturoplasty, which has the advantage of avoiding a blind-loop syndrome or stomal ulceration, has replaced bypass as the operation of choice for treatment of short obstructive duodenal Crohn disease. However, if the duodenal stricture is lengthy, multiple strictures are present, or the tissues around the stricture are too rigid or unyielding, then a stricturoplasty should not be performed, but rather an intestinal bypass procedure should be undertaken.

Ileoduodenal or coloduodenal fistulas may also complicate gastroduodenal Crohn disease. The fistula usually arises from a diseased ileocolic segment after a previous ileocolic resection or the transverse colon and drains into the duodenum or stomach secondarily. Most duodenoenteric fistulas are small in caliber and asymptomatic, and they are identified with preoperative small bowel radiography or discovered at the time of surgery. Larger fistulas may present with symptoms of malabsorption and diarrhea caused by the shunting of duodenal contents into the distal small bowel. Most duodenal fistulas are located away from the juncture of the duodenal wall at the head of the pancreas and, therefore, after adequate mobilization, resection of the primary segment with primary closure of the duodenal defect is often sufficient. Larger or complex fistulas that are involved with a significant degree of inflammation need to be handled with great care at surgery to limit the size of the duodenal defect resulting from resection of the fistula. When a large duodenal defect is present, a Roux-en-Y duodenojejunostomy or a jejunal serosal patch may be required for adequate closure. Duodenal resections are almost never necessary from gastroduodenal Crohn disease and should be considered the surgical option of last resort.

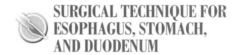

SURGICAL TECHNIQUE FOR ESOPHAGUS, STOMACH, AND DUODENUM

Gastrojejunostomy

A gastrojejunostomy and vagotomy are best performed though a midline incision. The vagotomy should be performed before the bypass to avoid any potential tension on the fresh anastomosis. The gastrojejunostomy can be performed either in an antecolic or a retrocolic fashion with either a handsewn or stapled anastomosis. If the colon is not involved, most surgeons prefer a simple side-to-side retrocolic approach in which a window is made in the avascular plane of the transverse mesocolon exposing the posterior wall of the stomach. Care is taken to identify the middle colic artery in order to avoid injuring it during the dissection. The most proximal loop of jejunum that lies tension-free next to the greater curvature of the stomach is selected. Two stay sutures are placed to hold the stomach and bowel together. In a stapled anastomosis, an enterotomy and gastrotomy are then made and the linear stapler is inserted and fired. The gastrotomy and enterotomy are then closed using two layers of interrupted 3–0 sutures. With a handsewn anastomosis, a posterior layer of interrupted 3–0 silk sutures is used to approximate the stomach and the seg-

ment of jejunum. An enterotomy and a gastrotomy are made and absorbable 3–0 sutures are used to make a continuous inner suture layer. An outer anterior layer of interrupted 3–0 silk sutures is then fashioned to complete the anastomosis and the defect in the mesocolon is closed.

Small Bowel

The small bowel is the most frequently affected gastrointestinal site in Crohn disease. Any portion of the small bowel may be diseased, but the terminal ileum is most commonly involved. Ninety percent of patients with Crohn disease of the small bowel experience abdominal pain caused by obstructive or septic complications, which may be associated with fevers, anorexia, or weight loss. Unremitting obstructive symptoms or an episode of high-grade obstruction indicate a severe degree of stenosis that will likely require surgical intervention. Crohn disease of the small intestine can also give rise to the formation of fistulas and abscesses. Patients may develop a palpable mass, usually located in the right lower quadrant, representing an abscess, a phlegmon, or a thickened loop of bowel. The differential diagnosis for small bowel Crohn disease includes irritable bowel syndrome, acute appendicitis, intestinal ischemia, radiation enteritis, pelvic inflammatory disease, endometriosis, and gynecologic malignancies.

Upper intestinal contrast studies, either small bowel follow-through or enteroclysis, are the best means of assessing the small bowel for Crohn disease. With early Crohn disease, a mucosal granular appearance with ulceration and nodularity can be identified radiologically. As the disease progresses, thickening of the mucosal folds and edema of the bowel wall becomes evident, eventually leading to the cobblestoning that is characteristic of advanced disease. Small bowel studies may occasionally demonstrate complications including high-grade strictures, fistulas, and abscesses, but are known to underestimate the extent of complicated Crohn disease. Small bowel studies may also be used to identify the location and length of involved intestine, to recognize whether the disease is continuous or discontinuous with skip lesions, and to determine whether areas of luminal narrowing are caused by acute inflammation or fibrostenotic scar tissue.

Surgical intervention in patients with Crohn disease of the small bowel is limited to the treatment of acute and chronic complications that do not respond to medical management. A study conducted at the

Cleveland Clinic found that with disease of 10 years' duration, 90% of patients with ileocolitis and 70% of patients with only ileal involvement required surgery. The researchers found that the indication for surgery was intestinal obstruction in 55% of patients and intestinal fistulas or abscesses in 32% of patients. Although the surgical approach may differ based on the indication for surgery and the site of disease, adherence to the principle of bowel conservation is preferred.

OPERATIVE TECHNIQUE FOR SMALL BOWEL

Small Bowel Resection

A planned small bowel resection is preceded by exploration of all four abdominal quadrants and of the entire small bowel for evidence of coexisting Crohn disease; this is mandatory, as up to 15% of patients will present with skip lesions. If areas of stenosis are suspected but not evident on serosal inspection, a Foley catheter with a balloon inflated to 2 cm and inserted through an enterotomy can be used to assess these sites. Before and after resection, the length of bowel should be measured and documented. The length of the diseased segment, the length of the resected segment, and the distance between strictures should be measured and recorded as well. The margins of macroscopic disease are then tagged with stay sutures and the diseased segment and its adjacent normal bowel are mobilized and isolated to minimize the possibility of contamination. In addition, the contents of the small bowel are milked either proximally or distally beyond the margins of the potential anastomosis. Matted loops of small bowel or omentum are often found adjacent to the diseased segment, especially if the terminal ileum is in-

volved. Care must be taken to adequately mobilize the affected areas, and mobilization of the ascending colon may even be required. The matted loops of bowel can then be separated with a combination of blunt and sharp dissection, and the area to be resected can be inspected. The length of the resection margin has been debated, but numerous randomized trials have reported that resection need only encompass grossly apparent disease and that wider resections do not improve surgical outcome.

Division of the thickened mesentery of the involved small bowel is often the most challenging aspect of the procedure. Because the extent of mesenteric dissection does not affect long-term results, the mesentery should be divided at the most advantageous level. It may be impossible to identify and isolate individual mesenteric vessels. Therefore, overlapping hemostatic clamps are commonly applied on either side of the intended line of transection and then the mesentery is divided between the clamps, with the tissue contained within the clamps suture-ligated using 0 or 1-0 absorbable sutures. Additional hemostatic mattress sutures may be needed to control bleeding (Fig. 1). Recently, newer sealing devices that employ bipolar technology have been developed for use in open and laparoscopic surgery that allow for safe control of vessels up to 7 mm in diameter. These instruments have reduced blood loss and the length of the procedure, and have simplified intraoperative management of the often thickened and friable mesentery of patients with Crohn disease. In spite of the technical challenges posed by the hyperemic and thickened mesentery, the risk of postoperative hemoperitoneum requiring surgical intervention has been reported to be less than 0.5%.

The bowel may be anastomosed in an end-to-end, end-to-side, or side-to-side

fashion using a handsewn or a stapled technique. In our practice, the bowel is anastomosed in a double-layered, handsewn, either end-to-end or side-to-side fashion. Recurrent Crohn disease after an ileocolic resection is likely to occur at the ileocolonic anastomosis or in the preanastomotic ileum. A side-to-side anastomosis is wider than an end-to-end or end-to-side anastomosis, and thus theoretically should lead to less fecal stasis and would require a longer period of time to stricture down to a critical diameter. However, clinical data have not demonstrated a significant clinical benefit for one configuration over another.

Resection with primary anastomosis can usually be performed with a high degree of safety, and small bowel anastomotic dehiscence rates can be kept to less than 1%. The decision to perform either a primary anastomosis or form a stoma depends on the overall condition of the patient and the conditions under which the procedure is performed. In the event that the procedure is emergent, the patient has suboptimal nutritional parameters, is on high-dose steroids or immunosuppressive agents, or diffuse peritonitis is present, formation of a stoma may be prudent. In these circumstances, the proximal end of the bowel may be brought out as a stoma.

When managing Crohn disease of the small bowel, it is important to consider the natural history of the disease. Reoperative rates have been reported to be as high as 60%, especially in patients undergoing resection of the small bowel. With each subsequent resection, the potential for intestinal insufficiency and short-gut syndrome increases. Therefore, nonresectional options such as stricturoplasty have gained popularity as an alternative to lengthy resections in the treatment of stricturing Crohn disease of the small intestine.

One of the earliest reports of intestinal stricturoplasty to treat ileal strictures secondary to intestinal tuberculosis was by Katariya et al. In the 1980s, Lee and Papaioannou began using this technique to treat fibrostenotic strictures in patients with Crohn disease. The advantage of a stricturoplasty lies in the preservation of the intestinal absorptive capacity of the normal segments of bowel located between strictures. Stricturoplasties can either be performed alone or in conjunction with a resection. However, they are best performed in the presence of either long segments of stricturing disease or multiple short strictures in which a resection would result in the loss of a lengthy segment of bowel or in patients with multiple prior resections. Stricturoplasties are also indicated when they

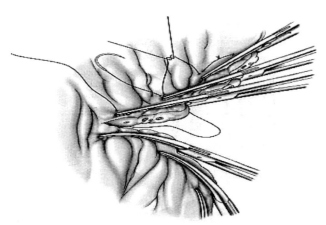

Fig. 1. Management of thickened Crohn mesentery. Hemostasis is obtained by placing overlapping hemostats across the bowel and then suture-ligating them.

fistulas typically heal well after fistulotomy and the risk of incontinence is low. In our experience 27 of 33 (82%) symptomatic low fistulas healed permanently with a superficial fistulotomy, a rate of success similar to the 79% reported by McKee and Keenan.

Surgical fistulotomies and cutting setons should not be used for suprasphincteric fistulas and should also be avoided for most transsphincteric fistulas. Medical treatment for extensive Crohn fistulas includes the use of 6—mercaptopurine, azathioprine, and cyclosporin. Probably the most effective agent at promoting healing of perianal fistulas related to Crohn disease is infliximab. With infliximab treatment, healing of the complex perianal fistulas is seen in 60% of cases. Recurrence of the fistula after infliximab, however, may be high. Additionally, persistent stasis or sepsis within the fistula tract can impede effective healing with medical treatment. To provide for adequate drainage throughout the fistula tract, many patients may benefit from placement of setons. The use of setons with infliximab therapy can improve the overall effectiveness of infliximab. Typically, the seton is placed prior to the initiation of infliximab therapy and then it is removed after the second or third treatment.

When adequate drainage of the tract has been achieved, and in the absence of rectal disease, a rectal advancement flap may be used to close the internal opening of the fistula. Kodner et al. reported a 92% success rate in patients with complex fistulas secondary to Crohn disease who underwent rectal advancement flaps, with primary healing reported in 17 of 24 patients and eventual healing in 5 of 24 patients.

Severe cases of perianal fistulas that do not respond to aggressive medical and surgical management may require fecal drainage with creation of an ileostomy. Diversion of the fecal stream often results in significant relief of local inflammation and can assist in the healing of perianal fistulas, but recurrences are common and intestinal continuity often cannot be restored. In a series of 69 patients with Crohn colitis who had undergone an ileostomy for fecal diversion reported by Lee et al., 22 (32%) eventually required a proctectomy and 25 (36%) remained defunctionalized. Restoration of intestinal continence was only achieved in 18 (26%) patients. Yamamoto et al. found that, in 31 patients who underwent fecal diversion for perianal Crohn disease, 81% (25) achieved early remission, but complete remission was only achieved in 26% (8) of patients, with 68% (21) even-

tually requiring proctectomy. Only 3 patients (10%) underwent restoration of intestinal continuity.

Proctectomy is indicated when perianal disease is unrelenting or results in damage to the sphincters, causing debilitating incontinence. However, a combination of catheter drainage, seton placement, and intensive medical therapy results in the avoidance of a proctectomy or a fecal drainage procedure in the majority of patients. At our institution, 224 of 717 patients with Crohn disease presented with anorectal complications. Of those, 139 patients (62%) retained anorectal function, with complete healing in 84 patients, control of sepsis in 25 patients, and observation in the remaining 30 patients. Eighty-five patients (38%) required a proctectomy with a permanent stoma. Patients with rectal involvement had significantly higher rates of proctectomy compared with patients with rectal sparing (77.6% vs. 13.6%, respectively). Therefore, although complete healing and control of sepsis can often be achieved in patients with anorectal Crohn disease, the presence of active rectal disease and multiple synchronous complications significantly increases the need for a rectal ablative procedure.

OPERATIVE TECHNIQUE FOR FISTULAS

Fistulotomy

The patient is placed in the prone jackknife position. A probe is carefully inserted into the external opening and advanced through the tract until it emerges from the internal opening. The probe should never be passed forcefully. If the path of the tract or the internal opening is difficult to find, methylene blue or dilute hydrogen peroxide can be injected into the external opening. Using electrocautery, the fistulotomy is performed over the probe, starting at the external opening and carried out to the internal opening while carefully maintaining meticulous hemostasis. If a significant portion of the sphincters are encountered in the fistulous tract, the fistulotomy is stopped and a seton is placed to drain the remainder of the tract. The unroofed fistulous tract is then curetted of all infected granulation tissue.

Rectal Advancement Flap

A rectal advancement flap can be used to cover the internal opening of a perianal fistulous tract or a rectovaginal fistula if the rectal mucosa is free of active disease.

The patient is placed in a prone jackknife position if the fistula's opening is anterior and in a lithotomy position if the opening is posterior. After making an incision at the dentate line, a thick, U-shaped flap inclusive of mucosa, submucosa, muscle fibers of the internal sphincter, and muscularis propria is elevated with the apex of the flap at the internal opening of the fistula. The flap is raised 4 to 5 cm cephalad. Using electrocautery, care is taken to obtain adequate hemostasis. The fistulous tract is then curetted and closed in layers with 3–0 or 4–0 absorbable sutures. The distal end of the flap is appropriately trimmed, elevated, pulled down over the repaired defect, and secured to the dentate line with a series of interrupted absorbable sutures. A temporary stoma may be considered for the difficult or recurrent repairs, although there are no data in the literature providing evidence that the healing rate is increased by fecal diversion.

Rectovaginal Fistulas

A rectovaginal fistula is a relatively rare complication of Crohn disease that is characterized by the discharge of stool or gas from the vagina. It is usually caused by a fistula that arises from the anorectum and eventually erodes through the vaginal wall, usually at the introitus. In one third to one half of patients, the rectovaginal fistula is either asymptomatic or presents with minimal symptoms and requires no treatment. However, symptomatic fistulas may result in dyspareunia, perineal pain, difficulty maintaining adequate hygiene, or repeated vaginal infections and must be treated aggressively. Fistulas may be initially treated with antibiotics and, if needed, the insertion of a noncutting seton. Once the infection is ablated, a transrectal advancement flap may be used to aid in the closure of the fistula in patients without significant anorectal disease.

CONCLUSION

Although significant advancements have been made in the medical management of Crohn disease, surgical intervention is still required in most patients to treat complications and palliate symptoms. As the investigation to elucidate the mechanism of Crohn disease and the development of more specific medical therapies continue, optimal treatment requires a team approach including surgeons, gastroenterologists, radiologists, pathologists, and nursing specialists. Although Crohn disease presents with varying clinical manifestations, requiring individualized treatment,

The Gastrointestinal Tract

the main goal of surgery in all individuals is to adequately relieve symptoms while avoiding excessive loss of bowel function or body disfiguration.

ACKNOWLEDGMENTS

This work was supported in part by an educational grant from Applied Medical, Rancho Santa Margarita, CA.

SUGGESTED READING

Crohn BB, GL, Oppenheimer GD. Regional ileitis: a pathological and clinical entity. *JAMA* 1932;99:1323.
Farmer RG, Hawk WA, Turnbull RB Jr, Indications for surgery in Crohn's disease: analysis of 500 cases. *Gastroenterology* 1976;71:245.
Fazio VW, et al. Effect of resection margins on the recurrence of Crohn's disease in the small bowel. A randomized controlled trial. *Ann Surg* 1996;224:563.

Fichera A, et al. Long-term outcome of surgically treated Crohn's colitis: a prospective study. *Dis Colon Rectum* 2005;48:963.
Greenstein AJ, et al. Spontaneous free perforation and perforated abscess in 30 patients with Crohn's disease. *Ann Surg* 1987;205:72.
Greenstein AJ, et al. Cancer in Crohn's disease after diversionary surgery. A report of seven carcinomas occurring in excluded bowel. *Am J Surg* 1978;135:86.
Hyman NH, et al. Consequences of ileal pouch-anal anastomosis for Crohn's colitis. *Dis Colon Rectum* 1991;34:653.
Lee EC, Papaioannou N. Minimal surgery for chronic obstruction in patients with extensive or universal Crohn's disease. *Ann R Coll Surg Engl* 1982;64:229.
Longo WE, et al. Outcome of ileorectal anastomosis for Crohn's colitis. *Dis Colon Rectum* 1992;35:1066.
Michelassi F, et al. Primary and recurrent Crohn's disease. Experience with 1379 patients. *Ann Surg* 1991;214:230.
Michelassi F, et al. Side-to-side isoperistaltic strictureplasty in extensive Crohn's disease: a

prospective longitudinal study. *Ann Surg* 2000;232:401.
Milsom JW, et al. Prospective, randomized trial comparing laparoscopic vs. conventional surgery for refractory ileocolic Crohn's disease. *Dis Colon Rectum* 2001;44:1.
Munoz-Juarez M, et al. Wide-lumen stapled anastomosis vs. conventional end-to-end anastomosis in the treatment of Crohn's disease. *Dis Colon Rectum* 2001;44:20.
Nugent FW, Roy MA. Duodenal Crohn's disease: an analysis of 89 cases. *Am J Gastroenterol* 1989;84:249.
Panis Y, et al. Ileal pouch/anal anastomosis for Crohn's disease. *Lancet* 1996;347:854.
Present DH, et al. Infliximab for the treatment of fistulas in patients with Crohn's disease. *N Engl J Med* 1999;340:1398.
Worsey MJ, et al. Strictureplasty is an effective option in the operative management of duodenal Crohn's disease. *Dis Colon Rectum* 1999;42:596.
Yamamoto T, Allan RN, Keighley MR. An audit of gastroduodenal Crohn disease: clinicopathologic features and management. *Scand J Gastroenterol* 1999;34:1019.

EDITOR'S COMMENT

Crohn disease is panenteric disease, with lesions that may occur from the oral cavity to the anus, the latter being quite common, the former being somewhat less common, although common enough that it is seen. Its cause remains obscure, with suggestions as far-ranging as the silica in tooth powder and toothpaste (the notion being that both toothpaste and the disease seem to have been discovered at the same time) to an autoimmune phenomenon, whatever that is, to an infectious cause. I have often wondered whether the disease itself is benign, and if the manifestations that we deal with are superinfection. When considering the cause, one should remember that Sir Kennedy Dalziel, a Scottish surgeon of great renown who was also surgeon to the Queen, in 1909 published an article in the *British Medical Journal* in which he resected nine patients with Crohn disease, without mortality, and noted atypical microbacteria in the extracted specimen. Although researchers have looked far and wide for these atypical microbacteria, it is only the occasional case in which microbacteria *Kansasii* has been noted. However, if the article had been remembered, we would have called it Dalziel disease, rather than Crohn disease, a name that should not be remembered as it was based on one of the greatest intellectual frauds of the 20th century. Crohn took the cases of Ginsberg and Oppenheimer without telling them, put their names on the article, and published it. This, in my view, should not be rewarded; therefore, the entity should be called *regional enteritis* rather than Crohn disease.

There are at least three different types of patients with regional enteritis, and we often lose sight of this. As far as I'm aware, there is only one article published pertaining to patients who never are hospitalized, with probably a mild form of regional enteritis. These are patients who are often 18 or 19 years old and who I will frequently see in the clinic, with tenderness in the right lower quadrant, a classic history of mucous-laden diarrhea 20 to 30 minutes

after meals, and on physical examination one could almost convince oneself that one feels a mass. I do not perform a barium enema on these people, nor do I perform a colonoscopy on them. I prescribe azulfadine, which to me is probably the most effective of the drugs for regional enteritis. In 6 months the symptoms are usually gone, and I do not see them again.

As for patients who require hospitalization and operation, Freund et al. (*Am J Surg* 1997;174:339) have pointed out in a very interesting article that patients who required operation because of serious complications are different from patients who do not want to be bothered with the symptoms of regional enteritis. They called these patients *lifestyle* patients. The two types of patients were different in outcome: lifestyle patients rarely had recurrences, were symptom-free after several years of follow-up of operation; whereas patients who were operated on for serious complications often had recurrences within 11 months, and required further therapy. The fact that there are several categories of this disease should not come as a surprise to anyone who deals with a chronic disease situation.

This chapter is a masterful chapter, written by someone who deals with this disease on a frequent basis, whatever one wants to call it, and is magnificently documented. Dr. Michelassi and his colleagues begin by telling us about gastroduodenal disease and that, despite the fact that one expects that this is a disease encompassing both the gastric antrum and the duodenum, duodenal disease is associated with gastric sparing in 40% of the patients. Should these patients require intervention, however, it is often intervention that is required for concomitant ileal disease. My experience is similar, and if one does see gastroduodenal or duodenal disease, it is in patients with very symptomatic ileal disease, and one picks up gastroduodenal disease because of the thorough investigation that should precede any therapy for regional enteritis.

The technical aspects of dealing with the thickened, often node-laden mesentery is well thought

out, and will result in far less difficulty with mesenteric bleeding by using the overlapping clamp technique. I often will score both sides of the mesentery, and then compress the edematous fat with the fingers prior to applying clamps, in addition to making certain that the clamps overlap. This is an added technique that enables one to resect these difficult mesenteries. It should be noted that it does not make a difference if one leaves the presumably inflammatory nodes at the base of the mesentery; the recurrence rate seems to be the same as with more radical excisions of the mesentery, which is technically difficult.

Much of the discussion in this chapter really deals with minimizing the short bowel syndrome, which is something that every surgeon who is experienced in dealing with regional enteritis knows. Originally, the concept of the "skimped resection," in which one merely wants to get to the point where one does not have gross ulceration of the bowel when doing the resection, which is necessary. I use the thickness of the mesentery near the bowel, as well as the absence of large nodes near the bowel, as my primary indication for what the resection margin should be. If one uses the absence of fat overgrowth, one takes out a great deal more of the bowel than is necessary, given the fact that margins that have absolutely no disease at all and margins that have microscopic disease both have the same rate of recurrence. However, as those patients who are referred to us have more and more severe disease, I agree with the contention of this chapter that strictureplasty should play a more significant role than it has in the past. One should remember, as the authors point out, that strictureplasty was originally proposed for those tight fibrotic strictures that were associated with inactive tuberculosis, the "cold strictures." And the cold stricture was the initial target in the strictureplasty in regional enteritis. As time evolved, surgeons became more adventuresome, and strictureplasty was applied not only to cold strictures, but also to

(continued)

warm strictures, although I don't think very many surgeons perform stricturoplasty for hot strictures. The fact that stricturoplasty is now being applied to warm strictures has led, in many instances, to a leak rate as high as 9% in some series.

Ileovesical or colovesical fistulas can be treated in a single stage. The diagnosis is often more difficult than the therapy. The history is specific enough, with pneumaturia and fecaluria, or vegetable material appearing in the urine. I have treated some patients who absolutely refuse operation for 8 or 9 years with intermittent antibiotics when they become symptomatic. The diagnosis is often more difficult than the therapy. Barium enemas and small bowel follow-throughs and enteroclysis will often not reveal the fact that there is a fistula. Cystoscopy often reveals a reddened area of inflammation in an area that one would expect would be a fistula, happily more often in the dome of the bladder, allowing one to deal with it expeditiously with a three-layer closure reinforced with omentum, rather than near the trigon, which would be more difficult. The best way of making the diagnosis is by having the patient ingest polyethylene glycol labeled with carbon 14 ([^{14}C]PEG), which of course is not absorbed, and [^{14}C]PEG then appears in the urine and can be counted. Trying to get an institutional committee to pass the ingestion of carbon 14 nowadays, however, is extraordinarily difficult.

Dr. Michelassi justifiably gets credit for introducing the side-to-side isoperistaltic anastomosis, often with a double Heineke-Mikulicz procedure, first described in 1996 (Michelassi F, *Dis Colon Rectum* 1996;39:345). This has been commented on by a number of authors. Sasaki et al. (*Dis Colon Rectum* 2004;47:940) described a modified isoperistaltic stricturoplasty associated, I believe, with intestinal resection in eight patients. In this study, which has more authors than patients, the technique is modified and, after partial bowel resection (it was not stipulated why resection was done), and if resection was done, it is not clear why the isoperistaltic side-to-side anastomosis had to be carried out. The article is confusing in that in one place the authors state they operated on eight patients, and in another place, 23 patients, and toward the end of the article, disease recurrence near the side-to-side anastomosis was confirmed during reoperation in 2 of 23 patients.

Because it is impossible to really know the outcome in this series, one then turns to Tonelli et al. (*Dis Colon Rectum* 2004;47:494), who reviewed a variety of operations in 31 patients, many of whom had additional concomitant bowel resection, and 17 patients—probably some in the same—received an additional stricturoplasty elsewhere in the bowel. Decreases of activity indices were observed in 62.3% of patients within 6 months after surgery, and after an average follow-up of more than 2 years, six patients required operation, but the recurrence involved the long stricturoplasty site in only one of these patients. The authors point out that, even in that case, the side-to-side isoperistaltic stricturoplasty was intact but without any inflammation or stenosis. Obviously, any patient in whom a stricture is 10 cm or longer and who is being operated on represents the severe extent of disease, so one really should expect patients to have very complex disease, requiring multiple operations.

Another reason for operation in patients with regional enteritis is toxic megacolon. True, most of us associate toxic megacolon with ulcerative colitis, and indeed Ausch et al. (*Colorectal Dis* 2006;8:195) reported on 70 patients with a mean age of 68 years and with surgically managed toxic megacolon. The older age of the patients gives credibility to the fact that toxic megacolon was the result of inflammatory bowel disease in only 48% of the patients. A variety of operations were done on these patients, including ileorectal anastomoses and ileal pouch-anal anastomoses. These results were taken from three academic colorectal units in Vienna, the University of Minnesota, and the Danube Hospital. In their series, toxic megacolon is present in up to 10% of patients admitted with ulcerative colitis, and only 2.3% of patients admitted with regional enteritis, which matches my own personal experience. Total mortality rate in the entire group was 16%, reflecting not so much the diagnosis of ulcerative colitis in 32 patients, but infectious colitis in 24, ischemic colitis in 8, iatrogenic toxic megacolon in 5, and cytotoxic medication in 3 patients.

A very nice pearl in this chapter is the statement that some patients with regional enteritis confined to the colon, and absolutely no indication of ileal regional enteritis, may be candidates for ileal-pouch and anal anastomosis. Indeed, having done approximately 400 of these operations, approximately 15% of the patients on whom I personally operated had indeterminate colitis (Robb et al., *Am J Sur* 2002;183:353). A number of them likely had regional enteritis. Dr. Michelassi and colleagues make the point that if there is no clear indication of small bowel involvement, it is probably safe to carry out an ileal-pouch anal anastomosis, and for the most part one will get away with it. Not on all patients, however, and a number of patients who turn out to have regional enteritis following ileal-pouch anal anastomosis will require pouch removal. Similar thoughts were expressed by Delaini et al. (*Tech Coloproctol* 2005;9:222), who focused more on continent ileostomy, but as only 15% of these patients underwent continent ileostomy for indeterminate colitis, they used the analogy that ileal-pouch anal anastomosis should also be acceptable. The follow-up was long: 27 and 24 years, respectively. The overall mortality rate was 22% in the continent pouch ileostomy and 19% in the conventional ileostomy. Deaths from postoperative complications were 9% in the patients who had continent ileostomy and 4% in the conventional ileostomy. The reasons for mortality are not mentioned, but the mortality clearly is high. Shen et al. (*Am J Gastroenterol* 2005;100:2796) reviewed complications of ileal-pouch anal anastomosis, including pouchitis, regional enteritis of the pouch, cuffitis, and irritable pouch syndrome, relying on biopsy and endoscopy as principal means of diagnosis. They, too, agree that patients with regional enteritis limited to the colon, with no small intestinal or perianal disease, are candidates for restorative proctocolectomy, as they call it, or ileal-pouch anal anastomosis, as most others call it (Panis Y et al., *Lancet* 1996;347:854). They do, however, point out that sometimes these patients will later present with clear regional enteritis of the pouch, years after having a pouch created after total proctocolectomy.

Although it is not emphasized in this chapter, it should be pointed out when one is discussing the status of the rectal segment, that patients who undergo operation for regional enteritis of the colon, and whose rectal segment is deemed unsuitable for anastomosis for any reason at the first sitting, will only undergo closure; in other words, takedown of ileostomy and ileorectal anastomosis between 3% and 7% of the time. Thus, if one does not think the rectal segment or the sigmoid segment is suitable for ileosigmoidostomy or ileorectostomy, one is better off doing a resection, as the authors claim, as it is highly unlikely that the patient will ever move the bowels through the rectum. However, it does occasionally occur; I recently carried out such a procedure on a gentleman after 4 years, although it is not clear why he was not connected in the first place. At the present time, 6 months after the procedure, he seems to be doing well, and the rectal segment does not show any evidence of renewed inflammation.

Stricturoplasty does seem to have become a staple of treatment of regional enteritis, perhaps much more so than resection in certain areas. Futami and Arima (*J Gastroenterol* 2005;16:35) reviewed 103 patients undergoing 293 stricturoplasties without operative mortality, although septic complications developed in 2 patients (1.9%). Mean duration of follow-up was more than 6 years, and the 5- and 10-year reoperation rate was 45% and 62%, respectively, of which 20% of patients had recurrence at the site of stricturoplasty. These patients were more traditional, with a mean age of 31.4 years, and 44 of the 103 patients had previous surgery, which emphasizes why they took such great pains to undergo stricturoplasty. Their experience seems to reinforce the emphasis placed on preservation of bowel in this chapter.

In most of the literature, neoplasia is usually associated with ulcerative colitis. However, neoplasia does occur on a regular basis in regional enteritis (Stahl et al., *Curr Prob Cancer* 1981;5:1). It is normally associated with small bowel adenocarcinoma, which has an entirely different pattern in regional enteritis than normal adenocarcinoma of the small bowel, which itself is rare. We are mostly familiar with a latency rate of approximately 15 to 20 years in patients who had undergone bypass rather than resection in classic regional enteritis affecting the terminal ileum and the secum. However, these patients are becoming rare as this operation was carried out mostly in the 1930s, 1940s, and 1950s, whereas resection is the treatment of choice at this time. The authors do emphasize that carcinoma of the large bowel also occurs, although at a much lower rate than ulcerative colitis. However, they argue for surveillance after 7 to 10 years, and biopsy of strictures, and if strictures prevent colonoscopic surveillance, the strictures should be resected.

Finally, a welcome article by Canavan et al. (*Aliment Pharmacol Ther* 2006;23:377) reviewed quality of life in patients with regional enteritis, as well as a meta-analysis of others' experience with the same questions. There are four categories of concerns, including (a) disease-related, e.g., financial difficulties, pain or suffering, dying early; (b) body stigma, loss of attractiveness, loss of bowel control, feeling dirty or smelly, having an ostomy bag; (c) the impact of Crohn disease on relationships, such as passing the disease on to others or being treated as different; and, probably the most difficult, (d) sexual intimacy, sexual performance, ability to have children, and loss of sexual drive. In general, patients who have undergone this surgery have lower quality of life than patients who have not, which is not surprising because the former are the more severe group. The authors point out something that is often forgotten in the treatment of patients with regional enteritis, which is our ability to make them comfortable and to restore quality of life. I agree.

J.E.F.

The Gastrointestinal Tract

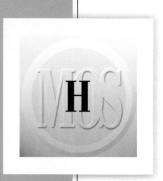

Surgery of the Colon

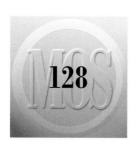

128 Anatomy of the Colon

RICHARD L. DRAKE

The large intestine consists of the cecum, the appendix, and the ascending, transverse, descending, and sigmoid colons (Fig. 1). Functionally, the large intestine is involved in the conversion of the liquid contents of the ileum into semisolid feces. Throughout its length, there is an alternating pattern of fixed and mobile components. The cecum and the transverse and sigmoid colons possess considerable mobility, whereas the ascending and descending colons are fixed to the posterior wall. The general characteristics of the colon are its large caliber; the presence of pendant-shaped bodies of fat enclosed by peritoneum, called *omental appendices;* and the longitudinal muscle in its walls, which forms three narrow, ribbon-like bands called *taeniae coli.* The locations of the taeniae are useful landmarks and are specific in relation to the position of the colon itself. The posterior taenia, or tenia omental, is found on the posterolateral border of the ascending and descending colons and the anterior border of the transverse colon. The anterior taenia, or tenia libera, is visible on the exposed or antimesenteric border of the cecum and the ascending, descending, and sigmoid colons, but it is located on the inferior surface of the transverse colon and covered by the attachment of the greater omentum. The lateral taenia, or tenia mesocolica, is located on the posteromedial side of the cecum and the ascending, descending, and sigmoid colons, and on the posterior border of the transverse colon at the attachment of the transverse mesocolon. Between the taeniae coli the colon is sacculated, forming the *haustra of colon.*

CECUM AND APPENDIX

The cecum is the saccular commencement of the colon. It is located in the right iliac fossa, where it lies on the iliacus muscle cranial to the lateral half of the inguinal ligament. At times, it may cross the pelvic brim to lie in the true pelvis. Anteriorly, it usually is in contact with the anterior abdominal wall. Superiorly, it is continuous with the ascending colon, and at some point along its medial border, the ileum enters it at the ileocecal ostium. This opening is surrounded by two flaps that protrude into the lumen and contain circular muscle derived partly from the ileal musculature and partly from the cecal musculature (Fig. 2). This structure is referred to as the *ileocecal valve,* but it is questionable whether the valve acts as a functional sphincter. The cecum has no mesentery, even though it is referred to as being an intraperitoneal structure in most individuals, because it has a considerable amount of mobility.

The vermiform appendix takes origin from the posteromedial border of the cecum and can be located by following the anterior taenia to its junction with the other two taeniae. Its size is variable, 5 to 10 mm in diameter and 8 to 10 cm in length; in most people, it is found in a retrocecal position. The attachment of the appendix is extended along the inferior border of the terminal portion of the ileum by its own mesentery, the mesoappendix (Fig. 3). The appendicular artery and vein are found in this mesentery. The appendix is involved in the formation of several recesses in

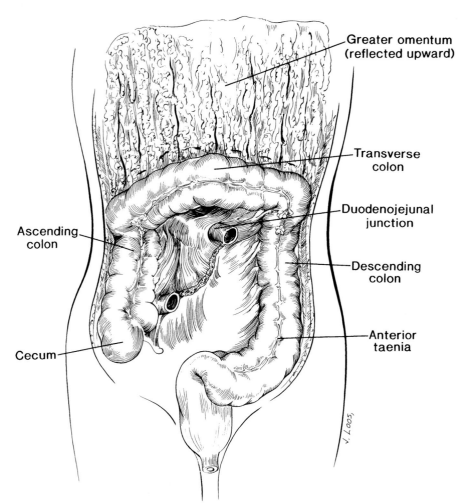

Fig. 1. The abdominal cavity opened to demonstrate the components of the large intestine, which consists of the cecum, the appendix, and the ascending, transverse, descending, and sigmoid colons.

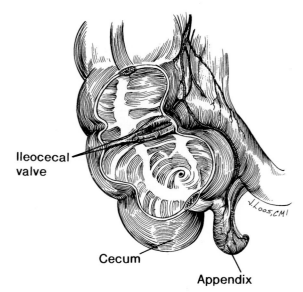

Fig. 2. The cecum is opened to show the ileocecal ostium. It is surrounded by two flaps that protrude into the lumen of the cecum and form the ileocecal valve.

association with the cecum (Fig. 3). The superior ileocecal recess (fossa of Luschka) lies anterior to the terminal ileum. It is formed by a peritoneal fold, the superior ileocecal or vascular fold, which extends from the mesentery of the terminal ileum, and, after crossing the ileum, it attaches to the lowest part of the colon and cecum. This fold contains the anterior cecal artery. Similarly, the inferior ileocecal recess lies between the mesoappendix and a fold of peritoneum referred to as the inferior ileocecal fold or the bloodless fold of Treves. This fold extends from the antimesenteric border of the terminal ileum to the base of the appendix or the anterior surface of the mesoappendix, or to both areas. The fold contains no sizable blood vessels. The surface projection of the base of the appendix lies at the junction of the lateral and middle third of a line joining the anterior superior iliac spine with the umbilicus, known as *McBurney point*. Patients who have acute appendicitis often describe a localized pain near this point.

ASCENDING COLON

The ascending colon begins at the superior end of the cecum. This part of the colon has no mesentery and is relatively fixed to the posterior abdominal wall. The upper part of the ascending colon is covered anteriorly by coils of small intestine, but the lower part may come into direct contact with the anterior abdominal wall. Posteriorly, the ascending colon is related to the lower pole of the right kidney and lies on the iliacus muscle and the aponeurotic origin of the transversus abdominis muscle. The kidney and branches of the lumbar plexus separate the ascending colon from the quadratus lumborum muscle.

Anterior to the right kidney and immediately inferior to the right lobe of the liver, the ascending colon makes a sharp bend to the left, forming the right colic (hepatic) flexure (Fig. 4). Structures posterior to this flexure include the descending or second part of the duodenum, which is covered by a layer of parietal peritoneum, and the renal, or Gerota, fascia surrounding the right kidney, since the posterior aspect of the hepatic flexure is not covered by peritoneum (Figs. 5 and 6).

Lateral to the ascending colon is the right paracolic sulcus, or gutter. This depression is formed by a reflection of the peritoneum after it crosses the ascending colon and before it continues onto the posterior abdominal wall. Material can move along this gutter from the appendix to the hepatorenal recess or from the liver

The Gastrointestinal Tract

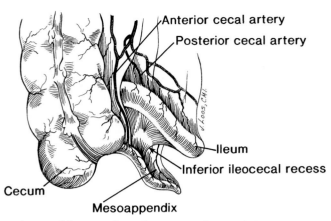

Fig. 3. The attachment of the appendix to the cecum and terminal ileum, which shows the superior and inferior ileocecal folds and the mesoappendix.

into the pelvis. Additionally, surgeons can incise the peritoneum along this border, the "white fascial line of Toldt," to mobilize the ascending colon. The blood vessels and lymphatics lie in the retroperitoneal connective tissue on the medial or posteromedial side of the ascending colon, which, during development, composed the mesentery of the ascending colon. Thus, by mobilizing the ascending colon on this lateral avascular border and raising it toward the midline, the retroperitoneal connective tissue containing the blood vessels and lymphatics can be lifted intact.

TRANSVERSE COLON

The transverse colon begins at the right colic flexure and passes to the left side, where it ends at the left colic or splenic flexure. It is intraperitoneal and suspended from the posterior abdominal wall by the transverse mesocolon. Although its posterior relationships can vary because of its mobility, the transverse colon is usually anterior to the hilus of the right kidney, the descending (second) part of the duodenum, and the head of the pancreas. Its cranial surface is in contact with the liver, the gallbladder, the greater curvature of the stomach, and the spleen. Its caudal surface is in contact with the small intestine, and its anterior surface contacts the anterior layers of the greater omentum and the abdominal wall.

Just inferior to the spleen, the transverse colon turns downward, forming the left colic or splenic flexure (Fig. 4). This flexure is higher and situated more posteriorly than the right colic flexure and is suspended from the diaphragm by the left phrenicocolic ligament, a distinct peritoneal fold. Structures posterior to this flexure include a portion of the spleen, the tail of the pancreas and the renal, or Gerota, fascia, which surrounds the left kidney (Figs. 5 and 6).

DESCENDING COLON

The descending colon begins at the left colic flexure where the intestine loses its mesentery. The upper part of the descending colon is separated from the anterior abdominal wall by the end of the transverse colon and by coils of the small intestine. The lower part frequently comes into contact with the anterior abdominal wall superior to the inguinal ligament. Posteriorly, as was the case with the ascending colon, the descending colon is related to the lower pole of the left kidney and lies on the iliacus muscle and the aponeurotic origin of the transversus abdominis muscle. The kidney and branches of the lumbar plexus separate the descending colon from the quadratus lumborum muscle. Posteromedially, the descending colon is in contact with the left psoas major muscle. As is the case with the ascending colon, the left paracolic sulcus (gutter) is immediately lateral to the descending colon. Because the major vascular and lymphatic channels are located on the medial or posteromedial side of the descending colon, a relatively bloodless mobilization is possible through incisions of the peritoneum along the gutter.

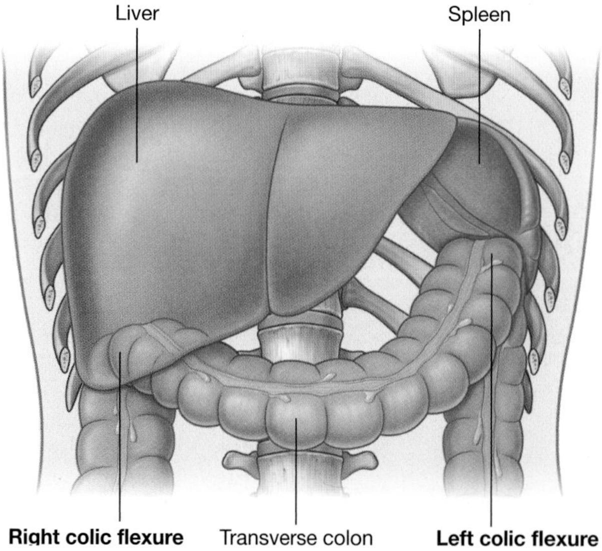

SIGMOID COLON

At or below the crest of the ileum, the colon acquires a mesentery and becomes the sigmoid colon. This section of the colon continues inferiorly until it loses its mesentery, usually anterior to vertebra S3, and becomes the rectum. This junction is indicated by a slight constriction caused by a functional rectosigmoid sphincter that controls the passage of the contents of the colon into the rectum. The sigmoid colon is attached at its junction with the descending colon and rectum, but mobile throughout its length. The mobile portion is suspended by a mesentery, the sigmoid mesocolon, whose inverted V-shaped attachment is to the pelvic brim and the posterior wall of the pelvis (Fig. 7). Structures posterior to the sigmoid colon include the left external and internal iliac vessels, the left gonadal vessels, the left ureter, and the roots of the

Fig. 4. Right and left colic flexures. (From Drake RL, Vogl W, Mitchell AWM. *Gray's anatomy for students.* Philadelphia: Churchill Livingstone [Elsevier], 2005.)

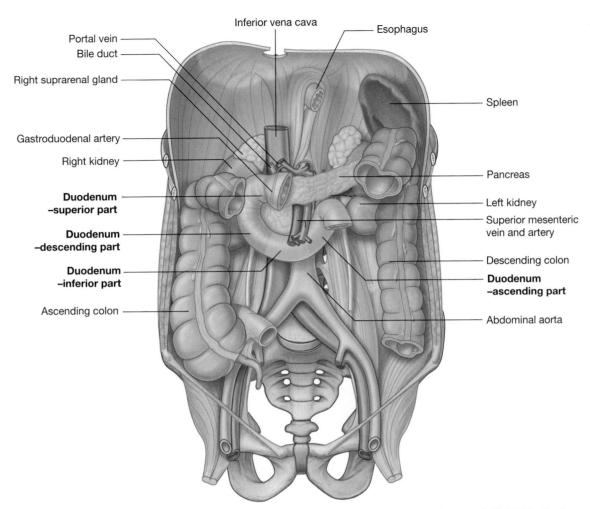

Fig. 5. Structures posterior to the right and left colic flexures. (From Drake RL, Vogl W, Mitchell AWM. *Gray's anatomy for students.* Philadelphia: Churchill Livingstone [Elsevier], 2005.)

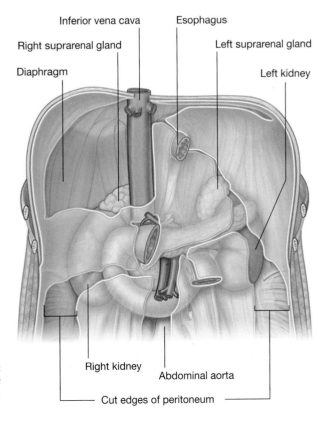

Fig. 6. Retroperitoneal positioning of the kidneys relative to the right and left colic flexures. (From Drake RL, Vogl W, Mitchell AWM. *Gray's anatomy for students.* Philadelphia: Churchill Livingstone [Elsevier], 2005.)

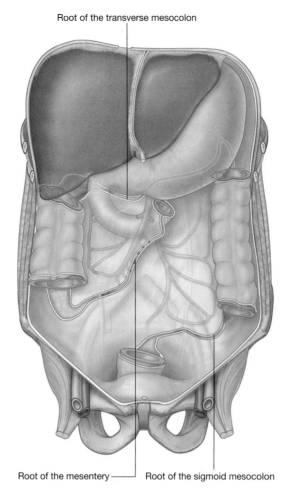

Fig. 7. Attachment or root of the sigmoid mesocolon along the posterior abdominal wall. (From Drake RL, Vogl W, Mitchell AWM. *Gray's anatomy for students.* Philadelphia: Churchill Livingstone [Elsevier], 2005.)

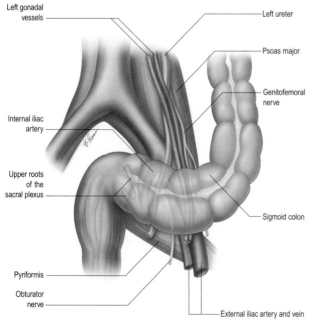

Fig. 8. Structures posterior to the sigmoid colon. (From Drake RL, Vogl W, Mitchell AWM. *Gray's anatomy for students.* Philadelphia: Churchill Livingstone [Elsevier], 2005.)

sacral plexus (Fig. 8). Care must be taken during any dissection in this area because of the relationship of these structures to the sigmoid mesocolon. Additionally, the left ureter lies along the lateral aspect of the inferior mesenteric vein throughout much of its long retroperitoneal course. Finally, because of the variable length of the sigmoid colon, it is separated from the bladder in the man and the uterus in the woman by coils of the small intestine.

VASCULAR SUPPLY

The vascular supply to the colon is through the superior mesenteric artery, the second ventral branch of the abdominal aorta, and the inferior mesenteric artery, the third ventral branch of the abdominal aorta (Fig. 9). The superior mesenteric artery arises opposite the lower border of vertebra L1 and descends in a groove on the posterior surface of the body of the pancreas. The artery crosses anterior to the left renal vein, the uncinate process of the pancreas, and the horizontal portion of the duodenum. It gives off three major branches to the colon. The first branch is the middle colic artery, which enters the transverse mesocolon and divides into right and left branches. These branches contribute to the marginal artery. The second branch is the right colic artery, which approaches the ascending colon retroperitoneally and divides into ascending and descending branches. These branches also contribute to the marginal artery. The third branch is the ileocolic artery, which runs directly toward the ileocecal junction along the root of the mesentery. As this branch approaches the ileocecal junction, it gives off several branches, including the ascending colic artery, which passes along the ascending colon and contributes to the formation of the marginal artery; the anterior cecal artery, which passes in the vascular fold to the cecum; the posterior cecal artery, which passes retroperitoneally behind the cecum; and the appendicular artery, which descends behind the ileum and enters the mesoappendix (Fig. 3). The appendicular artery often is a branch of the posterior cecal artery.

The second major artery supplying the colon, the inferior mesenteric artery, arises approximately 4 cm above the aortic bifurcation at the level of vertebra L3 (Fig. 9). Its major branches to the colon are the left colic artery, which runs retroperitoneally to the left, dividing into ascending and descending branches that contribute to the marginal artery, and the sigmoidal arteries, which consist of two to four branches.

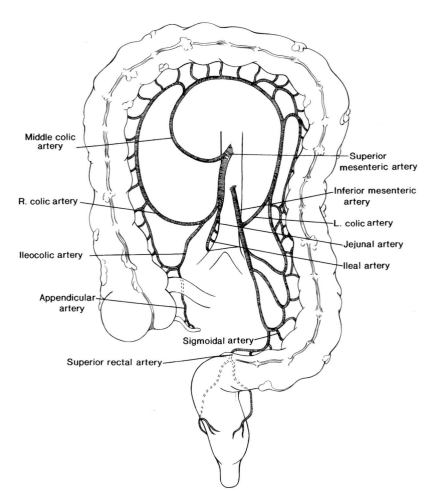

Middle colic artery

R. colic artery

Ileocolic artery

Appendicular artery

Superior rectal artery

Sigmoidal artery

Superior mesenteric artery

Inferior mesenteric artery

L. colic artery

Jejunal artery

Ileal artery

Fig. 9. The vascular supply to the colon is from the superior and inferior mesenteric arteries. The distribution of these arteries and their branches is shown.

All of the arteries mentioned previously contribute to the formation of a continuous arterial channel that runs on the inner margin of the colon, from the cecocolic junction to the rectosigmoid junction. Vessels involved in this arterial channel include the ascending branch of the ileocolic artery; the descending and ascending branches of the right colic artery; the right and left branches of the middle colic artery; the ascending, descending, and sigmoid branches of the left colic artery; the sigmoid branches of the inferior mesenteric artery; and the superior rectal artery.

When performing segmental resection for the treatment of colon cancer, the affected segment of colon is removed, along with its named blood supply (Fig. 9). For example, a cancer affecting the midascending colon would be removed after ligation of the right colic artery and the portion of the colon that it supplies (terminal ileum to midtransverse colon). When planning to remove the entire left colon, ligation of the left colic artery, or the ascending branch of the inferior mesenteric artery, would be performed, followed by removal of the midtransverse to sigmoid colon. Finally, resection of the sigmoid colon or rectum for the treatment of cancer should be done after high ligation of the inferior mesenteric artery.

Venous drainage of the colon passes through the superior mesenteric and inferior mesenteric veins, which contribute to the formation of the portal vein. The superior mesenteric vein receives drainage from the cecum, appendix, ascending colon, and most of the transverse colon. The inferior mesenteric vein receives drainage from the left part of the transverse colon, descending colon, and sigmoid colon.

LYMPHATIC DRAINAGE

Lymph from the colon reaches the superior or inferior mesenteric lymph nodes after passing through numerous groups of regional nodes. Therefore, a resection of a part of the colon must be accompanied by an extensive removal of the mesenteries and all associated lymph nodes. The superior mesenteric lymph nodes receive drainage from the ascending and transverse colons. The nodes communicate with the adjacent celiac and upper lumbar nodes. The inferior mesenteric lymph nodes receive drainage from the left end of the transverse colon, the left colic flexure, the descending colon, and the sigmoid colon. The nodes communicate with the lumbar nodes along the aorta. There is some dual drainage into the superior and inferior lymph nodes from the left third of the transverse colon and the left colic flexure. Lymph from these groups of nodes empties into the intestinal lymph trunk and continues into the cisterna chyli.

SUGGESTED READING

Drake RL, Vogl W, Mitchell AWM. *Gray's anatomy for students.* Philadelphia: Churchill Livingstone (Elsevier), 2005.

Standring S. *Gray's anatomy.* Edinburgh: Churchill Livingstone (Elsevier), 2005.

The Gastrointestinal Tract

EDITOR'S COMMENT

While anatomy has been de-emphasized in medical school, as most things that have to do with surgery have been de-emphasized, nonetheless, the knowledge of anatomy is critical for those who operate on patients. It is nice to know where things are because often they are distorted. I usually do operations by reviewing them beforehand and determining what I must not cut. Once I know where I am, and what I am being confronted with, then I can cut anything else and continue with the procedure. Somehow, I would find it difficult to comprehend how a surgeon or a surgical resident who does not know the anatomy and never had it taught in medical school would know what to cut and what not to cut if he or she never knew what the anatomy of the region is.

The taeniae, which are well described, are thought to be a source of increased strength in the colon. Thus, in doing an end-to-side anastomosis, for example, end of small bowel to the side of colon, one tries to do it through the taeniae.

(continued)

I do not know whether, in fact, the taeniae are stronger than the remainder of the colon, and wouldn't it be funny if, in fact, the taeniae were not stronger, but were instead weaker. However, we do not know that, and so I think generations of surgeons will continue to do anastomoses through the taeniae.

Not mentioned in this chapter is the additional fold lateral to the sigmoid. Ted Schrock said it best in Chapter 132 of the 4th edition, when he indicated clearly that if you are dissecting in fat when doing a sigmoid resection and mobilizing the sigmoid laterally, you are in the wrong place. There are two folds lateral to the sigmoid, and one must be careful to take the sigmoid down from the retroperitoneum, thus exposing, among other things, the ureter as it courses over the common iliac artery and vein. I usually make it a point to identify the ureter, and to place a vessel loop around it, leaving it long so that I

know where the ureter is. I usually identify it lower than where it courses along the inferior mesentery vein. This is somewhat different than the description that Dr. Drake uses.

The blood supply is obviously essential for a knowledge of the colon. The marginal artery, or arc of Riolan, forms, for the most part, a continual source of collaterals when one transects the blood supply of the colon as it emanates from either the inferior mesenteric artery or the superior mesenteric artery. In some of the recent colon and rectal literature, particularly relating to total mesenteric excision (TME), as proposed by Heald in Chapter 140, there has been remarkable consistency in the concept that taking an additional level of nodes does not result in any improvement in outcome. To my knowledge, there is only one paper that states that, written by Cole LJ et al. (Proc Natl Acad Sci 1961;47(4):594–602) in the 1960s, but this has never been duplicated.

This chapter does not extend to the rectum. Knowledge of the anatomy of the rectum as it is encompassed by and passes into the true pelvis is essential if one is to do a reasonable curative resection for carcinoma of the rectum. According to Heald, and I agree with this, staying within the proper plane, or the "holy plane," as he calls it, and not violating it (i.e., dissecting down to the rectum by sharp rather than blunt dissection) results in a 15% increase in salvage if one does a total resection of the rectal mesentery plus the rectum. In order to do this, one must feel comfortable with pelvic and rectal anatomy, which I'm quite certain is almost never taught in any medical school in the United States. It's a shame, with the stampede toward teaching science, that some of the basics as far as our ability to take good care of patients have been forgotten.

J.E.F.

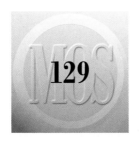

129 | Appendicitis and Appendiceal Abscess

STEPHEN F. LOWRY AND JOHN J. HONG

In 1997 in the United States, acute appendicitis accounted for over one million inpatient hospital days, at a cost of three billion dollars. Acute appendicitis remains one of the most common diseases treated by the general surgeon. Appendectomy is the most commonly performed emergency surgery in industrialized countries. Interestingly, the incidence of acute appendicitis is much lower in areas of Africa, Asia, and South America. Differences in diet, nutritional status, and alterations in colonic flora only partly explain this difference.

The pathophysiology of acute appendicitis has long been thought to be the result of luminal obstruction by a fecalith, hyperplastic lymphoid tissue, parasitic infestation, or tumor, with subsequent localized venous ischemia resulting in mucosal disruption followed by invasive bacterial infection; viral ulceration may also be the cause of mucosal ulceration in certain patients. Infection limited to the appendix itself results in localized inflammation and simple, or suppurative, appendicitis. Progression to full-thickness necrosis and gangrene of the appendiceal wall may result in complications of appendicitis, e.g., free perforation, abscess formation if the process is contained by adjacent structures, or even fistula formation if the inflammatory process continues unabated.

Mortality associated with acute appendicitis has decreased steadily during the 20th century, and in the United States, has been recently reported as 0.2 deaths per 100,000 cases. This most likely is attributable to improvements in perioperative resuscitation and monitoring, and antibiotic use. The majority of mortalities occur in the elderly, who have a much greater risk ratio for death compared with patients under age 65.

 DIAGNOSIS

Since the definitive description of the clinical findings of acute appendicitis made by Fitz in 1886, and McBurney's report to the New York Surgical Society in 1899, surgical removal of the diseased appendix has long been considered the standard of care for the treatment of acute appendicitis. With the exception of laparoscopic techniques, relatively little has changed in the surgical technique of appendectomy since the days of McBurney and Senn. However, since the advent of newer radiographic modalities, the diagnosis of acute appendicitis has become increasingly controversial, and continues to evolve.

Traditionally, obtaining a careful history and physical assessment has been the foundation of diagnosis. A "classic" clinical presentation of acute appendicitis starts

with the onset of poorly localized abdominal pain of a visceral nature that eventually localizes to the right lower quadrant; typically, the pain becomes increasingly severe and constant. Anorexia is a nearly universal finding. Nausea and vomiting are often present. On physical examination, localized right lower quadrant tenderness is the most specific finding, related to local irritation of the parietal peritoneum. The presence of rebound tenderness, a Rovsing, obturator, or psoas sign may be found, depending on the location of the inflamed appendix. Diffuse peritonitis is indicative of free abdominal perforation. An abscess may be suggested by the presence of a tender mass in the right lower quadrant. A low-grade fever and a moderate leukocytosis are frequently, but not invariably, present. Signs of severe systemic infection may accompany perforation or abscess formation. Other laboratory tests, e.g., urinalysis, serum amylase, urinary β-human chorionic gonadotropin, may be useful in identifying other disease processes mimicking possible acute appendicitis. Using Bayesian analysis, these historic, physical, and laboratory data have been incorporated into a variety of clinical scoring systems, several of which have been evaluated prospectively. The Alvarado or MANTRELS score is perhaps the most commonly used, and is actually a quantification of the most common signs, symptoms and laboratory findings typically associated with acute appendicitis.

Unfortunately, atypical clinical presentations are not uncommon. Women of childbearing age may have presentations difficult to differentiate from gynecologic disease. Abdominal tenderness may be absent or minimal in early appendicitis. Very young and very elderly patients are notorious for atypical or delayed presentation. Diarrhea or urinary symptoms related to inflammation of adjacent structures may mimic other disease processes. Measurements of serum levels of C-reactive protein, interleukins (IL-6, IL-8, and CD44) have been studied, but are of questionable clinical utility. With atypical clinical presentations, radiographic studies take on increased importance in the diagnosis of acute appendicitis.

A plain abdominal radiograph is helpful only if it demonstrates a fecalith. Other radiographic studies, such as ultrasonography, and scintigraphy using technetium-labeled white blood cells have been described, but typically are not routinely performed. In general, these tests are useful only if they clearly demonstrate appendicitis. Negative or equivocal studies do not rule out appendicitis.

Because of the significant increases in morbidity and mortality associated with perforation, surgeons historically have accepted a certain rate of "negative" appendectomies to ensure that they did not fail to operate on patients, especially those with atypical presentations, in a timely fashion. Rates of nontherapeutic appendectomies have been reported in the literature from as low as 5% to as high as 40%. With increasing reports of excellent (over 95%) accuracy rates associated with abdominopelvic computed tomography (CT), some have advocated routine use of CT for all patients with possible acute appendicitis, even questioning the utility of any clinical assessment. In response, others have questioned the need for routine use of CT on all patients, e.g., a young, healthy male patient with the classic presentation of acute appendicitis. A prospective randomized comparison of a scoring system using traditional clinical markers versus CT failed to show a statistically significant difference in accuracy rates. Clearly CT, if used, is most beneficial for those patients with an atypical presentation. Routine use of CT for all patients with possible acute appendicitis, although being done more frequently, especially in the United States, remains controversial.

TREATMENT

Antibiotics

Traditionally, the diagnosis of acute appendicitis is followed shortly thereafter with surgical treatment. Attempts at nonoperative management of acute appendicitis with antibiotic therapy alone have been associated with a high rate of clinical failure or recurrences. However, a single preoperative dose of antibiotics administered prior to skin incision clearly reduces postoperative wound infection rates. Single-agent therapy, typically with a second-generation cephalosporin, or a quinolone/metronidazole regimen is adequate. If the appendix is perforated, antibiotic therapy should continue in the postoperative period. The exact duration of antibiotic therapy should be mandated by the patient's clinical response, with antibiotics being administered for at least 1 week or until the patient's clinical infection has resolved; ongoing evidence of systemic infection 1 week after appendectomy implies pelvic or intra-abdominal abscess.

Surgical Technique

Incision

The classic McBurney incision is typically made at right angles to, and two-thirds along, the line between the umbilicus and the anterior superior iliac spine (Fig. 1). A transverse or Rockey-Davis incision may be used at the same location.

An incision made to lie in Langhans lines results in the best cosmetic result. The point of maximal tenderness found prior to induction of general anesthesia as well as palpation of the lateral border of the rectus abdominis may slightly alter the location of the incision, typically slightly lateral to McBurney's point. A lower midline incision may be necessary in morbidly obese patients, or in patients who have a strong possibility of having other pelvic abnormalities.

Irrespective of the skin incision, a muscle-splitting incision holds the least likelihood of dehiscence or hernia. The external oblique aponeurosis is sharply incised parallel to the direction of its fibers. The internal oblique fascia and muscle is then bluntly separated using large clamps spread at right angles until the transversalis fascia is identified. The transversalis fascia and peritoneum are identified and sharply divided. On entry into the peritoneal cavity, Army-Navy, appendiceal, or small Richardson retractors may be used to further bluntly separate the abdominal wall musculature (Fig. 2). If the incision needs to be extended, medial extension onto the superficial rectus sheath may be done, allowing for considerable medial retraction of the rectus abdominis

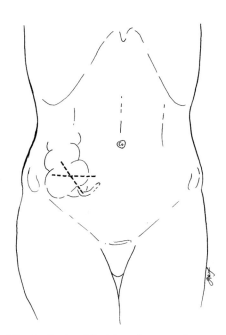

Fig. 1. Optional incisions for appendectomy (*dashed lines*). Either should be centered over the point of maximal tenderness on examination.

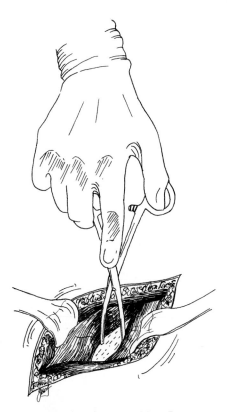

Fig. 2. Muscle-splitting incision. Retractors hold the skin, subcutaneous tissue, and external oblique fascia while a large hemostat is used to split the external oblique muscle to expose the transversalis fascia.

The Gastrointestinal Tract

muscle and exposure to the lower abdominal contents.

Usually, for simple cases, a small (2- to 4-cm) incision serves to keep viscera out of the operating field and yet is sufficient for mobilization of the appendix and its base into the wound. Because the pathogens are fairly predictable, and there is little likelihood that culture results will truly change clinical management, the value of culturing any fluid seen on entry into the abdomen is questionable.

Exploration and Mobilization of the Appendix

A finger placed into the peritoneal cavity may be sufficient to identify and then deliver the appendix into the wound. If necessary, the anterior tenia of the cecum can be followed by gently grasping the cecum with moistened gauze and delivering it into the wound, using a rocking motion, until the base of the appendix is identified (Fig. 3). If the appendix is retrocecal, medial mobilization of the cecum is necessary to access the appendix; this can typically be done bluntly, with a finger, combined with sharp or electrocautery division of the tissue along the white line of Toldt. Occasionally, in morbidly obese patients, or in cases with severe inflammation or aberrant anatomy, lower midline laparotomy may be necessary.

Removal of the Appendix

When the appendix has been mobilized sufficiently, the vascular arcade is divided between clamps and tied. This may be done in one step, at the base of the appendix, or, if the anatomy dictates, may be done in stepwise fashion along the

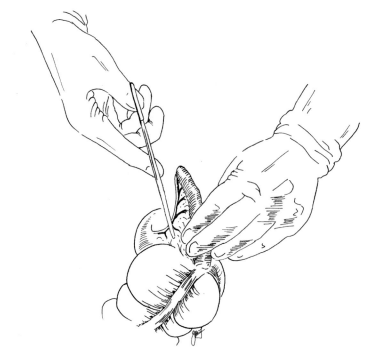

Fig. 4. The appendiceal vascular arcade is taken between clamps and subsequently ligated with a 3–0 silk suture.

mesoappendix, allowing for progressive mobilization along the length of the appendix until the base is reached. The base of the appendix must be definitively identified at the cecum to avoid partial appendectomy (as has been reported in the literature, particularly associated with laparoscopic techniques). The appendix is then crushed with a straight clamp approximately 3 mm from the cecum (Fig. 4). The straight clamp is then moved approximately 3 mm more distally onto the appendix and applied. The appendix is then ligated using a 2-0 or 0 ligature. A

scalpel is used to transect the appendix on the proximal side of the straight clamp, thus avoiding any spillage from the appendix. This same scalpel may be used to cauterize the exposed mucosa of the appendiceal stump, and then removed with the specimen off the surgical field, minimizing contamination. Inversion of the appendiceal stump is of questionable util-

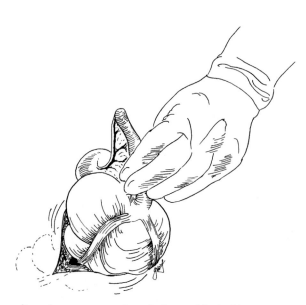

Fig. 3. The appendix and cecum are gently rocked out of the incision.

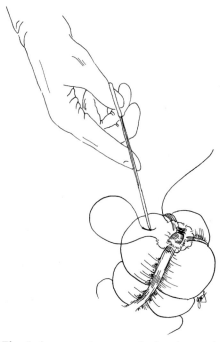

Fig. 5. A purse-string suture is placed around the appendix stump.

ity; when done, it can be simply accomplished using a purse-string or "Z" stitch placed around the base of the appendiceal stump (Fig. 5). Irrigation of the peritoneal cavity with normal saline is typically performed, especially in patients with murky abdominal fluid, gangrenous appendicitis, or frank perforation. There are little data in the literature supporting or refuting this practice. There is no role for prophylactic drainage of a simple case of acute appendicitis.

Closure

The wound is closed in layers. Depending on the anatomy, closure of the peritoneum and transversalis fascia may be performed. If a muscle-splitting incision was used, there is no need to approximate anything other than the external oblique aponeurosis. Following irrigation with normal saline, closure of the skin and subcutaneous tissues is routine for all cases of simple appendicitis. In cases of perforated appendicitis, closure of the skin is controversial. One recent prospective randomized study demonstrated an increased rate of wound infection in adult patients whose dirty abdominal wounds were closed.

APPENDICEAL ABSCESS

Although there is no role for prophylactic drainage in the management of appendicitis, therapeutic drainage is essential in the management of appendiceal abscess. Typically, patients who present with an appendiceal abscess have had a delay in presentation, a delay in diagnosis, or very rapidly progressing disease. The presence of a palpable tender mass in the right lower quadrant associated with other signs and symptoms of acute appendicitis, particularly if they have been present for over 48 hours, is consistent with an appendiceal abscess. A CT is diagnostic, and may be therapeutic if combined with guided percutaneous drainage of the abscess.

Controversy arises when the diagnosis of appendiceal abscess is known prior to induction of anesthesia. Most studies support the use of guided percutaneous drainage of the abscess as appropriate initial therapy, followed by interval appendectomy 6 to 8 weeks following catheter removal and clinical resolution of infection. Many authors advocate laparoscopic appendectomy as the best choice for interval appendectomy. If percutaneous drainage does not result in rapid clinical improvement, surgery is necessary. Patients with extensive disease may develop septic shock if not treated aggressively. Adequate debridement of devitalized tissue, elimination of all intra-abdominal and retroperitoneal loculations and collections, and adequate drainage are required. Severe cases may require ileocecectomy. Cases complicated by necrotizing soft tissue infection typically require multiple staged debridements to achieve surgical control of infection.

SUGGESTED READING

Alvarado A. A practical score for the early diagnosis of acute appendicitis. *Ann Emerg Med* 1986;15(5):557.

Davies GM, Dasbach EJ, Teutsch S. The burden of appendicitis-related hospitalizations in the United States in 1997. *Surg Infect* 2004; 5(2):160.

Hong JJ, Cohn SM, Ekeh AP, et al. A prospective randomized study of clinical assessment versus computed tomography for the diagnosis of actueacute appendicitis. *Surg Infect* 2003;4(3):231.

Rao PM, Rhea JT, Novelline RA, et al. Effect of computed tomography of the appendix on treatment of patients and use of hospital resources. *N Engl J Med* 1998;338(3): 141.

The Gastrointestinal Tract

EDITOR'S COMMENT

Appendicitis, as the authors state, is an extraordinarily common disease, and can result in a great deal of difficulty for patient and surgeon alike. This is a good review of the basic problems with acute appendicitis. First, the authors raise an interesting point as to why appendicitis is not as prone in Africa, Asia, South America, and other societies that are not as well developed as industrialized ones. The answer may be that appendicoliths are a source of obstruction of the appendix, and therefore if I were going to investigate this finding, I would probably look at the incidence of appendicoliths, and what it is it in our diets as opposed to those of the aforementioned societies, which probably does not result in as many appendicoliths as we have.

The syndrome of acute appendicitis involves either poorly localized or epigastric pain, depending on who you read and what patient you see. I prefer to believe that the epigastric pain is pylorospasm. Pylorospasm is a good, nonspecific sign that something is amiss in the abdomen, and may result in the diagnosis of carcinoma of the colon in patients with poorly localized symptoms. Weight loss and the feeling of malaise associated with pylorospasm, though, requires an investigation. I once made the diagnosis of carcinoma of the colon in the father-in-law of a close friend of mine; this had been missed elsewhere because of persistent pylorospasm as epigastric pain without any other symptoms. Alternatively, if one adopts the point of view that the prodrome is nonspecific, one could

explain these by the midline radiation of the delta nonmyelinated fibers that have very poor localization but tend to be perceived as being midline. When the parietal peritoneum becomes inflamed, then one perceives right lower quadrant pain and tenderness, and finally rebound when the alpha fibers of the parietal peritoneum are brought into play. Anorexia, in my experience, is present almost 100% of the time. If the patient is hungry, one should question the diagnosis of appendicitis.

I will not get into the tiresome controversy concerning CT scans in acute appendicitis. Given the cost of CT scans, it would be wise for us to restrict the use of this technology to women of childbearing age who are not pregnant, patients whose symptoms are somewhat atypical, and the elderly in whom a good history is not obtainable. However, usually the emergency medicine physicians order the CT scans even before they call a surgeon, at least in the university setting, so this yields overuse of CT scan in, for example, the young man in whom, in my opinion, history and physical examination is all that is necessary. Given the instance of evaluation of a young male patient, the diagnostic accuracy of CT scans versus physical examination in the hands of an experienced surgeon may approach 97% by both methods. However, the CT scan is not as readily available in all countries as it is in the United States.

Tzanakis et al. (*World J Surg* 2005;29:1151) have proposed the use of ultrasound as being more readily available than CT scanning, and a new scoring system,

and comparing it with nine other scoring systems, including those that have been commonly used in the United States. According to this scoring system, six points are given for ultrasound that demonstrates acute appendicitis, four points for tenderness in the right lower quadrant, three points for rebound tenderness (this is a separate point score), and two points for leukocyte count greater than 12,000. Several aspects of the study in this very complicated article reveal that a positive ultrasound finding with leukocytosis would give total score of eight points. According to both their external study and then a validating study, although the latter is a little more confusing, patients who had eight points had a diagnostic accuracy of 96.5%, similar to what we find with CT scan, even if right lower quadrant tenderness were absent. Among patients with moderate scores (five to seven points) in whom ultrasound was likely to be negative, in 150 patients only 4 (2.7%) had acute appendicitis. In patients who had four points or less (22 patients, or 7.3% of the total), none developed appendicitis. Thus, in a society in which CT scans are lacking, or perhaps some sanity had been added in the use of CT scans for evaluating acute appendicitis, ultrasound is a good substitution.

The diagnostic accuracy in other parts of the world leads one to wonder what, in actual effect, the diagnostic capabilities are. In a very involved study (Shum CF, et al. *Asian J Surg* 2005;28(4): 257), 518 patients underwent surgery for acute appendicitis,

(continued)

and the on-table operative diagnosis of surgeons was correlated with the histologic diagnosis of pathologists. Sensitivity for diagnosing normal appendices was low, at 51.3%, and surgeons weren't able to make an accurate on-table diagnosis in 14.3% of the patients. Thus, of 59 cases that the surgeon called normal, acute appendicitis was present on pathologic evaluation in 14 of these cases. The statistics in this article are staggering, but the overall conclusion seems to be that surgeons are not very good at judging acute appendicitis from the normal when the abdomen is open.

One thing to be concerned about is what to do when the appendix is perforated. There still is a school of thought that holds that individuals who have perforated appendicitis should not have their wounds closed primarily. I am not one of this group because of the pain and difficulty of having someone with a delayed primary closure. Besides, the incidence of wound infection in delayed primary closure is not 0%, it is closer to 5%. This has been studied extensively, particularly in Sweden. Surgeons in Sweden found that

patients who underwent primary closure without drainage had an incidence of wound infection somewhere in the 30% to 40% range in various studies. However, patients who had delayed primary closure had an incidence of 5%, as predicted. Patients who underwent primary closure and had wound drainage with a closed suction drain had an incidence of 11%. I believe that the latter method is preferable because even the 11% incidence of acute wound infection can be minimized by inserting a closed suction drain and leaving it for 10 days. The common error in closed suction drainage is to put a closed suction drain in and then remove it prematurely, let's say at 2 or 3 days, when it doesn't drain anything. The wound becomes suppurated later. If the drain is left in for a full 10 days, the incidence of wound drainage and wound infection decreases.

CT scan, although useful for the diagnosis of acute appendicitis, is less accurate in the diagnosis or characterization of abscesses. In children, this is especially important, and the incidence of perforation even with the CT scan is definitely not improving

(Hogan MJ. *Tech Vasc Interv Radiol* 2003;6(4):205). Hogan also states that this is even more important because the dose of radiation to children should be minimized. Clearly, in the pediatric population, relying on radiologic techniques has a long way to go.

Finally, Killelea and Arkovitz (*Pediatr Surg Int* 2006;22(3):286) reported a child with cystic fibrosis in whom there was an appendiceal umbilical fistula that was not operated on immediately but drained, and the drain perforated the cecum, requiring emergency laparotomy from which the child fortunately recovered after a prolonged postoperative course. They claimed that this is the second case of this that has been reported. I have seen a case of this in Crohn disease and I suppose that may not count, but one assumes that this is not as rare as the authors claim. In this case, the patient required cecectomy, and the case I dealt with also required ileocecectomy. I suspect this is quite a bit more common in Crohn disease than the authors are aware of, or were able to find in the literature that they reviewed.

J.E.F.

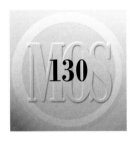

130   Laparoscopic Appendectomy

ZIAD T. AWAD AND W. STEVE EUBANKS

Acute appendicitis is the most common cause of acute abdominal pain that requires surgical treatment. There is an approximately 6% to 7% lifetime risk of appendicitis. Appendicitis is primarily a disease of adolescents and young adults with a peak incidence in the second and third decades of life. It is very uncommon in children younger than 5 years and by age 50, the risk of appendicitis is 1 in 35 for men and 1 in 50 for women. By age 70, the risk of appendicitis is less than 1 in 100. Among teenagers and young adults, males are more commonly affected than females with a male:female ratio of approximately 1.3:1, but the gender distribution becomes equal beyond these age groups. There have been reports of a wide variation in the incidence of appendicitis between countries, between regions of the same country, and between different racial and occupational groups. However, most attention has been directed to geographic variations in incidence that are probably due to differences in dietary fiber consumption. Appendicitis is relatively more common in industrialized nations where a highly refined, low-fiber diet is typically consumed. Appendicitis is rare in developing countries where a less-refined, high-

fiber diet that is characteristic of agrarian societies is generally consumed. It appears that the incidence of appendicitis has decreased in the past several decades. The reasons for the reduced incidence of appendicitis are not clear, but it may be due to the increase in dietary fiber consumption in industrialized nations.

 CLINICAL DIAGNOSIS

The clinical diagnosis of appendicitis remains difficult; there is 10% to 30% incidence of unnecessary surgical exploration for an incorrect diagnosis of appendicitis. The disease has a peak incidence in the third and fourth decades of life but can occur from infancy to old age. Clinical diagnosis hinges on the typical periumbilical pain spreading to the right lower quadrant (RLQ) as the localized inflammatory process causes peritonism in this area associated with mild leukocytosis and fever. However, with a retrocecal appendix, the condition may present as back pain or ureteric colic with evidence of cells in the urine. An inflamed appendix lying within the pelvis may produce pelvic symptoms, and an abscess in this

area can result in diarrhea as a result of irritation of the adjacent rectum.

The main diagnostic problem that arises is mistaking other benign conditions for appendicitis. This typically occurs in young women who have right-sided ovarian problems such as rupture of a hemorrhagic ovarian cyst, torsion of an ovarian appendage, endometriosis, hemorrhage into a fibroid, ruptured ectopic pregnancy, or pelvic inflammatory disease. This results in an up to 40% incidence of false-negative appendectomy in young women with RLQ pain. It is in these cases that a laparoscopic exploration may be of greatest benefit. Other conditions that may mimic appendicitis are regional adenitis, gastroenteritis in young children, Crohn disease, ulcerative colitis, terminal ileitis, urinary tract infection, torsion of an appendix epiploica, diverticulitis of the sigmoid colon lying in the RLQ, perforated duodenal ulcer, or cholecystitis. With such a variety of mimetic conditions, the surgeon may lack adequate access to other parts of the abdomen after having made a muscle-splitting RLQ incision for a mistaken diagnosis of appendicitis. This may even necessitate closing this incision and obtaining access to another part of the abdomen through another celiotomy. In this circumstance the ability to perform a complete exploration of the abdomen using the laparoscope becomes valuable.

Useful diagnostic modalities include a white blood cell count with evidence of increased polymorphonuclear lymphocytes and a radiograph of the abdomen, particularly looking for a fecalith in the appendix, which can be diagnostic of acute appendicitis and may be present in up to 10% of cases if carefully looked for. Foreign bodies, ranging from seeds of fruit to swallowed materials such as a lead shot, needles, or even a misplaced dental drill bit, can lodge in the appendix. A radiograph may reveal ileus of adjacent small bowel loops in the RLQ and the disappearance of the preperitoneal fat line on radiograph as a result of edema in the fatty tissues, making differentiation of this from the more solid intra-abdominal organs less clear. Similarly, the right psoas shadow may disappear radiologically because of edema of the retroperitoneal fat surrounding the muscle. In advanced cases a fluid level from an adjacent abscess may be evident.

Ultrasound has become valuable in making a diagnosis. The use of ultrasound as a diagnostic modality for appendicitis has several advantages and disadvantages. The disadvantages include the relatively low specificity of many of the findings on ultrasound and a lack of evidence-based procedures for conducting and interpreting appendiceal ultrasounds. Another disadvantage is that patients often complain of the discomfort evoked by the transducer pressure during ultrasound evaluation. As for the advantages, ultrasonography is relatively inexpensive, safe, and widely available. Other advantages include noninvasiveness, short acquisition time, lack of radiation exposure, and the potential for discovering other causes of abdominal pain. For these reasons, it is especially useful in pregnant women and children. It is also useful in women of childbearing age since ultrasound is an excellent modality for imaging of the reproductive organs.

As a diagnostic modality for appendicitis, the accuracy of computed tomography (CT) has been reported to be as high as 93% to 98% with sensitivity and specificity in the 87% to 100% and 95% to 99% range, respectively. The accuracy of CT relies in part on its ability to reveal a normal appendix more reliably and with greater consistency than ultrasonography. In a study of 210 helical appendiceal CT examinations in patients with oral and rectal contrast, an enlarged appendix with periappendiceal fat stranding was observed in 93% of patients

with appendicitis. In another study of 238 CT examinations with intravenous contrast, several CT characteristics of appendicitis were described. These findings include (a) enlarged appendix (diameter ≥6 mm) (sensitivity, 93%; specificity, 92%), (b) appendiceal wall thickening (sensitivity, 66%; specificity, 96%), (c) periappendiceal fat stranding (sensitivity, 87%; specificity, 74%), and (d) appendiceal wall enhancement (sensitivity, 75%; specificity, 85%). Other reports have also supported appendiceal diameter, wall changes, and fat stranding as being the top three CT findings suggestive of appendicitis.

In assessing the overall utility of CT, several authors have attempted to document its impact on the negative appendectomy and perforation rates for appendicitis. One study involving 908 patients noted a drop in the negative appendectomy rate from 20% to 7% and a drop in the perforation rates from 22% to 14%. The authors concluded that CT should be performed in nearly all female and many male patients. However, the high CT accuracy rates in literature reports are not duplicated at all hospitals. Naturally, decreased CT accuracy would reduce its potential impact on perforation and negative appendectomy rates. Thus, there is some controversy as to whether CT has positively impacted the perforation and negative appendectomy rates. In particular, Flum et al. showed no changes in the population-based incidence of negative appendectomy and perforation rate after the widespread use of CT and ultrasound imaging.

The advantages of CT over ultrasound include its higher diagnostic accuracy and operator independence. Additional advantages relating to accuracy include greater ability to detect the normal appendix, phlegmon, and abscess. In fact, CT is often used when ultrasound yields suboptimal or inconclusive results. The disadvantages of CT include possible iodinated contrast media allergy, patient discomfort from administration of contrast media (especially if rectal contrast media is used), exposure to ionizing radiation, and costs that generally range three to four times the cost of ultrasound.

PERIAPPENDICEAL ABSCESS

Periappendiceal abscess formation has been reported to develop in up to 10% of patients with appendicitis. The classic presentation is of a patient who experiences severe right lower quadrant pain for 1 to 2 days associated with fever and then resolves both the pain and fever. After 7 to 10 days,

the fever recurs and the patient notices mild to moderate right lower quadrant discomfort. Physical examination demonstrates a palpable mass in the right lower quadrant. Broadly speaking, any patient with a right lower quadrant mass and fever should be considered to have a periappendiceal abscess until proven otherwise. Imaging with ultrasound or CT will confirm the diagnosis in most cases.

Management depends on the patient's condition. If the patient is not toxic and signs of sepsis are absent, then it is preferable for the patient to undergo percutaneous drainage of the abscess with systemic antibiotic therapy. If adequate drainage can be achieved, then the abscess cavity will frequently collapse over 5 to 10 days and the inflammatory process will resolve. The patient can be discharged from the hospital once the infection is under control and undergo elective or interval appendectomy 6 to 8 weeks later. This approach avoids the morbidity associated with exploring a patient with a large abscess or phlegmon in whom it is often difficult even to locate the appendix, let alone remove it.

On the other hand, unremitting sepsis or inadequate percutaneous drainage should prompt operative intervention. Drainage should be as complete and dependent as possible. The surgeon should be prepared to encounter substantial inflammation and surgical therapy may be limited to abscess drainage alone. It may not be possible, nor should the surgeon aggressively pursue appendectomy. It is much safer to permit the abscess and surrounding inflammation to resolve before proceeding with a second-stage procedure to remove the appendix.

Recurrent and Chronic Appendicitis

Although surgeons debate their existence, both recurrent and chronic appendicitis appear to be real clinical diagnoses. Recurrent appendicitis refers to a pattern of symptoms in which the patient reports mild, self-limited attacks of right lower quadrant pain that typically last for hours before resolving spontaneously. Often, the symptoms are not severe and the patient may not seek medical attention. Eventually, the patient has a severe attack, the diagnosis of acute appendicitis is suspected, and appendectomy is performed. The diagnosis of recurrent appendicitis is a retrospective one in which the patient reports multiple attacks of pain of which all but the most recent one before surgery are mild in severity. Indeed, up to 9% of patients being evaluated for acute appendicitis report a history of similar symptoms. Similarly, if interval appendectomy after medical treatment of appendicitis is avoided, then the likelihood of recurrence is stated to be anywhere from 10% to 80%. Finally, after appendectomy for recurrent appendicitis, pathologic findings frequently include chronic as well as acute inflammation, providing further circumstantial evidence for the entity of "recurrent appendicitis."

Chronic appendicitis is considered to be even rarer and more difficult to diagnose than recurrent appendicitis. It refers to a patient who reports constant well-localized right lower quadrant pain and tenderness with no other identifiable pelvic or abdominal disease. If appendectomy completely relieves the pain and pathologic findings include chronic inflammation of the appendix, then the diagnosis of chronic appendicitis is secured. However, it is important to note that it is very difficult to make this diagnosis preoperatively and this explanation for a patient's abdominal complaints should be used sparingly.

Incidental Appendectomy

Removal of a normal appendix is contraindicated while carrying out a laparoscopic abdominal exploration for other conditions. Prophylactic removal of the appendix, such as was carried out in General MacArthur before the Pacific Campaign in World War II, remains contraindicated. Laparoscopy has not changed the indications for prophylactic removal of the appendix.

Laparoscopic Appendectomy

Laparoscopic appendectomy was first reported by Kurt Semm, a German gynecologist, in 1983, but it was not until the early 1990s that this approach gained wide acceptance. Since that time, there have been multiple prospective, randomized controlled trials, several meta-analyses, and nationwide database reviews comparing open to laparoscopic appendectomy. Despite the plethora of data, there is still controversy regarding laparoscopic versus open appendectomy. However, there appears to be an increasing trend in the use of laparoscopic appendectomy. A study of a large nationwide administrative database showed that the use of laparoscopic appendectomy in the United States has more than doubled,

from 20% of cases in 1999 to 43% of cases in 2003. In practice, the decision to perform appendectomy open or laparoscopically often depends on surgeon expertise and the availability of operative and hospital resources.

 ## INDICATIONS

The indications for laparoscopic appendectomy are the same as those for open appendectomy. A laparoscopic approach provides the surgeon with a tool not only to rule out appendicitis, but also to inspect other organs simultaneously to determine the true cause of the patient's symptoms. The visualization is often superior to the limited exploration that can be accomplished through a right lower quadrant incision. This is particularly important in the patient in whom the diagnosis is not clear and in women of childbearing age.

The indication for laparoscopic appendectomy in complicated or perforated appendicitis is controversial. There have been several studies that have examined the role of laparoscopic appendectomy in this setting, and they suggest that laparoscopic appendectomy can be performed safely in these patients. The overall complication rates are comparable and several studies suggest a lower wound infection rate and reduced hospital length of stay. As expected, the conversion rate in these patients typically ranges from 20% to 30%.

Given that a laparoscopic approach may be technically more challenging than an open approach, we believe that surgeons should exercise caution in performing laparoscopic appendectomy in the absence of sufficient training or expert assistance. Likewise, as with any laparoscopic procedure, conversion to an open operation should not be considered a complication, but rather an exhibition of sound surgical judgment.

 ## PREOPERATIVE PLANNING

The patient should be adequately hydrated with a balanced intravenous fluid. A meta-analysis of randomized or controlled clinical trials investigating the use of antibiotic therapy versus placebo for patients with suspected appendicitis who underwent appendectomy concluded that the use of antibiotics is superior to placebo in preventing wound infection and intra-abdominal abscesses, regardless of the pathologic state of the appendix. The optimal duration of treatment is un-

clear, although it is best to administer the first dose of antibiotics preoperatively. Finally, the choice of antibiotics should be governed by the bacteriology of appendicitis. Hence, it is best to use antibiotics that provide coverage for Gram-negative and anaerobic organisms. A nasogastric tube may be required in the presence of ileus, generalized peritonitis, or repeated vomiting. A Foley catheter is needed to decompress the bladder.

CONTRAINDICATIONS

The number of absolute and relative contraindications to performing laparoscopic appendectomy has decreased over the past 10 years as minimally invasive surgical equipment and surgical skills have improved. Perhaps the most common contraindication to performing laparoscopic appendectomy is lack of surgeon experience. As surgeons gain confidence in their laparoscopic skills and as the procedure becomes more common in residency training programs, this should not be a significant factor in the future. Absolute contraindications include the inability to tolerate general anesthesia, refractory coagulopathy, and diffuse peritonitis with hemodynamic compromise. Diffuse peritonitis with hemodynamic compromise represents a surgical urgency in which attempted laparoscopy is not prudent. Open laparotomy allows rapid determination of the cause and more expeditious management of the disorder. Relative contraindications include previous abdominal surgery with extensive adhesions, portal hypertension, severe cardiopulmonary disease, and advanced pregnancy.

LAPAROSCOPIC APPENDECTOMY TECHNIQUE

The patient is placed in the supine position on the operating table. After the induction of general anesthesia, a urinary catheter and an orogastric tube are placed. The surgeon and the first assistant may stand on the patient's left side. A single video monitor is used on the right side of the operating table. It is most convenient to place the initial port at the umbilicus. An open Hasson technique is used to gain access to the peritoneal cavity. The initial umbilical trocar can either be 5 mm or 10 mm, depending on the diameter of the laparoscope being used. An angled laparoscope, either 30 degrees or 45 degrees, is used. Once adequate CO_2 pneumoperitoneum is established, laparoscopic abdominal exploration is performed. The second port to be placed is a 10- to 12-mm port in the suprapubic area. This should be carefully placed to avoid injury to the urinary bladder. The choice of this larger port in the suprapubic area is so that a 10-mm telescope can be introduced if needed, to place a 12-mm stapling instrument, and for removal of the specimen. In addition, the larger port sites at the umbilicus and suprapubic area in the hairline allow for an excellent cosmetic result. The third port to be placed should be a 5-mm port in the left iliac fossa lateral to the inferior epigastric vessel. The reason for choosing this site is to allow an adequate distance from the first two ports and to allow for so-called triangulation toward the appendix. By this is meant the ability to have the two operating instruments approach each other at a 90-degree angle, which allows for much better tissue manipulation and ease of dissection. An additional 5-mm port may be placed in the upper midline or in the right upper quadrant. It is generally not advisable to have the port placed directly over the area of dissection.

Identification and Mobilization of the Appendix

The patient is rotated to a slightly left lateral decubitus position and mild Trende-lenburg to allow gravity to assist with operative exposure. In this position, the ascending colon is slightly suspended from the lateral wall and the small intestine falls away from the operative field. Once the cecum is identified, the base of the appendix is sought by determining the site of confluence of the tenia. The cecum may have to be mobilized by incising the peritoneum lateral to the cecum and lower ascending colon. This may be necessary in the event of a retrocecal appendix or a phlegmon. Gentle medial retraction of the cecum on the tenia coli allows the appendix to roll forward toward the operator and facilitate this part of the procedure. The appendix can then be manipulated into view.

Dissection of the Mesoappendix

With elevation of the appendix, the mesoappendix is usually easily identified. This may be easiest done by identifying the base of the appendix and dissecting the mesoappendix from this point. A window should be created at the base of the appendix in preparation for division of the mesoappendix. A GIA stapler can be fired across the mesoappendix. We prefer to use a linear stapling device with a 2.5-mm staple cartridge to ensure hemostasis. Alternatively, either metallic clips or the harmonic scalpel is used for this purpose.

After the mesoappendix has been secured, the base of the appendix is dissected to allow for clear visualization of its muscular circumference at the base and its attachment to the cecum to allow for accurate placement of the laparoscopic stapler.

Appendectomy

The appendix is transected with a laparoscopic linear stapling device with a 2.5-mm staple cartridge removing a short cuff of cecum to ensure complete removal of the appendix. The appendix is placed into a specimen bag and retrieved from the intra-abdominal cavity via either the umbilical or the suprapubic trocar site.

The staple line is examined carefully. The operative site is irrigated. The ports are removed under direct visualization. The fascia of the large and main access port site is closed with 0 or 1 absorbable suture material. The skin is closed with the subcuticular suture.

RESULTS OF LAPAROSCOPIC APPENDECTOMY

Multiple prospective, randomized trials and meta-analyses (Table 1) have been conducted to assess the value of laparoscopic appendectomy compared with open appendectomy. There is some

TABLE 1. SELECTED RANDOMIZED TRIALS OF LAPAROSCOPIC VERSUS OPEN APPENDECTOMY

Reference	n		OR Time (Min)		Conversion Rate (%)	LOS (Days)		RTNA		Wound Infection (%)		Complications (%)	
	L	O	L	O		L	O	L	O	L	O	L	O
Long et al. (2002) *Surgery*	93	105	107	91	16	2.6	3.4	14	21	18.2	16.2	28	28
Pedersen et al. (2001) *Br J Surg*	282	301	60	40	23	2	2	7	10	2.8	6.9	10.3	9.0
Ozmen et al. (1999) *Surg Laparoscop Endosc Percutan Tech*	35	35	28	38	—	1.6	3.7	—	—	5.7	8.6	18	52
Hellberg et al. (1999) *Br J Surg*	244	256	60	35	12	2	2	13	21	—	—	4.9	6.2
Heikkinen et al. (1998) *Surg Endosc*	19	21	31	41	5.3	2	2	10	19	0	4.8	—	—
Klinger et al. (1998) *Am J Surg*	87	82	35	31	0	3	4	14	15	6	7	—	—
Reiertsen et al. (1997) *Br J Surg*	42	42	51	25	0	3.5	3.2	15	19.7	2.4	0	40.5	28.6
Minne et al. (1997) *Arch Surg*	27	23	82	67	7.4	1.1	1.2	14	14	—	—	18.5	4.3
Macarulla et al. (1997) *Surg Laparosc Endosc*	106	104	55	45	8.3	3.4	4.8	—	—	0.9	4.8	5.6	7.7
Ortega et al. (1995) *Am J Surg*	167	86	68	58	6.5	2.6	2.8	9	14	2.4	12.8	4.2	20.9

L, laparoscopic appendectomy; LOS, hospital length of stay; O, open appendectomy; OR, operating room; RTNA, return to normal activity.

The Gastrointestinal Tract

variability in the results of these studies, but several generalizations can be drawn. Laparoscopic appendectomy was associated with longer operative times, usually about 15 to 20 minutes. Conversion rates to an open approach ranged from 5% to 25%, often depending on the presence of perforation or complicated appendicitis. Hospital length of stay was either not significantly different or favored a laparoscopic approach. In studies that demonstrated a significantly reduced length of stay for laparoscopic appendectomy, the advantage was typically 1 day. Most investigators observed a faster return to normal activities by approximately 5 to 7 days in patients who underwent laparoscopy. The results for overall complication rates were decidedly mixed, with no clear advantage for either approach. However, most studies demonstrated a reduced wound infection rate for patients who underwent laparoscopic appendectomy.

Several studies have accomplished cost comparison and the results are mixed. Some have demonstrated cost savings with laparoscopic appendectomy due to the reduced length of stay, whereas others suggest that laparoscopic appendectomy is associated with higher costs due to longer operative times and equipment costs.

Despite the rapid acceptance of laparoscopic cholecystectomy and other laparoscopic intra-abdominal procedures, there is no clear consensus regarding the use of laparoscopic appendectomy. The results of open appendectomy are reliable across the spectrum of hospitals and associated with highly satisfactory outcomes. The proponents of open appendectomy interpret the results of recent studies with the admonition that statistically significant differences are not necessarily clinically significant, and in the case of appendectomy, there is no clear indication that laparoscopy is the approach of choice. The proponents of laparoscopic appendectomy point out that multiple studies demonstrate an advantage in reduced morbidity and length of stay. Although the differences may not appear clinically significant to some, they are significant in light of the large number of patients who undergo the procedure annually in the United States. It is possible that eventually laparoscopic appendectomy may become the procedure of choice for appendicitis, but for the near future, open appendectomy is likely to predominate.

Special Clinical Circumstances

Pregnancy

Appendicitis occurs with equal frequency in pregnant and nonpregnant women, and the natural history is unaffected by the stage of pregnancy. The incidence is reported to be approximately 1 case in 1,500 to 6,600 pregnancies. When associated with perforation and peritonitis, there is considerable maternal morbidity and mortality, as well as significant fetal loss. Access to the appendix can be hampered by the presence of the enlarged uterus. Laparoscopic appendectomy in the pregnant patient has been controversial, and is considered a relative contraindication. If attempted, it should be performed only by experienced, advanced laparoscopic surgeons. Open access using the Hasson technique is a must; the intra-abdominal pressure should be kept at 10 to 12 mm Hg.

Necrosis of the Base of the Appendix

Necrosis of the base of the appendix with or without involvement of the cecal wall warrants limited cecal resection using the laparoscopic stapler.

Crohn Disease

Crohn disease limited to the appendix is a rare occurrence. Generally, medical treatment is instituted and the appendix is not removed to avoid appendiceal stump leakage or fistula formation if Crohn disease involves the cecum or base of the appendix. However, if the disease process involves the terminal ileum with sparing of the cecum, appendectomy is performed. If resection is warranted due to severe isolated Crohn disease and gross rupture, an ileocecectomy should be performed.

SUGGESTED READING

Andersen BR, Kallehave FL, Andersen HK. Antibiotics versus placebo for prevention of postoperative infection after appendicectomy. *Cochrane Database Syst Rev* 2004;4:1.

Bendeck SE, Nino-Murcia M, Berry GJ, et al. Imaging for suspected appendicitis negative appendectomy and perforation rates. *Radiology* 2002;225:131.

Choi D, Lim HK, Lee WJ, et al. The most useful findings for diagnosing acute appendicitis on contrast-enhanced helical CT. *Acta Radiol* 2003;44:574.

Chung RS, Rowland DY, Li P, et al. A meta-analysis of randomized controlled trials of laparoscopic versus conventional appendectomy. *Am J Surg* 1999;177:250.

Flum DR, Morris A, Koepsell T, et al. Has misdiagnosis of appendicitis decreased over time? A population-based analysis. *JAMA* 2001;286:1748.

Garbutt JM, Soper NJ, Shannon WD, et al. Meta-analysis of randomized controlled trials comparing laparoscopic and open appendectomy. *Surg Laparosc Endosc* 1999;9:17.

Golub R, Siddiqui F, Pohl D. Laparoscopic versus open appendectomy a meta-analysis. *J Am Coll Surg* 1998;186:543.

Guller U, Hervey S, Purves H, et al. Laparoscopic versus open appendectomy outcomes comparison based on a large administrative database. *Ann Surg* 2004;239:43.

Lane MJ, Liu DM, Huynh MD, et al. Suspected acute appendicitis nonenhanced helical CT in 300 consecutive patients. *Radiology* 1999;213:341.

Long KH, Bannon MP, Zietlow SP, et al. A prospective randomized comparison of laparoscopic appendectomy with open appendectomy clinical and economic analyses. *Surgery* 2001;129:390.

Minne L, Varner D, Burnell A, et al. Laparoscopic vs open appendectomy. Prospective randomized study of outcomes. *Arch Surg* 1997;132:708.

Nguyen NT, Zainabadi K, Mavandadi S, et al. Trends in utilization and outcomes of laparoscopic versus open appendectomy. *Am J Surg* 2004:188:813.

Ortega AE, Hunter JG, Peters JH, et al. Schirmer and Laparoscopic Appendectomy Study Group. A prospective, randomized comparison of laparoscopic appendectomy with open appendectomy. *Am J Surg* 1995;169:208.

Pedersen AG, Petersen OB, Wara P, et al. Randomized clinical trial of laparoscopic versus open appendicectomy. *Br J Surg* 2001;88:200.

Rao P, Rhea JT, Rattner DW, et al. Introduction of appendiceal CT impact on negative appendectomy and appendiceal perforation rates. *Ann Surg* 1999;229:344.

Temple LK, Litwin DE, McLeod RS. A meta-analysis of laparoscopic versus open appendectomy in patients suspected of having acute appendicitis. *Can J Surg* 1999;42:377.

EDITOR'S COMMENT

As one of the four most commonly performed operations, appendectomy is a staple of every general surgery practice. Nearly 10 years before the laparoscopic cholecystectomy revolutionized surgery, laparoscopic appendectomy had already been successfully performed in 1981 by K. Semm, a German gynecologist. Twenty-five years later, Dr. Eubanks summarizes lessons learned through randomized controlled outcome studies.

Too often today I am called to the operating room after CT scan confirms appendicitis, often before a proper abdominal examination. During my residency years we tolerated a 15% negative laparotomy rate and touted the advantages of laparoscopy for identifying other causes of abdominal pain mimicking appendicitis. Less commonly, appendicitis was found at operation for another presumed diagnosis. Not uncommonly, an inflamed or perforated appendix may be encountered during evaluation of pelvic or abdominal pain or it may be the surgical intent to electively remove the appendix. While many surgeons still advocate a small McBurney incision, proponents of the laparoscopic approach argue that abdominal examination through a scope allows more thorough visualization of the adnexa and intra-abdominal organs to exclude other causes of pain that mimic appendicitis. Gynecologic causes can be excluded. In one prospective randomized trial of 100 patients with the clinical diagnosis of appendicitis, 50 underwent open laparotomy and 50 underwent diagnostic laparoscopy. In the latter group, 19 patients,

or 38%, did not require appendectomy, and moreover, there were no complications from laparoscopy (Jadallah FA, et al. *Eur J Surg* 1994;160:41). With laparoscopy, there is a decreased incidence of wound infections because contaminated tissue is removed without coming into direct contact with the abdominal wound (Attwood SEA, et al. *Surgery* 1992;112:497).

Surgeons vary as to technique as reviewed by Dr. Eubanks. Using an open access technique, I will secure the Hasson port through a 10-mm infraumbilical incision. With the bladder decompressed, I will place a suprapubic 5-mm port at midline. A 5- to 12-mm radially expanding port is placed in the left lower quadrant and will be used to introduce the endoscopic stapler. Occasionally, I will place a 5-mm right flank port if another port is required to assist in the procedure. When staplers are not used, laparoscopic appendectomy can usually be performed through a 5- to 10-mm laparoscope and two 5-mm working ports as long as a 5-mm laparoscope is available.

Key to the operation is positioning the patient in steep Trendelenburg and the table rotated to the left. Obviously, the patient should be secured and well padded. The appendix is lifted and right cecum freed from lateral attachments until the base of the appendix can be clearly identified. While the mesoappendix and appendiceal artery can be ligated with a suture or taken with clips, I simply divide the mesoappendix with a vascular stapler and am done with it. The appendiceal stump may be divided with suture or endoloops, but another fire of the endolin-

ear stapler expedites the operation. Sometimes it is easier to divide the base of the appendix first. I always irrigate and aspirate copiously until return is clear to ensure no bleeding at the staple lines and minimize intra-abdominal contamination.

The necrotic appendiceal base is challenging even with an open approach. If there is significant inflammation around the cecum, closure of the stump is difficult. Whether open or laparoscopic, I will not hesitate to excise a portion of the cecum with a stapler. With laparoscopy, several time-honored rituals have proven unnecessary. We currently do not oversew the appendiceal stump or cauterize the mucosa after using a stapler.

If perforated, I will remove the appendix in an entrapment sack to minimize contamination of the abdominal cavity. The nonperforated appendix is brought into the port and removed with the port at the end of the case under laparoscopic visualization. The port sites are also irrigated and closed.

Numerous randomized prospective studies have shown that laparoscopic appendectomy decreases postoperative pain and expedites return to full activity when compared to conventional appendectomy. The laparoscopic appendectomy is commonly performed and gaining in popularity. While women and obese patients seem to benefit the most, thin men bounce back better after a laparoscopic appendectomy too and should not be denied a less invasive approach.

D.B.J.

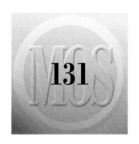

Technique of Colostomy Construction and Closure

IAN C. LAVERY

A colostomy may be constructed as an end colostomy or a loop colostomy. An end colostomy is usually permanent, constructed after removal or permanent exclusion of the distal bowel. A loop colostomy is usually constructed with an intention to reverse it at a later date after a definitive procedure is performed. The number of permanent colostomies has decreased in recent years, and intestinal continuity is being restored with increasing frequency. Modern stapling equipment allows the construction of a temporary loop stoma. For an operation to proceed well technically and for the stoma to function satisfactorily, there must be great attention to detail, including preoperative counseling of the patient and preoperative planning by the surgeon.

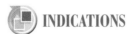 **INDICATIONS**

End colostomies are usually constructed in the sigmoid colon or the distal end of the descending colon. They are formed as part of the reconstruction after an abdominoperineal resection. Less commonly, they are constructed as a permanent diversion for radiation proctitis, incontinence, or perianal sepsis. A temporary end colostomy may be constructed in an emergency situation, such as after a resection for perforated sigmoid diverticulitis or trauma of the distal bowel.

Temporary loop stomas are constructed to relieve a distal obstruction or to prevent stool from flowing over a recently constructed distal anastomosis.

 PREOPERATIVE PLANNING

If a colostomy is to be made electively, preoperative counseling and psychological preparation of the patient are desirable. A visit with an enterostomal therapist or a specially trained visitor from a lay organization, such as the United Ostomy Association, is helpful.

The most common problems that occur after construction of a stoma relate to placement of the stoma or peristomal sepsis. A stoma located incorrectly predisposes the patient to problems that cannot be managed conservatively (i.e., with changes in the stoma equipment). The objective of stoma construction is to provide an anatomically stable opening that allows placement of an ostomy management

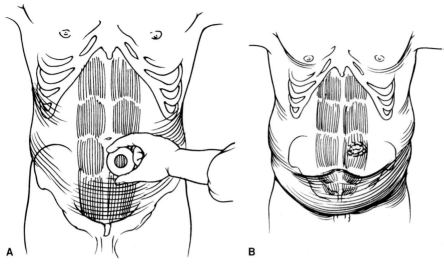

Fig. 1. Marking the site for the stoma. **A:** The usual site for a stoma is on the apex of the subumbilical fat roll. **B:** In obese patients, the stoma is located in the upper abdomen, where it is visible and on flat skin.

system that will maintain a seal for stool and gas for 5 to 7 days.

Most abdomens are not flat, muscular, and without scars. Most patients have some protuberance to their abdomen and lax musculature. Frequently, there are old incisions creating creases and weak musculature from neurovascular interruption. These circumstances make planning the location crucial to minimize postoperative problems. Locating the stoma is performed with the patient awake. An appropriately sized piece of equipment or a prepared disk of the same dimensions is used. The patient is marked while in supine, sitting, and bending positions. When the optimal site is determined, a tattoo is made with a sterile 27-gauge needle and indelible ink, so that when the abdomen is prepared and opened and the anatomic relationships are distorted, the site cannot be mistaken. The usual site in an average individual is on the apex of the subumbilical fat roll (Fig. 1A).

Primarily, the stoma must be constructed so that it is visible (i.e., not located on the inferior surface of a pendulous abdomen). The stoma should be away from the umbilicus, skin creases, scars, and bony prominences. Skin damaged by radiation or skin grafts should be avoided. In an obese individual with a pannus, the stoma is located in the upper abdomen, away from creases, where it is visible and the skin flat (Fig. 1B).

END COLOSTOMY

An end colostomy is usually constructed in conjunction with some other proce-

dure. If a stoma is to be constructed, my preference is to make the abdominal incision in the midline to avoid interfering with the rectus sheath or the rectus muscle and to preserve each quadrant of the abdomen for future use, should the need arise for relocation or revision of the stoma. One of the prerequisites to constructing an adequate stoma is to have sufficient bowel mobilized to bring the terminal portion to the skin level without tension. The left colon and the sigmoid colon must be mobilized, and the splenic flexure is taken down in certain circumstances. After an abdominoperineal resection, the sigmoid colon is mobilized as part of the primary procedure. Mobilization commences at the peritoneal reflection in the left paracolic gutter, and the dissection is carried medially in the avascular plane anterior to the gonadal vessels and the ureter. Mobilization is taken to the midline and medial to the duodenojejunal flexure. The more obese the patient, the more mobilization is necessary. Mobilization to the medial aspect of the duodenojejunal flexure allows the colon to be draped anterior to the small intestine *en route* to the stoma site in the rectus muscle. This avoids the need to close the mesenteric defect and essentially eliminates the possibility of a volvulus of the small intestine around the left colon. Mobilization should be sufficient to enable several centimeters of bowel to protrude without tension through the abdominal wall.

An adequate blood supply is an integral part of achieving the construction of a satisfactory end colostomy. When performed in

conjunction with an abdominoperineal resection, the inferior mesenteric artery is divided at its origin, proximal to the origin of the left colic artery. The left colic artery is divided proximal to its bifurcation into the ascending and descending left colic artery. As the inferior mesenteric artery is divided at its origin, the entire sigmoid colon must be resected because its arterial blood supply has been divided. The bowel is transacted at the junction of the descending and sigmoid colon, where it is perfused with blood from the middle colic artery through the marginal artery. A collateral blood supply is provided through the descending left colic and the ascending left colic arteries, through which the blood flow is reversed (Fig. 2). It is absolutely essential to check the blood supply, especially in the aged population, in which atheroma may be prominent, and diminish the blood supply through the marginal artery. If the end colostomy is being constructed for a condition that does not require resection of the sigmoid and rectum, there is less likelihood of a compromise of the blood supply. However, it is important to check the blood supply and ensure that the vasculature to the descending or sigmoid colon is not undercut during division of the mesentery. The blood supply is checked by observing the blood flow from the cut end of the bowel. If the blood flow is not bright and pulsatile, further bowel should be resected until this is achieved.

At the time of transection of the bowel, both ends of the colon are closed with a suture, or, more conveniently, with a stapling instrument. This maneuver minimizes contamination and allows the divided bowel to be brought through the site in the abdominal wall with minimal contamination.

PREPARATION OF OSTOMY SITE

Before the abdomen is opened, the optimal site for the stoma is marked, as discussed previously. The layers of the abdominal wall are oriented correctly and held in place with clamps attached to the edge of the rectal sheath and the dermis of the skin. While the layers of the abdominal wall are held in alignment, a circular disk of skin 2 cm in diameter (approximately the size of a quarter) is excised (Fig. 3A). Only the skin is removed, which preserves subcutaneous fat. This procedure is best performed with a scalpel to ensure that the opening is circular. A circular opening facilitates postoperative management. After the skin disk has been removed, while the abdominal wall is elevated and alignment of the layers of the abdominal wall is

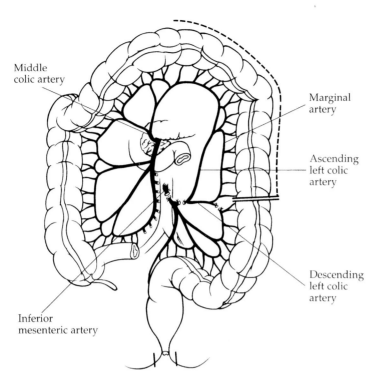

Fig. 2. The blood supply is defined and divided precisely to ensure a satisfactory blood supply at the terminal portion of the descending colon. The left colon is mobilized medially to the duodenojejunal flexure.

maintained, the fat is incised with a vertical incision down to the anterior rectus sheath. A linear incision is made in the anterior rectus sheath to expose the rectus muscle. The fibers of the rectus muscle are then split longitudinally by opening an instrument perpendicular to the line of the fibers (Fig. 3B). This procedure results in little or no bleeding unless the deep inferior epigastric vessels are encountered and divided deep to the rectus muscle. Caution should be taken to avoid this injury, as it can cause troublesome bleeding. If injury to the blood vessels occurs, hemostasis is secured by inserting an instrument through the opening in the abdominal wall and reflecting the medial part of the incision upward so that the vessel is exposed from the peritoneal aspect of the operative field, where it may be controlled with electrocoagulation or ligation.

After the rectus muscle is split and retracted, the posterior rectus sheath is divided (Fig. 3C). The opening in the abdominal wall should allow two average-sized fingers to pass through to the second phalanx (Fig. 3D). An opening of this size permits the construction of a colostomy through the strongest fascia and muscle of the abdominal wall, which minimizes the development of a hernia or prolapse, although with the passage of time, both these situations may develop. All muscle fibers

and the fibers of the anterior and posterior rectus sheath remain intact and help to support the intestine as it passes through the abdominal wall.

After preparation of the stomal opening, the terminal portion of the intestine is grasped with a noncrushing clamp and slowly maneuvered through the abdominal wall so that 3 to 4 cm protrudes without tension (Fig. 4A). With adequate medial mobilization of the left colon, it is unnecessary to attempt to close the mesenteric defect by suturing the mesentery to the parietal peritoneum. With the terminal portion of the intestine through the abdominal wall, the remainder of the intraperitoneal operation is completed. The abdominal wound is closed, and the skin adjacent to the stoma is approximated in the usual manner. In obese patients, or if the wound has been contaminated, it is desirable to leave the skin wound open or to close it loosely and hold it open with wicks. The wound is then protected, and the closed terminal portion of the intestine is excised (Fig. 4B). At this stage, it is important to be sure the blood supply is adequate by seeing pulsatile bleeding. If bleeding is not pulsatile, further resection is required. The maturation of the colostomy usually requires eight evenly spaced sutures in the circumference, which sutures the full thickness of the bowel to the dermis of the

abdominal wall (Fig. 4C). Sutures of 3-0 chromic catgut are used. After construction of the stoma, an appliance is placed over the stoma. If the stoma works in the early postoperative period, an appliance prevents the adjacent abdominal incision from being contaminated, and the patient is not subjected to the indignity of having feces on the abdomen.

SPECIAL CONSIDERATIONS

Obesity

The morbidly obese patient poses special problems when it comes to constructing a colostomy. The stoma must be located in the upper abdomen, where the skin is flat and the stoma is visible to the patient. Preoperative marking is essential. In a thin individual, location of the stoma in a less than perfect position can usually be managed, albeit with difficulty. In an obese patient, this is not possible, and any attempt to locate the stoma without previous marking inevitably leads to serious postoperative difficulties. With respect to mobilization of the colon, much more colon needs to be freely mobilized to allow the terminal portion to reach the skin without tension. The entire left colon needs to be mobilized. The distal transverse colon frequently needs to be mobilized with removal of the greater omentum from the colon to minimize the amount of tissue within the abdominal wall. It is sometimes necessary to divide the inferior mesenteric vein at the lower border of the pancreas to release the tethering action at this level. This maneuver provides an extra length of bowel that is quite remarkable and does not interfere with the blood supply.

It is unwise to have an opening in the abdominal wall so small that it is a struggle to bring the bowel through. The opening in the abdominal wall should be sufficiently large to allow easy transport of the intestine and the mesentery to the skin level. The incision in all layers of the abdominal wall, except the skin, needs to be enlarged considerably. Compression of the blood vessels as they pass through the wall results in ischemia and stoma necrosis. The incision is made as large as necessary by extending it cephalad and caudad through the anterior and posterior rectus sheath fasciae and the fibers of the rectus muscle. This maneuver is necessary to accommodate the thick mesentery of the left colon. If the incision in the abdominal wall is too small, attempts to bring the colon to the skin cause trauma to the mesentery and to the blood vessels to the bowel.

The Gastrointestinal Tract

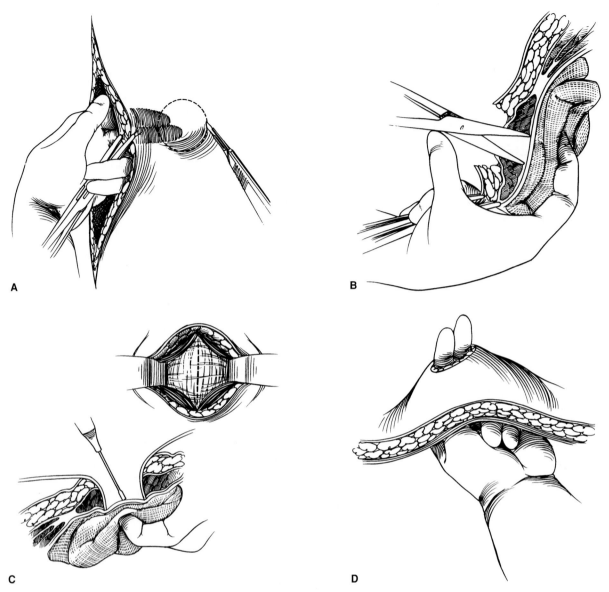

Fig. 3. Preparation of the stomal opening. **A:** While the layers of the abdominal wall are held in alignment, the left rectus muscle is elevated with a pad held by the left index and middle fingers as a disk of skin is excised at the previously marked site. **B:** The rectus muscle is continually elevated while the anterior rectus sheath is divided in a linear fashion and the rectus muscle is spread in the line of its fibers to expose the posterior rectus sheath. **C:** The opening of the wall is retracted with small right-angled retractors to expose the posterior rectus sheath being lifted with the pad on the fingers of the left hand. The sheath is then opened vertically with electrocautery onto the pad. **D:** The circular opening in the skin and the fiber-splitting incision in the deeper layers allow two fingers to pass through.

Once the bowel is positioned correctly, the defect in the abdominal wall is closed loosely around the bowel and the mesentery within the abdominal wall (Fig. 5). This should be done in a way that does not compress the blood supply. At this point, several interrupted chromic catgut sutures are placed between the fascia or parietal peritoneum of the abdominal wall and the seromuscular component of the bowel to help support the intestine within the abdominal wall until adhesions and healing occur. Theoretically, the sutures help to re-

duce the likelihood of a future peristomal hernia. In patients for whom maneuvers such as these are necessary, I believe we have to accept that a hernia will subsequently develop. This is preferable, however, to having an ischemic, or, at best, a stenotic, stoma in the immediate postoperative period.

Ascites

Because of the problem of leakage of ascitic fluid, every effort should be made to reduce its output. Leakage from around

the stoma is minimized by bringing the colon out through an extraperitoneal route. To achieve this, the peritoneum, if not already divided in the paracolic gutter, is divided, and, with blunt dissection, a tunnel is created in the extraperitoneal plane to the abdominal wall opening (Fig. 6A). The tunnel must be sufficiently large to accommodate the bowel and the mesentery loosely. Mobilization of the colon must be sufficient so that the extra distance involved is accommodated and no tension exists. One also needs to be sure

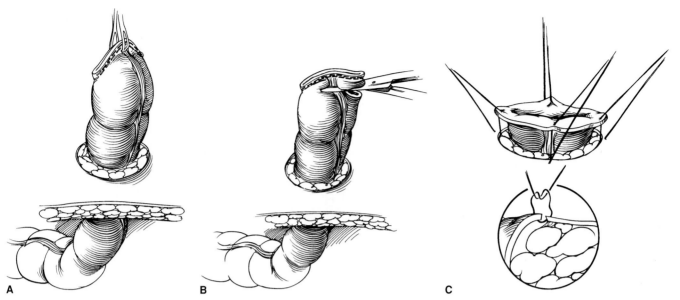

Fig. 4. Construction of end colostomy. **A:** The bowel is mobilized sufficiently so that 3 to 4 cm of the terminal portion can be brought through the opening without tension. The terminal portion is manipulated gently through the wall to avoid injury to the blood supply. **B:** The closed end of the bowel through the abdominal wall is excised in preparation for maturation of the stoma. Blood supply must be adequate. **C:** Primary mucocutaneous sutures are placed at the time of surgery, and an appliance is placed immediately.

that, as the mesentery passes under the cut edge of the parietal peritoneum, the blood supply is not compromised (Fig. 6B). With the bowel satisfactorily in position, the extraperitoneal tunnel is then closed by suturing the cut edge of the mesentery to the serosa of the bowel and the mesentery.

Radiation Injury or Rectal Stricture

When a colostomy is being constructed for radiation injury or a stricture in the rec-

tum, it is preferable to construct an end colostomy. With time, there is the potential for fibrosis and scarring to occur and cause retraction of a loop stoma. This allows spillover of stool and causes a recrudescence of symptoms, difficulty in maintaining an appliance on the colostomy, or both.

After the sigmoid colon has been mobilized and a site for the construction of

the colostomy has been selected in minimally irradiated intestine, the bowel is transected. Optimally, this is performed with stapling instruments that close the distal bowel and the proximal bowel. If it is not necessary to divide the marginal artery to allow the terminal portion of the proximal bowel to reach the skin, the artery should be preserved. If the distance is

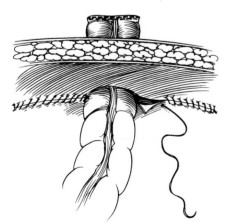

Fig. 5. In obese patients, the layers of the abdominal wall, except skin, are split longitudinally to make an opening large enough to accommodate the thick fatty mesentery. When the bowel is comfortably through the skin, the opening is closed loosely around the bowel and its mesentery.

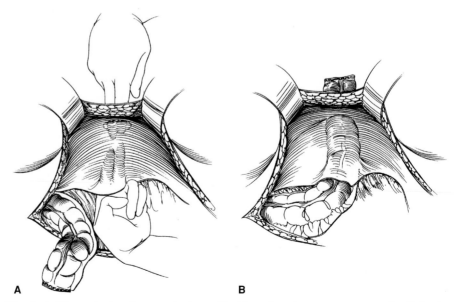

Fig. 6. A: The parietal peritoneum is elevated by blunt dissection to create a tunnel sufficiently large to accommodate the colon on its way to the stoma site. **B:** The cut edge of the mesentery in the left paracolic gutter is mobilized sufficiently to avoid compression of the blood supply to the distal bowel.

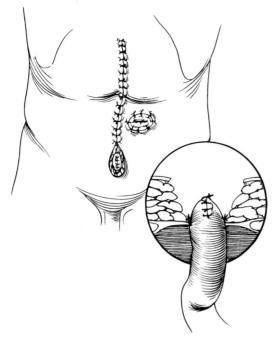

Fig. 7. After exclusion of a distal segment of irradiated bowel, the closed distal segment is attached in the subcutaneous location at the lower end of the wound. Sutures are placed between the anterior rectus sheath and the serosal surface of the intestine.

such that the marginal artery needs to be divided, care should be taken not to undercut the blood supply to the proximal or distal intestine. The mesentery is divided between the blood supply of the sigmoid vessels. The colostomy is then matured, as described previously for an ordinary end colostomy. The distal limb of the divided bowel is attached in the subcutaneous portion of the adjacent wound to obviate the possibility of a future pelvic abscess in the event there is a disruption of the closure of the distal loop of bowel (Fig. 7). Should this occur while the distal end is implanted in the subcutaneous portion of the wound, the worst that can happen is the development of an abscess in the lower end of the wound. Opening the abscess under local anesthetic may result in the development of a small low-output mucous fistula.

LOOP COLOSTOMY

Loop colostomies are constructed for diversion of a distal obstruction or a distal anastomosis. As with an end colostomy, it is desirable to have a potential site marked preoperatively. Although it is acceptable to construct a loop transverse colostomy through a midline abdominal wound and achieve a satisfactory long-term functional result, it is easier in the early postoperative period to manage a colostomy brought out through the rectus muscle

than through a midline abdominal wound. The site for the colostomy is prepared by making a 4- to 5-cm transverse incision in the right or left upper quadrant of the abdomen over the rectus muscle. The incision is extended down to the fascia, which is then divided in the same direction. The fascia is retracted to expose the rectus muscle. The lateral two thirds of the rectus muscle is then divided with

electrocautery. The superior epigastric vessels are identified and ligated. As the muscle is divided, it retracts and exposes the posterior rectus sheath. With a sponge held under the rectus sheath, the sheath is opened into the peritoneal cavity (Fig. 8).

The colon is mobilized by taking down the adjacent flexure and dividing the peritoneum at the base of the mesentery. The greater omentum is divided over the colon to allow the colon to be delivered through the omentum (Fig. 9). At this point, an opening is made in the mesentery of the colon approximately 1 cm from the bowel to avoid injury to the intestine. An umbilical tape is passed through the mesentery. Extreme care should be taken when placing the tape and rod through the mesentery, particularly in patients who are having the colostomy made to divert stool from a distal anastomosis. The tape and rod are placed between the marginal artery and the mesenteric border of the colon to avoid injury to the marginal artery, which is the sole vessel supplying the distal bowel after the inferior mesenteric artery has been divided. The tape is passed through the prepared site in the abdominal wall. With gentle traction on the tape passed through the opening and gentle manipulation from the intraperitoneal aspect, the loop of colon is delivered through the abdominal wall opening (Fig. 10A). The opening in the abdominal wall should accommodate the bowel and one finger without compression.

Once the colon is delivered without tension, the tape is replaced by a T-shaped

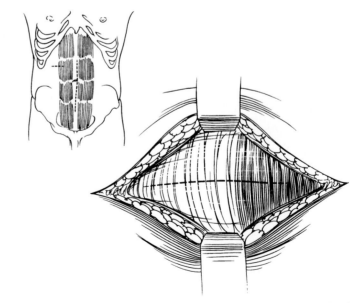

Fig. 8. A 4- to 5-cm incision is made over the lateral edge of the rectus muscle. The incision is extended down to the posterior rectus sheath, which is opened over a sponge to avoid injury to underlying viscera.

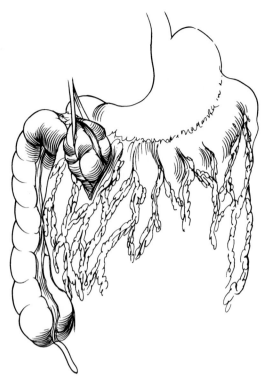

Fig. 9. The colon is brought through the greater omentum to allow the omentum to lie under the abdominal wound in its normal position. A tape is used as a retractor to help position the bowel where the loop will lie.

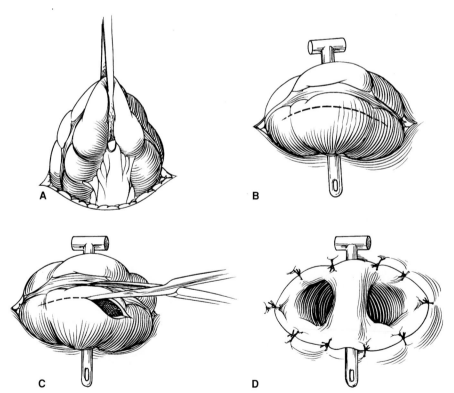

Fig. 10. Construction of loop colostomy. **A:** With gentle traction on the umbilical tape and manipulation of the colon intraperitoneally, the loop of colon is delivered through the prepared opening. Too vigorous traction may result in injury to the bowel. **B:** With the loop delivered through the abdominal wall, a rod replaces the tape to support the loop for 4 to 5 days. The rod helps create a spur of the posterior wall to help with diversion of stool. **C:** A longitudinal incision for the length of the loop is made in a convenient place (not necessarily along the taeniae coli). The incision is sufficiently long to allow the posterior wall to be easily seen. **D:** When matured, the proximal and distal limbs are separated. The stoma is diverted completely.

rod that rests on the skin and helps to support the posterior wall of the colon (Fig. 10B). The remainder of the procedure is performed as with an end colostomy, and the central abdominal wound is closed before maturation of the colostomy.

The loop of transverse colon is opened longitudinally for the entire length of the loop over the rod (Fig. 10C). This allows the posterior wall of the colon to act as a spur and be completely diverting (Fig. 10D). The colostomy is then matured by suturing the full thickness of the bowel wall to the dermis of the skin with interrupted 3-0 chromic catgut sutures. The rod is removed on the 4th or 5th day without complications. By this time, the rod is loose. If the patient is obese and difficulty was encountered in making the stoma, or if the patient's nutrition is poor, it may be necessary to leave the rod for a longer time.

If a small opening is made in the colon, a vent is created. The bowel ultimately drops back into the peritoneal cavity, and the stoma does not divert. If this happens early after the rod is removed, peritonitis may result as the bowel recedes into the peritoneal cavity.

CECOSTOMY

A cecostomy is a vent for the colon. It is no longer used to cleanse the colon in the presence of a distal obstruction. Cleansing is possible with a tube cecostomy, but it is messy, time-consuming, and, consequently, expensive. The most common use of a cecostomy today is in a patient who has an injury to the right colon or cecum or in a patient who has necrosis of the cecum in association with a cecal volvulus.

The stoma is constructed by making a skin-crease incision over the cecal opening and extending this into the peritoneal cavity by splitting the muscles in the line of its fibers until the peritoneum is encountered and opened. Seromuscular sutures are placed at an appropriate distance to allow the opened cecum to reach skin level. The opening in the cecum is made and the mucocutaneous sutures are placed (Fig. 11).

If a tube cecostomy is constructed, three concentric suture lines of 2-0 Vicryl are placed centered on the proposed tube site. The cecum is opened and the tube inserted. The tube is a large-bore (e.g., No. 30 French) Malecot-type catheter or a large Foley catheter. The sutures are then tied around the shaft of the tube in layers (Fig. 12). The catheter is brought out directly through the abdominal wall through a stab incision. The enlarged end of the catheter is

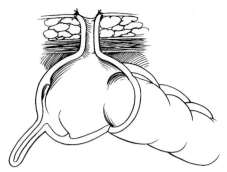

Fig. 11. An appropriately sized opening is made through the layers of the abdominal wall. This allows the cecal wall to be approximated to skin and primary mucocutaneous sutures to be placed.

pulled up to approximate the serosa to the parietal peritoneum. Eight 2-0 Vicryl sutures are placed from the peritoneum to the seromuscular layers of the cecum to maintain the approximation around the catheter (Fig. 13). The tube must be kept patent by irrigating at least three times a day. Leakage around the tube is a risk.

Once the need for the cecostomy has passed, removal of the tube allows the stoma to close by secondary intention. If a formal mucocutaneous suture line is made, formal closure may be required to rid the colocutaneous fistula.

CONSTRUCTION TECHNIQUES

During the construction of either an end or a loop stoma, it is not necessary to suture the parietal peritoneum to the seromuscular layers of the colon. If the colostomy is likely to be present for longer than 3 to 4 months, an

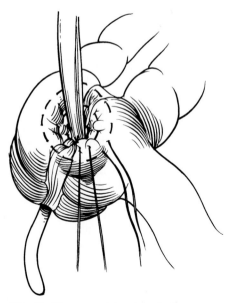

Fig. 12. The concentric sutures in the cecum, when tied around the catheter, imbricate the bowel wall in to help seal it and prevent leakage.

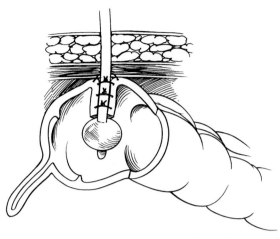

Fig. 13. The cecum is tacked to the abdominal wall. With the catheter withdrawn, the enlarged end in the cecum helps to maintain apposition of the serosa to the peritoneum and prevents leakage into the peritoneal cavity.

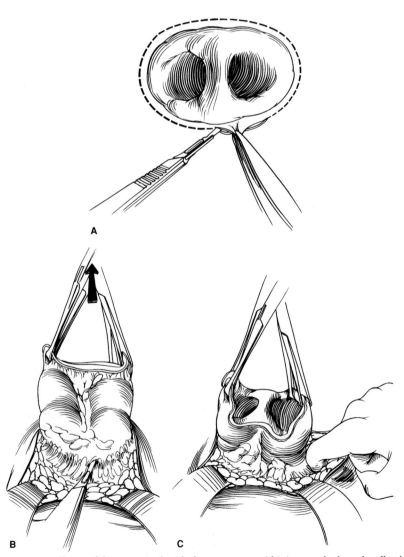

Fig. 14. A: A small rim of skin is excised with the stoma to avoid injury to the bowel wall, which must be anastomosed. Traction can be applied to the skin, which is removed later. **B:** With traction on the circumcised stoma and countertraction on the abdominal wall (*arrow*), the plane of dissection is demonstrated, and circumferential dissection frees up the bowel to the peritoneal cavity. **C:** When the peritoneal cavity is first entered, a finger is passed into the peritoneal cavity. This allows better demonstration of the remaining attachments between bowel and abdominal wall and permits safe division on the finger.

end colostomy or a diverting ileostomy may be preferable. Because prolapse occurs from the distal limb of the colostomy, this minimizes the potential for the development of prolapse of the colostomy or development of a parastomal hernia. A well-made ileostomy is easier to manage than is a flush loop transverse colostomy, which is larger than an ileostomy. The liquid output from a loop transverse colostomy is more difficult to contain in an appliance because the stoma is flush.

In the construction of either an end or a loop stoma, there is no place for delaying maturation of the stoma. With appropriate stoma equipment, contamination of the wound rarely occurs. Use of a second anesthetic or the procedure of opening the colostomy when the patient is on the hospital ward cannot be justified. The result is a poorly fashioned stoma after a long period of maturation by secondary intention.

If the loop colostomy is constructed to decompress bowel that is distended because of a distal obstruction, the technical aspects may be quite difficult. As a result, a trend in recent years is to perform a resection of the obstruction and construction of an end colostomy. However, there are circumstances in which construction of a loop stoma is optimal treatment, usually in patients who are not fit for the larger procedure. The site of the colostomy is selected according to the location of the obstructing lesion and the intended definitive procedure; for example, when the obstructing lesion is in the midrectum, the

choices are either sigmoid, left transverse, or right transverse colostomy. A sigmoid colostomy is constructed if the surgeon anticipates doing a definitive operation, one in which the colostomy is taken down and resected with the specimen. If it is predicted, however, that the anastomosis may require a temporary diversion, a right transverse colostomy should be chosen. If the colostomy is constructed in the left transverse colon, it may be necessary to take the colostomy down and close it to obtain sufficient length to perform a low colorectal or coloanal anastomosis. Subsequently, construction of a new right transverse colon or loop ileostomy for the diversion must be performed.

During construction of the colostomy, the enlarged colon is decompressed. Gas is removed from the colon by passing a large-bore (15- or 18-gauge) needle obliquely through the bowel wall at the site of the intended colostomy. The more solid contents are milked proximally and distally to reduce the bulk that must pass through the abdominal wall. The bulk to go through the wall is greater than the amount there is when one is dealing with a well-prepared and unobstructed colon. Inevitably, there are some contents, and the bowel wall is edematous or thickened by muscular hypertrophy, or both. The opening in all layers of the abdominal wall needs to be enlarged sufficiently to accommodate the bulk of the bowel without compressing the blood supply. Special attention must be given to passing a tape through the mesentery to avoid injury to

the marginal artery. The blood supply to the proximal end of a future anastomosis may depend on this, if the inferior mesenteric artery is divided as part of a cancer operation, or if mobilization of the descending colon is needed to reach a coloanal anastomosis. The colostomy is opened and matured over a rod, as described previously. The resulting stoma initially is edematous and larger than that made in unobstructed bowel. However, the stoma does reduce to a normal size and appearance during the next 3 or 4 weeks.

COLOSTOMY CLOSURE

A loop transverse colostomy is closed easily without opening the abdomen if sufficient time has passed since its construction. I prefer to wait 10 to 12 weeks before closing a colostomy. This allows time for edema and dense adhesions to resolve. Closing a colostomy earlier than this may be difficult because of adhesions of the bowel wall to the abdominal wall. The earlier the stoma is closed, the higher the complication rate.

The stoma is mobilized by making a circumferential incision in the skin approximately 2 mm from the mucosa (Fig. 14A). The excised skin is then grasped in each quadrant so that traction can be applied on the bowel. Countertraction is applied on the skin and subcutaneous fat to define the plane of dissection (Fig. 14B). The dissection is carried down circumferentially. As the dissection is performed, the

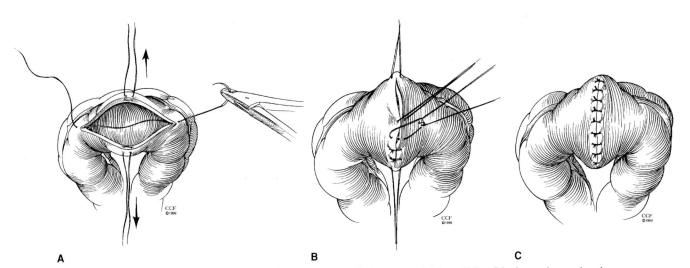

A   **B**   **C**

Fig. 15. A: The longitudinal incision is made transverse by placing sutures in the middle of the long edges and at the apex of the incision. The apical suture becomes the middle suture of the closure. **B:** Meticulously placed seromuscular sutures 4 to 5 mm apart approximate the wound edges. **C:** When closed completely, the sutures should approximate the wound edges. These should not be tied tightly to avoid ischemia and the potential for leakage. If there is conveniently located fat from adjacent epiploica or omentum, tack it over the suture line.

fascia is first exposed, followed by the muscle layers, until the peritoneal cavity is entered. Once the peritoneal cavity is entered, a finger is inserted between the bowel and the abdominal wall (Fig. 14C). The remainder of the peritoneal and serosal attachments are divided, and intraperitoneal adhesions are broken down by sweeping the finger. The need to enlarge the abdominal wall opening is unusual if 10 to 12 weeks have passed since construction of the colostomy.

Once the bowel is mobilized circumferentially into the peritoneal cavity, the skin is trimmed from the mucocutaneous junction. All skin and subcutaneous fat must be removed from the bowel wall before suturing. The initial longitudinal incision is closed transversely. Two sutures that will be part of the closure are placed in the middle of the colostomy. Traction is applied and a suture placed in the middle of the incision, now a transversely oriented incision (Fig. 15A). The colostomy is then closed with interrupted seromuscular sutures of 3-0 Vicryl (Fig. 15B,C). This closure needs to be performed meticulously. When closed, the bowel is irrigated and gently returned to the peritoneal cavity by methodically returning one limb of the bowel, followed by the second. Relaxation of the abdominal wall is helpful in returning the bowel to the abdominal cavity and in repairing the defect in the abdominal wall. The muscular and fascial layers are closed in the line of their fibers with a nonabsorbable suture. The skin is left open to avoid an infection. It heals quickly in a normal wound.

SUGGESTED READING

Abcarian H, Pearl RK. Stomas. *Surg Clin North Am* 1988;68:1295.

Hawley PR, Ritchie JK. The colon. 1. Complications of ileostomy and colostomy following excisional surgery. *Clin Gastroenterol* 1979;8:403.

Kodner IJ. Colostomy and ileostomy. Ciba Foundation Symposium, 1978;1:30.

Mileski WJ, Reg RV, Joehl RJ, et al. Rates of morbidity and mortality after closure of loop and end colostomy. *Surg Gynecol Obstet* 1990;171:17.

Rombeau JL, Wilk PJ, Turnbull RB, et al. Total fecal diversion by temporary skin-level loop transverse colostomy. *Dis Colon Rectum* 1978; 21:223.

Rutegard J, Dahlgren S. Transverse colostomy or loop ileostomy as diverting stoma in colorectal surgery. *Acta Clin Scand* 1987;153:229.

Turnbull RB, Weakly FL. *Atlas of intestinal stoma.* St. Louis: Mosby, 1967.

EDITOR'S COMMENT

As Dr. Lavery states in this very fine chapter, the most important aspect of the colostomy is the siting. This relatively small, or seemingly small, technical detail is probably the most important part of sustaining good function of a colostomy or an ileostomy. As Professor Lavery implies, it is important that a stoma nurse who does this daily should be involved in the siting of an ostomy before operation. The patient should be sitting and the folds, the beltline, and other previous scars should be taken into account. It should not be left to the most junior person on the team. Macdonald et al. (*Surgeon JR Coll* 2003;1:347) compared the siting abilities of two colorectal subspecialty interests; six trainees were asked to site an end colostomy in nine patients using an adhesive disc with a diameter of 1 cm. This was compared with the site selected by a stoma nurse, which was taken as the "gold standard." Colorectal specialists were much better at placing stomas than those with a general interest. The study concluded that there was no difference between consultants and trainees, including those that had been trained by a stoma nurse in their ability to site a stoma, although as only one stoma was made in the patient selected, this conclusion may not be accurate. However, the last statement of the article is reasonable: "Fashioning of the colostomy after an emergency laparotomy is frequently left to the most junior surgeon in theatre, as it is the easiest part to do. If the wrong site has been chosen, it has become the easiest part to do badly and the patient frequently has to live with the consequences." I agree.

Dr. Lavery states that, in temporary colostomies or ileostomies, one frequently does a loop, and permanent colostomies are done only when there is no intention to redo intestinal continuity. I disagree. In almost 400 temporary ileostomies from ileal pouch anastomoses, I have found it much better for the patient to do a standard end/Brooke ileostomy, to close the distal end and to attach it to the abdominal wall immediately below the ileostomy. One can then close the ileostomy in fashion similar to that done if one had a loop ileostomy just by making the incision around the ileostomy and retrieving the distal limb

where it is always in the same place. Similarly, with colostomies that are used to protect the patient following a very low rectal resection and chemotherapy and radiation, I do an end colostomy and attach the stapled end right to the underside of the colostomy and retrieve it in similar fashion. It may be slightly more time-consuming, but I think the results are better. This is becoming more of an issue especially because the shift in the colon and rectal practices is the preservation of rectal function, including resecting part of the rectal sphincter. Thus, these patients may have "temporary" colostomies for a long time, and we should make certain that they function.

Park et al. (*Dis Colon Rectum* 1999;42:1575) reviewed 1616 patients treated at the Cook County Hospital between 1976 and 1995 and found that there were complications in 34%. Of these, 553 patients had complications. In 448 patients, these complications occured early. In 105 patients, complication occured late complications. The most common complications were irritation and pain associated with stoma location, 12% and 7%, respectively, and partial necrosis, 5%. It was interesting that "the enteric stoma with the most complications was the loop ileostomy (74 percent). . . ." The enteric stoma with the least complications was the end transverse colostomy (6%).

A few words on technique: When I staple off a colon, for example to do an end colostomy, whether temporary or permanent, I usually use sutures of 4-0 or 3-0 silk immediately adjacent to the suture line and pull them up to help bring the colostomy through the abdominal wall most easily. This enables one to do this gently and without struggling. If the wound is contaminated, it is probably equally efficacious to put in closed suction drains and close the wound over the closed suction drain. They key is to leave the closed suction drains for 10 days to 2 weeks, because that is when suppuration occurs. The attraction of doing a delayed primary closure is that it avoids infection, but the problem is that it does not avoid infection 100% of the time. Wound infections following delayed primary closures occur in 5% of patients. Wound infection occurred in approximately 11% in a Swedish study in patients with primary clo-

sure over closed suction drains. Personally, I would rather take the chance on an 11% wound infection rate over the closed suction drains and avoid the pain and inconvenience of patients undergoing delayed primary closure. I also tend to do a classic Brooke ileostomy or colostomy closure with three-part sutures, and not including mucosa in either situation, for fear of getting a fistula between the skin and mucosa of the ileostomy or colostomy.

As far as closure of ileostomies or colostomies is concerned, I tend to wait for 4 months. This is particularly true of closing the ileostomy following an ileal pouch, anal anastomosis, or pull-through procedure, and I do this for two reasons: first, it is much easier to close the ileostomy after 4 months than after 3 because the adhesions have matured and become much more filmy; and second, the rectum functions better as the edema and the scarring and fibrosis has diminished considerably after 4 months following the closure.

Which type of patient gets a permanent colostomy? The commonly held point of view is that the elderly most often end up with colostomies following mid-to-low rectal resections. Law et al. (*World J Surg* 2006;30:598) attempted to answer this question by reviewing 612 patients who underwent curative resections for rectal cancer. One hundred thirty-three were older than 75 years of age. Ninety-six (15.7%) of the 612 patients ended up with a permanent end colostomy. In their study, only 21% of those patients who were more than 75 years of age underwent abdominal peritoneal resection, or the Hartman operation. There was a trend to treat elderly patients with surgery resulting with an end colostomy, but the difference did not reach statistical significance (*P* = 0.06). Thus, the old adage may be true.

The other situation in which patients may end up with temporary or permanent colostomies is following traumatic injuries. Murray et al. (*J Trauma* 1999;46:250) reviewed 140 patients from Los Angeles County at the University of Southern California Medical Center during a 5½ year period. These patients were selected from 720 patients with colonic injuries, but these patients required a

(continued)

resection. Twenty-eight of the 140 patients underwent a colostomy and the surgeon did not attempt an anastomosis. Forty-one percent of the 140 patients (57 patients) developed a colon-related complication: 28% had an abscess, an anastomotic leak rate of 13% in the colocolostomy group.

The authors concluded that right-sided injuries, not surprisingly, had fewer complications if an ileocolostomy was done, in which case there was a 4% leak rate (2 of 55). In right-sided injuries in which an ileocolostomy was not done, but rather a colocolostomy, the leak rate was 19%, confirming the ancient wisdom. Two of 7 patients

with colonic leaks died. With the left colonic injuries, the incidence of colonic leaks was 11%, and 6% (2 of 35) ended up with colonic fistulas. Thus, it appears that, with proper judgment, one can close colonic injuries but should be prepared for a number of complications.

Mahjoubi et al. (*Colorectal Dis* 2005;7:582) reviewed 330 patients with end colostomies and concluded that the highest complication rate was in psychosocial complications, which was found in 56% percent of patients. Those patients older than 40 years had a greater incidence of psychosocial complications than those younger than 40.

All of us who practice surgery know that patients who have colon cancer enter the office with fear concerning one aspect: that they end up with a permanent colostomy. In the contemporary practice of colon and rectal surgery, this does not happen very often, but if it does, or if a patient has to have a temporary stoma, siting of the stoma, the technique used in constructing it, and making certain to minimize the likelihood of pericolostomy hernias if and when patients end up with a colostomy are of vital importance for the comfort of patients.

J.E.F.

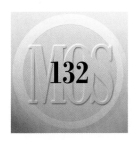

132 Care of Stomas

LAURIE MAIDL AND JILL OHLAND

This chapter will provide an overview on the management of ostomies. An intestinal stoma can be a life-altering event for many individuals. The location of the stoma on the abdomen, stoma construction, and appropriate appliance management are all key factors in the adjustment of the person with an ostomy.

ROLE OF THE WOUND, OSTOMY, AND CONTINENCE NURSE

Ostomy surgery significantly alters bowel function, necessitating physiologic and psychosocial adaptation. A wound, ostomy, and continence (WOC) nurse is a specialist who assists the patient and family with ostomy care during their adjustment to life with an ostomy. In the preoperative setting, the WOC nurse discusses the surgical procedure and lifestyle issues with the patient and his or her family, demonstrates various types of ostomy appliances, and marks the stoma site on the patient's abdomen.

Postoperatively, in the hospital, the WOC nurse assists the patient to learn management of the stoma using an appropriate ostomy appliance. Dietary advice, peristomal skin care, and resuming activities of daily living are discussed. Rehabilitation, focusing on body image, sexuality, and return to normal life activities such as work or school, is also discussed.

After hospital discharge, it is important for the patient to have regular contact with a WOC nurse to assist in management changes that may occur. These changes may include a decrease in stoma size, changes in

body contour, stabilization of weight after surgery, and increasing activity with return to normal lifestyle. The adjustment to a fecal diversion occurs over time. In the years following ostomy surgery, the WOC nurse is available to assist with problem solving of peristomal skin complications, ostomy appliance management difficulties, and psychosocial concerns. In addition, this allows the patient to remain current with ostomy appliances that are available.

STOMA CONSTRUCTION

A stoma may be constructed as an end, loop, or double-barrel stoma. An end stoma is created by dividing the bowel completely. The proximal end of the bowel is brought up to the abdominal wall at the premarked stoma site, everted, and sutured to the skin. The distal portion of the bowel may be removed or may be closed and left in the abdomen. If the bowel is left in the abdomen, the option of reanastomosis could be addressed at a future date. If any portion of bowel is left distal to the stoma, the patient will occasionally expel a mucous drainage per the anus. The mucous drainage is normal and will continue for as long as the patient is diverted.

A loop stoma is created by bringing a loop of bowel, either small or large intestine, to skin level. The bowel is partially divided and both openings are sutured to the abdominal wall. The proximal bowel may be everted and the distal bowel sutured below the proximal stoma. The distal bowel opening would represent a mu-

cous fistula. Mucous discharge would come from the distal stoma opening as well as the anus during the time the bowel is diverted. Management of the stoma may be more difficult with the flush distal loop as mucus is secreted and can undermine the appliance edge, resulting in skin irritation and appliance leakage. The appliance opening would need to be fit to allow both stomas to empty into the pouch.

A double-barrel stoma is similar to a loop stoma, except that the bowel is completely divided and both ends of the bowel are brought to the abdominal wall and matured. The proximal stoma is the functioning stoma and the distal stoma secretes mucus. The stomas may be placed close together and pouched in one appliance opening, or they may be placed at different sites on the abdomen. If they are placed at different sites, there should be at least 4 in. between the two stomas to allow for an adequate pouching surface. The proximal stoma would always be managed with an appliance. The distal stoma may be managed with a pouch initially, and if the amount of mucus decreases significantly, it may be possible to manage this stoma with a gauze dressing. It is important for the patient to know that there will always be some type of discharge from the distal stoma, even though the bowel is diverted.

When a stoma is constructed, it is important that it protrudes above skin level at least 2 cm. This would be true even with a descending or sigmoid colostomy. The stoma will be edematous for 6 to 8 weeks after surgery and will decrease in diameter as well as length during this time. As the stoma decreases in size, one that is adequately budded at the time of surgery should still have adequate protrusion when the edema resolves. Ideally the lumen of the stoma would be central, which would allow the effluent to empty into the pouch. If a stoma is flush with the skin or if the lumen empties near skin level, the effluent can undermine the appliance seal, causing appliance leakage and skin irritation.

TYPES OF STOMAS

Stomas typically managed with a pouching system are jejunostomy, ileostomy, colostomy, and urostomy. The anatomic location of the stoma provides information about the amount, consistency, and frequency of the output. This information will be used when choosing an appliance to manage the stoma.

A jejunostomy is an opening into the jejunum, which is the midportion of the small intestine. Crohn disease, trauma, or extensive bowel resections may result in a jejunostomy. There is a large amount of intestinal secretions from the jejunum, which aid in digestion. Therefore, the effluent from a jejunostomy is watery, clear, and dark green in color and usually begins within 48 hours after surgery. The volume of output can be over 2 L per day, so it is necessary to monitor the fluid and electrolyte balance for these patients. In addition, the absorption of nutrients, fluids, and electrolytes may be radically reduced in the patient with a jejunostomy. Absorptive capacity of the jejunum depends on the length and function of the proximal bowel. Therefore, nutritional management with hyperalimentation is not uncommon with jejunostomy patients.

An ileostomy is created from the ileum, or the distal portion of the small intestine. The most common reasons for an ileostomy are ulcerative colitis, Crohn disease, and familial polyposis. The initial effluent from an ileostomy usually begins within 48 to 72 hours after surgery and is liquid, but may thicken to a mushy consistency once the diet is advanced. In the first few weeks after surgery, the ileostomy output may exceed 1 L per day, resulting in the need to closely monitor fluid and electrolyte balance. Over time, the small bowel adapts and will absorb more fluid, reducing the volume of output to 500 to 1,000 mL and resulting in thicker stool. The consistency of the output will vary from day to day, depending on the amount of water in the stool.

A colostomy is an opening into a portion of the colon. A colostomy may result from cancer, diverticular disease, volvulus, incontinence, congenital anomalies, or trauma. A stoma may be created in any section of the colon, although cecal and ascending colostomies are rare. The output from the colostomy varies, depending on the stoma location. The more distal the location of the stoma in the colon, the thicker and less frequent the output from the colostomy is. Stoma function also is dependent on the extent of previous bowel resections, residual disease, medications, diet, and concurrent therapies, such as chemotherapy or radiation therapy.

A urostomy is an opening into the urinary tract. Cancer is the most common diagnosis resulting in a urostomy, but incontinence, interstitial cystitis, and congenital anomalies are also reasons a urostomy may be created. An ileal conduit, colon conduit, and ureterostomy are three types of incontinent urostomies and would require an ostomy appliance to contain the urine. The normal output of urine per day is dependent on fluid intake, but is about 1,000 to 1500 mL/d.

PREOPERATIVE TEACHING

Health care and the recovery from colon and rectal surgery have dramatically changed in the past years. Hospital stays are decreased, early discharge with follow-up care in the home is on the rise, and insurance coverage and payment restraints affect a person's ability to control and tailor health care to meet specific needs. All of these factors underline the need to have the patient receive preoperative education. Bass et al. conducted a study that concluded that patients who had preoperative education and stoma site marking by a WOC nurse had fewer stoma complications compared to a group that did not have education.

Preoperative education may include discussion of the proposed surgical option, demonstration of appliances, and description of the type of stoma and how it will be managed. It is helpful to describe the stoma appearance, the usual consistency and quantity of drainage, gas and odor control, diet, fluid and electrolytes, clothing, sexuality, recreation, and return to work.

STOMA SITE MARKING

There are two factors that are critical to patient satisfaction postoperatively with ostomy care: (a) stoma location and (b) surgeon skill in creating a budded stoma. A poorly sited stoma can increase the chance for appliance leakage and peristomal skin complications, which will further compromise the patient's adjustment and return to self-care. A well-sited stoma that allows for a secure appliance placement and that does not interfere with activities of daily living will allow the patient to rapidly gain confidence and adjust to life with a stoma.

A stoma site should be determined preoperatively for both temporary and permanent ostomies. Although the stoma may be in place only a few months, difficult appliance management due to poor stoma siting can lead to undue psychologic distress.

There are three factors critical to determining the ostomy site. The location of the site must be (a) within the rectus muscle, (b) outside of abdominal creases and scars, and (c) within the patient's line of vision. Siting the stoma within the rectus muscle will reduce the risk of hernia formation. Assessment of the abdomen in the supine, sitting, and standing positions is important for detection of changes in body contour. It is also important to have the patient bend at the waist when sitting and standing to evaluate for creases at the site. Bony structures are most evident when the patient is supine. Creases and skin folds are most prominent when the patient is sitting. Visualization of the stoma is very important in being able to return to self-care.

The most commonly accepted practice is to site the stoma on the apex of the infraumbilical bulge using the above three critical factors. Stoma sites in all the abdominal quadrants are shown in Figures 1 and 2. If a midline incision is used, it is best if the stoma can be located at least two to three fingerbreadths (about 2.5 in.) away from the incision, as this will allow for an adequate barrier to be placed around the stoma postoperatively. In the same manner, it is best to stay at least two to three fingerbreadths away from the iliac crest to avoid interference with appliance adherence. There has been much written in the literature about the controversial issue of marking the stoma site below the belt line. While most patients report that an ostomy site located below the belt line is easier to conceal within the clothing, the challenge is to find an adequate site on many patients, especially males, who wear their clothing well below the natural waistline of the body. Sites marked too close to the groin crease, too close to the iliac crest, or outside of the patient's line of vision are fraught with multiple appliance-fit issues. Often a site within the upper quadrant is preferable to the lower quadrant site if the patient can visualize this site and there is an adequate flat surface to adhere the appliance. Sites located within the natural waistline have a strong tendency to crease toward the umbilicus

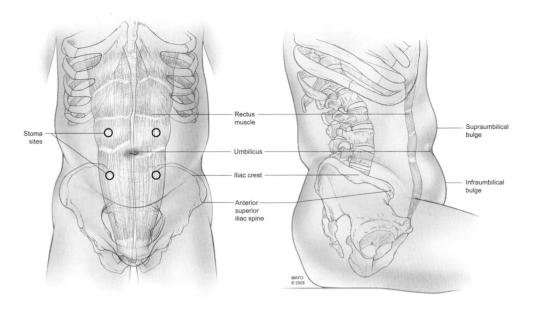

Fig. 1. Stoma site marking.

and are not suitable sites for stoma location. To assess for possible creasing of a stoma at a selected site, gently push in and up on the stoma site to visualize the natural tendency of the body to pull back on the bowel. Once the stoma site is located, it should be marked in a manner that will be visible after the surgical scrub. Often the site is marked with an indelible marker and later "scratched" with a sterile needle.

The ileostomy and ileal conduit are usually sited on the right side, whereas the colostomy is usually sited on the left side. Prosthetic devices, such as braces or belts, must also be assessed and the stoma site placed for continued use of these devices. When two stomas, such as a colostomy and ileal conduit, are needed, it is best if the stomas can be located on opposite sides of the abdomen, with sufficient

room between them for normal appliance barrier placement. If the rectus muscle needs to be removed for reconstruction reasons, both stomas can be located on the same side, usually one stoma in the lower quadrant and one in the upper quadrant. Adequate peristomal skin margins need to be left around each stoma for placement of the ostomy appliance.

 POSTOPERATIVE TEACHING

Ideally, postoperative teaching should be a continuation of the teaching already started preoperatively. Postoperative pain and surgical complications can impair the patient's ability to learn in the hospital setting. Short education sessions are usually better received than one long education session. Shorter hospital stays are prompting more of the ostomy education to be completed in the outpatient setting. Follow-up visits with a WOC nurse or home care nurse should be scheduled before the patient leaves the inpatient setting.

Educational goals should be set with the patient's input. Although it is ideal for each patient to learn ostomy care to become self-sufficient, many patients cope by having a spouse or family member initially learn the ostomy care. The patient then learns ostomy care at a later date.

Assessment of the patient/family learning styles and barriers is helpful in setting up an educational plan of care. Priority ostomy education focuses on the patient or family member learning how to empty the appliance and to do an appliance change. Upon discharge, the patient or family

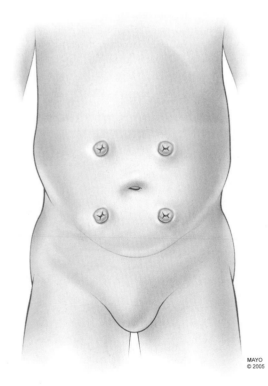

Fig. 2. Stoma sites in all four abdominal quadrants.

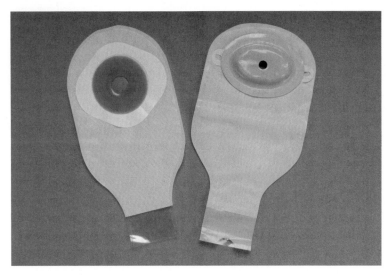

Fig. 3. Flat skin barrier **(A)** and convex skin barrier **(B).**

member should be able to demonstrate an appliance change and how to empty the ostomy appliance. Preoperative teaching, such as diet modification, fluid needs, and activity restrictions, also needs to be discussed.

Many changes occur in the stoma and abdomen within the first 2 to 3 months after surgery. These changes can affect the fit of the ostomy appliance on the abdomen. Also, the person with an ostomy has had some time to become familiar with the management of the ostomy, but may have questions or concerns about how to live a normal life with an ostomy. Teaching can be reinforced, as well as adjustment of the appliance fit and support and encouragement to the person with an ostomy.

OSTOMY APPLIANCES

The purpose of an ostomy appliance is twofold: (a) to protect the skin around the stoma from breakdown and (b) to contain the effluent in an odor-proof receptacle. There are numerous products on the market that have been developed to use in ostomy care. Ostomy appliances have three main components that need to be assessed when determining which appliance would work the best: (a) type of skin barrier, (b) type of pouch, and (c) type of pouch closure. The WOC Nurse Standards of Care series states that the average wear time for an ostomy appliance is 3 to 7 days. Generally, patients will change the ostomy appliance one to two times per week.

The skin barrier is the part of the appliance that protects the skin around the stoma. Skin barriers are available in standard wear and extended wear. The difference between these two barriers is in the amount of absorption of the product. The barrier with a delayed absorption provides a longer wear time and is considered extended wear. A stoma that has a high output or liquid output may get a better seal and skin protection with an extended-wear barrier. As a general rule, colostomies use a standard-wear barrier, whereas ileostomies and urostomies use an extended-wear barrier.

A skin barrier may also be flat or convex (Fig. 3). The peristomal skin plane will determine which type of barrier to use. The shape of the skin barrier should mirror the peristomal skin plane. Therefore, if there is retraction of the skin around the stoma, a convex skin barrier may be used. There are many additional skin barrier products that can be used on a skin barrier to provide all types of convexity (Fig. 4).

The skin barrier is available in cut-to-fit and precut options (Fig. 5). If the stoma is not completely round or is changing size in the immediate postoperative period, a cut-to-fit option may be best. For the patient with limited dexterity, the precut option may be used.

Skin barriers also come in paste and liquid forms. Paste is used as a caulk on the back of a solid skin barrier to fill in irregular areas. It should be noted that some pastes contain alcohol, which may cause temporary burning of denuded skin and will usually dissolve in 1 to 2 days due to contact with the effluent. For this reason, paste is not often used. Liquid and powder skin barriers may be used under a solid skin barrier to provide skin care to denuded skin (Fig. 6).

The pouch or "bag" is the part of the appliance that holds the effluent. Pouches are usually made from an odor-proof plastic. They are available in many shapes and sizes, and are either transparent or opaque. A pouch needs to be emptied when it becomes one-third to one-half full of gas or effluent.

The pouches come in three main styles: (a) drainable, (b) urinary, and (c) closed end (Fig. 7). The drainable pouch is used for fecal effluent. The effluent is drained out of the bottom of the pouch without having to remove the appliance from the body. The opening at the bottom is secured with a clamp or closure. The urinary pouch is used for urine and has a tap that can be easily opened to drain the urine from the bottom of the pouch without having to remove the appliance from the body. A closed-end pouch has no opening and must be removed either from the body or from the skin barrier to be

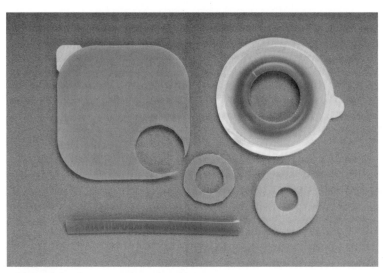

Fig. 4. Additional skin barrier products for adding convexity.

success for colostomy irrigation. Diarrhea or irregular bowel movements lend toward unsuccessful bowel control.

3. The patient must be willing to learn and perform the procedure independently.

4. It must be the patient's choice to perform colostomy irrigation as a method of bowel management.

Colostomy irrigation is contraindicated for people with stoma prolapse or peristomal hernia and for children. It is also a procedure that should be performed by the patient with an ostomy, not usually a significant other or caregiver, unless it needs to be done occasionally for management of constipation.

PEDIATRIC OSTOMY MANAGEMENT

The pediatric population requirements for an ostomy mirror those of the adult population, including inflammatory bowel disease, incontinence, cancer, and trauma. An additional category, congenital conditions, is more unique to this population. Congenital conditions include necrotizing enterocolitis, Hirschsprung disease, imperforate anus, prune belly syndrome, cloacal exstrophy, and myelomeningocele.

Care of the pediatric ostomy patient requires not only knowledge of ostomy care, but also knowledge in the areas of family dynamics, physical growth and development issues, and in some cases preterm infant skin care development. When an infant is born with an anomaly that requires medical attention, there is a period of adjustment for the family. Parents experience many emotions, including anger, fear, anxiety, and guilt. Parents may wonder if they did something that may have contributed to the condition of their infant. Also, they may be concerned about how they will be able to care for the child. They will need support, time to discuss their fears, and reassurance that they can care for their child.

A stoma requires an adjustment in body image. For infants, this adjustment is experienced by the parents since they were hoping for the "perfect" baby. Parents will be responsible for the care of the stoma and will need time to learn the care. Many times there may be additional surgeries to correct the physical problem. Parents will need a strong support system and encouragement as they care for their infant.

As the child grows, they will develop their own body image. If parents are accepting of the stoma and encourage the child in a positive manner, the child can develop a healthy body image. It is important to encourage the child to do normal activities, such as going to school, playing sports, and making friends. They want to lead a normal life and work toward independence. A school-age child can do much of the stoma care with some assistance from parents. Encouragement and positive reinforcement will help to promote independence.

Body image is very important for teen patients. They are still trying to develop their own identity. Teaching should be done directly with the teen, with the parents available for assistance and support as needed.

Physical growth occurs most significantly in infants. As the infant grows, there will be changes in the peristomal plane, body contour, and stoma size. The stoma should be measured about every 2 to 3 weeks and the appliance size will need to be adjusted as the infant grows. Physical activity will also increase with age, which can affect the wear time of the appliance. Discussion with parents about these expected changes will help them to understand the importance of contacting a WOC nurse to help with necessary appliance adjustments.

Parents may be concerned that their child is not growing at a normal rate. Physical growth is seldom delayed due to the presence of a stoma. It is helpful for the parents to understand that prematurity, other health problems, and nutrition may impact the child's development.

Premature infants have a less well-developed epidermal barrier, leaving them less equipped to deal with the outside environment. The preterm infant's skin is more permeable, and the infant may experience greater absorption to substances in contact with the skin. It is best to use minimal products on the skin and use products designed for infants to prevent increased absorption. The epidermis will usually be matured by about 1 month after birth.

Stoma site marking is not always possible in a newborn, as often the surgery is emergent. If it is possible to mark the site before surgery, there are some general factors to take into consideration. A site placed above the umbilicus will usually grow up with the body and stay in the same relative proximity to bony prominences. A site marked below the umbilicus will usually grow down and also stay in the same relative proximity to bony prominences. In older children and teens, the landmarks used for the adult population should be used.

Urinary and fecal stomas in infants can sometimes be managed with a diaper, depending on the location and output from the stoma. The option of diapering and pouching should both be discussed with the parents. Protection of the peristomal skin is the most important goal for the child with a stoma. If skin protection can be adequately achieved with a diaper, it is certainly an option.

As a child grows and becomes more active, pouching will be necessary to protect the skin and contain the effluent. There is a variety of infant and pediatric appliances available, in one- and two-piece styles (Fig. 10). Usually the appliance needs to be flexible for infants, due to the round contour of the abdomen. The skin barriers are thinner and less aggressive to prevent damage to the skin. This means that the barrier is less durable and usually needs to be changed every 2 to 4 days. Often when a child reaches 5 to 6 years of age, an "adult" appliance can be used.

A two-piece system may be preferred for an infant and toddler. This system allows the pouch to be removed from the body for emptying later and a second pouch to be applied. The flange system can also allow for easier release of gas, since infants produce a large amount of gas. If a one-piece system is used, the appliance can be placed at an angle, toward the hip, which may make it easier for the caregivers to empty. As the child grows, the appliance can be placed with the tail downward, so the child can assist with emptying.

Appliance changes should be scheduled at a time when the infant or child is quiet and happy. Initially, some assistance may be needed as stoma care is being learned and parents are becoming more comfortable with management. It is also important for the support people to learn ostomy care to share responsibility and to provide support for the caregivers.

Potential Complications for the Pediatric Patient

Dehydration

Dehydration is a potential risk for an infant or child with an ileostomy or high-output stoma. Monitoring the consistency and the amount of output from the stoma can help to identify problems. In addition to stoma output, fluids can also be lost from vomiting and perspiration. Parents should learn to recognize the early signs and symptoms of dehydration, such as decreased urine output, dry mucous membranes, and lethargy.

The Gastrointestinal Tract

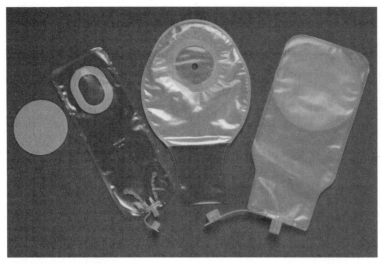

Fig. 10. Examples of pediatric pouches.

Fluids can be replaced using oral electrolyte solutions.

Stoma Prolapse and Peristomal Hernia

Stoma prolapse and peristomal hernias are common in infants. They do not have well-developed abdominal muscles to support the stoma. Crying produces increased intra-abdominal pressures, which can force the bowel through the fascial opening, creating a prolapse. Increased intra-abdominal pressures can also stretch the fascial opening to create a hernia. As in adults, the distal stoma, in a loop stoma, is more likely to prolapse.

It is beneficial to discuss these possible complications of hernia and prolapse with parents as it can be very frightening. The parents should be reassured that if the stoma color is red or pink, the stoma is functioning normally, and the infant appears comfortable, the prolapse is not a cause for concern. If the parents note any changes in stoma color or function, they need to seek immediate medical attention. The ostomy appliance should be flexible to fit the changes in abdominal contour and the appliance opening should be large enough to accommodate the prolapse. Parents can also be taught to reduce the stoma prolapse if needed. If the stoma is permanent, surgical intervention to repair the prolapse will be necessary at some point in time.

Skin Irritation

Skin irritation is most often caused by contact of effluent on the peristomal skin. This is usually due to an improperly fitting ostomy appliance, erosion of the skin barrier if the appliance is left in place too long, or skin sensitivity to products being used. The skin irritation can be treated by applying a skin barrier powder to protect the skin and absorb moisture from denuded skin. The most important step is to identify the cause of the skin irritation and correct it.

Teaching for the pediatric patient will involve primarily the parents and their support system. The family should be encouraged to participate in the child's care and to feel comfortable contacting health care professionals for questions or concerns.

The challenges of participating in the care of a child with a stoma includes working with the family, identifying the developmental age of the child and tailoring interventions to meet those specific challenges, understanding pouching principles that pertain to the pediatric population, and providing a nurturing, supportive environment to the child and family.

STOMA AND PERISTOMAL SKIN COMPLICATIONS

The primary goal for the person with a stoma is prevention of stoma and peristomal skin complications. Preoperative assessment and stoma site marking, postoperative education, and follow-up visits are helpful in preventing complications. When complications do occur, it is important to identify the cause to initiate the appropriate intervention until the problem is resolved. Follow-up is necessary to determine the effectiveness of the intervention.

Stoma Necrosis

Necrosis of a stoma is due to impaired blood supply to the stoma mucosa. This usually is evident within 24 hours after surgery. Stoma necrosis may result from surgical problems during stoma construction, such as excessive tension on the mesentery, or interruption of the blood supply to the stoma, compromising the blood supply. It can also occur in people with poor systemic circulation or a thick abdominal wall. The necrosis may involve the entire stoma or may involve only a portion of the mucosa. The stoma color will change from purple to gray to black and the surface of the stoma will become dry. As the stoma mucosa sloughs due to the lack of blood supply, there may be a strong odor evident from the tissue sloughing.

Interventions for a necrotic stoma include documenting the mucosa color and assessing the depth of the necrosis. This can be done by inserting a small lubricated test tube gently into the stoma and shining a flashlight into the tube to determine where the mucosa is pink and healthy. The stoma needs to be viable above fascia level to prevent peritonitis. As the nonviable tissue sloughs from the stoma, this tissue can be débrided. This will make it easier to do appliance changes and also reduce the odor from the sloughing tissue. Also, as the stoma mucosa sloughs, the skin edges will contract and may result in stoma stenosis. This may require surgical intervention if the stenosis causes problems with stoma function.

Mucocutaneous Separation

Mucocutaneous separation results when the suture line at the junction of the stoma and skin separates. This can occur when there is an oversized skin opening for the stoma, excessive tension at the suture line, insufficient suturing at skin level, or inappropriate sutures, or with patients who have compromised tissue healing, which may include those with diabetes, those taking high-dose steroids, those with malnutrition, or those receiving radiation therapy. Stoma necrosis can also cause a mucocutaneous separation as the necrotic tissue detaches from the skin.

Erythema or induration proximal to the mucocutaneous junction often precedes mucocutaneous separation. The separation may be partial or circumferential. There may be drainage present in the separation, usually serous or purulent in nature. Stool drainage could indicate a possible fistula in the separation.

The separation should be probed gently to determine the depth and access for tracts that may be present. A mucocutaneous separation should not be resutured. The defect can be irrigated gently and then packed with an absorptive wound

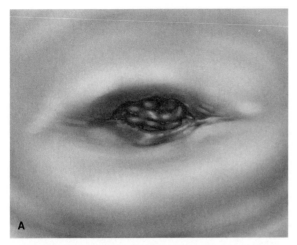

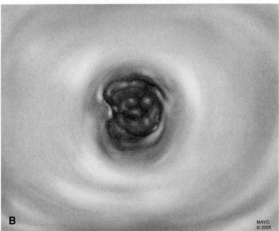

Fig. 11. Stoma retraction: Patient sitting **(A)** and patient lying **(B).**

a convex appliance, possibly with additional skin barrier rings to increase convexity, depending on the degree of retraction. The use of an ostomy appliance belt or a 4 to 5 in. support belt around the appliance will help to increase the convexity of the appliance and improve the appliance seal. Surgical intervention may be necessary if problems persist.

Stoma Stenosis

Stoma stenosis is described as a narrowing of the lumen of the ostomy at the skin or fascia level. The lumen contracts due to scar formation. Stoma stenosis can occur as a result of insufficient skin excision at the stoma site, excessive scarring due to stoma necrosis, peristomal abscess, or mucocutaneous separation. Significant stenosis can affect normal stoma function, resulting in discomfort when stool passes through the stoma. Also, the patient may experience explosive output with excessive gas as well as decreased caliber of stool.

Digital examination of the stenosed stoma reveals tightness at the skin or fascia opening. The patient with a stenosed colostomy may note symptoms of constipation and increased cramping with stoma function as well as effluent exiting the stoma under pressure.

Management of stoma stenosis would include a low-residue diet and stool softeners for the patient with a stenosed colostomy. This may ease evacuation of stool through the colostomy. Short-term stoma dilation may be performed, but when done over a long period of time, it may cause further stoma stenosis due to scar tissue formation. The ostomy appliance may need to be modified to allow for explosive stool to prevent appliance leakage. If stoma stenosis is severe, surgical revision of the stoma may be necessary.

Laceration (Stoma Trauma)

Stoma trauma or laceration is an injury or cut on the stoma mucosa. This can occur when the appliance opening is too small or is improperly placed over the stoma, with shaving, or as a result of direct injury to the stoma.

A laceration appears as a yellow to white linear discoloration in the mucosa where the injury occurred. Bleeding may occur at the site and there may be blood in the pouch. No pain is evident as there are no nerve endings in the mucosal layer of the bowel.

Management of a stoma laceration is to identify and correct the cause. The appliance

dressing if it is more than 1 cm in depth. Absorptive wound dressings, such as a hydrofiber or calcium alginate, would absorb drainage, prevent excessive soiling of the wound by stool, and promote healing of the separation. If the separation is shallow, the base can be filled with a skin barrier powder to absorb moisture. Once the separation is packed, the skin barrier of the pouching system is placed over the stoma and separation to provide protection from the effluent. It is important to note that the separation will heal even if exposed to stool. As the separation heals, it may be necessary to modify the appliance for improved fit on the peristomal area.

Retraction

Two types of retraction can occur with an ostomy: Stoma retraction or peristomal skin retraction. Stoma retraction (Fig. 11) occurs when the stoma does not protrude above the skin, but has pulled back to skin level or below skin level. It has been reported to occur in as many as 10% to 24% of all stoma patients. Skin retraction (Fig. 12) occurs

when the peristomal skin at the mucocutaneous junction pulls in, especially when the patient is sitting or standing. The patient may have a stoma that protrudes 1 to 2 cm or may have a flush stoma, but the skin retracts around the stoma. Retraction may be preceded by stoma necrosis or mucocutaneous separation. It can also result from excessive tension on the bowel due to obesity, edema, distention, inadequate stoma length, or short mesentery.

Evaluation of the stoma may reveal a stoma at or below skin level, although with skin retraction, the stoma may have adequate profile. There may be a receded or dimpled area on the skin due to the tension on the stoma. The stoma should be evaluated with the patient sitting and standing to determine the degree of retraction. Patients will present with problems with appliance leakage, decreased appliance wear time, and skin irritation from stool contact with skin.

The goal for management of stoma retraction is to maintain an adequate appliance seal to prevent effluent from causing skin irritation. This may require the use of

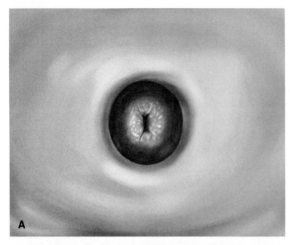

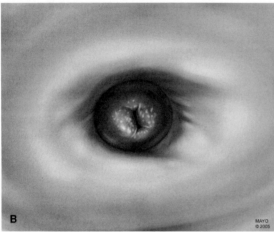

Fig. 12. Skin retraction around a budded stoma: Patient lying flat **(A)** and patient sitting **(B).**

should be altered to fit the stoma appropriately. If the stoma mucosa is bleeding significantly at the time of appliance change, direct pressure should be applied to the site until bleeding is controlled.

Peristomal Hernia

A peristomal hernia occurs when the fascial opening around the stoma becomes larger, allowing protrusion of the bowel or loops of intestine through the opening into the subcutaneous tissue around the stoma. This results in progressive bulging around the stoma. The bulging is usually more prominent with sitting and standing. Although there is no clear identified cause of peristomal hernias, siting of the stoma outside of the rectus muscle may be strongly implicated. They can also occur if there is a large fascial defect; an increase in intra-abdominal pressure, such as with excessive lifting or straining; placement of the stoma through an incision; aging; or excessive weight gain.

Peristomal hernias are visible when abdominal pressure is increased, such as when sitting or standing. The bulging is variable and may be on one side of the stoma or circumferential. Some patients note occasional pain or discomfort in the area of the hernia, which can worsen throughout the day.

Due to the changes in the abdominal contour when lying compared to sitting or standing, patients may experience difficulty maintaining the seal of the appliance. This can result in leakage and skin irritation as well as insecurity with the appliance. Patients who irrigate their colostomy and have developed a hernia may describe unpredictable or poor results with colostomy irrigation. Diagnosis of a hernia can be done by visual examination, having the patient cough or bear down to increase abdominal pressure. Digital examination allows the fascial defect to be felt as well. To confirm the presence of a hernia, a computed tomography scan with oral contrast or an upper gastrointestinal radiograph with small bowel or retrograde contrast study can be done.

Nonsurgical intervention is usually recommended if the patient is asymptomatic.

Hernia support belts or binders will provide support around the stoma, reducing the protrusion of the hernia, and can help with appliance adherence. The belt or binder should be put on when the hernia is reduced or when the patient is supine. It is best to use a flexible appliance to fit the changing contour around the stoma. The stoma size should be evaluated when the patient is sitting and standing as it will usually become larger when the hernia protrudes. It is necessary to seek medical attention if the stoma color becomes darker or there is significant pain around the stoma with change in stoma function.

Surgical intervention may include primary fascial repair, local repair with a prosthetic mesh, or relocation of the stoma to the opposite side of the abdomen. Surgeons differ in their preference for surgical intervention with a hernia. Also, the incidence of recurrence following peristomal hernia repair is high. Shellito reported the incidence of recurrence following a local fascial repair without mesh at 76%, a local repair with mesh at 50%, and stoma relocation at 33%.

Prolapse

Stoma prolapse is progressive elongation of the stoma through the skin opening. Prolapse can occur with each of the following scenarios: (a) the stoma has not been placed through the rectus muscle of the abdomen, (b) there is an excessively large opening in the abdominal wall at the time of surgery, (c) insufficient suturing to the abdominal wall, (d) weak abdominal musculature, (e) distended bowel, or (f) increased intra-abdominal pressure, possibly due to distention or crying in infants. Prolapses are seen most commonly in a loop stoma. Although either loop can prolapse, it is seen most often in the distal or nonfunctioning loop. It is important to note that a normal prolapse of 2 to 4 in. is common with stomas and is not considered abnormal or problematic.

The clinical presentation of a prolapse includes a stoma that is increased in size and length, is edematous, bleeds, and is easily traumatized. In severe prolapse, stoma obstruction and ischemia may result due to excessive tension on the mesentery. The stoma will appear dusky or purple. There may also be evidence of tiny ulcerations on the stoma mucosa. Stoma ischemia requires immediate surgical attention.

A prolapse can be managed conservatively if the stoma color and function remain normal. The prolapse may be manually reduced with the patient lying flat. Continuous pressure is applied to the distal portion of the stoma, or an ice pack or table sugar can be applied directly to the stoma to decrease the edema and aid in reducing the stoma. A binder or hernia support belt with prolapse flap may be used to keep the prolapse reduced, but in most people these are not effective because they do not apply enough pressure around the prolapse. It is common for the prolapse to recur when the person sits, stands, or coughs, as the intra-abdominal pressure is increased. The pouching system should be flexible, with sufficient length to accommodate the prolapsed stoma. The skin opening in the appliance should fit the stoma when it is at its largest diameter, usually with the person standing. Patients should be instructed to seek medical attention if the stoma becomes dark in color, stoma function decreases or stops, or the stoma becomes painful. Surgery may be necessary to resect the prolapse and revise the stoma.

Fistula

An enterocutaneous fistula is an abnormal communication between the stoma and the surrounding skin. It appears as an opening on the peristomal skin or at the mucocutaneous junction of a matured stoma. Stool may be evident at the fistula site and through the stoma.

Fistulas may occur when a suture is placed through the mucosa of the stoma at the time of surgery, but most commonly are due to recurrence of Crohn disease, poor healing, and mechanical trauma from the appliance being used.

Although some superficial enterocutaneous fistulas will heal spontaneously, surgical intervention may be needed to resolve the fistula. If surgical intervention is delayed or not indicated due to other medical problems, a pouching system that can accommodate both the stoma and the fistula should be considered. If the fistula is located close to the stoma, a convex appliance may provide a better seal for the skin.

PERISTOMAL SKIN COMPLICATIONS

Irritant or Contact Dermatitis

Irritant dermatitis of the skin results from contact with a chronic irritant, such as stool or chemicals. This may be due to poor stoma construction causing effluent to be in contact with the skin or from poor technique in appliance care. Effluent

may come in contact with the skin if the appliance is not the appropriate size, has not been applied appropriately, or has been left in place too long. Also, if the stoma is located in a poor location or is poorly constructed, this may contribute to leakage and dermatitis. Too many products used on the skin under the ostomy appliance may cause increased interaction of product ingredients, resulting in the development of sensitivity to products.

Skin damage correlates with the area that is exposed to the irritant. The effluent or chemical destroys or erodes the epidermis, resulting in pain and burning of the involved area. The skin initially shows erythema and swelling. It may progress to denudation, ulceration, bleeding, and weeping because of the loss of epidermis.

Treatment is directed at identifying and eliminating the cause. The goal is to protect damaged skin and avoid other irritants. The appropriate pouching system provides a secure, predictable wear time and protects the peristomal skin from effluent. Patch testing of the various products being used can be done to determine if the dermatitis is due to products being used on the skin. This can be done by applying a small amount of the various products being used on the skin, including the skin barrier, pouch, and any skin care products, and labeling them accordingly. The patches are applied to the skin on the abdomen, since it is most similar to the skin under the appliance. The patches should be removed in 48 hours and the sites evaluated for any skin reaction. If a product shows a positive reaction, it should be eliminated. Even after the product is eliminated, it may take several weeks for the reaction to resolve. Topical steroids may be used short term to reduce the inflammation and pain. Skin barrier powder can be applied to the skin to absorb moisture and provide a dry pouching surface.

Candidiasis

Peristomal candidiasis is an overgrowth of a *Candida* organism of sufficient magnitude to cause an inflammation, infection, or disease on the skin surrounding an ostomy. *Candida albicans* is the most frequent agent of candidiasis and thrives in dark, moist areas. A leaking ostomy appliance, body perspiration, and denuded skin, caused by too large of an appliance opening or prolonged wear time, all provide optimum environments for candidiasis to develop on the skin. Other predisposing conditions include long-term antibiotic therapy, diabetes mellitus, immunosuppression, myelosuppression, use of oral

contraceptives, topical corticosteroid therapy, and iatrogenic hypersteroidism.

Skin manifestations include papules, pustules, erythema, and pruritus. The lesions are extrafollicular, and satellite lesions, extending beyond the edge of the appliance, are common. Candidiasis may also be evident in skin creases, such as the axilla or groin.

Effective treatment of candidiasis begins with identifying the cause and eliminating it. A dry environment may be provided with an appropriately sized appliance, which fits the abdominal contour. Also, porous tapes and pouch covers or gauze under the pouch to absorb moisture may be used. A topical antifungal powder, such as nystatin or miconazole powder, should be applied sparingly to the affected area and rubbed into the skin, with the excess brushed off. This will not inhibit a secure appliance seal and treat the candidiasis. An antifungal powder should be used with each appliance change until the skin is completely clear. It is not recommended to use the powder prophylactically. Extended-wear skin barriers, which absorb moisture and keep the moisture in contact with the skin, may need to be eliminated if candidiasis recurs.

Allergic Dermatitis

Peristomal allergic contact dermatitis refers to hypersensitivity to chemical elements resulting in an inflammatory reaction. Damaged or inflamed peristomal skin is at increased risk for sensitization because the skin's immune system is overstimulated. The original skin problem may be denudation caused by an irritant dermatitis. The products used to treat the damaged skin may then create an allergic contact dermatitis. Once the sensitivity develops, it can last for months to years.

Management of allergic dermatitis consists of determining and eliminating the causative factors. An allergic dermatitis should be considered when the skin reaction is located in the area where a specific product is being used. Skin patch testing can be done to determine the causative agent. Treatment may also include the use of topical corticosteroids to reduce the inflammation, an appropriately fitting ostomy appliance, and the elimination of any unnecessary products on the skin to prevent further dermatitis.

Mechanical Injury

Damage to the peristomal skin may result from mechanical injury, such as trauma, shear, or pressure. Common causes include abrasive cleansing techniques and traumatic tape removal that results in epidermal stripping, shearing of the skin as the appliance moves on the skin, or continued friction or pressure from inappropriately fitting equipment. The affected skin is painful, and the moist, bleeding areas undermine the pouch seal, resulting in frequent pouch changes and further exacerbation of the problem. Lesions are typically shallow and irregularly shaped, and appear as a full- or partial-thickness skin loss located in the area of the trauma.

Mechanical injury can be prevented by educating the patient in appropriate appliance removal, which is gently pushing the skin away from the appliance instead of pulling on the skin. Adhesive removers may be necessary if the skin is thin or sensitive, but it is important to wash the adhesive remover off the skin before applying another appliance to prevent contact dermatitis. The appliance fit should be evaluated to determine if there is excessive pressure, possibly from a convex appliance or belt, especially with changes in body contour postoperatively or with a hernia, that may be causing an ulceration. This may necessitate the use of a softer or more flexible appliance or discontinuing the belt to prevent excessive pressure and promote healing of the ulceration. Skin barrier powder can be used to absorb moisture from the ulcer site, which will improve appliance seal.

Pseudoverrucous Lesions (Hyperplasia)

Pseudoverrucous lesions are raised areas located around the stoma, usually at the mucocutaneous junction. They are thickened epidermal projections with white, gray, brown, or dark red wart-like papules or nodules. These lesions are localized to areas of chronic exposure to moisture, usually stool or mucus, and can be extremely painful and bleed easily. The chronic irritation from moisture causes thickening of the epidermis, which may be due to the use of an appliance opening that is too large for the stoma or from chronic appliance leakage.

The primary treatment of pseudoverrucous lesions is to eliminate chronic exposure of effluent on the skin. The ostomy appliance should be resized to fit within one-eighth inch of the stoma and should fit the abdominal contour appropriately to prevent leakage or effluent undermining the skin barrier. The appliance skin barrier should cover the lesions to protect them from effluent. Silver nitrate may be used on large lesions to hasten healing and provide a flat surface for the pouching system. Appliance change intervals may need to be more frequent during the initial treatment, every 3 days, but once the lesions have resolved, a normal appliance change schedule may be resumed.

Folliculitis

Folliculitis is an infection of the hair follicles, usually caused by *Staphylococcus aureus.* Erythematous and sometimes pustular lesions are present around a hair follicle, which is helpful in the differentiation of folliculitis from candidiasis. Peristomal folliculitis generally results from traumatic hair removal, which may be the result of shaving hair from the peristomal skin too frequently. Other causes are indiscriminate shaving or dry shaving techniques and friction from careless pouch removal.

Management of folliculitis consists of determining the technique for peristomal hair removal. The patient should reduce the frequency of shaving to no more than once a week and shave lightly or clip the hair with a scissors to prevent skin damage.

Pyoderma Gangrenosum

Peristomal pyoderma gangrenosum (Fig. 13) is a rare, ulcerative skin condition of unknown cause that occurs in the area surrounding the stoma. It may start as one or more pustules that break open and form full-thickness ulcers with irregular, ragged, overhanging margins. A necrotizing inflammatory process extends peripherally from the primary lesion, resulting in a necrotic ulcer with undermined edges. The surrounding skin becomes red and purple, and the entire area is very painful, which may distinguish it from other types of ulcers. Peristomal pyoderma generally does not extend beyond the adhesive edge of the appliance system. Healing typically results in a cribriform scar. Ulcers that result from pressure are often misdiagnosed as peristomal pyoderma gangrenosum. One also must consider cutaneous Crohn disease, in which linear ulcers have undermined violaceous edges.

Peristomal pyoderma usually reflects underlying inflammatory processes rather than being a complication of ostomy construction. Diseases associated with pyoderma include ulcerative colitis, Crohn disease, arthritis, leukemia, polycythemia vera, and multiple myeloma. Diagnosis of pyoderma gangrenosum is a clinical one based on history and ulcer assessment. There are no diagnostic tests. Biopsy only serves to exclude disorders such as malignancy or vasculitis. The principles of management include decreasing the inflammatory process and maintaining the seal on the appliance for a predictable period of time. Screening for the presence of systemic active inflammatory bowel disease should be completed. Topical treatment may include anti-inflammatory agents such as steroid preparations or topical immunomodulators. Systemic medical therapy may be necessary if there is no improvement or worsening of symptoms using topical therapy.

The goals of pyoderma gangrenosum wound care include moisture control, maintenance of a clean wound base, protection of the wound base, delivery of topical anti-inflammatory/immunosuppressive preparations, and achievement of a predictable pouching system seal of at least 24 hours. Shallow ulcers may be filled with a skin barrier powder to absorb moisture and

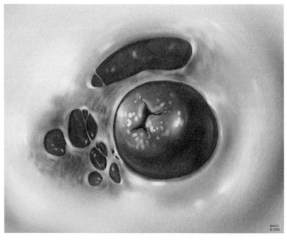

Fig. 13. Pyoderma gangrenosum.

promote a secure appliance seal. Hydrofiber or calcium alginate dressings can be applied over the ulcers to contain wound drainage. The frequency of appliance changes will be determined by the amount of drainage. When the ulcers heal, the area around the stoma may be uneven, resulting in the need to refit the pouching system.

FOLLOW-UP

Patients with ostomies must receive follow-up care after discharge as the stomas will change during the first 2 to 3 months after surgery. Change in stoma size, body contour, stabilization of body weight, and an increase in activity level may alter the fit of the appliance, making modifications necessary. Psychological support is also useful.

SUPPLIES

Ostomy supplies are available at ostomy supply centers, pharmacies, and medical supply stores, as well as through mail-order companies and online. Many insurance companies will reimburse for a portion or all of the cost of the supplies. The patient should inquire about this through his or her specific insurance agency. A prescription for ostomy prosthetics may be necessary for reimbursement. This is most often provided by the physician or WOC nurse.

ALTERNATIVE PROCEDURES

Continent Ileostomy (Kock Pouch)

The continent ileostomy (Kock pouch) is an internal pouch with a nipple valve constructed from the distal 18 in. (45 cm) of the ileum. This procedure is performed for patients with chronic ulcerative colitis or familial polyposis. The reservoir initially has a very small capacity. A 28 or 30 French catheter is placed through the nipple valve into the pouch at the time of surgery. The catheter is then clamped or removed from the pouch for increasing periods of time to allow the pouch to expand in size. Over time the capacity of the pouch can increase to hold 500 to 750 mL of stool. The pouch should be continent of gas and stool. To empty the pouch, the catheter is placed in the stoma every 4 to 6 hours. Patients with a continent ileostomy are able to wear a small waterproof pad or gauze over the stoma between intubations. This will absorb mucus from the stoma and protect clothing.

Problems with nipple valve dysfunction often result in the need for reoperation. The development of the ileal pouch–anal anastomosis (IPAA) procedure has resulted in a decreased use of the continent ileostomy as a procedure of choice. The continent ileostomy may still be performed for patients who are not a candidate for IPAA or who have a failed IPAA but would prefer not to wear an external ostomy appliance.

Ileal Pouch–Anal Anastomosis

The IPAA procedure is a procedure performed for people with chronic ulcerative colitis or familial polyposis. The IPAA procedure may be done in one, two, or three stages of surgery. An internal pouch is created from the ileum and sutured above the anus. A temporary loop ileostomy is frequently performed to allow the pouch to heal. The ileostomy is usually closed in 6 to 12 weeks.

Management of the temporary loop ileostomy is usually the most important focus for patients during the 6 to 12 weeks after surgery. Diet and fluid intake to maintain adequate nutrition and hydration are also very important. The loop ileostomy is located more proximal in the ileum, which can result in problems with high ileostomy output and dehydration. Intake of stool-thickening foods and the use of antidiarrheal medications prior to meals can help to reduce ileostomy output and maintain hydration.

Following closure of the ileostomy, when the internal pouch capacity is small, patients need to understand that they will have frequent stools with urgency. They may have up to 10 bowel movements per day initially. The internal pouch will gradually enlarge. As the patient starts to eat solid food, especially stool-thickening foods, the stool consistency will thicken, making it easier for the patient to hold back on the urge to have a bowel movement, increasing the size of the pouch capacity. The internal pouch will gradually adapt over time and after 6 to 12 months the patient may have only two to six bowel movements per day.

Frequent bowel movements and stool seepage between bowel movements can result in perianal dermatitis. Effective perianal skin protection should begin in the immediate postoperative period. After bowel movements, the perianal skin should be washed with a soft disposable cloth and the skin should be dried gently. A moisture barrier ointment is then applied to the perianal skin to protect the skin from stool drainage. Zinc oxide–based barriers are preferred over the petrolatum-based barriers. A protective dressing, such as a fluffed gauze, ARD dressing, or cotton ball, should be placed just at the anal opening. The dressing will absorb drainage to help protect the skin and should be used until there is no drainage between bowel movements.

Overall patient satisfaction following IPAA surgery has been high. The surgery eliminates the disease and the need for a permanent stoma. There is an adaptation phase that can take 6 to 12 months or even longer, and the functional results are not perfect, but patients appear to adapt without being restricted in their daily living.

CONCLUSION

Any patient with a possibility of needing an ostomy postoperatively should have preoperative education related to ostomy care. Marking the stoma site before surgery ensures that the stoma is in the best position for successful care by the patient. After surgery it is very important to continue ostomy education to fit the patient with an appropriate ostomy appliance. The abdominal contour changes during the postoperative period, so it is necessary to have the ostomy appliance assessed for appropriate fit 1 to 2 months after surgery. Yearly assessment of the ostomy and peristomal skin is needed to prevent ostomy complications that could occur over time. Proper ostomy care is necessary for the physiologic and psychosocial health of the patient.

SUGGESTED READING

Black PK. *Holistic stoma care.* Edinburgh, UK: Harcourt Publishers Limited, 2000.

Bryant RA. Skin pathology and types of damage. In: Bryant RA, ed. *Acute and chronic wounds: nursing management,* 2nd ed. St. Louis, MO: Mosby, 2000.

Colwell, J. Principles of stoma management. In: Colwell JC, Goldberg, MT, Carmel JE, eds. *Fecal & urinary diversions: management principles.* St. Louis, MO: Mosby, 2004:240.

Colwell JC. Stomal and peristomal complications. In: Colwell JC, Goldberg, MT, Carmel JE, eds. *Fecal & urinary diversions: management principles.* St. Louis, MO: Mosby, 2004:308.

Erwin-Toth P, Barrett P. Stoma site marking: a primer. *OWM* 1997;43(4):18.

Erwin-Toth P, Doughty DB. Principles and procedures of stomal management. In: Hampton BG, Bryant RA, eds. *Ostomies and continent diversions: nursing management.* St. Louis, MO: Mosby-Year Book, Inc., 1992:29.

Fleshman JW, Lewis MG. Complications and quality of life after stoma surgery: a review of 16,470 patients in the UOA data registry. *Semin Colon Rectal Surg* 1991;2(2):66.

Gordon PH, Rolstad BS, Bubrick MP. Intestinal stomas. In: Gordon PH, Nivatvongs S, eds. *Principles and practice of surgery for the colon, rectum and anus,* 2nd ed. St Louis, MO: Quality Medical, 1998.

The Gastrointestinal Tract

Hahnloser D, Pemberton JH, Wolff BG, et al. The effect of ageing on function and quality of life in ileal pouch patients. *Ann Surg* 2004:615.

Hampton BG. Peristomal and stomal complications. In: Hampton BG, Bryant RA, eds. *Ostomies and continent diversions: nursing management.* St. Louis, MO: Mosby-Year Book, Inc., 1992:105.

Harrison B, Boarini J. Pediatric ostomies: pathophysiology and management. In: Colwell JC, Goldberg, MT, Carmel JE, eds. *Fecal & urinary diversions: management principles.* St. Louis, MO: Mosby, 2004: 263.

Nugent KP, Daniels P, Stewart B, et al. Quality of life in stoma patients. *Dis Colon Rectum* 1999:1569.

Shellito PC. Complications of abdominal stoma surgery. *Dis Colon Rectum* 1998;41:1562.

White CA. Ostomy adjustment. In: Colwell JC, Goldberg, MT, Carmel JE, eds. *Fecal & urinary diversions: management principles.* St. Louis, MO: Mosby, 2004:326.

Wound, Ostomy and Continence Nurses Society. *Basic ostomy skin care: a guide for patient and healthcare providers.* Glenview, IL: Wound, Ostomy and Continence Nurses Society, 2004.

EDITOR'S COMMENT

As stated earlier in the introduction to the section on colonic surgery, the emphasis seems to have shifted between the fourth and fifth editions from the primary consideration being cure of cancer to some willingness to compromise on, or at least experiment with, previously held aspects of necessity for cure utilizing neoadjuvant therapy to prevent recurrence. Nonetheless, the nature of the procedures may involve, in a considerable percentage of them, the use of stomas, temporary to be sure; however, in some cases, even if only temporary, the period between the creation and removal of the stoma may be as long as 4 months, or even longer, depending on complications related to complex dissections in the presence of cancer and radiation therapy. Thus, quality of life of a patient with a temporary stoma may be an important concern for a prolonged period of time. It has generally been accepted in U.S. hospitals, especially those that have stoma nurses, that preoperative teaching is essential. They also participate in stoma marking before elective procedures, or in any procedure in which a temporary stoma may result. Apparently this has not been the case in the United Kingdom. A recent study from the Newcastle Upon Tyne Hospitals NHS Trust (*Dis Colon Rectum* 2005;48[3]:504) attempted to install a community-based stoma education study in which preoperative teaching would be carried out, as compared to the conventional postoperative stoma education teaching in a hospital. Forty-two elective patients were the subjects of this study, and they were randomized into two groups: Preoperative or postoperative. Every measure of outcome, including stoma proficiency, postoperative hospital stay, unplanned stoma-related interventions within 6 weeks of discharge, and anxiety and depression scores, resulted in a statistically significant improved outcome, including extraordinary increase in time to stoma proficiency (5.5 days vs. 9 days; $P = 0.0005$) and unplanned returns per patient (median 0 vs. 0.5; $P = 0.031$). The cost savings per patient was greater than \$2,100 ($£1,119$). Interestingly, despite the fact that stoma proficiency was achieved at 5.5 days, patients remained in the hospital for 8 days. This is a cultural difference, explaining in part the longer length of stay in the United Kingdom.

Irrigation, which long has been practiced in the United States, is now making its way across the world. Karadag et al. (*J Clin Nurs* 2005;14:479) taught colostomy irrigation to 25 patients, and followed them with quality-of-life questionnaires. In the irrigating group, scores improved significantly after stoma therapy ($P < 0.0001$), although the nonirrigating group improved significantly as well ($P = 0.009$). The irrigating group's quality of life improved significantly, as compared to that of the nonirrigating group. Once the stoma is in place, an important feature is appliance fit. Leakage is extraordinarily damaging to the skin around the ostomy. Hair may make the fit difficult, and may increase leakage. Shaving or clipping (which is preferable) may in fact damage the skin, thus making the fit more difficult.

Not mentioned in the chapter is the use of laser hair removal, which has been increasingly utilized, for example, in the treatment of pilonidal sinus, and which has become accepted as the treatment of choice, a marked shift from the fourth edition, in which excision was favored. Here, laser hair removal is reasonably expedient and it may take just a few treatments to make certain that there is little hair to interfere with the fit of the appliance.

There is also an increased appreciation for what pericolostomy hernia means and what prolapse consists of. Very much as the mylopectinate diaphragm has caused a reappraisal of the repairs, or at least the hypothetical repairs, for inguinal hernia and the hernia surrounding the mylopectinate diaphragm, the concept of bowel transiting the abdominal wall, when it is not protected by rectus muscles, which is the preferred site, has made one aware of the fact that there is an extraordinary recurrence of pericolostomy hernia and perileostomy hernia, as well as difficulties in prolapse. The best way to deal with these issues is to secure the ostomy around the opening through which the ostomy traverses by sutures to the peritoneum and, when possible, the fascia. One should take care to secure this because once a prolapse and/or hernia occurs, the recurrence rate is extraordinary, even with mesh repairs. Given the propensity of polyester to erode and shrink, I tend to use Vicryl mesh to reinforce the repair because it is my experience that it lasts for about 4 to 6 months, but afterward it gives

reasonably good scar. The long-term effects of Vicryl mesh in the repair of the pericolostomy hernia are not clear, but one is fooling oneself if one attempts to deal with a pericolostomy hernia without resiting the ostomy, preferably through the rectus on the other side of the abdomen. One could make an argument for using Vicryl mesh, for example, at the initial siting of the ostomy to try and discourage pericolostomy hernias.

The issue of pyoderma gangrenosum and recurrent Crohn disease around the ostomy is a very real problem. Recurrent Crohn disease around the ostomy is an extraordinarily troublesome situation that does not respond to the normal medications and types of therapies described in the text. Pyoderma, while it may not be as linear, certainly has the same violaceous look on the occasional case that I have seen. Telling the difference between these two is critical, and unfortunately there is little that one can do to help make that decision. Pyoderma is related to the activity of the disease, and therefore the therapy of how to deal with pyoderma probably depends on getting control of the disease itself. Finally, there is the issue of children. Olejnik et al. (*Rocz Akad Med Bialymst* 2005; 50[Suppl 1]:163) did a study of the ability of parents to care for 30 children, aged 0 to 2 with lower alimentary congenital defects, who had an intestinal stoma created in 2003. Hirschsprung disease (40%), anal atresia (37%), necrotizing enteral colitis (10%), and perianal fistula (10%) were the principal causes of a stoma, some of which apparently were to be permanent. It is interesting that, with help, 80% of the parents were able to care for their child, although it must have been an extraordinary burden. The most common complications were skin changes around the stoma (33%), hemorrhage (20%), prolapse (13%), and stenosis (10%). One feels a great deal of sympathy for parents of a child with a stoma. Every parent wants his or her child to be perfect, and this is a good example of when the child is not. The desire to care for the child, I'm certain, is overwhelming, but there must be extraordinary disappointment that the perfect baby did not result, and some of these children may be a burden for life.

J.E.F.

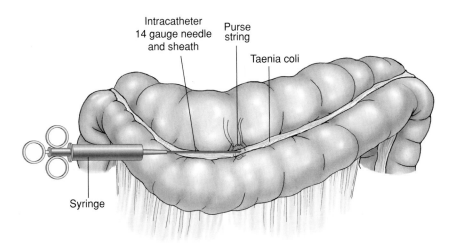

Fig. 3. Initial decompression of the colon is achieved by needle aspiration of air from the anterior aspect of the distended colon.

Colonic Decompression via the Ileum (Fig. 5)

A third technique to decompress the colon has been previously described by us. This method is especially useful when access to the distended colon is difficult and/or when the colon is more filled with semisolid material than with gas and liquid. The nondistended distal ileum is mobilized and two concentric 3-0 purse-string sutures are placed on its antimesenteric surface within 5 to 7 cm of the competent ileocecal valve. A noncrushing bowel clamp is placed across the ileum just proximal to the purse-string sutures. A soft but noncollapsible, large-diameter catheter with multiple holes cut in its distal 5 cm is connected to a large-bore Y-connector proximally. One limb of the Y connects to a noncollapsible tubing with a shut-off clamp and irrigation syringe and the other limb connects to wall suction. This catheter is then inserted via an ileotomy at the purse-string site and passed through the ileocecal valve into the right colon. Decompression is readily achieved. If the system gets plugged, the irrigation syringe is used to restore flow. The catheter can either be removed and discarded or pushed totally into the right colon and resected with the specimen. The ileal purse-string is tied. The ileotomy site ultimately is used for the ileostomy construction.

Decompression of Rectosigmoid via Proctoscopy

On occasion, it is useful to further decompress the rectosigmoid after accomplishing the more important task of decompressing

any manipulation of the colon. To minimize risk of iatrogenic colon perforation, we decompress the colon using one or several of the following four techniques.

Colonic Needle Decompression (Fig. 3)

If a massively distended portion of colon is easily accessible, moist laparotomy pads are placed gently around the area and a 4-0 purse-string suture using a fine, small-diameter, round needle is placed in a teniae coli. An intracatheter 14-gauge needle connected to a large syringe is inserted into the colon in the middle of the purse-string; air along the anterior surface of the colon is aspirated via the syringe. The needle is withdrawn, leaving only the flexible sheath within the colon, and the sheath is connected to suction. Often this dramatically deflates the colon as much of its distension is from excess gas. It is important not to stick the needle or sheath into solid stool or it becomes plugged so quickly that meaningful decompression is not achieved. If sufficient decompression is achieved, the sheath can be removed and the purse-string suture tied. Colectomy is then initiated.

Colonic Suction Decompression (Fig. 4)

Often, needle decompression lessens the danger of imminent perforation but does not achieve decompression to the point

necessary to safely manipulate the colon during resection. If this circumstance is present, the sheath can be removed and the needle colotomy extended slightly to accommodate insertion of a pool tip suction catheter within the purse-string–sutured area. By passing the catheter along the anterior surface of the colon, the surgeon can first decompress more gas and then begin to suction the liquid feces and blood from the colon. Care must be taken not to pass the suction catheter through the colonic wall. After decompression, the catheter can be removed as the purse-string suture is tied.

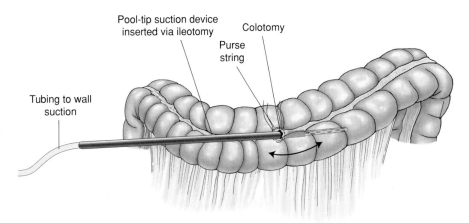

Fig. 4. Additional decompression of gas, liquid feces, and blood is achieved by passage of a pool tip suction catheter proximally and distally.

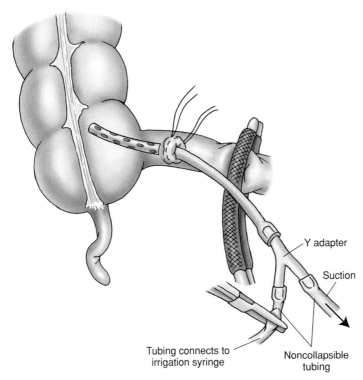

Fig. 5. Colonic decompression can be done via an ileotomy. (Modified from Khoo RE, Rothenberger DA, Way WD, et al. Tube decompression of the dilated cecum. *Am J Surg* 1988;156:214.)

the proximal and transverse colon. This can be done by having an assistant place a proctoscope via the anus while the sigmoid is gently compressed to push gas and feces distally. Flexible colonoscopes usually plug up if used for this purpose, but large-diameter proctoscopes can work well.

EXPLORATION AND PLANNING

Once the colon is decompressed, a full exploration is completed and any intra-abdominal pathology is noted. Serosal tears are sometimes noted, especially in the cecum, right, and transverse colon, and may be oversewn if it appears likely they could extend to a full-thickness tear during colectomy. Often, there is evidence of a walled-off perforation denoted by tight omental wrapping. This is especially noted in the left transverse colon–splenic flexure area. The status of the intra-abdominal rectum and sigmoid is especially important in planning the extent of distal resection and determining whether a mucous fistula or Hartmann pouch will be used. Self-retaining retractors are inserted and the colectomy commences.

COLON MOBILIZATION

If decompression was done via an ileotomy, we generally proceed to first mobilize the

cecum and right colon by dividing their lateral peritoneal attachments. As the hepatic flexure is approached, care is taken to identify and protect the duodenum. It is important to avoid excess traction on the colonic mesentery during mobilization of the hepatic flexure as troublesome bleeding from a branch of the mesenteric veins in the paraduodenal area can occur. If the omentum is free and easy to separate from the transverse colon, it can be preserved, but in most cases of toxic megacolon, the omentum is adherent to the serosal surface of the colon and may contain small perforations. If adherence is noted, we remove the omentum with the colon. The dissection is continued from right to left, entering the lesser sac and approaching the splenic flexure (Fig. 6). Because the splenic flexure can be difficult to dissect in the presence of colonic dilation and acute colitis with possible areas of walled-off perforation, we next mobilize the sigmoid and descending colon. The peritoneal attachments along the white line of Toldt are divided, beginning in the pelvis and working toward the splenic flexure. As we do so, the left ureter and gonadal vessels are identified and swept into the retroperitoneum. The risk of splenic traction injury is minimized by avoiding downward traction on the descending colon. Instead, we gently dissect upward in the retrocolic plane and then

sweep a hand laterally to expose and facilitate division of the remaining lateral attachments. Gentle simultaneous traction on the mobilized portions of the transverse and descending colon allows the splenic flexure to be taken down safely.

COLON RESECTION

Having mobilized the entire colon, we now divide the mesentery and proceed with the colectomy. If the mesentery is thick or difficult to secure, we utilize suture ligatures. The ileocolic mesentery is divided and tied. The distal ileum is transected with a linear cutter stapler near the cecum. As the remaining mesentery is divided, the right colic, middle colic, and left colic vessels are individually divided and ligated. At this point in the operation, the surgeon must decide how far the resection will be carried distally—that is, will the operation be a total colectomy or a subtotal colectomy? If the sigmoid colon appears significantly diseased from the underlying colitis, we divide the sigmoid vessels and resect the colon to the rectum at the pelvic brim. We proceed with a proctectomy only if there is evidence of perforation in the rectum, massive bleeding from the rectum, or such severe rectal disease that a secure closure cannot be ensured. If proctectomy is needed, it is usually possible to leave a short rectal stump for later ileal pouch anastomosis. If the sigmoid appears minimally involved from the colitis, a subtotal colectomy will restore the patient to health and the sigmoid can be safely retained. The colon is transected with a linear cutter stapler if possible and the specimen is submitted for pathology. If the upper rectum is too edematous to accommodate a stapler, it may be divided between bowel clamps and closed in a hand-sewn fashion. The abdominal cavity is irrigated with saline.

ILEOSTOMY CONSTRUCTION

After resection of the diseased colon, the ileostomy is constructed (Fig. 7). The goal is to create a round, symmetrically protruding, matured stoma that is 2 to 2.5 cm above the skin level at a site convenient for the patient to perform self-care. A 3.5 cm in diameter circle of skin is excised from the marked stoma site in the right lower quadrant. The subcutaneous fat is incised vertically and retracted to expose the anterior rectus abdominis fascia. A cruciate 2.5-cm incision is made with electrocautery, thus exposing the underlying muscle. As upward pressure is applied by the surgeon's hand placed inside the abdomen at the level

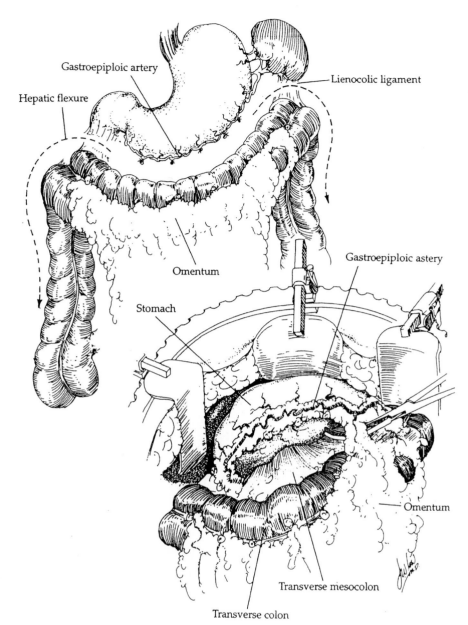

Fig. 6. The splenic flexure is usually the most difficult to mobilize, so it is approached after mobilization of the right and transverse colon and the sigmoid and descending colon. (From Nyhus LM, Baker RJ, Fischer JEF. *Mastery of surgery,* 3rd ed., vol. 2. Boston: Little Brown and Co, 1997:1534.)

suturing the mesentery, because doing so makes the subsequent ileostomy closure more difficult. In general, the risk of small bowel obstruction from twisting around the stoma is low in the immediate postoperative period. If obesity precludes the ability to create an end ileostomy that protrudes above the skin surface, a loop ileostomy should be considered. A loop of ileum just proximal to the stapled end of the bowel is brought through the abdominal wall defect. A rod or catheter may be placed through a small mesenteric window created just beneath the loop and used to support the stoma above the skin. Because a loop stoma requires mobilization of two limbs of bowel and the associated mesentery, it is thicker than an end stoma. As a result, the tunnel in the abdominal wall and the skin opening often have to be enlarged.

MANAGEMENT OF THE RECTUM OR RECTOSIGMOID

After preparing for the ileostomy, attention is focused on management of the rectum or rectosigmoid. In most cases, a total or near-total colectomy was performed and the retained large bowel stump is not long enough to create a mucous fistula or to leave it closed off in the subcutaneous tissues. Instead, a Hartmann pouch is created by oversewing the previously placed staple line on the end of the retained stump with interrupted absorbable sutures. It is useful to leave two long permanent sutures at the corners of the staple line to assist in identification of the rectal stump at a subsequent exploration. If the Hartmann pouch is long enough, the closed sigmoid can be sutured to the posterior fascia at the inferior aspect of the midline wound or to the back of the uterus or pelvic peritoneum, thus facilitating its later identification. More often, the Hartmann pouch consists of just the rectum or the rectum and a small segment of sigmoid colon and is simply left in situ at the level of the sacral promontory. We take several steps to minimize the small risk of a symptomatic leak or fistula from a "blowout" of the Hartmann pouch. An omental patch may be mobilized and placed over the closed stump. We decompress and irrigate the Hartmann pouch via proctoscopy before closing the abdominal wound. A soft drain may be placed into the rectum via the anus and left for 3 to 7 days postoperatively to minimize the risk of accumulations of mucus, blood, and gas that might cause the suture line to breakdown. If all of these maneuvers are done, the risk of

of the ileostomy site, a blunt Carmalt clamp or right-angle retractor is used to gently separate the muscle fibers and expose the posterior rectus fascia and peritoneum. Right-angle retractors are placed more deeply and used to retract the muscle fibers to each side. A cruciate incision large enough to accommodate passage of the distal ileum is made with electrocautery. Care is taken during this process to avoid injury to the inferior epigastric artery. If injured, it must be ligated. Two Babcock clamps are inserted into the abdomen through the abdominal wall defect created for the ileostomy and used to grasp the distal ileum at the previously placed staple line. With the

ileal mesentery oriented in a cephalad direction, the mobilized distal ileum is delivered through the abdominal wall defect. Intra-abdominal mobilization of the ileum and its mesentery should be done to allow the ileum to protrude 5 to 6 cm above the skin level. If necessary, the ileal mesentery may be thinned to allow passage through the abdominal wall aperture, but preservation of adequate blood supply to the distal ileum is paramount. For a permanent stoma, we suture the mesentery to the posterior fascia from the stoma site toward the liver to minimize the risk of a small bowel volvulus occurring around the stoma. If the ileostomy is temporary, we generally forego

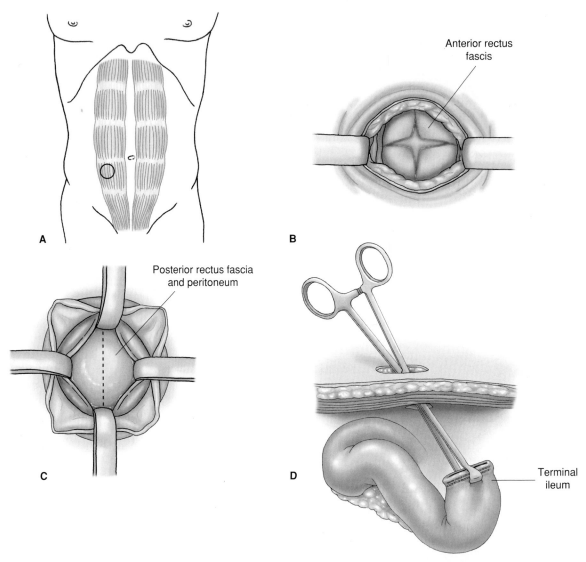

Fig. 7. A Brooke ileostomy is constructed. **A:** A 3.5 cm in diameter circle of skin is excised from the marked stoma site in the right lower quadrant. **B:** A cruciate 2.5-cm incision is made with electrocautery, thus exposing the underlying muscle. **C:** Right-angle retractors are used to retract the muscle fibers to each side and the posterior fascia and peritoneum are incised. **D:** The mobilized distal ileum is brought through the abdominal wall defect. (Modified from Gordon PH, Nivatoong S. *Principles and practice of surgery for the colon, rectum and anus.* St. Louis: Quality Medical Publishers, Inc., 1992.)

symptomatic breakdown of a Hartmann pouch closure is extremely rare, provided that the surgeon does not insist on closing a rectum that is so severely diseased that staples or sutures cut through the bowel. In such cases, it is better to proceed with proctectomy than to persist in trying to close the badly diseased rectal stump. Usually this requires a limited resection of several centimeters at the rectosigmoid junction to identify healthy tissues amenable to secure closure. If the entire rectum is severely diseased, a more extensive resection may be necessary, but for patients in whom a subsequent restorative ileal pouch procedure is appropriate, the anal canal can usually be left in situ. Subsequent removal or conversion to a pelvic pouch is more difficult but not impossible. If the anal canal is so diseased that it cannot be preserved, it is usually not going to be functional, and a total proctocolectomy is performed.

If a subtotal colectomy was performed and the retained rectosigmoid can be mobilized to reach the abdominal wall, our preference is to create a mucous fistula at a site remote from the midline wound, usually in the left lower quadrant of the abdomen. This does not require a large skin defect and the mucous fistula can be a flush stoma. If the sigmoid does not easily reach the skin and if it can be closed securely, it can be left closed off in the subcutaneous tissues adjacent to the ileostomy (Fig. 8).

WOUND CLOSURE AND STOMA MATURATION

After irrigation of the abdomen and confirmation of correct sponge and needle counts, the fascia is closed. In the absence of diffuse contamination, a closed suction round drain may be left in the subcutaneous space and the skin is closed with staples. Alternatively, the wound can be left open, packed with a sterile dressing, and closed at the bedside several days later (delayed primary closure). However, if diffuse contamination and/or fecal spillage was present, the skin should be left open and allowed to heal by secondary intention in order to prevent a wound infection. Whether or not to close the skin in the presence of colonic necrosis,

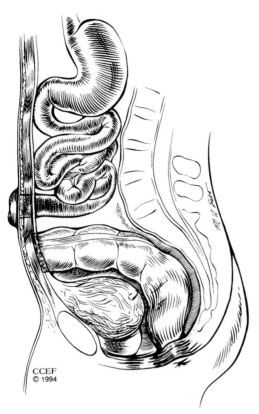

Fig. 8. The proximal end of the retained rectosigmoid is closed and left in the subcutaneous tissues near the ileostomy. (From Nyhus LM, Baker RJ, Fischer JEF. *Mastery of surgery,* 3rd ed., vol. 2. Boston: Little Brown and Co, 1997:1438.)

but without diffuse fecal peritonitis, remains controversial. In general, if there is any concern about a contaminated wound, leaving the skin open is considered the most conservative approach. The advent of vacuum dressing devices has simplified management of these open wounds and may make healing by secondary intention more appealing in this setting.

After protecting the midline wound with laparotomy pads, the staple line is removed from the distal ileum and the ileostomy is matured with 3-0 absorbable sutures (Fig. 9). Four anchoring sutures evenly spaced around the circumference of the stoma are placed to facilitate eversion of the stoma. These stitches incorporate a full-thickness bite of the ileal bowel edge, a seromuscular bite of the small bowel at the level of the skin edge, and the subcuticular tissues. We try to avoid placing the suture through the epidermis because this may result in bothersome mucosal implants and granulation tissue that can interfere with pouching. The stoma is everted and the anchoring sutures are tied. Intervening sutures are placed between the full-thickness edge of the ileum and the subcuticular tissues to provide a secure closure to the skin. If a mucous fistula is used, we remove the previously placed sigmoid staple line and mature a flush stoma by suturing the full thickness

The Gastrointestinal Tract

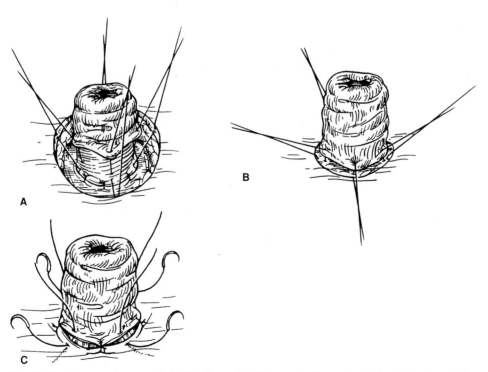

Fig. 9. The ileostomy is matured. **A:** The ileum should protrude above the skin level 5 to 6 cm before maturation. **B:** Four anchoring sutures are placed. **C:** Additional sutures are placed to complete the maturation process. (From Bell RH, Rikkers LF, Mulholland M, eds. *Digestive tract surgery: a text and atlas.* Philadelphia: Lippincott Williams & Wilkins, 1996:1278.)

of the colon to the skin edge with a running absorbable 3-0 suture. A temporary ileostomy appliance is secured, the mucous fistula is covered with a petroleum-impregnated gauze, and the midline wound is dressed. Postoperative care follows a standard postcolectomy protocol supplemented with additional therapy directed to the underlying cause of the colitis, prevention or management of infectious complications, and correction of associated conditions such as malnutrition.

CONCLUSION

Toxic megacolon is a life-threatening condition that may result from idiopathic inflammatory bowel disease, infectious colitis, or drug-induced colitis. Management of these patients is based upon adequate resuscitation, treatment of the underlying condition, frequent clinical evaluation to detect deterioration, and prompt surgical intervention if deterioration occurs. Intraoperatively, the diseased colon should be resected and a temporary ileostomy created. Several options exist for management of the retained rectosigmoid colon. Appropriate and judicious medical and surgical management may prevent the morbidity and mortality that has historically been associated with toxic megacolon.

SUGGESTED READING

Berg DF, Bahadursingh AM, Kaminski DL, et al. Acute surgical emergencies in inflammatory bowel disease. *Am J Surg* 2002; 184(1):45.

Caprilli R, Latella G, Vernia P, et al. Multiple organ dysfunction in ulcerative colitis. *Am J Gastroenterol* 2000;95(5):1258.

Carter F, McLeod R, Cohen Z. Subtotal colectomy for ulcerative colitis: complications related to the rectal remnant. *Dis Colon Rectum* 1991;34:1005.

Chua C. Surgical considerations in the Hartmann's procedure. *Aust N Z J Surg* 1996; 66:676.

Grant CS, Dozois RR. Toxic megacolon: ultimate fate of patients after successful medical management. *Am J Surg* 1984;147(1):106.

Heppell J, Farkouh E, Dube S, et al. Toxic megacolon. An analysis of 70 cases. *Dis Colon Rectum* 1986;29(12):789.

Khoo RE, Rothenberger DA, Wong WD, et al. Tube decompression of the dilated colon. *Am J Surg* 1988;156:214.

Kyle S, Steyen R, Keenan R. Management of the rectum following colectomy for acute colitis. *Aust N Z J Surg* 1992;62:196.

McKee R, Keenan R, Munro A. Colectomy for acute colitis: is it safe to close the rectal stump? *Int J Colorect Dis* 1995;10:222.

Morel P, Hawker PC, Allan RN, et al. Management of acute colitis in inflammatory bowel disease. *World J Surg* 1986;10(5):814.

Ng R, Davies A, Grace R, et al. Subcutaneous rectal stump closure after emergency subtotal colectomy. *Br J Surg* 1992;79:701.

Wojdemann M, Wettergren A, Hartvigsen A, et al. Closure of the rectal stump after colectomy for acute colitis. *Int J Colorect Dis* 1995;10:197.

EDITOR'S COMMENT

Toxic megacolon still remains a significant complication of inflammatory bowel disease. True, it is less common and, when it occurs, less lethal. Indeed, a recent review by Gan et al. (*Am J Gastroenterol* 2003;98[11]:2363) quoted rates between 1% and 6% (Grieco MB et al. *Ann Surg* 1980;191:75; Greenstein AJ et al. *J Clin Gastroenterol* 1985; 7:137) dealing with Crohn colitis (Grieco et al.) and both ulcerative and Crohn colitis (Greenstein et al.). A more contemporary study (Witte J et al. *Scand J Gastroenterol* 2000;35:1272) revealed no mortality from Crohn disease among 796 patients, separately documented in Jess et al. (*Gastroenterology* 2002; 122:1808). The deaths in the European study of 796 patients revealed a toxic megacolon–related death rate of only 0.2% over a 4-year follow-up. Whatever the cause, and, not surprisingly, nitric oxide and interleukins have recently been suggested as playing a pivotal role, earlier consultation is a necessity if these patients are going to be salvaged. In the past, when a gastroenterologist had a patient and had to refer him or her to surgery for ulcerative colitis, it was considered a defeat since permanent ileostomy was the usual outcome. Indeed, as a medical student, I remember a patient presented as a triumph by a gastroenterologist to our first-year class: This patient was blind and crippled from ankylosing spondylitis, and had all sorts of skin lesions, yet the presenting gastroenterologist said triumphantly that he had kept her from surgery for 40 years—some victory.

There still remain patients who are on anticholinergics and opiates who present with toxic megacolon. This is the result of a vicious cycle of diarrhea followed by more Imodium, Lomotil, or Paregoric, and then increased diarrhea, and then opiates are given until the bowel is paralyzed, at which point toxic megacolon occurs.

For the most part, in this country one would like to believe that mortality from toxic megacolon and surgery remains small—whatever the mortality there is, which it varies in various studies between 13% and 16% (D'Amico C et al. *Digestion* 2005;72:146; Ausch RD et al. *Colorectal Dis* 2005;8:195). Most of the time, the operation performed is an ileostomy and Hartmann turn-in, or sigmoid mucous fistula, which is rare in my experience. Every now and then, depending on the condition of the patient, I have carried out an ileal pouch–anal anastomosis with a diverting ileostomy. This is usually not done under acute conditions, but more often in the setting of a patient who comes in with toxic megacolon, improves somewhat, and then hits a plateau. At this point, if consulted, I would place the patient on parenteral nutrition; add intravenous chloramphenicol, a not-often-used drug that can actually be added to the total parenteral nutrition (Dr. Lester Martin, a noted pediatric surgeon, taught me this) in the dose of 3 g per 24 hours and allow the patient to improve; use rectal steroids; and carry out the ileal pouch–anal anastomosis during that hospitalization. This is not unreasonable. As reported in Greenstein's study (previously cited), 57% of toxic megacolon patients available for long-term follow-up, who were successfully managed with medical treatment alone, ultimately required a colectomy. In addition, followed on an average of 13 years in a study by the Mayo Clinic, 47% of the 38 toxic megacolon patients who had been successfully treated medically required a colectomy, 83% on an urgent or emergent basis (Grant CS, Dozois RR. *Am J Surg* 1984;147:106).

Following are some technical details. I prefer to make the incision as a lateral paramedian incision, keeping it well away from the placement of the ileostomy. I put in wound towels and sew them to the fascia prior to opening the peritoneum in case there is the opportunity for perforation of the colon. Antibiotic rather than sterile saline irrigation is most appropriate for the peritoneum, and peritoneal debridement with sponges and other devices to rid the peritoneum of solid stool may be necessary. I prefer kanamycin for the irrigation, or gentamicin if available.

The ileostomy sutures, in my view and as according to Brooke, should not go through the skin, which has already been mentioned, but nor should they go through the mucosa, as mucosal cells tend to grow along the suture if they are through the mucosa, as pictured here. With respect to the skin closure, delayed primary closure is appropriate, provided one understands that the infection rate for delayed primary closure is not 0%, but 5%. I prefer to close the skin primarily after irrigation and debridement of the subcutaneous fat, and leave closed suction drains in for 10 days, because that is when the wound suppurates. Irrigation with antibiotic solution to the subcutaneous tissue is perfectly appropriate. Primary closure and closed suction drainage is less painful, and if one leaves the drains in for a long period of time, one rarely gets a wound infection.

Newer, preferable methods of detecting toxic megacolon and irritable bowel disease include abdominal ultrasound. Maconi et al. (*Dig Dis Sci* 2004;49[1]:138) presented four cases followed by ultrasound. Quite honestly, while reading this paper I am not entirely certain how the presence of ultrasound benefited the patient since, in fact, the one pictured abdominal radiograph shown clearly revealed toxic megacolon.

Taken all together, I believe that toxic megacolon should alert the surgeon that surgical intervention is necessary. It would be best if the toxic megacolon were allowed to subside, if the opiates and the anticholinergics were removed, and if the patient was watched carefully, supported with parenteral nutrition, and allowed to get to a plateau where one could prepare the rectum for rectal stripping for those who carry out ileal pouch–anal anastomosis using that technique. There is little excuse for the patient perforating and having an abdomen full of stool. This implies inappropriately late consultation or error in diagnosis on the part of the consulting physician and surgeon.

J.E.F.

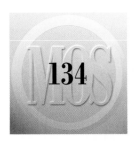

Ileoanal Pouch Procedure for Ulcerative Colitis and Familial Adenomatous Polyposis

FEZA H. REMZI AND VICTOR W. FAZIO

Restorative proctocolectomy with ileal pouch-anal anastomosis has been viewed as the most recent development in the evolution of continence-preserving procedures and has become the "gold standard" surgical treatment for the majority of patients with ulcerative colitis and familial adenomatous polyposis. It establishes gastrointestinal system continuity and anal continence, and avoids permanent stomas. Like so many surgical techniques, restorative proctocolectomy is not new in concept, and the origin of straight ileoanal anastomosis dates back to the 1940s. Functional outcome of this procedure was poor and was associated with a high frequency of defecation and urgency. Surgical techniques, however, continued to evolve, and to address these problems, ileal pouch-anal anastomosis was described first in experimental animals as early as 1955 by Valiente and Bacon. Finally in 1978, Sir Allen Parks from St. Marks Hospital in London reported the first application of S-shaped ileoanal pouch anastomosis in humans. At the same time, Fonkalsrud and Martin pioneered their method of ileoanal pouch formation, again based on the three-looped reservoir. These led to improvement of functional results related to frequency, urgency, continence, and less morbidity than the straight anastomosis. This technique began a new era in surgical management of ulcerative colitis and familial adenomatous polyposis. Many refinements of the ileoanal pouch procedure have occurred since the original description of total proctocolectomy, anorectal mucosectomy, hand-sewn ileal pouch-anal anastomosis, and diverting ileostomy. Some of these refinements include the introduction of different types of pouches and stapled anastomosis. However, the principles of the ileoanal pouch procedure have not changed and involve a conventional total proctocolectomy, construction of an ileal pouch, and ileal pouch-anal anastomosis. In most cases, a temporary diverting loop ileostomy is also constructed.

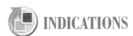

INDICATIONS

Ulcerative Colitis

Ulcerative colitis is the principal indication for restorative proctocolectomy with ileal pouch-anal anastomosis. Many patients with ulcerative colitis who are refractory to medical therapy and steroid dependent are suitable for this procedure. This constitutes the primary indication for the ileoanal pouch procedure in our institution.

Indeterminate Colitis

The dilemma and clinical difficulties of a diagnosis of indeterminate colitis relate to the concern surgeons express about performing pouch surgery in a patient whose final diagnosis is Crohn disease. Pouch failure rates are increased in patients with Crohn disease. A diagnosis of indeterminate colitis implies a significant chance that the ultimate diagnosis can be Crohn disease. This then mandates great circumspection by the surgeon when advising the patient about pouch alternatives for indeterminate colitis. In most cases, careful examination of gross and microscopic features will allow categorization of inflammatory bowel diseases as either mucosal ulcerative colitis or Crohn disease. About 10% of the cases will cause significant differential diagnostic problems by illustrating ambiguous features. Almost always, these cases are fulminant or toxic clinical disease requiring urgent or emergent colectomy in which pathologic features are ambiguous and do not permit precise separation of Crohn disease from ulcerative colitis. The histologic diagnosis of indeterminate colitis essentially indicates that the pathologist is unable to identify histologic features strongly in favor of either ulcerative colitis or Crohn disease. We believe it is safe to construct an ileal pouch-anal anastomosis in patients with indeterminate colitis. In our experience, functional results and the incidence of anastomotic complications and major

pouch fistulae have been the same in ulcerative and indeterminate colitis patients. Although indeterminate colitis patients were more likely to develop minor perineal fistulae, pelvic abscess, and Crohn disease, the rate of pouch failure was identical to that of ulcerative colitis patients. There was also no clinically significant difference in quality of life or satisfaction with ileal pouch surgery.

Late pouch complications are more common in the presence of preoperative clinical features suggestive of Crohn disease, such as perianal disease. The presence of perianal or small bowel disease indicates that the disease is likely to behave more like Crohn disease than ulcerative colitis. While functional outcome, quality of life, and pouch survival rates are equivalent after ileal pouch-anal anastomosis for indeterminate and ulcerative colitis, there is an increase in some complications and in the late diagnosis of Crohn disease.

Crohn Disease

In contrast, a proven diagnosis of Crohn disease is generally held to preclude ileal pouch-anal anastomosis. However, patients with ileal pouch-anal anastomosis for apparent mucosal ulcerative colitis who are subsequently found to have Crohn disease have a variable course. In our experience, patients who underwent ileal pouch-anal anastomosis for mucosal ulcerative colitis and who subsequently had that diagnosis revised to Crohn disease had favorable outcome. No pre–ileal pouch-anal anastomosis factors examined were predictors of the development of recrudescent Crohn disease. The overall pouch loss rate for the entire cohort was 12%, and was 33% for those with recrudescent Crohn disease during 46 months of follow-up. The secondary diagnosis of Crohn disease after ileal pouch-anal anastomosis was associated with protracted freedom from clinically evident Crohn disease, low pouch loss rate, and good functional outcome. We believe such results only can be improved by the continued development of medical strategies for the long-term suppression of Crohn disease, and our data support a prospective evaluation of ileal pouch-anal anastomosis in selected patients with Crohn disease.

Familial Adenomatous Polyposis

Restorative proctocolectomy is the preferred operation in older patients, especially those older than 30 years, because the risk for cancer rises with age. Restorative proctocolectomy removes all large bowel and mucosa, and theoretically eradicates the risk for colorectal cancer. The risk for polyps and cancer in the small bowel remains unchanged. There is controversy about the functional outcome comparing ileal pouch-anal anastomosis with total proctocolectomy and colectomy with ileorectal anastomosis. The previous studies showed that there was no functional outcome difference between these groups. Recently, several reports have challenged this notion, favoring the ileorectal anastomosis. At the same time, the risk of carcinoma developing in the rectal stump after an ileorectal anastomosis can be as high as 32% 20 years after anastomosis. However, this concern should be reconsidered in the postpouch era, since prior to the ileoanal pouch procedure, generally all patients were recommended for ileorectal anastomosis unless they had associated carcinoma. In our recent review, the risk of carcinoma developing in the rectal stump in the postpouch era was minimal.

Restorative proctocolectomy is a more complex surgical procedure than colectomy and ileorectal anastomosis and is associated with a higher morbidity. For this reason, in affected young adolescents, when the risk of cancer is low, colectomy and ileorectal anastomosis is a valuable option because of its simplicity, good function, and absence of need for a temporary stoma. We see the ileoanal pouch procedure as most suitable in young patients who present with diffuse multiple polyps in the rectum (>20 in proctoscopy) or in the patient with a late-onset disease and a malignancy in the upper rectum or colon. It is also an option in the patients who have previously had an ileorectal anastomosis and who have an unmanageable number of polyps in the rectum. Patients may choose restorative proctocolectomy because the cancer risk is lower than with ileorectal anastomosis. At the same time, the patient's wishes, extent of rectal involvement, availability of follow-up, and morbidity rate of restorative proctocolectomy should be considered before proceeding with this procedure.

In patients who have polyposis with an established colonic malignancy, or diffuse polyposis in rectum, the risk of further carcinoma developing is increased. Thus, unless the cancer is advanced or the distribution of polyps in the rectum is sparse, restorative proctocolectomy and ileoanal pouch-anal anastomosis is the surgical procedure of choice in patients with familial adenomatous polyposis.

Miscellaneous

Multiple polyps, multiple cancers of the colon and rectum, and functional bowel disease may also be indications for restorative proctocolectomy. The indication for functional bowel disease is controversial. The results are variable. It is reserved for patients in whom more conventional procedures have failed and when the patient refuses to have an ileostomy. In these circumstances, the procedure should be performed after extensive discussion with the patient, indicating limitations of the procedure. Motility disorder that causes a slow colonic transit may similarly affect the small bowel. Psychological assessment of the patient is important.

CONTRAINDICATIONS

Documented Crohn disease, advanced low-lying rectal cancer, and inadequate anal sphincter function are contraindications to pouch construction. There are no absolute contraindications to restorative proctocolectomy on the grounds of age at either extreme. However, resting and squeeze anal pressures tend to fall with age, especially in women older than 60 years of age. Serious co-morbid factors are also more common in the elderly.

TIMING OF SURGERY

Restorative proctocolectomy is an elective operation. In patients with a diagnostic dilemma of Crohn disease, requirement for high-dose prednisone (50 to 60 mg/d), signs and symptoms of toxicity, gross obesity, or malnutrition, staging the restorative proctocolectomy with initial subtotal or total abdominal colectomy with end ileostomy is our preferred approach (Fig. 1). We prefer suturing the stapled rectosigmoid stump to the distal aspect of the incision (Fig. 2). This places the suture line extraperitoneally, and if breakdown at the staple line occurs, drainage from the rectal stump can be controlled via a lower incisional fistula without the patient becoming septic. This technique also provides an easier identification of the rectal stump at the time of the second stage of the procedure when the ileal pouch is constructed.

This staged operation may be associated with a higher operative morbidity such as sepsis and small bowel obstruction than a colectomy and ileoanal anastomosis at a single operative setting. However, in the aforementioned patient population,

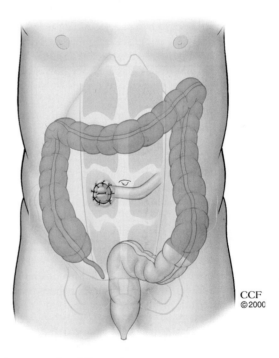

Fig. 1. Subtotal colectomy and end ileostomy.

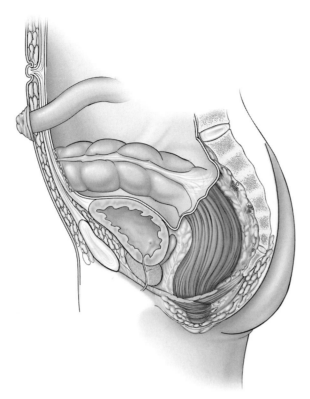

Fig. 2. The rectosigmoid stump is sutured to the lower aspect of incision extraperitoneally beneath the skin and subcutaneous tissue but above the fascia.

preliminary abdominal colectomy and end ileostomy with delayed ileal pouch construction are prudent. For these patients, ileal pouch-anal anastomosis is deferred 6 months because the adhesions can be extensive before that time. In over 90% of our cases, a temporary diverting loop ileostomy is constructed. This is closed 3 months later. Closure before that time is technically more difficult because of dense peri-ileostomy adhesions. We do routinely obtain a Gastrografin enema and pouch endoscopy prior to ileostomy closure to check for pouch and anastomotic integrity. If a laparotomy for adhesive bowel obstruction is necessary at any time, the ileostomy may be closed during the same procedure as long as the ileal pouch-anal anastomosis is intact and has the patency confirmed with Gastrografin enema and pouch endoscopy.

 PREOPERATIVE PLANNING

There are few operations where discussion with the patient and his or her family is so extensive. A complete and factual discussion of the indications for surgery, alternative treatments, sequelae, complications, and anticipated or possible outcomes is held. Preoperative preparation includes a preoperative assessment of the patient's fitness for surgery and assessment of the extent of colonic disease and anal sphincter function. A full colonoscopy with biopsies to determine Crohn disease or dysplasia is important. This is especially true where we commonly do serial biopsies from the lower and midrectum in patients with long-standing disease or known colonic dysplasia, since this may impact the type of anastomosis that will be used. An introduction to life with stoma by an enterostomal therapist is beneficial. A site for the temporary ileostomy is also marked preoperatively. Mechanical bowel preparation is provided by using polyethylene glycol or Fleet Phospho Soda.

At the time of the surgery, the patient is placed in the Trendelenburg position with the legs supported by Lloyd Davies Stirrups. Rectal washout with normal saline is performed in the operating room until the fluid return is clear. A urethral Foley catheter and a nasogastric tube are inserted after induction of anesthesia. Intravenous antibiotics, usually metronidazole and a third-generation cephalosporin, are given at induction and continued postoperatively for 2 to 5 days depending upon the degree of intraoperative contamination. Prophylaxis against deep venous thrombosis is also instituted.

 SURGICAL TECHNIQUE

The principles of restorative proctocolectomy and ileoanal pouch procedure involve a conventional total abdominal colectomy, proctectomy, construction of an ileal pouch, and ileoanal anastomosis.

Abdominal Dissection

A midline incision is made and a thorough laparotomy is performed to note whether there is any evidence of small bowel Crohn disease or any unsuspected neoplasm. The abdominal colectomy is performed in the standard manner with mesenteric vessels ligated and divided close to the bowel. However, in patients with a preoperative diagnosis of low- or high-grade dysplasia or cancer, or where the patient has longstanding disease of 10 or more years, we recommend a high ligation of the mesenteric vessels with a radical colectomy.

Proctectomy

The proctectomy should be done by avoiding any injury to the ureters and nervi erigentes. This can be accomplished by staying within the correct fascial planes. After identifying the ureters, the rectum is mobilized by first entering the presacral fascia between the investing layer of fascia propria of the mesorectum and presacral fascia (Fig. 3, *dotted line*). The presacral nerves are identified at the pelvic rim and preserved. The posterior pelvic dissection is continued midline posteriorly between the investing layer of the rectum and Waldeyer fascia to the level of the levator floor. It is important not to breech presacral fascia where nervi erigentes and presacral veins are vulnerable. Breaching this fascia may cause significant bleeding. Most of this dissection is usually done with cautery, is practically bloodless, and is expeditious, and the risk of impotence is low. After the posterior dissection is complete, anterior dissection is done starting about 1 cm above the peritoneal reflection (Fig. 3, *dotted line*). The plane of dissection is posterior to the Denonvilliers fascia and the seminal vesicles should not be seen. Beyond this level, a close rectal dissection is performed. This will ensure minimizing the risk of damaging the autonomic plexus that lies anterior to the Denonvilliers fascia. Lighted retractors allow good visualization of the pelvic structures. Throughout the pelvic dissection, firm traction on the rectum is essential. This is facilitated by placing the tissues

The Gastrointestinal Tract

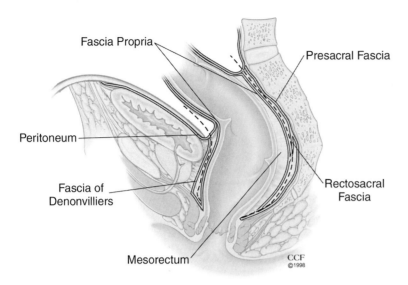

Fig. 3. Rectal dissection. Dotted lines point out the posterior and anterior dissection during the proctectomy.

under tension by using traction and countertraction. The lateral ligaments are divided close to the rectum with cautery. Occasionally, middle rectal vessels within the lateral ligaments may require suture or clip ligation. Anterior dissection close to the rectal wall is carried to the lower one third of the vagina, or to the lower border of the prostate gland. At this stage the rectum is fully mobilized down to the levators and an occluding tape is applied to the midrectum to avoid spillage. The next step, the transaction of the rectum, will depend on the plans for the type of the anastomosis, namely, stapled anastomosis or anorectal mucosectomy and hand-sewn anastomosis. After the transection, a pack is placed deep in the pelvis, abutting the levators to maximize the hemostasis; also, the specimen is opened and examined to rule out Crohn disease or associated colorectal cancer.

Pouch Design

The goal in restorative proctocolectomy and ileoanal pouch procedure is to construct a compliant sac of two or more loops of terminal ileum. Pouch construction has been shown to be superior to straight ileal anal anastomosis in terms of function. Several pouch designs using sutured or stapled techniques have been described. The foremost common pouch designs are the two-loop J-pouch, the triple-loop S-pouch, and the four-loop W-pouch with use of either sutured or stapled techniques. The functional results of these various pouch designs (Fig. 4) appear to be comparable, where the J-pouch

is easiest to construct and has functional outcomes identical to those of more complex designs. Factors other than pouch design, such as bacterial overgrowth, gut motility, and transit, probably play a more important role in deciding the functional outcome. There does not appear to be any correlation between ileal pouch capacity at the time of construction and functional outcome. However, the size of the pouch is of some importance. A very small pouch cannot fulfill its role as a reservoir, and a large floppy pouch may be associated with ineffective evacuation. In general, pouch capacity increases by two to four times at 1 year after construction.

The J-pouch is the pouch design of choice at the Cleveland Clinic Foundation. However, the S-pouch usually reaches 2 to 4 cm farther than does the J-pouch and is useful in patients with a short, fat mesentery and long, narrow pelvis, when the reach of the ileal pouch to the anal canal can be a problem. In our practice, this is especially true in patients where mucosectomy and hand-sewn anastomosis is indicated due to neoplasia.

Small Bowel Mobilization and Reach

The key to construction of an ileoanal pouch anastomosis is to mobilize the small bowel adequately so that it will reach to the levator floor without tension This can especially be a problem for obese patients, patients with extensive adhesions from previous surgery (such as in patients with familial adenomatous polyposis [FAP] and desmoids), patients with previous small resection, or patients necessitating mucosectomy and hand-sewn anastomosis. In order to accomplish this, the small bowel mesentery is totally mobilized as far as the third part of the duodenum and inferior border of the pancreas. In our practice, we ligate and excise the ileocolic artery and vein at the origin of the superior mesenteric artery. This provides a better mobility and tension-free anastomosis.

The segment of ileum requiring the greatest mobility varies with pouch design. For this reason, before transection of the rectum, we make sure the pouch reaches to the distal aspect of the anal

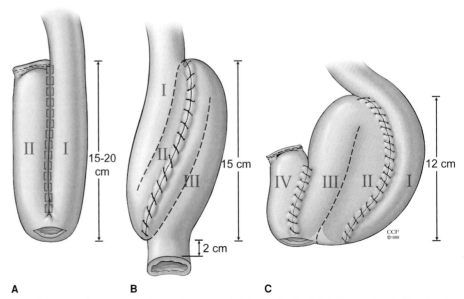

Fig. 4. Various designs of ileal pouch. **A:** Double J-pouch. **B:** Triple S-pouch. **C:** Quadruple W-pouch.

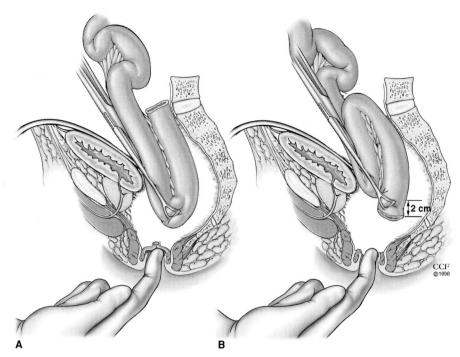

Fig. 5. Simulation of reach to pelvic floor. **A:** J-pouch. **B:** S-pouch.

canal either for planned stapled or muco-sectomy with hand-sewn anastomosis. The junction of the two loops of small bowel and the end-terminal ileum are the two points that require greatest mobility for the J-pouch (two loop) and S-pouch (three loop). The apex of the J-pouch is about 15 cm from the end of the ileum. That of the S-pouch is at the bowel end itself. The reach can be estimated by placing a Babcock clamp at the apex of the ileal pouch and grasping that and simulating the reach down to the levator floor. The reach is estimated by delivering the clamped apex into the pelvis and having the clamp abut the top of the levator floor or the index finger that is inserted into the anus (Fig. 5). The S-pouch usually reaches 2 to 4 cm farther than the J-pouch and can be helpful if there is likely to be tension with the anastomosis.

If these maneuvers fail to give clear indications that reach is tension free, which is especially true in obese patients or in patients who have had a previous small bowel resection, a number of maneuvers can be helpful. If further mobilization is necessary, excision of all peritoneal tissue to the right of the superior mesenteric vessels, leaving a very small edge of peritoneum lateral to these vessels, may provide added mobility (Fig. 6). Preservation of superior mesenteric vessels and their terminal arcades is important. Use of translumination facilitates identification of vessels that

must be preserved. A further maneuver that is helpful is the making of a series of transverse 1- to 2-cm peritoneal incisions over the superior mesenteric vessels anteriorly and posteriorly (Fig. 6). Formal mobilization of the duodenum with Kocher maneuver may also give additional mobility to provide a tension-free

anastomosis. These maneuvers usually add at least 2 to 3 cm to mobility.

Ileal Pouch Construction and Ileal Pouch-Anal Anastomosis

When an ileoanal pouch is performed, controversy exists about the technique to be used for the pouch-anal anastomosis. Techniques of anastomosis vary between a hand-sewn ileal pouch-anal anastomosis with mucosectomy of the anal transitional zone and a stapled ileal pouch-anal anastomosis at the level of the anorectal ring without mucosectomy of the anal transitional zone. Therefore, the optimal level of anorectal transsection is controversial after the rectal dissection. This controversy centers on the potential advantages and disadvantages of leaving a mucosal cuff of anal transitional zone ranging from 1 to 2 cm in length in order to allow transanal insertion of the stapler head. By transecting the rectum at the top of the anal columns (anorectal ring) as in stapled anastomosis, the anal sensory epithelium is preserved and tension on the pending ileoanal anastomosis is also minimized. Therefore, the potential advantages of stapled anastomosis include better functional results, lower rate of septic complications, and ease of construction; disadvantages include possible malignant or premalignant transformation of the columnar epithelial cells in the retained mucosal cuff and a longer, more difficult surgery.

The Gastrointestinal Tract

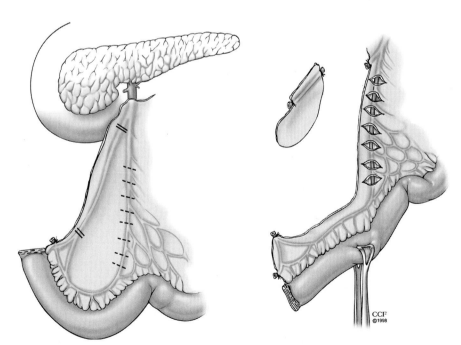

Fig. 6. Maneuvers for pouch to reach: Ligation of ileocolic artery and vein at its origin, excision of peritoneal tissue right of the superior mesenteric vessels, and transverse incisions over the superior mesenteric vessels.

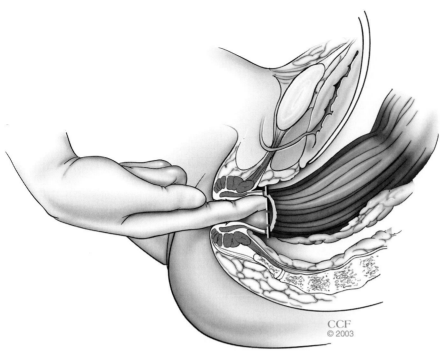

Fig. 7. With the proximal interphalangeal joint resting at the anal verge, the tip of the finger corresponds to the anorectal ring, and this corresponds to the level of linear staple for double-stapled or purse-string suture for the single-stapled linear staple for double-stapled anastomosis.

The prospective randomized trials have not shown a difference in functional outcome and septic complications between the two methods. However, these studies warrant careful analysis because of the relatively short-term follow-up, and the small number of cases studied makes them vulnerable to type II error. Our initial studies comparing the two types of techniques showed less septic complications and better functional outcome favoring stapled anastomosis. The most recent review from our institution of over 2,000 patients continued to show superior functional results in patients with stapled anastomosis, where the septic complications showed some increased trend in mucosectomy group, but this did not reach the statistical difference like the prior studies from our institution.

The estimated incidence of anal transitional zone dysplasia in our most recent study was 4.5% without any occurrence of invasive cancer in patients with a minimum of 10 years of surveillance. However, the risk of anal transitional dysplasia was significantly associated with cancer or dysplasia as a preoperative diagnosis or in the proctocolectomy specimen. More recently we had two cases of anal transitional zone cancer where both were successfully treated. Mucosectomy and hand-sewn anastomosis may decrease this concern but cannot fully eliminate the

neoplasia risk, because islands of colonic-type mucosa can be present even at the level of the dentate line or potential remnant columnar cells and left at the time of the mucosectomy dissection. These areas are later covered with the pouch itself where further surveillance of the muco-

sectomized anal transitional zone could not be as discrete as in stapled anastomosis. A very distal anal canal transsection also may lead to excision of some internal anal sphincter. In our practice, we favor mucosectomy with hand-sewn anastomosis in patients with a known diagnosis of rectal cancer or dysplasia in the lower two thirds of rectum before the surgery.

A stapled ileal pouch-anal anastomosis may be constructed using either a double-stapling technique or a single-stapling technique. Double-stapled ileoanal pouch anastomosis is our preferred technique at the Cleveland Clinic Foundation. If a stapled anastomosis is intended, the surgeon marks the level of planned anastomosis by transanal digital examination. With the proximal interphalangeal joint resting at the anal verge, the tip of the digit corresponds to the anorectal ring (Fig. 7). At this point the level is marked by use of cautery on the anterior surface of the rectum, and this corresponds to the level of linear staple for double-stapling anastomosis or purse-string suture for single-stapling anastomosis.

The double-stapling technique obviates the frustration of inserting purse-string sutures in the anorectum deep in the pelvis and minimizes intraoperative contamination. Disparity of the size of the bowel lumen is also avoided. With this technique, the distal anorectal stump is closed with a linear stapler. The PI 30 instrument (U.S Surgical Corp., Norwalk,

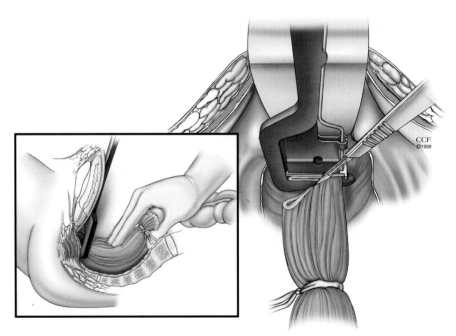

Fig. 8. A linear stapler is applied at the intended level of distal rectal transsection and a double row of staples placed. The rectum is divided along the cephalad edge of staples. An occluding tape is placed in the midrectum to minimize contamination.

CT) has a restraining pin to prevent extrusion of the tissues during staple closure. The linear staple line on the anorectum should rest at a level just below the superior border of the levator floor. In patients with a wide pelvis, there is a potential hazard that the linear stapler may be applied too distally, which could lead to excision of a significant amount of internal sphincter when subsequent ileal pouch-anal anastomosis is performed. Thus, the level of the intended ileoanal anastomosis should be determined and marked beforehand, as emphasized in Figure 7. Because of oblique positioning of the linear stapler on the anorectum, the posterior anastomotic line tends to be more distal than that of the anterior anastomotic line. After the stapler is fired, the specimen is divided above the linear staple line by using a long-handled knife (Fig. 8).

After the total proctocolectomy and the transection of the distal line of rectal resection, the terminal ileum is quarantined from the remaining peritoneal cavity. An occluding tape is applied in the midportion of the ileum. The distal portion is irrigated with normal saline and evacuated into a sterile bowl until the contents are clear. Care is taken to minimize contamination.

Our preferred technique at the Cleveland Clinic is the J-pouch because of its simplicity and no proven increased benefit of other various pouch designs. The J-shaped ileal pouch is constructed from the terminal 30 to 40 cm of small bowel folded into two 15- to 20-cm segments. Cutting cautery is used to make a linear 1.5-cm enterotomy at the apex. Both limbs are approximated on their antimesenteric surface; a 100-mm linear stapler is passed to its full length, the surgeon checks that no mesentery is interposed between the anvil and cartridge, and the instrument is fired. A second staple line is made similarly. Care is taken to leave no gaps between consecutive stapler lines. The end of the divided terminal ileum is closed by a linear stapler and oversewn with 3-0 polyglycolic acid sutures for reinforcement. If a stapled anastomosis is planned, a Prolene purse-string suture is applied to the apical enterotomy. The pouch is inflated with saline to check for leaks and the staple line is checked for hemostasis (Fig. 9). The stapled lines are also checked for hemostasis. The detached anvil of the circular stapler is then inserted into the pouch and the purse-string suture tightened.

After removal of packing from the deep pelvis and before construction of the anastomosis, total hemostasis is achieved in the pelvis. Double-stapled ileal pouch-anal anastomosis is then performed using a circular stapler, which removes an additional 1 cm of distal ring doughnut. A circular stapler (CEEA-31, U.S Surgical Corp., Norwalk, CT, or ILS- 29, Ethicon Endo-Surgery, Cincinnati, OH) with the anvil detached is introduced into the anus, and the trocar point is advanced just posterior to the linear staple line on the anorectum. This can be facilitated by putting the index finger into the anorectal staple line area from the abdominal side and guiding the trocar just posterior to the linear stapler line on the anorectal stump (Fig. 10).

The trocar of the circular stapler is then removed and the shaft of the circular stapler is mated with the anvil shaft emerging from the ileal pouch. The mesentery must be carefully inspected to ensure that no twisting has occurred. The ends are approximated, with care being taken to avoid extraneous tissue being included in the staple line (Fig. 11). It is important that the entire cartridge is inserted well within the anal rectal stump to avoid incorporation of the anal sphincters within the anastomosis. After the anastomosis is completed, both doughnuts are inspected for integrity and transanal insufflation with normal saline is performed to ensure that the anastomosis

The Gastrointestinal Tract

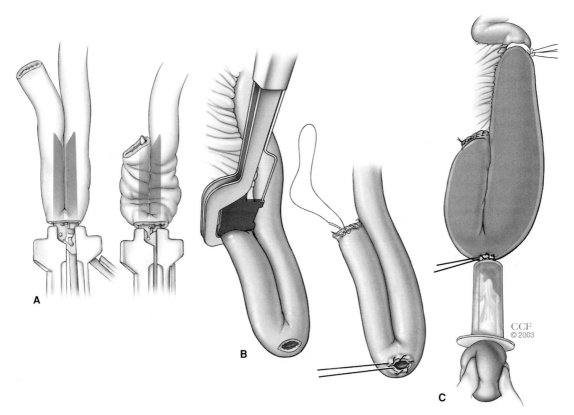

Fig. 9. A: Formation of J-pouch with two firings of a 100-mm linear stapler. **B:** The end of the divided terminal ileum is closed by a linear stapler and oversewn by running sutures. **C:** If a stapled anastomosis is planned, purse-string suture is applied to the apical enterotomy. The pouch is inflated with saline to check for leaks.

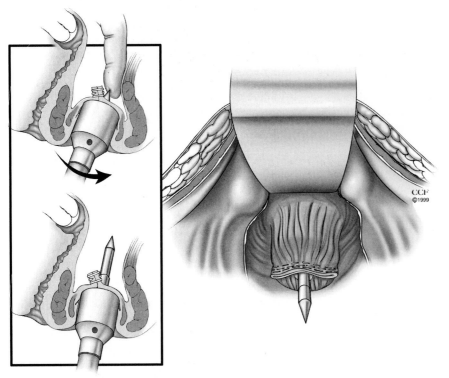

Fig. 10. In the double-stapling technique, the shaft/trocar should traverse posterior to the staple line. This can be facilitated by putting the index finger into the anorectal staple line area from the abdominal side and guiding the trocar just posterior to the linear stapler line on the anorectal stump.

is intact. This is our preferred anastomotic technique at the Cleveland Clinic.

Care must also be taken to avoid including the posterior vaginal wall within the anastomosis. This is a devastating complication that can be avoided in the creation of pouch vaginal anastomotic fistulae (Fig. 12). For this reason it is important to traverse the trocar of the circular stapler posterior to the linear staple of the anorectal stump. Although there are theoretic concerns about intersecting circular and linear staple lines, experimental and clinical experience attests to the safety of double-stapling techniques.

An S-pouch is constructed using three limbs of 12 to 15 cm of terminal ileum. The S-pouch usually reaches 2 to 4 cm farther than the J-pouch and is helpful if there is likely to be tension with the ileoanal anastomosis. The latter situation is more likely to arise in obese patients or in patients in whom mucosectomy and a hand-sewn ileal pouch-anal anastomosis is performed. The S-pouch is initially constructed with continuous seromuscular sutures of 3-0 polyglycolic acid by approximating the loops. Then an S-shaped enterotomy is made. The two posterior anastomotic lines later are closed from inside the pouch using running 3-0 polyglycolic acid sutures. The anterior wall is then closed with continuous seromuscular

sutures with reinforcement of the same type. It is important to leave the exit conduit no longer than 2 cm since a longer exit conduit is associated with evacuation

problems (Fig. 13). The S-pouch is also inflated with saline to check for leaks.

A hand-sewn ileal pouch-anal anastomosis is usually performed in conjunction with mucosectomy of the anorectal mucosa. If a mucosectomy and hand-sewn anastomosis are intended, the rectum is transected using a combination of cutting/coagulation current cautery at the anorectal ring around the upper border of the levator floor. Prior to transsection, we make sure the pouch reaches to the distal aspect of the anal canal for the anastomosis. If that is the case, mucosectomy of the anorectal mucosa is performed from the perineum. From a functional point of view, leaving a muscular sleeve of the rectum is not necessary. Most receptors for sensation in the neorectum do not lie in the rectal mucosa or muscle. In addition, preservation of a long muscular sleeve with a long mucosectomy is tedious and bloody, and has high septic sequelae. Some investigators, however, preserve the entire anal sensory epithelium and hand sew the end of the ileal pouch to the top of the columns of Morgagni.

The mucosectomy and hand-sewn anastomosis are usually recommended in our practice for patients with rectal cancer, dysplasia in the lower two thirds of the rectum, or large or carpeting rectal polyps of the anal transitional zone from familial adenomatous polyposis, or for patients in whom compliance for follow-up

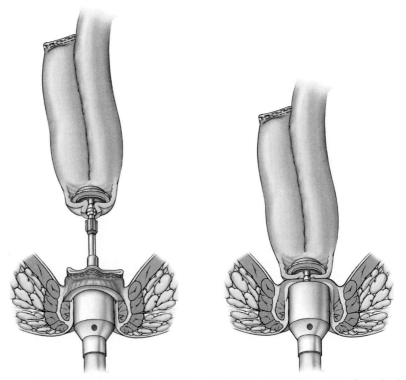

Fig. 11. The shaft of the circular stapler is mated with the anvil shaft emerging from the ileal pouch. The ends are approximated. Care is taken to avoid extraneous tissue being included in the staple line.

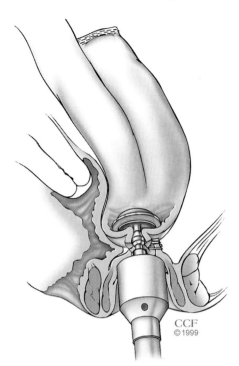

Fig. 12. Anastomosis pouch–vaginal fistula complication.

anastomosis with narrow pelvis where the levators are particularly prominent, the reach of the ileal pouch to the anal canal can be difficult. This can be overcome by a bimanual maneuver. A long Babcock clamp is passed transanally to grasp the apex of the pouch and the surgeon's hand is passed behind the pouch to gently coax and ease the pouch and its exit conduit to the level of the levator floor (Fig. 15).

Single-stapling anastomosis has been one of the earlier refinements of the ileal pouch-anal anastomosis after the initial description. It was commonly used until the

description and the safe application of double-stapled anastomosis. For a single-stapling anastomosis, a distal purse-string is applied to the anorectal stump. A small proctotomy is made at the anterior wall and stay sutures are placed. The purse-string suture is applied by hand, starting from the anterior wall with a 0-polypropylene, with small parts of muscularis and minimal parts of mucosa taken at small intervals across the anorectal ring. The proctotomy is gradually extended. Suture placement and cautery division of the bowel are performed sequentially to enable cephalad traction on

is unreliable. The anal verge is everted by radially placed 1.0 polyglycolic acid sutures in four quadrants as a first step to facilitate the exposure. A medium-sized lighted Ferguson anal retractor is placed in the anal canal to facilitate mucosectomy under direct vision. Excessive stretching of the anal canal should be avoided, since this may damage the anal sphincters and impair fecal continence. Here, the mucosa is stripped from the underlying sphincters from the dentate line to the level of the anorectal transection. An injection of 10 to 15 mL of 1/100,000 of epinephrine solution is used to elevate the anorectal mucosa starting at the dentate line. Mucosectomy is performed, with use of cautery. It is important not to leave any islands of large bowel mucosa that are not amenable to surveillance. Polyglycolic acid sutures (2-0) are placed radially at the dentate line and incorporate a small portion of internal anal sphincter. Care is taken not to take a stitch too deeply anteriorly in females because of the danger of anastomosis–vaginal fistula. The end of the exit conduit of the S-pouch or the apex of the J-pouch is delivered via a Babcock clamp on the anal verge. With the aid of the lighted Ferguson retractor, the previous sutures in the dentate line are now serially placed through the full thickness of ileum and tied after the retractor is removed (Fig. 14).

On occasion, in patients who have undergone mucosectomy and hand-sewn

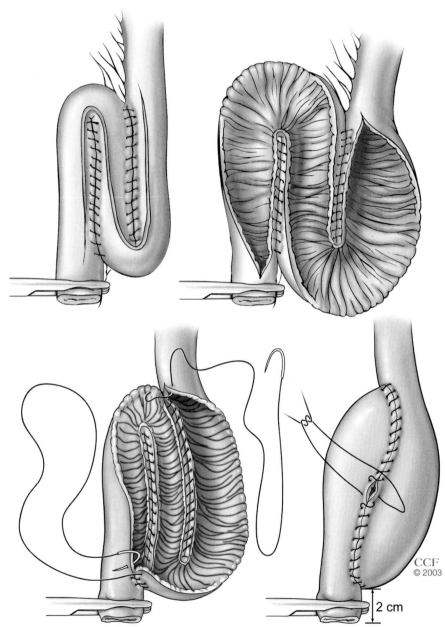

Fig. 13. An S-pouch is constructed using three limbs of 12 to 15 cm of terminal ileum. Continuous seromuscular sutures approximate the loops. An S-shaped enterotomy is made. The two posterior anastomotic lines later are closed from inside the pouch using running sutures. The anterior wall is then closed with continuous seromuscular sutures with reinforcement by the same type of suture. It is important to leave the exit conduit no longer than 2 cm, since a longer exit conduit is associated with evacuation problems.

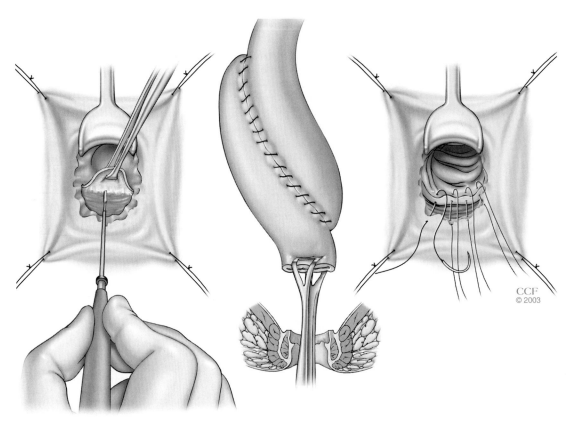

Fig. 14. Mucosectomy and hand-sewn anastomosis. The anal verge is everted by radially placed sutures in four quadrants as a first step to facilitate the exposure. A medium-sized lighted Ferguson anal retractor is placed in the anal canal to facilitate mucosectomy under direct vision. Mucosectomy is performed, with use of cautery. Sutures are placed radially at the dentate line. The end of the exit conduit of the S-pouch or the apex of the J-pouch is delivered via a Babcock clamp on the anal verge. The previously placed sutures in the dentate line are now serially placed through the full thickness of ileum and tied.

the rectum, which facilitates the accurate placement of the sutures. The surgical staple is inserted transanally, the shaft is advanced fully, and the purse-string is tightened snugly around the base of the shaft (Fig. 16). Ileal pouch–anal anastomosis is then completed by using the circular stapler as discussed above. Today we prefer to use single-stapled anastomosis in cases with technical difficulty with the double-stapled technique, such as misfiring or difficulty coming across the rectum with a linear stapler.

Anastomosis is then completed and integrity of anastomosis is checked by ensuring that two proximal and distal doughnuts are complete. For all types of anastomosis, it is our practice to do transanal insufflation with air to ensure the anastomotic integrity (Fig. 17).

Drains

We practice routine drainage of the presacral space using closed suction drains. The drain is left for 3 to 4 days or until drainage is less than 50 mL per day.

Ileostomy

Because of the large number of suture or staple lines involved in ileal anal-pouch anastomosis, because the operation is not always done under ideal circumstances, and because it is most often performed in steroid-dependent, malnourished patients, a temporary diverting ileostomy has traditionally been used. Our preferred technique is to bring out the most proximal loop of the ileum (usually 20 to 25 cm proximal to the pouch) to the preoperatively marked right lower quadrant of the abdominal wall without any tension. In some cases such as in obese patients with thick panniculus, a higher level of the ileum is used, which may be associated with excessive ileostomy effluent and even readmission for dehydration. Closure of loop ileostomy is performed 3 months later. In most cases, closure is performed through a peristomal incision.

The diverting ileostomy has its own morbidity. In addition, a second operation is necessary to close the stoma. Several surgical centers including our own have

evaluated omission of diverting ileostomy in restorative proctocolectomy. With increasing experience, there has been less trepidation about leaving the ileal pouch-anal anastomosis unprotected; some centers prefer to do this routinely and others do it only in selected patients (Fig. 18).

We prefer to omit ileostomy in selected patients with optimum conditions. In our practice, generally, no ileostomy is used with stringent criteria when the surgery is elective and the patient has high motivation, stapled anastomosis, minimal tension on ileal pouch-anal anastomosis, intact tissue rings, good hemostasis, absence of air leak, malnutrition, toxicity, anemia, or prolonged consumption of high-dose steroids (prednisone >20 mg). We would also consider omission of diverting ileostomy if its construction is likely to be problematic, as in obese patients. When a one-stage restorative proctocolectomy is performed, a pouch catheter (32 Fr.) is inserted transanally and left in place for 4 to 5 days. Our most recent study showed that omitting diverting ileostomy is a safe option in selected patients undergoing

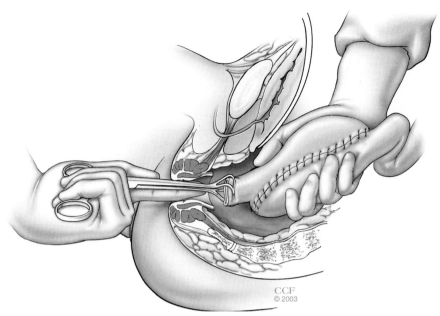

Fig. 15. A bimanual maneuver to bring the pouch to the level of the levators in patients with narrow pelvis and prominent levator muscles.

restorative proctocolectomy with the outlined stringent criteria. In general, we feel that a covering stoma is a safer option, especially in the early learning phase of the pouch surgeon.

PERIOPERATIVE AND POSTOPERATIVE MANAGEMENT

After ileoanal pouch procedure with diverting loop ileostomy, patients invariably have high ileostomy outputs from 1,000 to 2,000 mL per 24 hours. Effectively the "high" ileostomy bypasses 20% or more of the distal small bowel, and this sets the stage for dehydration. The following advice is given to our patients:

- Be aware of added risk factors for dehydration (hot weather, exercise, air conditioning).
- Be aware of the symptoms of dehydration—lassitude, fatigue, headache, and nausea.
- Maintain adequate intake of oral liquids, especially salty soups and electrolytes supplements.
- Avoid high solid fiber/indigestible foods for 6 weeks.
- Use liquid loperamide hydrochloride or diphenoxylate hydrochloride with atropine sulfate on a weight basis to thicken enteric output.

Use psyllium bulking agents in liquid form (e.g., Konsyl, Citrucel, Metamucil, and

FiberCon; usually no earlier than 6 weeks after the pouch procedure).

- Be aware of the fact that external ileostomy pouches may stay on for only 2 days or so (compared with 5 to 7 days for end ileostomies).
- Follow the steroid tapering schedule prescribed on discharge.

- Recognize symptoms of postoperative bowel obstruction.
- Recognize symptoms of postoperative steroid insufficiency.

Patients are seen in the office 4 to 6 weeks after surgery. The stoma site is remeasured so that new stoma appliances may be prescribed. Water-soluble contrast enema is done to rule out any occult leak prior to ileostomy closure. A digital examination of the pouch-anal anastomosis and a pouch endoscopy are also performed at that time. A web-like stenosis of the pouch-anal anastomosis is gently dilated with the finger. Digital dilation is easier at this time than later, when fibrosis ensues. Functional adequacy of the anal sphincters is evaluated by digital examination and evaluation of the patient's control of discharge of mucus from the pouch. If there is doubt, a more formal evaluation with enema challenge (ability to hold a 100-mL saline enema) and manometry is useful. In selected cases, sphincter muscle exercises with deferment of ileostomy closure may be considered. After the ileostomy is closed, a similar program as the one outlined above is instituted. However, antidiarrheal medications can and should be given more forcefully, often combining all three preparations of bulking agent, loperamide hydrochloride, and diphenoxylate hydrochloride with atropine sulfate. After 4 to 6 weeks, bowel function is

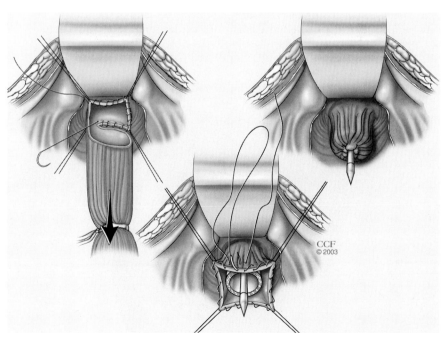

Fig. 16. For a single-stapling anastomosis, a distal purse-string is applied to the anorectal stump. A small proctotomy is made at the anterior wall and stay sutures are placed. The purse-string suture is applied by hand starting from the anterior wall. The proctotomy is gradually extended. Suture placement and cautery division of the bowel are performed sequentially to enable cephalad traction on the rectum, which facilitates the accurate placement of the sutures. The posterior rectal wall is then divided piecemeal and purse-string suturing completed in short stages.

The Gastrointestinal Tract

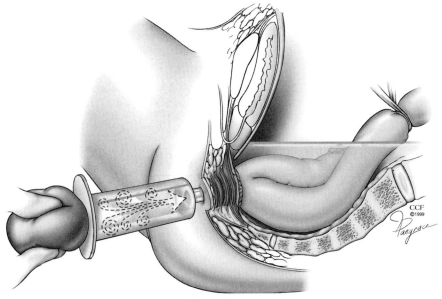

Fig. 17. Transanal insufflation with normal saline is performed to ensure that the anastomosis is intact.

usually satisfactory and a more liberal diet can be initiated.

In patients in whom the anal transitional zone is left behind, an anal pouch endoscopy and biopsy of the anal transitional zone are recommended. Neoplasia in the anal transitional zone is rarely encountered.

EXPERIENCE AT THE CLEVELAND CLINIC

Over 3,000 ileal pouch surgical procedures were performed at the Cleveland Clinic from 1983 to 2006. Ulcerative colitis is a primary indication for the pouch procedure. Despite the complex nature of the procedure, 30-day operative mortality was 0.2%. Morbidity averaged over 60%. However, serious complications such as anastomotic leak occurred in 5%. Most of the anastomotic stricture that occurred after the ileal pouch-anal anastomosis responded to simple dilation, performed in the physician's office. Small bowel obstruction affected approximately 20% of the patients, but only 6% needed surgery for obstruction.

Five-year ileal pouch survival was 95.6%. The ileal pouch was removed in 3.4% of patients and was nonfunctional in 1% of patients, making the pouch failure rate 4.4%. We recently developed a model to assess the risk factors that were associated with pouch failure. Data from 23 preoperative, seven intraoperative, and ten postoperative risk factors were recorded from 1,965 patients undergoing restorative proctocolectomy between 1983 and 2001. Primary end point was ileal pouch failure where the pouches were either excised or nonfunctional during the follow-up period of up to 19 years. Usual contributive risk factors found to be independent predictors of pouch survival were Crohn disease, prior anal pathology such as anorectal stricture or fistula, low resting pressures prior to ileostomy closure, patients' associated comorbidities, postoperative occurrence of pouch-perineal or pouch-vaginal fistulae, pelvic sepsis, and anastomotic stricture and separation. This model may play an important role in providing risk estimates for patients wishing to make informed choices on the type of treatment offered to them.

For patients who had ileal pouch-anal anastomosis failure caused by septic or functional complications, disconnection of an ileal pouch-anal anastomosis with repeat ileal pouch-anal anastomosis can be an option. In our recent review of 101 patients undergoing laparotomy, ileoanal disconnection, and repeat ileal pouch-anal anastomosis, 80 were referred from other

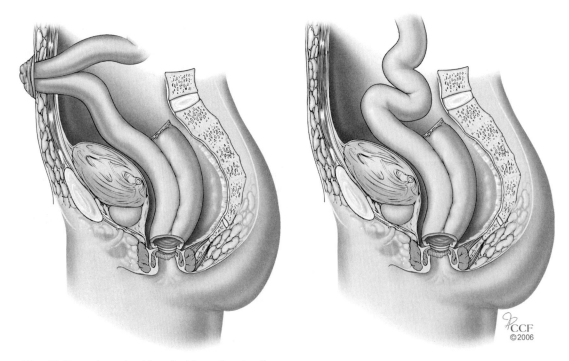

Fig. 18. Ileoanal pouch with and without diverting ileostomy.

institutions. Indications included chronic anastomotic leak (n = 27), perineal or pouch-vaginal fistula (n = 47), anastomotic stricture (n = 22), dysfunction/long efferent limb of S-pouch (n = 36), and previous ileal pouch-anal anastomosis excision or exclusion (n = 6). Five-year pouch survival was 74%, higher for ulcerative colitis (79%) than Crohn disease (53%). Patients had average bowel movements of six times per day and two per night. Thirty-five percent of patients never described urgency. Ninety-seven percent would undergo repeat ileal pouch-anal anastomosis again, and 99% would recommend it to others. Although pouch failure occurred more frequently than after primary ileal pouch-anal anastomosis, patient satisfaction and quality of life were high.

In approximately 90% of patients, a diverting ileostomy has been created at the time of ileal pouch-anal procedure in our series. A total of 1,504 patients underwent ileostomy closure after restorative proctocolectomy during a 19-year period. The median length of hospitalization was 3 days, and the overall complication rate was 11.4%. Complications included small bowel obstruction (6.4%), wound infection (1.5%), abdominal septic complications (1%), and enterocutaneous fistulae (0.6%). Hand-sewn closure was performed in 1,278 patients (85%) and stapled closure in 226 (15%). No significant differences in complication rates and length of hospitalization were found between hand-sewn and stapled closure techniques. Our results demonstrated that ileostomy closure after restorative proctocolectomy can be achieved with a low morbidity and a short hospitalization stay.

Pouchitis affected mainly patients with ulcerative colitis and occurred in 30% of our patients with inflammatory bowel disease. Rarely, it may also affect patients with polyposis. Pouchitis is a poorly defined and understood clinical syndrome consisting of acute diarrhea, urgency, rectal bleeding, abdominal cramps, malaise, fever, myalgia, and arthralgia. Pouchitis often is diagnosed based on symptoms alone. However, increased stool frequency, urgency, and abdominal pain could be due to other conditions such as irritable bowel syndrome. We recently did a study that was designed to assess the cause of bowel symptoms after ileal pouch-anal anastomosis using the Pouchitis Disease Activity Index (PDAI). Symptoms, endoscopy, and histology findings were assessed in 61 consecutive symptomatic patients with ulcerative colitis. Pouchitis was defined as

a PDAI score of greater than or equal to 7, cuffitis was defined as endoscopic and histologic inflammation of the rectal cuff and no inflammation of the pouch, and irritable pouch syndrome (IPS) was defined as symptoms with a PDAI of less than 7 and the absence of cuffitis. Thirty-one patients (51%) had pouchitis, four (6%) had cuffitis, and 26 (43%) had IPS. Increased stool frequency, urgency, and abdominal cramps were the most common symptoms in the three groups. Rectal bleeding was seen only in cuffitis. The majority of patients (87%) with pouchitis responded to a 2-week course of ciprofloxacin or metronidazole with a reduction in PDAI scores. All patients with cuffitis responded to topical hydrocortisone or mesalamine. Around 46% of patients with irritable pouch syndrome responded to antidiarrheal, anticholinergic, and/or antidepressant therapies, whereas the remaining patients had persistent symptoms despite therapy.

A substantial number of symptomatic patients after ileal pouch-anal anastomosis do not meet the diagnostic criteria for either pouchitis or cuffitis and have been classified as having IPS. There is an overlap of symptoms among patients with pouchitis, cuffitis, and IPS, and endoscopic evaluation can differentiate among these groups. Distinction between these three groups has therapeutic implications. Avoiding nonsteroidal anti-inflammatory drugs in patients with ileal pouch can decrease the risk for pouchitis. The cause of pouchitis is not clear. In most patients, the symptoms are brief and respond to oral antibiotics. However, with different causes of bowel symptoms after ileal pouch-anal anastomosis, if the patients are in close proximity to our center, we prefer to work them up in our pouch clinic rather than give them an empiric antibiotic therapy. In about one quarter of our patients with pouchitis, the symptoms are refractory or recurrent and may require long-term, low-dose metronidazole and occasional steroids. Underlying Crohn disease sometimes manifests as rampant pouchitis.

Infertility rates after ileal pouch-anal procedure has been recently recognized as an important concerning issue. In a recent study from our institution we evaluated the fertility rates before and after pouch procedure and compared them with the reproductive data of the general U.S. population to determine surgical parameters that might influence subsequent fertility. Out of 300 women, 206 attempted to conceive. Before operation, 48 (38%) of 127 patients were unsuccessful after 1 year of unprotected intercourse, whereas after

operation, 76 (56%) of 135 patients were unsuccessful. This infertility rate was statistically higher after operation than before. For the subgroup of 56 women who tried to get pregnant both before and after operation, the infertility rate was higher after operation than before (69% vs. 46%). This increased risk of infertility has been part of our preoperative counseling for patients who are of child-bearing age at the time of their pouch procedure. In patients who need the surgery and have a major concern of getting pregnant, we offer an initial subtotal colectomy with end ileostomy, followed by a staged pouch construction after a successful pregnancy. Our preferred type of delivery in patients who were able to conceive and successfully carry a full-term pregnancy has been the cesarean section, since vaginal delivery was associated with increased sphincter damage and decreased quality of life.

Functional results and quality of life improved with time and stabilized approximately 1 year after surgery. Functional outcome was good to excellent in 93% of our patients, and results were similar for patients with ulcerative colitis and familial adenomatosis polyposis. Bowel frequency ranges from four to nine per 24 hours, averaging six times per day. This, however, is not a good indication of success, as many patients will evacuate their pouches when it's convenient to do so rather than defer defecation. Continence for flatus and stool was achieved for 70% of patients during the night and 80% during the day. Major fecal incontinence was uncommon and occurred in less than 5% of patients. Functional results including anal sensation and nocturnal continence were significantly better after stapled anastomosis than after mucosectomy with anal hand-sewn anastomosis.

Our long-term follow-up of pouch function and quality of life indicates a very high degree of acceptance and happiness of the patients undergoing restorative proctocolectomy. This is on a par with age- and sex-matched U.S. citizens using the SF36 assessment tool. The standard operative option for the majority of patients with ulcerative colitis and familial polyposis remains restorative proctocolectomy and ileal pouch-anal anastomosis. For many patients, it is a more attractive surgical option than proctocolectomy and permanent end ileostomy. Most series in the literature demonstrate an acceptable complication rate with good to excellent functional and quality-of-life series. Surgical experience, peri- and postoperative care,

The Gastrointestinal Tract

and proper and competent intervention of complications affect surgical outcome and patient satisfaction. With increasing experience and better management of complications, an overall improvement in the results has been achieved. In addition to technical refinements, the surgery has been simplified, and it is now a relatively safe procedure.

ACKNOWLEDGEMENT

I would like to thank to Mr. Joe Pangrace for his help and expertise with the artwork.

SUGGESTED READING

Achkar JP, Al-Haddad M, Lashner B, et al. Differentiating risk factors for acute and chronic pouchitis. *Clin Gastroenterol Hepatol* 2005;3:60.

Baixauli J, Delaney CP, Wu JS, et al. Functional outcome and quality of life after repeat ileal pouch-anal anastomosis for complications of ileoanal surgery. *Dis Colon Rectum* 2004; 47:2.

Church JM, Burke C, McGannon E, et al. Risk of rectal cancer in patients after colectomy and ileorectal anastomosis for familial adenomatous polyposis. *Dis Colon Rectum* 2003; 46:1175.

Delaney CP, Fazio VW, Remzi FH, et al. Prospective, age-related analysis of surgical results, functional outcome and quality of life after ileal pouch-anal anastomosis. *Ann Surg* 2003;238:221.

Delaney CP, Remzi FH, Gramlich T, et al. Equivalent function, quality of life and pouch survival rates after ileal pouch-anal anastomosis for indeterminate and ulcerative colitis. *Ann Surg* 2002;23:43.

Fazio VW, Tekkis PP, Remzi FH, et al. Quantification of risk for pouch failure after ileal pouch anal anastomosis surgery. *Ann Surg* 2003;238:605, discussion 614.

Gunther K, Braunrider G, Bittorf BR, et al. Patients with familial adenomatous polyposis experience better bowel function and quality of life after ileorectal anastomosis than after ileoanal pouch. *Colorectal Dis* 2003;5:38.

Halverson AH, Hull TL, Remzi FH, et al. Perioperative resting pressure predicts long-term postoperative function after ileal pouch-anal anastomosis. *J Gastrointest Surg* 2002;6:316, discussion 320.

Hartley JE, Fazio VW, Remzi FH, et al. Analysis of the outcome of ileal pouch-anal anastomosis in patients with Crohn's disease. *Dis Colon Rectum* 2004;47:1808.

Remzi FH, Fazio VW, Delaney CP, et al. Dysplasia of the anal transitional zone after ileal pouch-anal anastomosis: results of prospective evaluation of prospective evaluation after a minimum of ten years. *Dis Colon Rectum* 2003;46:6.

Remzi FH, Fazio VW, Gorgun E, et al. Omission of temporary diversion after restorative proctocolectomy and ileal pouch anal anastomosis: surgical complications, functional outcome and quality of life analysis. *Dis Colon Rectum* 2006;In press.

Remzi FH, Gorgun E, Bast J, et al. Vaginal delivery after ileal pouch anal anastomosis (IPAA): a word of caution. *Dis Colon Rectum* 2005;48:1691.

Shen B, Achkar JP, Lashner BA, et al. Irritable pouch syndrome: a new category of diagnosis for symptomatic patients with ileal pouch-anal anastomosis. *Am J Gastroenterol* 2002;97:972.

Shen B, Fazio VW, Remzi FH, et al. Comprehensive evaluation of inflammatory and non-inflammatory sequelae of ileal pouch-anal anastomoses. *Am J Gastroenterol* 2005;100:93.

Shen B, Lashner B, Achkar JP, et al. Modified pouchitis disease activity index: a simplified approach to the diagnosis of pouchitis. *Dis Colon Rectum* 2003;46:748.

Wong KS, Remzi FH, Gorgun E, et al. Loop ileostomy closure after restorative proctocolectomy: outcome in 1504 patients. *Dis Colon Rectum* 2005;48:243.

EDITOR'S COMMENT

This procedure, which has become one of the standard procedures for ulcerative colitis, had its origins as early as the 1950s and with one report of what was an ileoanal anastomosis by Ravitch and Sabiston. For whatever reason, it did not catch on at that time, and it remained for several people to bring this into existence. Sir Alan Parks originated the S-pouch at St. Mark's Hospital, but the spout was too long, and these patients had difficulty with evacuation and had to catheterize themselves, the complication we still see when the efferent limb of the pouch is too long and needs to be shortened. The proper credit for the development of the operation as we now know it, at least as far as the S-pouch is concerned, belongs to Lester Martin, a brilliant pediatric surgeon and one of the last residents that Dr. Robert Gross trained. Lester, as he was called by everybody, was probably the best surgeon I have ever seen, and I have trained with and seen a lot of technically expert surgeons. He was truly ambidextrous, and was very good with either hand. He had a simple conception of operations, which often were very innovative, and he was a pleasure to work with. The first approach to ulcerative colitis was published in 1977, and there were several others since before one of our first series was put together and presented at the Southern Surgical in 1982 (Martin, Fischer JE. *Ann Surg* 1982;196:700). Whereas later in this commentary we will discuss a paper about a learning curve, when I came to Cincinnati, Lester was doing S-pouches single-handedly on both children and adults, and asked me if I'd be interested in working with him because he was uncomfortable taking care of the complications in adults. I agreed. The first operation we did was as a single team, and it

took 9 hours. I then suggested that we do it in two teams, with me doing the abdominal procedure for the most part, Lester doing the mucosectomy from below while I did the mucosectomy from above, and Lester doing the anastomosis. Once we started doing that, our time fell to about 3 hours and 15 minutes in young females, and a little longer in males. It was one of the high points of my professional life.

Essentially, the operation is done, or at least offered, to all patients with ulcerative colitis. As the authors detail, it may not be for everybody, depending on the circumstances. There is a group that has characteristics of both Crohn disease and ulcerative colitis, and a greater percentage of these patients, those with the so-called indeterminate colitis, finally show up with Crohn disease. However, with a good pathologist, this diagnosis should not occur in more than 10% to 15% of the patients. My impression, like that of Dr. Fazio's group, is that our patients with indeterminate colitis "did as well as" the patients with straightforward diagnosis of ulcerative colitis.

I once asked a resident who was in the lab if he would retrieve all of the indeterminate colitis diagnoses from our group of 400 patients that we had performed at that point. I then talked to Cecilia Fenoglia-Preiser, our chief of pathology and possibly the dean of gastrointestinal pathologists, and her response was that there is no such thing as indeterminate colitis, that there are only indeterminate pathologists. The review never got done. There was one characteristic of patients that basically told us that they probably had Crohn disease and we should stay away, and that was a history that was two perianal fistulas. In a previous version of this book, Professor Keighley suggested that there was a finite incidence of fistulas in ulcerative colitis, but I am not certain

this is the case because in this current edition, that statement is absent.

Regarding familial polyposis, in my own practice nowadays unless there is a carpet of polyps in the rectum or some of the other grave situations are present, such as severe dysplasia, it is my preference to do an ileorectal anastomosis and leave about 18 cm of rectum. I then fulgurate the polyps at 3-month intervals. For whatever reason, patients stop making polyps after an ileorectal anastomosis. I have never seen this fail. The question is, can they form cancers without first being polyps? Alvin Watne suggested that some of the kindreds in West Virginia had a cancer incidence of 34% following ileorectal anastomosis. I am not aware of any subsequent studies that suggest that this incidence is that high, and therefore I think with surveillance one can be safe in thinking that these patients will not form cancers. If patients have a previously established cancer in another part of the colon, the prognosis should be good, and ileorectal anastomosis is reasonable. I personally think that the outcome following ileorectal anastomosis may be as good as an ileal pouch-anal anastomosis, and therefore would go in the direction of something that was less complex.

Another indication for an ileal pouch-anal anastomosis is neuronal dysplasia, which is an adult form of Hirschsprung disease in which on pathology specimen there is a mass of disorganized fibers and no ganglia. These patients do quite well with an ileal pouch-anal anastomosis, or at least some of them do, probably those patients in which the disease has not totally affected the small bowel. For some reason, some of the patients have disease initially localized to the colon, but then the small bowel develops a motility disorder.

(continued)

Retention of the transitional zones is controversial. While almost all of the epithelium in the transitional zone is cuboidal, very much like the cuboidal epithelium of the transitional zone between columnar and squamous at the esophagogastric junction, there are obviously small nests of columnar epithelium that are subject to adenocarcinoma of the rectum. In truth, these remain quite rare. However, one can argue that it is now but 25 years since the initial operations were done in large numbers, and perhaps the wave of patients with anorectal carcinoma is yet to be seen.

I do think that when one is doing a mucosectomy from below, as portrayed in Figure 14, the Lone Star retractor offers better exposure than the four-suture technique, which is what I used to use but have since replaced it with the Lone Star retractor.

Intestinal obstruction is a problem, but I think it can be minimized by making certain that the bowel cannot loop around the ileostomy, which is one of the principal ways in which these patients get obstructed. I tend to sew individual loops of bowel to the anterior abdominal wall with fine silk, and thus wall off the right side of the abdomen, which theoretically should be empty from the left side, thus decreasing the incidence of intestinal obstruction. Our initial experience with intestinal obstruction was 22%, but after I started sewing the bowel both above and below the ileostomy to the anterior abdominal wall to prevent it from volvulizing, the incidence fell to 7%.

As opposed to the way the authors do their loop ileostomy, I do a formal divided Brooke ileostomy, oversewing the distal end so that it doesn't bleed since the staples are not necessarily hemostatic and we've had at least one episode of bleeding requiring six units, and sewing it to the underside of the ileostomy incision, in exactly the same place. I make certain that both the afferent and the efferent limbs of the ileostomy have a lot of slack, so for the closure one can circumscribe the ileostomy and, extending it slightly, find the other side of the loop on the distal segment and do a resection and anastomosis. I use a classical Brooke ileostomy because the appliance fits better than it does with the loop ileostomy, and there are some reports, initially at least, of loop ileostomies having a high incidence of complications.

The authors are correct in that pouchitis remains a difficult diagnosis to deal with. First, pouchitis is a syndrome; it is not a disease. It is a constellation of symptoms in which a previously well-functioning person with no diarrhea manifests watery diarrhea, which seemingly comes on suddenly. It may be associated with left lower quadrant pain, arthralgias malaise, and occasional fever. Quantitative cultures reveal a paucity of coliform organisms in a large number of patients, as compared to those patients who have done well and who are pair-matched for postoperative pouchitis. The biopsies were unrevealing; while the authors claim that biopsy reveals probably some of the worst patients from the standpoint of symptomatology of pouchitis, it also occurred in patients who were totally asymptomatic. The numbers of occurrence of pouchitis are not far off: of our total group of patients with pouchitis, approximately 18% had acute and chronic pouchitis, of which 12% were acute in that we treated them with only cyproflaxin, one tablet a day. Of the 18%, 6% were chronic and 12% had only one episode.

The problem of continence remains with us. Not being very strenuous in stretching the sphincter prior to doing the mucosectomy and during the anastomosis is extremely important. Continence to flatus takes the longest. I try to reassure patients that in time, they will be able to pass flatus without soiling. A good way to practice this is to assume the bird-dog position, that is, rear-end up and nose down, and practice. After approximately a year, patients are secure in their ability to pass flatus without soiling.

Tekkis et al. (*Ann Surg* 2005;241[2]:262) attempted to derive the learning curve for both senior staff and trainees by reviewing failed pouches. Of interest is the fact that the learning curve for trainees was 23, and for senior staff was 40. Only senior staff apparently did hand-sewn anastomoses and, in that group, the learning curve was 31. In my own situation, working with Dr. Lester Martin, I do not recall a learning curve, but then surgeons have very selective memories. We did lose a few pouches, but the only ones that I can remember were those with Crohn disease that we could not control. Larson et al. (*Dis Colon Rectum* 2005;48:1845) compared a relatively small series of 33 open and 33 laparoscopic ileal pouch-anal anastomoses. They found that the postoperative length of stay

was a little shorter in the laparoscopic group, with patients leaving the hospital in about 5.5 to 5.8 days. The control group, however, had a longer stay. Our own experience is that our open group, with a clinical pathway (Archer, et al. *Surgery* 1997; 122:699), also had a length of stay of about 5.8 days for those who adhered to the clinical pathway. The Cleveland Clinic in Florida had a postoperative length of stay of 5.8 days in a large number of patients (Ho KS, et al. *Colorectal Dis* 2005;8:235). In that paper, they also noted that age over 70 was not a contraindication to surgery, although the pouch loss was 12% in patients over 70 versus 1.2% in those under 70. This probably is significant, although not statistically so. In our own studies, a number of difficulties with septuagenarians had to do with extraneous factors, such as anxiety, loss of a mate, etc. Nonetheless, they do count as having to remove or leave the pouch in place, with permanent diversion.

A very pessimistic review of ileal pouch procedures and long-term follow-up has been proposed by Delaini et al. (*Technol Coloproctol* 2005;9:187) in which they questioned everything from long-term sepsis and loss of pouch to the risk of cancer formation, long-term complication rates, and pouchitis rates of 34% in the first year. I must say that they were so pessimistic that after reading it, I felt like crying. The only problem was that their experience is nothing like my own in doing 400 cases, especially as reviewed by Nussbaum (*Am J Surg* 2002;183:353). I do not know how they are doing the pouches or how they are selecting the papers that they quote. I would simply quote one of my great teachers, Dr. Robert Ritchie Linton, one of the early vascular surgeons, who said to me about vascular surgery: "You have to do it right."

Finally, Ozdogan et al. (*World J Surg* 2005; 29:1440) proposed that, in regard to chronic amebic colitis, it is possible that several patients qualified for the ileal pouch-anal anastomosis. In only two patients was the J-pouch constructed, and total colectomy and the Hartmann procedure performed in eight, with mild to moderate rectal involvement. They do propose that in time, these patients might be subject to ileal pouch-anal anastomosis with a successful outcome.

J.E.F

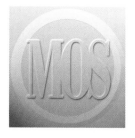

Introduction To Section On Colon Resections

JOSEF E. FISHER

As one reviews the colon resection section in the fourth edition of *Mastery of Surgery*, especially that of resection of rectal carcinomas, and compares it with this fifth edition, one notices a very substantial alteration in the attitudes of the authors. It is fair to say that in the fourth edition the focus seemed to be on cure of patients, particularly on the prevalence of the abdominal perineal resection in situations in which the lesion was below 5.5 cm from the anal verge. The statement concerning the actual length of

margin in carcinoma of the lower rectum was more or less absolute, and matched my own experience in patients who had had coloanal pull-throughs, in patients in whom the lesion was below 5.5 cm and for whom recurrence was seemingly inevitable.

All that has changed.

This section will emphasize preservation of rectal function, up to and including resection of segments of the internal sphincter in an effort to maintain long-term continence. The difference has been

the prevalence of neoadjuvant and postoperative chemoradiation therapy, much of it often focused, and, on occasion, localized brachytherapy. Whether the function is preserved to the extent that one is doing the patient a favor, and how much one sacrifices regarding long-term cure, remains in question. It is certainly clear that total mesenteric excision (Chapter 142) with a distal margin of 2 cm, or perhaps even 1 cm, has reasonable evidence to suggest that this is indeed a curative

The Gastrointestinal Tract

resection. The problem area probably is related to when one is performing intrasphincteric resection for preservation of function, and the extent of that function. In addition, neoadjuvant therapy very often leaves sphincters fibrotic, with inflammatory changes. The optimal time that resection and repair of the sphincter is reasonable—at 6 weeks, 8 weeks, 12 weeks, or longer—remains unresolved at present.

Suffice it to say that the emphasis from the fourth edition has been shifted to preservation of function. Whether the long-term gains of neoadjuvant or adjuvant therapy are first, curative, and second, provide sufficient preservation of function to make all of this worthwhile, is currently not clear.

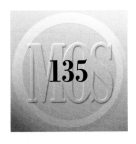

135

Laparoscopic Right, Left, Low Anterior, Abdominoperineal, and Total Colon Resections

MORRIS E. FRANKLIN JR, JORGE M. TREVIÑO, AND RICHARD L. WHELAN

INTRODUCTION

Approximately 130,000 new cases of colorectal cancer were diagnosed in 2000 in the United States, of which 75% occurred in people who have no predisposing risk factors. The remaining 25% occurred in patients with considerable risk factors compared with the general population. These risk factors are listed in Table 1.

Laparoscopic surgery has emerged as the procedure of choice for many intraabdominal disease processes. The earliest applications of laparoscopy, however, were primarily for diagnostic purposes. As surgical technology improved, more and more therapeutic interventions were developed. A large series of laparoscopic appendectomy was originally described by Semm in the early 1980s, though many surgeons remained skeptical of the value of this procedure. However, after the description of laparoscopic cholecystectomy by Mouret of France in 1987, and subsequent publications by Olsen and Reddick of the United States in 1988 as well as experience by B. McKernan, general surgeons took an active interest in learning diagnostic and therapeutic laparoscopy. The acceptance of laparoscopic cholecystectomy was quite rapid, fostering enthusiasm for additional applications for laparoscopy in the general surgical arena. Over the ensuing years, techniques for anti-reflux surgery, adrenalectomy, herniorrhaphy, splenectomy, hepatic resection, pancreatic surgery, and intestinal surgery have been developed.

One area that is of particular interest to surgeons is the role of laparoscopic colon surgery, which is now entering its second decade of practice. The first report in the literature was in 1990; since this early beginning, a multitude of investigators have confirmed the impressions of the early pioneers. This approach offers numerous advantages when compared with the open procedures, including less postoperative pain and ileus, reduced perioperative immunosuppression, decreased hospital stay, improved cosmesis, and earlier return to normal activity.

Controversy persists regarding the safety and efficacy of these minimally invasive procedures for the treatment of malignant disease, as well as whether they are appropriate in acute inflammatory or infectious processes. The equivalency in terms of length of the specimen, number of lymph nodes harvested, margins or resections, and adherence to oncologic principles has been well established by several authors. The issue of metastatic recurrence at the port site, first addressed in 1993 by Alexander et al., led many authors to back up and reconsidering using the laparoscopic technique in colorectal cancer. Some kept going and some prospective studies were begun, trying to show the feasibility and safeness of the laparoscopic technique for treatment of malignant disease of the colon. Recently, however, long-term reports have emerged with promising results; the Clinical Outcomes of Surgical Therapy (COST) Study Group was one of the first randomized, controlled trials to evaluate laparoscopic resections for colorectal cancer in the United States, and concluded that "the rates of recurrent cancer were similar after laparoscopically assisted colectomy and open colectomy suggesting that the laparoscopic approach is an acceptable alternative to open surgery for colon cancer." These and other results are encouraging and an emphasis on learning this surgery for the benefit of the patients is at hand.

PREOPERATIVE PREPARATION

This is a very important issue for a successful result in laparoscopic colon resection. A thorough history and physical examination with special emphasis on cardiac and pulmonary problems as well as previous surgeries are mandatory. The patient and the operating team must be adequately informed of the laparoscopic procedure. The patient should be informed that there is a possibility that the laparoscopic procedure may have to be converted to an open procedure. It is very important to perform a complete workup of the colon to allow the previous localization of the tumor by means of a barium enema, computed tomography (CT) scan, or colonoscopy when indicated. A baseline chemical profile including complete blood count, carcinoembryonic antigen (CEA), preoperative electrocardiogram, and chest radiograph should be performed as needed. Pulmonary function tests for patients with compromised respiratory function and additional tests for specific patients' problems are also in order. The bowel preparation must be modified from normal bowel preparation, as GoLYTELY frequently gives *inadequate* preparation and leaves *increased* fluid in the small bowel. The authors recommend 5 days prior to surgery a low-fiber diet, 3 days prior a full liquid diet, and 2 days prior clear liquids, adding 4 tablespoons of Milk of Magnesia in the middle of the day and another 4 tablespoons 6 hours later. The day prior to surgery we recommend continuing with clear liquids and adding neomycin (1 g PO q12h), erythromycin (500 mg PO q12h), magnesium citrate (60 mL PO q12h), and saline enema 8 hours previous to surgery.

TABLE 1. RISK FACTORS FOR COLON CANCER
Age more than 50 years
Colonic polyps
Family history of colorectal cancer
Familial colorectal cancer syndromes
Familial adenomatous polyposis
Hereditary nonpolyposis colon cancer
Ethnic background
History of colorectal cancer
History of intestinal polyps
Personal history of ulcerative colitis
Diet (lack of fiber intake, increased content of dietary fat)
Method of food preparation (deep frying, barbecuing, smoking food)
Physical inactivity
Obesity
Diabetes
Smoking
Alcohol intake
Occupational factors (dust inhalation, exposure to fumes, industrial employment)

TABLE 2. MONITOR POSITIONS	
Portion	**Monitors Placed**
Left, sigmoid, low anterior, or abdominoperineal resections	Monitor at the foot of the operating table
Left upper colon, splenic flexure, transverse colon, or hepatic flexure	Monitor toward the head of the table or at least at the level of the patient's shoulders
Cecum	Monitors at the foot of the table

ANESTHESIA

The cardiac and pulmonary status of the patient should be very carefully evaluated to ascertain the patient's ability to withstand a longer procedure and often a steep Trendelenburg position, with increased pressure on the diaphragm. Patients with extremely advanced chronic obstructive lung disease may not tolerate this well and reducing the CO_2 pressure will not appreciably reduce the pressure on the lungs. Placing an arterial line and central line in any patient undergoing laparoscopic colorectal surgery is also recommended, particularly in the presence of cardiac and/or pulmonary disease. Core temperature and CO_2 monitoring enables the anesthesiologist to identify the potential problems long before the patient has life-threatening arrhythmias or a decrease in blood pressure. Close discussion between the surgeon and the anesthesiologist is mandatory to prevent unsuspected problems and unwanted outcomes.

EQUIPMENT

Equipment required for laparoscopic surgery is basically the same as that required for laparoscopic cholecystectomy and advanced laparoscopic procedures, but recently staplers, ligation, and tissue handling devices have improved markedly. The equipment needed includes at least two monitors placed in accordance with the portion of the colon on which the operation is planned as shown in Table 2. No longer is the solitary stationary monitor used in laparoscopic cholecystectomy adequate; instead, it is highly recommended to have more than one monitor and that the monitors be mobile and can be moved from one position to another as the dissection proceeds. Many procedures, such as splenic flexure mobilization, transverse colon mobilization, and right hemicolectomy, are prolonged and require intense viewing by the surgeons and assistants, and a fixed monitor promotes fatigue, muscle spasm, and ultimately difficulties in the procedure. The operating table must allow for steep Trendelenburg positioning and for left and right tilting; additionally, anal access is frequently needed to ensure the endoscopic approach, and special staplers for lower resections, 0- and 30-degree scopes, a three-chip high-resolution video camera, and high-flow insufflator are very helpful. Trocars should be 5 mm, 10 mm, or universal 5/12 mm; these enhance the ability of a surgeon to place instruments of all sizes without changing reducers on the ports. A general rule is to "use as many trocars as needed." Generally, a half-circle around the target organ is the best setup for trocar placement. Standard graspers and special instruments including long bowel instruments, 5-mm laparoscopic scissors with cautery attachment, bipolar instrumentation, and those with cautery capabilities are needed, as are newer instruments for vessel control, such as the LigaSure coagulator (Valleylab, Boulder, CO). It is also important to have a harmonic scalpel (Ethicon, Cincinnati, OH) and argon beam available during all procedures to control excessive bleeding prior to its occurrence. Particularly effective suction and irrigation devices (5 mm and 10 mm) with extralong wands are recommended as well. Endo-GIA linear staplers with multiple reloads and circular intraluminal staplers of at least 28 mm in diameter and of appropriate width are in order. Clips may control smaller blood vessels; however, the authors prefer the use of LigaSure. Nevertheless, extracorporeal and intracorporeal knotting skills may be required. The availability of the colonoscope will aid in completing the procedure and testing the anastomosis as well as localization of small or occult lesions. An ultrasound device enhances evaluation of the liver as well as para-aortic nodes, and should be available in all cases. Other instruments include special dissectors to dissect and free individual vessels. Laparoscopic bulldog Glassman clamps for vascular and bowel content control are frequently helpful. An instrument table for opening of the patient also needs to be immediately available should encounters arise that could originate an open procedure.

Because of the technical nature of laparoscopic surgery, technique is everything. There is always an easy and a hard way to perform each kind of surgery. The purpose of this lecture is to demonstrate and discuss the indications, preparation, and technical tips the authors have found to be beneficial in the performance of laparoscopic colorectal surgery.

PATIENT POSITION AND PROTECTIVE DEVICES

Correct patient position can greatly enhance a laparoscopic procedure. A supine position with ready anal access with the legs slightly flexed, but not severely so, aided by Lloyd-Davis or Allen stirrups and the buttocks near the edge of the table is extremely helpful. The rectum can be elevated by placing the sacrum on a Gelfoam pad or tilting the rectum forward a slight amount. We have found that taping the patient about the shoulders without restricting the pulmonary function is a very adequate method of stabilizing the patient for the air-planning positional changes that will be needed; however, bean bags are also effective. Shoulder stripes or pads should be avoided as a sole means of preventing slippage as this can result in brachial plexus injury. It is also important to protect all exposed nerve surfaces, particularly those around the elbows and knees. The arms need to be secured by the patient's side to allow maximum tilt and mobility of the surgical team. Arms spread in the classic

The Gastrointestinal Tract

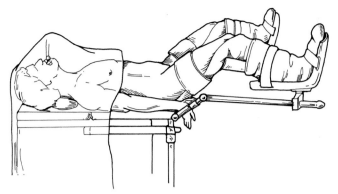

Fig. 1. Patient in Lloyd Davis modified position with anal access.

position may be an obstruction to movement around the operation table. Sequential compression devices are placed on the patient's legs to help avoid venous stasis and an increased risk of embolism. A warming blanket should be available to help prevent cooling of the patient, which may occur in longer procedures.

Provisions should be made for warming of intravenous fluid and irrigation fluids; the routine use of heparin (7,500 UI/Lt) in the irrigation fluid may be helpful in preventing large clots from forming as well as aiding in reducing tumor cell adhesion to instruments and trocars. With resections for cancer, povidone-iodine as an anticarcinogenic irrigation has been recommended to help reduce tumor cells and prevent tumor cell implantation on trocars and incisions.

Warming the inspired gas is strongly recommended, and many authors recommend also warming the CO_2, although no clear consensus is present for this. Wrapping the lower extremities in plastic bags is also recommended, and may prevent at least 1° temperature loss per hour in a 2-hour or longer procedure. (Fig. 1) A Foley catheter and a nasogastric tube are routinely inserted.

The surgeon should be positioned contralateral to the resection site with the camera holder in the same side; additional assistants may be placed between the legs for upper abdominal procedures or on the ipsilateral side for the right, sigmoid, and rectal procedures. (Fig. 2)

It is very important to emphasize that before embarking upon laparoscopic colon resection of any type, the surgeon should have a proper background in advanced laparoscopy that includes intracorporeal suturing, intra-/extracorporeal knot tying, good use of both hands, and experience with stapling devices to avoid unneeded conversions to open procedures. The surgeon and surgical team

should be thoroughly familiar with advanced laparoscopic techniques and have attended and practiced advanced laparoscopic colon resection techniques.

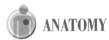 **ANATOMY**

Most surgeons are very familiar with the anatomy involved with virtually every type of colon resection performed. How-

ever, there is a different view of the anatomy with laparoscopy; while the anatomy does not change, the view through which the anatomy is seen does change. There are several critical areas that should be discussed in regard to anatomy; particularly important is the issue of the location of the ureters. It is the author's contention that the ureter should be identified very early in virtually every colon surgery, and the ureter should be used as a reference point whenever there is a doubt as to the anatomy during the course of the dissection. Avoidance of ureteral injuries is imperative and nonidentification of the ureters is an absolute indication to open as far as we are concerned. The duodenum should be clearly identified in transverse colon resection and right and total colectomies, and can be either as the colon is reflected inferiorly or through the mesenteric window of the hepatic flexure very early in this dissection. The spleen should be readily recognized, particularly with left colon resections, where the splenic flexure is mobilized. The middle

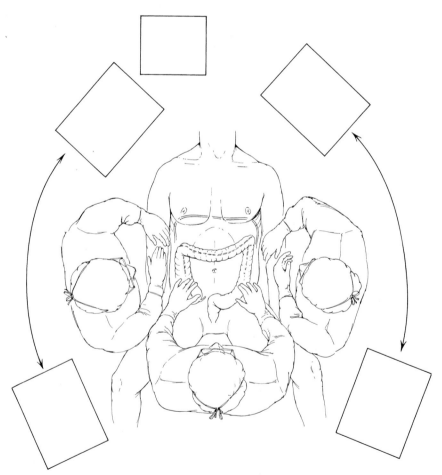

Fig. 2. Patient positioning and operating room setup. (Reprinted with permission from Fowler DL, Sonoda T, and McGinty JJ. "Laparoscopic Subtotal and Total Colectomy." In Mastery of Endoscopic and Laparoscopic Surgery 2e. Soper NJ, Swanstrom LL, Eubanks WS eds. Philadelphia: Lippincott Williams & Wilkins, 2005.)

hemorrhoidal vessels are frequently more clearly seen with laparoscopic surgery than with traditional open surgery. The key in recognizing the anatomy is if you get lost or if the camera is too close, back up, identify the anatomy that is clearly evident, and then work back down to the area in question. One useful key is indeed the ureter, and backing up to the ureter and tracing it down to an area where the anatomy becomes unclear almost inevitably will result in the recognition of the anatomy in this area.

MOBILIZATION

It is very important during the mobilization to use gravity to an advantage rather than a disadvantage. Frequent use of the Trendelenburg position, and often severe, reverse Trendelenburg, left and right tilt, can allow visualization and mobilization of almost any segment of the colon with much less effort than with nonuse of gravity. The table needs to allow left and right tilt as well as steep and nonsteep Trendelenburg. When grasping fat and the colon itself, we recommend the use of blunt instruments such as Glassman clamps and nonsharp Babcock clamps in colon mobilization. The scissors need to be sharp and allow electrocautery capability. We also prefer to push the colon and other organs out of the way rather than pull, as pulling, particularly with torquing, tends to injure the colon and other organs. We avoid very meticulously grasping the bowel that is not to be resected and very carefully avoid grasping the tumor in cancer cases. Blunt dissection is always better than sharp dissection unless one can actually see through the tissue being dissected. Remember, if you cannot see what are you dissecting, change the lens or the position of the lens until you can cleanly delineate what is being dissected.

SPECIMEN HANDLING AND REMOVAL

The specimen needs to be isolated as quickly as possible with stapling devices or with Endoloops (Ethicon Endo-surgery, Cincinnati, OH) around the proximal and distal segments of bowel prior to placing the segment of the colon in a bag. We try to avoid very hard direct manipulation of a tumor site when using laparoscopic surgery for cancer. We use a special bag for specimen removal, whether it is transanal or transabdominal. We believe that this prevents contamination, not only with stool but also with tumor cells in cases of

colon cancer. When we try to remove a large specimen through the rectum and in case of benign disease, we can cut the specimen into several smaller pieces, taking care to preserve the colon intact but debulk the omentum and pericolonic fat from a given specimen. This resulted in a successful rate of transanal removal without anal malfunction.

SPECIMEN REMOVAL

If the specimen is benign, it can be mobilized and delivered through the wound very easily, even unbagged.

Right Hemicolectomy

 INDICATIONS

The surgical treatment of diseases of the right colon has evolved dramatically over the past few years, particularly related to laparoscopy for these procedures of colon surgery. There have been few descriptions of the operative technique for laparoscopic colon resection, but a safe, time-efficient, and complication-free procedure should be performed. While there is a

staggering amount of literature focusing on laparoscopic surgery of the distal colon, there is a paucity of such regarding right-sided lesions approached laparoscopically. The reason for this relative underrepresentation is unclear.

The cecum and the ascending colon, along with the right mesocolon, are the most easily exposed segments of the colon during the laparoscopic approach, which allows for a very easy mobilization of the right colon (Fig. 3). The indications of a right hemicolectomy include adenomatous polyps not suitable by colonoscopy, inflammatory bowel disease, bleeding of arteriovenous malformations, obstruction, Crohn disease (and complications), ulcerative colitis, and any other condition suitable for resection. Based upon the recent reports in management of colon cancer, malignant disease can be performed safely including palliative resection for incurable carcinoma and potentially curable entities.

 SURGICAL TECHNIQUE

The patient is placed under general anesthesia and monitoring lines (central venous pressure, arterial pressure, pulse oximetry, electrocardiogram, blood pressure cuff, esophageal thermometer) are

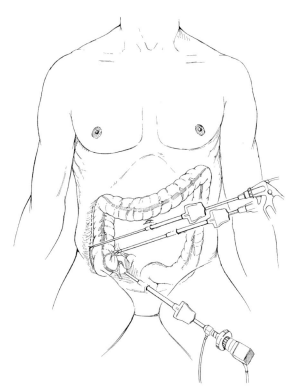

Fig. 3. Setup for dissection of the cecum and ascending colon. (Reprinted with permission from Fowler DL, Sonoda T, and McGinty JJ. "Laparoscopic Subtotal and Total Colectomy". In Mastery of Endoscopic and Laparoscopic Surgery 2e. Soper NJ, Swanstrom LL, Eubanks WS eds. Philadelphia: Lippincott Williams & Wilkins, 2005.)

The Gastrointestinal Tract

placed and secured as needed. A warm-air upper body warming device is laid across the patient's chest and arms to help prevent hypothermia. An orogastric suction tube, a urinary bladder catheter, and lower extremity pneumatic compression stockings are used in all cases.

The patient is placed in the modified lithotomy position, with the hips and knees slightly flexed to facilitate use of the flexible colonoscope intraoperatively and/or the placement of an assistant between the legs. The patient's arms are tucked at the side, and the shoulders are securely taped to the operating table to allow for the placement of the patient in steep Trendelenburg or air-planning as needed to aid in visualization.

After prepping and draping the patient in sterile fashion, the surgeon and the camera operator stand to the patient's left side, and the first assistant stands opposite them. A mobile video monitor is placed opposite the umbilicus to the patient's right side, and another to the left, usually at the left shoulder to ensure that the entire surgical team has good visibility.

Pneumoperitoneum is established by use of the Veress needle or Hassan technique, and the abdomen is insufflated with carbon dioxide gas to a pressure of 13 to 14 mm Hg. In most cases the Veress needle is placed in the left lower quadrant; however, an alternate site (upper midline, left upper

quadrant) is often selected in patients who have had prior abdominal surgery. Following adequate insufflation, a 5/12-mm port is placed and the 10-mm 0-degree video laparoscope is inserted. The abdomen is thoroughly inspected for signs of metastatic diseases or other disease processes, which may alter the anticipated procedure. Adhesions to the anterior abdominal wall are taken down carefully in a stepwise fashion, and the rest of the working ports are placed under direct visualization. The final configuration shows a 5-mm port in the upper midline, a 10-mm port in the right lower quadrant at the McBurney's point, another 5mm port in the left mid abdomen, and a 5-mm port at the umbilicus. (Fig. 4) Occasionally, additional ports may be placed in the left upper and right upper quadrants as needed (once placed, the trocars are secured to the abdominal wall with a suture to prevent dislodgement).

Once all trocars are placed and the diseased segment is identified, a careful "no-touch" technique for the tumor is rigidly enforced. Two options are available for right colon dissection (lateral-to-medial or medial-to-lateral dissection). In the case of lateral-to-medial dissection, the terminal ileum and cecum are mobilized first, followed by the ascending colon along the white line of Toldt. The mobilization is accomplished using medial and upward traction of the colon with a Babcock grasper

and mobilizing the abdominal wall attachments by sharp dissection with or without cautery, then continuing to the hepatocolic ligament including the gastrocolic ligament. When the right ileocolic ligament is approached, care must be taken to identify the right ureter and avoid injury should the terminal ileum be mobilized from its peritoneal attachments. Gravity is a very helpful tool to facilitate organ retraction, but manipulation and grasping of the bowel should be avoided except in special cases. We recommend grasping the mesentery or peritoneum to avoid unnecessary injury to the bowel or spread of tumoral cells in cases of colon cancer. If an injury to the wall of the intestine is eventuated during the mobilization (tearing, burning, etc.), it is recommended to repair with seromuscular inverting sutures immediately as this may not be found later. In the case of a lesion to the resected specimen, this can be closed with an Endoloop or any kind of suture with simple stitches, since it will be removed shortly.

The hepatic flexure and proximal transverse colon as far as needed are freed to ensure adequate distal margins and a tension-free anastomosis. Following this, the duodenum is identified behind the colon, and a window is created in the mesentery. (Fig. 5) At this point, this mesentery thickness should be one layer and should be expanded inferiorly to identify the colic vessels, immediately caudal to this opening. The ileocolic artery can be divided with staples, ligation, clips, or a coagulator device such as the harmonic scalpel or the LigaSure device. It is helpful to retract the mesentery of the ileocecal complex anteriorly, opposite the root of the mesentery, which will tent up, and the ileocolic vessels should be reactively mobile. Progressive dissection to the terminal ileum may be carried out with sharp dissection with scissors and controlling bleeding or with the use of the above-mentioned coagulation devices. Immediately superior to the duodenum is the right colic vessel either as a solitary branch or as a branch of the middle colic artery; this should be divided if a wide resection is needed.

At this point, patients who are to undergo totally intracorporeal anastomosis should have laparoscopic division of the colon at the distal end of the mesenteric window. This may be performed using the endoscopic stapling device after inspection of the region to ensure that an adequate blood supply is present (Fig. 6). The omentum is properly divided along the avascular plane between the omentum and the colon. This may be divided with

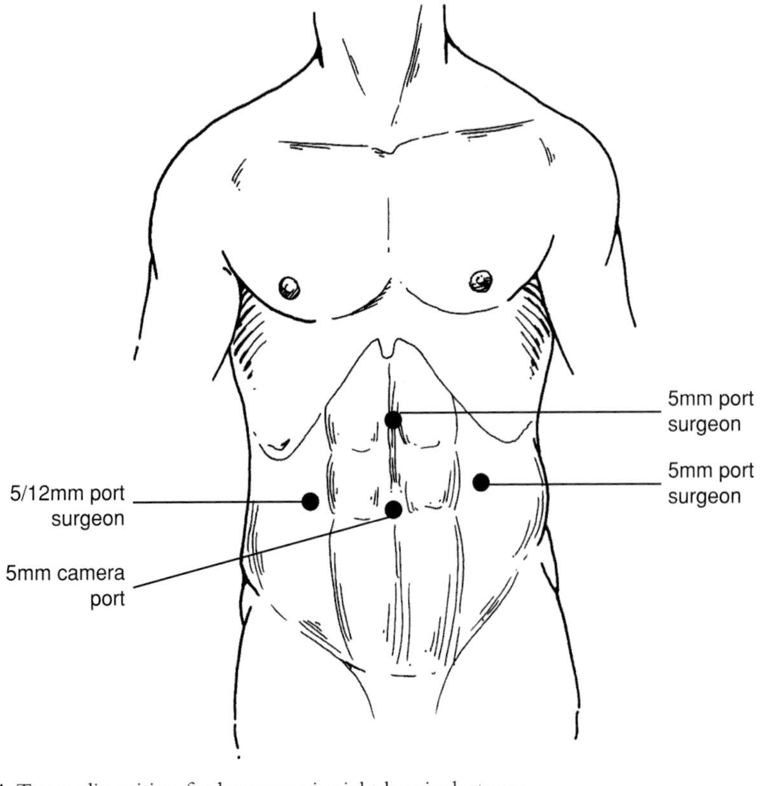

5mm port
surgeon

5mm port
surgeon

5/12mm port
surgeon

5mm camera
port

Fig. 4. Trocar disposition for laparoscopic right hemicolectomy.

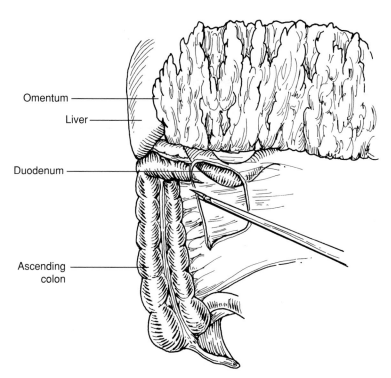

Omentum

Liver

Duodenum

Ascending
colon

Fig. 5. Medial to lateral dissection, with identification of the duodenum.

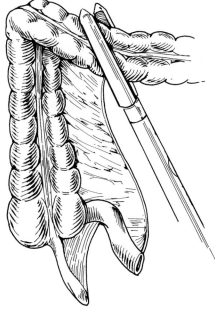

Fig. 6. Distal resection utilizing a laparoscopic linear stapler.

The Gastrointestinal Tract

the harmonic scalpel, LigaSure device, or scissors. The terminal ileum is divided at the desired level and the specimen is then placed in a large specimen bag, which is sealed and stored above the liver for extraction after intestinal continuity is restored. An ileotransverse colostomy is then constructed with the endoscopic stapling device in the following manner. First, a small enterotomy is made on the antimesenteric border of the colon at the edge of the previous staple line. This is then drawn over the staple side of the staples and held in place while this maneuver is repeated on the ileum side; while placing the anvil care must

be taken to ensure proper orientation of the bowel, and continuous checking of the mesentery protects the small bowel from rotation and ensures that the mesentery is not twisted. With the colon drawn over the lower jaw of the stapler and the terminal ileum in a similar position on the upper jaw, the stapler is closed, fired, and removed, creating a 6-cm anastomosis; if a longer anastomosis is required, a second firing could be performed in the same fashion (Fig. 7a). An additional firing of the stapler across the opening seals the enterotomy. (Fig. 7b) A laparoscopic hernia stapler may be used to repair the rent in the mesentery

if desired, but over the past 10 years this step has all but completely been abandoned. Next, a clamp is applied to the terminal ileum, utilizing intestinal bulldogs or handheld Glassman clamps. An intraoperative colonoscopy is performed to ensure that the target lesion has been removed, to inspect for synchronous lesions, and to check the anastomosis for leakage; in the eventual case of a leak, this should be repaired immediately. Colonoscopy is carried out prior to specimen transection in patients who present emergently and have therefore not undergone routine preoperative evaluation, or in any instance where the location of the target lesion is in question. Next, the right

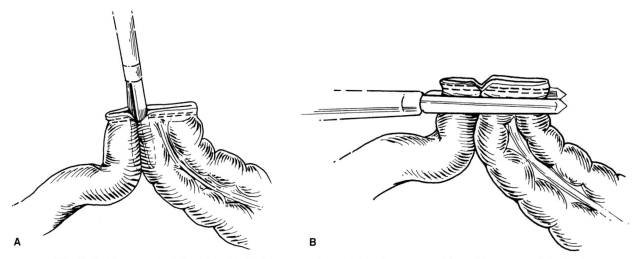

Fig. 7. A: Linear stapler is introduced in both enterotomies, and is fired to create a side to side anastomosis. **B:** Both enterotomies are closed using a new firing of the stapler.

lower quadrant trocar site (or alternate site selected for specimen extraction) is enlarged to 3 to 5 cm, and after placing a wound protector, the specimen is removed and the wound closed. The abdomen is then inspected a final time, with particular attention paid to previously inadverted lesion, leaks, and the integrity of the anastomosis. Thorough irrigation with dilute (3.5%) povidone-iodine solution is then performed to wash the anastomosis and all port sites and trocars. This is followed by saline irrigation and aspirating of all remaining fluid from the peritoneal cavity. Transfascial sutures are placed under direct visualization using the Carter-Thomason suture passer at all trocar sites greater than 5 mm. The insufflator is turned off and the pneumoperitoneum is released through the trocars while still in place, to further help prevent the "slosh phenomenon" of malignant cell migration. The trocars are then removed, and the fascial sutures are tied down securely without allowing fluid to pass into the trocar sites. Skin closure is accomplished with sutures or staples as desired.

For patients who are to undergo extracorporeal anastomosis, after mobilization of the terminal ileum, a right flank or midline incision is extended to a length of 3 to 5 cm. A wound protector is placed, and the specimen is delivered through the wound. The resection is completed either sharply or with a stapling device, and a handsewn or stapled ileotransverse colostomy is created. Again, proper orientation of the respective segments must be maintained by clamping or suturing the colon and small bowel. The anastomosis is then returned to the abdominal cavity, and after intraoperative colonoscopy, the final steps of the procedure are carried out as outlined above. This is the best opportunity to double-check for the integrity of the anastomosis limits.

Postoperatively, all patients have the orogastric tube removed when bowel sounds are present, usually postoperative day 1, and are allowed to have ice chips. On the second postoperative day patients are started on a clear liquid diet, and bladder catheters are routinely discontinued at this time. Diet is advanced as tolerated. The patients are discharged from the hospital when they have return of bowel function, can tolerate a regular diet, and have adequate pain control with oral analgesics.

Laparoscopic and hand-assisted left and sigmoid colectomy

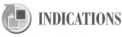 **INDICATIONS**

Indications for laparoscopic left and sigmoid colectomy are identical to the indications for open colectomy. Laparoscopy has

evolved into the preferred method for performing colectomy for most benign conditions. With regard to malignancy, results from randomized, prospective trials suggest that the laparoscopic method, in experienced hands, yields results that are at least equivalent, from an oncologic perspective, to traditional open methods. Factors that may hinder a laparoscopic approach include severe adhesions from prior abdomino-pelvic operations or inflammatory processes, cardiopulmonary insufficiency, morbid obesity, and cancer invading other structures.

PORT PLACEMENT

For left colon resections and sigmoidectomy, the Verres needle is placed in the right lower quadrant. In cases of colectomy for a polyp or tumor, an effort should be made after placing the first two or three ports to identify the lesion prior to placing additional ports as an unexpected location may alter port placement. At this time the abdomen should be surveyed for further pathology and metastatic disease and the feasibility of a laparoscopic resection should be addressed.

Attention to the inferior epigastric vessels during lateral port placement is important. If the operative plan calls for a Pfannenstiel incision to exteriorize the colon, it may be helpful to place a suprapubic port through a small transverse incision that can be extended later. This suprapubic port facilitates recto-sigmoid transection with a laparoscopic linear stapler. If a hand port is utilized, the trocar sites should be positioned at a sufficient distance from the "footprint" of the hand device such that the ports can be maximally utilized with the hand inside. For a left-sided colectomy, the hand port is usually placed through a Pfannenstiel or an inferior midline incision.

DISSECTING THE VASCULAR PEDICLE AND MOBILIZING THE COLON

There are three basic approaches to mobilization of the left colon and sigmoid mesentery. Medial-to-lateral mobilization can be carried out starting at the base of the rectosigmoid mesentery on the right side at the level of the sacral promontory. Lateral-to-medial mobilization usually starts at the level of the left iliac fossa or the descending colon. The third approach is to mobilize the inferior mesenteric vein (IMV) and the IMA in a medial to lateral direction starting at the IMV at the level of the ligament of Treitz.

Medial-to-Lateral Mobilization Starting at Sacral Promontory

This method begins at the level of the sacral promontory at the base of the rectosigmoid colon on the right side. The surgeon stands on the patient's right side and operates through the two right-sided ports. Exposure is facilitated by Trendelenburg positioning in order to retract the small bowel out of the pelvis. The IMA is exposed by grasping the sigmoid colon mesentery and elevating it cephalad, anterior, and to the left. With this exposure, it is possible to visualize the right ureter at the pelvic brim lateral to the area of interest. Palpate the sacral promontory to orient the pelvic inlet at the midline. Next the peritoneum is scored just dorsal to the main sigmoidal vessels at the level of the sacral promontory and carried into the pelvis a short distance. This plane runs transversely across the operative field. Typically an avascular plane can be entered dorsal to the sigmoid vessels. Develop a working space such that the sigmoid mesocolon is reflected ventrally and the retroperitoneum is pushed dorsally. The left gonadal vessels and ureter are identified from the right side of the pelvis. The gonadal vessels lie lateral to the ureter at this level. Keep in mind that the left psoas tendon can be confused for the ureter and if it is seen, signifies the dissection plane is too dorsal. If the ureter is not identified running along the floor of the dissection, the mesocolon should be inspected to determine if the ureter was reflected up during dissection. In this situation, carefully dissect the ureter down off the mesentery. The ureter must be clearly identified and protected prior to transecting the vascular pedicle when using the medial to lateral approach, because this mobilization leaves the peritoneal attachments of the left iliac fossa in place until later in the operation. If the ureter is not confidently visualized from the right side, then a standard lateral to medial dissection starting at the left iliac fossa should commence. If the ureter is still not visualized, then a hand port to help with the dissection or convert to an open approach is indicated.

The hypogastric nerves run in a superior to inferior direction dorsal to the superior hemorrhoidal artery. The plane of dissection used in medial to lateral mobilization of the mesentery stays immediately dorsal to this vessel in order to preserve the nerves.

The window beneath the sigmoid colon mesentery is enlarged by scoring the peritoneum at the base of the mesentery in the cephalad direction. This dissection will expose the origin of the IMA. If a high ligation is to be performed, the IMA is divided cephalad taking care not to injure the IMV. At this level, the course of the IMV diverges from the IMA and runs cephalad, parallel to the aorta.

If the superior hemorrhoidal artery is to be preserved then the proximal sigmoidal branches are dissected to allow individual ligation at their origin from the main vessel. The benefit to preserving the superior hemorrhoidal artery (leaving the rectum with a better blood supply) should be weighed against the risks of a more technically challenging dissection. When operating on patients with a post-inflammatory or otherwise foreshortened mesentery it may be prudent to avoid dissecting out the individual mesenteric vessels and to, instead, transect the main sigmoid vessels as for a cancer.

By taking the vascular pedicle as described above, the surgeon can then extend the retro-mesenteric plane and mobilize the descending colon. The plane of dissection for medial to lateral mobilization of the left colon is defined by the retroperitoneum dorsally, the mesentery of the sigmoid and descending colon ventrally, the aorta and its colonic branches medially, and the lateral peritoneal attachments along the left paracolic gutter. Elevation of the sigmoid colon mesentery with one instrument allows the use of a second instrument (or the fingers of the hand) to bluntly push the retroperitoneum posteriorly (including the ureter and gonadal vessels) to further develop the retro-mesenteric plane, which can be carried laterally as far as the abdominal sidewall and cephalad over Gerota's fascia towards the splenic flexure. This plane is relatively bloodless and can usually be dissected bluntly. If bleeding is encountered, it is usually because the plane of dissection has strayed ventrally into the mesentery or dorsally into Gerota's fascia. When the medial to lateral mobilization is complete, the final step is to divide the remaining lateral peritoneal attachments which are usually quite thin. If the left-sided pelvic peritoneal attachments have not yet been divided, they can be dealt with at this point.

Lateral-to-Medial Mobilization

The alternative to the various medial-to-lateral approaches is the lateral-to-medial mobilization of the left colon, which is the traditional approach that is used for open colectomy by most surgeons. With this approach, colon mobilization precedes ligation of the vascular pedicle. The sigmoid colon mesentery is retracted medially and the lateral peritoneal attachments are divided. As the colon is mobilized towards the midline, the colon is elevated up off the underlying

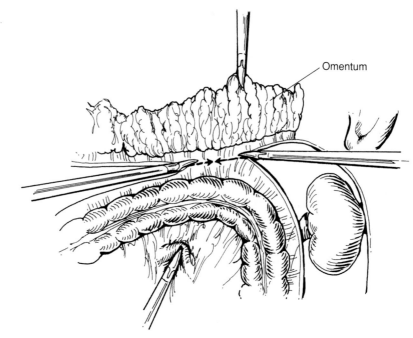

Fig. 8. Identify the ureter during medial to lateral dissection and continue the dissection toward the splenic flexure.

retroperitoneal structures. To identify and preserve the left ureter and gonadal vessels, continue the dissection up the left paracolic gutter towards the splenic flexure. Once the sigmoid colon is completely medialized and the crucial retroperitoneal structures are identified, the operation can proceed with identification and division of the vascular pedicle as previously detailed. (Fig. 8) One disadvantage to this approach is the loss of the natural retraction provided by the lateral attachments of the sigmoid colon.

To complete the descending colon portion of the splenic flexure mobilization, once the above steps have been accomplished, the patient is placed in the reverse Trendelenburg position with the right side down. The descending colon is retracted anteriorly and medially to expose the more proximal lateral attachments which are divided. Care is taken to find the correct plane between the colon mesentery and the anterior aspect of Gerota's fascia. If possible, at this time, the attachments between the spleen and the colon are carefully exposed and divided. If this proves too difficult, it is advised to shift attention to the transverse colon, enter the lesser sac and then approach the flexure from the transverse colon perspective.

Mobilizing the descending colon lateral to medial using hand-assisted methods is best accomplished with the surgeon standing between the legs with left hand in the abdomen retracting the descending colon medially and the right hand working via a left-sided port.

Medial-to-Lateral Mobilization Starting at the IMV

Beginning at the level of the ligament of Treitz, this dissection identifies and isolates the IMA, IMV, and left colic artery, and mobilizes the proximal descending colon off of the retroperitoneum. Using this method, it is possible to divide the left colon blood supply early in the case either at the IMA level or just distal to the left colic takeoff from the main trunk. In addition, the splenic flexure mobilization can also be completed rapidly and early in the case by separating the omentum from the distal transverse colon after completing the medial to lateral dissection.

For this dissection the patient is placed in the reverse Trendelenburg position with the right side tilted downward and the left-sided monitor is placed off the patient's left shoulder. The surgeon and the camera holder stand on the patient's right side with the first assistant positioned between the patient's legs. The first assistant grasps the distal transverse mesocolon via the upper left port and lifts cephalad and anteriorly while also retracting the proximal descending colon to the left via the lower left port, revealing the left colic artery running vertically or obliquely in the mesentery. The surgeon exposes the ligament of Treitz and the IMV by retracting the proximal small bowel to the right. The IMV is usually easily identified running parallel to the aorta at the base of the mesentery. The dissection begins by scoring the base of the descending colon mesentery for several centimeters either just dorsal or ventral to the IMV parallel to the IMV. The correct plane is bloodless. The most common error is to enter too deeply, so that the anterior aspect of Gerota's fascia is dissected off of the kidney. Dissection in this plane can result in bleeding. Once the correct plane has been established, the dissection is continued laterally beneath the mesentery and colon of the splenic flexure. The cephalad border of the dissection is the caudal edge of the pancreas. Vigorous retraction during this dissection can injure the marginal artery of the mesentery which can compromise the blood supply to the colon.

The same retromesenteric dissection plane is established and developed laterally after which the flimsy attachments separating the two retroperitoneal spaces are divided. Once completed, the proximal vascular division can be carried out at either the IMA or just distal to the left colic takeoff as described earlier.

Hand-Assisted Mobilization and Devascularization

The hand port can be used in several ways to accomplish this task. The surgeon, standing on the patient's right with the camera operator, places his right hand into the abdomen and utilizes a right-sided port to operate with his left hand. With the hand, retract of the sigmoid mesocolon to the left and cephalad to tent the IMA pedicle and visualize the infrasigmoidal sulcus on the right side. Score the peritoneum at the base of the mesentery and carry out the medial to lateral dissection as described above. A retromesenteric plane is created by using the fingers of the intra-abdominal hand to bluntly separate the mesentery from the retroperitoneum while the IMA pedicle is elevated with the left-handed instrument. An alternative approach is to have the first assistant, on the patient's left side, place a hand in the abdomen and use it to retract the sigmoid colon anterior and cephalad. The surgeon, standing on the right side, performs the dissection as described earlier. The intraabdominal hand can also be used to palpate and dissect once the plane of dissection has been established. Lastly, it is also possible to mobilize and devascularize without using a hand through the hand port. However, it makes sense to take advantage of the hand port access.

DISTAL TRANSECTION OF THE BOWEL

The distal margin is created by using the endoscopic stapler to transect the bowel,

assuring that the ureter and gonadal vessels are not in the vicinity of the instrument. Roticulating linear staplers and/or a suprapubic port for the linear stapler can facilitate division of the rectosigmoid. In cases where bowel transection requires more than one staple load, sequential staplers should be fired through the apex of the prior staple line in a plane perpendicular to the lumen. If the anatomy and mobilization are such that the stapler cannot be oriented in this plane, an arrow configuration is an acceptable alternative. A jagged or "crown" type staple configuration should be avoided because the resulting dog-ears may have an inadequate blood supply.

EXTERIORIZATION OF THE BOWEL

The extraction site can be made in a variety of locations. Some surgeons prefer to extend one of the port site incisions while others make a new and separate incision. One option is to transversely extend one of the left-sided port wounds. An alternative is to make either a suprapubic Pfannenstiel or low midline incision. Finally, some surgeons choose to enlarge the periumbilical port site. There are advantages and disadvantages for each location. A drawback to extending a lateral port incision is that should it become necessary to repair a leak at the anastomosis using open methods, an additional midline incision may be required. Meanwhile, exteriorizing through a low midline incision or a short Pfannenstiel incision usually requires an additional incision but allows better access to the pelvis and anastomosis. In cases in which a hand port has been utilized, the colon is exteriorized through this port.

Once an appropriate incision is made, a wound protector is used to help prevent tumor cell implantation and possibly reduce the risk of post-operative wound infection. In hand-assisted cases, the hand port may serve as the wound protector and does not need to be removed. With the wound protector in place, the mobilized colon is brought up to the skin incision using a previously placed anchor (i.e. a preformed loop tie or a locked laparoscopic grasping instrument). The colon is grasped through the incision and exteriorize it using a gentle rocking motion.

The exteriorized colon is then ready to be transected and delivered off the field. In the case of sigmoid colectomy the distal division will already have been done intracorporeally leaving only the proximal division to be done extracorporeally. For segmental resection of the descending colon it is likely that both the proximal and distal bowel transections will be done extracorporeally.

In either case, the point(s) of transection is chosen based on the desired surgical margin and the pathology in question. Quarantine the operative field to contain gross contamination, transect the bowel, and remove the specimen from the field.

For sigmoid colectomy, the size of the largest circular stapler that will fit into the cut end of the colon is determined and a full-thickness purse string is placed in the colon; the suture is secured around the anvil of the circular stapler. For segmental resection of the descending colon, extracorporeal anastomosis of the two ends of the colon is performed using open methods.

INTRACORPOREAL ANASTOMOSIS

For laparoscopic-assisted sigmoidectomy, replace the colon with the anvil in place into the abdomen, remove the wound protector, and close the fascia at the site of exteriorization. This method reestablishes pneumoperitoneum and provides easy access to the abdomen should the need arise. Reinsufflate, place the patient in the Trendelenburg position, and bring the proximal colon with the anvil into the pelvis. If it is difficult to locate the end of the colon, identify the cut edge of the mesentery and follow it back to the anvil.

Gently dilate the anus and pass the circular stapler up to the linear staple line in the rectum. To facilitate seating of the stapler, manipulate the rectum and the stapler so that the head of the stapler crowns appropriately at the linear staple line. Next, open the stapler and drive the trocar through the rectal wall. If necessary, separate and retrieve the pin. Confirm the colon is not twisted by inspecting the cut edge of the mesentery and by following the tenia libera. Join the anvil with the stapler and fire the stapler. Examine the two anastomotic rings and evaluate the integrity of the anastomosis under saline while occluding the descending colon proximally and gently insufflating the rectum.

In hand-assisted cases, the anastomosis may be performed with or without a pneumoperitoneum. Intracorporeal anastomosis is the authors' preference when feasible. In this case, the pneumoperitoneum is reestablished and the anastomosis performed intracorporeally with laparoscopic visualization as described above.

Laparoscopic Approach to Rectal Lesions

The approach to rectal cancer could be performed in two different ways: Low anterior resection and abdominoperineal resection. Which method to use depends on the localization of the tumor: The abdominoperineal resection (APR) is often performed for distal rectal cancer and is indicated for proctectomy for severe irritable bowel disease; lesions in the upper third of the rectum are treated with a low anterior resection (LAR) and primary anastomosis. The treatment of the carcinomas located in the middle and lower thirds of the rectum remains somewhat controversial. Local excision is an option to be considered in less than 5% of the population with carcinoma of the rectum. Such therapy is limited to patients with a small, mobile, well-differentiated lesion and no invasive tumors and with a normal CT scan and normal CEA levels. Salvatti et al. have reported electrocoagulation as another option to treat rectal cancer with an overall 5-year survival of 47%, with the best results in tumors of 4 cm or less in diameter. The most recommended treatment of rectal cancer is the surgical resection of the primary tumor and regional lymph nodes for localized disease. Local failure rates in the range of 4% to 8% following rectal resection with appropriate mesorectal excision (total mesorectal excision for low/middle rectal tumors and mesorectal excision at least 5 cm below the tumor for high rectal tumors) have been reported. On the other hand, the standard approach for lower rectal cancers is the abdominoperineal resection, first reported by Miles in 1908, the rationale being that after resection of the tumor, there is insufficient bowel remaining for re-establishment of intestinal continuity. In the abdominoperineal resection a double approach is employed, abdominal and perineal, often with two operative teams working simultaneously. The procedure chosen for midrectal carcinoma depends on different variables, the decision often not being made until during the procedure depending on the size of the tumor, localization, invasion, etc. If the lesion can be palpated easily on rectal examination, abdominoperineal resection is indicated (this is approximated at 3 to 7 cm from the anal verge). If at the time of the resection the remaining rectum is enough to perform an anastomosis, a low anterior resection could be safely performed.

Generally abdominoperineal resection is required for lesions distal to 7 to 8 cm from the anal verge. For lesions above 12 cm, anterior resection perhaps is always done. For lesions between 8 and 12 cm, the procedure may depend on the above-mentioned factors.

The approach to the tumor for a low anterior resection is similar to that used in abdominoperineal resection, including removal of ischiorectal fat and sigmoid mesentery and rectal mobilization to the level of the levator ani muscles. The low anterior resection with primary anastomosis below the level of the peritoneal reflection is completed if the distal margin is clear and enough rectal tissue is viable to perform an end-to-end anastomosis safely. However, if the surgeon believes that anastomosis cannot be completed safely, an abdominoperineal resection is recommended. The extent of the resection should not be affected by an understandable desire to preserve the anal sphincter.

A variety of special techniques have been proposed for use with resection of carcinoma of the colon and rectum. The laparoscopic approach adds a new exciting dimension to the treatment of colonic disease. Recently it has been demonstrated to be equivalent to open procedures in cancer, and it is gaining widespread acceptance; we firmly believe in all the benefits of the minimally invasive approach.

The indications for laparoscopic anterior resection are various and can be divided into benign and malignant. Benign includes complicated diverticulitis and prior complicated injuries to the rectum from different sources. Segmental Crohn disease and chronic volvulus, and in some cases colonic inertia, are also indications of low anterior resection. Malignant includes carcinoma of the rectum with or without previous radiotherapy, recurrent polyp carcinoma disease nonresponsive to transanal resection, and large villous adenomas and adenomatous polyps. APR includes epidermoid anal canal carcinoma not responsive to other means of treatment (radiotherapy, chemotherapy), recurrent adenocarcinoma after prior low anterior resection, or large carcinomas in the distal rectum.

The contraindications are numerous but related, primarily to expertise of the surgeon, anatomic considerations, and presence of concurrent or advanced disease. In our experience all patients are considered for laparoscopic surgery until it is shown that anatomic reasons preclude the laparoscopic procedure.

 SURGICAL TECHNIQUE

The operating room setup and trocar placement are the same for APR and LAR. It is very important place the trocar strategically to allow good mobilization of the sigmoid, rectum, and anus, as well as the potential need for splenic flexure mobilization and creation of an anastomosis and/or colostomy. We use the operating room disposition, with the surgeon on the left side of the patient and the assistant contralateral; usually we use five 5/12-mm trocars (two trocars for the surgeon and two trocars for the assistant). The camera is almost always placed at the umbilicus, although alternative sites may be used as needed.

We preferably use smooth trocars and avoid the screw-in type; these are secured to the abdominal wall to prevent dislodgement and the so-called "chimney effect" whereby possibly aerosolized viable tumor cells could pass through the naked skin edges and become adherent to the soft tissues, thus theoretically increasing the risk for port site metastases. It also prevents inadvertent loosening and extraction of the trocar with consequent loss of pneumoperitoneum and increased CO_2 absorption.

After insufflation with a Veress needle and placement of the initial trocar in a nonmiddle place, a 5mm scope is introduced and the remaining trocars are placed under direct vision as shown in Figure 9. After this we evaluate the abdominal cavity, looking for prominent lymph nodes, implantation of tumor cells in the omentum, and visualization of the colon, especially in the splenic flexure to ascertain the difficulty of its mobilization should it be required. The liver is thoroughly examined, and use of laparoscopic ultrasonography can accurately show the presence or absence of metastatic disease to the liver. This may indeed modify the extent of the dissection for a given patient.

The manipulation of the tumor is avoided by grasping the entire circumference of the bowel, with specific bowel handling instruments (e.g., laparoscopic Babcock).

It is preferable to hold the mesentery or appendices epiploica rather than the bowel itself if specific bowel instruments are not available. The use of smaller instruments frequently results in laceration of the bowel and can convert a clean, controlled case into a dirty, uncontrolled one.

MOBILIZATION

The initial maneuver is mobilization of the sigmoid and visualization of the left ureter. This can be performed in two fashions: Medial-to-lateral approach and lateral-to-medial approach. In the lateral-to-medial approach first we incise the peritoneum with a steady dissection of the sigmoid colon and the high portion of the rectum in a medial direction with care to avoid injury to the external iliac artery and hypogastric nerves (Fig. 10). Mobilization of the sigmoid should be performed until the

The Gastrointestinal Tract

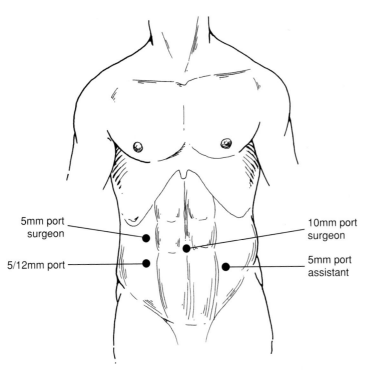

Fig. 9. Trocar disposition for low anterior resection and abdominoperineal resection.

ureter is identified and the peritoneum has been incised to the superior hemorrhoidal vessels. If the vessels can be readily identified on the left, they can be ligated. Frequently, however, the peritoneal dissection is extended down to the vessels. The right ureter is then identified, and with the sigmoid colon on anterior stretch, the peritoneum is incised on the right. This establishes a window through which the left ureter is identified. Laparoscopically this is quite easy, and frequently the CO_2 will help establish this dissection plane. Following this the inferior mesenteric artery and vein are identified 4 to 5 cm above the iliac bifurcation and can be ligated at the highest level possible with an ultrasonic device such as the LigaSure or harmonic scalpel (artery and vein separately). We also recommend a stepwise ligation first with 10-mm clips and then secured with a polydioxanone suture (PDS) pretied Endoloop; this provides a very secure permanent suture to the vessel. The artery should never be incised in one cut; rather, the artery should be partially incised and checked for residual back flow or additional bleeding. If this occurs, additional clips and/or ligation may be applied as needed. The inferior mesenteric vein is often medially adjacent to the artery, and care should be taken to identify this structure. In cases of colon cancer the inferior mesenteric vein can be traced to its origin at the splenic vein or at least to the ligament of Treitz, and ligation and division performed

at this point. (Fig. 11) Care should be taken to avoid injury of the ureter. The total mesorectal excision is moved downward into the pelvis along the endopelvic fascia. Lateral ligaments of the rectum are taken down along with the middle rectal and his branches, until the limit of the inferior hypogastric nerves. These nerves are preserved as far as possible. (Fig. 12) Anterior the Denonvilliers fascia is dissected, and posterior the rectosacral ligament and anococcygeal and pubococcygeal muscles are divided (Fig. 13). The mesorectum is excised completely. The anterior resection of the rectum should be reserved for last as this frequently results in additional bleeding, which drips into the posterior field. It is easy in most instances to continue the dissection to the levator ani muscle. If the posterior and lateral dissections have been adequately completed, the laparoscopist will have very little anterior dissection to perform. Care should be taken to avoid injury to the seminal vesicles in men and the vagina in women. In cases of colon cancer, if the disease process involves a portion of these organs, it will now be identified and a decision can be made as to the extent of bladder and/or vagina to be resected. After completion of this lower portion of the dissection, diffusion slowly from the periosteal surface of the presacral space may occur. This should be suction-dried, and a 4 × 4 gauze, or in several cases the argon beam coagulator, may be used to control this troublesome bleeding. Additional measures that can be used include the placement of bioabsorbable hemostat devices.

If a colostomy is to be constructed (in cases of rectal cancer with abdominoperineal resection), a higher resection and mobilization of the splenic flexure is not routinely needed. If an anastomosis is to be performed, the colon is cleaned for the distance of 1 to 2 cm circumferential for an intracorporeal anastomosis. This cleaning of the colon facilitates placing the anvil should a laparoscopically assisted procedure be used.

If a very low anterior anastomosis is to be performed, the dissection is completed and the splenic flexure mobilized. The patient should be placed in reverse Trendelenburg position with the left side rolled up.

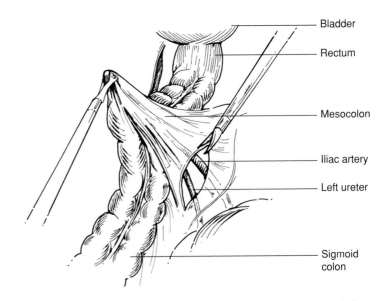

Fig. 10. Medial-to-lateral dissection, taking care to identify and preserve the left ureter.

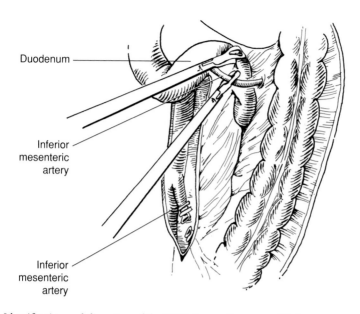

Fig. 11. Identification and dissection of the IMV close to ligament of Treitz.

Mobilization of the splenic flexure is easier to perform laparoscopically than open surgery because excellent visualization and identification of anatomic structures is possible with a laparoscope. The surgeon performs the dissection by placing the dissecting instrument in one of the trocars of the left. Concurrent procedures will work if the pneumoperitoneum is not broken before completion of the intra-abdominal resection. The perineal resection can now be completed, the specimen removed, and the levator ani muscles closed from below or above as indicated. The colostomy is brought up and matured, and a drain can be left in the sacrum if indicated. The area should be carefully reinspected for bleeding, the trocar site closed, and the operation terminated.

If a low anterior resection is to be performed, special attention must be given to the specimen. After complete dissection of the proximal portion of the colon, the point at which the resection is to be performed distally should be determined and the pericolonic tissue in this area cleaned circumferential for a distance of 1 to 2 cm. If an Endoloop is to be used to secure the head of the circular stapler, at least 2 cm is used. If an Endo-GIA is to be used, a lesser amount of dissection will be needed. If an anastomosis is to be performed and the anastomosis is to be done totally intracorporeally, we recommend using Endo-GIA

or sharp dissection to divide the colon at the predesignated site proximally and distally, controlling each end with a pretied Endoloop (if you are using sharp dissection) to prevent tumor or fecal spillage. Before division of the colon, an on-the-table colonoscopy should be performed to ensure and determine adequate margins, as well as to ascertain complete cleanliness of the colon. The colon is frequently irrigated with Betadine as an additional precautionary step. Before the colonoscopy, the proximal bowel should be clamped with a laparoscopic bulldog Glassman clamp or with an externally held conventional 10-mm instrument to prevent distension of the proximal colon and potentially the small bowel. The distal line of resection should be accurately determined with the colonoscope. After division of the distal portion of the colon, the rectum is left open. If a very low anterior resection has been performed (a distal resection line of <7 cm from the anus), care must be taken to keep the anus closed to prevent CO_2 loss from escaping through the open anus. Longer segments will almost always collapse and prevent CO_2 loss. The distal segment of the resected colon should now be encircled with a pretied Endoloop and the entire specimen now placed in an impermeable bag for subsequent removal. If the specimen is not too large, the anus can be dilated with two fingers. Most specimens up to 6 or 7 cm in diameter can be readily removed with the transanal route. (Fig. 14) If a laparoscopically assisted anastomosis is to be performed, the lower abdominal incision can be extended usually in the left side or a Pfannenstiel-type incision can be made to remove the specimen at this point. If the specimen will not fit through the anus and an intracorporeal anastomosis is to be performed, the bagged specimen can now be placed in the left upper quadrant and stored until the anastomosis is completed.

For laparoscopically assisted anastomoses the proximal end of the colon should be brought through the abdominal wall, a purse-string suture applied, and the anvil inserted, followed by the closure of the purse-string suture. Meticulous attention to detail is imperative for the successful completion of this portion of the procedure and care must be taken to leave a small rim of tissue rather than a large rim, which can interfere with the mechanics of the stapler. An Endo-GIA, if not previously used to divide the distal portion of the colon, can now be used to close the distal portion of the colon and the stapler spike brought through the closed rectum.

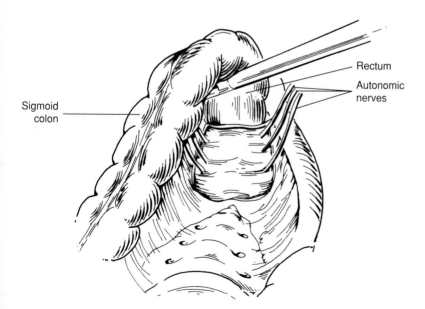

Fig. 12. Complete posterior dissection with identification of the autonomic nerves.

The Gastrointestinal Tract

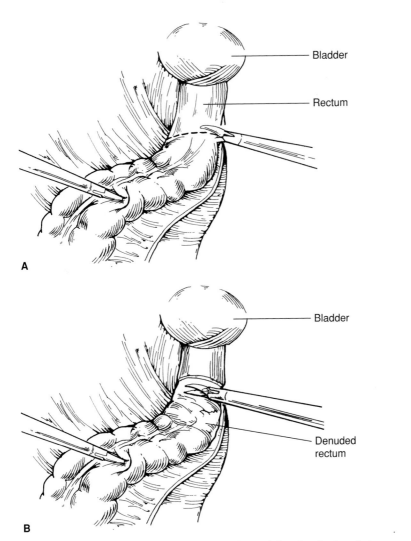

A

B

Fig. 13. A&B: Anterior rectal dissection with anterior traction and showing the denuded rectum.

The head and anvil of the stapler can now be joined and the anastomosis completed. It is strongly recommended that the tissue between the head and the anvil of the stapler be carefully inspected to ensure that adjacent tissue such as fallopian tubes or the ureter has not been incorporated.

If a totally intracorporeal anastomosis technique is to be used, the anvil should be introduced through the rectum either on the head of the stapler or on a separate introducing device such as a ring forceps (Fig. 15a). The anvil can be stored in the right or left ileac fossa for subsequent insertion into the proximal colon and the distal rectum can be stapled with an Endo-GIA 60 or similar stapling device (Fig. 15B). The anvil can now be inserted into the proximal portion of the colon and a second line of staples applied across the open end with subsequent protrusion and extraction of the point of the anvil through the staple line or adjacent to the staple line (Fig. 15C). Care should be taken using this technique to avoid losing the anvil in the proximal colon; the laparoscopic bulldog Glassman clamp works very well for this procedure. A secondary technique is that of application of a pretied loop, preferably of a strong suture such as PDS, around the anvil, again ensuring an adequate rim of tissue. Excising all redundant tissue affords a good mechanical working of the stapler. After securing the anvil, the proximal colon is brought into the pelvis and the spike in the head of the stapler is brought through the distal staple line and the two parts are joined. (Fig. 16) The stapler is carefully inspected to ensure that adjacent tissue such as a fallopian tube or ureter has not been incorporated. Again, care is taken to circumferentially inspect the staple line to ensure that additional extraneous tissue is present. (Fig. 17) After firing, the stapler is removed, and a colonoscopy is performed, exerting pressure into the rectum to test the anastomosis and to directly visualize the anastomosis internally. Most leaks can be controlled with simple suturing; however, if this is impossible, a protective ileostomy can be performed and brought out through a larger trocar site.

A drain is routinely left in the pelvis for excessive irrigation fluid. The entire area is irrigated with saline as well as 10% Betadine solution in the case of carcinoma. All ports are then irrigated with distilled water or Betadine. The trocar sites are individually closed with through-and-through 0 Vicryl using a suture passer Carter-Thomason. The patient is then returned to the recovery area for postoperative care.

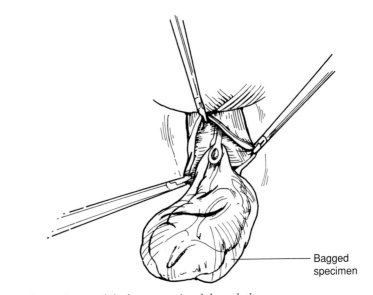

Fig. 14. The specimen and the bag are retrieved through the anus.

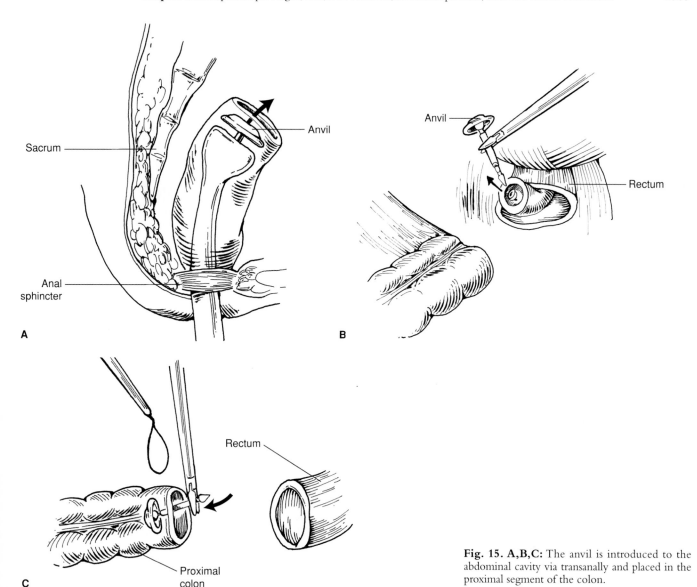

Fig. 15. A,B,C: The anvil is introduced to the abdominal cavity via transanally and placed in the proximal segment of the colon.

Laparoscopic Total Colectomy

Total or subtotal proctocolectomy with ileal pouch–anal (PCIP) has been performed since the 1970s and has become the most commonly performed procedure for ulcerative colitis and familial adenomatous polyposis. In recent years it has become thoroughly accepted in patients with hereditary nonpolyposis colorectal cancer syndromes and other entities involving colorectal cancer syndromes. The most frequent indications for total colectomy are listed in Table 4.

This procedure was initially performed for ulcerative colitis with a transanal mucosectomy beginning at the dentate line. Mucosectomy theoretically removes all columnar epithelium from the upper anal canal, thereby preventing inflammation in this area and eliminating

TABLE 4. INDICATIONS FOR LAPAROSCOPIC TOTAL COLECTOMY

Benign Disease
Familial adenomatous polyposis coli
Intractable or complicated inflammatory bowel disease
Bleeding arteriovenous malformations
Severe, chronic constipation
Ischemic colitis
Any other condition suitable for resection

Malignant Disease
Synchronous colon carcinoma

TABLE 3. CONTRAINDICATIONS OF LAPAROSCOPIC COLON SURGERY

Relative	Absolute
Advanced disease with frozen pelvis	Bleeding dyscrasias
Multiple operations with severe adhesions	Severe cardiopulmonary disease
Very large tumor	Intolerance to general anesthesia
Large abdominal aortic aneurism	Noncorrectable cardiovascular disease
Advanced cirrhosis	Inadequately trained surgeon
Prior gynecologic procedures	Intolerance to CO_2
Unprepared operating room	Dilated bowel

The Gastrointestinal Tract

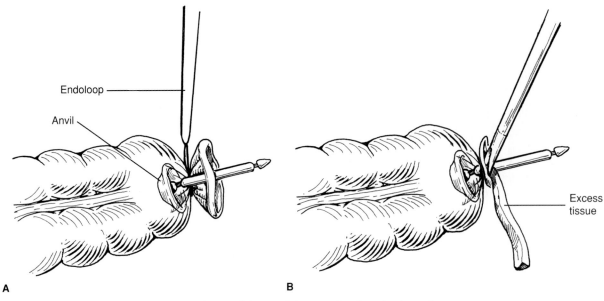

Fig. 16. A,B: The anvil is secured with an endoloop and the excessive tissue is trimmed.

the risk of dysplasia or carcinoma developing in residual rectal mucosa. However, mucosectomy is a time-consuming and technically demanding technique. Sphincter stretch and damage during the procedure may result in fecal seepage and soilage, and removal of the anal transitional zone may ablate the rectoanal inhibitory reflex and impair rectal sensation. Therefore, in recent years there has been a trend toward preserving the sphincter in these patients, lending a minimal amount of rectal mucosa.

The first report of a PCIP was in the 1980s and involves total colon resection from the abdominal approach, with division of the distal rectum between the *levator ani* usually 1 to 2 cm proximal to the dentate line using a linear stapler. A 12-cm longitudinal lumen pouch is constructed, and after the anvil of the stapler is inserted into the pouch, the anastomosis is constructed by placing the stapler transanally. In addition to avoiding prolonged retraction of the anal canal, this technique preserves the distal internal anal sphincter muscle and anal transitional zone, which may contribute to improved continence. Although there are exceptions, the majority of publications have demonstrated functionally superior advantages of this technique when compared to mucosectomy. These advantages

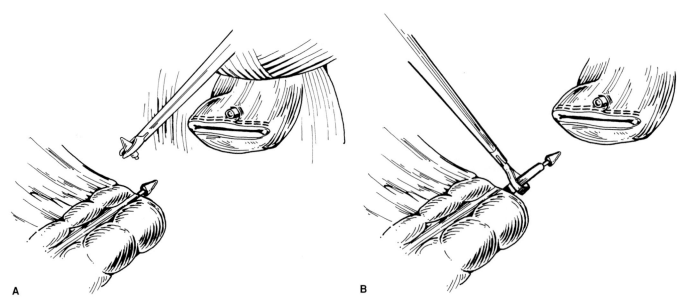

Fig. 17. A,B: Intracorporeal anastomosis for low anterior resection.

include increased anal resting pressure, preservation of the rectoanal inhibitory reflex, and improved continence. The use of double-stapled PCIP has also been shown in one large series to have fewer septic complications than the handsewn technique.

With the introduction of the PCIP, there were concerns regarding persistent inflammation in the retained strip of retained rectal and transitional zone mucosa, as well as the risk of developing dysplasia and carcinoma in the same area. Dysplasia in the anal transitional zone is extremely rare when there is no evidence of dysplasia or carcinoma in the colon and rectum, and develops in very few patients postoperatively. Some authors found low-grade dysplasia in 3% of 254 patients who underwent double-stapled PC for ulcerative colitis and were followed with annual postoperative biopsies of the anal transitional zone; they advocated completion mucosectomy when the dysplasia persisted on follow-up biopsy.

Mucosectomy has been reported as the preferred technique for patients with familial adenomatous polyposis and those with ulcerative colitis who have dysplasia or carcinoma elsewhere in the colon or rectum. However, residual nests of rectal mucosa have been found either outside the ileal pouch or adjacent to the pouch–anal anastomosis in up to 21% of patients undergoing mucosectomy. There have been at least three reports of patients developing rectal carcinoma after mucosectomy.

Laparoscopic total or subtotal colectomy is probably one of the most difficult, complex, and technically demanding procedures in laparoscopic colorectal surgery. This surgery requires mobilization of the entire colon and division of its mesentery, with management of all the major vessels of the colon, while exposing vital structures to be wounded and working in all four quadrants of the abdomen. Several technical factors are involved in the slow acceptance of this technique, which include the necessity of a complex bowel anastomosis (often deep in the pelvis), identification and division of large blood vessels, and the need for extraction of a bulky specimen.

PATIENT EVALUATION

Patients with an indication for a total or subtotal colectomy should undergo evaluation with colonoscopy and digital rectal examination. Rigid proctoscopy and transrectal ultrasound (TRUS) may be added if there is a suspicion of carcinoma. Before considering coloanal anastomosis,

sphincter function should be assessed. A detailed continence history and physical examination by an experienced surgeon are probably the most predictive of postoperative anal function. However, anal manometry may help in difficult cases. Despite the enthusiasm of many patients to restore intestinal continuity at all costs, it should be remembered that an abdominal colostomy is preferable to a perineal colostomy in cases where sphincter function is impaired either preoperatively or intraoperatively.

The presence of unresectable metastases makes an anastomosis ill advised. If a temporary diverting stoma is constructed to protect a line of anastomosis, the patient may never be fit enough to have the stoma closed. Even if the patient does not require a diverting stoma, the initial 6 to 18 months following coloanal anastomosis are often marked by frequent loose stools and occasional incontinence, and patients with metastatic disease may not survive long enough to benefit from the gradual improvement in function of the neorectum. If the patient is treated with chemotherapy postoperatively, the risk of diarrhea and fecal incontinence is increased further. Low anterior resection with Hartmann closure of the rectal stump may be a more prudent option for these patients. Similarly, if tumor invasion of pelvic structures makes complete resection impossible, low anastomosis should be abandoned because of the high risk of persistent tumor growth in the pelvis.

Some surgeons are enthusiasts of the combined transanal–transabdominal resection procedure, where the distal margin is defined and the distal dissection is performed from a transanal approach. If the tumor is so low that division in the proximal anal canal would not provide an adequate distal margin, then perhaps an abdominoperineal procedure would be safer from an oncologic standpoint. There may be a few patients who, because of a narrow pelvis or other aspect of body habitus, might benefit from such a technique.

Although a colonic pouch and pouch–anal anastomosis may be constructed entirely with suture, we consider performing this technique using surgical staplers safely. Although prospective randomized data are lacking, many surgeons feel that the risk of anastomotic or pouch leak with pelvic sepsis and subsequent fibrosis of the neorectum outweighs the benefits of avoiding temporary fecal diversion. In addition, a prolific number of patients undergoing proctectomy and coloanal anastomosis for rectal cancer will have stage II or

III lesions. Most of these patients will be treated with postoperative chemotherapy, and chemotherapy-induced diarrhea in a patient first adapting to a neorectum may cause fecal incontinence. Temporary fecal diversion may also be prudent in cases where neoadjuvant chemoradiation is used. Although dramatic reductions in tumor size can be achieved with the use of preoperative chemoradiation, it may predispose to anastomotic problems in patients not undergoing temporary diversion at the time of proctectomy and coloanal anastomosis. The most commonly used diverting stoma is the loop ileostomy, because its construction and subsequent takedown are straightforward, and the colonic mesentery is not threatened by such manipulation.

LAPAROSCOPIC TECHNIQUE

Under general anesthesia, the patient is placed supine in modified lithotomy position, with the arms tucked to the table, the thighs are kept in a straight line with the patient's body, and the legs are placed in semiflexure to permit a better approach to the anus and instrument manipulation. The surgeon should stand between the patient's legs with the assistant/camera holder on the patient's right and an assistant on the left. The nasogastric tube and bladder catheter are placed with additional monitoring devices as needed. The abdomen is prepped and draped in the usual manner, with care taken to preserve anal access to facilitate intraoperative colonoscopy and specimen extraction in cases of subtotal colectomy. The abdomen is insufflated with a Veress needle in an alternative location (usually left lower and often upper quadrant) to avoid possible small bowel injury due to adhesions in the midline. Typical trocar placement is shown in Figure 18. Usually we use four to six trocars to facilitate the approach to all four quadrants. Initially the surgeon is stationed between the legs of the patient and the abdominal cavity is surveyed to evaluate the anatomy of the colon and to perform adhesiolysis if required. The first step is to elevate the omentum over the top of the transverse colon to gain access to the transverse resection. The transverse colon is then elevated and sharp dissection is carried out in the area of the mesotransverse colon until the middle colic artery is identified and isolated from surrounding tissue. Elevating the transverse colon could frequently allow staging of the vessels and facilitate the identification. This artery is then controlled and coagulated using Endoclips, an Endoloops, or coagu-

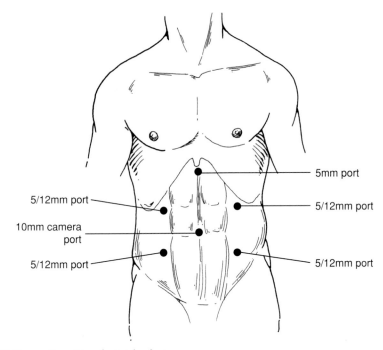

Fig. 18. Trocar disposition for total colectomy.

lator devices; another option is to use an energy device such as a harmonic scalpel or a vessel sealing system such as LigaSure. Many other devices are now becoming available. The lesser sac is then entered above the superior margin of the pancreas, and dissection is carried out primarily to the left side of the transverse colon in a stepwise fashion, with care taken to identify and control all vessels in the mesentery including the left colic (which will be identified approximately 3 cm to the left of the middle colic). The splenic flexure will have be easily reached and freed from the mesenteric side. Dissection to the patient's right frees the hepatic flexure above the duodenum. At this point the surgeon moves to the left side of the patient and dissection is carried out on the right side, taking the right colic artery and several additional branches in this area. With the mesentery thus taken and the duodenum clearly identified, a window is developed in the preperitoneal space to Toldt fascia. Dissection is then carried out inferiorly until the ileocolic artery and vein are identified, isolated, and eventually coagulated. The cecum is lifted up to identify the terminal ileum and in a stepwise fashion division of the mesentery of the small bowel is then carried out to the ileocecal valve at a previously determined point of resection. Care must be excessive in this area to preserve as much blood supply to the terminal ileum as possible. The right colon is then liberally mobilized from the lateral to the medial aspect

using sharp dissection, connecting the two dissection planes and mobilizing the colon readily in this fashion. The surgeon then moves to the right side of the patient and the omentum is taken down from the colon in a stepwise fashion, starting from the middle portion of the transverse colon and dissecting from the right side initially and then working to the left, coagulating all bleeding points as they appear with a harmonic scalpel. Dissection at the splenic flexure is carried around this plane, freeing it completely. A brief dissection may be carried out along the gutter of the descending colon until the entire splenic flexure of the colon is completely mobilized. Attention is now turned to the sigmoid colon, lifting up the sigmoid colon and dissecting the mesentery until the inferior mesenteric artery is identified. Care must be taken with multiple anatomic variations in the area and all the branches should be divided most expeditiously with the LigaSure device. A retroperitoneal dissection is carried out superiorly connecting the previously dissected space to the new space coming from the inferior portion. The entire descending colon and sigmoid are dissected free from the lateral pelvic attachment and mobilized medially. The sigmoid colon is then mobilized from its lateral attachments and the ureter is clearly identified and preserved. Dissection is carried out along the pelvic floor, identifying and preserving the parasympathetic nerves. Posterior dissection is carried out in the avascular plane

until deep in the pelvis, and then lateral dissection is carried out to identify the middle hemorrhoidal vessel when present. Dissection is continued to the left from a posterior approach, being mindful of the location of the left ureter; staying in the correct plane ensures protection of the ureter. The colon is then elevated and posterior dissection is continued to the levator ani level in the avascular presacral space. Dissection is then carried along the right aspect of the rectum mobilized from the right. Reflecting the rectum to the right allows rapid dissection of the left peritoneal reflection. With the colon thus mobilized and the peritoneal reflection taken down, we place two endoscopic bulldog Glassman clamps in the terminal ileum using a laparoscopic bulldog clamp applier, and a colonoscopy may be performed to ensure the margin of resection. The distal margin should be double-checked in the case of subtotal colectomy to ensure adequate clearance. At this same time the rectum is irrigated with saline and Betadine by colonoscopy. In the laparoscopic approach we utilize a 45- or 65-mm multifire Endo-GIA stapler in the spot previously selected for the divided resection line.

LAPAROSCOPICALLY ASSISTED

In the case of an ileal pouch construction, an incision of approximately 4 to 6 cm is performed in the right lower quadrant, and using a wound protector the specimen is taken out along with terminal ileum. The small bowel is then divided at the ileocecal valve and a reservoir is constructed by folding into a J configuration with an 11-cm limb length. The apex of the pouch is opened and a linear cutting stapler is used to create the lumen of the pouch. This can be accomplished by a single fire of a 75- or 90-mm stapler but may require more than one firing to create an adequate pouch length. A purse-string suture is placed around the opening of the pouch apex and the anvil of a 25-mm circular stapler is inserted. Alternatively, if the distal margin of resection has previously been determined by transanal dissection, the pouch can be passed to the anus and a handsewn anastomosis performed.

After the pouch is constructed, the ileum is reintroduced into the abdominal cavity and the incision is closed, the pneumoperitoneum is re-established, and the ileoanal anastomosis is then completed by reuniting the anvil and the stapling device in the anastomosis and firing the device. Testing the anastomosis with the colonoscope providing air pressure with the anastomosis under water seems to be the most efficient method to prove any leaks.

TOTALLY LAPAROSCOPIC

The decision for an ileoanal anastomosis without reservoir is extensively explained above; however, if an ileoanal anastomosis has been changed, the distal end of the rectum at the desired level is resected using scissors. The lumen is again immediately irrigated with Betadine supplied from the standard irrigation sources. The distal end of the resected specimen is immediately closed with an Endoloop to protect the abdominal cavity from spillage. The proximal line of resection is then identified and transected using a linear stapler. It is important to emphasize that minimal amount of bowel should be cleaned to protect against ischemia and a subsequent higher risk of stenosis at the anastomosis. In cases of colon cancer, first we introduce a specially designed bag with a purse-string suture that allows easy closure around the bag. This bag can be introduced through a 5- to 12-mm trocar or through the anus, and the colon is deposited inside the bag and closed with the purse-string and also using and extra Endoloop. The specimen and the bag are then turned around so that the Endoloop end of the bag is facing the rectum. A ring forceps is brought through the rectum and the size of the rectum is compared with the size of the tumor. An exceptionally large tumor obviously cannot be removed transanally, but most tumors up to about 5 cm can be readily removed through this route. The anus in these patients is carefully dilated until two fingers can be easily reached. The bag and the colon are then grasped and slowly "snaked" out through the rectum and anus using the bag as a sheath in the rectum and not pulling directly on the bag. To have a bag that is strong enough to sustain very strong traction, the size of the bag is increased significantly, which diminishes the size of the tumor that can be removed transanally. Thus, the bag is used more as a sheath, and the colon is literally "snaked" out of the bag through the rectum. The bag is then removed, and the pelvis is inspected for bleeding or tearing. It is irrigated with Betadine solution as is the remainder distal ileum.

The circular stapler is then brought into the rectum. The size of the proximal end of the ileum has been previously determined and an appropriately sized stapler chosen. We have found that a 28-

or 29-mm stapler usually allows passage of the anvil and results in a very adequate lumen. The EEA circular stapler can be used to introduce the anvil into the abdominal cavity through the rectum; this anvil is detached from the stapler and is washed with Betadine solution again and then placed in the proximal margin of the previous open terminal ileum.

Then the rectal stump is closed using a 35 or 45 Endo-GIA linear stapler and the rim of tissue thus separated is removed through the right lower quadrant trocar; the area is checked again for bleeding and a colonoscopy is performed to ensure the impermeability of the rectal stump. The anvil is placed in the ileum and secured using an Endoloop, and the excess tissue surrounding the anvil is trimmed to ensure a complete exposure of the tissue with the staples.

In both cases, totally laparoscopic or laparoscopically assisted, the EEA stapler is introduced through the rectum and the spike is slowly extruded through the center of the rectal stump; the spike is deattached from the EEA stapler with a 5-mm grasper and pulled out through the right lower quadrant trocar (5/12-mm trocar); and then the anvil and the stapler are united and the stapler is fired in a conventional manner.

The amount of tension is then double-checked, and a second colonoscopy is performed to ensure the absence of leaks or bleeding in the anastomotic ring. We fill the pelvis with saline solution and inject air through the colonoscope into the bowel lumen. Any leaks should be repaired immediately by sutures placed intracorporeally. The clamps on the colon that were left in place during the resection are removed after the colonoscopy is completed. These clamps serve not only to prevent leakage of the small bowel contents upstream, but also to help orient the ileum because they were applied initially on the antimesenteric surface and still should be in the same position. The clamps prevent rotation of the bowel and a 180- to 360-degree misplacement of the staple line.

After we ensure the absence of leaks, the entire cavity and particularly the trocars are irrigated with Betadine solution, we aspirate all the solution, and a 10-mm flat Jackson-Pratt drain is then placed in the pelvis and brought out through the left lower quadrant trocar. All trocars larger than 10 mm should be closed using 0 Vicryl and a Carter-Thomason suture passer. The entire abdominal cavity is reinspected; all Betadine is washed free with normal saline, and the peritoneal cavity is

suctioned dry. The patient is placed in a slight reverse Trendelenburg position, and the abdomen is deinsufflated. After the trocars are removed, all port sites are immediately closed. The subcutaneous tissue is irrigated thoroughly with Betadine solution and closed; the skin is closed with staples or sutures in a subcuticular fashion and Steri-strips. In cases of anastomosis with high risk of dehiscence, such as difficulty performing anastomosis, previous radiation, leaks repaired transoperatory, or other entities, we recommend the construction of a protective ileostomy.

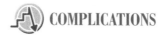

COMPLICATIONS

Because of the nature of the procedure and the fact that the patients frequently are under steroids or have other medical problems, the morbidity rate of this procedure is relatively high; however, this has a low mortality rate of less than 0.5%.

The most common complication in these patients is an intestinal obstruction, which is very important to detect and treat early because of the risk of loss of small bowel.

The most frightening complication is a leak with peritonitis, especially when a protective ileostomy is not used. This is most often partial and secondary to tension on the anastomosis. It is very important to keep in mind this serious complication to detect it early and treat it adequately. Another complication is anastomotic bleeding, which should be detected with colonoscopy. This is rare but can be difficult to manage.

In Table 5 we show probably the most frequent complications expected with respective time of occurrence.

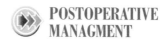

POSTOPERATIVE MANAGMENT

In all our patients the postoperative medications are the standard agents used in colon resections. The patients are under intravenous fluids dependent on their requirement, adjusting IV fluids to maintain urine output of 1 mL/kg/h. A nasogastric tube may or may not be left in place depending in the manipulation of the bowel, length of the surgery, age of the patient, and so on. This determination can only be made intraoperatively by the surgeon. The patient is usually given IV antibiotics for 24 hours; we prefer antibiotics that cover colon flora such as cefotaxime, metronidazole, or cefepime. Additional

TABLE 5. COMPLICATIONS OF TOTAL COLECTOMY

Timing	Complication	Percentage
Early postoperative period	Staple line hemorrhage	<2
	Anastomotic leak	<2
	Pelvic abscess	5–10
	Pelvic hematoma	5
	Intestinal obstruction	13
	Ileostomy dysfunction	5
	Urinary disturbance	5
Late-after Hospital Discharge	Pelvic sepsis	5
	Intestinal obstruction	10
	Ileostomy dysfunction	<5
	Anastomotic dehiscence	<5
	Sexual or bladder problems	<4
After Ileostomy Closure	Peritonitis related to stoma closure	<2
	Peritonitis—delayed anastomotic failure	<3
	Intestinal obstruction	9
	Pouch malfunction	5–12

medications include analgesics, in restriction but enough to obtain good control of the pain, especially narcotics, as well as medication for the undesirable postoperative nausea. Obviously, other previous medical conditions need to be treated, and medications don't need to be suspended, such as antihypertensives, antiseizure medications, diabetic medications, and cardiac medications.

We recommend waiting at least 6 hours to start a diet, but in aging patients the waiting time recommended is 12 hours; most of the patients can tolerate clear liquids the next day. The indication for a full diet is passage of gas.

The patient's progress determines the evolution of the patient. The requisite for a satisfactory discharge is that the patient be able to tolerate the regular diet and have regular bowel movements. Also their medical problems need to be under control, no fever can be registered at least 24 hours previous, they must ambulate satisfactorily if they were able to do so, the pain must be under control, the wounds must be clean and healing, and all drains must be removed. This time period averages 3.5 days for patients less than 50 years and 5.5 days for patients over 50 years for most of the colon surgeries.

We recommend the closure of the protective ileostomy 6 to 8 weeks after surgery, after confirming the integrity and total healing of the coloanal anastomosis by visual examination and contrast imaging studies with water-soluble agents in cases of J-pouch construction. The timing to return to normal activity is a gray area and is very loosely determined depending on the individual practitioner. Most of the patients are able to return to normal activity within 7 to 10 days, but this depends on the type of activity obviously. We do not recommend return to work any sooner than 5 to 10 days after surgery unless the patient has a sedentary occupation. Most patients are able to tolerate returning to full activity and/or work within 7 to 10 days. Some patients may not be able to return to work for 2 weeks. Patients with very heavy labor-related occupations require at least 10 days to 2 weeks before they can return to full, unrestricted work activities.

It is very important to advise the patient about fecal urgency and frequency; to help diminish this we recommend the use of bulky or high-fiber supplements.

CONCLUSIONS

In conclusion, laparoscopy has opened a new arena for the treatment of most colon and rectal diseases; however, multiple issues are present in this exciting field. These include technique, training, and the approach to carcinoma. There is no doubt that an extremely high level of skill is needed to successfully complete this procedure. Recent reports recommended as a prerequisite that experience should include at least 20 laparoscopic colorectal resections with anastomosis for benign disease or metastatic colon cancer before using the technique to treat curable cancer. We believe that perhaps 40 cases is a reasonable number before one can perform a safe and highly curable surgery for colon cancer; also, hospitals may base credentialing for laparoscopic colectomy for cancer on experience gained by formal graduate medical educational training or advanced laparoscopic experience and participation in hands-on training courses and outcomes.

SUGGESTED READING

Clinical Outcomes of Surgical Therapy Study Groups. A comparison of laparoscopically assisted and open colectomy for colon cancer. *N Engl J Med* 2004;350(20):2050.

Croce E, Olmi S, Azzola M, et al. Laparoscopic colectomy: indications, standardized technique and results after 6 years experience. *Hepato-Gastroenterol* 2000;47:683.

Daniels LJ, Chekan EG. Laparoscopic cholecystectomy. In: Pappas TN, Chekan EG, Eubanks E, eds. *Atlas of laparoscopic surgery,* 2nd ed. Philadelphia: Appleton & Lange, 1999:13.1.

Franklin ME Jr, Berghoff KE, Arellano PP, et al. Safety and efficacy of the use of bioabsorbable seamguard in colorectal surgery at the Texas endosurgery institute. *Surg Laparosc Endosc Percutan Tech* 2005;15(1):9.

Greznlee RT, Murray T, Bolden S, et al. Cancer statistics, 2000. *CA Cancer J Clin* 2000; 50:7.

Franklin ME, Kazantsev GB, Abrego D, et al. Laparoscopic surgery for stage III colon cancer: long-term follow-up. *Surg Endosc* 2000;14:612.

Kockerling F, Rose J, Schneider C, et al., for the Laparoscopic Colorectal Surgery Study Group (LCSSG). Laparoscopic colorectal anastomosis: risk of postoperative leakage: results of a multicenter study. *Surg Endosc* 1999;13:639.

Maxwell-Armstrong CA, Robinson MH, Scholefield JH. Laparoscopic colorectal cancer surgery. *Am J Surg* 2000;179:500.

Muckleroy SK, Ratzer ER, Fenoglio ME. Laparoscopic colon surgery for benign disease: a comparison to open surgery. *J Soc Laparoendosc Surg* 1999;3:33.

Nishiguchi K, Okuda J, Toyoda M, et al. Comparative evaluation of surgical stress of laparoscopic and open surgeries for colorectal carcinoma. *Dis Colon Rectum* 2001; 44:223.

Schlachta CM, Mamazza J, Seshadri PA, et al. Defining a learning curve for laparoscopic colorectal resections. *Dis Colon Rectum* 2001;44:217.

Siriser F. Laparoscopic-assisted colectomy for diverticular sigmoiditis: a single-surgeon prospective study of 65 patients. *Surg Endosc* 1999;13:811.

Whelan RL. Laparotomy, laparoscopy, cancer, and beyond. *Surg Endosc* 2001;15:110.

EDITOR'S COMMENT

Dr. Franklin is truly one of the pioneers in laparoscopy, having guided thousands of surgeons through their "learning curve." Throughout his career he has advanced the field of laparoscopic colon surgery with his technical mastery, ingenuity, and steadfastness. Over the years, I have embraced several of his pearls. This chapter describes proven techniques that will compel even the most experienced laparoscopic surgeon to reflect upon one's training and current operative technique.

In general, I prefer integrated Endosuites for all advanced laparoscopic procedures. Multiple high-definition flat screens suspended by booms provide optimal visualization from several vantage points for both the surgeon and assistants. Patients are secured on a beanbag and the table checked for extremes in positioning (reverse Trendelenburg, steep Trendelenburg, rotate right and left). For laparoscopic colectomy, the operating room should have readily available a colonoscope, laparoscopic ultrasound, LigaSure, ultrasonic shears, convection warming blanket, and sequential compression device. Colonoscopy localizes the lesion and tests the anastomosis. Ultrasound checks the liver for possible metastatic disease. Ureteral catheters are used liberally in inflammatory diverticulitis.

Dr. Franklin has downsized many of his ports to 5 mm and boasts the view he gets from a 5-mm laparoscope. He utilizes 5-mm ports in the umbilicus and another 5-mm port at the subxiphoid area to facilitate dissection. An additional port in the left upper quadrant facilitates mobilization around a particularly large transverse colon. While liberal use of additional ports can be very helpful, for less experienced surgeons using all 10- to 12-mm ports in an anchor pattern allows for the versatility of 10-mm instruments and may be simpler as the surgeon establishes a routine. Furthermore, I find that my 5-mm scopes are frequently mishandled and consequently of variable image quality.

If the lesion is not tattooed, Dr. Franklin locates the lesion with an on-the-table colonoscopy. The medial-to-lateral approach has gained popularity for identifying and isolating the blood vessels prior to lateral dissection. As with open right colectomy for cancer, the vessels are taken very near the origin of the superior mesenteric artery. Dr. Franklin avoids clips, staplers, and the harmonic scalpel, and instead recommends the LigaSure for its faster and better seal of the vessels. After mobilization, I will usually deliver the right colon through a small midline incision for a laparoscopic-assisted approach.

For sigmoid and left colon resection the medial-to-lateral approach is also used. The splenic flexure is approached from two directions. He extends the retroperitoneal dissection going from medial to lateral to the left gutter and to the splenic flexure. Dr. Franklin advises taking the omentum first after the retroperitoneal dissection to facilitate safe mobilization of the splenic flexure.

During sigmoid colectomy for diverticulitis, the distal bowel is transected below the sacral promontory to allow complete removal of diverticula. However, at this level, constructing an extracorporeal anastomosis is more difficult. In this case, Dr. Franklin recommends an intracorporeal, or at least partially intracorporeal, anastomosis utilizing an EEA stapling device. He removes the specimen transanally to avoid the morbidity of an abdominal incision.

For mobilizing the sigmoid colon, Dr. Franklin starts medially just below the inferior mesenteric artery and extends the initial dissection into the pelvis. Careful dissection down to the levators helps preserve the parasympathetic nerves. For the rectal dissection in a female patient, Dr. Franklin suggests suspending the uterus with Keith needles inserted on each side of the midline and passing the suture around the ligaments and body of the uterus. During abdominoperineal resections, Dr. Franklin completes the entire rectal dissection down to the levators laterally and anteriorly prior to division of the colon. Division of the colon and construction of the colostomy is completed after the rectum is fully mobilized. The dissection plane must start posteriorly, work laterally, and be kept below the seminal vesicles.

Many surgeons have adopted the use of a hand port to simplify laparoscopic-assisted colectomy. A gloved hand retracts tissue while standard laparoscope instruments complete mobilization of the colon. The hand port, it is argued, is approximately the same size as the incision that would be required to complete an extracorporeal anastomosis. Placing the hand-assist device early allows for the benefits of tactile feedback, while still achieving a much smaller incision than would usually be required for an open colectomy. Operative time using the hand-assist device tends to be less than the totally laparoscopic approach. The laparoscopic hand–assisted colectomy has also been advocated as a bridge to intracorporeal anastomosis or as a salvage maneuver with markedly inflamed tissue.

Convincing data from the Clinical Outcomes of Surgical Therapy (COST) Study Group showed that laparoscopic-assisted colectomy is equivalent to open colectomy for colon cancer (*N Engl J Med* 2004;350:2050). The incidence of postoperative complications, local recurrence, and survival was comparable. Clinical data from Europe (*Lancet* 2002;359:2224) demonstrated that disease-free survival rates were actually higher for patients whose colon cancers were removed by laparoscopic techniques, leading some to suggest that laparoscopy may influence tumor biology and immunology. Based on the best evidence, the American Society for Colorectal Surgery (ASCRS) and the Society for American Gastrointestinal and Endoscopic Surgeons (SAGES) have endorsed laparoscopy for cancer.

Proper utilization of laparoscopy requires mastery of advanced laparoscopic skills and expertise in management of colonic disease. Despite COST requiring surgeons to do 20 cases prior to entering data into the study, 21% of cases were converted to open. This raises real concerns for training, as typical residency programs do not offer trainees even this minimal exposure in laparoscopic colectomy. While many MIS fellowships and Colorectal fellowships are able to provide sufficient experience, most general surgeons entering practice directly after completing residency will find it difficult to obtain formal in-depth training in laparoscopic colectomy. Challenges with adequate training notwithstanding, laparoscopic colectomy is an acceptable alternative to open colectomy for many, if not most, colonic lesions.

D.B.J.

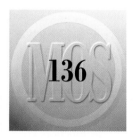

136

Total Colectomy and Ileorectal Anastomosis

FRANK G. OPELKA

Total colectomy (sometimes referred to as *subtotal colectomy*) is the removal of the entire colon and preservation of the rectum. Intestinal continuity is restored by ileorectal anastomosis, also known as *ileoproctostomy* or *ileorectostomy*.

The role for total colectomy and ileorectal anastomosis continuous to evolve in the treatment of colonic diseases. Improved understanding of the cause of surgical conditions and the availability of alternative procedures redefines the role of removing the entire colon, the rectum, and restoring intestinal continuity with an ileal rectal anastomosis. At one time, total colectomy served patients with ulcerative colitis who presented with presumed "rectal sparing" of their disease. The rectal involvement of ulcerative colitis is common and the presumed sparing may have come from therapeutic enemas. Now, restorative proctocolectomy has replaced total colectomy in these patients. In the past, the cause of massive lower gastrointestinal hemorrage escaped definition and unstable patients' condition forced surgeons to perform total colectomies. Still, colorectal cancer and polyposis syndromes are found in a subset of patients who could benefit from a total colectomy. Hereditary nonpolyposis colorectal cancer syndromes find some experts calling for a prophylactic colectomy and lifelong surveillance of the remaining rectum. Patients with Crohn disease or those suffering from colonic inertia are also candidates for a total colectomy.

Total colectomy is an operative procedure used for both elective or emergent care. Emergent care challenges surgical judgment to consider a one- or two-stage procedure. In urgent situations, a total colectomy and ileal rectal anastomosis is proven safe despite the lack of a preoperative mechanical bowel preparation. Current literature has begun to question the value of a bowel preparation even in elective colon operations. Proper antibiotic prophylaxis remains a staple in limiting postoperative complications. Fulminant colitis, severe inflammatory disease of the rectum, frank pus in the pelvis, malnutrition, and severe concomitant disease are reasons to delay the ileal rectal anastomosis. In the two-stage procedure, the operation concludes with a resection of the colon, the construction of an end ileostomy, and closing the rectal stump with staples or sutures. Alternatively, the distal end can be exteriorized as a mucous fistula. The rectum does not reach the abdominal wall without extensive mobilization, which may be unwise in this situation; therefore, usually the rectosigmoid or even the distal sigmoid is brought to the abdominal wall as a mucous fistula.

Surgeons are now skilled in performing laparoscopic or hand-assisted laparoscopic total colectomy with ileorectal anastomosis. Typically, the colonic mobilization and part of the mesocolic ligation are carried out laparoscopically. Once the surgeon has mobilized the entire colon, a small incision is made in the lower abdomen to deliver the intestine and gain access to any remaining mesocolon that needs division. With control of the mesocolon, you may transect the specimen and perform the anastomosis. A few surgeons have the skills to do the entire procedure intracorporeally, extracting the specimen through the rectum before performing a stapled anastomosis. Laparoscopic total colectomy is difficult to master, but it is likely that more surgeons will use this approach in the future.

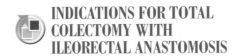

INDICATIONS FOR TOTAL COLECTOMY WITH ILEORECTAL ANASTOMOSIS

Crohn Colitis

Crohn colitis is a segmental colitis that may deteriorate despite intestinal rest and aggressive medical therapy. Patient's condition with colitis will vary from nutritionally replete to severely malnurished and immune dysfunction, additionally related to medical therapy. In patients with severe or fulminant disease, close coordination of care between the medical and surgical disciplines leads to the best outcomes for the patient. Designing surgical options for a patient must include information about anorectal aspects of Crohn disease to assess the rectal compliance and anal sphincter function. Usually, the history and physical examination are sufficient to make this assessment, but anorectal manometric studies to quantify sphincter function may be helpful. It is essential that the rectum be distensible for the operation to have a good functional result; distensibility can be judged by insufflation of air through a sigmoidoscope. If the rectum is nondistensible because of inflammation or scarring, it is best to remove it. An abscess or fistula should be resolved before ileorectal anastomosis can be considered. A history of anorectal abscess or fistula does not absolutely contraindicate ileorectal anastomosis, but it should make one cautious; the complexity of the fistula is a guide. An ileal rectal anastomosis may exaccerbate the fistulous disease. Of course, if previous fistulotomy damaged the sphincters, ileorectal anastomosis may be contraindicated. Finally, Crohn colitis creates patients with a long history of chronic diarrhea. Patient tolerance for diarrhea is less of an inconvenience to these patients than to others. They have accommodated their lifestyle to this situation and improved their anorectal sphincter function. The patients may be willing to live with mild-to-moderate diarrhea rather than have an ileostomy. Unfortunately, the risk of subsequent proctectomy for dysfunctional or Crohn disease progression may be as high as 60% to 70%. Patients will require a completion proctectomy and end ileostomy.

Occasionally, patients present with a unclear picture of indeterminant colitis. For example, the colonic biopsies reveal clear ulcerative colitic features, but the patient has a long history of stable chronic anal fistulae. Patients with indeterminant colitis seem to behave more like they have ulcerative colitis and are reasonable candidates for a restorative proctocolectomy with an ileal anal pouch. Alternatively, patients with indeterminate colitis may be suitable for total colectomy with ileorectal anastomosis. Examination of the resected colonic specimen helps make a definitive diagnosis, and, if rectal disease subsequently requires proctectomy, the choice between an ileoanal pouch and a permanent ileostomy may be more clear with this information.

Neoplasia

Family history of colon cancer and advances in genetics brings into the light three different risk groups for colorectal cancer. These are familial adenomatous polyposis, hereditary nonpolyposis colon cancer syndrome, and genetic mutations that lead to sporadic colon cancer. Additionally, synchronous or metachronous colorectal cancers represent high-risk patients and suggest patients should undergo a total or completion colectomy with ileal rectostomy. Familial adenomatous polyposis (FAP) accounts for less than 1% of cases of colorectal cancer in the United States. FAP is an autosomal dominant disorder that exists because of a mutation on the long arm of chromosome five (5). In families suspected of having FAP, surveillance begins early in the teen years because most of these patients develop polyposis and malignancies younger than age 40. Surveillance includes genetic testing and flexible sigmoidoscopy. Once polyps are identified, patients should undergo colectomy to remove the risks of cancer.

Patients with FAP who have rectal involvement require a restorative proctocolectomy. If the rectum has a few easily controlled polyps, these can be removed and the rectum spared from resection by performing a total colectomy and ileal rectal anastomosis. Rectal preservation in FAP patients preserves pelvic nervi ergenti and limits risk to altered sexual function in young patients. Also, ileal rectostomy patients had improved quality of life with reasonable bowel function. These patients had less perineal soilage or nocturnal seepage.

FAP patients with rectal sparing require sigmoidoscopic surveillance every 3 months after ileorectal anastomosis, and compliance is a problem. Currently, total restorative proctocolectomy with a pelvic pouch–anal anastomosis is the preference of most surgeons because it eliminates the at-risk mucosa while preserving the sphincters.

Hereditary nonpolyposis colorectal cancer or Lynch syndrome represent several genetic mutations, such as DNA-mismatch repair gene MSH2, with an 82% cumulative risk of colon cancer. Hereditary nonpolyposis colon cancer may account for approximately 5% of cases of cancer of the large bowel. In 1997, Henry Lynch was one of the earliest providers to suggest the need for a prophylactic colectomy as the risk of colon cancer approached the same risk as patients with familial adenomatous polyposis. Unlike FAP, the rectum involvement is more limited, making total colectomy and ileal rectal anastomosis an ideal procedure. Not everyone has been so willing to agree to a prophylactic colectomy alone as these patients also carry risks of 60% and 12% for endometrial and ovarian cancer, respectively.

The diagnosis of hereditary nonpolyposis colon cancer currently depends on the family history (modified Amsterdam criteria): (a) three or more relatives with histologically proven colorectal carcinoma, one of whom is a first-degree relative of the other two people; (b) colorectal carcinoma involving at least two generations; and (c) one or more cases of colorectal carcinoma diagnosed before the age of 50 years. In addition to endometrial and ovarian cancer, kindreds have shown malignancies of the small intestine, ureter, hepatobiliary system, and stomach. Molecular genetic testing assesses mismatch repair genes and can report on microsatellite instability.

Obstructing cancer of the left colon may be seen with a dilated proximal colon, which is unsuitable for a primary resection and anastomosis. These patients can be treated by total colectomy and ileorectal anastomosis in one stage. Alternatives are a staged approach or the use of on-the-table washout with primary colonic or colorectal anastomosis. Nonobstructing cancer of the distal transverse or proximal descending colon can be treated by total colectomy with ileorectal anastomosis. This procedure avoids anatomically awkward attempts to restore continuity of the hepatic flxure to the sigmoid colon or rectum. In addition, a broad resection assures adequate nodal resection for proper tumor staging.

Lower Gastrointestinal Hemorrhage

Severe bleeding from the colon can be massive and uncontrollable without sur-gery. Typically, these patients are elderly and their struggle develops from hemorrhagic diverticulosis coli or angiodysplasia, also called an arterial venous malformation. Oftentimes, the hemorrhage spontaneously stops, possibly associated with the resultant hypotension. Fortunately, surgeons today are seldom faced with an operative decision in these patients. If bleeding continues, aggressive preoperative diagnostic evaluation, including colonoscopy, radionuclide scanning, and angiography, usually localizes the bleeding to a segment of the colon. Clinical resuscitation and selective nonoperative treatment usually controls the hemorrhage. Patients may receive selective embolization or selective vasopressin infusion of the distal colonic vessels. Unstable patients who fail medical therapy must undergo surgery. Intraoperative colonoscopy may assist in pinpointing the bleeding site and thus limit the resection to one segment. Rarely, patients present with a primary hemorrhage or recurring episodes, with two possible sources (typically, angiodysplasias in the right colon and severe diverticulosis in the left colon). These patients are candidates for total colectomy to eliminate both potential sources of bleeding.

Chronic Constipation and Colonic Inertia

Severe chronic constipation refractory to vigorous medical management may be an indication for total colectomy with ileorectal anastomosis. These conditions are referred to as *intestinal motility disorders.* When the motility disorder resides within the colon, it is termed *colonic inertia.* Other conditions such as diabetes mellitus or collagen vascular disorders may manifest themselves as gastroparesis, small intestine motility dysfunction or colonic inertia. Medical conditions fare poorly with surgical therapy. Disorders in motility could be related to specialized neural ganglion in the intestine such as Meissner or Auerbach plexus, or the cells of Cajal. Small intestinal contrast imaging may demonstrate multiple, scattered true diverticula, which may represent sequelae of and underlying panenteric motility disorder.

To isolate segmental enteric inertia, first perform a simple study of colonic motility with the use of radiopaque markers. In candidates for total colectomy, the markers are scattered throughout the colon after 5 days, an indication of a diffuse colonic motility disorder. Markers that have migrated to the rectosigmoid without passing through the anus may portend difficulties in rectal emptying. Anorectal functional assessment includes cinedefecography to evaluate rectal function and exclude pelvic outlet dysfunctions such as nonrelaxing puborectalis syndrome. Patient selection for functional disorders is a vital part of the surgical decision. Patients are candidates for total colectomy with ileal rectal anastomosis in cases with isolated colonic inertia, and with a normal rectum and pelvic floor function.

TECHNIQUE OF RESECTION

Position

Although total colectomy certainly can be accomplished with the patient supine, the lithotomy position has the advantage of access to the anus for intraoperative colonoscopy or sigmoidoscopy, stapling maneuvers if desired, and inspection of the anastomosis for integrity. Proper positioning should include placement of intermittent compression stocking or other means for deep venous thrombosis prevention. Compression stocking may also assist in preventing sural nerve damage in patients placed in lithotomy. With the patient in Lloyd-Davies or Allen stirrups, the rectum can be examined and a triple-lumen irrigation catheter is positioned for use with rectal irrigation with a balanced salt solution before skin preparation and draping.

The positions of the surgical team depend on the experience and the anticipated role of the assistants. If the first assistant is capable of dissection under guidance, it is advantageous for the surgeon to stand on the patient's left side. The surgeon thus has control of retraction and exposure of the right and transverse colon. The description of technique here assumes this arrangement. When the left colon is dissected, the assistant retracts with one hand and dissects with the other while the surgeon displays the tissues to be incised laterally. In a teaching case, sometimes there is shifting of positions around the table.

Incision

A midline incision is standard. A transverse incision below the umbilicus is feasible in slender patients and those with long-standing inflammatory bowel disease, which often shortens the colon and mesocolon. Some prefer a transverse incision with the thought that it lowers the

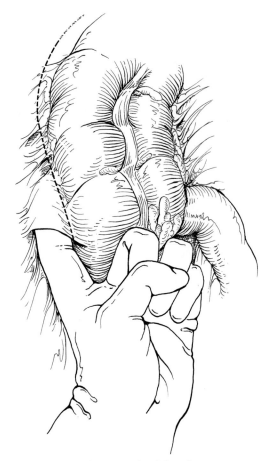

Fig. 1. Finger beneath peritoneum adjacent to the right colon.

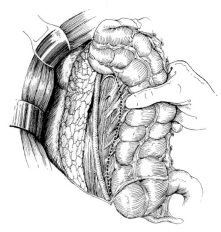

Fig. 2. Duodenum and ureter exposed behind the right colon.

incidence of incisional hernias. However, transverse incisions can be too low and they will not always facilitate the perisplenic dissection.

Mobilization of the Colon

After inspection of the abdomen, mobilization of the colon begins right side. The surgeon pinches the peritoneal surfaces together lateral to the cecum to protect the bowel from injury, and the peritoneum is incised close to the cecal wall. Electrocautery of tiny peritoneal vessels minimizes blood loss, but scissors can be used as well. Once the lateral peritoneal leaf is opened, the surgeon inserts the left index finger into the defect, retracting the cecum and ascending colon medially while the lateral peritoneum is incised (Fig. 1). The counter traction applied by the exposing surgeon tolls the cecum medially and cephalad along the ileocolic arterial axis. A dissection in the retroperitoneum, immediately adjacent to the meocolon, will expose the gonadal vessels and the right ureter. The ureter should remain untouched in the retroperitoneum. By pulling the colon to the patient's left

and dividing the lateral peritoneum close to the colonic wall, the amount of bare area is minimized. A tendency to extend the plane of dissection too laterally leads to unnecessary exposure of the Gerota fascia or toward the posterolateral aspects of the pancreas and doudenum.

As the hepatic flexure is approached, the anterior surface of the duodenum appears, and the mesocolon is separated from it by division of filmy tissue containing tiny vessels (Fig. 2). Full mobilization up to the pancreas is unnecessary in most cases. In cases of cancer, one needs to mobilize fully to ligate the vessels close to their origin. Hepatic flexure lateral attachments contain vessels of varying size, some large enough to require ligature. Careful medial traction at the hepatic flexure will avoid tearing of the middle colic vein near the superior mesenteric vein. A venous tear in this region is often difficult to control and requires prompt attention. It is important to isolate and control the vessel to avoid injury to the superior mesenteric vein.

At this point, a decision must be made about preserving or removing the greater omentum. If it is to be preserved, the

omentum is detached from the transverse colon, and if it is to be removed, the gastrocolic ligament is serially divided and ligated outside the gastroepiploic vessels. Although the omentum is a valuable "ally" after most abdominal operations, it can become a source of adhesions. It adheres to small bowel loops and the abdominal wall. It often becomes fenestrated, and these strands are a common source of more adhesions. Some authors report a higher incidence of postoperative adhesive bowel obstructions when the omentum remains.

If the omentum is to be excised, the lesser sac is entered to the left of the midline before the hepatic flexure is taken down completely. Once in the lesser sac, adhesions of stomach to the transverse mesocolon are lysed, the gastrocolic ligament is serially divided and ligated outside the gastroepiploic vessels (Fig. 3), and the hepatic flexure is approached from the left.

The mesocolon is left intact until it is fully separated from the gastrocolic, duodenal, and pancreatic attachments. At this

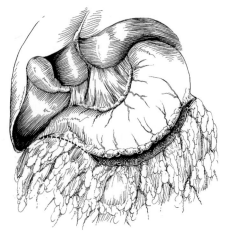

Fig. 3. Dividing and ligating the gastrocolic ligament between the stomach and transverse colon.

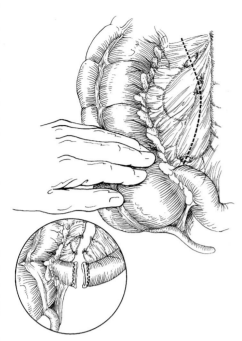

Fig. 4. Dividing vessels to right colon and dividing the ileum with stapler.

point, I prefer to return to the ileocecal area and to divide the ileum from the cecum, typically using a linear cutting stapler. Once divided, the dissection moves along the ileocolic mesentery to the root of the ileocolic vessels. One can then divide and ligate the ileocolic, right colic (if present), and middle colic vessels at the appropriate level defined by the operative condition (Fig. 4). I preserve the ileal

branches of the ileocolic vessels in non-malignant cases to preserve the vasculature for an ileoanal pouch, even though I may later divide these vessels at the time of pouch construction. If the pouch is deferred to a later time, preserving these vessels may protect the essential arcades needed for the future reservoir. Securing the right colic and middle colic vessels with ligatures leaves the right and proximal transverse colon mobilized.

Once the dissection has reached the distal transverse colon, it is my preference to mobilize the sigmoid colon to approach the splenic flexure from the left. The sigmoid colon and mesocolon are retracted to the right by the exposing surgeon, who remains standing on the patient's right side. Congenital or acquired adhesions of the appendices epiploicae, colon, and mesocolon to parietal peritoneum are divided in a bloodless plane. When mobilizing the sigmoid colon, do not cut fat! There is no fat in the proper plane; therefore, cutting into fat in this location signifies that one is in the wrong plane—an appendix epiploica, the mesocolon, or the retroperitoneal tissues (Fig. 5). After these congenital adhesions have been divided, the sigmoid colon is rolled in a medial and slight cephalad fasion. The dissection along the mesosigmoid and the retroperitoneum should again expose the ureter, now on the left side

medial to the left ureter. The peritoneal incision is carried longitudinally, parallel to the course of the ureter, and the ureter is swept laterally in its lower third, to avoid injury. The surgeon should remember the presence of the sympathetic nerves on the surface of the aorta, approximately 1 cm posterior to the superior hemorrhoidal vessels. In men with benign disease, it is unnecessary to risk impairing ejaculatory function by injury to these nerves, so once the ureter is seen, dissection in the vicinity should be minimized. The mesocolon is incised at its base on the right side (Fig. 6).

The splenic flexure is approached from the left, from below, and from behind (Fig. 7). When the spleen sits in a deep fossa and the colon lies with it, I often will lift the entire spleen and place a surgical sponge behind it to bring the spleen and colon more anterior. The hope is that this will further limit unnecessary traction on the splenic capsule. Traction on the distal transverse colon or omentum from the left upper quadrant to the right or inferiorly are common reasons for avulsion injuries or tears to the splenic capsule and underlying parenchyma. The lateral peritoneal attachments of the descending colon are incised directly lateral to the colon to avoid overextension of the dissection into the retroperitoneum. It is important that the dissection remain within

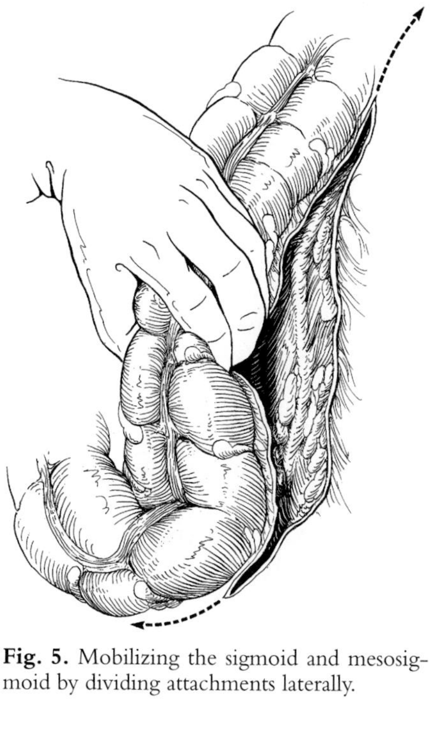

Fig. 5. Mobilizing the sigmoid and mesosigmoid by dividing attachments laterally.

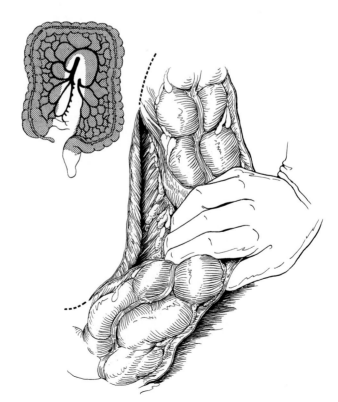

Fig. 6. Incising the sigmoid mesocolon at base on the right.

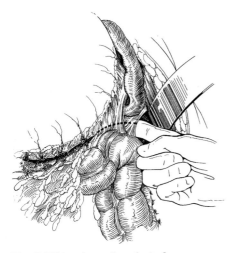

Fig. 7. Taking down the splenic flexure.

a few millimeters of the colon as the flexure is taken down. This is the plane of attachment of the omentum and is relatively avascular. If one divides the tissue a greater distance from the colonic wall, larger vessels are encountered that require ligation. These maneuvers separate the omentum from the colon, and, if the omentum is to be removed, the remaining portion of gastrocolic ligament requires division and ligation to connect with the plane established earlier.

It is necessary to incise the anterior layer of the peritoneum of the transverse mesocolon to get the splenic flexure down. Behind this thin layer, of course, lie the mesocolic vessels, and they require ligation. In patients with malignancy, the inferior mesenteric artery and vein are divided and ligated, usually separately, after the left colic vessels are taken. In men with colitis or other benign disease, it is preferable to divide the left colic vessels

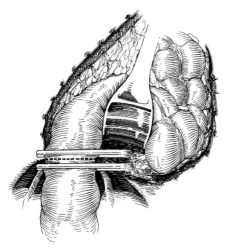

Fig. 8. Dividing the rectum between clamps.

and then the sigmoidal branches, leaving the inferior mesenteric vessels intact to avoid dissection in the vicinity of the sympathetic nerves. If the vessels must be taken, dissection is carried out as close to them as possible to minimize the risk of nerve injury.

The vessels at the rectosigmoid are divided close to the rectal wall in men with benign disease, and the proximal rectum is prepared for transection by division of the mesorectum. The rectosigmoid is a 4-cm long transitional zone at the sacral promontory; here, the taeniae coli merge into a confluent circular muscle coat and the lumen widens. The rectum is divided between clamps or with a linear stapler (Fig. 8).

ANASTOMOSIS

Hand-sewn ileorectal anastomoses are preferred by many surgeons. One can perform an end-to-end or end-to-side stapled anastomosis (Fig. 9). Because the ileal lumen is smaller than the rectal lumen, an end-to-end anastomosis is facilitated by making an antimesenteric slit in the ileum to enlarge it. The problem of discrepancy between the lumens is obviated by constructing a stapled side-to-end ileorectal anastomosis, and that technique is described later. I prefer a hand-sewn side-to-end ileal rectal anastomosis in a single layer, absorbable monofilament suture. The ileum is arranged so that the cut edge of the mesentery is to the patient's right.

For a double-stapled anastomosis, two stay sutures are placed on the lateral aspects of the stapled rectal stump. The ileal side is prepared by placing a noncrushing clamp proximal to the anastomosis. A purse-string suture of 0 polypropylene is placed around the ileum at the site of the insertion for the head or anvil of the circular stapler (Fig. 9). A divot large enough to accommodate the intraluminal stapler is excised from the ileal staple line and extended as needed along the antimesenteric wall of the ileum with scissors. I prefer the largest stapler (31 or 33 mm, depending on manufacturer), but sometimes the next size down seems to fit better. A purse-string suture of 2-0 polypropylene is placed on the ileal defect. The end-to-end or intraluminal stapler is inserted through the anus. To facilitate placement of the transanal intraluminal stapler, I place Fansler anoscope into the anus and pass the stapler through the anoscope. The slot in the anoscope allows it to be removed from the stapling instrument. The intraluminal stapler must be advanced under

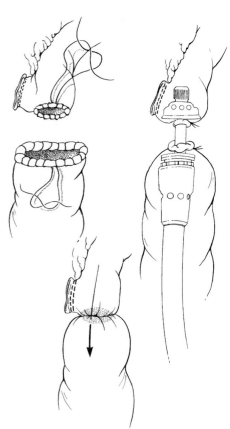

Fig. 9. Side-to-end ileorectal anastomosis with intraluminal stapler.

direct inspection of the remaining rectum from within the abdomen. The rectal stay sutures facilitate proper alignment of the stapler in the midpoint of the rectal staple line.

Once the stapler is in position, the trocar of the instrument is advanced to pierce the stable line. The trocar is removed and the proximal anvil in the ileum is docked into position with the rectal stapler. The device is closed, fired, and removed. Two intact "donuts" should be obtained. The anastomosis is checked for integrity by inserting a rigid sigmoidoscope through the anus and insufflating air, with the pelvis filled with saline.

The edge of the ileal mesentery is sutured to the retroperitoneal surface to eliminate the potential hernia defect. Drains are not required. Diverting-loop ileostomy is rarely necessary with total colectomy and ileorectal anastomosis.

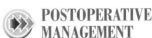

POSTOPERATIVE MANAGEMENT

Ileus can be prolonged after total colectomy. Once intestinal function returns, patients suffer from postoperative diarrhea, sometimes with urgency and even minor incontinence. Bulking agents and loperamide hydrochloride are an effective antidiarrheal agent, but its use should be deferred for a day or so until stool passage is well established. Incontinence should not be a lingering problem once stools slow and thicken, provided that preoperative assessment of sphincter adequacy was correct.

RESULTS

Anastomotic leak is more common in patients with inflammatory bowel disease than in people with other indications for total colectomy. The incidence of this complication should be less than 4%. Large leaks require reoperation and resection of the anastomosis, closure of the rectal stump, and end ileostomy. After a reasonable recovery, the patient may consider another attempt to restore continuity. Small leaks can be managed nonoperatively.

Function depends on the indication for the operation, presence of rectal disease, age, and co-morbid factors. Generally,

otherwise normal persons who undergo total colectomy with ileorectal anastomosis have from three to five stools per day for the remainder of their lives. This stool pattern does not interfere with physical activities or daily routine.

SUGGESTED READING

Biondo S, Martí-Ragué J, Kreisler E, et al. A prospective study of outcomes of emergency and elective surgeries for complicated colonic cancer. *Am J Surg* 2005;189:377.

Boardman L. Heritable colorectal cancer syndromes: recognition and preventive management. *Gastroenterol Clin North Am* 2002;31:1107.

Delaney CP, Pokala N, Senagore AJ, et al. Is laparoscopic colectomy applicable to patients with body mass index 30? A case matched comparative study with open colectomy. *Dis Colon Rectum* 2005;48:975.

Pocard M, Pomel C, Lasser P. Laparoscopic prophylactic surgery for HNPCC gene mutation carrier: has the time come? *Lancet Oncol* 2003;4:637.

McShane MS, Bax T, MacFarlane M, et al. Outcomes for a laparoscopic approach for

total abdominal colectomy and proctocolectomy. *Am J Surg* 2006;191:673.

Nieuwenjuijzen M, Reijnen MM, Kuijpers JH, et al. Small bowel obstruction after total or subtotal colectomy: a 10-year retrospective review. *Br J Surg* 1998;85:1242.

Papa MZ, Karni T, Koller M, et al. Avoiding diarrhea after subtotal colectomy with primary anastomosis in the treatment of colon cancer. *J Am Coll Surg* 1997;184:269.

Pfeifer J, Agachan F, Wexner SD. Surgery for constipation: a review. *Dis Colon Rectum* 1996;39:444.

Rao S. Constipation: evaluation and treatment. *Gastroenterol Clin North Am* 2003;32:659.

Reemst PH, Kuijpers HC, Wobbes T. Management of left-sided colonic obstruction by subtotal colectomy and ileocolic anastomosis. *Eur J Surg* 1998;164:537.

Rieger N, Collopy B, Fink R, et al. Total colectomy for Crohn's disease. *Aust N Z J Surg* 1999;69:28.

Rivadeneira DE, Marcello PW, Roberts PL, et al. Benefits of hand assisted laparoscopic restorative proctocolectomy: a comparative study. *Dis Colon Rectum* 2004;47:1371.

Rodriguez-Bigas MA, Vasen HF, Pekka-Mecklin J, et al. Rectal cancer risk in hereditary nonpolyposis colorectal cancer after abdominal colectomy. International Collaborative Group on HNPCC. *Ann Surg* 1997; 225:202.

The Gastrointestinal Tract

EDITOR'S COMMENT

Total colectomy and illeorectal anastomosis is not an operation looking for its place. There are a number of legitimate uses of total abdominal colectomy and illeorectal anastomosis. Among these are patients with familial adenomatous polyposis. A number of patients with familial adenomatous polyposis do not have tremendous rectal involvement and there are sufficiently few polyps that can be removed. These patients can undergo surveillance. Although patients do not normally wish to undergo repeated flexible sigmoidoscopy or rigid sigmoidoscopy for a period of 3 to 6 months, my experience with this disease is that after awhile, something about the illeal contents going directly into the rectum, leads to a decrease in the production of polyps in these patients, and then the period of surveillance can be decreased. Another reasonable use of subtotal colectomy or total colectomy in illeorectal anastomosis is the Lynch syndrome or hereditary nonpolyposis colorectal cancer, in which there frequently is rectal sparing. The problem is convincing patients that they are prone to colorectal cancer when they are already worried about endometrial and ovarian carcinoma. However, in properly selected patients, this procedure does decrease the incidence of carcinoma in the colon.

Another situation in which one might want to look at total abdominal colectomy and ileorectal anastomosis is in segmental Crohn disease of the colon. As we all know, Crohn disease of the colon has a much worse prognosis than small bowel Crohn disease, particularly as far as recurrence is concerned. Tekkis et al. (*Colorectal Dis* 2006;8:82) focus on a meta-analysis of 488 patients subjected to resection for colonic Crohn, including 223 with

total colectomy and ileorectal anastomosis, and 265 with segmental colectomy. It is not clear that any of these were randomized prospective trials. In brief, the authors found that patients with two or more colonic segments involved, were associated with a lower reoperation rate in the ileorectal anastomosis group; although this did not reach statistical significance. One difference was the recurrence rate. The recurrence-free interval of 4.4 years favored the ileorectal anastomosis group, which was statistically significant at $P < 0.01$. There was no difference in the need for permanent stoma, unlike studies reviewed in other chapters, in which it does appear that more distal resection for Crohn disease resulted in an increased likelihood of a permanent stoma. The total surgical recurrence in this group was 66% during 10 years. Perianal disease seemed to be an indicator of future difficulty and surgical recurrence, a finding that is not surprising.

One other area of usefulness for ileorectal anastomosis and total colectomy is in ulcerative colitis in female patients. Mortier et al. (*Gastroenterol Clin Biol* 2006;30:594) reviewed female patients, 40 years old and younger, who underwent ileorectal anastomosis. They were interviewed by telephone. Of 40 eligible patients, 15 wished to have children after ileorectal anastomosis. Sixty-six percent or 10 became pregnant. Five were sterile. They compared this with reduced rate of fecundity, which has recently been shown after ileal pouch anal anastomosis; although in my own personal experience carefully done ileal pouch anal anastomosis reduces fecundity to some extent, but not to a great extent. However, this is not the common view.

Finally, another useful outcome of total colectomy in patients with ulcerative colitis involves regulatory T

cells, which were suppressed prior to total colectomy. However, the incidence of T-regulator cells was increased shortly after total colectomy, with significant differences between postoperative day 1 and postoperative day 7, and then again between postoperative day 7 and postoperative day 20. The authors claim that this shows that the T-regulator cells may play a pivotal role in the pathogenesis of ulcerative colitis, but it is more likely that their diminished presence is the result of a chronic illness, which may trigger immunologic consequences (Furihata et al. *World J Surg* 2006;30:590).

The technique that Dr. Opelka describes is fairly classic, with the exception of emphasis on taking the line of Toldt closer to the colon so as not to leave Gerota's fascia and the rest of the retroperineum as widely open as is traditional. I agree that this is primarily a blunt dissection. On the left side, the adhesions for the sigmoid colon make it imperative that one does not dissect fat while taking down the sigmoid colon. I too agree that it is not necessary to mobilize the right ureter, as one can usually see it through the peritoneum, somewhat higher on the pelvic wall than the left ureter. The left ureter, however, often passes close to the sigmoid vasculature and the inferior mesenteric, and it is very easy to include the ureter in the ligature, particularly if it is a mass ligature, when one is dividing the superior hemorrhoidal. Thus, I take the trouble to dissect out the left ureter and place a vessel loop around it, leaving it hanging loosely, so that one can always find the ureter as the operation proceeds.

Not surprisingly, laparoscopy, laparoscopic total colectomy, and ileorectal anastomosis have received a lot of attention, especially in regard to

(continued)

comparison with open operation. In a series of ileal pouch anal anastomoses, in the early 1990s, Dr. Mike Nussbaum and I used laparoscopic colectomy in taking down both the hepatic and the splenic flexures. We did set a time limit and found that it might be useful, but that in time, especially in thin patients, we could use a left lower quadrant transverse incision, both for removing the colon and for creating the pouch, even without laparoscopy, and so our interest diminished.

Yet, it seems that a number of groups have analyzed and compared, not necessarily in a full comparative randomized clinical trial, laparoscopic colectomy with open colectomy. Belizon et al. (*Surg Endosc* 2006;20:947) studied the effects of conversion of operation more than 30 minutes after the procedure had begun. They found that perioperative morbidity was significantly higher in laparoscopic procedures converted to open procedures more than 30 minutes into the case. Predictive factors were inflammatory process beyond the sigmoid and obesity. Operative predictors, not surprisingly, were adhesions and bleeding. They proposed earlier conversion and better selection, so that conversion greater than 30 minutes could not take place. This does not seem very logical because if one starts out to do a laparoscopic colectomy, one persists until it becomes clear that it is not going to work. Earlier conversion is not likely to change the rate of increase in postoperative mor-

bidity, seen in the 20% (28 of 143 patients) of laparoscopic colon resections.

Tilney et al. (*Colorectal Surg* 2006;8:441) compared laparoscopic with open colectomy for benign and malignant disease. They carried out meta-analysis of studies comparing laparoscopic and open subtotal colectomy. It is not clear that any of these are randomized clinical trials. The conversion rate in 143 (43%) of 333 patients was 5%. The differences seen here, which are fairly consistent, are that operative time was longer by 1.5 hours and length of stay was shorter by almost 3 days. In answer to the question of whether postoperative intestinal obstruction, either immediate or remote, was present in these groups, as proposed by Gurland and Wexner (*Inflamm Bowel Dis* 2002;8:46), they found no evidence that this was the case.

A case match study—although, again, I am not certain that this was a randomized clinical trial—was reported by Pokala et al. (*Surg Endosc* 2005;19:531), in which the operating times were 136 minutes in a laparoscopic group and the length of stay shorter by 3 days. This is similar to what the previous study reported. Again blood loss was somewhat less in the laparoscopic group.

Ausch et al. (*Colorectal Dis* 2005;8:195) reviewed the cause and surgical management of toxic megacolon. This was a retrospective review in which 70 patients during 20 years were surgically managed. The median age was 63 years, which seems old for a group in which almost half of the patients with inflamma-

tory bowel disease underwent resection. Only two patients had an ileal pouch anal anastomosis at that time. It is true that one wants to prepare the rectum, in my case with steroid enemas, so that the mucosal stripping is carried out more easily. If there is comparative sparing of the rectum, I have not hesitated to do an ileal pouch anal anastomosis in the presence of toxic megacolon, provided that the patient is not unstable, that there has not been a subclinical leak or abscess, and that one can do the operation with minimal blood loss, which is sometimes possible. Interestingly, in this study only 26 of the 70 patients had their continuity restored, despite the fact that 70% of the patients, initially, had subtotal colectomies and an additional 20% had total abdominal colectomies that left the rectal intact.

McNevim et al. (*Am J Surg* 2006;191:673) reviewed a total of 51 patients, mean age of 40 years, treated for a variety of diseases, including eight with toxic megacolon, or toxic colitis as they refer to it. Open conversion was present in five patients, including three of the eight with toxic colitis. There were 10 complications (20%) including 5 intra-abdominal abscesses. This seems rather high for a group of 51 patients. The authors of this study promote laparoscopic approach for colectomy, but it does seem as if the incidence of severe complications is somewhat high, and surgery is not an adventure in "look at me and see what I can do."

. J.E.F.

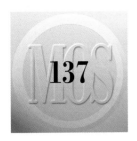

Segmental Resection for Diverticulitis

ROBERT D. FRY, NAJJIA N. MAHMOUD

Diverticular disease of the colon is a disease of Western civilization; its emergence as an important clinical entity roughly coincides with the onset of the Industrial Revolution. It is hypothesized that the dietary changes associated with the introduction of roller milling of wheat and refinement of sugar contribute to irregularities in intestinal motility that result in the pathologic anatomic findings associated with the disease. Diverticula are mucosal herniations that protrude through the colonic wall at vulnerable sites traversed by nutritional arterioles (Fig. 1). These diverticula are composed only of mucosa and serosa, and absent a muscular layer are actually pseudodiverticula. True diverticula contain all normal layers of the colon (mucosa, muscularis, and serosa), are thought to be congenital rather than acquired, and are seldom a cause of infection or bleeding.

Diverticulosis (the presence of colonic diverticula without inflammation) is usually associated with hypertrophy and brittleness of the affected colonic musculature

(mychosis); this muscular abnormality often precedes the appearance of diverticula. The condition is thought to be caused by chronic segmental contractions of the circular muscle of the colon, which in turn causes increased intraluminal pressure (especially in the sigmoid colon), muscular hypertrophy, and herniations of mucosa through the weak areas in the colonic wall. It is generally assumed that the low-residue diet favored by many Americans and northern Europeans is a major causative factor. Advancing age is certainly another associated risk factor, but diverticulosis is not rare in Americans in the fourth decade of life. At least 75% of Americans over the age of 60 will harbor sigmoid diverticula, and the prevalence of diverticulitis across all age groups in the United States is approximately 60 per 100,000.

The mere presence of colonic diverticula would be of little concern except for two serious events that may accompany the condition: bleeding and perforation. It is noteworthy that these two problems

seldom occur at the same time; it is distinctly unusual for major colonic hemorrhage to occur simultaneously with an attack of diverticulitis.

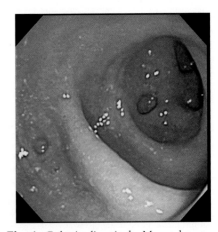

Fig. 1. Colonic diverticula: Mucosal protrusions through the muscular layer of the colon at the site of arteriolar penetration, most commonly on the mesenteric side of the antimesenteric tenia.

Although this chapter will deal only with the surgical treatment of diverticulitis and its complications, it is interesting to consider the pathogenesis of bleeding from a diverticulum. The diverticulum protrudes through the colonic musculature often in intimate contact with the nutritional artery (Fig. 2). With the passage of time the artery undergoes pathologic changes characterized by eccentric muscular thickening and intimal thinning. Occasionally this affected artery will bleed into the diverticulum and then into the colonic lumen; the arterial bleeding can be massive in volume and yet difficult to localize. Although the affected artery is associated with the diverticulum that protrudes to the serosal surface of the colon, the bleeding is virtually always into the colonic lumen. It is extremely rare that an artery associated with a diverticulum will bleed into the peritoneal cavity. This is in contrast to the inflammation associated with diverticulitis, which is actually an extraluminal, paracolic infection.

PATHOGENESIS

DeQuervain recognized that the condition we commonly call diverticulitis would more properly be designated as "peridiverticulitis." It is an infection of the paracolic tissues caused by a perforation of a diverticulum. The cause of the perforation is conjectural (increased luminal pressure, ischemia, microtorsion, etc.), but the result is extravasation of feces through the colonic wall. Since most diverticula are located on the mesenteric side of the colon, the perforation is often contained or confined within the mesentery. Still, this is an intra-abdominal infection that may well require the attention of the surgeon. Unfortunately, not all diverticular perforations are immediately contained by the mesentery or omentum; a perforation into the peritoneal cavity may cause life-threatening peritonitis, and even if the infection associated with a perforation is contained by the abdomen's natural defenses (omentum and adjacent organs), an abscess cavity may rupture into the free peritoneal cavity or into adjacent organs, causing peritonitis or creating a fistula.

The paracolic contamination resulting from the perforation of a diverticulum may vary tremendously, and it is not possible to recommend a simple treatment plan that will apply to all cases of diverticulitis. Hinchy described a clinical classification that is somewhat useful in describing and categorizing the clinical severity of the disease:

> Stage I: Microperforation (phlegmon) contained by paracolic tissues
> Stage II: Abscess
> Stage III: Perforation of an abscess into the peritoneal cavity
> Stage IV: Fecal peritonitis

The clinical scenario and appropriate treatment plan are obviously different for each stage of this disease. But the overall treatment goal for any case of diverticulitis is to control the infection, assess the chance for persistent or recurrent disease, and formulate a treatment that will control the infection and minimize the chance of recurrence.

DIAGNOSIS

History and physical examination remain the cornerstones for the diagnosis of diverticulitis. By far the most common location of diverticula is the sigmoid colon, and this is the most common site of colonic diverticulitis. The clinical manifestations of paracolic inflammation caused by a perforated sigmoid diverticulum correspond to the location of the perforation and the severity of the infection. The typical clinical presentation is one of left lower quadrant abdominal pain and fever. Examination of the abdomen may reveal guarding and tenderness in the left lower quadrant, sometimes associated with a palpable mass. In elderly patients a redundant, tortuous sigmoid colon may reside in the right lower quadrant, and diverticulitis can mask appendicitis by presenting with right lower quadrant abdominal pain and tenderness. Leukocytosis is common, and significant infection can be associated with ileus or small bowel obstruction secondary to involvement of adjacent loops of intestine by the inflammatory process.

It is necessary to establish the diagnosis and exclude other causes of abdominal pain that might require a different treatment, such as colonic ischemia, appendicitis, or perforated sigmoid carcinoma. The preferred test to confirm the suspected diagnosis of diverticulitis is computed tomography of the abdomen. The computed axial tomography (CAT) scan typically reveals inflammatory changes in the region of the perforation, with stranding of the mesentery and thickening of the paracolic soft tissues. The CAT scan is particularly useful in detecting the presence and location of an abscess (Fig. 3). Such abscesses in the abdomen or pelvis can then be drained percutaneously with the aid of radiologic guidance.

Barium enema is relatively contraindicated in patients suspected of having diverticulitis; the hydrostatic pressure during administration of colonic barium risks causing extravasation of barium through the perforated diverticulum; barium combined with feces results in peritonitis of greater severity than that caused from exposure to either alone. Some authors have

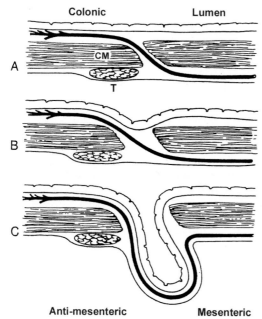

Fig. 2. Demonstration of the relationship of a diverticulum to the intramural vessel. **A:** The colon wall is penetrated obliquely by vasa recta through the circular muscle (CM) typically on the mesenteric side of the tenia (T). **B:** The blood vessel becomes stretched and attenuated as it is drawn along with the forming diverticulum. **C:** The vasa recta are draped over the apex of the diverticulum and are prone to intraluminal rupture. (From Meyers, MA, et al.: Pathogenesis of bleeding colonic diverticula. Gastroenterology, 71: 577, 1976.

The Gastrointestinal Tract

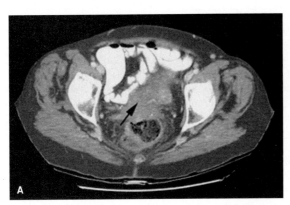

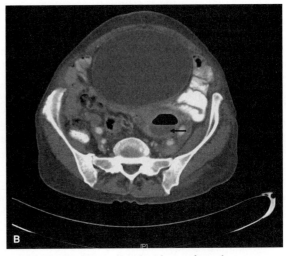

Fig. 3. CT scans of mesenteric phlegmon (**A**) and a pelvic abscess (**B**) associated with a perforated diverticulum.

recommended water-soluble contrast enema to confirm the diagnosis of diverticulitis, but this still risks aggravating the situation with increased intraluminal pressure.

INITIAL TREATMENT

Initial treatment depends upon the severity of the infection; this can range from a small perforation into the mesentery that is immediately contained and sealed to an uncontrolled intraperitoneal fecal spillage with generalized peritonitis. A small contained perforation may resolve with no therapy, but antibiotics are indicated once the diagnosis is established. Oral antibiotics may suffice for a small contained perforation, but with significant tenderness, fever, and leukocytosis, broad-spectrum intravenous antibiotics should be administered. If an ileus or small bowel obstruction is present, nasogastric decompression and intravenous fluids are required. If an abscess is detected by computed tomography, it should be drained percutaneously under radiographic guidance (either by computed tomography [CT] scan or ultrasound). The goal of initial therapy is to support and stabilize the patient and contain and control the infection.

EMERGENCY RESECTION FOR SIGMOID DIVERTICULITIS

In the relatively rare case of free intraperitoneal perforation and generalized peritonitis, immediate celiotomy is obviously required. In such circumstances, the goal is to resect the diseased, perforated sigmoid

colon and fashion a colostomy from the descending colon. While it is relatively unusual, in my experience, to have to perform the Hartmann operation as an emergency for diverticulitis, recent experience has shown that only 56% of colostomies fashioned for diverticulitis are subsequently reversed. Therefore, the operation should be conducted in such a fashion that the function of the stoma is optimal. Prior to induction of anesthesia, the patient should be examined in both the supine and sitting position, with the intent of selecting the best site for the stoma. Generally the best position is at the summit of the infraumbilical fat mound over the left rectus muscle. However, in obese patients an abdominal crease at this site may prevent the secure application of a colostomy face plate, and a better site will usually be cephalad to the abdominal crease.

In emergency operations for diverticulitis I usually explore the abdomen through a midline incision, preserving both sides for possible placement of a stoma. During initial exploration of the abdomen I verify that the sigmoid colon is the site of contamination, but I try to avoid manipulating the sigmoid or entering the pelvis (which often harbors an abscess) until I have mobilized the splenic flexure adequately to allow normal-appearing, pliable descending colon to reach the abdominal skin at the anticipated stoma site. This is accomplished by incising the peritoneum of the left colic gutter cephalad to the sigmoid with electrocautery, reflecting the left side of the omentum from the distal transverse colon in the area of the splenic flexure, and dissecting the retroperitoneal surface of the descend-

ing colon from Gerota's fascia. At times it is necessary to divide the inferior mesenteric vein close to the edge of the pancreas to gain sufficient mobility for the descending colon to reach the left lower abdomen without tension, but this is not invariably so (Fig. 4).

After adequate mobility of the descending colon has been achieved, attention is directed to the diseased sigmoid colon. There is almost invariably a phlegmon present, composed of the sigmoid, its mesentery, and adjacent organs, usually small bowel, bladder, or uterus. The sigmoid is separated from the adjacent organs by blunt dissection, often pinching the sigmoid from the adjacent organs (Fig. 5). Any abscesses are unroofed, and any interloop collections of pus within folds of the mesentery are freed. It is not uncommon for the left ureter to be involved with the phlegmon, and in such circumstances the ureter should be identified in its proximal course as it emerges from the kidney under the area from which the descending colon was reflected. The ureter can then be traced distally as the inflamed sigmoid and its mesentery is reflected medially by a combination of electrocautery and blunt dissection.

As mentioned earlier, the sigmoid musculature is often thickened and brittle because of the pathologic process associated with diverticulosis, and it is necessary to excise all abnormal, thickened colon. This often means carrying the dissection to 1 or 2 cm distal to the sacral promontory, where soft, pliable rectum will virtually always be found. I don't divide the inferior mesenteric artery close to the aorta in patients with diverticulitis (in contrast to patients with colorectal cancer) in order to avoid injury to the hypogastric

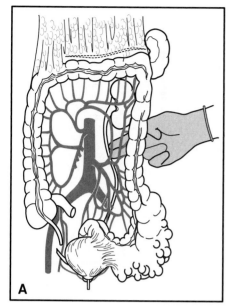 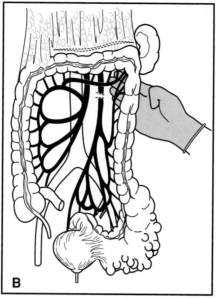

Fig. 4. A: The descending colon is mobilized and separated from the prerenal (Gerota's) fascia. The avascular fusion of the omentum to the left transverse colon is divided. If the ureter is difficult to appreciate in the region of the phlegmon, it can be identified as it exits the kidney under the descending colon and traced caudally. **B:** The inferior mesenteric vein may tether the descending colon and prevent it from reaching the anterior abdominal wall (or pelvis) unless divided.

scending colon at the beginning of the operation becomes obvious: It is not necessary to dissect the retroperitoneum in the left upper abdomen after dissecting the phlegmon or draining abscesses, and the risk of contaminating the subdiaphragmatic space is lessened. Since the mesentery of the descending colon has been mobilized from Gerota's fascia, the entire descending colon and its mesentery can be brought to the abdominal wall anterior to the small intestine. There is no mesenteric attachment to the posterior abdomen for the small bowel to twist around after the operation. It is not necessary to "close the lateral gutter" by sewing the edge of the colonic mesentery to the lateral and anterior peritoneum .

To create the aperture for the colostomy a disk of skin 2.5 cm in diameter is excised, the subcutaneous fat and anterior rectus fascia are incised longitudinally, the rectus muscle fibers separated with a Kelly clamp, and the posterior rectus fascia incised longitudinally. The size of this aperture permits easy passage of the index and middle fingers. The colon is then drawn through the abdominal wall and maintained in this position with a

plexus (the disruption of this sympathetic plexus would result in ejaculatory dysfunction). The sigmoid mesentery is serially clamped, divided, and ligated with absorbable sutures (Fig. 6). A site to transect the normal-appearing descending colon is then selected, with care taken to ensure that the intestine is well vascularized, soft, and pliable. Incidentally, the presence of some diverticula in a soft, pliable descending colon is not an indication to excise that segment. It is generally accepted that the cause of recurrent diverticulitis after sigmoid resection for the condition is not from diverticula in the unresected descending colon, but from abnormal sigmoid colon retained adjacent to the rectum. The descending colon is transected with a linear cutting stapling device (Fig. 7).

The rectum is then transected with a TA stapling instrument (Fig. 8). If the dissection is carried down to normal rectum, the proximal rectum will readily accept the staples and it is not necessary to invert or oversew this staple line. After the specimen has been resected, the operative field is irrigated with saline containing neomycin and Polysporin.

At this point in the operation the advantage afforded by mobilizing the de-

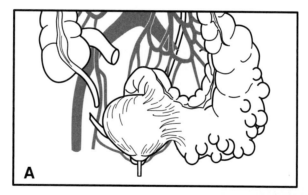 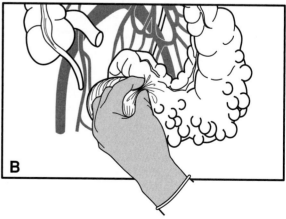

Fig. 5. A: The inflamed sigmoid colon is attached to the bladder. **B:** The phlegmon is separated from the bladder by pinching the organs apart.

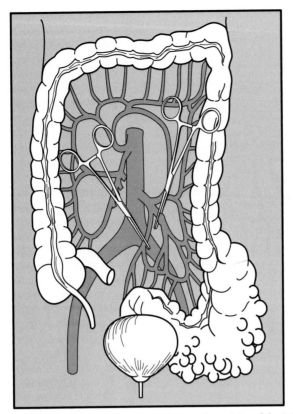

Fig. 6. Division of the sigmoid mesentery. Dissection close to the origin of the inferior mesenteric artery is avoided to prevent injury to the sympathetic hypogastric plexus.

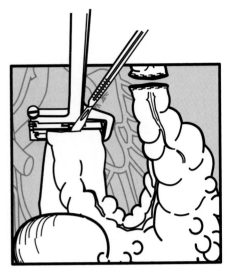

Fig. 8. Transecting the rectum with a TA stapler.

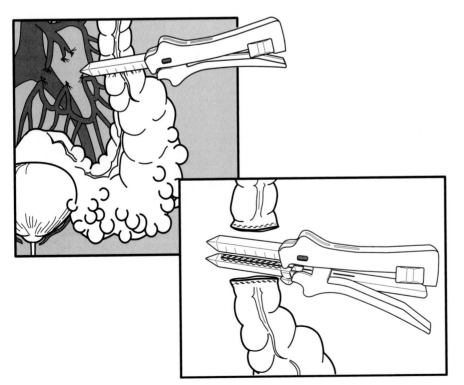

Fig. 7. Transecting the descending colon with the GIA stapler.

Babcock clamp until the incision has been closed. After closure, the incision is protected with a sterile towel and the colon matured by excising the staple line and approximating the full thickness of the colon to the skin (Fig. 9). I have no hesitancy to sew the colon to the abdominal wall skin with absorbable sutures; unlike ileal mucosa, colonic mucosa will not transplant into the suture tract. (While fashioning an ileostomy, I suture the ileal wall to the subcuticular layer of the integument, since ileal mucosa may grow at the suture sites on the peristomal skin if the suture is placed through the full thickness of the skin, a feature that occasionally hinders the maintenance of an ileostomy appliance.) Intestinal continuity can be restored approximately 10 weeks later with an anastomosis between the descending colon and the rectum. Since all of the diseased sigmoid was removed at the initial operation, minimal dissection or mobilization of the rectum will be required during the second operation, and the anastomosis is easily accomplished using the circular stapler.

TREATMENT OF PATIENTS NOT REQUIRING EMERGENCY OPERATION

Most patients experiencing an attack of diverticulitis will respond favorably to nonoperative treatment. As discussed earlier, this treatment varies depending upon the severity of the disease and specific circumstances, ranging from oral antibiotics to bowel rest, nasogastric decom-

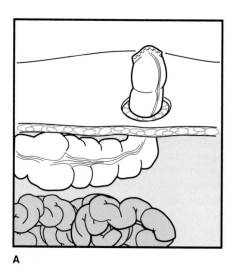
A

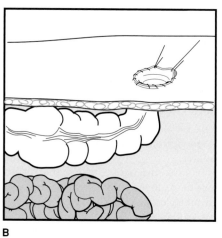
B

Fig. 9. **A:** The descending colon has been completely freed from the posterior abdominal wall, and lies anterior to the small intestine as it is brought through the anterior abdomen to form the colostomy. **B:** Sewing the colon to skin following excision of the staple line.

The Gastrointestinal Tract

pression, intravenous antibiotics, and percutaneous drainage of intra-abdominal or pelvic abscesses. Diverticulitis that responds readily to antibiotics is considered to be uncomplicated. A patient who experiences a single uncomplicated attack of diverticulitis that responds to antibiotic treatment has approximately a 20% chance of having a subsequent attack, with patients under the age of 50 years being more likely to suffer recurrences than older patients (27% vs. 17%). However, the risk of a subsequent attack requiring emergency surgery and a colostomy is less than 6%. Taking these factors into consideration, most physicians feel that a single episode of uncomplicated diverticulitis is not an indication for operation. However, the risk of more attacks (and complicated attacks) does increase with each subsequent attack, although the exact risk of such attacks is difficult to assess. Nevertheless, most surgeons recommend elective sigmoid resection after two documented but uncomplicated attacks of sigmoid diverticulitis, and after a single attack of complicated diverticulitis (with abscess requiring drainage, small bowel obstruction, or fistula formation).

PREPARATION FOR SIGMOID RESECTION FOR DIVERTICULITIS

The goal of initial treatment of a patient with diverticulitis is to convert a complicated emergency situation into a simple elective one. Infection should be con-

trolled, abscesses drained, fistulas assessed, cancer excluded, and nutrition optimized. The initial approach to control infection has already been discussed. Percutaneous drainage of abdominal or pelvic abscess under radiographic guidance has been a great boon to the treatment of diverticulitis. In the past, laparotomy with open drainage of an abdominal or pelvic abscess was often undertaken in conjunction with the Hartmann operation. Unfortunately, draining the abscess via an abdominal incision exposed the uninfected regions of the peritoneal cavity to the contents of the abscess, an unavoidable event that often spread rather than contained the infection.

After an abscess is drained percutaneously, it is not rare for an enterocutaneous fistula to form along the drainage tract. Fistulas complicating diverticulitis may also involve the bladder, uterus, vagina, or small bowel. A fistula between the sigmoid colon and bladder may cause pneumaturia, fecaluria, and recurrent urinary tract infections. A CAT scan may demonstrate air in the urinary bladder in such circumstances (Fig. 10).

It is important to exclude a sigmoid cancer in patients with signs and symptoms suggestive of diverticulitis. The surgeon should be especially wary of the case of presumed diverticulitis that does not respond favorably as anticipated to nonoperative treatment with antibiotics, percutaneous drainage, etc., because a perforated cancer can mimic diverticulitis, and the appropriate operative treatment is markedly different for the two diseases.

Whereas colonoscopy is of little use (and may actually be detrimental) during the acute attack of diverticulitis, after the infection is controlled this examination should be done prior to elective sigmoid resection. Every measure should be taken to exclude colon cancer prior to operation, because appropriate oncologic surgery requires en bloc resection of all adherent organs, whereas the operation for diverticulitis entails the blunt separation of the affected colon from adherent organs and the disruption of fistula tracts, maneuvers that would result in the loss of any chance to cure a patient with cancer. On the other hand, oncologic principles applied to an operation for diverticulitis would demand an unacceptable resec-

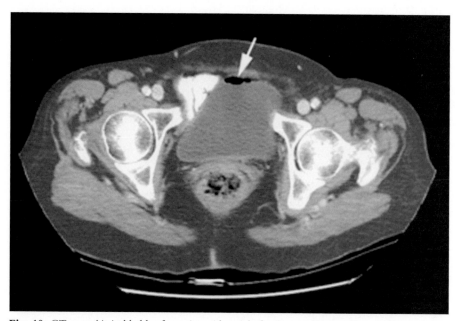

Fig. 10. CT scan: Air in bladder from sigmoid-vesicle fistula complicating diverticulitis.

tion of normal organs, such as adherent bladder, uterus, ureter, and small bowel.

The patient's nutrition should be optimal. Usually this is not a problem in a patient appropriately treated for diverticulitis, but the occasional patient who does not rapidly respond to antibiotics and bowel rest will benefit significantly from total parenteral nutrition. In such circumstances the nutritional requirements of the patient can be satisfactorily maintained until the infection is controlled, and a situation that would have required a colostomy can be converted to one that can be treated by resection with anastomosis.

ELECTIVE RESECTION FOR DIVERTICULITIS

Most operations for diverticulitis are elective procedures, with the most common indications being repeated attacks, recovery from a single complicated attack, or presence of a fistula (fistula may occur between the sigmoid colon and the skin, bladder, uterus, vagina, or small intestine).

The operations should be timed after sufficient recovery from the preceding attack has allowed resolution of inflammation of paracolic tissues and organs. Usually 6 weeks is sufficient time, but there is always a risk that another attack can occur during this recovery period. However, that risk is relatively small, and the advantages gained by waiting until the inflammation has subsided are great. As the operative date approaches, a colonoscopic examination should be done to exclude other colonic pathology. If the schedule can be arranged for the colonoscopy to be done the day prior to the operation, one bowel cleansing can suffice for both procedures.

If circumstances during the prior episode of diverticulitis suggest that the left ureter may be involved in the inflammatory process, it is helpful to have a cystoscopic examination and placement of a stent in the left ureter after induction of anesthesia. However, ureteral stents are not immune to complications, the left ureter is usually readily identified, and I find myself using ureteral stents only if I expect to encounter significant pelvic inflammation.

The patient is positioned in the dorsal lithotomy position with the lower extremities supported by Yellow Fin stirrups (Fig. 11). Care is taken to ensure proper positioning of the legs to prevent pressure on the peroneal nerves. This position provides excellent exposure of the abdomen, pelvis, perineum, and anus, facilitating transanal introduction of the stapling in-

strument and proctosigmoidoscope later in the course of the operation.

If the patient is relatively thin I usually explore the abdomen through an infraumbilical incision, dividing both rectus abdomini and extending the incision slightly farther laterally on the left side. This incision allows excellent exposure to the pelvis; the major concern from many surgeons is inadequate exposure for mobilization of the splenic flexure. However, should there be a problem with access to the splenic flexure, the left edge of the incision can simply be extended in a lateral and cephalad direction without major consequence.

If the patient is obese, a midline incision will provide better access to the entire abdomen, including the splenic flexure.

I protect the wound with a ring drape placed immediately after completing the incision. While there has been no convincing evidence that this barrier decreases the incidence of wound infections, it does facilitate exposure during the operation and seems to prevent desiccation of the exposed wound edges.

The operative findings will, of course, vary considerably, depending upon the site of the perforation and the extent of the infection. It is not unusual for the thickened sigmoid colon to be adherent to the bladder and to appear to extend deeply into the pelvis. However, separating the sigmoid from the bladder and retracting it back into the peritoneal cavity will invariably reveal the normal, noninvolved pelvic rectum.

After assessing the situation and the extent of persistent inflammation, I usually begin the dissection by dividing the peritoneum lateral to the descending colon and reflecting the colon medially from Gerota's fascia. The omentum is separated from the distal transverse colon with electrocautery. Care should be taken during this stage of the operation not to apply excessive downward traction on the omentum or transverse colon; it is during this portion of the operation that the capsule of the spleen can be torn, and this is almost always due to excessive traction on the omentum. The colon is actually dissected from the omentum, leaving the omentum in place. After the distal transverse colon is separated from the omentum, electrocautery is used to further dissect the space between the retroperitoneal surface of the splenic flexure and Gerota's fascia. At this point the inferior mesenteric vein at the level of the lower edge of the pancreas is the only significant structure that prevents the descending colon

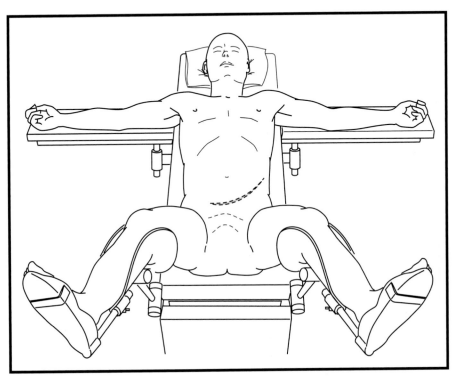

Fig. 11. Dorsal lithotomy position.

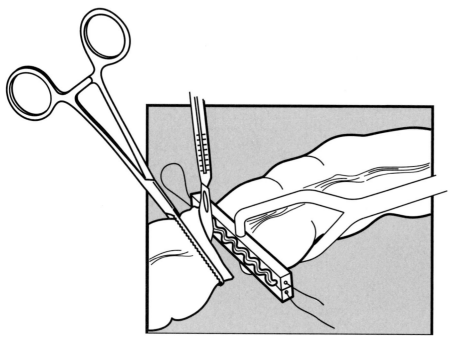

Fig. 12. The descending colon is divided between a Kocher clamp and a purse-string clamp.

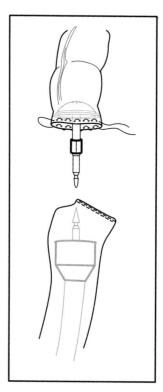

Fig. 13. Anvil head of the circular stapler inserted into the lumen of the descending colon and the purse string tied about the post of the anvil head.

from being able to reach deep into the pelvis. However, I wait until later in the operation to assess the ability of the descending colon to reach the pelvis before deciding whether or not to divide the inferior mesenteric vein.

The next stage of the operation is mobilization of the sigmoid colon. Unlike an operation for cancer, this portion of the operation is conducted in a fashion to preserve all adjacent organs that may be adherent to (or form fistulas with) the sigmoid, and to resect the entire sigmoid, leaving normal, nonthickened, nonconstricted rectum and descending colon for the anastomosis.

If the sigmoid is adherent to the bladder, the organs are separated by blunt dissection, often developing the plane by pinching the tissues between the thumb and index finger. The lateral peritoneum is then incised, taking care to identify the left ureter. The ureter lies medial to the genital vein, and can usually be readily identified crossing the left iliac artery. If the ureter is involved in an incompletely resolved inflammatory process, and a ureteral stent has not been placed to aid in its identification by palpation, I usually search for it along its more proximal course, in the region that has been developed during the mobilization of the descending colon.

After the ureter is identified and displaced laterally, the mesentery to the sigmoid is serially divided between Kelly clamps, and hemostasis is obtained with absorbable suture ligatures. The sigmoid

mesentery is often contracted, but it is not necessary to resect any more of the mesentery than will permit complete removal of the sigmoid. There is no need to risk injury to the hypogastric nerves by dissecting the inferior mesenteric artery close to the aorta.

After the sigmoid has been mobilized and its vascular supply divided, I select the site in the descending colon for the proximal component of the anastomosis. It is important that the colon at this site not be thickened or constricted. The descending colon is divided between a large Kocher clamp and an autosuture purse-string device; the edges of the colon are carefully inspected to ensure the integrity of the purse-string suture (Fig. 12). If there are any gaps between the staples holding the purse string, I simply close them with a 4-0 suture. It is worthwhile to inspect the site where the knot will be tied to complete the purse string—often the stapling instrument will leave too large a space between staples at this point, and a suture is required to ensure complete encompassment by the purse string.

The next step is to place the anvil head of the circular stapler into the descending colon. It is preferable to use the largest diameter of stapler that the descending colon will accept, but too large a stapler runs the risk of tearing the musculature of the colon wall and causing ischemia at the staple line. If the colon is obviously of a large diameter, I use the 31-mm stapler, but more often

I use the 28-mm size (Fig. 13). After the purse string has been tied about the post of the anvil head, I return the descending colon to the peritoneal cavity, placing it in the left lateral abdomen, taking care to avoid compromising its blood supply by twisting or kinking it.

Attention is then directed toward selecting the proper site to transect the rectum. It is absolutely mandatory that the rectum be transected distal to the thickened sigmoid colon—incorporating the distal sigmoid into the anastomosis risks the complications of anastomotic leak, stricture, and recurrent diverticulitis. It is seldom necessary to dissect deeply into the pelvis to reach normal rectum, but it is likely that an appropriate site for the anastomosis will be at least 2 cm distal to the sacral promontory. The rectum is skeletonized at the selected site and transected with a TA-55 stapler.

Attention is now redirected to the descending colon. If the site selected for the anastomosis easily reaches the top of the rectum, the anastomosis can be fashioned. However, if the descending colon does not reach, it will be necessary to divide and ligate the inferior mesenteric vein as it crosses under the fourth portion of the

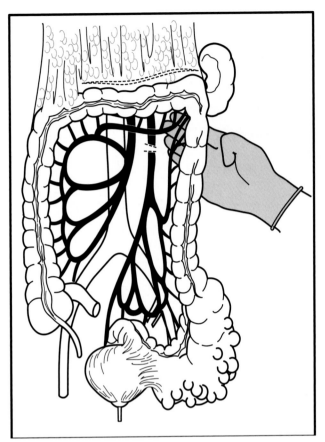

Fig. 14. The inferior mesenteric vein is divided if necessary to permit the descending colon to reach the pelvis without tension.

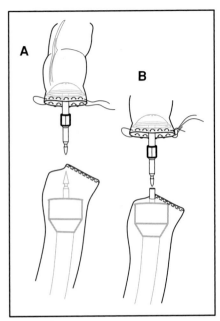

Fig. 15. A: The rectum is positioned so that the trocar is positioned to extend through one of the TA staple line corners. B: The trocar is removed and the stapler is engaged and activated resulting in the excision of one of the TA corners and creation of an end-to-end anastomosis.

duodenum. This maneuver will permit the necessary mobility to allow the descending colon to descend to the level of the upper rectum (Fig. 14).

The lubricated cartridge comprising the base of the circular stapler is then inserted through the anus and gently guided to the stapled end of the proximal rectum. I find that direct visualization of the pelvis by the surgeon inserting the stapler is essential—the cartridge can be visually detected as it moves along the rectum and insertion is continued until the shape of the cartridge is seen (and felt) at the TA staple line.

The areas of the anastomosis that are most tenuous with this technique are the intersection of the TA staple line with the circular staple line. If the circular stapler is placed in the center of the TA staple line, there are often two such potential danger areas. Therefore, I often will position the base of the circular stapler in such a fashion as to completely excise one corner of the TA staple line, leaving only one intersection of staples (Fig. 15).

The trocar is extended from the base of the instrument, penetrating the rectal wall adjacent to (but not through) the TA staple line. The trocar is removed, the post of the anvil head of the stapler is inserted into the receptacle in the base, and the instrument is closed—a maneuver that approximates the descending colon to the rectum. The descending colon is again inspected to ensure that there has been no torsion of the mesentery, that its color verifies excellent arterial blood supply to the level of the anastomosis, and that there is sufficient length as to avoid tension.

The instrument is then activated, creating the anastomosis while simultaneously excising a portion of the TA staple line from the rectum and the purse-string suture from the descending colon (Fig. 16). The stapler is opened and withdrawn from the rectum, and the "donuts" of rectum and descending colon that have been formed are inspected to ensure that the rings are intact. An incomplete "donut" suggests that the anastomosis has not completely formed.

A rigid proctosigmoidoscope is now inserted through the anus into the rectum, the anastomosis is inspected through the scope, and the rectum is gently distended with air insufflated through the proctoscope after the pelvis has been filled with saline to a level above the anastomosis (Fig. 17). Any defects in the anastomosis will be detected by bubbles

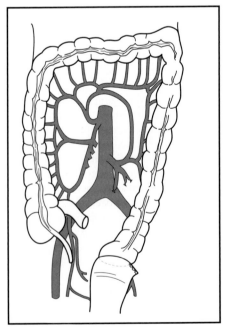

Fig. 16. Anastomosis between descending colon and rectum.

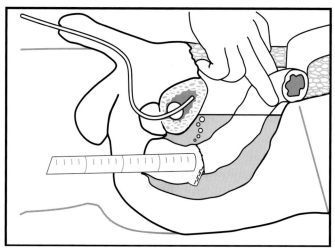

Fig. 17. The rectum is distended with air insufflated through a proctoscope to demonstrate the integrity of the anastomosis.

nus at the level of the infraumbilical fat mound. After the patient recovers from the operation, the integrity of the colorectal anastomosis is verified by proctosigmoidoscopy and a contrast enema, and the ileostomy can be safely closed. An interval of approximately 10 weeks from the sigmoid resection is the preferred time to close the ileostomy.

SUGGESTED READING

Bartus CM, Lipof T, Shahbaz Sarwar CM, et al. Colovesicle fistula: not a contraindication to elective laparoscopic colectomy. *Dis Colon Rectum* 2005;48:233.

Chapman J, Davies M, Wolff B, et al. Complicated diverticulitis: is it time to rethink the rules? *Ann Surg* 2005;242:576.

Chapman JR, Dozois EJ, Wolff BG, et al. Diverticulitis: a progressive disease? Do multiple recurrences predict less favorable outcomes? *Ann Surg* 2006;243:876.

Janes S, Meagher A, Frizelle FA. Elective surgery after acute diverticulitis. *Br J Surg* 2005; 92:133.

Rafferty J, Shellito P, Hyman NH, et al., for the Standards Committee of the American Society of Colon and Rectal Surgeons. Practice parameters for sigmoid diverticulitis. *Dis Colon Rectum* 2006;49:939.

Salem L, Veenstra DL, Sullivan SD, et al. The timing of elective colectomy in diverticulitis: a decision analysis. *J Am Coll Surg* 2004; 199:904.

Schoetz DJ. Diverticular disease of the colon: a century-old problem. *Dis Colon Rectum* 1999;42:703.

escaping from the staple line. Should a small defect be identified, it is easily closed with a Lambert suture.

The abdomen is closed by approximating the peritoneum with running suture of chromic catgut for transverse incisions. For midline incisions, the peritoneum from the inferior pole to the arcuate line is approximated with running chromic catgut. The fascia of either transverse or midline incision is approximated with a running suture of Maxon. The subcutaneous tissue is irrigated with a solution of neomycin and bacitracin, and the skin is approximated with stainless steel staples.

One of the reasons for delaying the operation after an episode of diverticulitis is to permit a single-stage resection and avoid a colostomy, and this is usually possible. However, if there is still a significant amount of inflammation present at the time of sigmoid resection, or if any of a number of technical difficulties should give rise to concern of an increased risk of anastomotic leak, I protect the anastomosis with a temporary loop ileostomy, brought through the right rectus abdomi-

EDITOR'S COMMENT

In this direct and no-nonsense approach to diverticular disease, Dr. Fry covers the extent of the controversies that currently exist regarding diverticulitis and, indeed, the field is changing. It seems well accepted that the absence of fiber in the Western diet in industrialized countries will develop a movement disorder that will ultimately lead to the colonic diverticula, which are false diverticula, as the author states. By age 80, over 65% of patients have chronic diverticula. It is also true that the amount of time it takes for those immigrating into a Western culture to develop symptoms and be hospitalized for diverticular disease is relatively short. This concept was put forward by Hjern et al. (*Aliment Pharmacol Ther* 2006;23:797). Working in Sweden out of the Karolinska Institute, they used the excellent Swedish database of their entire population to track the risk of diverticular disease and related death in a total of 4.4 million Swedish inhabitants, including 3.9 million native Swedes and 536,000 immigrants. They were able to track the origin of the immigrants, their degree of acculturation, and their tenure in Sweden. Remarkably, following the incidence of hospitalization, and tracking patients for their origin in countries of Western Europe, North America, Eastern Europe,

The Balkans, the Middle East, and as far away as Asia, they were able to show that the degree and the period of acculturation was relatively short, as low as under 5 years for non-Western immigrants who had come to Sweden. Further, they showed that the prevalence of diverticular disease increased only slightly among Jews from Europe and America (16% to 17%), but a sevenfold increase was seen in Arabs over this period of time. Levy et al. (*Dis Colon Rectum* 1977;20:477, and *Dis Colon Rectum* 1985;28:416) used barium enemas with a 10-year interval in Israel. The take-home message is that the Westernized diet does appear to bring on diverticular symptoms and hospitalization in a very short period of time once immigrants get to a Westernized country.

Once the diverticula are established, patients usually complain of pain, either in the left lower quadrant or a remarkable number in the right lower quadrant. To me, this pain is not caused by inflammation, although some authors have recently stated that the early nonspecific crampy pain of diverticulitis is chronic inflammation rather than simply cramping and thickening of muscles. One can find a number of patients with pain in the right lower quadrant, while it is commonly thought that the reason for this pain is that, when the colon is so redundant, the sigmoid in

such patients allows it to go over to the right, and thus what they are really complaining about is sigmoid inflammation. My own hypothesis is that the pain has to do with the nerve fibers. Delta-fibers, localized to the midline, are nonmyelinated and only respond to distention and spasm. The alpha-fibers, on the other hand, which are in the anterior parietal wall of the peritoneum, are what respond to inflammation and localize well. I do believe that what we are seeing in regard to right lower quadrant pain associated with diverticular disease is simply a manifestation of spasm and crampy abdominal pain of diverticular disease regardless of where the colon actually is. Ever since Griffen so stated at a symposium in the 1970s (*Dis Colon Rectum* 1976; 19:293), the dictum has chronically been that patients with two attacks of diverticulitis had an increased incidence of complications and are likely to get into more difficulty, thus requiring surgical therapy. The author disagrees (having presented a paper last year that is quoted in this manuscript), saying that patients who have had two diverticular episodes only had a 6% incidence of perforated diverticulitis. This concept has also been challenged by Chapman et al. (*Ann Surg* 2005;242[4]:576), who concluded that 53% of patients presented with complicated

(continued)

diverticulitis (perforated) as their first manifestation of the disease. Further, they noted that the mortality in this disease, to the extent of 60%, occurred in patients who were immunosuppressed, and that immunosuppression and other treatments for co-morbidities were responsible for the lion's share of mortality and the morbidity of 41%. In a presentation at the American Surgical, those authors argued that perhaps the old criterion of "two strikes and you're out" possibly was not contemporarily correct in deciding the need for surgery. Indeed, the management of uncomplicated diverticular disease has recently changed significantly with the advent of probiotics, a mixture of bacteria with supposedly beneficial effects, or at least bacteria that would compete with the potential pathogenic bacteria within the colon. It makes sense to finally pay attention to what bacteria there are on the other side of the gut barrier. To assume that potentially pathogenic bacteria are totally harmless when present in great numbers is perhaps disingenuous. In addition to seeing probiotics as being useful in the management of asymptomatic or minimally symptomatic diverticular disease, mesalazine, an anti-inflammatory drug typically used in a patient with inflammatory bowel disease, has been gaining increasing credibility as an alternative treatment option in patients with uncomplicated diverticular disease. Looking at it as an action appears to be topical rather than systemic, reducing inflammation by blocking cyclooxygenase and inhibiting some prostaglandin production at this point in the colon. If chronic mucosal inflammation, rather than hypertrophy of muscle and inflammation around the diverticular disease, is the cause of diverticular disease, conceivably it might be to the patient's advantage to take a combination of medications including mesalazine. For example, Brandimarte and Tursi (*Med Sci Monit* 2004;10:170) treated 90 patients with rifaximin (400 mg b.i.d.) plus mesalazine (800

mg daily) for 10 days followed by mesalazine alone (800 mg b.i.d.) for at least 8 weeks, and saw an 81% reduction in their symptomatology, although reduction in symptoms was 96% as observed by the authors.

Finally, questioning whether or not diverticular disease is a disease of the muscle or a disease of chronic mucosal inflammation—somewhat more similar to inflammatory bowel disease—is a current subject. A number of investigators have questioned a possible role for the interstitial cells of Cajal (ICC) in the propagation of the slow waves, as important in the cause of diverticular disease. Bassotti et al. (*J Clin Pathol* 2005;58:973) reported that patients with diverticulosis have significantly reduced numbers of all types of colonic ICC and enteric glial cells, but their enteric neurons compare well with those of healthy controls.

Now, as to the chapter, I agree with the author that a barium enema, either with water-soluble dye or with thin barium, is contraindicated. A CT scan seems to be used rather freely without too many complications in this group of patients, including ingestion of large amounts of oral dye. Why this does not provoke a complication is beyond me, but thus far I have not seen many complications from this technique.

Once the patient's abscess has been drained percutaneously and a respectful interval has resulted, an elective procedure may be carried out. I prefer a lateral left paramedial incision, in which a good swatch of muscle is retracted laterally, and then during the closure sutured back to the midline so as to have the advantage of the staggered layers. I agree that median paramedian incision has no advantage over the midline. The incision pictured by Dr. Fry is used by some, and seems to work well, but does transect both rectus muscles with some disability there.

I agree with Dr. Fry that the splenic flexure should be taken down initially, even if one doesn't need it, so that after draining the abscess in doing the resection, one does not put contaminated material in the left upper quadrant. I agree wholeheartedly that

one can leave an occasional diverticulum provided that one goes back to soft pliable bowel. Remember that this is a lifelong disease and that, unless there is a significant change in management or in the actual food intake of Western society, a long resection in which one goes back to very thin normal bowel with no muscular disability, one might get a reasonable amount of mileage in relatively young people. I tend to put on a barrier drape, but not plastic, of wound towels soaked in antibiotic and sewn to the peritoneum to protect the wound. Others like Dr. Fry tend to use a pliable plastic drape with a ring, which tends to hold the wound apart, and that also prevents contamination and presumably cuts down on the incidence of wound infection.

One must find the ureter. Once I find it, I place a vessel loop around it, so that I can pull on the hung vessel loop when I'm wondering where the ureter is as I go down into the pelvis. It also is useful to find the right ureter through the peritoneum so one knows where it is; it is usually farther lateral and away from the superior hemorrhoidal artery, so that one need not damage the ureter during either the pelvic dissection or the anastomosis. Lastly, in mobilization, taking the inferior mesenteric vein at the fourth portion of duodenum certainly does give one length that one didn't have before.

The wisdom of taking down the splenic flexure and the area around the splenic flexure initially, and thereby not liberating pus inadvertently from an area in the phlegmon, is that the left upper quadrant will be well protected, as will the wound, thus obviating the necessity to worry about a delayed primary closure.

In short, the world of diverticulitis is changing. Long-held tenets are being challenged, as well they should be. The cost of diverticular disease in the United States is almost $3 billion a year. It is about time somebody is thinking about it.

J.E.F.

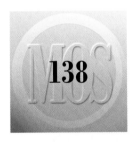

138

Right Hemicolectomy for Treatment of Cancer: Open Technique

BRUCE G. WOLFF AND DAVID W. LARSON

Open right hemicolectomy is the standard of care for the surgical treatment of malignant neoplasms of the right colon. This technique has set the standard by which all other techniques (laparoscopy) are measured. Pathologic findings of the right colon include a number of benign and malignant conditions. For the purpose of this chapter, malignant neoplasms will be our focus. Other pathologic entities would include, however, adenomatous polyps that cannot be endoscopically addressed, carcinoid, irritable bowel disease (namely Crohn disease), and various tumors of the appendix.

Adenocarcinoma of the right colon too often presents with little warning. When

signs or symptoms exist, they often take the form of occult bleeding and/or anemia, partial obstruction, and, on occasion, a palpable mass in the right lower quadrant. The tumor-node-metastasis (TNM) classification of malignant colon cancer is the standard staging system that we use. According to this system, adenocarcinoma invading the submucosa is classified as T1, invading the muscularis propria is T2, invading serosa or pericolic fat is T3, or invading into adjacent organs is T4. Although malignant neoplasms begin locally, they can, over time, spread through regional lymph vessels or by hematogenous dissemination. Carcinomatosis occurs if the tumor has spread

beyond surgical cure to involve multiple separate areas within the abdominal cavity. Adjuvant therapies such as chemotherapy and radiation therapy in general serve only as adjunct to the mainstay of treatment, which remains surgical resection. These adjuvant therapies are based on surgical and pathologic stage.

 PREOPERATIVE PLANNING

EVALUATION

Because right colon cancer rarely presents with obstruction, the surgeon and primary care physician have the luxury of time to complete the proper staging and workup for most patients. Routine workup for planning treatment of a right colon cancer includes complete colonoscopy to confirm pathologic diagnosis and clear the rest of the colon, which has a 3% to 5% rate of synchronous cancer. Additional workup should include a chest radiograph, complete blood count, liver function tests, and carcinoembryonic antigen measurement. As laparoscopic surgery becomes more prevalent, computed tomography (CT) of the abdomen and pelvis have become more useful to fully evaluate patients for abdominal metastasis, locally advanced disease, and liver metastasis. Considerations must also be given to the possibility of familial syndromes (hereditary nonpolyposis colorectal cancer) and the need for genetic and microsatellite instability tests in selected patients with strong family history, early onset, and right-sided lesions.

PREPARATION

Patient preparation includes mechanical cleansing of the bowel prior to surgery. Included with this oral preparation, typically 2 L of a lavage solution such as GoLYTELY, many chose to use preoperative oral antibiotics such a neomycin and Flagyl as part of the preparation. We do not believe it is necessary to administer both preoperative and intraoperative broad-spectrum antibiotics unless an infectious complication is present at time of surgery. The lavage solution is administered to the patient the evening prior to surgery in an outpatient setting for most patients. However, if the patient is elderly or frail, this procedure may be performed in the hospital setting on the night before the operation. Oral intake is usually restricted the night prior to surgery. Therefore, once the patient is admitted to the hospital it is important that the patient be hydrated as the bowel preparation and "nothing by mouth" status can affect patient intravascular volume significantly. As long as the patient has no evidence of obstruction, this preoperative treatment should always be employed. Having said this, if the patient is obstructed, primary anastomosis is not contraindicated for a right colon cancer. Gross contamination or tenuous tissues, however, may prevent the surgeon from performing a primary anastomosis.

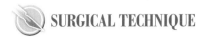

SURGICAL TECHNIQUE

RIGHT COLECTOMY

All operations begin with positioning. It is our practice to position patients on the table in a supine position. Ankle straps are often used to allow for Trendelenburg position. The surgeon stands on the patient's left and across from the first assistant on the right. If a second assistant is needed, it will be most helpful if that assistant is on the surgeon's left early in the case and then on the other assistant's right later in the case as the hepatic flexure is mobilized.

Once the patient has been placed under general anesthesia, prepared, and draped, a midline incision is made centering on the right side of the patient's umbilicus. Incision length is in direct proportional to the body habitus of the patient. Once the abdomen is entered, a thorough exploration of the abdomen is the first order of business. The liver is palpated, the gallbladder assessed for stones, and the surrounding organs of the upper and midabdomen are examined. The small bowel is run from the ligament of Treitz to the ileocecal valve. The stomach, kidney, pancreas, spleen, aorta, and iliac vessels are palpated and examined for evidence of disease. In women, the uterus and ovaries are inspected for any abnormalities. After assessing the abdomen for metastatic disease and surgical resectability, the tumor and surrounding structures are addressed.

Special consideration should be given to locally aggressive tumors such as those that involve adjacent organs (T4). If adjacent organs such as duodenum, small bowel, omentum, and retroperitoneal structures such as the ureter or gonadal vessels are involved, every attempt must be made to complete an en bloc resection. At no time should a surgeon attempt to surgically separate intra-abominal structures from the tumor, as this would violate oncologic surgical principles and potentially adversely affect patient outcome. An R0 resection is the goal of every operation. Rarely, a primary tumor is found intraoperatively to have unresectable metastatic disease despite preoperative workup. In general, our practice has been to resect the primary tumor to prevent the future possibility of hemorrhage or obstructive complications. If the surgeon believes the primary tumor cannot be removed safely, a bypass procedure should be performed to prevent future obstruction.

Vascular Anatomy

The avascular window between the right branch of the middle colic artery and the right or ileocolic artery, as well as between the ileocolic and the last ileal branches, are important anatomic landmarks. It is well known that the right colic artery rarely branches directly off the SMA. It is most often (90% of the time) a branch of the ileocolic artery, and therefore rarely requires separate ligation. The vessels that must be ligated for a right colon resection include the ileocolic, right colic, and right branch of the middle colic.

SURGICAL DISSECTION: OPEN TECHNIQUE

The line of resection for a right colon cancer depends somewhat on the location of the tumor. For those tumors located in the cecum, a 10-cm margin of terminal ileum is generally taken. On the other hand, if the tumor is located in the ascending colon, only a few centimeters of ileum is required as a margin. This line of resection should extend to the right side of the transverse colon at the level of the right branch of the middle colic vessels (Fig. 1). Care must be taken to preserve the main branch of the middle colic vessels. The right colic and ileocolic vessels are taken at their origins to ensure proper lymph node harvest. Omental attachments to the right colon are generally removed with the specimen.

Mobilization of the right colon begins by separating the retroperitoneal structures (gonadal vessels and ureter) from the terminal ileum and cecum. This is performed by incising the peritoneal attachments to these structures laterally and rotating the cecum anteriorly and medially (Fig. 2). Once this mobilization is completed, the medial and inferior attachments to the cecum and terminal small bowel are incised up toward the junction of the third and fourth portions of the duodenum. A sponge is often helpful to gently separate the filmy adhesions to the retroperitoneum posteriorly as mobilization continues in the superior direction. Of course care is taken during this dissection to identify and posteriorly displace the gonadal vessels and ureter. Mobilization of the ileocolic vessel is complete once the surgeon has identified the middle colic as it crosses the duodenum. Continuing the lateral dissection up and around the hepatic flexure, the surgeon's index finger provides the plane of dissection for cauterization by

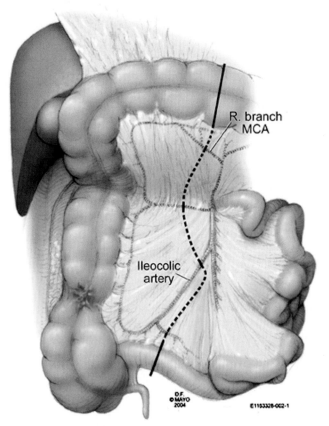

Fig. 1. Line of resection for a right hemicolectomy for treatment of cancer. MCA, middle colic artery.

where it crosses the lateral or inferior edge of the duodenum. The peritoneum overlying the ileocolic vessels is incised and then the vessels are doubly ligated and divided. Next, the marginal branches to the ileum are divided, thus preparing the proximal line of resection. The final step divides the right colic artery, if needed, and the right branch of the middle colic artery. After this, the distal bowel margin is cleared of fat and prepared for an anastomosis.

ANASTOMOSIS

Hand-sewn

Two categories of anastomosis can be employed in a right colon resection, either hand-sewn or stapled. There are numerous techniques within each category. The hand-sewn anastomosis most often performed in our practice begins by placing crushing bowel clamps across the colon a few centimeters distal to the area to be divided on the ileum and a few centimeters proximal to the line of transection on the colon. Noncrushing clamps are then placed straight across the colon and ileum. At this point, the ileum and colon are divided and the specimen is sent for pathologic evaluation. If the diameter of the

the first assistant (Fig. 3). Retracting the midtransverse colon inferiorly, one can complete the exposure of the hepatic flexure. The thin plane between the mesocolon and the gastrocolic ligament can be developed bluntly and dissected to complete the flexure mobilization. As one mobilizes the gastrocolic ligament, there may be a few vessels which need ligation.

By placing gentle traction on the transverse colon, one can complete the remaining mobilization of the proximal transverse colon. It is important to perform this with a gentle touch in order to avoid avulsing a branch of the middle colic vein off its origin, especially in obese patients. Once this has been completed, the right colon is retracted superiorly and medially, exposing the anterior edge of the duodenum and the head of the pancreas. Release of these filmy attachments is the last remaining step in the dissection.

At this point, vascular ligation may commence. The avascular area between the ileocolic and right branch of the middle colic vessel is incised down to the base of the ileocolic vessels at about the level

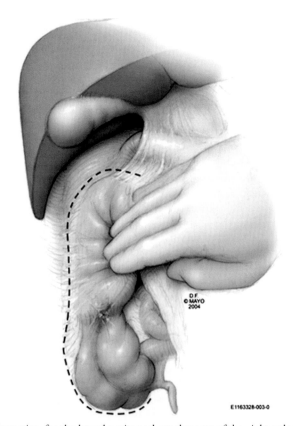

Fig. 2. Line of resection for the lateral peritoneal attachments of the right colon.

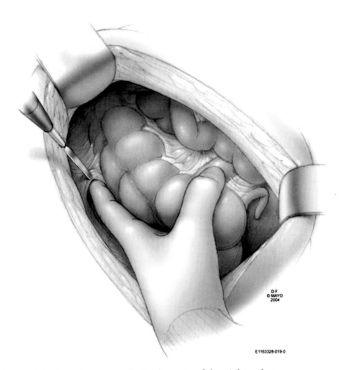

Fig. 3. Release of the lateral peritoneal attachments of the right colon.

transected ileum is small, it can be enlarged by dividing it longitudinally along its antimesenteric boarder (the so-called cheatle cut). Three standard anastomotic techniques can be performed: end-to-end, side-to-side, or end-to-side. An open two-layered anastomosis performed in an end-to-side fashion is illustrated in Figure 4. First, the two ends of the bowel are approximated, making sure there are no twists. We use 3-0 stay sutures in the corners of the bowel to aid with approximation. A posterior row of Lembert sutures is placed first. These sutures should be placed deep enough to incorporate most of the muscle layer. If the suture can be seen through the serosa, then the stitch has been placed too superficially and a deep needle passage is required. The sutures are tied to approximate tissues, not to strangulate them. Next an inner layer of running 3-0 suture is used to approximate the mucosal and submucosal layers. The corner of the bowel is secured first, and the running suture is then advanced along the posterior aspect of the anastomosis. This suture is continued around the opposite corner to complete the anterior mucosal approximation. The suture is then tied to itself at the corner. The occluding

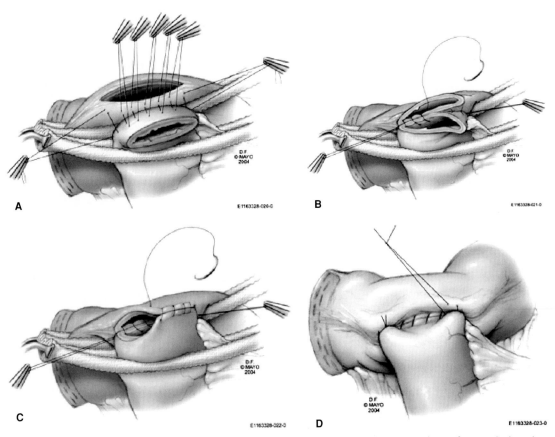

Fig. 4. Hand-sewn anastomosis. **A:** Posterior row of interrupted suture. **B:** Posterior running layer of suture. **C:** Anterior running layer of suture. **D:** Anterior row of interrupted suture.

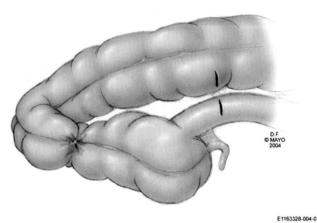

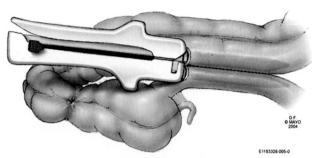

Fig. 6. Stapled anastomosis.

Fig. 5. To begin a stapled anastomosis, l-cm transverse incisions are made on the antimesenteric borders of the ileum and colon.

bowel clamps are removed from the bowel to allow blood flow to return to the ends of the bowel. The final step includes the anterior second layer of 3-0 Lembert sutures, approximating the serosal layer and thus bolstering the anastomotic line.

Stapled Anastomosis

In the conventional stapled functional end-to-end anastomosis, one or two firings of a linear cutting stapler and a linear noncutting stapler are used. However, the standard technique we employ is that of a simplified procedure using only two firings of a disposable linear cutting stapler.

This anastomotic technique begins with the clearing of the terminal ileum and transverse colon of mesenteric fat for approximately 2 cm. One-centimeter transverse incisions are made on the specimen side of these cleared areas on the antimesenteric borders of the ileum and colon (Fig. 5). Placing one of the two sides

of the linear cutting stapler into each of the holes in the small bowel first, and then the colon, the stapler is gently closed, approximating the small bowel and the colon along the antimesenteric border (Fig. 6). Once it is assured that the mesentery is clear and the stapler is in good position, it is fired and then removed. On doing this, the previously separate ileal and colonic enterotomies become joined into a single enterotomy, and a pair of Babcock clamps is used to grasp opposite borders of this enterotomy at the anterior and posterior staple lines. A reloaded, long (75- to 100-mm) linear cutting stapler is then placed across the ileum and transverse colon, at a right angle to the previous

staple line (Fig. 7). By retracting the previous enterotomy, the stapler is fired, completing the surgical resection and anastomosis.

It is our practice to imbricate the corners and cross staple line of our anastomosis with four 3-0 sutures. One is placed at the distal end of the longitudinal (first) staple line between the ileum and colon to add mechanical strength to this end of the anastomosis. Two sutures are placed to invert each end of the transverse (second) staple line. Finally, one inverting suture is placed at the point where the two staple lines intersect (Fig. 8). The mesenteric defect can be closed or left open, depending on the surgeon's preference. Omentum, if available, can be placed over the anastomosis to provide further protection against postoperative anastomotic leak.

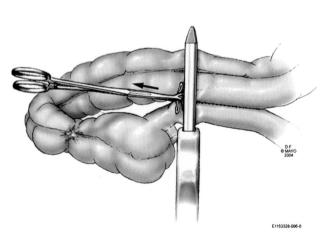

Fig. 7. Completion of a stapled anastomosis.

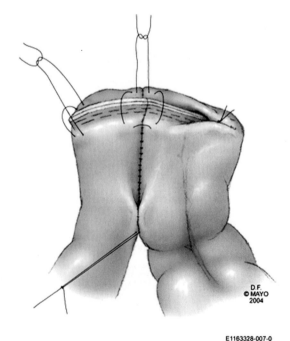

Fig. 8. Oversewing the staple line with interrupted suture.

CLOSURE

Prior to closure, the abdomen is checked for adequate hemostasis and thoroughly irrigated with saline irrigation. Drains are used only in cases of infection or abscess. Interrupted or running sutures are then used to close the facial layer, and a running subcuticular suture or skin staples approximate the skin.

CONCLUSION

Surgical resection of the right colon is a classic standard operation in the training of all surgeons. The importance of surgical technique and anatomic dissection are the keys to successful oncologic outcome and postoperative patient success. Following these principles will allow continued excellent outcomes.

SUGGESTED READING

Devine R, Pemberton JH. Right and left hemicolectomy. In: Donohue J, Van Heerden J, Monson J, eds. *Atlas of surgical oncology.* Cambridge, MA: Blackwell Science, 1995:215.

Meagher AP, Wolff BG. Right hemicolectomy with a linear cutting stapler. *Dis Colon Rectum* 1994;37:1043.

EDITOR'S COMMENT

As depicted by Professors Wolff and Larson, open right hemicolectomy is established as the standard technique for the surgical management of malignant tumors of the right colon. Thus, as indicated by the authors, the open method remains the "gold standard" to which all techniques will be compared. The authors have therefore been assigned the task of evaluating technical and therapeutic outcomes for the surgical management of lesions of the right colon, inclusive of neoplastic disease, adenomatous polyps, carcinoid, inflammatory bowel disease, and tumors of the appendix.

The use of flexible sigmoidoscopy remains one of the principal screening tools for colorectal carcinoma. Flexible sigmoidoscopy provides direct visualization of the left colon and rectum, with identification of suspicious lesions that may be biopsied for histologic validation. Its disadvantage is that it only examines the lower third of the colon; thus, to properly examine right colon lesions requires colonoscopy and/or barium contrast enemas, although the latter has lower sensitivity and specificity than direct visualization by endoscopy. For open or laparoscopic surgical resection of the right colon, tissue procurement is essential by endoscopy, with the exception of the rare obstructing lesion. The considerable early enthusiasm for virtual endoscopy, which is based on acquisition of cross-sectional images, can be provided by using CT or magnetic resonance imaging (MRI). Recent studies suggest that both techniques are effective to detect clinically relevant disease. Svensson et al. (*Radiology* 2002;222:337), evaluating more than 100 patients having both virtual and conventional endoscopy, noted favoring of the virtual technique by 82% of the patients. However, virtual colonoscopy based on acquisition of CT data is associated with high doses of ionizing radiation. The recent report by Lauenstein et al. (*Magn Reson Imaging Clin N Am* 2005;13:349) of Germany characterizes the preferable application of MRI for virtual colonography. The actual sensitivity and specificity of this technique will almost certainly improve, and interventional diagnosis will move to the less-invasive diagnostic procedure with favor over endoscopic approaches. Its future role for management of right colon, transverse, left colon, and rectal lesions remains unanswered.

Although this chapter focuses on open technique, laparoscopic surgery for colon cancer remains an acceptable alternative to the open approach. However, there are small, albeit measurable, short-term benefits of the laparoscopic approach, which include earlier return of bowel function, shorter length of hospital stay, and the decreased usage of postoperative narcotics. It would appear from contemporary studies that recurrence and survival are not compromised by the laparoscopic technique approach. In the large, multi-institutional, randomized

trial in the United States by the Clinical Outcomes of Surgical Therapy (COST) Study Group (*N Engl J Med* 2004;350:2050), similar outcomes for the two procedures were reported among participating surgeons in high-volume centers of excellence. It is unclear if the excellent results of the COST trial outcomes can be achieved in the majority of national clinics; further monitoring and study will be essential to answer this important question. Conventional colonoscopic approaches remain of the highest accuracy for procurement and diagnosis in the evaluation of colorectal masses or inflammatory bowel disease. This procedure does require conscious sedation, and there may be poor patient acceptance and incomplete preparation by the patient preoperatively to assure an adequate unlimited examination as a screening tool. Further, the presence of a stenotic site or elongated bowel segments may abrogate the colonoscopic approach to visualize the entire colon and the ileocecal valve in certain patients.

In contrast to the left colon, the larger circumference and surface area of the right colon is infrequently obstructed in the cecal, ascending, or right transverse segments; thus, a period of time for workup, procurement of tissue, and bowel preparation for associated lesions of the organ is routine. For any patient presenting with documented lesions of the right colon, careful family history should be established and, when appropriate, genetic counseling completed in the perioperative period. Differentiation of the autosomal-dominant colorectal cancer syndrome, familial adenomatous polyposis (FAP), initiated by a germline mutation of the APC gene (chromosome 5q21), is characterized by hundreds of adenomatous colorectal polyps that invariably progress to colorectal carcinoma between the ages of 35 and 40. Gardner syndrome is characterized by osteomas, abnormalities of dentition, soft tissue tumors, and epidermal cysts. Other specific variants of the FAP syndromes include Turcot syndrome that has heritable desmoid disease and is associated with CNS malignancies. The establishment of this syndrome would mitigate against the selective right colectomy described by the authors in that a total abdominal colectomy and proctocolectomy is appropriate. Similarly, the treatment of ulcerative colitis with its chronicity and risk of debilitating bowel disease and colorectal carcinoma is inappropriately treated by the right colectomy described herein. Rather, the authors focus on the management of a specific segment of the colon with abnormalities that have no pancolonic features.

Similar to the authors, we opt for a resection margin of approximately 10 cm for the terminal ileum; the line of resection is inclusive of the right transverse colon that sacrifices the right branch of the middle colic artery, together with the ileocolic artery (Fig. 1). Also similar to the authors, we advocate stapled anastomoses for its technical speed and the integrity of the

result. When hand-sewn anastomotic technique is chosen, we too place a posterior row of Lembert sutures using 3-0 silk, with placement deep enough to incorporate much of the muscularis. An inner row of running 3-0 Vicryl or chromic gut is used to approximate the mucosal and submucosal layers. Finally, the anterior second row of 3-0 Lembert silk sutures is used to approximate the serosal layer and to bolster the anastomotic line integrity. Defects in the mesocolon are closed with 2-0 Vicryl or silk to avoid internal herniation and/or rotation of the colonic segment anastomosis.

The accurate pathologic staging of cancer of the right colon is essential and requires diligence by the pathologist on removal of the right colonic segment. Comprehensive assessment including total (quantity) nodes, as well as final histologic status, is essential. Metastatic nodal disease remains the most important prognostic factor for patients with colorectal carcinoma. Patients with node-negative disease have a 5-year survival rate of 75%; patients with node-positive disease experience a 5-year survival rate of 30% to 60%. Further, the number of nodes resected bears on the survival of patients with node-negative and node-positive disease; completeness of resection and staging accuracy therefore translates into a potential survival benefit. Thus, the en bloc lymphadenectomy has both a diagnostic and therapeutic role in the management of right colon, as well as left colon and rectal cancer. The historic contribution by Cabañas in 1977 (*Cancer* 1977;39:456) established the importance of lymphatic histology with sentinel node mapping of patients with penile carcinoma. This approach identified the sentinel lymph node (SLN) as the first site of regional nodal metastasis, and is predictive of the nodal status of the remaining nodal basin. Thereafter, in 1989 Morton et al. (Second International Conference on Melanoma 1989:131) established the importance for use of this technique using blue dye for clinical stage I melanoma to assess the regional nodal basin. Such techniques have been extensively applied to breast lesions.

A recent review by Stojadinovic et al. (*J Am Coll Surg* 2005;201:297) reviewed the published results of colorectal SLN mapping with isosulfan blue dye alone, demonstrating high success rates for identification of at least one sentinel node in those centers with extensive technical experience with the technique. These authors suggest that the SLN reflects the status of the remaining nodal basin with 92% to 96% accuracy with a low risk of "skipped metastasis" (negative SLN/positive non-SLN; 4% to 8%) in these studies. Additional techniques to ultrastage colorectal carcinoma sentinel nodes are highly variable with multilevel step sectioning using hematoxylin and eosin stains or combinations using cytokeratin, carcinoembryonic antigen-IAC, or reverse transcriptase polymerase

(continued)

The Gastrointestinal Tract

chain reaction. The differentiation in outcomes for this early phase of prospective studies to assess the advantage of rectal versus colonic lymphatic mapping is unclear; early data would suggest the techniques are similar in outcomes.

The establishment of histologically positive (by hematoxylin and eosin) lymphatics advances the stage of disease and emphasizes the importance for the addition of adjuvant chemotherapy to improve outcomes and survival. Vascular endothelial growth factor (VEGF) has emerged as an important therapeutic target; various strategies remain in evolution to inhibit VEGF. The recent Food and Drug Administration (FDA) approval of bevacizumab, a recombinant humanized monoclonal antibody with specificity to VEGF, marks a new therapeutic approach for cancer therapy. With its approval by the FDA in 2004, the phase III randomized clinical trial noted an improvement of overall survival. This is one of the first major contributions in years to the adjuvant therapy of this organ-site cancer, and validates the application of a targeted molecule to VEGF; this drug has opened the panorama of opportunities for other studies with combination therapies. This phase III study for patients with untreated metastatic colorectal carcinoma received combination therapy with irinotecan, 5-fluorouracil, and leucovorin, with and without bevacizumab. The bevacizumab added to the combination triple therapy enhanced response rates by 10%, increased progression-free survival by 4 months, and increased median survival by nearly 5 months, compared with the chemotherapy arm alone. Use of anti-VEGF and antiepithelial growth factor receptor monoclonals may be the future for treatment of regional and metastatic colon cancer.

Despite the advancement for application of targeted molecular therapies in the treatment of colorectal cancer, the combination of 5-fluorouracil and leucovorin remains the reference treatment. Sun and Haller (*Semin Oncol* 2005;32:95) consider that capecitabine may be considered an alternative to 5-fluorouracil and leucovorin for the therapy of stage III colon cancer. The therapeutic benefit of adjuvant therapy for localized node-negative disease (stage II disease) is evident, but small. Thus, the application of evolving molecular and biologic-agents hold great promise as adjuvant and therapeutic modalities.

K.I.B.

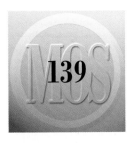

139 Left Hemicolectomy for Treatment of Malignancy

MARTIN R. WEISER

Surgical resection remains the primary curative treatment modality for left colon cancer and includes removal of the primary lesion with clear margins and locoregional lymph nodes. Determining the extent of lymphadenectomy can be the most challenging aspect of an oncologic resection. For colorectal cancer, evaluation of at least 12 lymph nodes optimizes staging and outcome. More extensive resection does not necessarily translate into prolonged survival and can be associated with increased morbidity. For example, "extended" left hemicolectomy, with ligation of the inferior mesenteric artery at the level of the aorta, increases the risk of autonomic nerve injury, has not been show to reduce recurrence, and should therefore be used selectively.

This chapter will emphasize left hemicolectomy for cancer in which the extent of colon resection is defined by adequate lymphadenectomy. The successful execution of an oncologic left hemicolectomy requires a clear understanding of the regional anatomy and lymph node drainage pattern.

LEFT COLON ANATOMY

The blood vessels and regional lymphatics of the left colon reside in the mesentery. In general, the distal transverse colon is supplied by the middle colic pedicle, which is the first branch of the superior mesenteric artery as it emerges from beneath the pancreas. The left colic artery supplies the left colon distal to the splenic flexure, which is the first ascending branch of the inferior mesenteric artery. The left colon has a relatively well-developed marginal artery and vein, which form a mesenteric vascular arcade adjacent to the colon. This collateral circulation may be underdeveloped in some patients, resulting in a potential watershed area at the splenic flexure, which should be considered if the inferior mesenteric artery is divided at its origin. The superior hemorrhoidal artery is the most distal branch of the inferior mesenteric artery and gives rise to multiple sigmoidal arteries prior to becoming enveloped in the mesorectum at the sacral promontory. The venous return from the left colon runs with the arteries in the mesentery and coalesces to form the inferior mesenteric vein just lateral to the duodenum, before uniting with the splenic vein and superior mesenteric vein to form the portal vein.

The majority of lymphatic channels run in the submucosa of the colon wall. Invasive colon neoplasm requires extension of dysplastic glands beyond the muscularis mucosa into the submucosa of the intestinal wall. It should be noted that this definition is distinctly different from other gastrointestinal malignancies in which carcinoma is defined by dysplastic cell invasion beyond the epithelial basement membrane. The rationale for this definition stems from the edict that metastatic disease is not possible unless dysplastic glands penetrate into the submucosa where the majority of lymphatics reside.

The efferent colonic lymphatic channels pass from the submucosa to the intramuscular and subserosal plexus of the bowel to the epicolic nodes, which are adjacent to the large intestine. Paracolic lymph nodes are located adjacent to the marginal vessel along the mesenteric side of the colon, and these and the epicolic lymph nodes are usually the first sites of nodal metastases. Intermediate nodes are found along the major arterial branches in the mesocolon, and principal nodes are located at the origin of the vascular pedicles.

The bidirectional lymphatic flow from colonic tumors has been well documented in classic studies of cleared colon specimens (Fig. 1) that form the basis of oncologic resection. Specifically, lymph node metastases are noted along major vascular pedicles both proximal and distal to the lesion. For example, as noted in Figure 1, lesions at the splenic flexure metastasize along the left colic artery and left branch of the middle colic artery in 93% and 20% of cases, respectively. Therefore, proper lymphadenectomy includes resection of principal vessels above and below the lesion with en bloc removal of epicolic, paracolic, and intermediate lymph nodes.

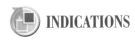 INDICATIONS

Left hemicolectomy is indicated for patients with (a) malignant lesions, (b) a history of prior malignant polypectomy with

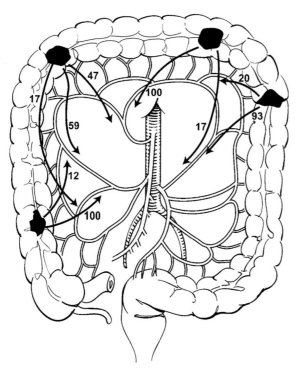

Fig. 1. Tumors can metastasize to lymph nodes bidirectionally along major vascular pedicles. The numbers in the figure signify the percentage of metastasizing carcinomas that have demonstrated positive nodes along a given vascular pedicle. For example, node-positive tumors in the left colon metastasize along the left colic in 93% of cases and along the left branch of the middle colic pedicle in 20% of cases. Lymphadenectomy at time of colon resection should include the vascular pedicles at risk for nodal metastases. (Adapted from Herter FR, Slanetz CA. Patterns and significance of lymphatic spread from cancer of the colon and rectum. In: Weiss L, Gilbert H, Ballon S, eds. *Lymphatic system metastases.* Boston, MA: GK Hall,1980:275.)

high-risk pathologic features such that there is a significant possibility of lymph nodes metastases, and (c) high-risk premalignant polyps not amenable to endoscopic removal. High-risk pathologic features include poor differentiation, lymphovascular invasion, involvement of the base of the polyp (Haggitt level 4), and margin less than 2 mm. The rationale for performing colon resection with lymphadenectomy for potentially benign polyps is to obviate the need for reoperation if invasive cancer is ultimately diagnosed. Therefore, patients with relatively high-risk adenomas not amenable to endoscopic polypectomy, large or sessile lesions, and those with significant dysplasia are advised to undergo formal hemicolectomy.

 PREOPERATIVE PLANNING

A thorough preoperative workup is required to optimize an oncologic resection. This includes a history and physical examination, pulmonary and cardiac evaluations as indicated, and a complete extent of disease workup. The colon should be fully evaluated for additional lesions. Synchronous polyps and invasive cancers are noted in 30% and 3% of cases, respectively. If the primary lesion was detected by a "noninvasive" fashion such as virtual colonoscopy (computed tomographic [CT] colography), full endoscopy evaluation for histologic confirmation is indicated. Multiple site (three- or four-quadrant) tattooing of small lesions or polypectomy sites can be helpful to localize disease at time of resection.

For obstructing lesions, endoscopic stenting is a useful bridge to colectomy. Once stented, the colon can be decompressed, cleared of solid material with a mechanical bowel preparation, and evaluated by colonoscopy for synchronous lesions. In some cases, this can obviate the need for subtotal colectomy.

A thorough workup for metastatic disease, including a CT scan with oral and intravenous contrast, is advocated to optimize treatment planning. Identification of metastatic disease prior to surgery allows for patient counseling and consideration of synchronous liver resection. In patients with asymptomatic primary colon lesions and metastatic disease, initiation of chemother-apy is a viable alternative to immediate colectomy. This approach is theoretically advantageous as it allows for rapid treatment of the often survival-limiting systemic disease as well as identification of patients with chemoresponsive tumors who may be candidates for aggressive surgical debulking at the time of colectomy.

Recent reports have indicated that bowel preparation is not mandatory for successful colon surgery. Indeed, we have known for some time that primary closure of traumatic colotomy is a viable, even preferred, treatment option. However, in the setting of elective colectomy for cancer, a bowel preparation remains advantageous. Removal of solid stool from the colon allows for easy intestinal manipulation, assessment of synchronous disease by palpation, and intraoperative colonoscopy when necessary.

Preoperatively, patients are instructed to follow a clear-liquid diet at home, beginning the morning prior to surgery. The mechanical bowel preparation begins that afternoon, and can be achieved with either 4 L of polyethylene glycol solution (GoLYTELY) or two doses of an oral sodium phosphate solution (Fleet Phospho-Soda, 1.5 oz at 2 PM and at 6 PM), followed by several glasses of water. Oral phosphate solution is generally avoided in patients with renal insufficiency or congestive heart disease. Currently, patients are only rarely admitted for bowel preparation with intravenous hydration and monitoring of electrolytes. In addition, an oral antibiotic bowel preparation generally consists of a modification of the Nichols-Condon preparation, including 500 mg of neomycin and 500 mg of metronidazole given at 3, 7, and 10 PM on the day prior to surgery. A second-generation cephalosporin (for example, 2 g of cefotetan) is administered intravenously within 1 hour of incision. In patients with penicillin allergies we use an aminoglycoside, such as gentamicin (1.5 mg/kg), and clindamycin (900 mg). In patients who require endocarditis prophylaxis, ampicillin (2 g), clindamycin (900 mg), and an aminoglycoside are administered preoperatively. Lastly, for penicillin-allergic patients who require endocarditis prophylaxis, vancomycin (1 g), metronidazole (500 mg), and an aminoglycoside are used.

DETAILS OF SURGICAL PREPARATION

After induction of general anesthesia, the patient is placed in the supine position, with the arms abducted on armboards and the legs in a low (modified Lloyd-Davis)

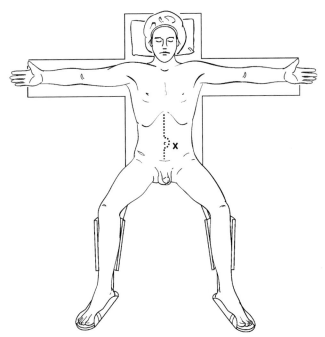

Fig. 2. Recommended positioning of a patient for left hemicolectomy. Note that the arms are in the abducted position to allow placement of a self-retaining retractor. The patient is marked preoperatively for the optimal placement of a colostomy, should this be necessary. Access to the rectum should be available to facilitate a stapled low anastomosis.

lithotomy position (Fig. 2). The pelvis is elevated on gel pads, allowing easy access to the perineum. The rectum is then irrigated with 1 L of saline to remove any residual fecal material if a colorectal anastomosis is anticipated. Prophylaxis against deep vein thrombosis is accomplished by intermittent pneumatic compression devices placed at the time of anesthesia induction. In high-risk cases, preoperative unfractionated heparin or low molecular weight heparin is administered prior to induction as well. Postoperatively, both pneumatic boots and heparin are used. The abdomen and perineum are prepared with an antibacterial wash and then draped. A sterile Foley catheter is inserted.

After squaring the abdomen with towels, a sterile plastic covering is placed over the abdomen to secure the draping. The patient is explored through a midline incision and the extent depends on the location of the lesion. Cephalad extension to the xiphoid process is used for splenic flexure lesions, and caudad extension to the pubis is advantageous for lower sigmoid lesions. Moist laparotomy pads and a plastic wound protector are used to contain any intestinal spillage that may occur and to keep the abdominal wall moist. A thorough abdominal exploration is performed with particular attention to the liver, omentum, and peritoneal surfaces. In women, the ovaries are carefully inspected to rule out metastatic disease and ovarian

cancer. Routine prophylactic oophorectomy is generally not recommended unless the patient is postmenopausal or the patient has a significant family history of ovarian cancer. The intestine is evaluated by palpation to rule out synchronous disease, especially in those cases in which a satisfactory colonoscopy could not be performed. Intraoperative colonoscopy is occasionally necessary if the lesion cannot be identified by palpation or visualization of serosal tattoo markings. In such situations, it is helpful to occlude the colon proximal to the area of interest to limit bowel distention. Newer techniques such as carbon dioxide insufflation during colonoscopy appear to be advantageous because the gas is rapidly absorbed at the time of the procedure.

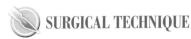 **SURGICAL TECHNIQUE**

Lymphadenectomy and Intestinal Resection

The length of intestine resection is determined by the extent of intestinal devascularization required for proper lymphadenectomy (Fig. 3), and obtaining a 5-cm margin of normal colon proximal and distal to the lesion is rarely an issue. In general, tumors located at the splenic flexure and left colon require resection of lymph nodes along the left branch of the

middle colic, left colic, and first sigmoidal pedicles (Fig. 3A). Lesions in the sigmoid colon generally require lymphadenectomy along the inferior mesenteric artery (Fig. 3B). The pedicle is generally ligated distal to the left colic artery at the level of the superior hemorrhoidal artery. Routine high ligation of the inferior mesenteric artery at the level of the aorta does not improve survival, is associated with injury to sympathetic trunks, and therefore should be performed selectively. The rare lesion located at the junction of the left and sigmoid colon (Fig. 3C), which lies in the narrow area between the left colic and first sigmoidal pedicles, may benefit from ligation of the inferior mesenteric artery at its origin to include lymphadenectomy along all the left colic and superior rectal pedicles.

Tumors of the Splenic Flexure and Left Colon

The operating surgeon stands on the patient's left side, and the assistant on the right. Optimal exposure is initially obtained by retracting the small bowel cephalad and to the right in a moist laparotomy pad, using a self-retaining retractor, such as a Bookwalter or Thompson retractor (Fig. 4). The sigmoid colon is first mobilized off the lateral side wall and retroperitoneum: the assistant retracts the sigmoid colon medially, and the lateral attachment of the colon is meticulously dissected with cautery by the operating surgeon. This maneuver exposes the peritoneal reflection, which often extends onto the sigmoid mesentery. It is important to dissect the parietal peritoneum off the sigmoid mesentery to ensure entry into the correct avascular plane. This maintains the lateral position of the gonadal vessels and ureter. The left ureter is identified medial to the gonadal vessels in the retroperitoneum. The peritoneal reflection is then incised along the white line of Toldt proximally to the splenic flexure to mobilize the left colon. Care must be taken to continuously sweep the gonadal vessels and ureter laterally during this maneuver to avoid lateral retroperitoneal bleeding. Bleeding from injury to the gonadal vessels is cautiously controlled with clips or cautery with attention to the location of the ureter at all times.

After the sigmoid and distal left colon is mobilized, the self-retaining retractor is repositioned to allow visualization and mobilization of the splenic flexure. Lateral colonic dissection is continued along the white line of Toldt to the lower pole of the spleen. For splenic flexure lesions, the distal omentum is resected with the colon

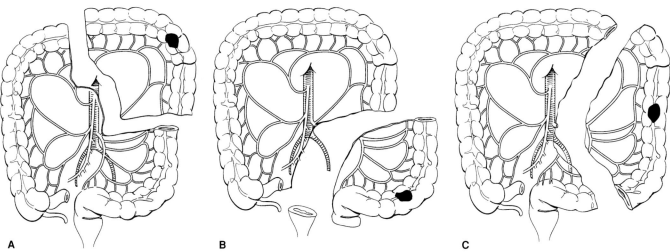

A   B   C

Fig. 3. The recommended lines of resection for tumors within the various areas of the left colon. Note that the resections are based on the vascular supply to the tumor. **A:** Tumors located at the splenic flexure and left colon require resection of lymph nodes along the left branch of the middle colic, left colic, and first sigmoidal pedicles. **B:** Tumors in the sigmoid colon generally require lymphadenectomy along the inferior mesenteric artery. **C:** Rarely, there may be lesions at the junction of the left and sigmoid colon, which lies in the narrow area between the left colic and first sigmoidal pedicles; these may benefit from ligation of the inferior mesenteric artery at its origin to include lymphadenectomy along all the left colic and superior rectal pedicles.

by dividing the gastrocolic ligament and gastroepiploic arcades with entry into the lesser sac. For descending colon or sigmoid lesions, the distal omentum does not necessarily need to be resected with the specimen, and the gastrocolic omentum is dissected off the distal transverse colon, which allows entry into the lesser sac.

Next, with simultaneous gentle inferior tension on the transverse and descending colon, the renocolic and splenocolic ligaments are divided with cautery. These maneuvers mobilize the splenic flexure colon off the retroperitoneum, including the tail of the pancreas. Care must be taken to avoid excessive retraction on the colon as

the splenic flexure is often closely applied to the inferior aspect of the spleen and undue tension can cause a splenic capsular tear, resulting in considerable hemorrhage. If spleno-omental adhesions are noted, they should be initially divided to prevent a capsular tear when tension is applied to the omentum. Should hemorrhage occur from splenic capsular tears, hemostasis can usually be attained with a variety of methods including argon beam coagulation and use of hemastatic agents.

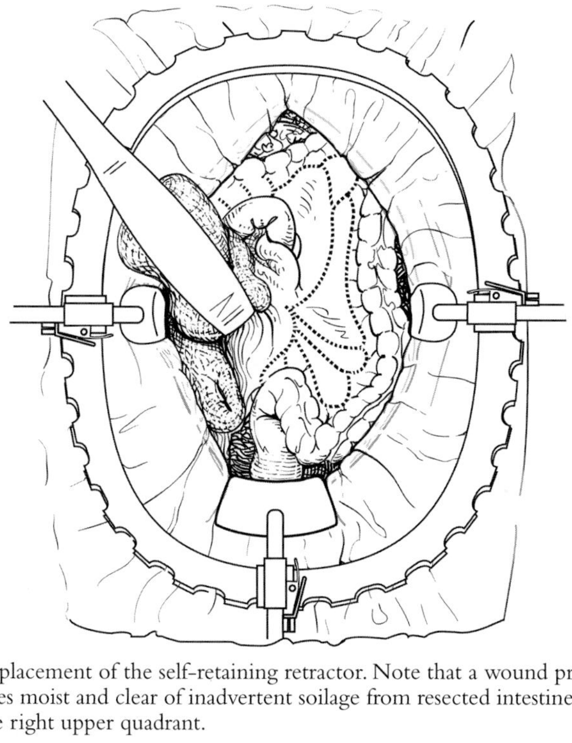

Once the splenic flexure, left, and sigmoid colon are fully mobilized, the mesentery can be evaluated and the extent of resection determined (Fig. 5). The left branch of the middle colic, left colic, and proximal sigmoid pedicles are isolated by dividing the overlying peritoneum and sweeping any lymph nodes distally along the pedicle. The vessels are ligated at the base with 2-0 Vicryl suture, vascular staples, or sealing devices such as Ligasure. I generally prefer to doubly ligate large, named vessels. Care must be taken to again identify the left ureter before dividing any left colon mesenteric pedicles. The extent of colon resection is then determined by the remaining vascular supply, providing a minimum of 5 cm of normal intestine proximal and distal to the lesion is included in the specimen. The mesentery is divided to the selected colon resection sites with care to secure the marginal vessel. After resection, restoration of intestinal continuity can be performed by suturing or stapling, either in

Fig. 4. Optimal placement of the self-retaining retractor. Note that a wound protector is used to keep wound edges moist and clear of inadvertent soilage from resected intestine. The small bowel is retracted in the right upper quadrant.

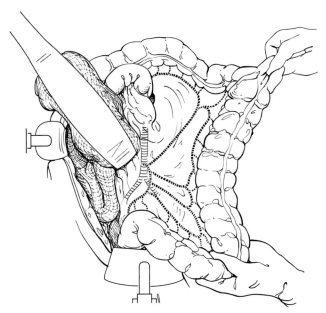

Fig. 5. After splenic flexure mobilization, the major vascular pedicles are identified and margins of resection are determined.

an end-to-side, side-to-side, or end-to-end manner. This depends on colon mobility, intestinal caliber, and surgeon preference. A sutured anastomosis can be performed with a single layer or double layer. Whether stapling or sewing, the principles of creating an anastomosis are similar and include maintaining adequate blood supply, absence of tension, gentle handling of tissues, absolute hemostasis, and precise apposition of tissues.

In general, I perform a stapled anastomosis in continuity. The tumor is isolated using bowel clamps and the sites of colon transaction are juxtaposed. Moist laparotomy pads are then placed around the site of future anastomosis to collect any inadvertent spillage of intestinal contents. Adjacent to the area of cleared mesentery, two colotomies are performed on the antimesenteric borders of the proximal and distal colon, in portions of intestine to be resected (Fig. 6). A GIA 80-mm stapler is inserted into both limbs of intestine and closed (Fig. 7). The surgeon confirms that the mesentery has not been included in the instru-

ment, the stapler is deployed, and the staple line is inspected for hemostasis as the GIA is removed. Bleeding along this staple line is best controlled with suture. Allis clamps are then used to oppose the intestinal wall, and a linear stapler (usually a TA-90) is placed below the common colotomy in the area corresponding to cleared mesentery on the proximal and distal colon (Fig. 8). The linear stapler is deployed and the intestine is divided above the stapler, allowing removal of the specimen from the field. Minor bleeding from the staple line is controlled with cautious use of electrocautery or suture. Excessive cautery is not advocated as the current can be readily transmitted along the staple line. The base of the anastomosis is then reinforced with 4–0 PDS or Vicryl interrupted suture.

For hand-sewn anastomosis, I prefer a two-layered technique. The proximal and distal colon is divided between bowel clamps and the specimen is removed from the field. The ends of colon to be anastomosed are placed in direct apposition to create continuity. The bowel clamps are slightly rotated and an outer row of seromuscular 4–0 silk Lembert sutures is placed. Sutures are tied and trimmed (except for the corners), then bowel clamps are released. The inner continuous row of sutures is then placed for mucosal opposition and hemostasis. Two separate 4–0 Vicryl sutures are placed in the center of the posterior wall (Fig. 9). The sutures are then bidirectionally advanced in an interlocking and running fashion, taking full-thickness colon wall, with care to stay above the deep silk

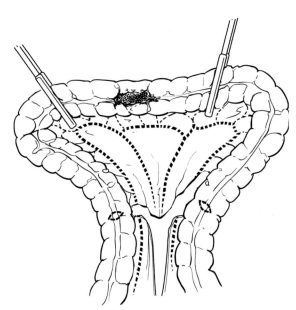

Fig. 6. The tumor is isolated with bowel clamps, and proximal and distal colotomies are created in the devascularized colon.

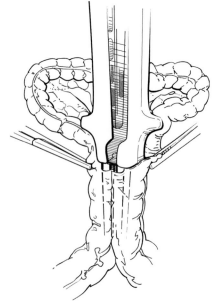

Fig. 7. The stapling device is inserted and deployed along the antimesenteric border of the colon.

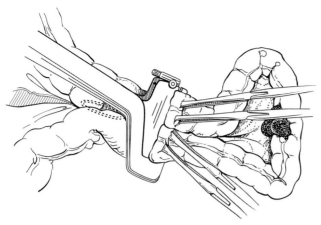

Fig. 8. The common colotomy is reapproximated with Allis clamps and closed with a linear stapling device.

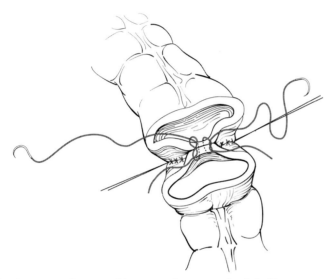

Fig. 9. Following a posterior row of interrupted seromuscular 3-0 silk sutures, two 3-0 Vicryl sutures are placed to form the inner, posterior layer.

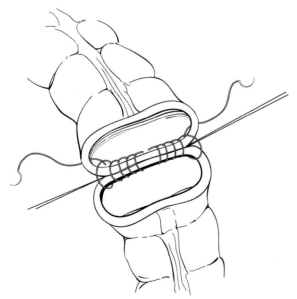

Fig. 10. The mucosa is opposed and hemostasis is achieved by running and interlocking the Vicryl suture.

layer (Fig. 10). At the corner on each end, one or two nonlocking sutures are placed again from inside to out until the corner is turned (Fig. 11). At this point, the suture is passed from the mucosal side of one of these segments of bowel through its wall to the serosal side. Now, with the suture on the outside, a Connell suture is used to invert the anterior layer of the inner closure. The "outside-in, inside-out" technique is used on alternating sides of the anastomosis and from each end, such that the suture lines are joined in the midportion of the anterior layer of the intestinal wall (Fig. 12). The ends are securely tied and trimmed. Completion of the outer wall anteriorly is then performed in a manner similar to that of the posterior row, using interrupted Lembert 4–0 silk sutures (Fig. 13).

After wound irrigation, the abdominal fascia is closed with No. 1 PDS. Interrupted No. 2 internal retention Vicryl sutures are used selectively. Skin is reapproximated with staples.

TUMORS OF THE SIGMOID COLON

Lymphadenectomy for lesions in the sigmoid colon include ligation of the inferior mesenteric artery just distal to the left colic artery (Fig. 3B). The entire sigmoid colon is resected and an anastomosis created between the left colon and rectosigmoid/upper rectum.

The procedure is begun as previously outlined with dissection of the lateral attachments of the sigmoid colon, identification of the gonadal vessels and left ureter in the retroperitoneum, and mobilization of the left colon. The inferior mesenteric pedicle is then isolated by incising the peritoneum at the base of the sigmoid mesentery on the right. The dissection proceeds just inferior to the superior rectal pedicle with care to avoid lifting of the sympathetic trunks from the retroperitoneum. The sympathetic nerves run deep to pedicle and, if raised unintentionally, feel like strings pulled on tension. If the nerves are inadvertently elevated, dissection is redirected to immediately below the superior rectal artery, to allow the nerves to retract to the retroperitoneum.

The inferior mesenteric artery is isolated just distal to the left colic artery by identifying the clear area in the mesentery just below the left colic artery. This can be performed by a technique in which the surgeon passes a finger beneath the pedicle and palpates the mesenteric clear space between the left colic artery above and first sigmoidal pedicle below (Fig. 14).

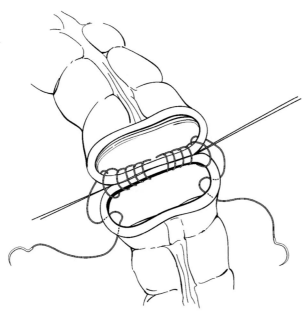

Fig. 11. At the corner on each end, one or two nonlocking sutures are placed again from inside to out until the corner is turned

The superior rectal artery is isolated and lymphatic tissue is swept distally along the pedicle for excision with the specimen. The pedicle is ligated and divided.

The left intestinal mesentery with any collateral vessels is divided to the junction of the left and sigmoid colon. The intestine is stapled and divided using a GIA device. With caudal retraction on the divided distal colon, the sigmoid mesentery is further dissected off the retroperitoneum, again remaining mindful of the sympathetic nerves. Dissection is continued into the retrorectal space between the visceral and parietal layers of the endopelvic fascia. Distal dissection is performed to the rectosigmoid junction, which is defined by coalescence of the tinea coli to form a complete muscular layer on the upper rectum. For low sigmoid lesions, dissection is taken 5 cm below the lesion onto the upper rectum. The mesentery of the rectosigmoid and upper rectum is well developed and contained within an enveloping fascia. Dissection is taken close to this layer to avoid injury to the sympathetic nerves, which lie inferior and then lateral to this fascial layer at the pelvic brim. At the proposed distal margin, the mesorectum

is divided first by incising the visceral layer of the endopelvic fascia, and then dividing lymphatic, vascular, and adipose tissues. This can be performed using a variety of methods including unipolar cautery, ties, or sealing instruments such as Ligasure device. Prior to rectal division, a bowel clamp is placed below the lesion and the distal rectum is irrigated with 1 L of saline. A 45- or 60-mm right-angle linear stapler is positioned and deployed (Fig. 15). The rectum is divided above this staple line, and the specimen is removed from the field.

After pelvic irrigation, the left colon is assessed for anastomosis in the pelvis. If additional length is required, partial or complete splenic flexure mobilization is performed as outlined. My preferred method of anastomosis at this level is a double-stapled technique, with a circular stapler passed per anus. The circumference of the descending colon determines the size of the circular stapler used. The left colon staple line is removed and a 2-0 Prolene purse-string suture is placed. The anvil is removed from a circular stapler and secured in the left colon by tying the purse-string suture. The stapler is then passed per anus to the stapled end of the upper rectum with care to follow the natural cure of the sacrum (Fig. 16). If prominent rectal folds make passage of the stapler shaft difficult, removal of the stapler and insertion of EEA sizers can be useful to help direct the path. Once the stapler head is correctly positioned, the pin is then advanced adjacent to the linear stapler line of the rectum. The anvil is engaged to the circular stapler, which is closed with care to correctly orient the descending colon mesentery (Fig. 17). The stapler is deployed, removed, and the surgical tissue rings or "donuts" are inspected for completeness.

The upper rectal anastomosis is then visualized with rigid proctoscopy and checked for hemostasis. A test for air leak is performed by filling the pelvis with fluid and insufflating the rectum with air while the descending colon is occluded. A continuous stream of air bubble in the pool of irrigation signals an anastomotic leak and should be investigated. The anastomosis should be inspected and repaired, usually with 4-0 PDS or Vicryl suture. A diverting ileostomy should be liberally used if necessary. A complete disruption of the staple line requires repeat anastomosis, which is not a difficult issue as there is usually ample length of colon and rectum for either repeat stapling or creation of a hand-sewn anastomosis.

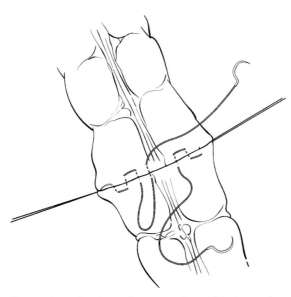

Fig. 12. A Connell suture is used to invert the anterior layer of the inner closure.

The Gastrointestinal Tract

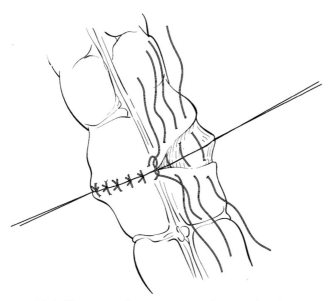

Fig. 13. Interrupted 3-0 silk seromuscular sutures are used to complete the outer, anterior layer.

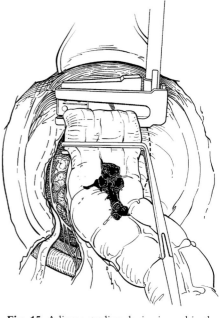

Fig. 15. A linear stapling device is used in the pelvis. Note the location of the ureters and sympathetic nerves.

A primary hand-sewn anastomosis, either end-to-end or end of left colon-to-side of rectum is also feasible. When there are significant size discrepancies, an end-to-side anastomosis can be advantageous. I prefer a double-layer technique, as previously described.

There are occasions in which ligation of the inferior mesenteric artery is reasonable for complete lymphadenectomy. For example, if the colon lesion lies between the left colic artery and first sigmoidal pedicle, lymphadenectomy including all branches of the inferior mesenteric artery is reasonable (Fig. 3C). In this case, the base of the inferior mesenteric artery is visualized by incising the posterior parietal peritoneum superiorly along the left colon mesentery overlying the aorta. The pedicle is cleared for ligation by sweeping lymphatic tissues along the vessel. Because high ligation can be associated with sympathetic nerve injury, care is taken to divide the vessel 1 to 2 cm distal to the aorta to avoid injury to the autonomic nerves. There is a potential watershed area at the splenic flexure when the inferior mesenteric artery is ligated, so the left colon should be evaluated for adequate blood supply. If visualization of the left colon or palpation of the marginal artery does not indicate adequate blood supply, resection should be extended to include the splenic flexure colon, with anastomosis between the distal transverse colon and rectosigmoid.

SPECIAL CIRCUMSTANCES: OBSTRUCTION, PERFORATION, AND LOCALLY ADVANCED TUMORS

Obstructing left colon cancers pose surgical planning and technical challenges as many confounding issues may apply: the proximal intestine usually has not been evaluated for synchronous disease, the colon can contain significant amounts of solid fecal material, and the proximal intestine can be greatly dilated and not amenable to anastomosis. If at all possible, conversion of an emergent case to an elective one is highly advantageous. Recent use of colonic stenting is one method of decompressing the proximal intestine, clearing the colon of synchronous disease, and fully preparing the bowel for surgery. Other options include subtotal colectomy and ileosigmoid or ileorectal anastomosis, which are reasonable options in young patients with significant family history or known synchronous disease. Some

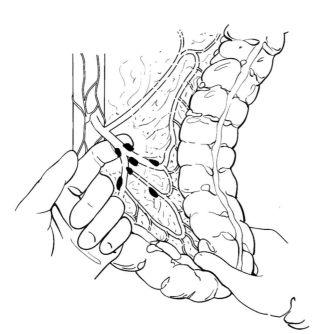

Fig. 14. The inferior mesenteric pedicle is isolated distal to the left colic artery by palpating the clear space in the left colon mesentery. Care is taken to keep the sympathetic trunks in the retroperitoneum.

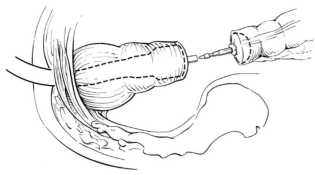

Fig. 16. The anvil is secured in the descending colon with a purse-string suture and the shaft of the stapler placed per anus and advanced to the stapled end of the rectum.

surgeons advocate on-table lavage, which I find cumbersome and does not address the associated proximal bowel dilatation that may be present. Other options include initial diverting stoma or a Hartmann procedure. In general, I prefer to use colonic stents when feasible.

Operations on perforated cancers usually require the use of a stoma because of fecal contamination. Perforation can occur either at the site of the lesion or more proximally, when complete obstruction has occurred. In the setting of perforation at the site of the cancer, a standard resection is required, followed by left colostomy and Hartmann turnin. If the dissection planes are obscured, the surgeon should start the dissection above or below the mass, in an area relatively free of inflammation, where appropriate tissue planes can be identified. Ureteral stent placement preoperatively or intraoperatively can be useful when there is excessive retroperitoneal inflammation or fibrosis. If the tumor has invaded into the abdominal sidewall or retroperitoneum, surgical clips can be placed at the site of resection to guide possible postoperative radiation.

Locally advanced tumors with involvement of adjacent structures require radical en bloc resection. Organs most commonly involved include spleen, uterus, dome of bladder, abdominal wall, adjacent small bowel colon, and ureter. It is often impossible to determine if adherent structures represent tumor infiltration or inflammatory adhesion. Because dissection of a malignant fistula is associated with tumor spillage and poor outcome, en bloc resection of adherent organs or structures is preferred.

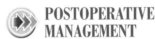

POSTOPERATIVE MANAGEMENT

Orogastric tubes are removed on patient extubation as postoperative ileus occurs in 10% to 20% of cases, irrespective of feeding pattern or use of nasogastric tubes. Diet advancement is directed by the patient's progress. Clear liquids are given when perioperative nausea has passed, and low-fat, low-fiber diet is offered thereafter. Postoperative antibiotics are limited to 24 hours or less unless there was obvious fecal spillage or other mitigating circumstances.

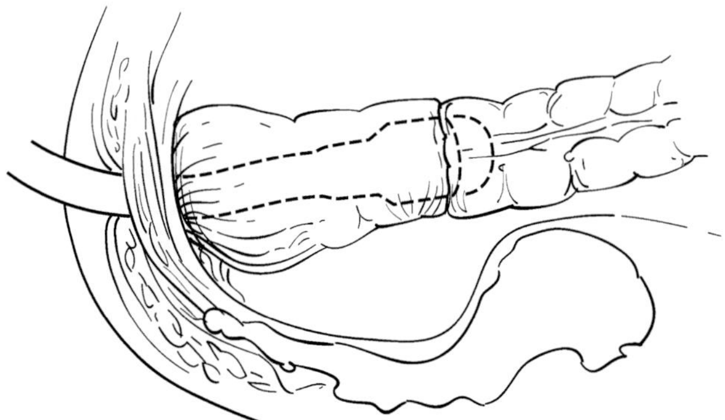

Ambulation is begun on postoperative day 1, and deep vein thrombosis prophylaxis with low molecular weight heparin is begun the day of surgery or the first postoperative day. Pneumatic compression boots are maintained until the patient is capable of ambulation without assistance four to six times a day.

Postoperative ileus requires observation if the patient is clinically stable. Reduction of narcotics, increased ambulation, and correction of electrolytes are advocated. In rare cases, parenteral nutrition is initiated if an ileus is prolonged more than 14 days, or earlier if the patient had evidence of preoperative nutritional deficit.

Postoperative fever should raise the concern of a possible anastomotic leak, although other sources such as pulmonary, urinary, intravenous lines, and wound infection are more common. Computed tomographic scans with gentle rectal contrast or contrast enema studies with Gastrografin can diagnosis an anastomotic leak. Small leaks may be treated conservatively with parenteral nutrition and percutaneous drainage; however, significant anastomotic disruptions or persistent sepsis often require re-exploration, with creation of a temporary diverting stoma.

Follow-Up

Follow-up is performed most intensely for the first 2 to 3 years because 80% of tumor recurrences will occur during this time. After left hemicolectomy, most patients should be evaluated every 3 to 4 months with physical examination and carcinoembryonic antigen serum studies. Rectal anastomosis can be evaluated by flexible sigmoidoscopy. Colonoscopy should be repeated 1 year from the time of surgery, and then at 3- to 5-year intervals if no additional adenomatous polyps are identified. If the colon was not completely evaluated with endoscopy prior to surgery, a colonoscopy should be performed approximately 3 months following resection. The CT scans and chest radiographs are obtained on an individual basis, usually every 6 to 12 months on high-risk, stage III patients. Following 2 to 3 years, patients are evaluated every 6 months until 5 years and then yearly thereafter.

SUGGESTED READING

Herter FP, Slanetz CA. Patterns and significance of lymphatic spread from cancer of the colon and rectum. In: Weiss L, Gilbert H, Ballon S, eds. *Lymphatic system metastases.* Boston, MA: GK Hall, 1980:275.

Fig. 17. The anvil is secured to the shaft of the stapler, closed, and deployed.

EDITOR'S COMMENT

The chapter provided by Professor Weiser of Memorial Sloan-Kettering Cancer Center in New York emphasizes surgical approaches to carcinoma of the left hemicolon and focuses on extent of regional resection, which is "defined by adequate lymphadenectomy."To provide en bloc resection requires surgical knowledge of regional anatomy with emphasis on lymphatic nodal drainage patterns to execute the proper oncologic left hemicolectomy. The author provides graphic depiction (Fig. 1) of bidirectional lymphatic flow along major vascular pedicles and provides the frequency for expectation of metastatic disease relative to its given vascular pedicle with portal to the systemic circulation.With the high frequency of metastatic disease to hepatic parenchyma via the portal venous system, it is the liver that has the highest frequency of distant spread (>60%) to a solid organ from colon carcinoma. Thus, as emphasized by the author, proper lymphadenectomy with left hemicolectomy requires an intraoperative identification of the vascular pedicle at greatest risk for nodal metastasis and its proper inclusion in the resected specimen. As the left colon has an identifiable, well-developed marginal artery and vein to form the mesenteric vascular arcade that parallels the colonic inner wall, its location should be sought in the resection. In some patients, this collateral circulation is incompletely developed, and as emphasized by the author, results in a potential "watershed area" at the splenic flexure.

We agree with the author that thorough preoperative workup is essential to optimize the proper oncologic resection. Besides routine laboratory and chemistry examinations, a familial and genetic history is appropriate. The colon must be fully evaluated for synchronous lesions and, as noted by the author, synchronous polyps and invasive cancers are evident in 30% and 3% of cases, respectively. The evolving application of virtual colonoscopy (CT colography) represents a noninvasive method to evaluate right colon, transverse, and left colon lesions. However, full (comprehensive) endoscopic evaluation with histologic confirmation of associated lesions is indicated with detection of the new or synchronous primary. With identification of small cancerous lesions evident at the time of colonoscopy in which polypectomy is completed, multisite "tattooing" of these small lesions is appropriate to correlate margins of resection. The use of preoperative CT evaluation with oral and intravenous contrast is advocated by the author; although highly criticized by many surgeons for its overuse, it is often uncompensated by insurance carriers as a diagnostic tool. However, we concur with Professor Weiser that CT contrast evaluations of the entire abdomen and chest are appropriate for histologically confirmed carcinoma of the left colon. Such tests will identify potential metastatic sites, including extensive nodal disease and extension of the primary with solid organ metastasis, which has high metastatic frequency to the liver and lung. Moreover, the CT examinations often initiate extension of an operation to evaluate intra-abdominal metastatic sites not evident with cursory examination at the time of opening the patient.

Similar to the author, our preference is to do complete mechanical bowel preparation, beginning with clear-liquid diet prior to the day of surgery with additional usage of polyethylene glycol solution (GoLYTELY) or use of oral sodium phosphate solution (Fleet Phospho-Soda) followed by rapid hydration with water. It makes little sense to avoid the use of this mechanical preparation, and we concur with the author's use of oral antibiotic bowel preparation with use of second-generation cephalosporins administered within 1 hour of the operation to diminish systemic sepsis and wound infection.

The accurate pathologic staging of cancer of the right colon is essential and requires diligence by the pathologist on removal of the right colonic segment. Comprehensive assessment including total (quantity) nodes, as well as final histologic status, is essential. Metastatic nodal disease remains the most important prognostic factor for patients with colorectal carcinoma (Le Voyer TE et al. *J Clin Oncol* 2003;21:2912). Patients with node-negative disease have a 5-year survival rate of 75%; patients with node-positive disease experience a 5-year survival rate of 30% to 60%. Further, the number of nodes resected bears on the survival of patients who are node-negative and node-positive; completeness of resection and staging accuracy therefore translates into a potential survival benefit.Thus, the en bloc lymphadenectomy has both a diagnostic and therapeutic role in the management of right colon, as well as left colon and rectal cancer. The historic contribution by Cabañas (*Cancer* 1977;39:456), in 1977, established the importance of lymphatic histology with sentinel node mapping of patients with penile carcinoma.This approach identified the sentinel lymph node (SLN) as the first site of regional nodal metastasis, and is predictive of the nodal status of the remaining nodal basin.Thereafter, Morton et al. (Second International Conference on Melanoma 1989:131), in 1989, established the importance for use of this technique using blue dye for clinical stage I melanoma to assess the regional nodal basin. Such techniques have been extensively applied to breast abnormalities.

A recent review by Stojadinovic et al. (*J Am Coll Surg* 2005;201:297) reviewed the published results of colorectal SLN mapping with isosulfan blue dye alone, demonstrating high success rates for identification of at least one sentinel node in those centers with extensive technical experience with the technique. These authors suggest that the SLN reflects the status of the remaining nodal basin with 92% to 96% accuracy with a low risk of "skipped metastasis" (negative SLN/positive non-SLN; 4% to 8%) in these studies. Additional techniques to ultrastage colorectal carcinoma sentinel nodes are highly variable with multilevel step sectioning using hematoxylin and eosin stains or combinations with cytokeratin, carcinoembryonic antigen-IAC, or reverse transcriptase polymerase chain reaction. The differentiation in outcomes for this early phase of prospective studies to assess the advantage of rectal versus colonic lymphatic mapping is unclear; early data would suggest the techniques are similar in outcomes.

Many left colon lesions are detected by flexible sigmoidoscopy as it provides direct visualization of the colon and the ability to procure polyps and diagnose frankly invasive disease. Flexible sigmoidoscopy has advantage over colonoscopy in that it does not require that the patient be given sedation or anesthesia. Further, it can be achieved with a single enema that can be self-administered. The limitation of the flexible sigmoidoscopy is its length for passage into the level of the left colon and distal aspects of the transverse colon. The use of flexible sigmoidoscopy remains one of the principal screening tools for colorectal carcinoma. The procedure provides direct visualization of the colon and suspicious mucosal lesions that may be biopsied for histologic validation. Its disadvantage obviously is that it only examines the lower third of the colon; thus, to properly examine right colon lesions requires colonoscopy and/or barium contrast enemas, although the latter has lower sensitivity and specificity than direct visualization by endoscopy. For open or laparoscopic surgical resection of the *right colon*, tissue procurement *is essential* by endoscopy with the exception of the rare obstructing lesion.

Although this chapter focuses on open technique, laparoscopic surgery for colon cancer remains an acceptable alternative to the open approach. However, there are small, but measurable, short-term benefits of the laparoscopic approach, which include earlier return of bowel function, shorter length of hospital stay, and decreased necessity of postoperative narcotic administration. It would appear from contemporary studies that recurrence and survival are not compromised by the laparoscopic approach. In the large, multi-institutional, randomized trial in the United States, by the Clinical Outcomes of Surgical Therapy (COST) Study Group (*N Engl J Med* 2004;350:2050), the results for participating surgeons in high-volume centers of excellence suggested similar outcomes. The applications of laparoscopic colectomy for cancer are included in Chapter 130. Since the first application of laparoscopic colonic resection in 1991, this minimally invasive resection approach has not been readily adopted. Within the past 2 years, in addition to the COST trial, two international trials are currently being conducted, one in Europe and the second in the United Kingdom. Laparoscopic surgery for colorectal carcinoma is currently accepted as an *alternative* to open resection; the open left hemicolectomy for carcinoma is considered the "gold standard" on which all comparisons must be made. Of interest, the COST trial performed by experienced laparoscopic surgeons with a minimum of 20 laparoscopic resections in high-volume centers of excellence, had similar morbidity and mortality results to the open approach. Whether these results can be transferred to achieve outcomes and long-term survival similar to the open technique will require future prospective study.

Conventional colonoscopic approaches remain among the highest accuracy available for diagnosis and procurement of tissue for detection of colorectal masses or inflammatory bowel disease.This procedure does require conscious sedation, and there may be poor patient acceptance and incomplete bowel preparation preoperatively to assure an adequate unlimited examination as a screening tool. Further, the presence of a stenotic site or elongated bowel segments may abrogate the colonoscopic approach to visualize the entire colon and the ileocecal valve in certain patients. The considerable early enthusiasm for virtual endoscopy that is based on acquisition of cross-sectional images can be provided by using CT or magnetic resonance imaging. Recent studies suggest that both techniques are effective to detect clinically relevant disease. Svensson et al. (*Radiology* 2002;222:337), evaluating more than 100 patients having both virtual and conventional endoscopy, observed favorable outcomes with the virtual technique by 82% of the patients. However, virtual colonoscopy based on acquisition of CT data is associated with high doses of ionizing radiation.The recent report by Lauenstein et al. (*Magn Reson Imaging Clin N Am* 2005;13:349) of Germany characterizes the preferable application of magnetic resonance imaging for virtual colonography.The final sensitivity and specificity of this technique will almost certainly improve and move the science to a less-invasive interventional diagnostic procedure than the endoscopic approaches. Its future role for management of right colon, transverse, left colon, and rectal lesions remains unanswered.

Finally, as colorectal is one of the most common gastrointestinal malignancies worldwide,

(continued)

especially in North America and Europe, the therapy of regional nodal metastasis is pivotal to producing superior outcomes of local control and survival. Further, surgical resection remains the only curative maneuver for its treatment; thus, efforts during the past decades have centered on measures to enhance survival rates with the use of systemic chemotherapy in the adjuvant setting; such studies have been extensively explored in randomized prospective trials. Combinations of 5-fluorouracil (5-FU) and leucovorin (LV) currently remain the reference therapeutic approach. The advantage of infusion of 5-FU/LV with additive oxaliplatin (FOLFOX) was compared bimonthly in a European trial (Mosaic) for patients with stages II and III colon cancer. These results were published by Andre (48 Sun) et al. (*N Engl J Med* 2004;350: 2344). In this European trial of 2,248 patients, results confirmed that FOLFOX was safe, feasible, and effective to prevent relapse with minimal associated toxicity. Compared with the 5-FU//LV arm alone, the combination FOLFOX sustained a 3-year disease-free survival of 78.2% versus 72.9%

($P < 0.002$), representing a risk reduction of 23%. This represents the first study to demonstrate that combination chemotherapy is superior to the current 5-FU/LV standard, and was also superior to irinotecan. Many medical oncologists advocate combination chemotherapy with FOLFOX for high-risk cancer patients following curative surgery (stage II) and for all stage III disease.

Studies await maturation from the Mosaic trial and confirmation of additional studies using 5-FU/LV (Mayo Clinic/Roswell Park regimen) compared with Xelox (capecitabine plus oxaliplatin). Currently planned is a trial that compares infusional 5-FU/LV plus irinotecan (FOLFIRI) to surgery alone for the therapy of stage II disease. Before therapeutic decisions are made for patients with stage II and III disease, detailed and careful discussion between patient and surgeon regarding benefits/risk ratios of adjuvant therapy is necessary. Such discussions must also include the anatomic and biologic risk factors of the primary neoplasm, as well as the potential toxicities related to chemotherapy. Such considerations are strongly evident in the current

evolution of effective antiangiogenic strategies that use vascular endothelial growth factors (VEGF) and that have emerged as important therapeutic targets for their inhibition. The principal anti-VEGF agent used has been bevacizumab, which has been used for untreated metastatic colorectal carcinoma. Bevacizumab was approved for use in colorectal cancer by the Food and Drug Administration based on data from a phase III study comparing combination chemotherapy with irinotecan, 5-FU/LV with and without bevacizumab. These data confirm that the additive effect of bevacizumab to this chemotherapy combination enhanced response rates by 10%, increased progression-free survival by more than 4 months, and enhanced median survival by nearly 5 months compared with the chemotherapy alone. Additional studies of this anti-VEGF agent alone and additional prospective studies using other chemotherapeutic combinations are essential to formulate prospective effective strategies for treatment of colorectal carcinoma.

K.I.B.

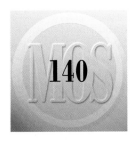

Rectal Cancer in the 21st Century— Radical Operations: Anterior Resection and Abdominoperineal Excision

140

R.J. HEALD

BASIC PRINCIPLES

"Even at its scientific best medicine is a social act." Certainly the social implications of the decisions made in rectal cancer management are grave indeed—cure of cancer, local control of one of Nature's cruellest malignancies, the necessity for a permanent stoma, the preservation of sexual function, and much more. Furthermore, in the new century, decisions regarding both radiotherapy and chemotherapy now present major challenges in a field of ever-increasing complexity.

For so many reasons, therefore, we must recognize that "even at its most scientific, *surgery* is the act of an artisan or, at best, a *craftsman*." Surgery is not amenable to study by the same methods as those applicable to drugs or medicines or to measurable interventions such as irradiation, yet surgical technique has by far the greatest impact on rectal cancer outcomes. The randomized, controlled clinical trial has so far contributed remarkably little to the development of surgical techniques because, in the difficult and complex surgery of cancer, "the devil is in the details." As a basic principle of any cancer operation, however, the block of tissue to be removed should be

precisely defined and subjected to scrutiny. Thus, surgical anatomy and histopathologic audit should become exact sciences in their own right and a meaningful judgment on the oncologic quality of the specimen made by an independent pathologist after every surgical excision.

HISTORICAL CONSIDERATIONS

Most of the literature in the Western world has paid scant attention to detail of how the actual dissection around a rectal tumor should be carried out. The diagrams in current textbooks bear witness to the crude manual extraction techniques that bedevil "conventional" surgery for rectal cancer (Fig. 1). However, the Japanese with their special interest in the detailed vascular and neuroanatomy of the pelvis, and we, with our total mesorectal excision (TME) initiative, have both attempted to improve on the simplistic concept of abdominoperineal excision, an operation originally described in 1907 by the Englishman Ernest Miles. His concept of a cylinder of maximal size that "empties the whole pelvis" was at least an attempt at defining in advance the block of tissue to be excised by the surgeon. This idea, illustrated in Figure 2,

has dominated the minds of doctors throughout the 20th century. Indeed, if surgeons had really produced perfect "oncologic cylinders," there would have been far fewer local recurrences and failures, though the morbidity in terms of sexual and pelvic autonomic function would have been formidable while the deadspace would have required packing for many months. The famous John Goliger used to comment, "If you haven't made the patient impotent, you probably haven't cured him of rectal cancer."

Miles considered that spread occurred, particularly in the lymphatics, in all directions and included very clearly in his diagrams his perception of why he had seen 31 perineal recurrences in the wound of his operations (Figs. 2 and 3). He believed that the reason for these was that he had failed to encompass by his operation spread that had occurred into the ischioanal fat via nodes around the inferior hemorrhoidal (rectal) vessels. The same diagram also shows many nodes sitting on the surface of the levator muscles within the imagined "cylinder" of spread. He clearly also believed that, for this reason, only the widest possible clearance at this level had any hope of curing the patient

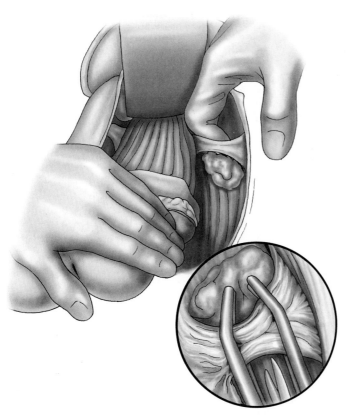

Fig. 1. This would make a patient impotent.

where the satellites of cancer commonly occur since the ideal radical cancer operation should encompass only the common fields of spread that do not exact too high a penalty from the patient. The design of the optimal operation that modern surgery can now offer should take into account the field of spread amenable to surgical removal with the primary tumor, the disabilities inflicted by each component of the surgery, and the point in time at which cure becomes impossible by local surgery because metastases have already become established.

The first major steps toward minimizing mutilation can be attributed to many surgeons who embarked upon anterior resection (AR) to avoid sacrifice of the anal sphincters. Initiated on both sides of the Atlantic before and after World War II, the proportion of rectal cancers undergoing sphincter-preserving surgery has risen steadily to a current level of 90% in specialized units and around 70% in most general hospitals.

Modern rational surgical planning should consider each of the possible fields of spread of rectal cancer in turn, and the disabilities and sacrifices paid by the patient for their removal. In each case we should, to give the patient what we would wish for ourselves, try to balance the benefit of an extra chance of cure against the functional and anatomic price to be paid. At the time of going to press this implies that preoperative assessment should supplement full clinical and endoscopic appraisal with a computed tomography (CT) scan of the whole body for metastatic spread and a specialized magnetic resonance imaging

and it was commonplace for tumors as high as 15 to 25 cm to suffer the same fate. So it is that permanent colostomy became established as the necessary price for cure and became a very common and widely dreaded association of bowel cancer in the public mind. Similar thought processes about spread govern most extended surgical lymphadenectomies, but careful studies of ischioanal fossa node involvement to justify this heavy price have never been undertaken. Furthermore, long surgical experience teaches us that multiple nodes on the surface of the levators or in the ischiorectal fat such as those in the diagram are simply never seen.

Such studies were certainly not attempted by Miles, who simply regarded the whole of the surrounding cylinder of tissue as "highly dangerous tissues"—particularly "the levators, the ischio-anal fat and the perianal skin."

The background then to all our current attempts to move toward an optimal cancer operation is a standard but empirical procedure that was designed almost a century ago. Virtually no detail of how the actual dissection should be effected appears in the literature. The Miles operation was certainly radical in the sense that it appeared in the diagrams to remove the cancer with much of the surrounding tissue. It was also an operation that could be completed at great speed—often in less than an hour. In the early years of the last century such speed often meant the difference between a live patient and a dead one at the end of the operation! However, the term radical refers to *radix,* a root in Latin. Leave part of the root and the plant regrows. In cancer terms this implies a need for real understanding of

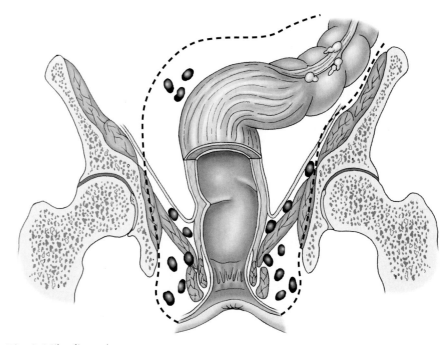

Fig. 2. Miles diagnosis.

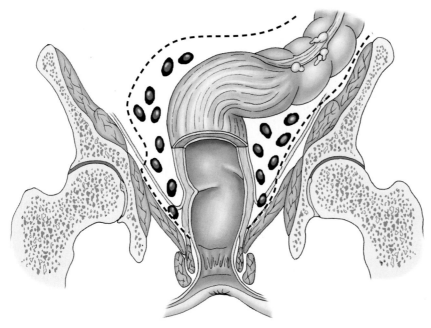

Fig. 3. Our concept of the field of spread.

(MRI) scan for appraisal of the primary cancer within the pelvis.

EMBRYOLOGY

Conceptually TME has a basis in scientific thought, which is attractive to all members of the modern multidisciplinary team with background training in basic science. The theory behind it is that cancer spread will tend, initially at least, to remain within the embryologic hindgut "envelope." The gut, after all, spent its early fetal existence actually outside the abdomen. When secondarily rectum and mesorectum became "plastered" back onto the retroperitoneal structures and into the developing pelvis, they retained their midline lymphovascular integrity and remained separate from the surrounding paired organs and parieties. Their adherence to them is by a collagenous cobweb of areolar tissue, which allows a degree of movement, is recognizable by the surgeon as a "surgical plane" and is almost entirely avascular. In a number of publications, the author has drawn attention to this "holy plane of rectal surgery" and attempted to point out the value of painstakingly following the perimesorectal avascular plane around the midline hindgut into the depths of the pelvis as a practical surgical policy. This was eventually shown to improve local recurrence rates. Straying into the field of cancer spread within the mesorectum was, and still is, in conventional practice, an extremely common cause of involved surgical margins and

residual pelvic disease: straying out can damage the autonomic nerve layers and is a common cause of impotence. Some workers in the past postulated a physical barrier to the spread of cancer at this interface: it seems intrinsically more probable, in the light of Judah Folkman's work, that

tumor angiogenesis is impeded by the avascular nature of the areolar interface between midline hindgut and surrounding parieties.

So it is that embryology is the true key to defining the *oncologic package* that will encompass the *relevant* field of spread. The surgeon should bear in mind that the tapering hindgut "package," surrounded by the "holy plane," is inserted into the funnel-shaped sloping levators, which become the parietal external sphincters distally.

THE MESORECTUM FOR THE SURGEON

Surgical Anatomy

The original idea for TME was born from the practice of surgery. The mesorectum only becomes a reality for each individual surgeon from enthusiasm for slow, meticulous, painstaking dissection in difficult but achievable planes. These, once recognized and identified, become the defining objectives of the surgery and the redefined building blocks of the anatomy.

Once the surgeon has grasped the new system of anatomy, as Stelzner originally did from his diagram, it also becomes clear that the basis for the planes does indeed lie in the embryology (Fig. 4).

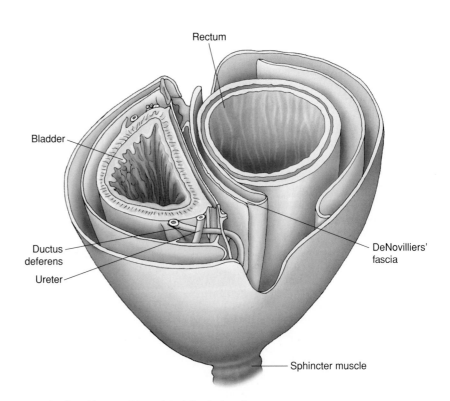

Fig. 4. The fascial layers of the pelvis (after Stelzner).

The innermost "holy plane" is that which surrounds the midline hindgut within its lymphovascular envelope—the core—while the two surrounding lamellae comprise a neural layer and a wolffian ridge layer, which develop from the paired structures outside the hindgut. This concept has been made relatively simple to comprehend by the Japanese suggestion of comparing pelvic anatomy with the layers of an onion.

Much of surgery of the whole gastrointestinal tract is a question of pursuing the planes between embryologically separate organs or tissues. The careful and thoughtful surgeon who is mobilizing any part of the large intestine by sharp dissection becomes aware of a choice of two relatively avascular and therefore surgically satisfying planes, which are of special value as in his or her journey down into the pelvis. The innermost "holy plane" envelopes the integral visceral mesentery of the hindgut or "mesorectum." This "safety margin" is a complete fatty and lymphovascular surrounding on all aspects in the middle third of the rectum, which constitutes the greater part of the organ and the commonest site for cancer. In the upper third the anterior aspect is covered only by the peritoneum with "mesorectum" at the back and the sides as the peritoneal reflection tapers forward toward the "cul-de-sac." In the lower third of the rectum virtually no fatty tissue intervenes between the anterior aspect of the rectum and the back of the prostate. Posteriously the prostate has an important fascial attachment to the lowest extremity of the shiny front surface fascia (Denonvilliers fascia) of the encircling midrectal mesorectum. The surgeon has to divide this layer to enter the plane between the rectum and the prostate. In the female the middle third has a rather thin and tenuous fatty layer between the rectum and vagina with Denonvilliers fascia being often scant and difficult to identify. I use the term Denonvilliers fascia to describe this shiny anterior surface of the excised middle third of the specimen and its forward continuation to fuse with the back of the prostate. This seems logical because Denonvilliers fascia is recognized by some embryologists as the downward prolongation of peritoneum, which has become obliterated as a cavity. Fritsch has preferred to call it the "rectogenital septum," which certainly conveys the reality of a rectangular or trapezoidal "bib" between hindgut behind and vesicles and prostate in front. Just as peritoneum is the integral surface of the anterior aspect of the upper intraperitoneal third of the rectum, Denonvilliers fascia is integral to the

fatty anterior mesorectum in the middle third in the male. Posteriorly and posterolaterally the areolar plane is well defined around the globular expanding bilobed mesorectum. A condensation of the fascia called the rectosacral ligament often presents a barrier to the surgeon posteriorly below the promontory. It is essential that this be positively divided either with diathermy or scissors. Beyond it the plane is easy to recognize except that the forward angulation demands strong anterodistal retraction to facilitate direct visualization.

THE MESORECTUM FOR THE PATHOLOGIST

The pathologist Quirke identified that there is a high positive predictive value of circumferential margin involvement (CRM) for the subsequent development of locally recurrent cancer. This implies that completeness and intactness of the specimen are crucial factors—ideally that it should be one recognizable block of tissue whose orientation and former relations can be identified. While "specimen-orientated surgery" has become the established practice in our unit, recognition of the features of the TME specimen and the freedom of its margins from cancer involvement become the key factor of audit. In most cases naked-eye inspection provides the initial necessary quality control, with microscopic examination of the suspected areas of margin involvement as a logical primary objective for the surgeon. Visual inspection of the front of a well-performed TME specimen should show three clear landmarks (Fig. 5):

1. The cut edge of the peritoneal reflection
2. The smooth shiny anterior surface of the anterior mesorectum of the middle

third—Denonvilliers fascia—or the rectogenital septum
3. The almost bare anterior aspect of the anorectal muscle—in the lowest anterior resections or abdominoperineal excision (APE) specimens only

Laterally the fatty mesorectum expands distally beyond an anteroposterior groove made by the nerve erigentes, whilst posteriorly a perfect specimen exhibits perfectly curved "buttocks" with a central groove corresponding to the anococcygeal raphe (the pubococcygeus muscle).

MODERN IMAGING—FINE-SLICE HIGH-RESOLUTION MRI

The great step forward of the new millennium is the establishment by Brown, Blomquist, and others that specialized fine-slice high-resolution MRI can visualize this "holy plane" before the surgery and thus predict the detail of the oncologic specimen that the surgeon endeavours to remove and its probable contours around the tentacles of tumor. TME principles are now more readily comprehended by nonsurgeons because of the development by these specialist MRI radiologists of images that are far superior to anything previously achievable. The fine-slice high-resolution methods are demonstrably superior to any x-ray–based modality, which inevitably suffers limitations in differentiating tumor tissue from muscle wall. MRI demonstrates, for the first time, the contours of the mesorectum and the distribution of the cancer within it. The recent "Mercury" study from the Pelican Center in Basingstoke has demonstrated reliable equivalence between MRI prediction and histopathologic reality (Fig. 4). It also demonstrates that a 1-mm mesorectal

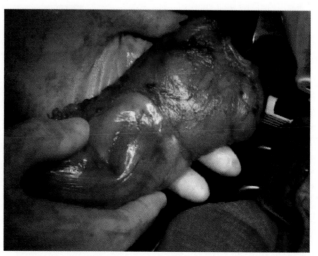

Fig. 5. Front of a total mesorectal excision specimen.

clearance on MRI between cancer within and mesorectal fascia without can reliably be used to predict the need for neoadjuvant "downstaging" because the mesorectal margin is in danger of being breached during surgery. It can also provide a "workshop guide" for the detailed surgery, whether this be performed laparoscopically or open. This may become particularly crucial as a "route map" for laparoscopic surgeons as they increasingly extend their dissections into the challenging depths of the true pelvis where the inability to feel the cancer can be a serious disadvantage.

Critical MRI Decisions in Lower-third Cancers

One focal area of current controversy centers on the anatomic and embryologic fact that the mesorectal envelope tapers down in this (infralevator) lower third to appear very thin indeed—particularly on the crucial coronal MRI cuts on which decisions in modern multidisciplinary teams (MDTs) are made. On such an MRI it is extremely tempting to predict that this tapering and narrowing area of the mesorectum will constitute a hazardous margin: thus, a decision may be made to administer preoperative downstaging neoadjuvant therapy or even choose abdominoperineal excision for fear of margin involvement. In such cases, where the cancer is below the levator origins on MRI, it is essential that an *experienced surgeon* examines the patient to establish *free mobility of the tumor* in the conscious patient (with muscle tone). In the author's opinion this clinical observation does almost invariably mean that a TME will be an achievable surgical objective. It does not confront the other tendentious issue of the higher incidence of internal iliac and particularly obturator node involvement in tumors less than 4cm from the anal margin.

MULTIDISCIPLINARY TEAM MANAGEMENT

MDT management is now mandatory for all major malignancies in the United Kingdom and is increasingly standard practice in many institutions throughout the world. For the reasons outlined above, the focal point of the decision-making process is becoming the MRI images, which can be readily understood by all.

The TME concept can now be extended to embrace a multidisciplinary six-stage process:

1. Phased-array-coil fine-slice MRI
2. MDT planning

3. Preoperative neoadjuvant therapy in cases selected on the basis of preoperative MRI staging of the pelvis plus whole-trunk CT for the detection of metastases
4. Detailed precision surgery—TME or "TME plus." "TME minus" or "partial TME" for upper one-third cancers implies that the mesorectum is divided 5 cm below the tumor and a rectal and mesorectal remnant remain.
5. Detailed audit of the specimen after removal with special emphasis on naked-eye assessment of mesorectal integrity and microscopic evaluation of the margins.
6. MDT assessment and decision regarding postoperative therapy.

TME for the surgeon comprises six basic principles:

1. Perimesorectal "holy plane" sharp dissection by monopolar diathermy and scissors under direct vision. Three-directional traction and countertraction is a vital principle for diathermy dissection as it is essential that the areolar tissue be "on stretch" if "holy plane" dissection is to be accurate (Fig. 6).
2. Specimen-orientated surgery and histopathology, of which the object is an intact mesorectum with no tearing of the surface and no circumferential margin involvement (CMI)—naked eye or microscopic
3. "Quirke-style pathology" audit for CMI as the principal immediate outcome measure. Combined with objective assessment of the whole specimen, this confirms the optimal planning and execution of the surgery. Surgeons and oncologists may also base postoperative therapy on this pathology report.

4. Recognition during surgery of, and preservation of, the autonomic plexuses and nerves, on which sexual and bladder function depend
5. A major increase in anal preservation and reduction in the number of permanent colostomies
6. Stapled low pelvic reconstruction, usually using the Moran triple stapling technique, plus creation of a short colon pouch anastomosed to low rectum or anal canal

BEFORE THE OPERATION— BIMANUAL PELVIC EXAMINATION

CT scans and colonoscopy report should always be at hand in the operating room. Never commence surgery without examining the patient digitally when awake plus performing bimanual examination under anaesthesia. This is especially true in the female so as to establish whether the tumor is fully mobile on the posterior vaginal wall. The decision as to whether to excise a part of the posterior wall is finally made at this time by a combination of rectal and vaginal examination, and the latter must never be omitted. Sometimes, if anterior resection is possible, a disc of the posterior wall may be circumscribed around an area of tethering using the angled-point diathermy from below. This is often best performed before the abdominal dissection is started. Routine excision of the posterior vaginal wall is not usually necessary unless it is involved.

Steps of the Operation

The key principle is that dissection should only proceed in the areolar tissue plane

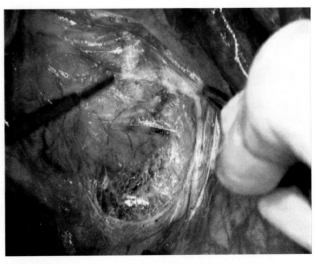

Fig. 6. Areolar dissection.

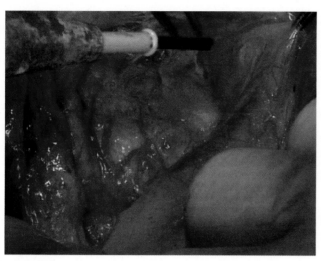

Fig. 7. Pedicle package.

(the "holy plane") within (and thus sparing) the autonomic nerve plexuses, the nonvisceral presacral fat pad (when present), the parietal sidewall fascia of the small pelvis, the hypogastric plexus, the vesicles, and the prostate in the male, and the vagina in the female. All of the dissection should be performed sharp with diathermy or scissors under direct vision with good light (Fig. 6). Throughout, the dedicated assistants should provide three-directional traction to open up the planes for the operator—diathermy can only be used safely when the areolar tissue is on stretch. Compared with traditional methods of manual extraction, the difference in time can be considerable. A careful TME plus pouch to anus reconstruction takes 3 to 5 hours according to the detail of the patient's build and the particular cancer; a conventional APE was often completed in 1 hour.

The Incision

A long midline incision is made from the symphysis pubis to within a few centimeters of the xiphisternum. If possible, at least 5 to 7 cm is best left at the top as this facilitates tidy packing away of the small intestine in the right upper quadrant.

Some young ladies may prefer a suprapubic skin crease incision combined with a vertical midline between the rectus muscles

Laparoscopic Anterior Resection

The author takes a major interest in this area of extending laparoscopic practice but continues to perform *open* surgery for rectal cancer as detailed below. The principles remain the same and there is no doubt that excellent clearance of relatively small cancers can be achieved laparoscopically. The author would suggest that only very experienced laparoscopic gastrointestinal surgeons

should embark upon the deep dissection for cancer and that special caution, if not total avoidance, is appropriate for very large cancers, especially in narrow male pelvises. The elevation of an intact mesorectal package, safely encompassing a large cancer, requires carefully applied but substantial *upward traction,* which is very difficult to achieve with laparoscopic instruments. At present the author would counsel great caution with tumors greater than 7 cm in any dimension, but most importantly in axial diameter. A further area of limitation is the cross clamping and washout of the anorectal muscle tube for which laparoscopic instrumentation remains imperfect.

Manual Palpation and Inspection—Laparotomy

This must be thorough, with particular emphasis on liver and peritoneum. Careful assessment of the para-aortic nodes in

the lesser sac is easy to forget. At this stage it is a good routine to review the CT and the colonoscopy report and to palpate the whole gastrointestinal tract carefully.

Packing

Careful packing and retraction of the intestines upward and to the right is crucial to provide clear access to the pelvis. Adhesions in the right lower quadrant commonly require division.

"Starting Right"—The Pedicle Package—The Clue to the Top of the "Holy Plane" (Fig. 7).

Starting correctly involves three-directional traction on the colon and retroperitoneum to identify the plane between the back of the pedicle package and the gonadal vessels, ureter, and preaortic sympathetic nerves—all of which must be carefully preserved. The key to this phase is the recognition of the shiny fascial-covered surface of the back of the pedicle—like a tapering longitudinal "sausage" with the inferior mesenteric vessels within, which must be gently lifted forward. It is usual in open surgery to start on the left of the sigmoid mesocolon. It is equally satisfactory, as commonly performed in laparoscopic surgery, to start on the right. In either case the identification of the shiny fascial envelope behind, what I like to call the "pedicle package," is crucial to proper entry into the pelvis.

High Ligation of the Inferior Mesenteric Vessels (Figs. 8 and 9)

With the pedicle package lifted gently forward the dissection behind it can be extended up to its proximal end; separate high ligations of the inferior mesenteric artery and vein can be performed with the

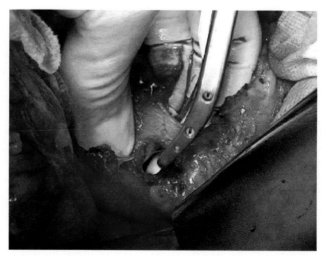

Fig. 8. High ligation of artery.

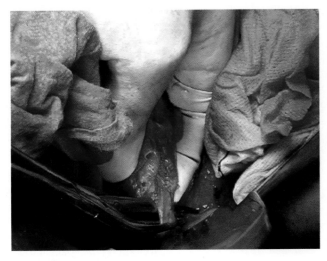

Fig. 9. High ligation of vein.

pedicle controlled by the left index finger. The artery is taken 1 to 2 cm anterior to the aorta so as to spare the sympathetic nerve plexuses; the vein is divided above its last tributary close to the pancreas. These two high ligations are an integral part of the otherwise avascular planes, which need to be developed upward extensively for a full mobilization of the splenic flexure.

The ascending left colic artery and either the accompanying inferior mesenteric vein or its last tributary from the left colon may also need to be divided separately to complete the vascular isolation of the specimen with full mobilization for ultra-low pouch anastomosis.

In a minority of cases a particularly long and healthy sigmoid may obviate the need for this full mobilization process, which is not entirely without risk (e.g., to the spleen itself). Thus, it is logical, if a decision is made to use such a long healthy sigmoid and thus avoid the splenic flexure, to ligate the inferior mesenteric artery just distal to the ascending left colic, which is essentially a part of its primary blood supply.

The "Division of Convenience" (Fig. 10)

The sigmoid mesentery and the sigmoid colon are divided well above the cancer. This is an important step in every cancer dissection as optimal mobility of the top of the specimen facilitates gentle opening of the perimesorectal planes by traction and countertraction in any direction throughout the pelvic dissection. After the division, there is also the best possible visualization of the pelvis with all of the gut to be retained drawn upward and to the right.

Commencing the Pelvic Dissection

The surgeon is now optimally placed to identify the key planes that must be developed circumferentially around the mesorectum. He or she starts at the back and then follows identifiable areas of the "holy plane" at various points on the mesorectal circumference in a stepwise manner. If bleeding in one area is troublesome, it is sensible to tackle the opposite circumference so that pressure is applied while progress continues.

High Posterior Dissection

Forward traction demonstrates the shiny posterior surface of mesorectum within the bifurcation of the superior hypogastric plexus. This plane is extended downward toward and eventually beyond the tip of the coccyx, step by step as other sectors of the circumference are developed.

Division of the Rectosacral Ligament or Fascia (Fig. 11)

This condensation may constitute an apparent barrier to downward progress posteriorly, requiring positive division with scissors or diathermy. Just in front of it, within the mesorectum, the superior rectal vessels can often be seen through the back of the mesorectal fascia, and around them cancerous nodes are likely to occur only millimeters away. This poses one of the greatest dangers of blunt manual extraction or of any haste or roughness, since the rectosacral ligament may be stronger than the surface fascia over the nodes. Thus, tearing into the lymphatic field by the inserted hand becomes a real risk. Sharp dissection under direct vision is crucial. A further safety factor in identifying positively the "holy plane" posteriorly in front of the presacral fat pad (when present) is that one avoids the risk of tearing thin-walled presacral veins. These will never become a problem if the correct plane is followed and tearing is avoided; if they should be torn, a small pack and a considerable period of anterior dissection will provide the safest way forward

Lateral Pelvic Dissection

This involves forward extension of the plane around to the sides, gently easing the adherent hypogastric nerves laterally off the mesorectal surface under direct vision. The freedom to lift the divided rectosigmoid forward often means that the tangentially running hypogastric nerves are first positively identified at this stage, the superior hypogastric plexus itself only becoming obvious proximal to the nerves after they have been dissected away from the mesorectal surface on each side.

These nerves are far more important than hitherto appreciated because they

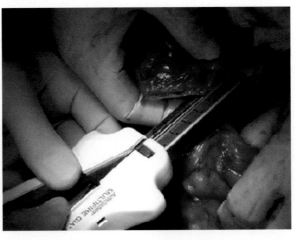

Fig. 10. Division of convenience.

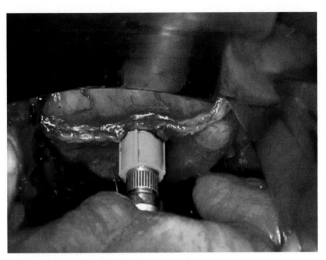

Fig. 22. Linear plus circular stapling.

staple line is thus eliminated and the second TA-45 or TA-30 is fired through the washed bowel while the anatomy is distorted by upward traction on the first (pathologist's) stapler. This process, in our view, justifies the cost of a second stapler because of the greater security against spillage of potentially malignant bowel contents. Only this washed staple line remains within the patient.

The first of these two linear staple lines should be safely clear of the palpable distal edge of the cancer. This is usually, though not absolutely invariably, the microscopic edge. Downward spread along the muscle tube is not a significant factor in recurrence—a 2-cm clearance is more than adequate and 1 cm plus the "donut" is acceptable.

The Colon Pouch (Fig. 23) or Coloplasty?

Several variations of pouch construction are available—typically a GIA-60 is inserted 5 cm from the end of the fully mobilized colon to create a J pouch. The anvil of the CEEA-31 staple anvil is inserted into the same colotomy, which is "purse stringed" around the shaft with 00 Surgipro. The body of the circular stapler, usually the CEEA-31, is inserted from below transanally. It is essential with ultra-low anastomoses to be certain that only the internal sphincter is purse stringed into the instrument. To this end it must be confirmed that only one thickness of muscle can be felt around the periphery of the cartridge. Adequate length from the splenic flexure mobilization is essential for the pouch to lie without tension in the hollow of the sacrum, and demonstrably pulsatile blood supply is the essence of success. Two low-suction Abdovac drains are used for 48 hours unless there is copious drainage when they may need to be left for longer.

The objective is to avoid hematoma in the hollow of the sacrum, which may become infected, form an abscess, and point into the bowel at or near the anastomosis—thus creating a "late leak" around 10 to 20 days later.

The "Building Blocks" of the Cancer Specimen
The Mesorectum (TME)
From the tapering pedicle at the top down the globular bilobed expansion at the bottom, this core specimen is the objective of cancer surgery for all middle and lower-third cancers.

"TME Plus"
Where directly involved by visible and palpable cancer spread, or indeed when adherence implies the possibility of such adherence to the adjacent mesorectal margin, it may be necessary to excise in continuity with the TME the following, in selected cases. In modern practice these extra building blocks can usually be predicted on MRI and appropriate plans made in advance.

TME PLUS—THE LEVATORS, ISCHIORECTAL FOSSA, AND PERIANAL SKIN

Abdominoperineal Excision

This is the equivalent of a conventional APE but with the extra care to perform the perimesorectal dissection that is inherent in TME—at least as far distally as the origin of the levator muscles from the obturator internus muscles. Exposed circumferential margins are, however, almost twice as common after conventional APE than after AR, which implies that the operation is often less well done. We believe that the conventional performance of APE, particularly involving synchronous combined excision by two surgeons, has often been less precise than a fastidious AR performed from above—largely because the planes cannot be readily defined. Optimal performance of an APE, especially when undertaken for a laterally spreading cancer, probably should incorporate a disc of levators and the surgeon should avoid the lowermost "holy plane" dissection (i.e., to avoid dissection in the lowest part of the plane where it is in contact with the levators). In this way a more cylindrical and wider clearance may be achieved and the commonly observed "waist" on the specimen avoided.

THE PRONE JACKKNIFE POSITION FOR THE PERINEAL DISSECTION

The views into the pelvis from below are considered by many surgeons to be superior

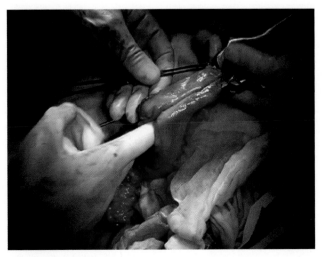

Fig. 23. Short 2 × 5 cm colon patch.

to those in the conventional steep Trendelenburg position. In particular, spectacular access is provided if the coccyx is excised with the cancer

STARTING THE OPERATION FROM BELOW

There are considerable advantages in commencing the operation from below with the patient in the prone jackknife position. This is particularly true if there are likely to be major problems with the abdominal surgery—as, for example, when performing APE for a local recurrence after AR. Commencing from below has the advantage that the patient does not need to be turned completely twice (i.e., at the end of the major procedure). The disadvantage is that the pneumoperitoneum necessary for a laparoscopic "top end" may not be achievable. Starting at the perineal end, however, is in the author's view a crucial advantage if APE is being performed for low local recurrence as it provides optimal tissue planes for the dissection around the cancer.

THE POSTERIOR VAGINAL WALL (FIG. 24)

Bimanual examination via the rectum and the vagina in the anesthetized patient is essential. If there is free mobility of the cancer on the posterior vaginal wall, then it need *not* be excised. If tethered over a small area, a disc of vagina may be taken with the tumor, or in a case that requires APE, because of proximity to the sphincters, the whole or most of the posterior wall from the perianal skin upward may

need to be removed. We now only perform this once standard procedure when there appears no alternative due to the anterior extension of the cancer, as ultimate vaginal function may be much impaired. When it does have to be excised, it is not essential for the vagina to be resutured though the long-term function must be in some doubt.

OTHER ORGANS OCCASIONALLY REQUIRING EN BLOC REMOVAL ON ACCOUNT OF DIRECT INVASION

Seminal Vesicles

These can sometimes provide an extra anterior safety margin, and the most anterior "layer" of vesicles sometimes has a dissectible, though vascular, plane between it and the adherent or invaded posterior vesicles.

One or Both Ureters

Ileum
The Folded-over Sigmoid
With advanced sigmoid cancer when the colon is folded down and invading the anterior aspect of the upper rectum, an extensive en bloc resection of both may be required. A large tumor mass blocking the upper true pelvis is a formidable undertaking for which ureteric stenting is a wise precaution. Neoadjuvant chemoradiotherapy may be considered

One or Both Hypogastric Plexuses
Parts of the neural lamella may have to be removed.

Other Pelvic Sidewall Structures
Appendix
Uterus, ovaries, and adnexal structures
Bladder

Block dissection of an internal iliac compartment is possible, but has not been part of our routine. When there are obvious extramesorectal lymph nodes, we will usually excise these as cleanly as possible, preferably without damaging the autonomic nerves.

THE BASINGSTOKE EXPERIENCE OF TOTAL MESORECTAL EXCISION 1978–1997

In 1998 we published data on 519 consecutive surgical patients with adenocarcinoma of the rectum receiving surgical treatment for cure or palliation under the direct supervision of or performed by one surgeon. These may be important data as follow-up approached 20 years and use of radiotherapy and chemoradiotherapy had been so minimal and recent that they can be regarded as "virtually pure" surgical results. Cancer-specific survival of all surgically treated patients, including those with metastases on presentation, was 68% at 5 years and 66% at 10 years. The local recurrence rate was 6% (95% confidence interval, 2% to 10%) at 5 years and 8% (95% confidence interval, 2% to 14%) at 10 years. In 405 "curative" resections (no obvious residual disease), the local recurrence rate was 3% (95% confidence interval, 0% to 5%) at 5 years and 4% (95% confidence interval, 0% to 8%) at 10 years. Disease-free survival in this group was 80% at 5 years and 78% at 10 years. An analysis of histopathologic risk factors for recurrence indicated only the Dukes stage, extramural vascular invasion, and tumor differentiation as variables in these results.

CONCLUSION

Rectal cancer surgery is probably the most rewarding of all the challenges to the aspiring gastrointestinal surgeon. Arguably there is no cancer operation where proper decisions, the judicious selective use of adjuvant therapy, and, most of all, surgical skill of the highest order can bring so much benefit to the patient. Cancer cure, normality of bowel function, avoidance of a lifelong stoma, sexual function—all of these hang in the balance for the patient. The profession still has a long way to go in using its resolves to deliver what is possible and affordable to each person who hopes for an optimal outcome.

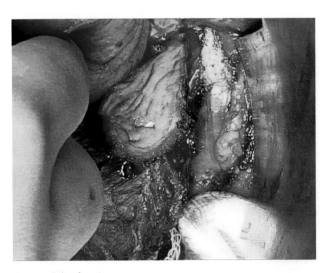

Fig. 24. Sometimes a disk of vagina.

REFERENCES

Adam IJ, Mohamdee MO, Martin IG, et al. Role of circumferential margin involvement in the local recurrence of rectal cancer. *Lancet* 1994;344:707.

Birbeck K, Macklin C, Tiffen N, et al. Rates of circumferential resection margin involvement vary between surgeons and predict outcomes in rectal cancer surgery. *Ann Surg* 2002;2354:449.

Dukes CE. The classification of cancer of the rectum. *J Pathol Bacteriol* 1932;35:323.

Heald RJ. The 'holy plane' of rectal cancer. *J Royal Soc Med* 1988;81:503.

Heald RJ, Moran BJ, Ryall RDH, et al. The Basingstoke experience of total mesorectal excision 1978-1997. *Arch Surg* 1998;133:894.

Hermanek P, Wiebelt H, Staimmer D, et al. The German Study Group Colorectal Carcinoma (SGCRC). Prognostic factors of rectal carcinoma—experience of the German Multicentre Study. *Tumori* 1995;81:60.

Jass JR, Atkin WS, Cuzick J, et al. The grading of rectal cancer: histological perspectives and multivariate analysis of 447 cases. *Histopathology* 1986;10:437.

Karanjia ND, Schache DJ, North WR, et al. 'Close shave' in anterior resection. *Br J Surg* 1990;77(5):510.

MacFarlane JK, Ryall RD, Heald RJ. Mesorectal excision for rectal cancer. *Lancet* 1993; 341(8843):457.

Miles WE. A method of performing abdomino-perineal excision for carcinoma of the rectum and terminal portion of the pelvic colon. *Lancet* 1908;35:320.

Moran MR, James EC, Rothenberger DA, et al. Prognostic value of positive lymph nodes in rectal cancer. *Dis Colon Rectum* 1992;35(6):579.

Moriya Y. The 'onion rings' of rectal fascia. In: Heald R, ed. 2002.

Quirke P, Durdey P, Dixon MF, et al. Local recurrence of rectal adenocarcinoma due to inadequate surgical resection. Histopathological study of lateral tumour spread and surgical excision. *Lancet* 1986;2(8514):996.

Quirke P, Scott N. The pathologist's role in the assessment of local recurrence in rectal carcinoma. *Surg Oncol Clin North Am* 1992;1:1.

Silen W. Mesorectal excision for rectal cancer. *Lancet* 1993;341.

Wolmark N, Wieand HS, Rockette HE, et al. The prognostic significance of tumor location and bowel obstruction in Dukes B and C colorectal cancer. Findings from the NSABP clinical trials. *Ann Surg* 1983;198(6):743.

EDITOR'S COMMENT

This is a wonderful chapter, combining as it does the various alternatives in high, middle, and low rectal cancer. We are privileged to have Professor Heald, who is the originator of the concept of total mesenteric excision, write it. It is rare that as significant an advance in surgery has such a clear attribution, but in this case, it does, and it has changed the nature of the way rectal cancer is cared for. As with all great contributions, it is based, to a considerable extent, on a thorough knowledge of the embryology and the development, the blood supply, the nodal drainage, and, most of all, the anatomy of the rectum in its various portions. This leads to an anatomic approach to carcinoma of the rectum. Unfortunately, anatomy has been downgraded in most medical schools in favor of cell biology, and I'm certain that there are few medical schools in which the anatomy of the rectum, its blood supply, and lymph node drainage even receive scarce coverage. This is something that we must incorporate in our surgical residencies and other training programs in order to derive the most benefit for our patients.

The introduction is delightful, and it is philosophical in its base. It is, to my way of thinking, one of the essences of surgery, and why surgery remains attractive as a career. The philosophy is something with which I think no one can argue, especially regarding the nature of the *craft* of surgery. No one talks about craft anymore. The competencies, which I introduced to the American Board of Surgery when I was vice chair, have been altered beyond belief so that the initial attempt to get the Board to declare that one is not certified, but competent, has been completely lost. This is not surprising in view of the fact that the individuals who worked it out hadn't seen a patient, and wouldn't recognize a patient if they tripped over one, for 30 years. So instead of a simple statement that someone's competent to take care of a patient, what we have is a mélange of education speak, in which some, such as "systems-based learning," remain completely undecipherable, even several years after the hallowed six competencies have been put into place. In our program, we add two additional competencies, which was my original intent: (7) Can a resident actually do the operation? and, (8) Can a resident actually conceive of the operation before the operation begins? That, to a surgeon, is the essence of competency, and that is what Professor Heald has put forth.

The Miles operation was quite simple. There was a large cylinder, which contained a tumor, and one must sacrifice normal function in order to achieve a cure. What one was faced with previously was urologic and sexual dysfunction versus survival. It was probably not as simple as that, but the question asked of the patient—Would you rather be potent and dead, or impotent and alive?—could not be simpler. The delineation of total mesenteric excision as well as what must remain encompasses the concept that taking out a rectum—whether it is to do a low anterior anastomosis or complete the abdominal perineal resection, sparing the nerves that are involved with potency, ejaculation, and urologic function—is much easier, now that it has been explained to us that one can achieve all of these goals if one knows the anatomy; is familiar with the territory; and, under sharp, not blunt, dissection, excises the draining lymph nodes of carcinoma of the rectum at various levels.

In order to do this, and in order to understand what one is confronted with, the critical nature of the MRI, and three-dimensional reconstruction when possible, is all-important. In institutions such as ours where it is possible to have a postanesthesia care (PAC) system in every operating room, which we do, surgeons are enabled to re-examine the MRI while the case is going on. In addition, one of the pearls in this chapter, and there are many, is that the mobility of the rectum, and of the tumor, in the conscious patient in whom there is muscle tone generally indicates that total mesenteric excision is achievable. There is meticulous description of craftsmanship and a description of the nerves, where they can be found, how they can be exposed, and the pitfalls thereof. The lateral stalks are a particularly illuminating anatomic discussion.

Does all of this make any difference? The answer is a resounding yes. The Basingstoke experiences detailed in this chapter illustrate an important milestone in what can be achieved, even with disease that is considered somewhat advanced, and is excellent because of the knowledge of the anatomy, physiology, nodal drainage, and blood supply, as well as the technical precision of not violating the rectal mesentery, which TME brings with it. Other surgeons have been able to duplicate these results, which is significantly indicative that craftsmanship is not completely absent. A very persuasive paper by Piso et al. (*J Surg Oncol* 2004;86:115) comes from a series of departments, including Hannover Medical School in Germany, Royal

Prince Alfred Hospital in Sydney, University of Regensburg Department of Surgery in Germany, and the Department for General and Visceral Surgery at the Clinic of Oldenburg in Germany. They reported 337 patients, largely performed at Hannover by individuals obviously trained by Professor Piso. Of these patients, 212 had lower rectal carcinomas and 125 had middle rectal carcinomas. The rate of resections completed with TME was 96%. Of these patients, 223 were treated by anterior rectal resection and 92 underwent abdominal perineal resections. A few others, 10 in all, were treated by a Hartmann resection. Postoperative morbidity was 35%, a leakage of anastomoses in 9%, and mortality was a respectable 4%. The rate of local recurrence was 86%, but more importantly, the 5-year survival rate after curative resection was 69.3%, thus indicating that the superb results, even with advanced disease, were achievable in other settings. Papers from Italy, including that from La Sapienza, which is a little more difficult to understand with the principal surgeon being Di Matteo (Di Matteo et al. *Panminerva Med* 2000;42[3]:201), have discussed the local recurrence issues. Professor Di Matteo published a personal series done between January 1985 and December 1997, with a variety of techniques, including nerve-sparing technique (NST), with a curative (R0) TME including 47 patients and TME plus lateral pelvic lymphadenectomy and NST in 7, sacrificing the pelvic autonomic nervous system only in case of neoplastic infiltration. The local recurrence rate was 8.5% and 0%, respectively, at mean follow-up of approximately 4 years. Reresection was not possible, and the survival of the recurred group was 50% at 14 months. In contrast, in another group treated between January 1985 and December 1988 with partial mesorectal excision, again an R0 extirpation, the incidence of local relapse was 22% (9 of 41 cases). Thus, the authors concluded, and I agree that the number of relapses can be minimized by total mesorectal excision, if the holy plane is not violated.

However, this comes with a price. Daniels et al. (*World J Surg Oncol* 2006;4:6) reviewed by questionnaire 18 women (of 23 sent) with a mean age of 65.5 years (range 34 to 86) at follow-up of 18.8 months (range 3 to 35). Preoperatively, 28% (5 of 18) were sexually active. Seventeen percent (3 of 18) described urinary symptomatology, and stress incontinence was reported by 39% (7 of 18) *prior to*

(continued)

surgery. Postoperatively, all previously sexually active patients remained active, although dyspareunia with penetration was described by some. Two of the sexually active patients described decreased libido, which they blamed on the stoma—not unreasonable. However, postoperative urinary symptoms developed in 59%, who reported new development of nocturia, and 18% developed stress incontinence, with one patient requiring a permanent catheter. Of those with symptoms, 80% persisted longer than 3 months. The symptoms were predominant in those with low rectal cancers, particularly those undergoing abdominal perineal resection, which is not sur-

prising. How to deal with the perineal wound in its closure and not get a septic complication is still an issue being discussed. For example, Meyer et al. (*Technol Coloproctol* 2004;8:S230) described a method of closing the wound that is not unfamiliar, including muscle ischiorectal closure and subcutaneous fat, with local administration of carriers releasing antibiotics and closed suction drainage. Using this approach, the rate of septic perineal wound complications fell from 18% to 5% in a multicenter trial.

Finally, the occasional patient with anorectal melanoma was discussed by Weyandt et al. (*Br J Cancer* 2003;89:2019), who reviewed 19 patients with

melanoma of different sizes and different depths. They concluded that wide local incision was not appropriate for anything beyond 4 mm in thickness, and they required total mesenteric excision and abdominal perineal resection, up to and including, for the most part, the Miles operation as described in this chapter. In those patients, local recurrence was lower after abdominal perineal resection, even for patients with less favorable tumor, as compared with wide local excision alone. They concluded that wide local excision has no place in the management of anorectal melanomas thicker than 4 mm.

J.E.F.

Chapter 140A, see www.masteryofsurgery.com

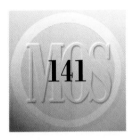

141

Anterior and Low Anterior Resection of the Rectum

WARREN E. ENKER, ANTONIO I. PICON, AND JOSEPH MARTZ

INTRODUCTION

Anterior resection of the rectum is defined as the removal of the proximal portion of the rectum (e.g., the upper third) with reanastomosis of the colon to the peritonealized portion of the rectum, and low anterior resection implies reanastomosis to the extraperitonealized portion of the rectum. Which operation is performed largely depends upon the height of the lesion (i.e., the distance from the anal verge), but the location of the peritoneal reflection may vary considerably, especially in women, making the definition quite subjective. Both procedures are performed transabdominally, share the same techniques and concepts, and involve the anastomosis of the sigmoid or descending colon to the rectum to preserve intestinal continuity. In both cases, mobilization of the splenic flexure and the descending colon may be required. In patients with rectal adenocarcinomas, total mesorectal excision (TME) must be performed to achieve adequate oncologic results. The sine qua none of TME, an adequate resection for rectal cancer, is the complete mobilization of the rectum. We will review these procedures in stepwise fashion.

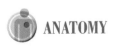

ANATOMY

The splenic flexure is defined by the junction of the transverse colon and descending colon, usually ending in an acute angle, and often, the distal end of the transverse colon

overlaps the first portion of the descending colon. The splenic flexure is attached to the stomach via the gastrocolic ligament, to the diaphragm by the phrenocolic ligaments, and to the spleen by the splenocolic ligament. Retroperitoneally, it is adherent to the Gerota fascia. The descending colon begins at the splenic flexure and ends at the inlet of the false pelvis. Peritoneum covers all but its retroperitoneal or posterior surface. Structures behind the descending colon are subcostal vessels and nerve; iliohypogastric and ilioinguinal nerves; the lumbar arteries; the lateral femoral cutaneous, femoral, and genitofemoral nerves; the gonadal vessels; and the external iliac vessels. The left kidney and the ureter are an important part of this anatomic backdrop.

The sigmoid colon occupies the false pelvis and is more of an intraperitoneal organ. It forms a variable loop that may be as long as 30 to 40 cm and that can reach the right lower quadrant. This loop of sigmoid returns to the midline of the pelvis anywhere between S-1 and S-4, and at this point the sigmoid colon blends with the rectum. The sigmoid mesocolon, planar in its orientation, diminishes its length and becomes cylindrical as it approaches the rectum, where it disappears.

The relationship of the sigmoid to surrounding structures will depend on many variables including length; mobility of the mesocolon; degree of distension; condition of the rectum, bladder, uterus, and ovaries; and gender or racial variation. A practical landmark that identifies the transition from the colon to the rectum is

where the three separate teniae coli become confluent with the rectum.

The rectum is a pelvic organ situated along the sacrococcygeal concavity, following the curvature of the sacral hollow, and making a 90-degree angle at the upper end of the anal canal. The anorectum is about 16 cm long. The first 2.5 to 4 cm from the anal verge comprise the anal canal and the next three sections make up the lower, middle, and upper thirds of the rectum. The American College of Surgeons includes all lesions between 0 and 15 cm in the classification of rectal cancer; however, most cooperative groups (e.g., the Gastro-Intestinal Tumor Study Group, (GITSG), ECOG, and RTOG) employ a definition of 0 to 12 cm based on the patterns of recurrence of pelvic cancers above and below 11 to 12 cm as described by Pilipshen et al. The rectosigmoid junction can be estimated at approximately 12 to 18 cm from the anal verge, but it may vary between individuals. The upper third to half of the rectum may be covered by peritoneum, mostly on its anterior and lateral aspects, and lower down only the anterior aspect is covered by peritoneum, from which it is reflected onto the anterior pelvic structures. The level of the peritoneal reflexion is about 7 to 8 cm from the anus in males, and is generally lower in female patients at about 6 to 7 cm from the anus. During dissection of the rectum, knowledge of the fascial planes becomes important, especially in the resection of rectal neoplasm (Fig. 1).

The endopelvic fascia at the level of the sacral promontory divides into two

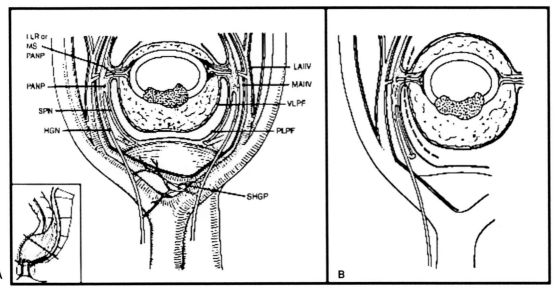

Fig. 1. Anatomy of the pelvis. **A:** A transverse coronal cross-section through the pelvis at the level of the midrectum. Emphasis is given to the fascial layers of the pelvis surrounding the posterior visceral compartment of the true pelvis. These layers define the surgical planes of dissection: VLPF and PLPF, visceral and parietal layers of the pelvic fascia; LAIIV and MAIIV, lateral and medial adventitia of internal iliac vessels; LLR, lateral ligament of the rectum, and MSPANP, medial segment of the pelvic autonomic nerve plexus (PANP), according to Sato K et al.; SPN, sacral parasympathetic nerve; HGN, hypogastric nerve; and SHGP, superior hypogastric plexus. **B:** Sharp dissection under direct vision is to be performed between the VLPF and the parietal layers of the pelvic fascia (PLPF) along the dotted line, medial to the autonomic nerves and plexuses.

thin, transparent but histologically distinct layers. The visceral layer of the endopelvic fascia (VLPF) envelopes the rectum, but it is most prominently developed along its posterior aspect. The parietal layer of the endopelvic fascia (PLPF) is known as the presacral fascia in the midline, but it invests or envelopes the autonomic nerves, the vessels, and the musculoskeletal structures of the pelvic sidewalls. It is the sharp dissection between these layers that maintains the integrity of the mesorectum. Posterolaterally and distal to S-4, the VLPF and the PLPF extend together and fuse with the attenuated mesorectum for the remaining few centimeters above the levator ani. This fusion of the VLFP and the PLPF constitutes Waldeyer fascia.

Laterally, and mostly peripheral to the PLFP, the mesorectum is surrounded by the hypogastric (sympathetic) and the sacral parasympathetic nerves and pelvic autonomic nerve plexuses and the internal iliac blood vessels medial to the pelvic sidewalls. The so-called "lateral ligaments" are simply bilateral neurovascular structures carrying the autonomic nerves and middle hemorrhoidal vessels to the rectum. Anteriorly, the rectum distal to the peritoneal reflection is bound by the rectovesical fascia, also known as Denonvilliers fascia. It separates the rectum from the seminal vesicles and prostate in males and from the vagina in females.

Much of the blood supply of the distal third of the transverse and descending colon derives from the left branch of the middle colic artery, with some contribution as well from the left colic artery. The sigmoid colon and upper part of the rectum derive most of their blood supply from the inferior mesenteric artery (IMA). The IMA may be ligated at its origin or beyond the takeoff of the left colic artery during anterior resection. When the IMA is divided, the blood supply of the descending colon is maintained through the left branch of the middle colic artery and the marginal artery of Drummond. In a small group of patients the marginal artery of Drummond is discontinuous at the level of the splenic flexure, the watershed area. Although it is rarely needed, the left colic artery may be preserved, ensuring blood supply to the descending colon.

After resection of the upper rectum, circulation to the mid- and lower rectum is maintained through the middle rectal and inferior rectal arteries. This systemic blood supply results in an important difference between rectal and colon cancer patterns of spread; in rectal cancers, 50% of distant spread takes place to the lungs instead of to the liver due to the direct exposure of the rectum to the systemic or internal iliac circulation.

Autonomic Nerves and Nerve Pathways

The sympathetic innervation of the hindgut comes from the thoracolumbar part of the trunk. The superior hypogastric plexus diverges around either side of the inferior mesenteric artery and continues retroperitoneally, anterior to the abdominal aorta. The parasympathetic supply comes from the pelvic splanchnic nerves (nervi erigentes) from which rami pass from the sacral foramina anterior and laterally to the inferior hypogastric plexus (also known as the pelvic autonomic nerve plexus [PANP]) to supply the other pelvic viscera. Some fibers may ascend to the superior hypogastric plexus to supply the transverse, descending, and sigmoid colon, following the route of the named blood supply. Sympathetic nerves to the rectum and upper anal canal come partly via the superior and inferior hypogastric plexuses and along the inferior mesenteric and superior rectal arteries. Lubrication and emission and part of the ejaculatory functions are dependent on sympathetic input from the hypogastric nerves. Parasympathetic nerves come from the pelvic splanchnic nerves (S-2, S-3, and S-4) and pass forward as long strands from the sacral nerves and join the inferior hypogastric plexus (PANP) that interfaces with the hypogastric nerves along the lateral aspect of the rectum, forming the lateral segment of the lateral ligaments. Erectile function depends on the preservation of intact parasympathetic pelvic plexuses and nerves.

At the confluence of the inferior mesenteric and superior rectal arteries and overlying the aortic bifurcation, the superior hypogastric plexus may be recognized and the hypogastric nerves may be identified as distinct structures coursing anterolaterally toward the inferior hypogastric plexus. The midline hypogastric nerves divide in the retrorectal space just below the bifurcation of the iliac arteries, into somewhat of a "horseshoe" pattern (Fig. 2). Along the pelvic sidewalls, each hypogastric nerve becomes enmeshed with the pelvic plexus helping to form its distal branches. These run anterolaterally from the pelvic sidewalls to the prostate, seminal vesicles, vagina, bladder, and urethra. The surgeon's knowledge of this pelvic neuroanatomy is essential if one is to avoid injury to the autonomic nerves and plexuses as one performs a TME with autonomic nerve preservation (ANP). Low anterior resection is a cancer operation, first and foremost. As such, these autonomic structures should be sacrificed if the lateral extension of a tumor presents a problem of obtaining uninvolved (R0) circumferential margins, a definition of an oncologically adequate result. Even under the best of circumstances, occasional injury to these nerves will take place despite the best of precautions.

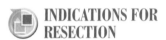

INDICATIONS FOR RESECTION

Patients with benign or malignant disease of the distal sigmoid and proximal rectum may require an anterior resection. Pathology involving the middle and even the lower third of the rectum may require a low anterior resection.

Benign Diseases

The most common benign pathology that requires anterior resection is diverticular disease of the sigmoid colon. It is important that the distal resection margin is below the confluence of the teniae coli, avoiding anastomotic complications and the risk of recurrence. Often, this is below the peritoneal reflection where the bowel wall is free of diverticula. The proximal resection margin will vary between the splenic flexure and the junction of the descending sigmoid colon, depending on the extent of the disease. In addition, the blood supply of the healthy bowel wall must

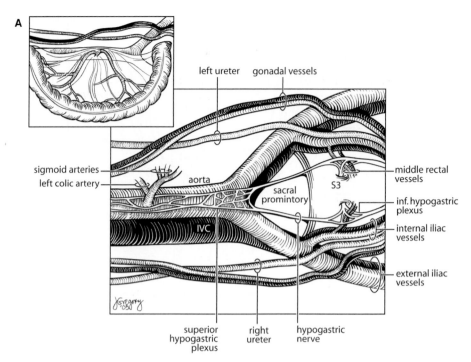

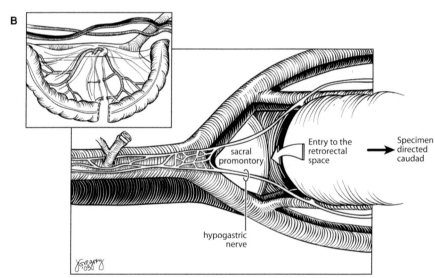

Fig. 2. Pelvic anatomy. **A:** Mobilization of the descending and sigmoid colon. The colon is reflected into the midline with detailed anatomy of retroperitoneal and pelvic structures. **B:** Once the sigmoid colon and mesenteric vessels are divided, the sigmoid colon and the upper part of the rectum are retracted upward and caudad, revealing the presacral space between the mesorectum and the presacral fascia. The hypogastric nerves are intimately located posterolaterally to either side.

appear to be unaffected by the prior episodes of inflammation and the resulting scarring, avoiding the complications of anastomotic leak or of late stricture formation.

In the case of rectal prolapse, one of the abdominal procedures associated with low recurrence rate is anterior resection with or without rectopexy. Whether open or laparoscopically, the rectum is mobilized by dissecting posteriorly down to the pelvic floor with minimal lateral mobilization.

The sigmoid and upper rectum is resected and fixation of the rectum occurs by the perianastomotic fibrosis or by suturing the posterolateral aspect of the mesorectum, fixing it to the sacral promontory or below.

In the case of polyps of sigmoid colon or upper rectum that cannot be removed endoscopically, or if the polyp is endoscopically excised but contains an invasive cancer, resection is indicated. Given the risks of local recurrence or of lymph node involvement, resection of the segment of colon and its mesentery should be performed, applying the same techniques used to treat proven invasive malignant disease (vide infra). Other indications include the presence of other pelvic malignancies (e.g., ovarian cancer) invading the rectum or rectosigmoid that requires en bloc resection to obtain adequate oncologic results.

Malignant Diseases (Resectable)

Adenocarcinoma is the most common malignant lesion of the distal colon and rectum that requires anterior or low anterior resection. Among many issues, the most important factor influencing the selection of patients for anterior or low anterior resection is the location of the tumor, generally designated as the distance of the lowest edge of the tumor from the anal verge. Tumors located in the upper third of the rectum are managed by anterior resection. Tumors in the lower two thirds of the rectum can be more difficult to manage and require a low anterior or an abdominoperineal resection depending on the location of the tumor in relation to the anorectal ring and the anal verge. Tumors infiltrating the sphincter complex posterolaterally as well as the sphincter muscles and prostate gland anteriorly will require abdominoperineal resection for adequate oncologic results. Locally advanced tumors (i.e., extremely large, bulky, and/or tethered tumors and those at risk of adjacent organ invasion or those with obvious mesorectal lymph node involvement on imaging) are better treated preoperatively with neoadjuvant chemoradiation therapy. Part of the treatment goal is that patients should be candidates for restorative resection. Tumor fixation to adjacent pelvic structures should not necessarily contraindicate the operation as long as an en bloc resection can be performed with uninvolved (i.e., tumor-free) circumferential margins of resection. In a very selected group of patients (T1, <3 cm, well to moderately differentiated tumors without lymphovascular invasion, involving <25% of the circumference), transanal excision may be indicated with the caveat of 17% to 35% local recurrence rates in T1 and T2 disease.

In male patients, particularly those with a very narrow pelvis, an enlarged prostate, or both, all technical aspects of the operation, from dissection to anastomosis, will prove much more difficult. Under these circumstances, the principles of traction and countertraction, sharp dissection, exposure, direct visualization, and good lighting may be severely put to the test. After describing the technique of the operation, various reconstructive methods will be considered.

Patient-related contraindications to the procedure are extremely rare. They include individuals who are too medically incapacitated to tolerate the procedure and those with pre-existing severe fecal incontinence. Advanced age is not a contraindication per se, although comorbidities should be taken into account in assessing risk. Disease-related contraindications include advanced locoregional disease (i.e., pelvic peritoneal implants) and the likelihood of an R1 to R2 resection. Distant metastatic disease is only a relative contraindication to low anterior resection depending on the extent of the distant tumor burden. If the patient has a predictable longevity, the procedure may be performed for palliation or for local control of the primary tumor. This group of patients often benefits from an initial trial of systemic treatment. Patients presenting with an obstructing sigmoid lesion may undergo diverting colostomy or, preferably, the placement of a stent as a "bridge" to resection. Alternatively, these patients may need to undergo a Hartmann resection. Colonic stents are rarely tolerated in the rectum.

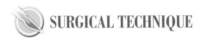

SURGICAL TECHNIQUE

Positioning and Preparation

Prior to an anterior or low anterior resection, consent should be obtained for a possible permanent end left-sided colostomy or a temporary diverting right-sided colostomy or ileostomy. The location for either of these stomas is marked by the surgeon while the patient is sitting in an upright position just prior to the operation. Once in the operating room and under general anesthesia, the patient is positioned in the extended Trendelenburg-lithotomy position, on Allen hydraulic stirrups. The legs are separated adequately to allow access to the anorectum either to introduce a stapling device or to perform an abdominoperineal resection, if needed. There should be appropriate padding to the sacrum and the peroneal nerves, and sequential compression stockings are placed on both legs. A Foley catheter is inserted sterilely. The arms are generally at right angles to the body to avoid hyperextension and brachial plexus palsy. The rectum is irrigated with up to a liter of saline using a mild solution mixed with alcohol (about a 1:5 solution) or povidone-iodine until the effluent is clear.

Abdominal Exploration and the Dissection

An infraumbilical abdominal midline incision is made and can be extended above the umbilicus depending on the needs for access to the splenic flexure and to the rest of the abdomen. The peritoneal-abdominal cavity is entered and explored, searching for liver metastases, peritoneal implants, and mesenteric or extramesenteric (e.g., retroperitoneal lymphadenopathy) and locoregional or adjacent organ spread. Any lesions that are suspicious for metastases are biopsied at this point. A Thompson self-retaining retractor system (Thompson Surgical Instruments, Traverse City, MI) and a plastic wound protector are routinely employed. The small bowel is packed away into the upper abdomen under moist laparotomy pads, and the pack is held in place using either a large blade from the self-retaining retractor or a wide ribbon retractor. With lateral and caudad body wall retraction, the entire true pelvis is under direct vision.

The surgeon, if right-handed, stands on the left side of the patient, the first assistant on the right side and the second assistant between the legs. At all steps, the surgeon and the first assistant create a balance of traction and countertraction guiding the dissection. Good lighting is essential. The sigmoid is retracted medially, and the mobilization of the colon is started by the surgeon using either scissors or the electrocautery, freeing the sigmoid and the left colon by the dividing along the paracolic attachments and/or adhesions between the colon and the abdominal wall (i.e., the line of Toldt). In the pelvis, the peritoneum is incised lateral to the visible mesorectal fat. This will expose the retroperitoneum, and care must be taken to dissect the plane between the mesenteric fat and the retroperitoneal fat. A minimal number of small vessels encountered during this dissection may be coagulated directly by grasping each vessel with forceps and applying diathermy. The extent of mobilization will depend on the length of the colon required to achieve both a radical mesenteric resection and a tension-free anastomosis.

Mobilization of the Splenic Flexure

Mobilization of the splenic flexure may involve several components. In an open operation, access may require that the upper pole of the abdominal incision be extended. In a "hybrid operation," this step may be performed laparoscopically. The

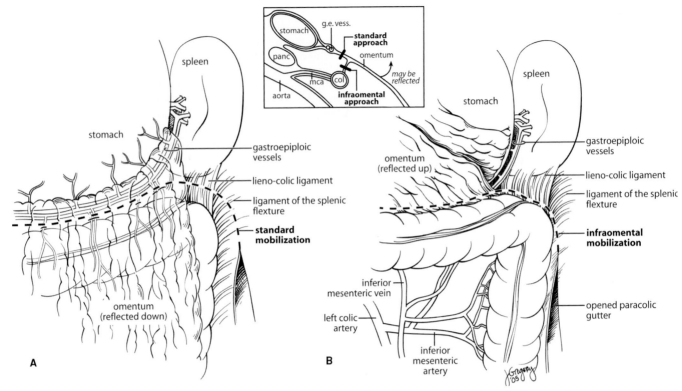

Fig. 3. Dissection of the splenic flexure. Mobilization of the splenic flexure may be performed using several anatomical pathways. **A:** The standard mobilization of the splenic flexure achieved by dividing each of the splenic flexure ligaments. **B:** The infraomental mobilization of the splenic flexure, immediately adjacent to the colonic wall. The latter is our preferred method, in most cases.

splenic flexure may be mobilized using several anatomic pathways. We prefer the "infraomental" mobilization that follows the embryologic plane of the splenic flexure (immediately adjacent to the colonic wall), as opposed to having to divide each of the formally named splenic flexure ligaments (Fig. 3). In the event that tension remains a factor (e.g., when performing a low anterior resection with a coloanal anastomosis), the inferior mesenteric vein may have to be divided just below the pancreas to obtain adequate length. The criterion that indicates a tension-free anastomosis is the complete sacralization of the colonic segment as it descends into the pelvis.

Dissection of this plane allows identification of the gonadal vessels and left ureter that are identified as the colon and its mesentery are drawn into the midline (Fig. 2). Dissection is carried out medially toward the base of the sigmoid mesocolon until the hypogastric nerves are identified. Next, the sigmoid mesentery is retracted toward the left side, and the peritoneum on the right side at the base of the sigmoid mesocolon is incised, taking care not to damage the hypogastric nerves, the left and right ureters, and the right iliac vessels. The division of the peritoneum

continues from the right common iliac artery along the anterior aspect of the distal aorta until the inferior mesenteric artery is encountered (Fig. 2A). At this point the artery is cleaned, double ligated, and divided above or below the takeoff of the left colic artery. The inferior mesenteric vein is identified, ligated, and divided most often at this same level, but as previously indicated, in a difficult mobilization, it may be divided as high up as the inferior border of the tail of the pancreas.

The mesentery of the sigmoid colon is divided up to the wall of the colon at the level of the desired division. The colon is divided using a linear cutter stapler; the distal end is grasped with a straight Kocher clamp and used as a handle for the specimen. The descending colon is packed into the left upper quadrant behind one of the retractor blades.

The specimens (i.e., the sigmoid colon and the upper part of the rectum) are retracted upward and caudad (toward the feet), and this maneuver reveals the presacral space between the mesorectum anteriorly and the presacral fascia with the hypogastric nerves lying posterolaterally to either side (Fig. 2B). The correct plane of dissection is between the visceral layer of

the pelvic fascia, or the fascia propria of the mesorectum, and the presacral fascia, or the parietal layer of the pelvic fascia (Fig. 1). This areolar plane is developed with upward and caudad traction of the specimen, and with the dissecting scissors or the electrocautery, this plane will ultimately be developed along the concave shape of the sacrum down to the coccyx (Fig. 4A). The hypogastric nerves may actually enter the visceral fascia briefly, requiring careful dissection to avoid injuring these nerves early on in their dissection, before they continue anterolaterally on to the inferior hypogastric plexus along the lower lateral wall of the pelvis. When the posterior midline dissection has been accomplished to the point that retraction and visibility are no longer optimal, midline or posterolateral dissection to the right or to the left side of the rectum is carried out, making effective use of a St. Marks retractor.

The rectosacral fascia that is located in the midline and is thicker than the areolar tissue is encountered at about the level of S-3 and S-4 and is divided with either the electrocautery or with long scissors while maintaining anterior retraction on the rectum (Fig. 4B). One must appreciate the sacral curvature at this point to stay in the

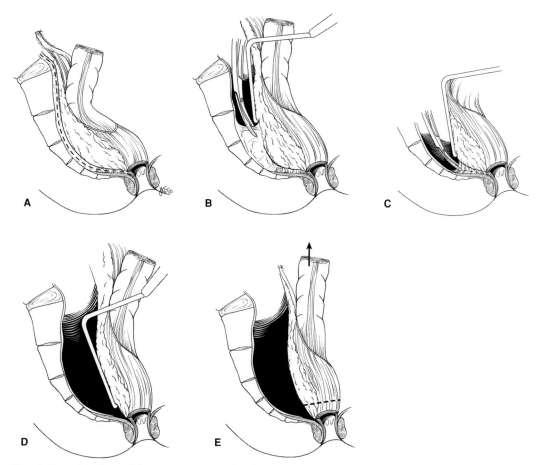

Fig. 4. Posterior plane of dissection. Sequential mobilization of the rectum by sharp dissection of the posterior plane between the visceral layer and parietal layers of the pelvic fascia. **A:** Plane of the posterior dissection between the visceral and parietal layers of the pelvic fasciae. **B:** Sharp division of the rectosacral fascia. **C:** Division of the Waldeyer fascia, completing the posterior dissection to the anal hiatus. **D:** Complete mobilization of the rectum down to the levators. **E:** A typical level of distal level of transection.

correct plane of dissection, in order to avoid entering the presacral fascia with serious bleeding consequences. In general, the first phase of the posterior dissection ends at this level to avoid suboptimal exposure, blunt dissection, or dissection "in a hole."

Attention is now turned to the anterior dissection. In female patients, the uterus and fallopian tube are retracted upward and forward with a heavy stitch from the fundus of the uterus to the anterior abdominal wall or to the lower bar of the Thompson retractor. The anterior peritoneum is then incised at the level of the "cul-de-sac" either above or at the level of the rectouterine or rectovesical pouch (Fig. 5A). The St. Marks retractor is placed in the space drawing the vagina or the prostate anteriorly, and the surgeon's nondominant hand retracts the rectum downward and backward. In female patients the rectovaginal plane is developed between the anterior mesorectum and the posterior wall of the vagina, while in male patients Denonvilliers fascia is left attached to the anterior

rectal wall, as the anterior boundary of the visceral layer of the rectal fascia, defining the mesorectum. This dissection takes place between the fascia and the seminal vesicles, and is carried down below the prostate

(Fig. 5B). Care must be taken to dissect anterior to the Denonvilliers fascia, particularly when dealing with an anterior or a circumferential tumor of the rectum, in order not to compromise one's margins.

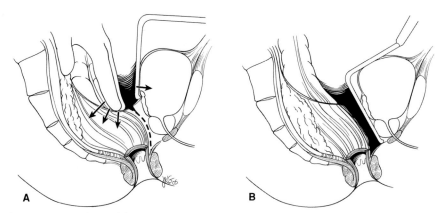

Fig. 5. Anterior plane of dissection. Sequential mobilization of the rectum by sharp dissection of the anterior plane between the Denonvilliers fascia and the anterior pelvic structures (seminal vesicles and prostate in men and posterior wall of the vagina in women). **A:** Plane of anterior dissection along the rectoprostatic plane distal to Denonvilliers fascia. **B:** Complete mobilization of the rectum down to pelvic floor.

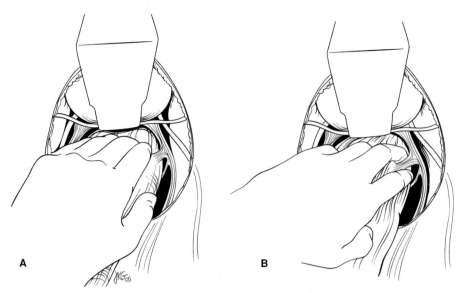

Fig. 6. Lateral plane of dissection. Left lateral and posterior traction applied to the rectum for better visualization of the "lateral ligament" and lateral pelvic structures. This step of the operation is generally performed after the anterior dissection has been completed. Traction for the anterior dissection is nearly the same.

After the posterior and anterior dissections have been completed to the level of S-4, the so-called "lateral ligaments" are developed and then divided. The surgeon here endeavors to obtain wide (i.e., tumor-free) margins on the one hand, and to preserve the autonomic nerve supply to the genitourinary system on the other. The "lateral ligament" is first developed by defining an anterolateral space as traction with the non-dominant hand pulls the rectum posterolaterally (Fig. 6A). As a hole develops anterior to the ligament, the second and third fingers may be used to create lateral traction around the medial segment of the ligament (Fig. 6B). Using medial retraction, it becomes evident that the portion headed toward the rectum is the medial segment of the lateral ligament that contains only an autonomic nerve and the middle rectal vessels. The lateral segment (i.e., the inferior hypogastric plexus) remains attached to the pelvic sidewall. Also known as the pelvic autonomic nerve plexus, the lateral segment contributes both the sympathetic and the parasympathetic nerve supplies to the genitourinary tract (Figs. 1 and 6). To preserve the lateral segment, one only divides the medial segment. Bleeding from the middle rectal arteries can be easily controlled with electrocautery, and deep sutures are eschewed because they may damage the autonomic nerve supply and function.

As soon as the so-called lateral ligaments have been divided, the levator fascia becomes visible. The remaining mobilization involves the dissection of the very distal junction of the visceral and parietal fascia layers (i.e., Waldeyer's fascia) in the posterior midline (Fig. 4C) and areolar tissue anteriorly and laterally (Fig. 4D). Once this is accomplished, the rectum has been circumferentially mobilized beyond the lesion and down to the pelvic floor to guarantee a total mesorectal excision. By pulling the specimen upward and away from all other structures, the rectum may be divided at the correct level in preparation for an anastomosis (Fig. 4E).

The Distal Margin of Resection

Many authors have demonstrated that distal intramural spread is generally not present for more than 1 cm, and that further distal spread is generally limited to cases of poorly differentiated disease or with other adverse features. If the issue of the distal margin was limited only to the wall of the bowel, a 1- to 2-cm distal margin would suffice. However, the resection of the cancer is a regional issue, and it has been demonstrated that the repository of concern for distal disease is not the rectal wall, but the mesorectum. In a series of 168 cleared surgical specimens, Hida et al. demonstrated that 22% of patients with T3 lesions harbored lymph node metastases as far as 4 cm distal to the lowest palpable edge or border of the primary rectal cancers. Based on these data, the distal margin of concern is the margin of mesorectum to be taken in a total mesorectal excision. We therefore strive to remove 5 cm of the mesorectum distal to the lowest palpable edge of the tumor, dividing the rectum at

right angles at that same level. In the fully mobilized and straightened rectum, the sine qua none of a TME resection, the choice of a 5-cm distal margin of mesorectum almost never interferes with sphincter preservation because of the additional elevation approaching 5 cm that accompanies the upward traction or straightening of the completely mobilized rectum. Because they are not situated along the curve of the sacral hollow, anterior midrectal lesions do not rise up quite as much with mobilization and traction as do posteriorly situated midrectal cancers. With the 5-cm guideline kept in mind, the selected margins help to ensure no compromise to the resection of all mesorectal pathology.

ANASTOMOTIC METHODS OF RECONSTRUCTION

Four methods of reconstruction are generally considered: A straight (i.e., end-to-end) colorectal anastomosis, a side-to-end colorectal anastomosis, a stapled or hand-sewn coloanal anastomosis; or any of the above with a colonic J-pouch.

When the distal margin of resection is selected, the rectum is divided, preferably using a linear stapler. Generally, the single firing of a 30-mm stapler (standard or thick tissue) will suffice for either the distal rectum or for an adequately cleaned off midrectal site of division. The 45-mm staplers often cannot negotiate the narrow confines of the male pelvis. If needed, two firings of a 30-mm stapler are easier and just as sound a means of getting across the rectum. When two firings are employed, the first firing is applied at a slight "upward" angle and the second firing is at a slight "downward" angle to incorporate the defect created by the passage of the "pin" through the apical midpoint of the rectal wall. Before firing the stapler we verify that the stapler is positioned low enough to obtain the described adequate distal margin. If the pelvis allows adequate room, the bowel may first be occluded with a right-angle bowel clamp, before applying the stapler. If not, the distal end of the specimen may first be occluded with a linear stapler that remains in place. This first stapler is used as a "handle" for traction, and a second stapler that defines the apex of the rectal stump is applied distally. Some surgeons choose to irrigate the rectal stump with povidone-iodine solution either for cleansing effect or to destroy the exfoliated malignant cells that have been shed in the distal rectum prior to applying the distal linear stapler. Except in the case of a very friable tumor, where whole clumps of a tumor might be

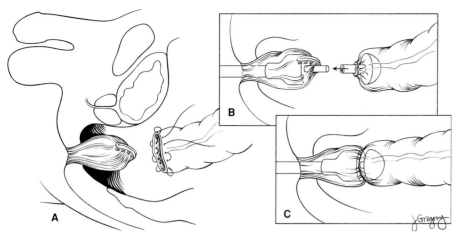

Fig. 7. Double-stapled anastomosis. **A:** The rectum is transected with a linear stapler and the proximal bowel is prepared by applying a purse-string suture. **B:** The anvil is placed in the proximal end of the bowel and the purse-string suture is tied. The shaft of the circular stapler is advanced through the anus and remaining rectum. **C:** Both ends of the circular stapler are connected and the stapler is closed, fired, and gently withdrawn.

fractured by handling, irrigation just prior to using the stapler has not been our practice, as the theoretic cause of pelvic recurrence has little if anything to do with exfoliated intraluminal cells.

The rectum is then divided either between the right-angle bowel clamp and the stapler or between the two stapling devices. In rare instances, this second stapling device cannot be negotiated within a tight pelvic space, and the rectum may be divided distal to a right-angle bowel clamp, and a hand-sewn purse-string suture is required deep in the pelvis. As a backup to stapling devices, this art of achieving a hand-sewn purse-string along the proximal edge of the rectal stump must be mastered if patients are going to end up with an appropriately restored continuity. In addition, the coloanal anastomosis is available where no other method of sphincter preservation may be accomplished, and where sphincter preservation is oncologically appropriate. But from the standpoint of bowel function, preserving the distal rectum, wherever possible, is preferred.

The Proximal End of the Anastomosis

In most cases, we prefer the double-staple technique (Fig. 7). After the rectum has been divided with the linear stapler the proximal end of the bowel is prepared. A 2-0 polypropylene purse-string suture is placed over and over the open edge of the proximal colon. The stitches are full thickness, but are placed close to the edge of the bowel to avoid including excessive amounts of tissue that may interfere with tying or gathering the bowel around the post of the anvil head. The

other option is to use an automatic purse-string applier on the proximal end of the bowel. The anvil head is placed in the proximal colon and the purse-string is tied. For a side-to-end anastomosis, we

gently advance the blunt, pointed end of the shaft proximally and bring it out through the taenia libra about 7 cm proximal to the open end of the bowel. The 7 cm guarantees a good blood supply and does not compromise the principle of avoiding tension. The distal end is then closed with a linear stapler.

Colonic J-Pouch

In the event that we are creating a colonic J-pouch, a 6-cm length of the bowel is turned back and the two limbs of the J-pouch are sutured along the edges of the free taeniae. An apical colotomy is created after the bowel is cleaned of fat, and the 75-mm linear stapler is used to cut and divide the pouch via the colostomy (Fig. 8-A). The purse-string suture is then sewn to the edge of the colotomy, and the anvil is inserted and tied down in place. The anastomosis is then completed (Fig. 8-B). We strive for the use of a 31-mm stapler wherever possible, affecting capacity and reducing the likelihood of mucosal bridging and stricture formation.

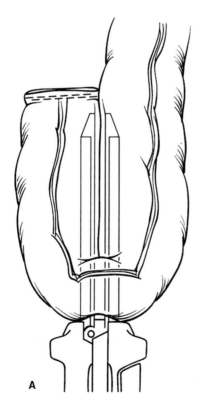

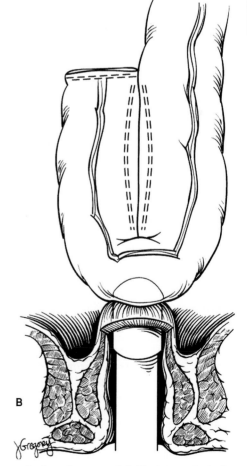

Fig. 8. Colonic J-pouch. **A:** The 75-mm linear stapler is used to cut and divide the pouch via the colostomy. **B:** The anvil is placed in the proximal end of the bowel and the purse-string suture is tied. The anastomosis is completed as show in Figure 7.

The Gastrointestinal Tract

Stapling the Anastomosis

The anal canal is gently dilated with fingers, prior to the easy insertion of the cartridge of the well-lubricated stapler as it is introduced into the rectum. The abdominal surgeon feels and carefully guides the stapler until it is adjacent to the staple line. Gentle rotation of the head is often helpful during advancement and withdrawal. Under direct visualization, the circular stapler is slowly opened and the trocar is advanced through the rectal wall either in front of or behind the staple line, but as close to the center of staple line as is possible. The trocar with its sharp point is then removed. The abdominal surgeon orients the proximal colon and its mesentery, making certain they are not twisted, and engages or "docks" the post of the anvil head onto to the center rod of the stapler. The perineal surgeon slowly closes the stapler to the appropriate tissue thickness firing range and fires it. The stapler is then opened, angled slightly to either side of midline, and gently rotated and withdrawn. The full-thickness tissue donuts are checked for integrity. We generally do not submit the rings to pathology as they do not represent the real proximal and distal margins of resection.

Checking the Anastomosis

The bowel should appear bright pink, with a good blood supply. The anastomosis should be without tension. The proximal colon should rest comfortably along the sacral hollow with no gaps between the mesocolon and the sacrum. If tension does exist, it can be addressed by the methods previously described: Mobilizing the splenic flexure or ligating the inferior mesenteric artery at its origin and the inferior mesenteric vein at the inferior border of the pancreas. Occasionally, the solution is as simple as incising a small area of sigmoid mesenteric peritoneum. After completion of the stapled anastomosis, the integrity of the anastomosis should be checked. The surgeon's hand or a bowel clamp occludes the lumen of the colon proximal to the anastomosis. The perineal surgeon introduces a Toomey syringe and insufflates air while the anastomosis is submerged in saline solution. Alternatively, a rigid sigmoidoscope may be introduced into the anorectum, visualizing the anastomosis. In the presence of two complete donuts and no air leak during insufflation, the anastomosis is considered intact and complete. Incomplete donuts or evidence of a definable air leak indicates an incomplete anastomosis and requires reinforcement with interrupted silk sutures. If the air leak cannot be addressed, or if the surgeon is not satisfied with the integrity of the anastomosis for any reason, a proximal diverting stoma should be created.

In the event of or in the anticipation of tension, mobilization of the splenic flexure is performed as previously described (vide supra) (Fig. 3). It is a common and safe practice to mobilize the splenic flexure from both proximal and distal approaches. During dissection of the splenic flexure, it is important to avoid excessive traction that can cause splenic avulsion. Laparoscopic mobilization is associated with a low incidence of splenic injury.

If the surgeon decides to perform a hand-sewn anastomosis, we favor the two-layer anastomosis with interrupted silk or polyglycolic acid sutures. Any mesentery, perirectal, or pericolic fat should be trimmed back at least 1 cm from the distal edge. Stay sutures on each side of the colon and rectum are placed. The posterior outer row of inverting sutures that penetrate into the submucosal layer (Lembert sutures) are placed, followed by the posterior and anterior inner row of interrupted or running full-thickness sutures. The anastomosis is completed with the anterior outer row of Lembert sutures.

In a hand-sewn anastomosis, the Baker side-to-end anastomosis may be necessary or easier to perform than an end-to-end anastomosis. The distal end of the colon is closed with the linear stapler. Stay sutures may be placed to align both segments and to avoid leaving a long blind segment of the colon. Rarely, the latter may dilate over time causing a blind loop or an inflammatory syndrome that may require a further resection. Both segments are opened to a desired length and the anastomosis performed following the same suture technique described above.

Pelvic Drains

We prefer to drain the pelvis routinely, especially in either distal anastomoses or in patients who have undergone preoperative radiation. Two closed suction drains are left posterolaterally between the sacrum and the reconstituted rectum. The drains are placed to evacuate serosanguineous fluid from the pelvis and to prevent abscess formation. These drains are left in place for up to 4 to 6 days, but in view of increasingly earlier hospital discharges, they are most often removed much earlier (i.e., when drainage significantly diminishes and the bowel is functioning). If an anastomotic leak occurs in the absence of peritonitis, these drains may play a role in the management of the leak.

SUGGESTED READING

Principal References

Coller FA, Kay EB, MacIntyre RS. Regional lymphatic metastasis of carcinoma of the rectum. *Surgery* 1940;8:294.

Enker WE, Kafka NJ, Martz J. Planes of sharp pelvic dissection for primary, locally advanced, or recurrent rectal cancer. *Semin Surg Oncol* 2000;18(3):199.

Enker WE, Thaler HT, Cranor ML, et al. Total mesorectal excision in the operative treatment of carcinoma of the rectum. *J Am Coll Surg* 1995;181(4):335.

Griffen FD, Knight CD Sr, Whitaker JM, et al. The double stapling technique for low anterior resection. Results, modifications, and observations. *Ann Surg* 1990;211(6):745.

Heald RJ, Ryall RD. Recurrence and survival after total mesorectal excision for rectal cancer. *Lancet* 1986;1(8496):1479.

Hida J, Yasutomi M, Maruyama T, et al. Lymph node metastases detected in the mesorectum distal to carcinoma of the rectum by the clearing method: justification of total mesorectal excision. *J Am Coll Surg* 1997;184(6):584.

Additional References

Abcarian H, Pearl RK. Simple technique for high ligation of the inferior mesenteric artery and vein. *Dis Colon Rectum* 1991;34(12):1138.

Chambers WM, Mortensen NJ. Postoperative leakage and abscess formation after colorectal surgery. *Best Pract Res Clin Gastroenterol* 2004;18(5):865.

Cirocco WC, Brown AC. Anterior resection for the treatment of rectal prolapse: a 20-year experience. *Am Surg* 1993;59(4):265.

Enker WE. Mesorectal excision (TME) in the operative treatment of rectal cancer. *Int J Surg Investig* 1999;1(3):253.

Enker WE. Potency, cure, and local control in the operative treatment of rectal cancer. *Arch Surg* 1992;127(12):1396.

Enker WE, Havenga K, Polyak T, et al. Abdominoperineal resection via total mesorectal excision and autonomic nerve preservation for low rectal cancer. *World J Surg* 1997;21(7):715.

Eriksen MT, Wibe A, Norstein J, et al. Anastomotic leakage following routine mesorectal excision for rectal cancer in a national cohort of patients. *Colorectal Dis* 2005;7(1):51.

Griffith CD, Hardcastle JD. Intraoperative testing of anastomotic integrity after stapled anterior resection for cancer. *J R Coll Surg Edinb* 1990;35(2):106.

Havenga K, Enker WE. Autonomic nerve preserving total mesorectal excision. *Surg Clin North Am* 2002;82(5):1009.

Havenga K, Enker WE, McDermott K, et al. Male and female sexual and urinary function after total mesorectal excision with autonomic nerve preservation for carcinoma of the rectum. *J Am Coll Surg* 1996;182(6):495.

Hojo K, Vernava AM III, Sugihara K, et al. Preservation of urine voiding and sexual function after rectal cancer surgery. *Dis Colon Rectum* 1991;34(7):532.

Kessler H, Hohenberger W. Laparoscopic resection rectopexy for rectal prolapse. *Dis Colon Rectum* 2005;48(9):1800.

Leong AF. Total mesorectal excision (TME)—twenty years on. *Ann Acad Med Singapore* 2003;32(2):159.

Lindsey I, Guy RJ, Warren BF, et al. Anatomy of Denonvilliers' fascia and pelvic nerves, impotence, and implications for the colorectal surgeon. *Br J Surg* 2000;87(10):1288.

Maeda K, Maruta M, Hanai T, et al. Irrigation volume determines the efficacy of "rectal washout". *Dis Colon Rectum* 2004;47(10):1706.

Moreira LF, Hizuta A, Iwagaki H, et al. Lateral lymph node dissection for rectal carcinoma below the peritoneal reflection. *Br J Surg* 1994;81(2):293.

Nagtegaal ID, Marijnen CA, Kranenbarg EK, et al. Circumferential margin involvement is still an important predictor of local recurrence in rectal carcinoma: not one millimeter but two millimeters is the limit. *Am J Surg Pathol* 2002;26(3):350.

Nicholls RJ, Zinicola R, Binda GA. Indications for colorectal resection for adenoma before and after polypectomy. *Tech Coloproctol* 2004;8 Suppl 2:s291.

Paty PB, Nash GM, Baron P, et al. Long-term results of local excision for rectal cancer. *Ann Surg* 2002;236(4):522.

Peeters KC, Tollenaar RA, Marijnen CA, et al. Risk factors for anastomotic failure after total mesorectal excision of rectal cancer. *Br J Surg* 2005;92(2):211.

Pilipshen SJ, Heilweil M, Quan SH, et al. Patterns of pelvic recurrence following definitive resections of rectal cancer. *Cancer* 1984;53(6):1354.

Rothenberger DA, Wong WD. Rectal cancer—adequacy of surgical management. *Surg Annu* 1985;17:309.

Sato K, Sato T. The vascular and neuronal composition of the lateral ligament of the rectum and the rectosacral fascia. *Surg Radiol Anat* 1991;13(1):17.

Sugarbaker PH, Corlew S. Influence of surgical techniques on survival in patients with colorectal cancer. *Dis Colon Rectum* 1982;25(6):545.

Surtees P, Ritchie JK, Phillips RK. High versus low ligation of the inferior mesenteric artery in rectal cancer. *Br J Surg* 1990;77(6):618.

Tocchi A, Mazzoni G, Lepre L, et al. Total mesorectal excision and low rectal anastomosis for the treatment of rectal cancer and prevention of pelvic recurrences. *Arch Surg* 2001;136(2):216.

EDITOR'S COMMENT

This succinct but very nicely done chapter explores some of the issues in anterior and low anterior resection quite well. The technique is very well described. It does appear that all have agreed that total mesorectal excision carried out by sharp dissection under direct vision is a sine qua non of a curative dissection for cancer of the upper and especially the middle and lower rectum. There is a particularly good explanation of Waldeyer fascia made up of a fusion of the visceral layer of the endopelvic fascia as well as the parietal layer of the endopelvic fascia joining together below the level of S4 and fusing with the attenuated mesorectum for the remaining few centimeters above the levator ani.

Enker et al. (*World J Surg* 1997;21[7]:715) take issue with the commonly held supposition that the distal margins need to be only 2 cm because of the fact that the distal spread is rarely downward. The explanation, in addition, that 50% of distal spread takes place to the lungs instead of the liver is based on the middle rectal and inferior rectal arteries and veins going to the iliac circulation rather than the portal circulation, and thus the spread is to the lungs rather than the liver.

Diverticular disease is dealt with simply by saying that one must come below the peritoneal reflection or at the very least where the taenia fuse in order to avoid recurrence. I would simply add that proximally, one must go to the thin bowel and not bowel that has already been affected by the muscular disorder, which is the basis of diverticular disease and the same applied distally. Not to do so invites long-term recurrence of the symptoms of diverticular disease.

For prolapse, Dr. Enker et al. differ somewhat from some of the prolapse chapters as far as lateral mobilization. They do, however, hold, as do the other authors, that anterior rectal resection in prolapse actually aids in the prevention of recurrence in the sense that the fibrosis of the anastomosis and the suturing of the mesorectum following resection actually aid the securing of the anterior rectosigmoid to prevent further recurrence of prolapse.

As for the techniques of resection, I agree entirely in using the rectosigmoid as a handle and placing it distally under tension over the pubic symphysis. Dr. Enker uses a plastic ring to wall off the wound; I happen to use antibiotic-dipped towels sutured to the wound, but the effect is the same. The anterior dissection in the male is well described, including what Denonvilliers fascia actually is, which is difficult to transmit to residents especially. Getting down to the level of the prostate and the seminal vesicles, one must be very careful not to get into bleeding during the anterior resection of the rectum. This requires, as Dr. Enker states, use of the St. Marks retractor (especially the one with the lip) and traction and countertraction with the assistant hauling mightily to try to enable the surgeon to see. Similarly, the use of lighting, traction, and countertraction in the sharp dissection, which is essential for total mesorectal incision, is important. If one gets into bleeding in the area of the seminal vesicles and the base of the prostate, one must be very careful because damage to the nerves here results in retrograde ejaculation or impotence, depending on the degree of the damage.

My own prejudice is that a hand-sewn anastomosis is better than a stapled anastomosis because of the incidence of late stricture. All stapled anastomoses have a tendency to stricture, and Dr. Enker et al. attempt to prevent this by the use of a 31-mm EEA stapler so that even if it does stricture, one does not have to revise the anastomosis or dilate it. Stapled anastomoses, particularly in gastrojejunostomies, are responsible for a large number of the revisions of gastrojejunostomies that my practice performs in postgastrectomy or postgastric procedures.

In the past, I did essentially all Joel Baker–type anastomoses, that is, side of colon to end of rectum. However, I've recently had three cases of the enlargement of what I call the proboscis, which is the end of the proximal rectum, and some resulting inflammatory changes. I've tended to use more and more end-to-end anastomoses, which do not have this problem. The anastomosis I prefer is a two-layer hand-sewn 4.0 silk anastomosis that does not stricture and usually gives excellent results.

There is little question that the use of neoadjuvant therapy, especially in patients with large bulking tumors, some stage 2, but all T3 and T4 tumors, has resulted in disease-free intervals and increases in the long-term incidence of cure, and in those that recur, lengthening of disease-free intervals. It does, however, come with a cost. First, as Pollack et al. have shown (*Dis Colon Rectum* 2005;49:1), there is diminished anal function after neoadjuvant therapy. They reviewed 64 patients who answered by questionnaire, after a total study of 528 patients originally treated with low anterior resection in the Stockholm I and II trials. Of these, 119 were still alive and 64 patients were alive without a stoma. A number of patients did not wish to participate in the study because of physical and other infirmities. Of these 64 patients, 21 had received preoperative radiotherapy and 43 had been treated with surgery alone. Irradiated patients had significantly more symptoms of fecal incontinence (57% vs. 26%, $P = 0.01$), soiling (38% vs. 16%, $P = 0.04$), and significantly more bowel movements per week (20% vs. 10%, $P = 0.02$). There were physiologic counterparts to this impaired anorectal function in that irradiated patients had significantly lower resting pressure (35 mm Hg vs. 62 mm Hg, $P < 0.001$), lower squeeze pressure (104 mm Hg vs. 143 mm Hg, $P = 0.05$), and on endoanal ultrasound, more scarring of the anal sphincters (33% vs. 13%, $P = 0.03$). Unless there was soilage, there was no difference in the quality of life, but patients who reported soilage obviously did have an inferior quality of life as evidenced by the questionnaire.

Buie et al. (*Dis Colon Rectum* 2005;48:1868) commented on the increased risk of pelvic sepsis, both leakages and abscesses, after neoadjuvant chemoradiation. In this series, 5,040 Gy were given with three cycles of 5-fluorouracil–based chemotherapy. Of 246 patients, 60 patients (24%) had neoadjuvant chemoradiation. Nine (15%) of them developed pelvic sepsis, including three leakages and six abscesses, compared with 9 out of 186 (4.8%) after primary surgery (six leakages, three abscesses, $P = 0.01$).

J.E.F.

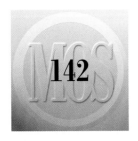

142

Radical Groin Dissection

DANIEL G. COIT

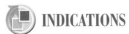

INDICATIONS

Groin dissection is a procedure performed in the treatment of a number of cutaneous malignancies, including melanoma, squamous cell carcinoma, Merkel cell carcinoma, and other skin-appendage tumors metastatic to that nodal basin. Other primary tumor sites potentially metastatic to the superficial groin include the vulva, anus, and penis. Visceral sites potentially metastatic to pelvic nodes include cervix, endometrium, prostate, and bladder. This chapter will deal specifically with lymphadenectomy for metastatic disease to regional nodes, and will not specifically address resection of benign or malignant soft tissue neoplasms of the groin region. Furthermore, it will focus on the technical details of open surgical lymphadenectomy, rather than the minimally invasive laparoscopic approach.

Through the 1980s, perhaps the most common indication for groin dissection was in the elective setting for intermediate-thickness melanomas of the trunk or lower extremities. However, the overall incidence of groin dissection for melanoma has decreased dramatically during the last 20 years. In the absence of prospective data to support routine application of elective lymph node dissection, and with the advent and subsequent widespread application of sentinel lymph node biopsy, the principal indications for this procedure in melanoma have evolved to either selective or completion lymph node dissection in patients with positive sentinel nodes, or therapeutic lymph node dissection for those with clinically positive regional nodes, both in the absence of known distant metastatic disease. The procedure may be unilateral or, in the case of midline primary tumors, bilateral. The procedure may entail removal of inguinofemoral nodes in the superficial groin, that is, those nodes superficial to the inguinal ligament, the ileo-obturator nodes in the deep groin, or both.

Although never formally confirmed in the context of a prospective randomized trial, in the absence of distant disease, few would argue with the therapeutic value of complete lymph node dissection in patients with clinically positive nodes; a substantial proportion of these patients are cured with no further treatment beyond complete surgical resection. On the other hand, the therapeutic value of completion lymph node dissection in patients with a positive sentinel lymph node from melanoma is unknown, and is currently the focus of an ongoing prospective randomized study, the Multicenter Selective Lymphadenectomy II trial.

In patients with known distant metastatic disease, palliative groin dissection may be indicated to achieve control of symptomatic regional disease in the nodal basin. Given the substantial morbidity of the procedure, groin dissection to control potential future symptoms in the presence of known systemic metastases should be done sparingly if at all, and if so, only on a case-by-case basis.

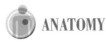

ANATOMY

The anatomy of the groin is quite constant. The superficial groin is defined by the femoral triangle, consisting of the sartorius muscle laterally, the adductor magnus and pectineus muscles medially, and the inguinal ligament superiorly. The transition from external iliac to common femoral vessels occurs as they traverse the femoral canal from the pelvis into the thigh. Medially in the femoral canal there are lymphatics containing Cloquet's lymph node. Proceeding laterally, we encounter the common femoral vein, the common femoral artery, and more laterally, the common femoral nerve. The saphenous vein enters the inferior apex of the femoral triangle at the junction of the adductor magnus and sartorius muscles, and courses through the middle of the triangle, through the fossa ovalis, to drain into the common femoral vein at the saphenofemoral junction. Branches of the saphenofemoral junction include the lateral femoral circumflex, medial femoral circumflex, external pudendal, superficial circumflex iliac, deep circumflex iliac, and superficial epigastric veins. The exact anatomy and caliber of these veins varies from one patient to the next; most of these veins have corresponding arteries. As all of these small vessels traverse the lymphadenectomy specimen, each requires division at both the periphery and center of the lymphadenectomy.

Working cephalad, just above and deep to the inguinal ligament, the common femoral vessels become the external iliac vessels. Laterally, we see the deep circumflex iliac branches, and the inferior epigastric branches arise medially. There are few if any branches of the external iliac vessels. Working cephalad further, we encounter the bifurcation of the common iliac into the internal and external iliac vessels. The internal iliac vessels branch widely. The first branch is the superior gluteal, which traverses the sciatic notch to the buttock, and represents an important source of collateral circulation to the lower leg in the event of external iliac interruption. Other branches include the inferior and superior vesical, the internal pudendal, the obturator, and the superior and middle hemorrhoidal vessels. Not all of these branches can be traced out in every pelvic lymphadenectomy. Traversing the triangle between the external and internal iliac vessels is the obturator nerve, which joins the obturator artery and vein to exit the obturator foramen. Medial to the deep pelvic node compartment is the peritoneum and its contents, including the ureter, rectum, and bladder. The lateral aspect is bordered by the endopelvic fascia.

SURGICAL TECHNIQUE

Anesthesia

Groin dissection is most commonly performed under either regional or general anesthesia. If pelvic lymphadenectomy is to be undertaken, muscle relaxation is important to achieve adequate exposure, and general endotracheal anesthesia is preferred. Bladder catheterization is generally not necessary unless a prolonged and difficult procedure is anticipated.

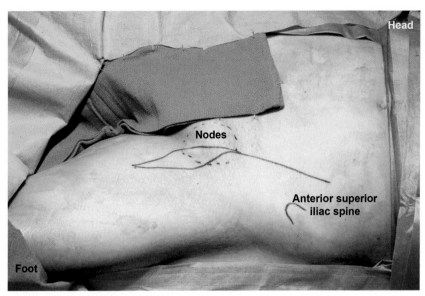

Fig. 1. Incision for en bloc superficial and deep groin dissection. An ellipse of skin over the femoral triangle is removed to minimize postoperative skin-edge necrosis.

Positioning

The patient is generally positioned supine on the operating room table, with the ipsilateral hip slightly abducted and the knee flexed. This opens up the femoral triangle. The knee can be rested on a pillow for support. The surgical field may be prepared and directly squared off, or the entire lower extremity may be prepared and draped into the field, at the discretion of the operating surgeon. We employ compression boots on one or both legs, depending on whether the ipsilateral leg has been prepared into the field.

Incision

There is a variety of incisions that can be used to performed groin dissection. Many of the short-term wound-related complications associated with the superficial groin dissection are a consequence of a vertically oriented incision, which traverses the groin crease. This incision is subject to a great deal of motion and stress, and often fails to heal primarily. Modifications of the vertical incision include the oblique incision oriented along lines of skin tension, either above or below the groin crease. In the case of pelvic lymphadenectomy, exposure can be achieved by extending the vertically oriented incision cephalad to a point 3 to 4 cm medial to the anterior superior iliac spine (Fig. 1). Although this incision does traverse the inguinal crease, division of the inguinal ligament over the femoral vessels affords the potential for an en bloc dissection

of both superficial and deep node compartments. This approach also provides excellent access for a more thorough dissection of the most distal external iliac nodes. An alternative to this approach would be a skin crease-infrainguinal incision for the superficial groin and a parallel suprainguinal skin crease or transplant-type incision for the deep groin. These parallel incisions generally heal quite well, but the main disadvantage is the relative lack of access to the most distal external iliac nodes.

If a vertically oriented incision is to be used, it is important to excise an ellipse of skin overlying the femoral triangle, approximately 3 to 4 cm in width. This shortens the length of flaps that need to

be dissected, and dramatically diminishes the likelihood of skin-edge necrosis and subsequent superficial wound dehiscence.

Superficial Inguinofemoral Lymphadenectomy

Once the skin incision has been selected and made, skin flaps are raised in the plane just deep to Scarpa's fascia, circumferentially around the lymph node basin. These flaps should not be too thin because if they are, they will be devascularized, inevitably leading to skin-edge necrosis and delayed wound healing. Branches of the saphenofemoral junction with their corresponding arteries are clipped and divided as they are encountered at the periphery of the lymphadenectomy. Flaps are raised laterally to the sartorius muscle (Fig. 2), medially to the adductor magnus muscle, and inferiorly to the point where these two muscles cross, where the saphenous vein is traditionally identified, clamped, divided, and ligated. Superiorly, skin flaps are raised to include 5 to 6 cm of fatty and lymphatic tissue overlying the inguinal ligament, medially to the level of the external ring, where the spermatic cord (or ligamentum teres) is exposed and preserved. The dissection proceeds to the pubic tubercle, then on down to the pectineus and adductor magnus muscles (Fig. 3). We prefer to take the fascia of the sartorius, adductor magnus, and pectineus muscles, although the therapeutic value of this maneuver is unknown. Some authors have described preservation of the muscle fascia to minimize postoperative morbidity; no strong data exist to support or refute either approach.

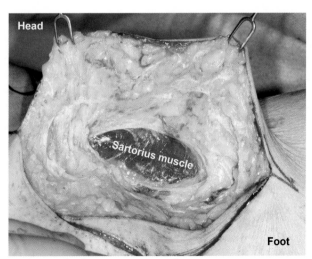

Fig. 2. The lateral skin flap is raised first, down to and including the sartorius fascia (muscle). Preservation of the fascia is optional.

The Gastrointestinal Tract

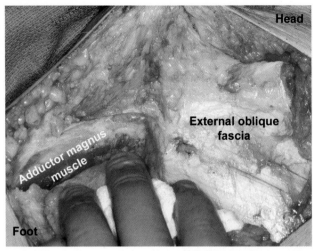

Fig. 3. The medial flap is raised down to the adductor and pectineus muscles. The fatty and lymphatic tissue is dissected off the external oblique fascia, medially to the external inguinal ring, and spermatic cord (ligamentum teres). In this instance, the nodal disease involves the ligamentum teres, and that structure is taken with the specimen.

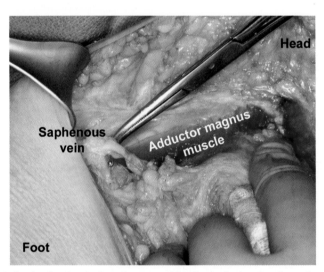

Fig. 4. Inferiorly, the flap is raised to the apex of the femoral triangle, where the adductor and sartorius muscles cross. In the classic superficial groin dissection, the saphenous vein is taken at this point, although saphenous vein preservation has been proposed to minimize postoperative morbidity.

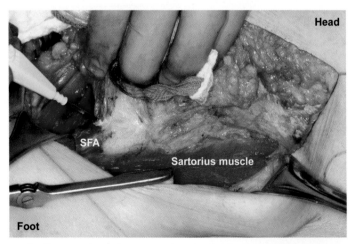

Fig. 5. Once the flaps are elevated, exposure is maintained with a large self-retaining retractor, and the lymphatic tissue is dissected off the superficial femoral artery (SFA) and vein.

At the inferior apex of the femoral triangle the saphenous vein is encountered. In the classic inguinofemoral dissection, the saphenous vein is clamped, divided, and ligated at this point (Fig. 4). Again, in an effort to decrease postoperative morbidity, a modification of the procedure that preserves the saphenous vein has been described, and will be discussed later.

Once the skin flaps have been raised, exposure is maintained with a self-retaining retractor (we prefer a Gelpi or Beckman retractor). We then begin dissection of the nodes from the inferior apex of the femoral triangle working cephalad, in the adventitial plane along the superficial femoral artery and vein (Figs. 5 and 6). Care is taken to clip longitudinally oriented lymphatics as they are encountered. Approaching the femoral vessels, the fascia of the adductor and sartorius muscles is once again transected to get into the correct plane. Small arterial branches and venous tributaries are clipped and divided as they are encountered. Working up toward the common femoral vessels, we take the fatty and lymphatic tissue off the inguinal ligament at the lateral aspect of the femoral triangle and dissect this medially off the sartorius muscle. Overly aggressive use of the electrocautery at this point will result in stimulation of the motor branches of the femoral nerve, and should be avoided. The fatty and lymphatic tissues are swept medially, off the common femoral artery. At this point, the saphenofemoral junction is identified and is clamped, divided, and suture-ligated (Fig. 7). The lymphatic tissue is then dissected off the medial aspect of the femoral vein, up toward the femoral canal, together with the fascia of the adductor magnus and pectineus muscles. If the procedure is to be terminated, the superficial inguinofemoral contents are removed and submitted for appropriate pathologic examination (Fig. 8).

At this point, the femoral canal is entered, and an attempt made to identify the so-called node of Cloquet. This maneuver starts by inserting a finger through the femoral canal and manually palpating for enlarged external iliac or obturator nodes. We find that placing a small loop retractor on the inguinal ligament, then reaching under and gently grasping and delivering Cloquet's node with an Allis clamp works well (Fig. 9). Once removed, Cloquet's node is submitted for frozen-section examination.

Although Cloquet's node may not be a reproducible anatomic entity, the concept is that the lymph node lying within the femoral canal represents a bridging node

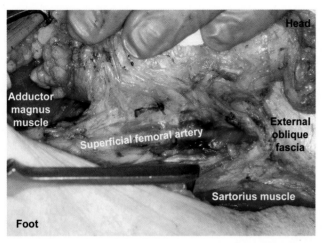

Fig. 6. This dissection proceeds from caudad to cephalad, and from lateral to medial.

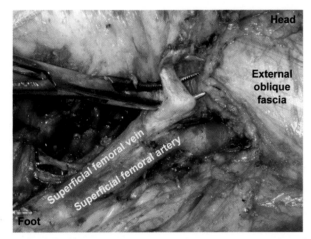

Fig. 7. When the saphenous vein is being taken with the specimen, the saphenofemoral junction is exposed, clamped, divided, and suture-ligated.

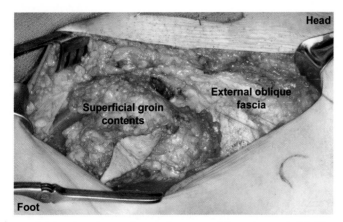

Fig. 8. The superficial groin contents about to be removed from the surgical field.

between the superficial and deep node contents. The status of this node has been used by many to guide a decision as to whether to proceed to elective deep pelvic node dissection. In melanoma at least, many, but not all, believe that if this node is positive, there is a significant likelihood of deep pelvic node involvement, and the operation should be extended. On the other hand, if this node is negative, there is a low likelihood of clinically occult pelvic nodal involvement, and the operation may be concluded at this point.

If the procedure is concluded, the incision is closed. The first step is to close the femoral canal to prevent postoperative femoral hernia. For a secure repair, this involves approximating the inguinal ligament to the lacunar ligament (rather than the pectineus muscle) with one or two interrupted figure-of-eight nonabsorbable sutures (Fig. 10). It is important not to narrow the femoral canal too much with these sutures, to avoid occlusion and/or thrombosis of the common femoral vein. Closed suction drains are placed to deal with postoperative lymphorrhea (Fig. 11). The incision is then closed in layers. We prefer closely spaced interrupted sutures to Scarpa's fascia to achieve an airtight closure, followed by either a subcuticular suture or clips to the skin.

Deep Ileo-obturator Lymphadenectomy

If pelvic lymphadenectomy (ileo-obturator lymphadenectomy) is to be performed—and this is anticipated ahead of time based on imaging studies—Cloquet's node need not be sampled, and the entire lymph node package, both superficial and deep, can be removed in continuity by extending the incision cephalad and dividing the inguinal ligament (see following discussion). If the superficial groin contents have been removed previously, then the pelvic nodes can be approached through a suprainguinal skin crease type of incision. That incision should be placed low enough to enable access to the distal most external iliac nodes, and should be long enough to provide adequate exposure and access to the more proximal pelvic nodes.

If Cloquet's node is positive on frozen section, and the deep pelvic portion of the lymph node dissection is to be done in continuity, the skin incision is extended cephalad, up toward a point 3 to 4 cm medial to the anterior superior iliac, as previously described. The skin and subcutaneous tissues are divided. The fascia of the external oblique muscle is divided lateral to the

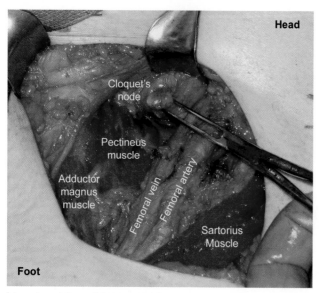

Fig. 9. Cloquet's node is delivered through the femoral canal, medial to the femoral vein, with an Allis clamp.

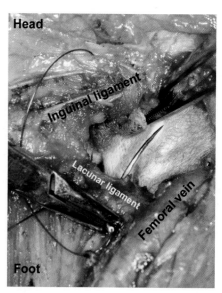

Fig. 11. After the femoral canal is reconstructed, closed suction drains are placed and the superficial groin dissection wound is closed in layers.

rectus abdominus muscle in the direction of its fibers, bringing that incision down toward the inguinal ligament at the level of the femoral vessels. Prior to dividing the inguinal ligament, the retroperitoneum is entered. This is done by grasping the internal oblique muscle lateral to the rectus muscle and dividing it in the direction of the previous incision. An areolar plane is entered just deep to the transversalis fascia. Great care is taken at this point not to violate the peritoneum. The peritoneum and its contents are then bluntly dissected off the undersurface of the transversalis muscle laterally and the femoral vessels in the depth of the incision. We prefer to retract

the inferolateral aspect of the abdominal wall with Kocher clamps to facilitate this access to the retroperitoneum.

The incision is then developed more cephalad, dividing the abdominal wall muscles to the level of the anterior superior iliac spine, and caudad down toward the femoral canal. A finger is placed through the femoral canal to protect the femoral vessels as the ligament is divided at this level. At this point, complete exposure of the pelvis can be achieved, as the peritoneum and its contents are bluntly dissected and retracted superomedially. We find that a multiblade self-retaining retractor (such as Bookwalter or Thompson) at

this point is invaluable to provide and maintain exposure (Fig. 12). Deep Richardson-type blades are placed to retract the peritoneum superiorly and medially, to retract the bladder medially, and to retract the abdominal wall laterally. This generally affords excellent exposure to the lower retroperitoneum and pelvis. As with all self-retaining retractors, care must be taken at this point to avoid sustained pressure on the femoral nerve so as to prevent postoperative nerve palsy.

We initiate the pelvic lymphadenectomy at the level of the common iliac artery and vein. The lateral aspect of the dissection is the ileofemoral nerve, a nerve that has often been divided distal to the inguinal ligament in the course of the superficial groin dissection. The fatty and lymphatic tissue is gently dissected off the distal common iliac vessels. It should be noted that the lymphatics completely encircle the external iliac vessels, and the specimen may need to be bivalved to remove it completely. This dissection may be facilitated by gentle retraction of the external artery and/or vein using soft-rubber vessel loops. Care should be taken not to occlude the vessels during the course of this retraction. Proceeding from cephalad to caudad, and from lateral to medial, we then dissect all of the nodal tissue down along the hypogastric (internal iliac) vessels. In so doing, the origin of the obturator nerve is encountered as it courses through the triangle formed by the internal and external vessels (Fig. 13). In a thin patient, one can often visualize

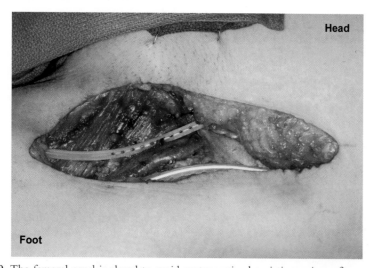

Fig. 10. The femoral canal is closed to avoid postoperative herniation, using a figure-of-eight nonabsorbable suture to approximate the lacunar ligament to the inguinal ligament. Care is taken not to narrow the canal too much, to avoid narrowing the femoral vein. The sponge is helpful for exposure and is removed prior to tying the suture.

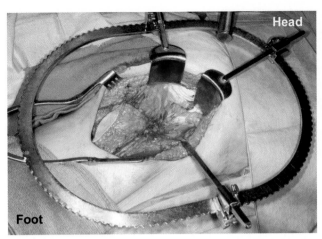

Fig. 12. When an en bloc superficial and deep groin dissection is to be performed, the incision is extended superolaterally, and the retroperitoneum entered. The peritoneum and its contents are retracted superomedially with a multiblade self-retaining retractor, affording excellent exposure to the lower retroperitoneum and pelvis.

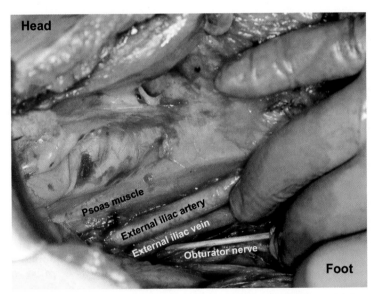

Fig. 13. As the pelvic node dissection proceeds from cephalad to caudad, the nodal tissue is swept down off the internal and external iliac vessels, exposing the obturator nerve.

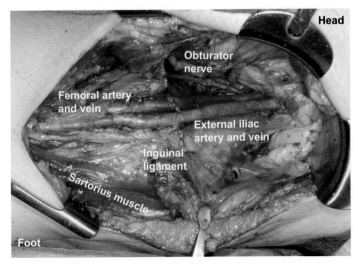

Fig. 14. The surgical field after en bloc removal of the superficial and deep groin contents.

the superior gluteal, superior vesical, and obturator vessels. The hemorrhoidal vessels can be quite difficult to see because of limited exposure. All of the fatty and lymphatic tissue is dissected off the endopelvic fascia, preserving the named vessels insofar as possible, and preserving throughout the structure and function of the obturator nerve. In the absence of grossly involved nodal disease, much of this portion of the dissection can be done bluntly, as the nodal tissue easily separates from the neurovascular structures.

Next, the nodes are dissected off the bladder medially, down toward the obturator foramen, and then up toward the external iliac vessels and inguinal ligament (Fig. 14). In many instances, particularly when combined superficial and deep dissection is anticipated, the entire lymph node specimen can be removed en bloc. The specimen should be marked to assist the pathologist with orientation, and then submitted for appropriate pathologic examination (Fig. 15).

Once hemostasis is verified, the wound is closed. Deep pelvic drains are not necessary. The retractor is removed and the peritoneum and its contents are returned to the pelvis. The internal oblique and transversus abdominal muscles are closed with a running No. 0 absorbable suture down as far as closure can be completed without undue tension. Care is taken in closing this layer not to violate the peritoneum medially. The external oblique muscle is closed with a similar running No. 0 absorbable suture. This often leaves a very large femoral canal (Fig. 16). Medially, the femoral canal is closed with figure-of-eight sutures of nonabsorbable suture to approximate the inguinal ligament to the lacunar ligament, as previously described for closure of the superficial groin dissection.

At this point, a judgment needs to be made as to whether the residual defect through which the iliac vessels exit the pelvis into the thigh is snug enough to avoid a postoperative hernia. If not, a useful method to prevent peritoneal herniation through an incompetent femoral canal after pelvic lymphadenectomy is to transpose the sartorius muscle over the femoral vessels, under the inguinal ligament (see following discussion). An alternative to sartorius muscle transposition would be to insert a piece of nonabsorbable mesh, fixed to the undersurface of the abdominal wall, then tucked up into the retroperitoneum, over the iliac vessels.

Once the deep pelvic closure is complete, closure of the superficial groin is completed as previously described (Fig. 17).

The Gastrointestinal Tract

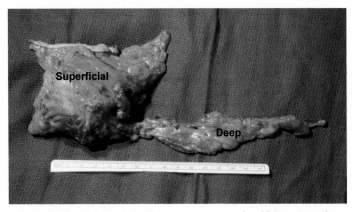

Fig. 15. The superficial and deep groin dissection specimen should be oriented to assist in the pathologic examination.

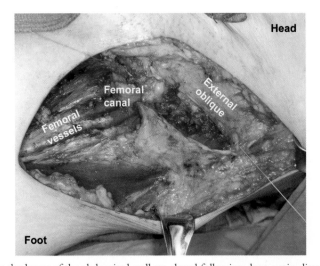

Fig. 16. After the layers of the abdominal wall are closed following deep groin dissection, there is often a large defect at the femoral canal. If this cannot be closed by approximating the lacunar ligament to the inguinal ligament (Fig. 10), either sartorius muscle transposition or prosthetic mesh can be employed.

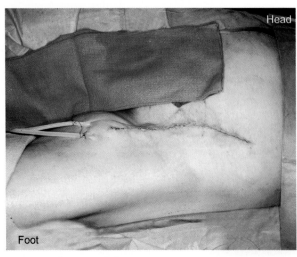

Fig. 17. Final appearance after wound closure.

Local Muscle Flaps

The sartorius muscle can be exceedingly useful in certain instances. In the case of an obese patient with a high likelihood of wound failure, the sartorius flap is helpful in covering the femoral vessels so as to minimize their exposure should the wound break down. This can be particularly important in patients who have had radiation to the groin. Additionally, the sartorius flap can be used to fill the femoral canal following closure after pelvic lymphadenectomy when simple closure is insufficient. Although some have suggested sartorius muscle transposition may increase the incidence of postoperative edema, this observation has not been subject to rigorous evaluation.

The sartorius flap is easily developed and quite reliable, with minimal donor site morbidity. The muscle's origin is on the anterior superior iliac spine, and it courses down to the medial knee, to insert on the anterior tibia. Its blood supply is segmental, proximally derived from the deep femoral circulation. The flap is developed by encircling the muscle origin with a finger, taking care to protect the underlying femoral nerve and iliopsoas complex. The muscle is detached from the anterior superior iliac spine as high as possible, and then freed up for a length sufficient to permit its rotation over to cover the femoral vessels. This usually entails sacrifice of no more than one of the segmental vascular branches. It is important not to devascularize this muscle flap in the course of mobilization because its vitality is essential to protect the underlying vessels. Once adequately mobilized, the muscle flap is rotated over the vessels, and then secured to the undersurface of the inguinal ligament and to the adductor magnus muscle with interrupted absorbable sutures. This very nicely covers the vessels and fills the femoral canal.

In instances where very bulky ulcerated nodal metastases have been removed with significant amounts of skin over the femoral triangle, or in instances of groin dissection following nodal basin irradiation, more extensive myocutaneous flaps may be required. Very reliable flap coverage can be achieved with either the rectus abdominus flap or the tensor fascia lata flap, depending on which feeding vessels are available following lymphadenectomy. When such flaps are anticipated, it is imperative that the operating surgeon work closely with the plastic surgeon preoperatively to plan to preserve the necessary blood supply to these myocutaneous flaps.

Surgical Variations

Saphenous Vein Preservation

A number of authors have advocated saphenous vein preservation as a way to minimize postoperative morbidity of this procedure, especially lymphedema. Although it is not clear that sacrifice of the saphenous vein improves the oncologic results of most groin dissections, unless the vein itself is intimately associated with malignant lymphadenopathy, neither has it ever been shown in any prospective fashion that preservation of this vein leads to substantial diminution in the morbidity of the procedure. Thus, preservation of the saphenous vein becomes almost a matter of personal style and preference, rather than a recommendation to be embraced with strong conviction.

Minimally Invasive Approaches

Addressing the concern that at least a component of the morbidity of superficial groin dissection is related to the incision used, at least one group has reported on a small experience performing this procedure using minimally invasive techniques. They showed that this is a feasible technique in experienced hands, but there has been no formal comparison of this to the more conventional open approach, to quantify differences in cost, length of stay, short- and long-term morbidity, and perhaps most importantly, the adequacy of the operation in terms of locoregional control.

Although laparoscopic staging and treatment of pelvic nodes is becoming much more widely accepted in the management of patients with prostate, bladder, and gynecologic malignancy, this approach has not yet been widely adopted in the treatment of metastatic pelvic lymphadenopathy from cutaneous malignancy. A few reports have appeared describing a combination of open superficial groin dissection with laparoscopic deep pelvic lymphadenectomy for melanoma, confirming the feasibility of this approach, without long-term follow up. The abdominal incision required to achieve retroperitoneal exposure in patients undergoing pelvic lymphadenopathy clearly results in longer length of hospital stay and ultimate recovery. If the laparoscopic approach to pelvic nodes can be shown to be comparable with the open operation in other respects, then it would seem to be an entirely reasonable alternative.

Perioperative Care

Many unsubstantiated recommendations have been made regarding the perioperative care of patients undergoing groin dissection, in an effort to make impact on short- and long-term complications.

Most patients receive at least preoperative if not also postoperative prophylactic antibiotics, despite findings from at least one small and probably underpowered prospective randomized trial that was unable to demonstrate any benefit. If antibiotics are given, most evidence suggests that they should be limited to a single preoperative dose, given within 1 hour prior to skin incision. Repeated and long-term use of antibiotics is to be discouraged.

Many patients also receive perioperative prophylactic heparin to minimize the probability of deep venous thrombosis (DVT). An older small, prospective, randomized trial evaluating the impact of prophylactic unfractionated heparin was unable to demonstrate any reduction in DVT, at the expense of a slightly increased risk of bleeding complications. No comparable trial using low molecular weight heparin has been performed. In the absence of a specific contraindication, it would seem reasonable to use the same DVT prophylactic regimen as employed in other major surgical procedures.

We prefer early ambulation, either on the day of or the morning after surgery. Patients undergoing superficial groin dissection are usually discharged on the day of or the day after surgery, and those undergoing pelvic lymphadenectomy usually require 3 or 4 days in hospital to achieve adequate pain control and to resume a normal diet. Prior to discharge, patients are instructed in drain management as the amount of drainage usually determines when the drains are ready for removal. Closed suction drains are left in until the output is consistently less than 50 mL/day for a few consecutive days, usually 2 to 3 weeks. In rare cases of persistent high drain output exceeding those guidelines, drains may generally be safely removed at 4 to 5 weeks, once the flaps are firmly adherent to underlying muscle, without significant adverse sequelae.

We instruct the patients to keep their legs elevated when they are not walking to avoid short-term edema. Others have advocated early institution of elastic compression stockings. The impact of these recommendations on the ultimate degree of lymphedema is unknown. In the long term, once the drains are out and the wound is healed, we encourage patients to resume their normal activities.

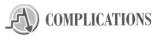 COMPLICATIONS

Adverse events following superficial and deep groin dissection can be separated into short- and long-term events. In the short term, the most common complication recorded following groin dissection is wound infection. The severity of infection can range from a mild cellulitis to infection of an underlying seroma with abscess formation. Wound infection may be associated with skin-edge necrosis from devascularized flaps. If the infection does not respond to oral or parenteral antibiotics, the wound may need to be formally opened and drained. These complications can be quite devastating, particularly in obese patients, those who are most likely to experience them. Large open wounds may be treated with repeated wet-to-dry gauze packing, or by application of a vacuum wound care system. Fortunately, virtually all of these wounds will heal within 3 to 6 weeks with aggressive local wound care, no matter how bad they look initially.

Any surgical procedure is associated with a small but finite incidence of bleeding and/or DVT. The latter can be quite difficult to detect clinically because the ipsilateral leg is often somewhat swollen. The clinician should have a low threshold for obtaining a Doppler ultrasound study of the venous circulation if there is any clinical suspicion of DVT.

Another inevitable sequela of this operation is sacrifice of some of the cutaneous nerve branches enervating the anterior thigh. This often leads to a troubling sense of numbness. Patients should be counseled prior to surgery to expect this so they are not surprised by it.

The most universal and troubling long-term complication of groin dissection is lymphedema. Although the true incidence of lymphedema is impossible to quantify based on retrospective studies, in large part because of inconsistent definitions of the condition, it is my observation that virtually everyone who has a groin dissection will develop some degree of lymphatic stasis in the leg. This can range from quite mild, almost unnoticeable, to quite severe and disabling. Significant lymphedema is often predicted by the amount of lymphatic drainage retrieved by the postoperative suction drains. Identified risk factors for lymphedema consistently include patient obesity and older age, and less consistently include operative factors such as thin skin flaps, transverse incisions, sacrifice of the saphenous vein or muscle fascia, and transposition of the sartorius muscle. It is not clear that deep groin dissection contributes much to the overall incidence/severity of lymphedema. The incidence/severity of lymphedema is increased if adjuvant radiation therapy is to be used as a component of treatment. Although techniques such as omental flap transposition have been proposed, unfortunately to date there are no proven prophylactic strategies to minimize the incidence/severity of lymphedema.

Management of lymphedema ranges from simple maneuvers, including leg elevation and compression stockings, to more aggressive and time-consuming lymphedema regimens, including sequential pump therapy and manual massage. In cases of moderate-to-severe lymphedema, there is some evidence to suggest that these more intensive regimens may reduce some of the long-term sequelae. Diuretics are generally ineffective in ameliorating lymphedema following lymph node dissection.

Patients who develop chronic long-term lymphedema are more susceptible to cellulitis, presumably because of impaired lymphatic clearance of bacteria. These patients should be vigilant about breaks in the skin, including trauma and even fungal foot infections. Any episodes of cellulitis should be treated aggressively.

SUMMARY

Groin dissection is an operation performed for malignancy involving inguinofemoral and/or ileo-obturator lymph nodes. With the advent of sentinel lymph node biopsy, this procedure is being undertaken much less commonly for cutaneous malignancies, no longer for the 80% of melanoma patients with histologically negative nodes. Nonetheless, in the patients who require the procedure, it still results in very substantial and almost inevitable short- and long-term morbidity, morbidity for which there is no known preventive maneuver. The likelihood of long-term lymphedema is not clearly related to technical details of the procedure, proponents of individual techniques notwithstanding. Patients should be fully informed about these expectations preoperatively to help them cope with them following this procedure.

SUGGESTED READING

Benoit L, Boichot C, Cheynel N, et al. Preventing lymphedema and morbidity with an omentum flap after ilioinguinal lymph node dissection. *Ann Surg Oncol* 2005;12:793.

Bevan-Thomas R, Slaton JW, Pettaway CA. Contemporary morbidity from lymphadenectomy for penile squamous cell carcinoma: the M.D. Anderson Cancer Center Experience. *J Urol* 2002;167:1638.

Bouchot O, Rigaud J, Maillet F, et al. Morbidity of inguinal lymphadenectomy for invasive penile carcinoma. *Eur Urol* 2004;45:761.

Dardarian TS, Gray HJ, Morgan MA, et al. Saphenous vein sparing during inguinal lymphadenectomy to reduce morbidity in patients with vulvar carcinoma. *Gynecol Oncol* 2006;101:140

Gaarenstroom KN, Kenter GG, Trimbos JB, et al. Postoperative complications after vulvectomy and inguinofemoral lymphadenectomy using separate groin incisions. *Int J Gynecol Cancer* 2003;13:522.

Karakousis CP. Surgical procedures and lymphedema of the upper and lower extremity. *J Surg Oncol* 2006;93:87.

Kehoe SM, Abu-Rustum NR. Transperitoneal laparoscopic pelvic and paraaortic lymphadenectomy in gynecologic cancers. *Curr Treat Options Oncol* 2006;7:93.

Klemm P, Marnitz S, Kohler C, et al. Clinical implication of laparoscopic pelvic lymphadenectomy in patients with vulvar cancer and positive groin nodes. *Gynecol Oncol* 2005;99:101.

Micheletti L, Bogliatto F, Massobrio M. Groin lymphadenectomy with preservation of femoral fascia: total inguinofemoral node dissection for treatment of vulvar carcinoma. *World J Surg* 2005;29:1268.

Milathianakis C, Bogdanos J, Karamanolakis D. Morbidity of prophylactic inguinal lymphadenectomy with saphenous vein preservation for squamous cell penile carcinoma. *Int J Urol* 2005;12:776.

Nelson BA, Cookson MS, Smith JA Jr, et al. Complications of inguinal and pelvic lymphadenectomy for squamous cell carcinoma of the penis: a contemporary series. *J Urol* 2004;172:494.

Picciotto F, Volpi E, Zaccagna A, et al. Transperitoneal laparoscopic iliac lymphadenectomy for treatment of malignant melanoma. *Surg Endosc* 2003;17:1536.

Ramirez PT, Slomovitz BM, Soliman PT, et al. Total laparoscopic radical hysterectomy and lymphadenectomy: the M. D. Anderson Cancer Center Experience. *Gynecol Oncol* 2006;102:252.

Rouzier R, Haddad B, Dubernard G, et al. Inguinofemoral dissection for carcinoma of the vulva: effect of modifications of extent and technique on morbidity and survival. *J Am Coll Surg* 2003;196:442.

Schneider C, Brodersen JP, Scheuerlein H, et al. Combined endoscopic and open inguinal dissection for malignant melanoma. *Langenbecks Arch Surg* 2003;388:42.

Scribner DR Jr, Walker JL, Johnson GA, et al. Laparoscopic pelvic and paraaortic lymph node dissection: analysis of the first 100 cases. *Gynecol Oncol* 2001;82:498.

Starritt EC, Joseph D, McKinnon JG, et al. Lymphedema after complete axillary node dissection for melanoma: assessment using a new, objective definition. *Ann Surg* 2004;240:866.

Wu LC, Djohan RS, Liu TS, et al. Proximal vascular pedicle preservation for sartorius muscle flap transposition. *Plast Reconstr Surg* 2006;117:253.

EDITOR'S COMMENT

The excellent chapter provided by Professor Coit of the Memorial Sloan-Kettering Cancer Center in New York provides our reader an excellent treatise on the management of cutaneous neoplasms metastatic to the inguinal (groin) lymph node basin. Such primary tumors have origin from skin and skin appendages, penis, anus, vulva, and other remote sites that are inclusive of prostate, endometrium, cervix, and bladder. Dr. Coit provides a visual review in the excellent figures that accompany the chapter, which properly depict the three-dimensional anatomic relationships and specific areas of caution that are essential to recount and avoid intrinsic injury to contiguous neurovascular structures. As this chapter has focused on lymphadenectomy of metastatic disease, he has specifically excluded the detailed, differential management for tumors of soft tissue origin (benign and malignant variants) that are inclusive of connective tissue tumors.

The author has properly characterized the importance of groin dissection as a *therapeutic intervention* that is principally applied and of great consequence to outcomes for the management of the aforementioned tumors. Specifically, the principal management of groin metastatic disease to lymphatics is surgical therapy and, in itself, may be curative of regional metastases. However, as the author has properly and concisely noted, the frequency of inguinal nodal dissection has dramatically decreased in the past 20 years because of the selectivity for dissection for melanoma metastases of the trunk and the lower extremities. With the application of the sentinel lymph node biopsy championed by Morton et al. (*Arch Surg* 1992; 127:392), following the original report by Cabañas (*Cancer* 1977;39:456) for penile carcinoma, dissection, specifically for melanoma, has decreased for the intermediate thickness and most superficial lesions. Moreover, the selective application of groin dissection for the intermediate-thickness melanoma of the trunk and lower extremity now allows only approximately 20% to 30% of such patients to require the necessity of a groin dissection, thus accounting in great part for the decrease in the application of the procedure for melanoma.

In all circumstances, regardless of thickness, grossly palpable disease that is histologically confirmed by a fine-needle aspiration or open biopsy

(continued)

requires dissection. On occasion, the necessity for removal of ileoinguinal nodes in the superficial groin and/or the ileo-obturator nodes in the deep groin, or both, may be essential for regional control of disease in the presence of known metastatic disease. Further, regardless of the metastatic staging of distal sites, presentations with ulceration skin fixation and bleeding in a physiologically suitable patient should have dissection of the regional nodal basin, which may require the transfer of myocutaneous flaps and/or split-thickness skin graft coverage. The author emphasized that *palliative groin dissection* is indicated in patients with known metastatic disease when control of symptomatic regional disease (bleeding, ulceration, skin fixation) is observed. Such cases should be made on a case-by-case evaluation, but again, only in the physiologically appropriate presentation.

Professor Coit has enumerated the reports using combination open superficial groin dissection with laparoscopic deep pelvic lymphadenectomy for melanoma, as has been described by Picciotto et al. (*Surg Endosc* 2003;17:1536), Schneider et al. (*Langenbecks Arch Surg* 2003;388:42), as well as Trias et al. (*Arch Surg* 1998;133:272). None of these reports provide long-term follow up for outcomes. However, laparoscopic staging and therapy of pelvic nodes increasingly has been accepted in the management of prostate, bladder, and gynecologic tumors, as indicated by the author; the approach is currently being evaluated for metastatic cutaneous tumors, but at present, such studies are immature.

As observed by Nathansohn et al. (*Arch Surg* 2005;140:1172) of the Sackler School of Medicine, Tel Aviv, when there are "previous interventions" (excisional biopsy, incomplete dissection) in a nodal drainage basin for melanoma, this privileged and selective surgical procedure site will enhance the probability for recurrence of melanoma in the surgical field. These authors note that open interventions in a lymph node basin in which there is incomplete clearance of the dissected site represented the only independent prognosticator of failure in the field. This event was evident in 10 (83%) of 12 patients who had failure in the surgical field as compared with only 6 (10%) of 62 patients with other sites of first failure (*P* < 0.001). This effect does not translate into a survival difference; moreover, failure in the surgical field does not appear to be related to patients who have previously undergone sentinel lymph node biopsy for melanoma.

The surgeon must also be cognizant of the possibility of synchronous involvement of the popliteal basin with distal lower extremity melanoma. Such was recently observed by Menes et al. (*Arch Surg* 2004; 139:1002), in which they note that the popliteal basin represents the first site of drainage in approximately 90% of all patients with concurrent drainage to the groin. These authors identify three distinct patterns of drainage to the popliteal region, which may impact overall surgical therapy and the necessity for treatment of the popliteal basin when this site was not properly evaluated in the original surgical management. Thus, the reader should be aware that synchronously palpable popliteal and groin metastases require nodal dissections of *both* areas with presentation of cutaneous tumors/lesions below the knee.

Radical groin dissection and radiotherapy are commonplace for management of advanced squamous cell neoplasms of the pelvis, the vulva, contiguous skin of the anus, and groin, and represent the current standard of care; however, morbidity is significant in both short- and long-term follow-up. The recent report by Janda et al. (*Int J Gynecol Cancer* 2004;14:875) from Australia depicts the grave concern of a diminished vulvar cancer-specific quality of life score that has been developed from a functional questionnaire that follows semistructured interviews for patients treated with vulvar cancer (International Federation of Gynecology and Obstetrics stage 0–III). Patients experienced reduction in several aspects of their quality of life that includes emotional function, physical function, social function, sexuality, and body image. This study brings in focus the grave concern of the impact on quality of life for vulvar cancer-specific reduction in lifestyle.

Although the principal management of histologically confirmed lymphatic metastatic cutaneous malignancies is regional lymphadenectomy, many controversies exist regarding the extent of the surgical intervention. These controversies have included the consideration of lymphatic dissection of unusual locations and the role of adjuvant radiation therapy. Thus, relative to the groin, burden of disease, comorbidity issues, imaging techniques, and the status of Cloquet's node must be considered. Specific to irradiation, perhaps most controversial is the addition of adjuvant radiation therapy following lymphadenectomy. As noted by Balch et al. (*J Clin Oncol* 2001;19:3635), only a small proportion of high-risk patients will benefit from groin dissection should distant metastasis be evident as these patients have a universally poor overall prognosis. Ballo et al. (*Int J Radiation Oncol Biol Phys* 2002; 52:964) note a 29% risk of lymphedema following adjuvant axillary radiation, of which approximately half of the patients are asymptomatic or transient. Further, Stevens et al.

(*Cancer* 2000;88:88) suggest a 58% risk of lymphedema following adjuvant axillary irradiation, while adjuvant inguinal radiation has been recommended less frequently because of the great concern of lymphedema. Thus, the application of adjuvant radiation therapy is controversial as there remains a paucity of phase III trial data as suggested by Ridge (*Ann Surg Oncol* 2000; 7:550) and Mack and McKinnon (*J Surg Oncol* 2004;86:189) to confirm its value.

The surgical dogma regarding excessively radical procedures to dissect lymphatic metastasis of the groin (distal to the inguinal ligament) remains entrenched in our literature for all tumors metastatic to inguinal sites. All accept, however, that the morbidity of the extensive en bloc dissection is significant, thus the need for a procedure of this magnitude has been challenged on the basis that a deep nodal dissection cannot extend distally greater than the saphenofemoral junction. The recent study by Hudson et al. (*Int J Gynecol Cancer* 2004;14:841) of the University of London, targeted anatomic groin dissections from cadavers and observed no nodes deep to the deep fascia that is distal to the saphenous opening. These authors suggest that the cribriform fascia that covers the saphenous opening have nodes of the superficial group evident within fenestrations of the fascia and has accounted for the historic descriptions of deep femoral nodes that are distal to the saphenofemoral junction. These authors conclude that an inguinal lymphadenectomy that is confined to the superficial fascia may fail to include all those nodes that are normally regarded as being within the superficial inguinal group. The authors conclude that neither removal of deep fascia in the femoral triangle, nor its incision with consequent stripping of the femoral veins in the thigh, is necessary in a radical groin dissection. These authors therefore make a strong case for full evaluation of the fascia with preservation techniques as described by Borgno et al. (*J Reprod Med* 1990; 35:1127) for surgical removal of deep (as well as superficial) inguinal lymph nodes. These authors suggest that when there is intent to remove *only* superficial inguinal nodes, the fossa ovalis should be cleared and the saphenofemoral junction dissected. As suggested by Poierier et al. (*Les Lymphatiques* [translated and edited by Leaf CH]. London: Constable, 1903) in his 1903 dissertation, incomplete surgery is relevant as it is a direct correlate of local recurrence.

K.I.B.

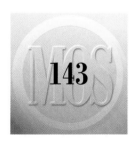

Total Proctectomy with Sphincter Preservation for Distal Rectal Cancer

143

ROBERT W. BEART, JR.

This chapter differentiates itself by dealing with tumors of the lowest part of the rectum. In particular, it deals with the difficult decision-making as when to preserve the rectum and when the patient is best served by removing the rectum, the anus, and surrounding tissues.

Technically, we can restore intestinal continuity in virtually any situation. Even if the sphincter muscles are partially involved, studies have shown that partial resection of the sphincter muscles is consistent with long-term local control. Nevertheless, implied in this chapter

is the fact that the technical ability to do something is not the same as it being in the patient's best interest, and we hope we can shed some light on the techniques and difficult decision-making involved in dealing with very low rectal cancers.

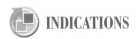 **INDICATIONS**

The rectum is typically defined as the last 12 to 15 cm of the colon. The exact site of measurement for this, however, is unclear. Most studies measure from the anal verge. This measurement is confounded by the fact that the anal canal can be from 1 to 7 cm in length. Therefore, the amount of rectum involved may be from 1 to 8 cm in length. Most people think of the rectum, however, as being 12 to 15 cm in length, and are actually measuring in a cephalad direction from the puborectalis. At best, however, this is an indirect measurement.

The rectum is divided into three portions. The lower third would be considered the distal rectum, the measurement above the puborectalis from 5 to 10 cm would be considered the middle third, and from 10 to 15 cm above the puborectalis would be considered the upper third of the rectum. Increasingly, it is recognized that the patterns of recurrence following the management of these different segments of the colon varies. In current literature, this is influencing the recommendations to use adjuvant and neoadjuvant therapy as well as surgical techniques.

For lesions of the distal third of the rectum, traditionally it has been said that an abdominal perineal resection should be performed. Current surgical techniques allow us to remove virtually any tumor in this area without removing the anal canal. The entire oncologic dissection for a rectal cancer takes place through the abdomen. All of the perirectal and hypogastric lymph nodes to be removed are removed through the abdomen. The only incremental tissue that is removed with an abdominal perineal resection includes a portion of the anus, the anal canal, a portion of the levator muscles, and ischiorectal fat. These are unusual sites for local recurrence in patients who have a low anterior resection. Therefore, it is only when these structures are directly involved that they need to be removed. Rather than using the traditional "5-cm rule" to determine which patient should have an abdominal perineal resection, during the last 15 to 20 years we have relied on the anatomic relationships to predict whether an abdominal perineal resection should be performed. If the tumor is distinct from the puborectalis muscle, usually within a distance of 1 to 2 cm, we are comfortable in counseling the patient preoperatively that they will not require a permanent colostomy. We may choose to perform a temporary diversion, particularly in patients who have had

neoadjuvant therapy. However, the surgeon who is technically adept at operating in this area can routinely use one of several techniques to remove the tumor and all of the lymph node-bearing tissue. There is no oncologic advantage to removing the anal canal in this situation.

Recent articles have even suggested that if a portion of the puborectalis or anal canal is involved, this can be resected en bloc with the tumor, and the anal canal can be reconstructed to preserve intestinal continuity. We have done this and found it not particularly difficult technically, but still think it should be considered an experimental procedure. It is important that patients come to understand that the need for a colostomy is rare today. A previous study by the American Cancer Society suggested that upward of 80% of people in this country believe that if they get colon cancer it means they need a colostomy. This deters many patients from seeking screening and early detection. This is analogous to the period of time when women thought they automatically would lose their breast for breast cancer. It is important for surgeons to develop the surgical techniques to avoid colostomies and let their patients know that it is rare that a colostomy should be required.

 PREOPERATIVE PLANNING

Bowel Preparation

Beginning in 1964 with the publication by Washington and Judd, bowel preparation has been the standard of the management of patients scheduled for colonic resection. More recent studies, however, suggest that the bowel preparation may not only be unnecessary, but in fact may be harmful. Our own experience during the last year suggests that bowel preparation is not routinely necessary. We have not used it in any of our elective cases, and have not recognized an increase in any infectious complications. This would decrease the discomfort to the patient. Occasionally, we have encountered patients with excessive bulky stool in the colon. This is usually milked into the resected segment. However, even leaving firm stool behind has not posed a problem in our practice. Our preoperative bowel preparation then consists only of a Fleet enema given shortly before surgery in patients whom we think will need a stapling device. In addition, we use preoperative second-generation cephalosporins for systemic coverage.

Counseling the Patient

It is very important to counsel patients preoperatively in order that they can handle the postoperative events. In particular, because a rectal reservoir is being removed, the patient will undergo an adjustment period characterized by stool frequency and urgency. If they recognize this preoperatively, they are more likely to accept its inconvenience. The symptoms during this period can be minimized through the use of fiber and antidiarrheal agents such as Lomotil. We have also found that, in some patients who have multiple urgent bowel movements, hycosamine has been helpful in relieving the symptoms of this irritable bowel.

The patient should similarly be counseled as to how long he or she will be in the hospital, whether or not drains will be used, and the possibility that a stoma may be required. It should be the exception that patients are not given good advice as to whether intestinal continuity can be restored. As indicated, this is a decision that can be made routinely based on the physical findings prior to surgery and the tumors relationship to the anal canal.

Stoma Siting

All patients should be seen by an enterostomal therapist prior to surgery. Even if a stoma is not anticipated, it is good practice to have the patient seen and have a stoma discussed. If anastomotic complications develop postoperatively, the patients will be prepared and enlightened as to the need and mechanisms of a stoma. If a stoma is placed intraoperatively, it is important that it be sited to minimize postoperative morbidity. Stomas sited in skin creases or beltlines are a perpetual nuisance and compromise appliance function. This is a totally avoidable problem if the patients are seen preoperatively.

Although we counsel all patients having colonic surgery about stomas and ask the enterostomal therapist to site the stomas on both sides of the abdomen, the use of stomas is variable in our practice. We do not believe proximal diversion is mandated for all rectal anastomosis. The local conditions dictate whether we recommend diversion. Other surgeons, however, believe that all patients with anastomoses in this area should have diversion. This clearly is an individual preference as there are no data that scientifically prove that one decision is better than the other. In particular, however, for patients who have had radiation therapy, we frequently think the tissues are less healthy and there is a recognized increase in leak rate following neoadjuvant therapy.

Obstructing Tumors

If the patient presents with an obstructing tumor, we would prefer to stent this tumor, then carry out neoadjuvant therapy, and then proceed with surgery. Stenting allows the bowel to be more completely cleansed, but also allows the dilated bowel proximally to contract down to its more nearly normal size, which is often unhealthy and does not heal well. Some would advocate neoadjuvant therapy because it shrinks the size of the tumor. We find that neoadjuvant therapy does not alter our margins of resection, and only rarely does it shrink the tumor in a way that makes the operation any easier.

Neoadjuvant Therapy

Recent studies have suggested that preoperative radiation and chemotherapy is more effective than postoperative radiation neotherapy. Although statistically significant in a large number of patients, it is a very small significance when dealing with an individual patient. I think either of these approaches will benefit the patient. There is clearly an increasing trend to use neoadjuvant therapy. However, in large studies, only about 5% of the patients truly benefit from the neoadjuvant therapy. This means most patients do not benefit and this provides an opportunity to be selective in the use of neoadjuvant therapy. Clearly, for T1 and T2 tumors, we would not use neoadjuvant therapy. Even for T3 tumors in the upper rectum, we would not think that it is necessary. However, for lesions in the lower rectum, there seems to be a higher local recurrence rate and we tend to use it more aggressively. In addition, it is conceptually attractive to radiate the rectum, then remove this radiated tissue and replace it with nonradiated bowel from higher in the abdomen. This should function better in the long run and develop a better reservoir, as well as have fewer problems such as stool frequency and anastomotic dehiscence.

Basic Principles

There are two parts to this operation. The first is removing the bowel and the second is putting things back together again.

The removal of the bowel is done the same regardless of which techniques are being used to restore intestinal continuity. The entire dissection is done through the abdomen and includes a total mesorectal excision deep into the pelvis. Landmarks in our practice include exposure of Waldeyer's fascia posteriorly. This is a few cell layers wider than the standard fascia propria dissection described by Heald. I think either dissection level is fine, but it is important to recognize that this is an avascular plane without lymphatics and can be rapidly dissected sharply or bluntly. As one moves around to the lateral aspects of the rectum, it is important to stay outside the fascia propria. Perhaps an even better margin, which we try to use routinely, is to expose the hypogastric vessels laterally. This plane is easy to dissect, it is avascular, and it is only as you get deeper into the pelvis that you encounter vascular structures. It has also been demonstrated that lymphatics traverse this tissue in the lower third of the rectum. Staying medial to this plane, deep in the pelvis, it is important to avoid the nervi erigentes. These can be identified and preserved.

Anteriorly, one dissects the rectum from the vagina in the female patient. If the vagina is involved, we would recommend taking a portion of the vagina. This does not necessarily imply removing the anal sphincter mechanism. If the anal sphincter mechanism is involved, clearly this should be removed as well and an abdominal perineal resection should be performed. In either case, the vagina can be closed primarily, or it can be closed with a rectus abdominus flap. In the male patient, there is debate as to whether one should stay ventral or dorsal to Denonvilliers' fascia. In most of our patients, we will stay dorsal to this. We find this plane to be easier to dissect and have fewer risks of bleeding from the prostate. There has been no proven oncologic benefit to one dissection or the other.

Nerve preservation has become increasingly important, particularly in male patients. As the rectum is mobilized off the sacral promontory, the sympathetic nerves can be identified visually. If one has lifted the tissue right off the sacral promontory, then the nerves will go with the specimen and one can palpate them along the posterior wall of the mesorectum. These can be dissected free and followed deep into the pelvis. Staying just medial to these sympathetic nerves is consistent with a mesorectal dissection.

Patient Selection

Enough has been discussed already about proper patient selection. It has been demonstrated that continence preservation can be extended beyond what has been historic criteria. If there is an obstructing lesion and diversion preoperatively is necessary, we would favor a right transverse loop colostomy or an ileostomy. If the stoma is placed in the left transverse colon, the descending colon, or the sigmoid, then mobilization of this portion of the bowel may be compromised and the ability to restore intestinal continuity can be limited. Increasingly, diversion preoperatively is less necessary with the use of endorectal stenting, and we have found this to be a very satisfactory alternative.

Oncologic Considerations

As previously indicated, neoadjuvant therapy is increasingly common. This is usually given as a combination of radiation and chemotherapy. The exact nature of the chemotherapy is evolving and there are multiple major studies looking at different regimens. It is important to emphasize, however, that the majority of patients will not benefit from neoadjuvant therapy and the surgeon should become selective in offering it only to those patients who are at increased risk for needing the therapy. Offering it to low-risk patients in whom the risks of local recurrence are low increases morbidity to no advantage of the patient.

The philosophy of resection is based on an understanding of the patterns of recurrence. Recurrence after the removal of a low rectal cancer almost never occurs along the levator muscles or in the ischiorectal fat unless an abdominal perineal resection is performed. Rather, the tumors tend to recur in the presacral space or along the hypogastric lymph nodes. The hypogastric lymph nodes are not routinely removed in the United States for a low anterior resection. Randomized prospective studies from Japan have strongly suggested that there is improved survival if these lymph nodes are removed in patients with stage 3 disease. Because the anal canal, ischiorectal fat, and distal levator muscles are rarely involved with recurrence, routine removal of these structures should not be necessary.

It is recognized that the distal-third cancers seem to behave differently than tumors in the proximal two thirds of the rectum. They tend to have more lateral spread, and they have a higher local recurrence rate. Whether this is from technical problems with the operations or differences in biologic behavior is not clear. Our published studies, however, suggest that local recurrences of 5% are achievable in this area and without routine neoadjuvant therapy.

Physiologic Considerations

Physiologically, there are three important considerations.

Nerve Preservation

Nerve preservation was previously discussed, and we strongly advocate nerve preservation in the male patient. This does not totally obviate postoperative impotence and urinary retention, particularly if neoadjuvant therapy is used. The combination of radiation and surgery seems to have an increased risk of injury to these nerves. Nevertheless, the ultimate goal of the surgery is local control, and this clearly should take precedence over concerns about physiologic dysfunction.

Postoperative Sphincter Function

A second concern is postoperative sphincter function. If the anus is dramatically dilated by using traditional anal retractors, sphincter function has been shown to be compromised. Postoperative continence will be a function of not only reservoir function, but also sphincter function, and efforts should be made to minimize this trauma. Use of the Lone Star (Lone Star Medical Products Inc. Stafford, TX) retractor seems to be one way of minimizing the trauma to the anal canal and helping to preserve continence, and we have found this to be a very good retractor, particularly for the coloanal anastomosis.

Rectal Reservoir Function

Probably more important than preserving anal sphincter function is preserving rectal reservoir function. For tumors in the lower rectum, attention should be paid to the reservoir. Many people have advocated the routine use of a pouch in this area. Although the J pouch would be the most common type of pouch, we find this very difficult to bring low into the pelvis, and particularly into the anal canal. In these patients, we have tended to use a proctoplasty as described by the Cleveland Clinic. This has been shown to help with stool frequency and certainly fits in the anal canal better than a J pouch. However, it is recognized that reservoir function is similar after 6 months whether a pouch has been used or not. Some patients with a pouch find after 6 months that they are bothered by obstipation. It would seem that these patients are unable to empty their pouches well. Therefore, we recommend a selective approach. If the bowel being sewn into the distal rectum or anal canal is large enough to accept a 33-mm

stapler, then we do not routinely incorporate a reservoir. We think these patients develop a good reservoir over time and think they may be harmed by creating a reservoir. Management of obstipation in these patients is very difficult, and anatomic relationships that cause it should be avoided.

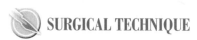

SURGICAL TECHNIQUE

There are two fundamental procedures that are performed in patients with distal rectal disease.

The abdominal dissection will be the same regardless of the continence-preserving technique to be used. First, I would like to describe the abdominal dissection.

Abdominal Dissection

The surgery is performed under general anesthesia with the patient in the modified lithotomy position. The legs should be slightly elevated so that the ankles are above the heart in the prone position. The patient will subsequently be placed in Trendelenburg position, which will keep blood flow from the legs, minimizing postoperative clotting. We favor the placement of sequential compression devices around the calf during the surgery. The legs should be slightly bent. If they are too bent, they will tend to interfere with the arm of the surgeon during the pelvic dissection. The gluteus area should be placed just over the distal end of the table. This helps to keep the patient from sliding when placed in Trendelenburg, and also assures adequate access to the anus for continence-preserving procedures. The entire abdomen is prepared from above the costal margin down to perineum and then to the legs, and draped. The vagina should similarly be prepared in anticipation of a potential access to the vagina. A Foley catheter is placed and drapes are placed over the abdomen and legs during the entire sterile field. Some surgeons choose to irrigate the rectum with Betadine, and this would be a good time to do that to minimize contamination at a later point.

Antibiotics are used preoperatively. Recent controversy has evolved as to whether a bowel preparation is necessary, as has been previously discussed. We have not used a bowel preparation for about 1 year, and have not recognized any adverse consequences. A second-generation cephalosporin should be used. Broader spectrum antibiotics are acceptable, but should be used for only 24 hours. Even if there is some contamination, that is all that is generally necessary. For excessive

contamination, the antibiotics may be continued for up to 5 days.

A midline infraumbilical incision is all that is generally necessary. Occasionally, we extend the incision to the side or slightly above the umbilicus in those patients whose xiphoid-to-pubic distance is short. We prefer to keep the anterior abdominal wall intact. This allows us to pack the small intestine out of the way. After the incision is made, care should be taken to extend it all the way down to just above the pubic bone. The abdomen is inspected in the usual fashion. The patient can then be placed in slight Trendelenburg. A self-retaining retractor can be used to maintain the incision in an open position, and a moist towel is used to pack the small intestine up into the upper abdomen. This gives excellent exposure to the pelvis. At a later point, it may be necessary to extend this incision if the splenic flexion needs to be mobilized. The dissection is initiated along the left lateral border of the sigmoid, which is completely mobilized. The ureter is identified and the sigmoid is then placed back into its original position. The sigmoid is then placed on traction and an incision is made along the right side of the peritoneum, right at the base of the mesorectum and sigmoid mesentery. This should not be made too far lateral to the right as it will increase the risk of injury to the ureter, and it should not be made high on the mesentery of the rectum and sigmoid as this increases the risk of getting into the sigmoid mesentery and bleeding.

With the rectum on traction, the presacral space is entered bluntly and the rectum can be reflected bluntly out through the sacrum and pushed forward. This is an avascular space, which allows for ease in mobilization. There are no lymphatics or blood vessels going across this space and you can proceed with aggressive dissection at this point. This should be carried out until it is no longer easy and visibility is compromised; then the dissection begins with movement around the rectum. The peritoneum is incised on both sides of the rectum and sharp dissection is used along the fascia propria of the rectum. The fascia propria of rectum is defined posteriorly and a midline sulcus or groove can be seen, which helps to assure the surgeon that the fascia is intact. The same fascia extends laterally and can be dissected sharply from the surrounding structures. The nerves should be identified prior to beginning the lateral dissection. The sacral sympathetic nerves are easy to identify. They may have been left on the sacrum if the dissection was slightly above the sacrum. Alternatively, they may have been lifted up with the rectal specimen. If they are, they can be palpated along the posterior rectal mesentery and sigmoid mesentery, and should be dissected free laterally. Dissection is generally carried out medial to these nerves. We do like to expose the hypogastric vessels on both sides. We think this is an even more reliable and definable plane than just trying to stay close to the fascia propria. As exposure is compromised laterally, the dissection is continued anteriorly by incising the peritoneum and then bluntly dissecting between the rectum and vagina. Once the plane is clearly identified, sharp dissection is used to complete the dissection.

The dissection then proceeds in a circular fashion around the rectum, cutting the tissue that is on tension. When the tissue is no longer on tension, another area should be dissected where there is tension. This dissection is carried down posteriorly until the coccyx is reached. Then a sharp transection of the inner coccygeal ligament is carried out, and an additional 3 to 4 cm of dissection can be carried out posteriorly to the point where the rectum meets the puborectalis muscle. Similarly, the dissection is carried out laterally to the puborectalis muscle and anteriorly under the vagina as far as possible or to a point below the level of the prostate gland. Once the mobilization has been completed, the decision needs to be made as to how to proceed with transection of the rectum. If the tumor is palpable and the mobilization has resulted in the tumor being lifted up to a point where a TA stapling device (Ethicon Corp. Cincinnati, OH) can be placed below it, this is desirable. Several centimeters of tissue should be excised below the tumor. This is usually a position well below the mesentery of the rectum, resulting in a total mesorectal excision. Generally, only a TA-30 stapler will fit in this position. A 45 stapler is usually too large to fit deeply into the pelvis. The rectum can then be transected distally.

After the presacral space is entered, attention should be turned to ligating the inferior mesenteric artery. This tissue can be dissected up above the bifurcation of the aorta, which is the point of transection. It is not necessary to go through the origin of the inferior mesenteric artery routinely. There is always a vascular bundle and a clear space to the patient's left of this vascular bundle. With the left hand placed around the bundle, the forefinger can be brought to this clear space, isolating the bundle. A right-angled clamp can then be placed in one or two bites across the pedicle, and the pedicle is divided. Care should

be taken after clamping, but before dividing the pedicle, to reinspect the ureter to make sure that it is not being grasped in the clamp. The ureter runs about 1 cm away from this pedicle, and if not careful, it can be caught in the clamp. After the pedicle is transected, we continue the mesenteric dissection up into the distal, descending, or proximal sigmoid colon. There has not been any proven value for removing a large portion of the sigmoid. It is most important to get this inferior mesenteric pedicle and the associated lymph nodes. Therefore, it is sometimes prudent to identify a point in the midsigmoid and dissect the mesentery to that point and ligate the vessels.

After the rectum is transected, the sigmoid can be divided similarly at the previously identified point. If the sigmoid is large enough to accept a 33-mm stapler, we tend to not want to fashion a pouch. It has been our experience that patients with a larger sigmoid tend to develop a good reservoir. A pouch tends to cause the patients to become obstipated with time. If, however, the sigmoid or descending colon is small and does not accept a 33-mm stapler, we would recommend doing a proctoplasty at this point. This is usually carried out approximately 4 cm proximal to the transected margin. We then use a 29-mm circular stapler to reanastomose the descending colon to the rectum. If necessary, this is the point at which the left colon and splenic flexure can be mobilized to get adequate length. In mobilizing the mesentery of the descending colon, the usual tension point will be along the medial aspects of the mesentery. Both the left colic artery and inferior mesenteric vein tend to be the limiting factors. These need to be ligated.

Following the ligation of these vascular structures, it is important to assess the vascularity of the cut end of the sigmoid or descending colon. It would be nice to see active arterial bleeding from this surface. A 29-mm circular stapler can then be placed into the proximal bowel, and this can be anastomosed to the rectum under direct vision. Care must be taken not to include the vagina or seminal vessels in this anastomosis. Following the anastomosis, we must evaluate whether there is any tension on the bowel. If there is, additional mesenteric and left colon mobilization should be carried out until the bowel lies in the hollow of the sacrum.

Coloanal Anastomosis

If, on the other hand, there were not several centimeters of bowel below the tumor, then a mucosal dissection and coloanal

anastomosis should be performed. Following the complete mobilization of the rectum and transection of the bowel, attention is turned to the perineum, where a Lone Star retractor is placed in the perineum and the anal mucosa is exposed. The anal mucosa can be dissected from the underlying sphincter complex easily. Some choose to inject epinephrine containing saline. I have generally not done that and have not had any difficulty. The mucosa is sharply dissected from the anal canal. This dissection is facilitated if a lap pad is placed deep behind the rectum, which can easily be palpated from below, through the rectum. Once the mucosal dissection is carried through to this level, the rectum can be transected as one is assured that they are above the sphincter mechanism. The lap pad can then be removed, the finger can be placed through the hole in the posterior rectal muscle, and the finger can then be placed along the right side of the rectum, which can be brought down into the clear vision. This can be divided with cautery. In a similar way, the left side of the rectal muscle is divided with cautery under direct vision. The hand can then be placed through the anus and above the rectum, between the rectum and the vagina or the prostate, and traction can be placed into the anal canal, and the anterior rectal muscle can be divided.

At this point, the rectum should be completely free and can be withdrawn through the anus, minimizing the risk of any spillage into the pelvis. A long Allis clamp is then placed through the anus. The proximal bowel is grasped and brought down into the anal canal. Care must be taken to make sure there is no tension on this bowel. We anchor the bowel into the anal canal with four 2-0 Vicryl sutures (Ethicon Corp. New Brunswick, NJ), placed approximately 1 cm above the cut end of the rectum, and into the anal muscle. We then use 2-0 Vicryl sutures to suture the full-thickness rectum into the dentate line. This is generally done with about four sutures in each quadrant. That complete, the Lone Star retractor can then be removed. One technical note is that we use a UR-6 needle on our sutures. This is a 5/8 circle needle, which makes rotating it within the relatively narrow anal much easier. We then turn our attention to the abdomen.

The anastomosis is now completed. Care is taken to make sure that there is no tension on the bowel, that it is laying in the hollow of the sacrum, and that there it is no bow-stringing across the pelvis. Although controversial, we tend to place drains in the pelvis for at least a short period of time. This is based on work that suggests that at least 50% of anastomotic leaks will be controlled by the drains and may minimize the need for further surgery.

Postoperative complications after this surgery are real. One should recognize the potential for increased risk of embolic disease, and prophylactic anticoagulation should be considered. Anastomotic leaks are increased in the lower third of the rectum. We do not routinely divert these patients with a stoma, but if there is evidence of pelvic scarring or any unfavorable anatomic features, then we would favor a temporary loop ileostomy. We would allow patients to recover, regain their health, and cease taking all medications; we would anticipate closing the loop ileostomy approximately 6 weeks following their resection. Patients are encouraged to resume a liquid diet on the 2nd postoperative day, and the diet is advanced as the patient tolerates it. Drains are removed when the fluid is serous, generally on the 5th day. The Foley catheter is generally left in place because of the patient's limited ambulation until about the 5th day, at which time that is also removed. Urinary retention is increased, particularly in male patients, following this surgery. If urinary retention occurs, we teach patients to self-catheterize and send them home on that regimen. During several weeks to months, we would expect that they begin to urinate more easily, with a lower residual of urine. Once the residual of urine is less than 100 mL, we discontinue the self-catheterization.

SUGGESTED READING

Camilleri-Brennan J, Ruta DA, Steele RJ. Patient generated index: new instrument for measuring quality of life in patients with rectal cancer. *World J Surg* 2002;26:1354.

Dimick JB, Cowan JA Jr, Upchurch GR Jr, et al. Hospital volume and surgical outcomes for elderly patients with colorectal cancer in the United States. *J Surg Res* 2003;114:50.

Faerden AE, Naimy N, Wiik P, et al. Total mesorectal excision for rectal cancer: difference in outcome for low and high rectal cancer. *Dis Colon Rectum* 2005;48:2224.

Gastinger I, Marusch F, Steinert R, et al., and Working Group 'Colon/Rectum Carcinoma.' Protective defunctioning stoma in low anterior resection for rectal carcinoma. *Br J Surg* 92: 2005;1137-1142, 2005.

Guillem JG, Chessin DB, Cohen AM, et al. Long-term oncologic outcome following preoperative combined modality therapy and total mesorectal excision of locally advanced rectal cancer. *Ann Surg* 2005;241:829.

Heald RJ, Smedh RK, Kald A, et al. Abdominoperineal excision of the rectum—an endangered operation. Norman Nigro Lectureship. *Dis Colon Rectum.* 1997;40(7):747–751.

Ho YH, Brown S, Heah SM, et al. Comparison of J-pouch and coloplasty pouch for low rectal cancers: a randomized, controlled trial investigating functional results and comparative anastomotic leak rates. *Ann Surg* 2002;236:49.

Jeong SY, Chessin DB, Guillem JG. Surgical treatment of rectal cancer: radical resection. *Surg Oncol Clin North Am* 2006;15:95.

Laurent A, Parc Y, McNamara D, et al. Colonic J-pouch-anal anastomosis for rectal cancer: a prospective, randomized study comparing handsewn vs. stapled anastomosis. *Dis Colon Rectum* 2005; 48:729.

Marusch F, Koch A, Schmidt U, et al. Value of a protective stoma in low anterior resections for rectal cancer. *Dis Colon Rectum* 2002;45:1164.

Marusch F, Koch A, Schmidt U, et al. Impact of age on the short-term postoperative outcome of patients undergoing surgery for colorectal carcinoma. *Int J Colorectal Dis* 2002;17:177.

Renehan AG, Egger M, Saunders MP, et al. Impact on survival of intensive follow up after curative resection for colorectal cancer: systematic review and meta-analysis of randomised trials. *BMJ* 2002;324:813.

Rullier E, Laurent C, Bretagnol F, et al. Sphincter-saving resection for all rectal carcinomas: the end of the 2-cm distal rule. *Ann Surg* 2005;241:465.

Sauer R, Becker H, Hohenberger W, et al., and German Rectal Cancer Study Group. Preoperative versus postoperative chemoradiotherapy for rectal cancer. *N Engl J Med* 2004;351:1731.

Wasserberg N, Kaiser AM, Nunoo-Mensah JW, et al. Preservation of bowel and urinary continence in the management of locally recurrent rectal cancer. *J Surg Oncol* 2005; 92:76

EDITOR'S COMMENT

As Professor Beart states in his clear exposition of carcinoma of the rectum, the emphasis in carcinoma of the low rectum has now completely changed from extirpation of the entire rectum, such as was proposed by the Miles operation of abdominal perineal resection, to preservation of both rectal continence and the sphincter itself, thus obviating the need for a permanent colostomy. Indeed, in every survey concerning colonic surgery, it is clear that the greatest fear of patients is to "wear a bag." In my own practice, one has to reassure patients undergoing right colectomy that they will not end up with a permanent colostomy. Moreover, one does not know how many patients delay presenting for obvious symptoms of carcinoma of the colon because of their abhorrence of wearing a bag. Most studies of patients with carcinoma of the colon reveal that the average duration of symptoms prior to presenting for medical and surgical care is approximately 8 months, a delay partly from physicians not even doing a rectal examination for rectal bleeding and from patients ignoring symptoms for fear of a colostomy. Thus, the emphasis here is well placed.

Things have changed dramatically in the past decade, largely because of the presence of neoadjuvant and postoperative radiochemotherapy. Early experiences with a coloanal anastomosis, notably at Memorial and elsewhere, revealed that the coloanal type of anastomosis should be limited to patients whose lesions were above 5.5 cm in the stretched state from the anal verge. Indeed, my own experience with numerous coloanal anastomoses was that patients below this level almost invariably had a recurrence and died a rather painful death. However, this was before neoadjuvant therapy. Now, maintenance of continence has enabled one to excise cancers of the rectum even when they impinge or actually invade the rectal sphincter, and to carry out not only coloanal anastomoses but, by excising the rectal and anal margins thus leaving the sphincter intact, also what is basically perineal colostomy. The other aspect of this with small lesions is local excision, probably for which between 10% and 15% of patients presenting or being found on screening colonoscopy qualify. Here again, postoperative adjuvant therapy with both radiation and chemotherapy may enable one to "get away with" local excision without compromising long-term survival.

Dr. Beart also touches on the question of colonic preparation. Recent studies, notably from the colon and rectal groups, indicate that the time-honored mechanical preparation (the Nichols preparation is seemingly becoming extinct rather rapidly) has been questioned, with good data suggesting that patients undergoing a mechanical preparation actually do less well than patients in whom this is omitted. It is difficult to find in the literature what one is talking about with a mechanical preparation. Dr. Beart is one of the few people who is specific, saying that he uses no mechanical preparation except, perhaps, an enema for rectal lesions.

The issue of whether colonic J pouches empty better or worse, or actually facilitate normal recovery to a state more resembling the preoperative resection of carcinoma of the rectum, is the subject of numerous articles. The first thing that one must remember is normal rectal physiology. The area above the columns of Morgagni consists of columnar epithelium. Pain is obviously absent, but there is deep proprioception, and the normal physiological function of this area for approximately 5 cm above the tops of the columns is to relay the urge to defecate. This obviously is excised during operations for cancer of the rectum, in my experience, this is what patients following low anterior anastomoses take longest to establish, perhaps as long as 2 or 3 years, not surprising in view of the complicated neural nets that are necessary to be re-established.

An early analysis of coloanal anastomosis was reported by Velez et al.(*Am J Surg* 1999;177:467), who summarized 52 patients operated on for a low-lying rectal lesion with an "external coloanal anastomosis" (perineal colostomy). Fecal continence was apparently normal in 70%, 18% had mild incontinence, 6% had moderate incontinence (defined as frequent episodes of incontinence causing important interference in normal activity), and 6% were completely incontinent. Five patients receiving preoperative chemotherapy and radiation did not, in

(continued)

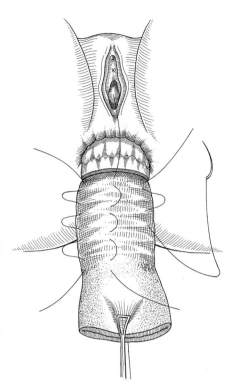

Fig. 8. After the mucosal sleeve is stripped from the muscularis, plication of this layer is performed using longitudinal sutures.

placed in the four quadrants (Fig. 10). Once the anastomosis is complete it usually is pulled back spontaneously into the anal canal (Fig. 11).

This treatment strategy may represent a good alternative for patients with small rectal prolapse or internal prolapse. Sphincteroplasty can be added to the Delorme

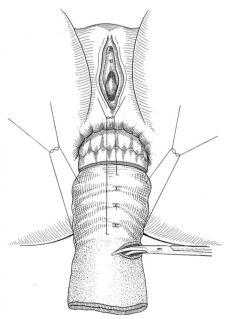

Fig. 9. Plication of the muscular layer is followed by resection of the excess of stripped mucosa.

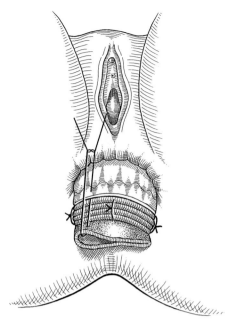

Fig. 10. Mucosal coloanal anastomosis is performed with interrupted absorbable sutures

procedure in patients with fecal incontinence to improve results. Complications may include bleeding, leakage, stricture, and fecal incontinence.

Perineal Rectosigmoidectomy with Coloanal Anastomosis (Altemeier Procedure)

Prolapse Delivery

The rectal prolapse is delivered through the anus using Babcock clamps (Fig. 12). Once everted, the prolapsed segment consists of an outer tube of rectum attached to the dentate line and an inner tube of rectum attached to the sigmoid colon. Epinephrine solution (1:200,000) is injected circumferentially in the submucosal layer, 1.5 cm proximal to the dentate line to minimize bleeding.

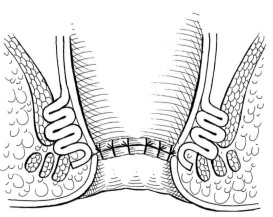

Fig. 11. Final aspect of the anastomosis and underlying muscular plication.

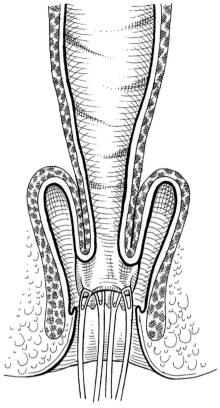

Fig. 12. Rectal prolapse is delivered through the anus by Babcock clamps.

Incision

A circumferential incision is initiated with the posterior outer rectal wall, 1.5 to 2 cm from the dentate line, preserving the entire transitional zone of the anal canal. To obtain symmetry of the incision, marking it with electrocautery may be helpful (Fig. 13). Our preference is to begin by sectioning the posterior wall first (Fig. 14). The incision is made through all layers of the outer rectal wall and deepened until the perirectal fat is encountered and the mesorectum identified. Care should be taken not to damage the mesorectal vessels and to

The Gastrointestinal Tract

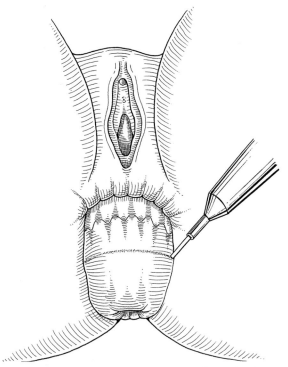

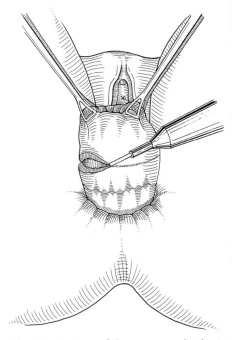

Fig. 13. Incision is circumferentially marked 1.5 cm cranially to the dentate line by electrocautery.

Fig. 14. Incision of the outer rectal tube is made, initiating at the posterior aspect.

avoid simultaneous transection of the inner rectal wall.

Rectal Mobilization

Mobilization of the rectum proceeds cranially with careful isolation and ligation of mesorectal vessels close to the intestinal wall. Division of the mesorectal vessels is continued until there is resistance to gentle traction. At this point, a sliding hernia of peritoneum (cul-de-sac) is visible and should be opened to facilitate sigmoid mobilization and allow palpation of intraperitoneal contents (Fig. 15). Division of the mesorectum and mesosigmoid continues until the redundant rectum and sigmoid are adequately mobilized. Careful control of the mesentery with vessel ligation is imperative to prevent retraction of bleeding vessels into the pelvis (Fig. 16). If there is excessive hernia sac tissue, resection should be performed to avoid anterior intussusception. Closure of the hernia sac is not routinely performed; however, some surgeons prefer to close it with a continuous absorbable suture.

Levatorplasty

The colon is drawn anteriorly to enable appropriate visualization of the levator ani muscles. These posterior muscles are approximated with interrupted 2-0 nonabsorbable sutures; usually only two to three stitches are necessary (Fig. 17). Anterior levatorplasty can also be associated to the

posterior levatorplasty to further narrow the opening of the anal canal. The rectum should fit loosely in the opening, allowing a finger to be inserted along its side. This modification to the Altemeier procedure proposed by Prasad et al. restores the angles of the pelvic floor, which may reduce recurrence and improve incontinence.

Anastomosis

Before sectioning the proximal colon, arterial patency is tested by dividing the

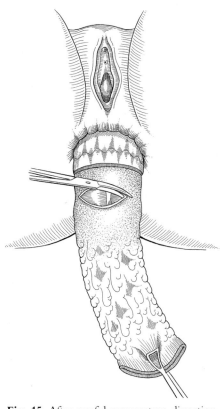

Fig. 15. After careful mesorectum dissection, the Douglas pouch is opened transversally, facilitating full rectosigmoid mobilization and allowing the intraperitoneal contents to be palpated.

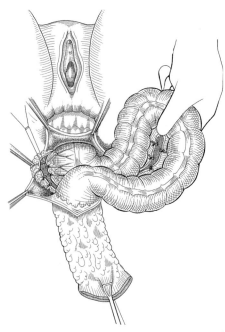

Fig. 16. Mesocolic vessels are ligated until mobilization of the redundant bowel is complete.

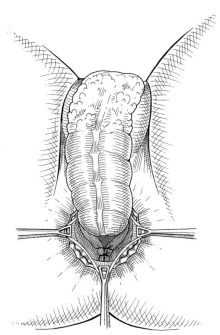

Fig. 17. Posterior levatorplasty is performed with 2-0 nonabsorbable suture (two to three stitches) until bowel fits loosely in the opening.

ting the anterior half of the proximal bowel and initiating the anastomosis using interrupted 4-0 absorbable sutures. Once the anterior half is complete, the remaining posterior wall is transected and the anastomosis to the anal canal is completed (Figs. 18 and 19). Circular staplers can also be used to perform the anastomosis (Figs. 20 and 21).

 POSTOPERATIVE MANAGEMENT

Patients are offered a clear-liquid diet in the immediate postoperative period and are advanced to a regular diet on the following day. The urinary catheter is removed on the first postoperative day. Patients are discharged once they tolerate a regular diet without vomiting, nausea, or fever, usually in the first or second postoperative day. Fiber supplementation, sitz baths, and nonopioid analgesia are usually recommended.

Recurrence rates following perineal rectosigmoidectomy with levatorplasty are similar to those reported after transabdominal procedures and may include full-thickness or exclusive mucosal recurrences.

However, specific technical aspects of the perineal rectosigmoidectomy are of paramount importance on improving outcomes such as the opening of the Douglas pouch, extension of resection of

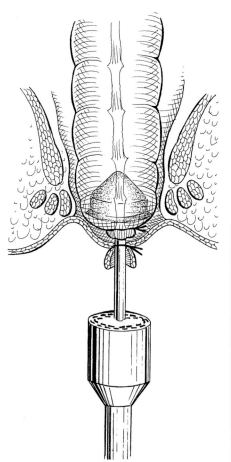

Fig. 20. Coloanal anastomosis using circular stapling devices.

the usually redundant sigmoid colon, and the association of levatorplasty. Association of this latter procedure has reduced recurrence rates without significant increase in operative time.

terminal branches before clamping them, as we performed in all our intestinal anastomoses. The level of the redundant rectum or sigmoid colon that will be transected is identified and marked circumferentially using electrocautery to avoid irregularities or recess formation by sutures placed in different levels on each side. We start by cut-

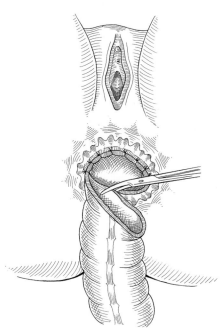

Fig. 18. Once the anterior half has been cut and sutured, the posterior wall is sectioned and the anastomosis is completed with interrupted suture.

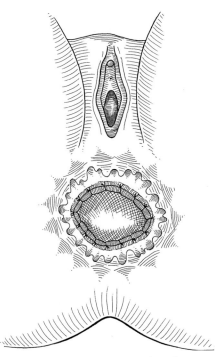

Fig. 19. Final aspect of the coloanal anastomosis.

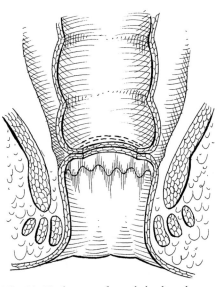

Fig. 21. Final aspect of a stapled coloanal anastomosis.

Recurrent Rectal Prolapse

Perineal rectosigmoidectomy and levator-plasty may also be the recommended treatment option for recurrent rectal prolapse initially managed by abdominal approach. In such cases, the perineal procedure is preferred as potentially adhesive areas due to a prior abdominal surgery are avoided, thus obviating potential injury to the nerve plexuses or presacral fascia. A contraindication to this procedure includes patients with previous resection of the left or sigmoid colon in which perineal resection may leave a devitalized colonic segment, increasing the risk of anastomotic dehiscence. In this setting, the Delorme procedure may be an option. Results associated with this perineal approach for recurrent rectal prolapse seem to be similar to those following management of primary disease.

SUGGESTED READING

Altemeier WA, Culbertson WR. Technique for perineal repair of rectal prolapse. *Surgery* 1965;58:758.

Brown AJ, Anderson JH, McKee RF, et al. Strategy for selection of type of operation for rectal prolapse based on clinical criteria. *Dis Colon Rectum* 2004;47:103.

Felt-Bersma RJ, Cuesta MA. Rectal prolapse, rectal intussusception, rectocele, and solitary rectal ulcer syndrome. *Gastroenterol Clin North Am* 2001;30:199.

Gregorcyk SMD. Perineal proctosigmoidectomy: the procedure of choice for rectal prolapse. *Clin Colon Rectal Surg* 2003:263.

Kim DS, Tsang CB, Wong WD, et al. Complete rectal prolapse: evolution of management and results. *Dis Colon Rectum* 1999;42:460; discussion 466.

Madiba TE, Baig MK, Wexner SD. Surgical management of rectal prolapse. *Arch Surg* 2005;140:63.

Madoff RD, Mellgren A. One hundred years of rectal prolapse surgery. *Dis Colon Rectum* 1999;42:441.

Prasad ML, Pearl RK, Abcarian H, et al. Perineal proctectomy, posterior rectopexy, and postanal levator repair for the treatment of rectal prolapse. *Dis Colon Rectum* 1986;29: 547.

Watts AM, Thompson MR. Evaluation of Delorme's procedure as a treatment for full-thickness rectal prolapse. *Br J Surg* 2000;87:218.

EDITOR'S COMMENT

Rectal prolapse is a very troublesome problem, and is increasingly so because of the increase in age and in the frequency of patients who live into their 80s and 90s. While the prolapse itself is somewhat of an issue, the associated incontinence and constipation tend to make significant prolapse an important issue for these patients. Difficulty in defecation, of course, will cause a greater prolapse, as well as discomfort. While previous obstetric injuries, pelvic floor relaxation, loss of muscle tone, and dietary habits that are dependent on cathartics for evacuation all contribute to the cause of rectal prolapse, it is not clear that we know everything about the cause of rectal prolapse. Professor Habr-Gama et al. raise the issue of remote pudendal nerve injury as perhaps causative, but we know nothing about the cause of such pudendal nerve injury. Likewise, the observation that psychiatric patients may have an increased incidence of rectal prolapse leads one to question whether the liberal use of phenothiazine in psychiatric hospitals somehow, because it results in constipation, leads to an increased incidence of rectal prolapse. Finally, the cause of the constipation and difficulty in defecation, which seem to accompany rectal prolapse, is not clear. Suffice it to say that following repair, constipation continues in many patients, although excuses are given as to a taut rectal segment, or the fact that there is a stricture at the anastomosis following rectosigmoid resection. It is difficult to believe that these factors alone contribute to the constipation, which appears chronic.

Because it is not entirely clear what the cause of rectal prolapse is, and it is not entirely clear what steps are needed to fix the rectal prolapse, it would be the sum total of the exposition one is talking about: That abdominal repairs in general have a lower recurrence than perineal repairs, that the addition of prosthetic material posterior to the rectum probably helps a little bit, if not too much, and that resection probably adds something to the repair because the anastomosis tends to scar down when it is folded in the rectum and is likely to hold the rectum proximal, which will straighten out the path of the rectum and make it follow the curve of the sacrum and thus prevent constipation.

As for deciding which procedure is appropriate, Marzouk et al. (*Surg Radiol Anat* 2005;27:414) describe "the hook test," which is basically a digital assessment of lower rectum fixity in rectal prolapse. In determining which is appropriate, if the hook test actually reveals that the mobile lower rectum is pulled downward against the sacrum by the flexed index finger, then a perineal approach is appropriate. Conversely, if the index finger is successfully inserted in the furrow outside the prolapsed rectum and a high prolapse is assessed, then the abdominal procedure is more appropriate.

I'm afraid that I disagree with the author on some of the techniques of the perineal rectosigmoidectomy, or the Altemeier repair. I was Dr. Altemeier's successor, and Bill Culbertson, who was the author of many of the papers on the results of the Altemeier procedure, took me through my first few Altemeier repairs. Although I thought I knew how to do the repair, but had never done it, it was very helpful to have Dr. Culbertson, a true Virginia gentleman, present at the procedure. One aspect of the procedure that is not emphasized in this chapter, although it is mentioned, is the presence of the sliding hernia and the necessity for exploration and closure of the sac. Dr. Culbertson thought that this was extremely important, and that the presence of an enterocele was an important feature in which successful repair was carried out. He further told me that if an enterocele was present and if it was not repaired, recurrence would be likely. The other nice technical detail that may prevent a stricture at the anastomosis, which is mentioned in the chapter as a complication, is to do the anastomosis between the remnant mucosa at the top of the columns of Morgagni, which is the appropriate level of lower resection, and the remaining rectum in quadrants with interrupted sutures, thereby guaranteeing that the anastomosis is less likely to stricture.

My own experience with the perineal sigmoidectomy is that the recurrence rate is quite low when done properly. I must say that I was initially skeptical of the perineal approach, being a devotee of anterior resection and fixation to the sacrum in one way or another, and I was corrected by its success in a number of elderly patients that I operated on. I would still tend to use it on the elderly, but would seek some abdominal procedure in patients who are young and who, as the author points out, are quite rare candidates for this condition.

The lack of clear cause for fecal incontinence enables one to try different repairs for neurogenic fecal incontinence, with the expectation that successful results may be present. Österberg et al. (*Br J Surg* 2000;87:1546) carried out a prospective study to evaluate the results of anterior levatorplasty on 31 patients with idiopathic (neurogenic) fecal incontinence and 20 patients with traumatic anal sphincter injury who underwent anal sphincteroplasty. In the levatorplasty group, 18 of 31 patients reported continence to solid and liquid stools 1 year after operation, a great improvement over the 2 out of 31 who were continent before surgery. In the sphincteroplasty group, the incontinence was improved from 2 of 20 to 10 of 20. If, in fact, the defect following sphincter injury was clearly identified on ultrasound, it is difficult to comprehend why incontinence is not present in greater percentiles. I have absolutely no idea why levatorplasty was successful in neurogenic fecal incontinence other than, as the authors suggest, that the repair may result from the stenosing effect on the anal canal.

Others (Lamah et al. *Colorectal Dis* 2001;3:412) utilized anterior levatorplasty for rectocele. They found that the operation was rated as good or excellent in 82% (27 of 33 patients with rectocele only and 11 with rectocele and fecal incontinence, reporting 7 out of these 11 pronounced themselves continent). I'm not certain of exactly what the purpose of this paper is. Anterior levatorplasty, in addition to the imbrication of the rectocele, is part and parcel of every rectocele repair I carried out, so I'm not sure what the news is, but I probably missed something.

Hirst et al. (*Colorectal Dis* 2005;7:159) retrospectively reviewed 82 patients in whom obstructed defecation was the chief complaint. The cause was thought to be rectocele, and transanal repair (plication of the rectocele) was carried out in 42 women, transperineal plication and levatorplasty in 33, and a mesh repair in seven. Seventy-seven percent of the women (63 total) were pleased with the result, although recurrence resulted in a return of symptoms in 17 of the 63 patients, or 27%. Ten of these patients with recurrences finally ended up with a stoma, and five of these ten had undergone two subsequent operations without improvement.

Two recent reviews listed a number of approaches and the end-report results in the collective

(continued)

series. Of these, the review by Schiedeck et al. (*Langenbecks Arch Surg* 2005;390:8) is less authoritative as the listing of procedures carried out by others is not as complete. In addition, they reviewed their own series of 150 attempted laparoscopic approaches for second- and third-degree prolapse. A laparoscopic procedure without conversion in 147 patients, of which resection rectopexy was carried out in 73% (108 patients), followed by suture rectopexy alone (N = 32, 21.8%) and sigmoid resection alone (N = 17, 11.9%). They are less sanguine about the Delorme procedure, with a higher recurrence rate, or perineal rectosigmoidectomy. However, they do not report their own results.

A more extensive and very nice review by Madiba et al. (*Arch Surg* 2005;140:63) lists the extensive results in collective series of all the known approaches to repairing rectal prolapse, and includes the number of patients; the design of the study; the mortality; the improvement of incontinence, if any; the improvement in constipation, if any; the recurrence; and the number of months of follow-up. The authors concluded that the abdominal approach is superior to the perineal approach, but that they reserve the perineal approach, in which they favor

the rectosigmoidectomy as opposed to the Delorme procedure, mostly for elderly infirm patients.

The anterior sling rectopexy (known as the Ripstein procedure) is not favored because of the incidence of rectal obstruction with whatever kind of mesh is put in anterior to the rectum. One of the reasons why they do not favor this approach is because of an absolutely horrendous report from the Lahey Clinic, in which Roberts et al. (*Arch Surg* 1988;123:554) reported a 52% complication rate, of which the most serious is a presacral hematoma in 8% of the cases, and an overall recurrence rate in 10%, which is equaled in only one other study. In addition, Ripstein himself has given up on completely encircling mesh, which he acknowledges does cause postoperative rectal obstruction. Suture rectopexy seems to have almost as good a result as placing a mesh behind the rectum and suturing it to both the rectum and the sacrum. The Ivalon sponge appears to come in for criticism as having a slightly higher infection rate, especially when combined with resection, than the other prosthetic materials, although the results do not appear to me to be statistically significant (3.7% vs. 3%). The addition of sigmoid resection to rectopexy (Frykman-Goldberg

procedure) combines the advantages of mobilization of the rectum, sigmoid resection, and fixation of the rectum, most of which is carried out through suture rectopexy to avoid the added risk of infection with a prosthetic material. They do not advocate division of the lateral ligaments in addition to rectopexy.

The results of the Delorme procedure, in which an attack on the basic cause does not occur, only in mucosa resection and the reefing up of the musculature, are fraught with a relatively large number of complications, mostly recurrence ranging from 4.2% to 38% in a small series. The table on perineal rectosigmoidectomy (the Altemeier procedure) reproduces only the earliest Altemeier paper and, for some reason, disregards the three later papers with recurrence rates that are considerably lower, presumably as the learning curve enabled Dr. Altemeier and his co-workers to do a better operation.

Whether or not one agrees with all the conclusions of the paper, the paper is very well researched and the tables are very complete and can be read with great profit.

J.E.F.

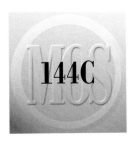

Laparoscopic Treatment of Rectal Prolapse

DENNIS L. FOWLER AND AKUEZUNKPA O. WELCOME

INTRODUCTION

Over 100 procedures have been described to treat rectal prolapse, or procidentia. Since the first descriptions of laparoscopic procedures for the treatment of rectal prolapse in the early 1990s, a substantial body of literature has accrued that compares open to laparoscopic techniques, as well as the various laparoscopic techniques to each other. The benefits of laparoscopic over open surgery have been demonstrated in virtually all major abdominal surgical procedures, including those for rectal prolapse. The benefits include decreased postoperative pain and narcotic use, decreased length of postoperative ileus, decreased hospital length of stay, improved cosmesis, and high patient satisfaction. The benefits of laparoscopy have extended the more durable transabdominal approaches to patients who may not have been considered candidates for an abdominal approach in the past. This chapter shall outline the most common laparoscopic techniques described in the current literature.

EPIDEMIOLOGY AND PATHOPHYSIOLOGY

Procidentia has a bimodal incidence and is most frequently seen at the extremes of life. Rectal prolapse in children is primarily mucosal. Unlike procidentia in the pediatric population, adult rectal prolapse is not a self-limiting disease. The more common version is acquired and predominantly affects elderly women. Patient complaints include mucous discharge, pain, tenesmus, and a sensation of incomplete evacuation.

Rectal prolapse has been conceptualized as either a sliding hernia or an intussusception of the rectum. The various classification systems have been based on these two causes. In general, both systems classify prolapse according to the layers that form the intussusceptum (full thickness vs. mucosal) and whether the intussuscipiens–intussusceptum complex passes through the anus (complete vs. partial). Complete (fullthickness) rectal prolapse is an indication for an antiprolapse operative repair. False or incomplete (mucosal) prolapse may benefit from a hemorrhoidectomy or banding

(Fig. 1). The anatomic abnormalities in patients with rectal prolapse include a redundant sigmoid, an elongated mesorectum with loss of the rectosigmoid angle, atrophy and separation of the levator ani, a patulous anus, and a deep cul-de-sac (Fig. 2).

There are functional abnormalities as well. The condition is commonly associated with constipation and anal incontinence. In patients with rectal prolapse, the rectum requires smaller volumes of stool to stimulate the urge to defecate. At the same time, the resting pressure of the internal sphincter is decreased but squeeze pressures remain normal. This suggests that the internal sphincter alone is dysfunctional. The combination of a weak internal sphincter and a rectum that is hypersensitive to distension provides a plausible explanation for the high incidence of incontinence in this patient population.

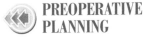 PREOPERATIVE PLANNING

The most important part of the preoperative evaluation is the patient's history.

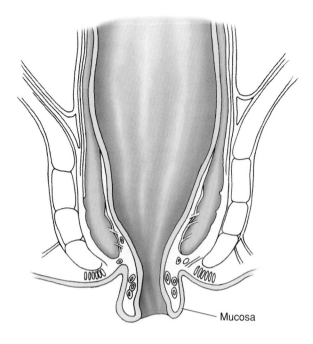

MUCOSAL PROLAPSE

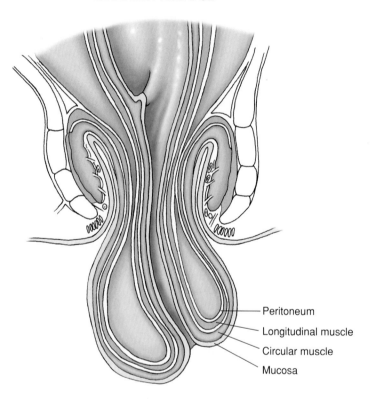

COMPLETE RECTAL PROLAPSE

Fig. 1. Complete **(top)** versus mucosal **(bottom)** rectal prolapse.

Specific questions should address the presence and degree of constipation. This can be evaluated by asking about the number of successful defecations per week, the amount of time spent straining, the duration and quantity of laxative or suppository use, and the need for digita- tions. The review of systems should gauge the patient's degree of incontinence using one of several validated scales. The physi- cal examination must include not only a digital rectal examination to assess rectal tone and rule out the presence of a sig- moidocele, a mass, or sphincter defects,

but also an examination of the patient's anus while he or she strains on the toilet.

Authors differ on the number and type of preoperative imaging and functional studies that are required prior to operat- ing. Most tests are ordered based on the patient's constellation of symptoms. How- ever, a screening colonoscopy or flexible sigmoidoscopy with barium enema is im- perative to evaluate the colon for other abnormalities. If no protrusion of rectum is seen during the physical examination, defecography may be needed to diagnose a more proximal intussusception. In addi- tion to these studies, some authors obtain colonic transit studies to evaluate for slow transit, electromyography, and measure- ment of pudendal nerve terminal motor latency to rule out neurologic problems and/or anal manometry to measure sphincter pressures.

It is imperative to distinguish patients with morphologic disorders (such as a rec- tocele or sigmoidocele) from those with functional disorders such as anisum or pu- dendal nerve neuropathy. These results may impact the decision to operate, choice of operation, and the surgeon's ability to offer the patient prognostic information regarding the recovery of continence and the resolution of his or her constipation. Different reports have presented contra- dictory results regarding the degree of cor- relation between these test results and pa- tients' pre- and postoperative symptoms. For example, patients with slow transit will benefit from a resection; very low preoper- ative resting pressures may prolong or pre- clude the restoration of continence. Nonetheless, different reports have pre- sented contradictory results regarding the degree of correlation between these test results and patients' pre- and postoperative symptoms. All authors agree that it is im- portant to identify patients with anisum, for they most certainly will not benefit from a surgical procedure and are best served by biofeedback training.

SURGERY

The goals of surgery are twofold: To cor- rect the anatomic abnormalities associated with prolapse and to provide the patient with functional improvement of his or her symptoms. As many as 75% of patients with rectal prolapse suffer from anal in- continence, and 25% to 50% report con- stipation. Any assessment of the success of an operation would be incomplete if it did not document the efficacy of the pro- cedure in resolving these symptoms. To that end, all procedures involve one or

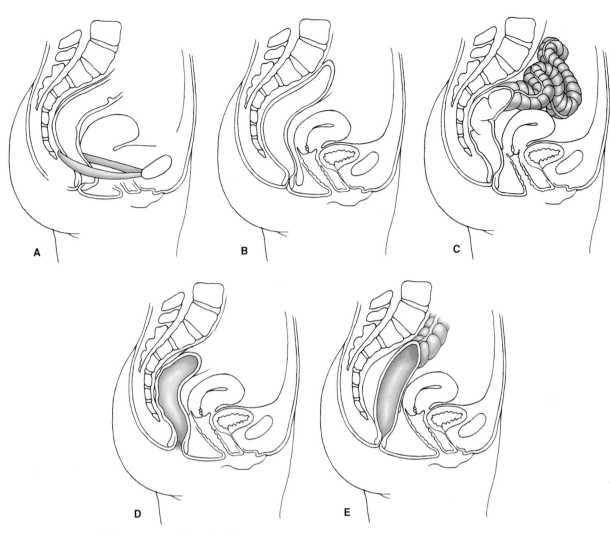

Fig. 2. Pathologic anatomy of rectal prolapse.

more of the following steps: Resection of redundant sigmoid colon, fixation of the rectum to the sacrum, and a reconstruction of the pelvic floor. The various nonlaparoscopic approaches to rectal prolapse have been described in earlier chapters. The laparoscopic approaches that will be described mimic the abdominal approaches. In patients whose medical conditions preclude the administration of general anesthesia, the perineal procedures provide adequate relief of symptoms, but are associated with a shorter duration of relief and a higher recurrence rate.

The laparoscopic surgical options include rectopexy with or without mesh, sigmoid resection alone, or a combination of the two. No one operation is suitable for all prolapse patients; therefore, the operation must be tailored to the patient and his or her individual symptoms. A resection with rectopexy is indicated in patients who have sigmoid diverticular disease, a sigmoidocele, a redundant sigmoid

colon, slow transit time, and/or constipation. A rectopexy alone is relatively contraindicated in patients with constipation due to the high rates of persistence or worsening of constipation following this procedure. An absolute contraindication to a laparoscopic repair is the patient's inability to tolerate general anesthesia, while relative contraindications include prior abdominal surgery and irreducible prolapse (Fig. 3).

Preoperative Preparation

Patients start a clear liquid diet 2 days before surgery. On the day prior to surgery, the patient should take two doses of an over-the-counter phosphosoda preparation. If antibiotic prophylaxis is desired, the patient should take 1 g metronidazole and 1 g neomycin at 2 p.m., 3 p.m., and 11 p.m. The patient is NPO the night before surgery. Preoperative parenteral antibiotics (a third-generation cephalosporin or a

fluoroquinolone and metronidazole for patients with penicillin allergies) are given prior to the induction of general anesthesia. The patient is positioned supine on a beanbag atop a split-leg table and sequential venous compression stockings are placed on both lower extremities.

Patient Positioning and Port Placement

After induction, a urinary catheter is placed in the bladder and the patient is repositioned on the table so the buttocks extend slightly into the space between the separated legs. The legs are abducted by separating the legs of the table. If no split-leg table is available, candy cane stirrups or other types of stirrups may be used to achieve the same goal. There should be enough room to allow access to the anus for endoscopy and the insertion of a stapling device. Both arms are tucked at the patient's sides and the beanbag is hardened

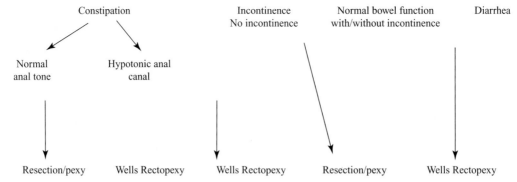

Fig. 3. Clinical algorithm for choosing a laparoscopic approach to rectal prolapse. (From Senagore AJ. Management of rectal prolapse: The role of laparoscopic approaches. *Semin Laparosc Surg* 2003;10:197.)

to prevent the patient from slipping off the table when in it is the steep Trendelenburg or reverse Trendelenburg positions. The surgeon stands on the patient's right side and the assistant stands on the left. Two monitors are positioned at the foot of the bed (Fig. 4).

The surgeon may use either a Veress needle or the Hassan technique to access the peritoneal cavity at or superior to the umbilicus. A carbon dioxide pneumoperitoneum of 15 mm Hg is created, a 30-degree laparoscope is inserted, and the abdominal cavity is inspected. Two additional ports are placed on the right, a 5-mm port just lateral to the rectus sheath slightly cephalad to the camera port and a 12-mm

port in the right iliac fossa at the McBurney point. The 12-mm port is used in resection cases for the introduction of stapling devices and in rectopexy cases for intracorporeal suturing. A 5-mm port is placed on the left that mirrors the right upper port location. If needed, an additional port may be placed in the left iliac fossa if a second port for the assistant is needed.

The patient is then placed in steep Trendelenburg position and the small bowel is lifted out of the pelvis into the upper abdomen. Atraumatic bowel graspers are used for retraction and the 5-mm LigaSure (Tyco, Norwalk, CT) is used for dissection and coagulation. Additional instruments that will be used include an occluding

bowel clamp, 45- or 60-mm endoscopic linear cutting staplers, a circular stapling device, a wound protector, a suction irrigator, a right-angled clamp, laparoscopic needle holders, and a flexible sigmoidoscope.

Rectopexy without Mesh

A complete mobilization of the rectum from the sacral promontory to the coccyx remains the most critical part of any rectopexy. To begin, the assistant retracts the sigmoid anteriorly and slightly to the left as the surgeon incises the posterior peritoneum to the right of the sigmoid. After the peritoneum is cut down the rectosigmoid fossa toward the anterior peritoneal reflection, the plane posterior to the mesosigmoid and mesorectum but anterior to Toldt fascia is entered and developed. As the surgeon moves from the right iliac fossa toward the left, the assistant maintains tension by retracting the sigmoid toward the anterior abdominal wall. In the course of developing this plane, the right and left ureters are identified, and the hypogastric nerves are kept with the retroperitoneal tissue posterior to the rectum. Once the posterior plane has been developed, the rectum is mobilized to the level of the levators anteriorly and posteriorly. The assistant must continuously reposition the grasp on the rectum to provide adequate tension by alternatively retracting the rectum anteriorly as the mesorectum is separated from the presacral fascia and pulling the rectum posteriorly as the anterior rectal wall is separated from the bladder and vagina or prostate. Many authors advocate preservation of the lateral rectal ligaments to prevent disruption of the parasympathetic supply to the rectum, arguing that the high rate of constipation after rectopexy alone may be caused by disruption of these nerves.

Once the rectum has been fully mobilized, the surgeon performs the rectopexy.

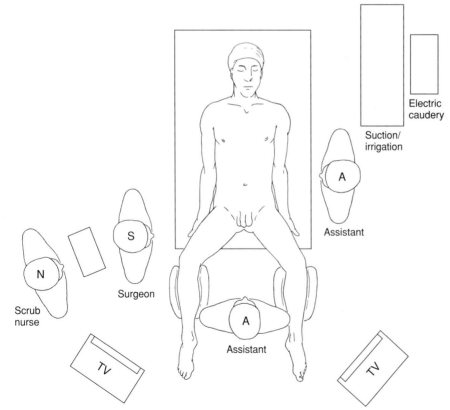

Fig. 4. Operating room setup.

As the rectum is placed on cephalad tension, two or three nonabsorbable stitches are used to secure it to the presacral fascia at the level of the sacral promontory. These lateral rectal stitches are placed on both sides and should include the submucosa but not the mucosa. The presacral stitches should engage the fascia without piercing the presacral venous plexus. After the pelvis is examined for hemostasis, the ports are removed, the pneumoperitoneum is evacuated, and the incisions are closed with an absorbable subcuticular stitch.

Rectopexy with Mesh

After rectal mobilization, as outlined above, sacral fixation can be achieved with the use of mesh place anteriorly (per Ripstein) or posteriorly (per Wells). The Ripstein procedure consists of an anterior, circumferential fixation of the rectum by a piece of polypropylene mesh. Most surgeons have abandoned this procedure because the postoperative fibrotic reaction is often dense and leads to varying degrees of obstruction. We prefer to use a posterior, partial mesh wrap. The construction of a posterior rectopexy begins with the creation of a T-shaped piece of mesh. The long part of the "T" is sutured with nonabsorbable suture (or stapled with a hernia tacker) to the presacral fascia so that the junction of the "T" is at the level of the sacral promontory. The "arms" of the "T" are sewn to the lateral rectal walls with two or three nonabsorbable stitches. The arms do not completely encircle the rectum, and the final product resembles a hotdog (rectum) in a bun (mesh). The ports are removed and closed as in the previous section. Although the "T" shape for the mesh is the classic description, it is not essential for the mesh to assume a "T" configuration since a rectangular piece works just as well.

Sigmoid Resection with Rectopexy

Sigmoid resection without rectopexy or anterior resections have been largely abandoned in favor of sigmoid resection with rectopexy.

After complete rectal mobilization as outlined in an earlier section, the sigmoid colon must be dissected free from its lateral attachments. While the patient is in the steep Trendelenburg position, the table is tilted with the right side down. The assistant grasps the sigmoid colon and retracts it medially. The surgeon incises the white line of Toldt from the pelvic brim toward the splenic flexure as he or she also retracts the sigmoid medially. By staying adjacent to the colon in this part of the dissection, the sigmoid mesocolon is lifted away from the retroperitoneum. Once again the left ureter is identified and a proximal margin of resection is chosen based on the ability of the colon to easily reach the rectum (which is placed on tension to eliminate redundancy). This area can be marked with a suture or clips. It is often unnecessary to fully mobilize the splenic flexure because the sigmoid colon is redundant in this patient population. The sigmoidal branches of the inferior mesenteric artery are divided close to the bowel with the LigaSure device (Tyco, Norwalk, CT).

An articulating, linear, endoscopic stapler is used to divide the proximal rectum at the distal line of resection. The distal end of the specimen is eviscerated via a left lower quadrant muscle–splitting incision and the proximal line of resection is divided extracorporeally. After dividing the bowel, a purse string is placed using a 3-0 monofilament, nonabsorbable suture, and the bowel is divided just distal to the purse string. The anvil of an appropriately sized circular stapler is inserted into the proximal end of the bowel and the purse string is tied. The bowel is then returned to the peritoneal cavity and the incision is closed. Once the pneumoperitoneum is re-established, the assistant moves to the foot of the bed and irrigates the rectal stump with a dilute Betadine solution. He or she then inserts the circular stapling device into the rectal stump and passes the spike through the rectal wall at a site that is proximal to, but not through, the linear staple line. The surgeon connects the anvil to the circular stapler docket. The assistant then closes and fires the stapler as the surgeon maintains the colonic mesentery in its proper orientation.

The stapler is not removed after firing the device, but rather it remains in the rectum and is used to maintain tension in the posterior direction as an anchoring stitch is placed in the presacral fascia and the lateral rectal wall. Once this first stitch has been placed, the stapler is removed from the rectum and additional stitches are placed on the right and then the left side of the rectum as outlined in the rectopexy section. A mesh rectopexy is not recommended after a bowel resection for fear of infection of the mesh.

After removing the stapler from the rectum and inspecting the anastomotic rings for completeness, the pelvis is filled with irrigation fluid, and a flexible sigmoidoscope is used to inspect the anastomosis for hemostasis and integrity. If there are no air bubbles present upon insufflation of the rectum, the air is evacuated and the scope is withdrawn. A single absorbable suture is used to close the right lower quadrant 12-mm port site using a suture passer device. After a final inspection of the abdominal cavity, the 5-mm ports are removed as the pneumoperitoneum is evacuated. The skin is closed as described in previous sections.

Results

Rectopexy with or without mesh has been demonstrated to be just as efficacious and safe as open rectopexy. The complication rates range from 0% to 30% in most series. Reoperation is rarely performed for bleeding (1% to 2%) or fecal impaction (<1%). Rectopexy alone is associated with higher rates of postoperative constipation than resection rectopexy. The creation of an acute angle between the point of posterior fixation and the mobile sigmoid has been implicated as a possible cause. Another potential cause is increased rectal wall thickness in response to the presence of mesh, or dissection alone.

A recent article has described excellent results with a partial anterior rectopexy after a limited anterior rectal dissection. The authors hypothesized that the decreased rates of constipation in their series could be explained by avoiding the disruption of the rectal nerves in the lateral ligaments and the smaller degree of rectal thickening that results from a circumferential dissection. Their medium-term results were excellent, but long-term durability of the repair remains to be seen.

Resection with rectopexy has become the preferred approach for rectal prolapse repair in patients, especially those who are relatively young and healthy and suffer from constipation. Reported leak rates remain in the 1% to 2% range. Anal incontinence rates decrease by 40% to 60%, and constipation improves in 60% to 90% of patients after resection rectopexy. Resection with rectopexy is as efficacious as rectopexy alone in resolving incontinence, but has decreased postoperative constipation rates. Not only does it eliminate the creation of an acute angle at the rectosigmoid junction by removing redundant colon, but it also preserves the rectal reservoir and avoids damage to sphincters as opposed to the perineal approach. Reported recurrence rates of both rectopexy with and without resection are low and range from 0% to 7% over 2 to 4 years of follow-up.

The Gastrointestinal Tract

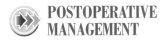
POSTOPERATIVE MANAGEMENT

Early postoperative pain is controlled with parenteral narcotics and parenteral nonsteroidal drugs. On the day of surgery, patients are encouraged to ambulate and are allowed clear liquids.

The average length of stay for rectopexy patients is 1 to 2 days, but patients who have undergone a resection remain hospitalized for longer. Most patients begin to mobilize third-spaced fluids between postoperative day 1 and 2 and their diet is advanced with the passage of flatus. The parenteral narcotics are replaced on postoperative day 2 with an oral narcotic/acetaminophen combination. Most patients are discharged on postoperative day 3. Resolution of incontinence may take as long as 6 months, so patients may need reassurance to defer contemplation of any additional procedures to restore continence.

SUMMARY

Rectopexy is associated with the least number of postoperative complications and the shortest length of stay. Mesh rectopexy also has fewer complications than resection, which has the added risk of a 1% to 2% leak rate. Bleeding, especially in the presacral plane, is a potentially worrisome complication, but an anatomic dissection that preserves the presacral fascia will avoid any bleeding from this area. All three procedures are effective at curing incontinence with rates reported from 70% to 92%. The improvement in anal continence is thought to be due to improved internal sphincter function.

Some advocates of perineal approaches argue that a reoperation is easily performed for patients with recurrent prolapse after perineal repair. Advocates of the laparoscopic approaches argue that a prior laparoscopic operation for rectal prolapse is also not a contraindication to repeat surgery. If a patient has a recurrence after a suture rectopexy, then a mesh rectopexy or a resection may provide improved protection against recurrent prolapse. Reoperative pelvic surgery is not easy open or laparoscopically and should be undertaken only by those with extensive laparoscopic surgical experience.

The laparoscopic options for treating full-thickness rectal prolapse have evolved over time from rectopexy to resection with rectopexy as laparoscopic skills and equipment have improved. Each patient's preoperative workup and ultimate operation is guided by his or her overall medical condition and constellation of symptoms. The three most common procedures have been shown to be equivalent to the open variants in terms of safety, effectiveness, and recurrence rates. In centers with the necessary expertise in laparoscopic pelvic surgery, recurrences can be treated laparoscopically as well. For patients with no contraindications to general anesthesia, laparoscopic approaches combine decreased surgical stress with equivalent rates of symptomatic and functional improvement along with decreased lengths of stay, postoperative pain, and high patient satisfaction.

SUGGESTED READING

Baker R, Senagore AJ, Luchtefeld MA. Laparoscopic-assisted vs. open resection: rectopexy offers excellent results. *Dis Colon Rectum* 1995;38:199.

Benoist S, Taffinder N, Gould S, et al. Functional results two years after laparoscopic rectopexy. *Am J Surg* 2001;182:168.

Boccasanta P, Rosati R, Venturi M, et al. Comparison of laparoscopic rectopexy with open technique in the treatment of complete rectal prolapse: clinical and functional results. *Surg Lap Endosc* 1998;8:460.

Cuschieri A, Shimi SM, Vander Velpen G, et al. Laparoscopic prosthesis fixation rectopexy for complete rectal prolapse. *Br J Surg* 1994;81:138.

D'Hoore A, Cadoni R, D'Hoore A, et al. Laparoscopic ventral rectopexy for total rectal prolapse: long term outcome. *Br J Surg* 2004;91:1500.

Eu KW, Seow-Choen F. Functional problems in adult rectal prolapse and controversies in surgical treatment. *Br J Surg* 1997;84:904.

Gordon PH. Rectal procidentia. In: Gordon PH, Nivatvongs S, eds. *Principles and practice of surgery for the colon, rectum and anus.* St. Louis, MO: Quality Medical Publishers, 1999:503.

Heah SM, Hartley JE, Hurley J, et al. Laparoscopic suture rectopexy without resection is effective treatment for full-thickness rectal prolapse. *Dis Colon Rectum* 2000;43:638.

Kairaluoma MV, Viljakka MT, Kellokumpu IH. Open vs. laparoscopic surgery for rectal prolapse: a case-controlled study assessing short term outcome. *Dis Colon Rectum* 2003;46:353.

Madbouly KM, Senagore AJ, Delaney CP, et al. Clinically based management of rectal prolapse. *Surg Endosc* 2003;17:99.

Rose J, Schneider C, Scheidbach H, et al. Laparoscopic treatment of rectal prolapse: experience gained in a prospective multicenter study. *Langenbeck's Arch Surg* 2002;387:130.

Senagore AJ. Management of rectal prolapse: the role of laparoscopic approaches. *Semin Laparosc Surg* 2003;10:197.

Solomon MJ, Young CJ, Evers AA, et al. Randomized clinical trial of laparoscopic versus open abdominal rectopexy for rectal prolapse. *Br J Surg* 2002;89:35.

Stevenson ARL, Stitz RW, Lumley JW. Laparoscopic-assisted resection-rectopexy for rectal prolapse: early and medium follow-up. *Dis Colon Rectum* 1998;41:46.

Xynos E, Chrysos E, Tsiaoussis J, et al. Resection rectopexy for rectal prolapse: the laparoscopic approach. *Surg Endosc* 1999;13:862.

EDITOR'S COMMENT

Rectal prolapse is a benign, common, debilitating disorder that predominantly affects elderly women. While numerous open surgical options for treatment are available, laparoscopic techniques to correct the deformity are preferable in most cases. In this chapter, Dr. Fowler nicely outlines the preoperative evaluation, minimally invasive treatment options, and his operative technique.

Patients may present with complaints of mucous discharge, tenesmus, incomplete evacuation, constipation, and anal incontinence. Digital examination will assess resting and squeeze pressures, and the leading point of the anorectal intussusception may be felt when the patient strains. Prolapse may be achieved with the patient bearing down in the left lateral or squatting position. Proctoscopy, defecating proctography, endorectal ultrasound, and manometry may be indicated to exclude other prolapsing lesions, delineate associated pelvic floor functional disorders, and assess sphincter integrity.

Dr. Fowler identifies two goals of the operation. First, the anatomic abnormality of prolapse must be corrected. Second, the patient should experience a functional improvement in symptoms such as constipation and incontinence. Whether open or laparoscopic, the operation should specifically (a) resect redundant sigmoid colon, (b) fix the rectum to the sacrum, and (c) reconstruct the pelvic floor.

Patients undergoing laparoscopic treatment must tolerate a general anesthetic. For patients not suitable for general anesthesia, rectal prolapse can be treated successfully with other perineal procedures well described previously; however, Dr. Fowler cautions that these approaches may have a shorter duration of relief and higher recurrence rate.

Rectopexy requires circumferential mobilization from the sacral promontory to coccyx, and good assistance is essential to separating the mesorectum from the presacral fascia and the anterior rectal wall from the bladder, vagina, or prostate. In women, a uterine manipulator used by an assistant from between the legs can be helpful.

(continued)

Occasionally, the large uterus can be lifted to the anterior abdominal wall with a Keith needle through the abdominal wall to improve laparoscopic visualization. As the assistant retracts colon cephalad, several permanent sutures fix the rectum to the presacral fascia at the level of the sacral promontory.

While suture fixation is effective, most surgeons prefer rectopexy with mesh. While I have experience only with a flat 3 × 8 cm Marlex mesh, Dr. Fowler recommends a T-shaped mesh sutured or tacked first to the presacral fascia and then sewn to the lateral rectal walls. Dr. Fowler describes his mesh wrap like a hotdog bun. However, after sigmoid resection mesh should be avoided because of the risk of mesh infection.

Rectopexy alone can worsen constipation; therefore, sigmoid resection with sutured rectopexy is frequently performed in patients with redundant sigmoid, slow transit, and constipation. Redundancy is assessed, and the sigmoid mobilized. Care needs to be taken to preserve parasympathetic supply to the rectum in the lateral rectal ligaments and sacral sympathetic fibers at the level of the sacral promontory. The left ureter is also at risk and should be identified and traced down to the level of pelvic dissection. Distal division is performed intracorporeally with endoscopic staplers. We favor a laparoscopic hand-assisted approach through a 6-cm incision to secure the anvil; however, an alternative is a Pfannenstiel incision, which obviates laparoscopic intracorporeal division altogether. The circular stapler is passed

through the rectal stump for a double-stapled anastomosis. Proctoscopy and air insufflation test for leaks.

Rectopexy with and without sigmoid resection is an ideal laparoscopic procedure. Compared to other laparoscopic colorectal procedures, resection of redundant colon and rectopexy is very straightforward and should be well within the skill set of most fellowship-trained laparoscopists. Despite the longer operative time, patients will often benefit with less postoperative pain and narcotic use, decreased length of postoperative ileus, decreased hospital stay, improved cosmesis, faster recuperation, and higher patient satisfaction compared to traditional open approaches.

D.B.J.

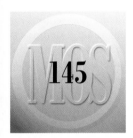

145

Management of Rectal Foreign Bodies

FRANK G. OPELKA

The Gastrointestinal Tract

Historically, in research regarding rectal foreign bodies, the literature begins with some individuals resorting to use of the anus and rectum for heinous crimes. One such tale begins with King Edward II, when he was assassinated on September 21, 1327, in Berkley Castle near Gloucester, England. In an effort to murder the king without leaving a trace, the queen convinced her partner to design an undetectable method. With His Majesty adequately sedated, the king's rival inserted a bull's horn into the royal anus. He passed a hot poker through the horn, which resulted in a perforation of the king's intestine without leaving an external trace of any assault. When the king awoke, his peritonitis seemed spontaneous and led to his ultimate demise. If the king had been obviously murdered, civil rebellion would have ensued. With no outward signs of trauma, the tragic civil unrest never occurred.

Today, patients suffering from rectal foreign body injuries, entrapments, or impactions more commonly participate in the process. The majority of retained rectal foreign bodies are related to anal sexual eroticism. Undoubtedly, history has long reported patients who experimented with rectal foreign bodies throughout the centuries. In open, liberal societies, reports of sexual conduct with anal eroticism experimentation leads to retained foreign bodies in an effort to discover new and different forms of stimulation or gratification.

Alternative lifestyles involving self-mutilation, illicit drugs, trauma, or torture have provided a series of reports displaying a wide range of foreign bodies. These include sexual erotic instruments or vibrators, illicit drugs, vegetables, cups and glassware, rounded objects, light bulbs, pistols, flashlights, metal containers, concrete, thermometers, and enema tips. Oftentimes, patients afflicted with a retained foreign body have lifestyles that promote co-morbid conditions. The astute clinician would prudently explore the patient history for associated conditions. Drug abuse, human immunodeficiency virus, and associated infections further complicate the care and management of these patients. Urine toxicology may expose drug use such as amphetamines, cocaine, or other street agents. Necessary precautions are vital in providing safe and effective care.

CLINICAL PRESENTATION AND HISTORY

Patients afflicted with a retained foreign body commonly present with a delay in clinical presentation. Social stigmata or embarrassment hinder patients from seeking immediate attention for clinical care. The afflicted remain hopeful that the normal, antegrade peristalsis may lead to a prompt resolution without medical intervention. The angulations of the pelvis often will not cooperate with large objects

that have traversed the levator plate. The provider must obtain a patient's personal and sexual history to generate a complete differential diagnosis and note associated conditions without further patient embarrassment. A proper choice of language in an interview is vital to conveying a sense of professional empathy and understanding. Questions may focus on the problem but it might be wise to avoid asking, "Are you a practicing hetero- or homosexual? Do you engage in anoreceptive activities? Are your partners male, female, both, or neither?" "Do you have a therapist helping you address any needs you may have?" These questions can be saved for another day.

Rape evaluations must not be excluded and, if suspected, the proper authorities brought forward to assist in patient care. It is noteworthy that the definition of rape has changed to a more inclusive definition in recent years. Once, the English common law definition described rape as the involuntary penetration of a woman by a male sex organ. The law is now more inclusive with the addition of involuntary penetrating acts against a man or a woman. Thus, physicians treating patients with anorectal trauma or rectal foreign bodies must be aware of the potential psychosocial and legal implications of the clinical setting. Busch and Starling suggest that the victim should be seen in a private room and that consent forms are needed for the examination, treatment, collection of evidence, and photography. The physician should follow standard rape protocols.

Once a provider suspects a history that highlights anal eroticism, it would be a helpful reminder to consider proper precautions for specific risk factors for sexually transmitted diseases. Ultimately, some patients may offer the information; most do not. Each patient differs in his or her willingness to provide highly personal information often associated with a social stigma. Given the social implications, the embarrassment, and the potential for criminal assault, providers must be keenly aware and sensitive to the needs of the patient. As well, it is important to approach these patients with precautions for sexually transmitted diseases. Some physicians unfortunately develop a personal bias toward patients with aberrant sexual activity. Their viewpoints are derived from societal stereotypes and prejudices. Tainted viewpoints cloud clinical judgment, which could further delay diagnosis and treatment. Early recognition of a personal bias should cause a physician to refer the patient to another competent physician.

If the patients are minimally symptomatic, they often resist medical intervention in the hope that, with your reassurance, they will evacuate the device. Once the object passes proximal to the puborectalis muscle, its orientation and size may prevent expulsion without medical assistance. Some patients, as in King Edward's case, will not volunteer that a foreign object resides within the rectum. Others provide outlandish fables of falling or sitting on an object that accidentally passed through the anus into the rectum before they could prevent its entry.

When a physician suspects anorectal trauma or a retained rectal foreign body, all such patients should be assessed for active bleeding, bowel perforation, infraperitoneal injury, and peritonitis. Patients require hospitalization if they present with unstable vital signs, tachycardia, fever, hypovolemia, acute anemia, leukocytosis, a potential deep laceration, or perforation. During initial evaluation and resuscitation, patients with significant pelvic or abdominal complaints require an upright chest roentgenogram or acute biplanar abdominal films. The radiograph will identify opaque foreign bodies or intraperitoneal free air. If the diagnosis of perforation cannot be established, the rectum should be examined endoscopically, once the object has been extracted. Most perforations from foreign bodies occur on the anterior wall of the rectum. Still, if the clinical situation remains uncertain, the rectum can be imaged with water-soluble contrast imaging.

Initial inspection and examination must exclude acute peritonitis. After excluding any abdominal finding, further examination typically requires conscious sedation and possibly anesthesia. The anesthetic options include a local anal sphincter block to enhance anorectal relaxation. Spinal anesthetics may provide adequate perineal relaxation while keeping the patient awake. The conscious patient can assist in extraction by providing increased abdominal pressure through Valsalva maneuvers, on demand.

Perineal inspection for external trauma may suggest a tormented patient and raise awareness of abnormal patient discomfort prior to a more probing examination. A digital rectal examination should assess the sphincter tone and identify the presence of a foreign body. The examination must note the absence or presence of hematochezia. A false-negative examination rate is reported to be as high as 30%, with an incomplete examination accounting for half of all missed injuries. Objects in the middle and lower rectum, up to 10 cm, are usually rescued through a transanal approach. Once in the upper rectum, the extraction may often require a transabdominal component.

A complete examination notes any physical or chemical trauma to the anoderm, anal canal, and sphincters. Physical forces used to insert rigid or semirigid devices can create superficial lacerations or deep sphincter injuries. Chemical agents include suppositories, toxic materials, or the deliberate insertion of illicit drugs. Physical or chemical trauma can lacerate the mucosa and generate hematomas, mucosal proctitis. or intraperitoneal trauma. A patient history suggesting a high risk of sexually transmitted diseases calls for a careful assessment of the anorectum to exclude infectious causes. When an infectious cause is considered, cultures of suspicious areas should include specifics for gonorrhea, *Chlamydia*, herpes simplex, dark-field microscopy, and appropriate serology.

Prior to attempting extraction of a retained foreign body, it is important to evaluate the patient for anal sphincter injury. An injured sphincter may be prone to further damage during the actual extraction of the object. Mild dilation and transient dysfunction are common after anal eroticism. Minimal disruption and limited inflammation may be primarily repaired after the foreign body has been removed. Complete disruption is often associated with hematoma, significant edema, and inflammation. Confirmation with water-soluble contrast enemas assist in mapping the injury and determining the operative approach. These patients may need a transanal primary repair or a transabdominal approach. Removal of all gross contamination and appropriate aerobic and anaerobic antibiotics, along with close observation, are critical. With extensive injuries, the surgeon may consider a temporary fecal diversion, as is reported in the anal sphincter repair associated with other traumatic or severe obstetric-related, sphincter repairs.

FOREIGN BODY EXTRACTION

Although most rectal foreign bodies can be removed safely under conscious sedation at the monitored bedside, some require removal in the operating room. Good results can be achieved if basic principles in the management of colorectal injuries in general are applied to colorectal perforations by foreign bodies. Lake et al. recently reported on 93 patients; bedside extraction was performed in 75% of their cases, which is slightly higher than the 60% reported by Barone et al. by Cohen and Sackier. In the case of a small palpable foreign body, a digital examination without dilation would safely remove a retained foreign body. These small objects may include a small cap for an enema bottle. Regardless of size, sharp objects, jagged edges, and glass objects should be removed in the operating theater under controlled conditions. For larger objects identified on digital examination, Yaman et al. advise a strategic assessment of the object to assure a safely planned extraction. The larger objects require imaging to establish location, shape, and consistency of the foreign body. Goligher notes that injury from irregular and sharp foreign bodies is more likely to occur during unskillful attempts at removal. These large retained objects require a variety of supportive care in order to remove them. Surgical approaches are not immediately necessary in stable patients. Admission to the hospital, followed by a period of observation and reattempted transanal extraction under spinal anesthesia, are appropriate measures. If the object still cannot be extricated, abdominal exploration may be necessary.

Anatomic stratification may define a method for management and ultimate extraction of the implanted item. Nohme-Kinsley and Abcarian described anatomic position relative to the divisions of the rectum. Foreign objects engaging the low and middle rectum are typically removed from a transanal approach, often with out regional or general anesthetic. Objects within the upper rectum have slipped proximal to the anorectal angle. When rectal foreign bodies migrate proximal to the anal sphincters, the objects change their axial position, induce edema in the bowel, or become trapped in the natural concavity of the sacrum. Such changes make it more difficult to extract the foreign body from a transanal approach alone. Devices caught above the sphincters or in the sacral hollow could require an abdominal or combined abdominal perineal approach to facilitate extraction.

Selecting the best method to remove a retained rectal foreign body challenges the ingenuity of the physician. The process involves dilation of the anal sphincters and delivery of the object without further injury. The literature is replete with creative methods for object extraction. Morand reported to the Academy of Paris the story of a monk with a retained bottle in the rectum. The device was retrieved by a boy with a small hand. Others have commented that the small hands of female surgeons can pass beyond the sphincters through the sacral curvature to retrieve more proximal retained objects. When a transanally placed frozen porcine tail finally thawed, its bristles curled and clung to the mucosa, leading to retention of the tail. Unable to pass the tail, it was ultimately extracted by proctoscopically placing a hollow reed over the top of the tail, leading to its safe extrication. Glass objects need careful attention to avoid breakage. Hollow objects with a caudally placed opening can be filled with plaster around an embedded tongue blade or an instrument that can harden in the plaster and serve in the extraction process (Fig. 1).

Foreign bodies that fill the lumen and span the entire mucosal surface create a vacuum that seals the object against the mucosa and prevents pulling the device in a caudal direction, thus impairing its ultimate delivery. Diwan and Graves et al. suggest placing a Foley catheter across the device to break the vacuum (Fig. 2). Others have had success with a Sengstaken-Blakemore tube. These can be placed transanally and extend proximal to the device. Expansion of the catheter balloon can aid in the traction when you attempt to tug the object toward the anal opening. Many have suggested that endoscopy can assist in the extraction of these objects, but Sohn and Weinstein note the contrary. Endoscopy may displace the object into the proximal bowel and confound its subsequent removal. If the lesion is visible using rigid anoscopy, a tenaculum could grasp the object and coax it below the pelvic floor. Lake et al. noted that size was not predictive of success with bedside ex-

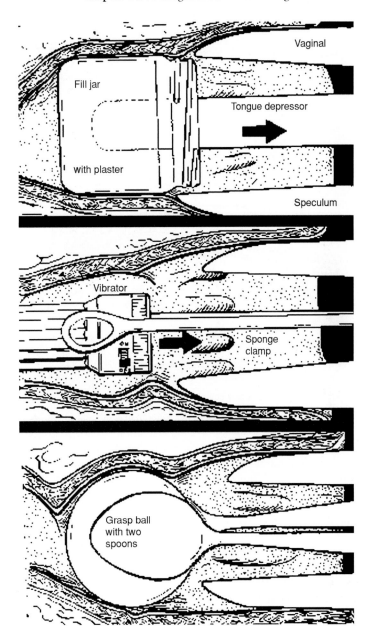

Fig. 1. *Arrows* depict the vectors of force involved in the extraction of rectal foreign bodies. Numerous methods may be used in the extraction process.

traction. They found that lesions located in the sigmoid had a higher likelihood (55%) of requiring operative intervention when compared with 24% of patients with objects in the rectum.

If extraction at the bedside fails, then removal is best performed under anesthesia in an operating room setting. When bedside extraction fails because of a high lying position, Nohme-Kingsley and Abcaraian suggest that patients without peritonitis can be observed for 12 to 24 hours with the hope of distal migration of the object. Similarly, Lake et al. found no association between the length of time of retention and the ultimate need for a surgical extraction or further patient injury.

Once the decision to operate has been reached, the patient's anesthesia is delivered and the patient is placed in the lithotomy position. Lithotomy provides for bimanual manipulations of the object and may convert a high-lying object to a low-lying position.

Once the patient is in the lithotomy position, the surgeon should assess the patient's anal sphincters and carefully dilate the anus. A Fansler anoscope or operating anoscope will centrally apply radial forces and dilate the anus for examination. Surgeons will be able to visualize the lower rectum and approach the retained object. Surgeons have deployed numerous instruments, some fashioned specifically for this

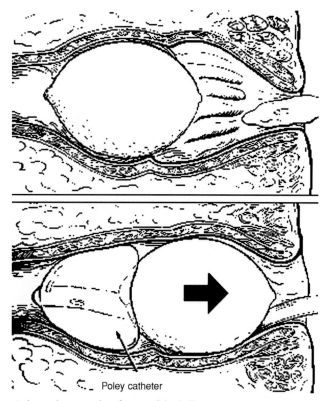

TABLE 1. CATEGORIES OF ASSOCIATED INJURIES WITH RECTAL FOREIGN BODIES	
Category	**Clinical Assessment**
I	Retained foreign body without injury
II	Retained foreign body with mucosal laceration
III	Retained foreign body with sphincter injury
IV	Retained foreign body with rectal perforation

Poley catheter

Fig. 2. A large Foley catheter, with inflation of the balloon, may be used to extract an object.

unique therapy, including obstetric forceps, tenaculum, suction, shoe horns, spoons, and a child's suction dart (Fig. 1).

Once the extraction was completed, Lake et al. performed endoscopy on 43% of their patients. They noted that only 38% had no injuries to the mucosa. Postextraction mucosal abrasions were noted in 43% and mucosal lacerations were noted in 16%. Similarly, nonperforating mucosal lacerations from retained rectal foreign bodies occurred in 16% of patients reported by Barone et al. in 55 patients with rectal trauma associated with anal sexual eroticism. Furthermore, Barone et al. assigned prognostic categories based on the levels of injury (Table 1).

Simple lacerations with minimal bleeding can be observed. Sphincter injuries are not always readily obvious. In this instance, watchful waiting and close follow-up are necessary. When a grossly apparent sphincter injury occurs, a primary repair can be performed. For rectal perforation, the injury requires a controlled rectal washout, primary repair, and local drainage. Only injuries with extensive damage require fecal diversion and presacral drainage.

The treatment of patients with retained rectal foreign bodies can be challenging. The surgeon may need ingenuity, an index of suspicion of foul play, and an unusual amount of patience.

SUGGESTED READING

Barone JE, Yee J, Nealon TF. Management of foreign bodies and trauma of the rectum. *Surg Gynecol Obstet* 1983:156:453.

Busch DB, Starling JR. Rectal foreign bodies: case reports and a comprehensive review of the world's literature. *Surgery* 1986;100:512.

Cohen JS, Sackier JM. Management of colorectal foreign bodies. *J R Coll Surg Edinb* 1996;41:312.

Diwan VS. Removal of 100 watt electric bulb from the rectum [letter]. *Ann Emerg Med* 1982;11:643.

Grasberger RC, Hirsh EF. Rectal trauma: a retrospective analysis and guidelines for therapy. *Am J Surg* 1983;145:795.

Graves RN, Allison EJ Jr, Bass RR, et al. Anal eroticism: two unusual foreign bodies and their removal. *South Med J* 1983;76:667.

Hicks TC, Opelka FG. The hazards of anal sexual eroticism. *Perspect Colon Rectal Surg* 1994;37–57.

Kingsley AN, Abcarian H. Colorectal foreign bodies: management update. *Dis Colon Rectum* 1985;28:941.

Lake JP, Essani R, Petrone P, et al. Management of retained colorectal foreign bodies: predictors of operative intervention. *Dis Col Rectum* 2004;47:1694.

Manning PC, Pratt JH. Fecal incontinence caused by lacerations of perineum *Arch Surg* 1964;88:569.

Sohn N, Weinstein MA. Foreign bodies of the rectum. In: Fazio VW, ed. *Current therapy in colon and rectal surgery*. Philadelphia: BC Decker; 1990:105.

Wagner J. Foreign bodies in the rectum. *Am J Surg* 1937;36:266.

Yaman M, Deitel M, Burul CJ, et al. Foreign bodies in the rectum. *Can J Surg* 1993;36:173.

EDITOR'S COMMENT

The emphasis of this chapter is on the cooperation of the patient. Many of these patients are subject to societal abuse because of sexual preferences. In order to successfully traverse the minefields of removal of rectal foreign bodies, one must be sensitive to sexual orientation and other difficulties the patient may have because the patient's cooperation is essential. I am continually surprised by what can traverse the rectal canal and get above the curve, making removal very difficult. Clarke et al. (*Colorectal Dis* 2005;7:98), writing from Durban, South Africa, reported a really varied series of colorectal objects that needed to be removed under various circumstances. Another example of a rather large, bulky, endorectal object was reported in a review by Low and Dillon (*Australas Radiol* 2005;49:400) in which five subjects, who were mules in the trafficking of heroin and cocaine, were retained by authorities who obtained radiographs showing as many as 107 small objects containing the drug ecstasy (3,4-methylenedioxymethamphetamine, MDMA),

(continued)

which were subsequently removed. Others may not give any report at all. Ooi et al. (*Aust N Z J Surg* 1998;68:852) reported 30 cases, only 10 of whom admitted cooperatively that the foreign body was inserted in the rectum. The rest had to be elicited from careful physical examination and radiology. Nine of the 20 who did not admit to rectal manipulation had objects that could be felt digitally. There were only two injuries in the 30

patients. Finally, ingenuity continues to fill this field. Humes and Lobo (*Gastroint Endosc* 2005;62:610) removed a rectal foreign body by using a Foley catheter passed through a rigid sigmoidoscope. Associate Editor Lawrence J. Brandt, MD, commented that a similar result could have been achieved using flexible sigmoidoscopy.

Not surprisingly, laparoscopic-assisted rectal foreign body removal has been reported at least once.

Berghoff and Franklin (*Dis Colon Rectum* 2005;48:1975) used laparoscopy and Glassman clamps to push the foreign body down toward the rectum or, at least, prevent it from going superiorly in the manipulation. In fact, the transanal grip was occasionally lost during the extraction, but the combination of pushing and pulling finally got rid of what appears to be at least a 5.5-inch foreign body.

J.E.F.

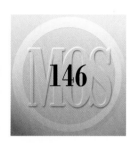

146

Anorectal Disorders

MICHAEL R. B. KEIGHLEY

The Gastrointestinal Tract

Fissure in Ano

 CLINICAL PRESENTATION

The principal clinical presentation of fissure in ano is intense anal pain during defecation, often associated with a small amount of bright red bleeding noticed on the toilet paper. There may be perianal swelling from a skin tag and discharge of mucus. There is often a sensation of tearing during defecation, and there may be a dull ache in the perineum 3 to 4 hours after bowel evacuation.

Women are more commonly affected than men, in a ratio of approximately 58% to 42%, respectively. Most patients are in the third decade of life, but fissure can occur at any age and is well recognized as a cause of pain and constipation in children. Fissure may be exacerbated by a recent episode of constipation and straining. It commonly occurs in women after vaginal delivery. It may occur as a complication of severe diarrhea.

Inspection of the perineum reveals a small, shallow anal ulcer with a sentinel pile and edema, usually in the posterior aspect of the anal margin, particularly in men. Fissures occur anteriorly in 40% of women.

CAUSES

The causes of fissure in ano are unknown. Primary fissure is often associated with alteration in bowel habit, particularly an episode of constipation. Postpartum fissure may be a result of tearing of the anterior aspect of the anal canal during childbirth. Local trauma is believed to be

responsible for the initial skin defect that leads to a boat-shaped ulcer, resulting in chronic symptoms.

Primary fissure in ano may be acute. If healing does not occur, the fissure becomes chronic, in which case the ulcer enlarges in size. There is edema around the fissure associated with an anal skin tag. In 10% of chronic fissures, there is a low intersphincteric anal fistula communicating between the base of the fissure and the dentate line.

Anal fissure is associated with increased resting anal canal pressures. Motility studies reveal ultraslow waves indicative of increased internal anal sphincter activity. Some data suggest that anal fissure is associated with a local reduction in blood flow. Healing of anal fissures is associated with a return to normal anal canal pressures with normal blood flow measurements.

Secondary fissure in ano may occur as a complication of Crohn disease, anal tuberculosis, or acquired immunodeficiency syndrome (AIDS). Occasionally, fissure in ano may complicate a previous operation on the anal canal. Fissures complicating Crohn disease and tuberculosis are often painless. By contrast, anal fissures and ulcers complicating AIDS are often intensely painful and are associated with incontinence and local sepsis.

 DIAGNOSIS

Diagnosis of anal fissure can usually be achieved by inspection. Gentle parting of the buttocks reveals an edematous skin tag and a shallow anal ulcer, usually situated

posteriorly in men but anteriorly in women. There is puckering of the perianal skin as a result of intense spasm of the anal sphincters. Digital examination is often impossible and should not be attempted in patients with severe pain, because the diagnosis can be made by inspection. In patients with chronic anal fissure, digital examination and proctoscopy are often well tolerated. The fissure has edematous margins and is boat shaped, with the transverse fibers of the internal anal sphincter seen at the base of the fissure.

Sigmoidoscopy to exclude a primary cause for fissure in ano and to exclude any rectal pathology should be performed in patients who can tolerate a rectal examination.

 TREATMENT

Medical Therapy

As much as 40% of chronic anal fissures heal by conservative therapy alone. If patients have a history of chronic constipation, treatment should include a bulk laxative, such as methylcellulose or psyllium hydrophilic mucilloid, with a mild laxative, such as bisacodyl or docusate sodium. Patients should be told to avoid straining and be instructed in basic anal hygiene.

Application of local nonsteroidal preparations to control pain may be helpful. Local anesthetic agents may be effective, particularly for acute anal fissure. Steroid preparations may be used to reduce inflammation. A wide variety of commercially available ointments and suppositories exist, which consist of local anesthetic and steroid preparations. The cumulative relapse rate after medical treatment for chronic anal fissure is approximately 50% at 12 months.

SURGICAL TECHNIQUE

Most patients with anal fissure can be treated during an office visit or in an outpatient surgical unit. The purpose of surgical treatment is to reduce excessive activity in the internal anal sphincter by anal dilation or sphincterotomy. Anal dilation results in disruption of the fibers of the internal sphincter and also causes some damage to the external sphincter. The procedure is therefore less specific than internal sphincterotomy, which divides a part of the internal sphincter but leaves the external sphincter intact. Sphincterotomy may be performed as a subcutaneous blind technique or may be performed as an open operation. Preoperative treatment involves use of a disposable phosphate enema. Postoperatively, the patient should be prescribed adequate analgesics and local anesthetic creams, as well as a mild laxative to avoid postoperative constipation. Patients should be warned that there is a 3% risk of postoperative bleeding, and that local pain may continue for 2 to 3 weeks. Incontinence is usually transient, lasting only 2 to 3 months, and may occur in 3% to 5% of patients. Long-standing incontinence is recognized in patients treated by anal dilation, particularly in women and in patients who have had more than one anal dilation. Long-standing incontinence rarely complicates internal sphincterotomy, unless a part of the external sphincter has been inadvertently divided.

Anal Dilation

The patient is anesthetized in a left lateral position. A gentle dilation is undertaken initially using two fingers and slowly stretching the anal canal to accommodate four fingers. A circumferential movement is required, so that the dilation is directed to all parts of the sphincter muscle. The procedure should be performed for 2 to 3 minutes. Forceful dilation should be avoided. A small tampon should be placed in the anal canal after the procedure to prevent hematoma.

Lateral Subcutaneous Internal Sphincterotomy

This procedure may be performed with local or general anesthesia. The intersphincteric groove is identified. Twenty

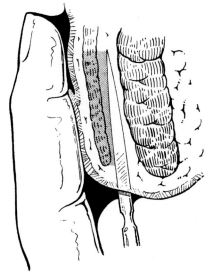

Fig. 1. Lateral subcutaneous sphincterectomy under general anesthetic. (From Keighley MRB, Williams NS. *Surgery of the anus, rectum, and colon.* Philadelphia: WB Saunders, 1993, with permission.)

milliliters of a local anesthetic with a weak adrenaline solution is infiltrated in the submucosal and the intersphincteric planes. A fine cataract blade is inserted in the intersphincteric groove with the blade lying parallel to the circular fibers of the internal sphincter. The cataract blade is then rotated, so that the blade faces the lumen of the anal canal. With the surgeon's index finger in the anal canal, the cataract blade is advanced toward the index finger so as to divide the internal sphincter, but not the anal mucosa (Fig. 1). A small tampon is placed in the anal canal to prevent hematoma.

Open Internal Sphincterotomy

This is my preferred surgical procedure. The patient may be placed in the prone jackknife or the lithotomy position, depending on the surgeon's preference. The lateral aspects of the submucosal and intersphincteric planes are infiltrated with a local anesthetic and a weak adrenaline solution. An anal speculum is inserted to expose the lateral aspect of the anal canal. A transverse incision is made just inside the anal canal and below the dentate line for a length of approximately 1.0 to 1.5 cm. Scissors are used to develop the submucosal plane so that the anal mucosa can be lifted from the internal sphincter and to develop the intersphincteric plane so that there can be no damage to the external sphincter. Once the lower fibers of the internal sphincter have been clearly

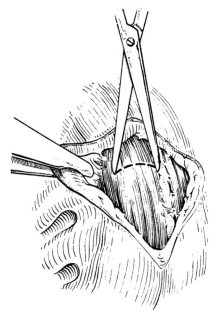

Fig. 2. Open internal sphincterectomy. (From Keighley MRB, Williams NS. *Surgery of the anus, rectum, and colon.* Philadelphia: WB Saunders, 1993, with permission.)

separated from other structures, internal sphincterotomy consists of dividing the internal sphincter with scissors for a length of approximately 2 cm (Fig. 2). Occasionally, for patients with recurrent anal fissure refractory to all other methods, bilateral internal sphincterotomy may be performed.

We never advocate posterior sphincterotomy or excision of the anal fistula, because these operations may be complicated by a gutter deformity in the anal canal and thus result in soiling and impaired continence.

Anorectal Abscess

CLINICAL PRESENTATION

Anorectal sepsis usually presents with anal pain, swelling, and fever. There may be associated swelling and discharge around or within the anal canal. Approximately 30% of patients give a history of a previous episode of anorectal sepsis that has spontaneously discharged or required surgical drainage. Constitutional symptoms are common, and swelling is obvious in patients with ischiorectal abscess, because large volumes of pus under tension give rise to fever, malaise, anorexia, and weight loss. By contrast, swelling may not be evident in patients with intersphincteric and submucous abscesses; similarly, patients

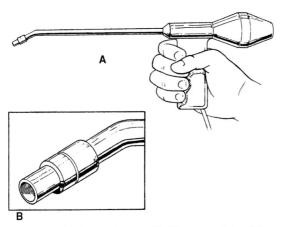

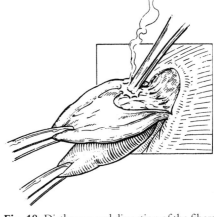

Fig. 16. A: Infrared photocoagulation equipment. **B:** Close-up of tip of photocoagulator. (From Keighley MRB, Williams NS. *Surgery of the anus, rectum, and colon.* Philadelphia: WB Saunders, 1993, with permission.)

Fig. 18. Diathermy and dissection of the fibers of the muscularis submucosa ani. (From Keighley MRB, Williams NS. *Surgery of the anus, rectum, and colon.* Philadelphia: WB Saunders, 1993, with permission.)

Hemorrhoidectomy

Hemorrhoidectomy remains a painful operation, but for most patients is extremely successful as a means of controlling symptoms from third-degree piles. Patients should be counseled before the operation and told that there is a small risk of reactionary or secondary hemorrhage, scarring from excessive skin loss, and of incontinence or soiling from damage to the internal anal sphincter or the formation of a gutter deformity. Rare complications include postoperative fissure or fistula, as well as submucous abscess. In the majority of patients, the operation is successful at controlling prolapse and bleeding.

There are two techniques for hemorrhoidectomy. The operation may be performed as an open procedure so that any discharge of blood, serum, or pus can drain easily, or a closed hemorrhoidectomy may be performed in which the mucosa and the skin defect are closed, which leaves an intact anal canal. We have compared these two techniques and find that the degree of postoperative pain is identical. Physiologic studies also indicate that internal and external sphincter function are equally well preserved by the two operations. Thus, the choice of technique is entirely personal. This author has practiced both techniques but tends to favor the open operation, because the risk of postoperative hematoma is reduced.

Open Hemorrhoidectomy

The operation may be performed in the lithotomy or prone jackknife position. We prefer lithotomy for open hemorrhoidectomy. We also prefer to use general anesthesia. The patient is placed with the feet in stirrups, and the anal canal is gently dilated.

A proctoscope is inserted to identify the site of the three principal hemorrhoids. A weak adrenaline solution (1:200,000) in saline is infiltrated around the skin adjacent to each primary hemorrhoid, and further injection is made in the lower part of the intersphincteric space and in the submucosal plane under the hemorrhoid.

Tissue forceps are then applied to each pile and to the skin adjacent to the hemorrhoid (Fig. 17). I prefer to start with the 7 o'clock hemorrhoid, followed by the 3 o'clock hemorrhoid, and finish with the 11 o'clock hemorrhoid, so that the operation field is not obscured by bleeding. The tissue forceps holding the hemorrhoid and its adjacent skin is grasped in the left hand. A V-shaped incision is made in the surrounding perianal skin with scissors. The cut is deepened toward the anal canal to reveal the lower fibers of the internal anal sphincter. The sphincter is gently swept away with tissue forceps from the hemorrhoid (Fig. 18).

The scissors are then used to excise the hemorrhoidal tissue within the anal canal, which leaves the apex of the hemorrhoid with its arterial supply and venous drainage intact for ligature. The pedicle of each hemorrhoid is then enclosed in an arterial clip, and the pedicle is transfixed using nonabsorbable suture material (Fig. 19). Hemostasis is then secured from the bed of the hemorrhoid by use of cautery. Only then is the pedicle ligated. The ligature is left long so that if any further bleeding occurs, the pedicle can be easily identified and delivered into the operative field. Each hemorrhoid is dealt with in the same manner; however, well-established skin bridges between each V-shaped segment of excised skin must remain. At the end of the operation, an anal speculum is inserted to be absolutely certain that there is complete hemostasis. Gauze dressings are then applied to each hemorrhoidal area.

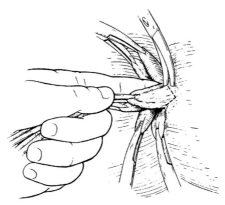

Fig. 17. A V-shaped incision is made over the anoderm at the base of the hemorrhoid. (From Keighley MRB, Williams NS. *Surgery of the anus, rectum, and colon.* Philadelphia: WB Saunders, 1993, with permission.)

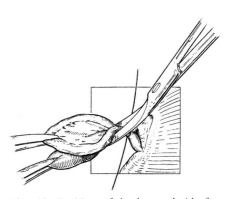

Fig. 19. Excision of the hemorrhoid after transfixion and ligature of its base. (From Keighley MRB, Williams NS. *Surgery of the anus, rectum, and colon.* Philadelphia: WB Saunders, 1993, with permission.)

The Gastrointestinal Tract

Closed Hemorrhoidectomy

We perform closed hemorrhoidectomy with the patient in the prone jackknife position with the buttocks strapped apart and with 40 degrees of hip flexion. A Fansler proctoscope is crucial to the success of the operation. First, the proctoscope is inserted so that the three sites of the primary hemorrhoidal disease are identified. A maneuver that helps to identify the primary hemorrhoids is the insertion of a soft gauze swab into the anal canal. The swab is withdrawn from the anus after removal of the proctoscope. Removal of the swab usually brings with it the hemorrhoids, which can be readily identified.

In our clinic we use general anesthesia for this procedure, but some prefer caudal or regional anesthesia. Even when general anesthesia is used, we strongly advise infiltration with a local anesthetic and a weak adrenaline solution, such as bupivacaine with 1:200,000 adrenaline. Ten milliliters of infiltrate is introduced into the submucosal and subcutaneous planes of each hemorrhoid, so that the hemorrhoidal tissue can easily be separated from the fixed fibers of the internal anal sphincter. Short, curved scissors are used for the excision. The anal skin tag is lifted up with tissue forceps and, by use of the heel of the scissors, the skin tag is cut away from the underlying internal anal sphincter. With a second cut of the scissors, the hemorrhoidal tissue is divided from the wall of the anal canal, which leaves the circular fibers of the internal sphincter readily displayed at the base of the wound (Fig. 20). With an adrenaline solution, there is minimal bleeding. The next maneuver is to dissect any residual hemorrhoidal tissue

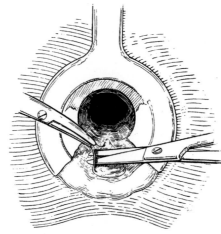
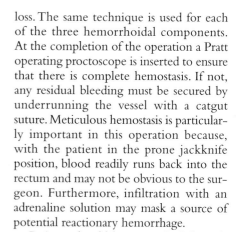

Fig. 21. Additional vascular tissue beneath the anoderm on either side of the incisions is removed. (From Keighley MRB, Williams NS. *Surgery of the anus, rectum, and colon.* Philadelphia: WB Saunders, 1993, with permission.)

from beneath the cut edge of the mucosa on either side of the defect (Fig. 21). This also facilitates creating two mucosal flaps for subsequent closure of the defect. Closure is achieved starting at the apex of the mucosal defect in the depth of the anal canal. We use a plain catgut suture on a cutting needle. The apex of the mucosal defect is anchored to the internal anal sphincter at the apex, and a running suture is then used to approximate the cut mucosal edges (Fig. 22). At the anal verge, a subcuticular technique is used to approximate the skin to avoid leaving a knot at the perianal apex of the wound. The catgut suture is thus continued backward into the anal canal, and a knot is tied just below the dentate line. The process of closure usually completely controls blood

loss. The same technique is used for each of the three hemorrhoidal components. At the completion of the operation a Pratt operating proctoscope is inserted to ensure that there is complete hemostasis. If not, any residual bleeding must be secured by underrunning the vessel with a catgut suture. Meticulous hemostasis is particularly important in this operation because, with the patient in the prone jackknife position, blood readily runs back into the rectum and may not be obvious to the surgeon. Furthermore, infiltration with an adrenaline solution may mask a source of potential reactionary hemorrhage.

Patients should be warned of the risk of bleeding. They must be given liberal supplies of analgesics and laxatives. If fever develops, patients should return to the doctor as quickly as possible because submucosal and intersphincteric abscesses are a recognized complication of closed hemorrhoidectomy.

COMPLICATIONS

The following complications may occur after hemorrhoidectomy, and patients should be warned of them:

1. Reactionary hemorrhage
2. Secondary hemorrhage
3. Pain
4. Retention of urine
5. Postoperative fissure (may be complicated by fistula)
6. Anal stenosis
7. Incontinence
8. Anorectal sepsis

Anorectal Warts

CLINICAL PRESENTATION

Patients present with small, discrete, papuliferous warts around the perineum or at the anal margin. Some anal condylomata coalesce to form large sessile edematous swellings with hyperkeratinization and discharge of mucus. Anal condylomata may bleed or may give rise to pruritus ani. Associated lesions are common and may occur in the vulva and vagina in women, and on the penis or on the scrotum in men. They may also occur within the urethra and the anal canal, and they may be found on the face and hands.

CAUSES

Anorectal warts are caused by the human papillomavirus. They are usually, but not

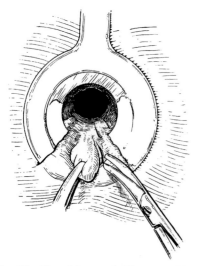

Fig. 20. Closed hemorrhoidectomy. (From Keighley MRB, Williams NS. *Surgery of the anus, rectum, and colon.* Philadelphia: WB Saunders, 1993, with permission.)

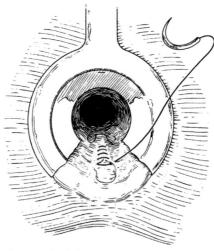

Fig. 22. The defect in the anal canal mucosa is closed. (From Keighley MRB, Williams NS. *Surgery of the anus, rectum, and colon.* Philadelphia: WB Saunders, 1993, with permission.)

exclusively, acquired by sexual transmission. Inoculation may occur from the finger or the penis. Homosexual patients may have associated sexually transmitted disease. Thus, many of these patients should be counseled and screened for the human immunodeficiency virus, as well as for gonorrhea, syphilis, chlamydia, hepatitis, *Giardia,* herpes, cytomegalovirus, and lymphogranuloma venereum.

The human papillomavirus is responsible for malignant change; long-standing anal condylomata should be biopsied. The urethra and the anal canal are important sources of reinfection, and so treatment must be directed for the patient or the patient's partner to such potential sources of reinfection.

 ## DIAGNOSIS

Anal warts are obvious on clinical inspection of the perineum. Women should undergo a full speculum examination so as to exclude lesions in the vulva and vagina. All patients should undergo proctoscopy to exclude condylomata within the anal canal. In male patients, the penis, scrotum, and urethra should be inspected.

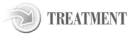 ## TREATMENT

Patients with anal condylomata should be screened in a clinic for sexually transmitted diseases for the reasons given previously. The lesions may be treated by topical application of podophyllum resin, by chemo- or immunotherapy, or by surgical excision.

Podophyllum resin is usually applied as a 10% or 20% solution in benzoin. Long-term studies, however, indicate that only 25% of all patients treated with podophyllum resin achieve complete resolution.

Chemotherapy with colchicine, thiotepa, or fluorouracil (5-FU) has been used. Today, these methods are rarely recommended. There was a vogue for immunotherapy, but long-term studies do not substantiate the early claims of resolution in more than 80% of patients.

Surgical treatment is by cautery, laser ablation, cryotherapy, or scissor excision. We do not advocate cryotherapy. Laser treatment is highly specific to each lesion and causes less tissue destruction than fine-point high-frequency cautery. However, we prefer scissor excision and recommend the technique of subcutaneous and submucosal infiltration with a weak adrenaline solution, which lifts the condylomata away from the normal skin

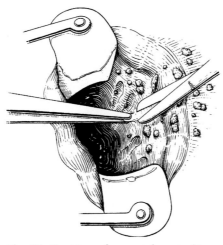

Fig. 23. Excision of anorectal warts. (From Keighley MRB, Williams NS. *Surgery of the anus, rectum, and colon.* Philadelphia: WB Saunders, 1993, with permission.)

so that the condylomata themselves can be excised and leave the surrounding skin or mucosa intact (Fig. 23). This technique is tedious, but it causes infinitely less tissue destruction than excision by cautery and probably less than that from laser excision. In confluent lesions, it may be necessary to treat patients in more than a single visit. Despite the use of a weak adrenaline solution, bleeding can be quite troublesome after multiple scissor excisions. We do not recommend the use of cauterization to control bleeding, but prefer pressure tamponade. Any lesions in the anal canal must be thoroughly cleared by scissor excision as well as removal of the perianal lesions. Follow-up is absolutely essential, because some patients require treatment more than once, and recurrence is common. The overall recurrence rate is approximately 40%. Many recurrences are caused by reinfection. Hence, patients must be carefully counseled and their partners screened.

Pilonidal Sinus

 ## CLINICAL PRESENTATION

Pilonidal sinus is associated with small midline pits behind the anal canal over the sacrum and coccyx. There may be lateral openings, particularly if the disease is complicated by sepsis. These sinuses often discharge purulent material that causes pruritus. Alternatively, the disease may be complicated by acute infection presenting as an abscess. The midline pits often contain hair. The condition principally affects young people after puberty, is more com-

mon in men than in women, principally affects whites, and is rare in black or Asian patients. The condition may be completely asymptomatic and may disappear with age.

CAUSES

There are two theories about the cause of pilonidal sinus: That the disease is caused by a developmental abnormality, or that it is acquired. The developmental theory proposes that there are epidermal rests with hair embedded below the dermis in the midline as a result of failure of fusion. Occasionally, implantation dermoids are seen, but they are quite distinct from pilonidal disease. Most authorities now believe that pilonidal disease is acquired.

The acquired theory suggests that hair is shed from around the perineum or from the head, and that the distal ends of the hair act as drills into small sebaceous or hair follicles. In this manner, hair penetrates or is sucked into the dermis and subcutaneous tissues, which creates minute pits. Subsequently, the pits become infected by skin organisms and give rise to suppuration. The fact that pilonidal disease is more common among barbers and that it can occur between the web spaces of the fingers strongly supports the acquired theory.

 ## DIAGNOSIS

Pilonidal disease is easily diagnosed by the typical location of the midline pits behind the anus overlying the sacrum and coccyx. Occasionally, pilonidal disease may form small subcutaneous fistulae around the anal canal, but this is rare. Most sinuses are directed cephalad, and lateral openings are characteristic if previous episodes of sepsis have occurred. Broken hairs can often be seen exuding from the midline pits.

 ## TREATMENT

Management of Pilonidal Abscess

Pilonidal abscess presents as a swelling just lateral to the midline over the sacrum. There is a hot, tender, fluctuant swelling that may exude pus through the midline pit and also may spontaneously discharge at its apex. Treatment in the emergency room is by incision and drainage. Any further treatment is meddlesome at this stage. Thereafter, treatment of the underlying disease is as described in the following sections.

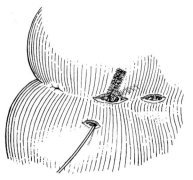

Fig. 24. Excision of midline sinuses and their lateral tracks. (From Keighley MRB, Williams NS. *Surgery of the anus, rectum, and colon.* Philadelphia: WB Saunders, 1993, with permission.)

Elective Treatment of Pilonidal Sinus

Elective treatment of pilonidal sinus can be divided into three major categories: (a) minimal surgery, (b) opening of sinus tracks, and (c) excision with or without rotational skin flaps. Before any form of surgical treatment is begun, serious consideration must be given as to whether treatment is likely to cause more morbidity than does the underlying pilonidal disease itself. In many instances, surgical treatment leaves the patient worse, not better. For many patients, treatment involves a chronically discharging open wound for months or even years and necessitates frequent hospital admission for surgical curettage, as well as repeated office appointments. Furthermore, the natural history of pilonidal disease in untreated patients suggests that, in some, the disease disappears with time.

Minimal Surgery

The principle of minimal surgery is simply to remove hair from midline pits and to keep the buttocks shaved. Many patients with pilonidal disease are not particularly meticulous about personal hygiene. Thus, some form of counseling is necessary to explain the importance of washing the area regularly and to teach how to shave the area. A fine wire brush may be used with local anesthesia to clear the pits and any lateral openings of granulation tissue and hair (Fig. 24).

Opening of Sinus Tracks

If minimal surgery does not control episodes of suppuration, the sinuses themselves may be opened as in fistulotomy (Fig. 25). A probe is passed through the pilonidal sinuses, and the tracks are carefully opened by dividing the skin with a scalpel blade or by cautery. The granulation tissue at the base of the sinuses is curetted. The edges of the skin are excised so that there is an open granulating wound that must be kept meticulously clean and free of hair by the methods described in the previous section. The superficial wounds may heal completely. If they do not, a skin graft or advancement flap may be used to close the defect.

Excision

Wide excision of the pilonidal area, including all affected skin and subcutaneous tissues down to the presacral fascia, may be needed if all other methods of treatments fail. The excision has traditionally been by midline incision to enclose all the disease process. The wound may be left open, allowed to marsupialize, or closed as a primary procedure. There is a high breakdown rate, mainly because of the shearing forces around the buttocks in young, active patients. The shearing forces can be minimized by placing the incision

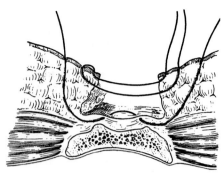

Fig. 26. Excision and primary closure of pilonidal sinus. (From Keighley MRB, Williams NS. *Surgery of the anus, rectum, and colon.* Philadelphia: WB Saunders, 1993, with permission.)

off the midline. There is some evidence to suggest that the avoidance of midline incisions reduces the risk of nonhealing.

If the wound is infected at the time of excision, no attempt should be made to primarily close it. The wound may be left open to granulate and secondary suture may be performed, or a technique of marsupialization may be used, whereby the skin surrounding the defect is sutured down to the presacral fascia.

Primary closure, if it is to be performed, should ensure that there is no dead space and that some form of pressure dressing is maintained to prevent hematoma that may become secondarily infected. Suction drains may be used. Alternatively, compression dressings can be applied within the sutures used to close the defect (Fig. 26).

Occasionally, there are patients whose primary excision site has never healed. These postoperative ulcers can cause considerable morbidity, and their closure may prove difficult. Techniques that may be used to cover such defects include Z- plasty, the use of the rhomboid flap, or the use of myocutaneous flaps based on the superior gluteal artery and nerve. Under these circumstances, most coloproctologists require the help of a plastic surgeon. However, Z-plasty and rhomboid flap techniques may be used during primary excision and suture.

Hidradenitis Suppurativa

 CLINICAL PRESENTATION

Hidradenitis suppurativa never occurs before puberty. Women are affected more commonly than men. The disease presents with skin suppuration and superficial fistulae associated with brawny edema and

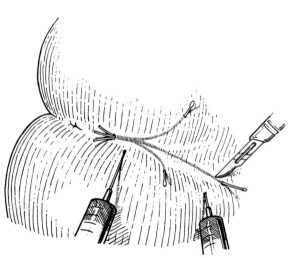

Fig. 25. Laying open of multiple pilonidal sinus tracks. (From Keighley MRB, Williams NS. *Surgery of the anus, rectum, and colon.* Philadelphia: WB Saunders, 1993, with permission.)

induration in areas of the body in which there are apocrine glands. One of these areas, the perineum, may give rise to extensive disease that can be difficult to differentiate from perianal Crohn disease, anorectal fistulae, tuberculosis, and anogenital cancer. The typical presentation is of boils, furuncles, induration, and discharging sinuses on the perianal region, the vulva, the groin, or the axilla. The discharge is thin, watery, and offensive. The condition is often associated with acne.

CAUSES

It is presumed that there is a hormonal basis for this disease, because it never occurs before puberty. The principal abnormality is the occlusion of apocrine ducts by keratin. Obstruction leads to retention of secretions, and secondary infection resulting in fibrosis, sinus formation, and induration.

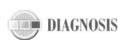

DIAGNOSIS

Diagnosis of hidradenitis is made by the typical appearance in association with lesions in the groin or the axilla. If there is difficulty in making a diagnosis, excision biopsy may prove necessary.

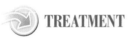

TREATMENT

Treatment depends mainly on the severity of disease. Some patients with chronic induration and only occasional discharge prefer to accept the morbidity of the disease rather than the morbidity of surgical treatment. Surgical treatment is often extensive, is not always successful, and may be associated with extensive morbidity and prolonged hospital stay. Low-dose antibiotics may be used for prolonged periods to prevent secondary infection, but under these circumstances there is inevitable risk of bacterial resistance and superinfection. Alternatively, intermittent courses of antibiotic may be used to treat acute exacerbations of the disease or for secondary infective complications. Localized collections of pus may need drainage. With time, the disease often slowly disappears, leaving fibrosis without infection.

Surgical treatment, to be effective at all, requires total ablation of the apocrine area. Hence, all skin and subcutaneous tissue involved in fibrosis, sinus, and fistulae are excised. For perianal disease, this may involve extensive saucerization, which leaves only perianal skin. The defect may be left to granulate, and elastomer foam dressings have proved extremely helpful, particularly for deep cavitating wounds, to keep the area clean and for ease in subsequent skin grafting, if this should be necessary. A variety of commercially available preparations may also be used to reduce infection and stimulate granulation tissue. Once the area is clean, secondary skin grafting may prove useful. Alternatively, myocutaneous flaps may be used to cover the defect. For extensive perianal disease requiring wide excision, a defunctioning stoma is often necessary to keep the area clean, allow healthy granulation tissue to form, and facilitate subsequent skin grafting.

Rectovaginal Fistula

CLINICAL PRESENTATION

The principal symptom for a patient with a rectovaginal fistula is of the passage of pus or feces through the vagina. Symptoms may be intermittent or continuous and may result in impaired vaginal hygiene or lead to frank fecal incontinence. Small fistulae are often associated with intermittent symptoms, amounting to a small amount of vaginal discharge sometimes accompanied by the passage of gas through the vagina. Small, low rectovaginal fistulae can be extremely difficult to diagnose, whereas large rectovaginal fistulae are clinically obvious with perianal soiling, fecal incontinence, and severe pelvic sepsis and necessitate urgent surgical management.

CAUSES

Rectovaginal fistulae are classified into three broad anatomic groups: (a) forniceal fistulae, (b) septal fistulae, and (c) perineal fistulae.

Forniceal Fistulae

Fistulae entering the posterior fornix of the vagina arise from disease in the pouch of Douglas or from the upper rectum. The common causes are diverticular disease, carcinoma of the large bowel, Crohn disease of the ileum or large bowel, postirradiation fistulae after treatment of gynecologic malignancy (particularly after hysterectomy), and postoperative fistulae after an intestinal anastomosis in the pouch of Douglas.

Septal Fistulae

Fistulae running through the rectovaginal septum, that is, within the middle third of the vagina, are often large, are usually direct, and are invariably caused by rectal or gynecologic conditions. The rectal causes include rectal carcinoma, rectal Crohn disease, and postirradiation rectovaginal fistulae. Gynecologic causes include carcinoma of the cervix or vagina and severe postobstetric fistulae resulting from pressure necrosis from the fetal head in obstructed labor.

Perineal Fistulae

Perineal fistulae often pursue a tortuous course. They run through a part of the perineum or sphincter mechanisms. The fistulae may be small and cause minimal symptoms. Causes of perineal rectovaginal, rectovulvar, and anovulval fistulae include cryptoglandular infections, as in anorectal abscess and fistula (see previous sections); postobstetric fistulae from sphincter damage associated with a defect between the two viscera; iatrogenic fistulae caused by previous surgical treatment; and fistulae complicating perianal Crohn disease (often cryptoglandular).

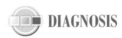

DIAGNOSIS

Identification of large fistulae is often not difficult. By contrast, small, tortuous perineal fistulae may prove exceedingly difficult to positively identify. Large rectovaginal fistulae causing fecal incontinence are associated with intense excoriation of the perianal skin and a red, raw vagina, obvious clinically. Vaginal speculum examination for smaller fistulae is necessary to identify the site of the vaginal opening. Perineal fistulae may be difficult to see, but septal and forniceal fistulae are usually obvious. Examination should also include proctoscopy, particularly for perineal fistulae, to identify whether there is an opening at the dentate line, which is characteristic of a cryptoglandular origin. Proctosigmoidoscopy is necessary to exclude rectal malignancy, Crohn disease, and irradiation damage.

Special investigations may be helpful in delineating the cause and the course of the fistula. Barium enema examination may be necessary to identify inflammatory bowel disease, but the examination is relatively limited in defining the course of the fistula. Likewise, colonoscopy is useful in identifying inflammatory or malignant disease of the large bowel but rarely demonstrates the internal opening unless it is large. Vaginography is a helpful method of identifying forniceal fistulae that cannot be demonstrated by speculum examination.

Examination with the patient anesthetized may be necessary to demonstrate certain fistulae, particularly those that are cryptoglandular in origin or that are postoperative fistulae. The use of fistula probes and injection of dyes may also facilitate identification. Rectal ultrasound is disappointing in the identification of rectovaginal fistulae except in the septal region, in which they are already obvious clinically. Perineal MRI is particularly helpful in identification of obscure fistulae. Any suspicious fistula should be biopsied to exclude malignancy.

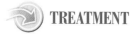

TREATMENT

Preliminary Fecal Diversion

Preliminary fecal diversion is absolutely essential for patients with severe fecal incontinence or where a fistula is complicated by pelvic sepsis.

Definitive Treatment

Disease in the Pouch of Douglas

Disease in the pouch of Douglas causing a fistula through the posterior fornix of the vagina should be treated by resection, when possible. Thus, resection is indicated for Crohn disease associated with fistulae, for diverticular disease causing a rectovaginal fistula, and for malignancy, but in these cases radical hysterectomy and partial excision of the vagina may be necessary. Rectal cancer associated with rectovaginal fistulae certainly requires radical resection of the rectum and the uterus and vagina. High postirradiation fistulae should be treated by sleeve coloanal anastomosis and covering loop ileostomy.

Surgical Treatment of Septal Fistulae

A carcinoma of the middle third of the rectum that causes a rectovaginal fistula is usually treated by abdominoperineal excision, hysterectomy, and partial vaginectomy. Occasionally, sphincter-saving procedures are possible with a coloanal anastomosis and covering loop ileostomy. In patients with a rectovaginal fistula complicating severe rectal or perianal Crohn disease, proctocolectomy and end ileostomy are the treatment of choice. Septal fistulae resulting from radiation damage require rectal excision and an end stoma or a sleeve coloanal anastomosis after excision of the fistula with a covering loop ileostomy (Fig. 27).

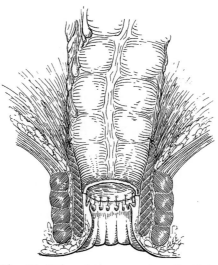

Fig. 27. Coloanal reconstruction of a high rectovaginal fistula. (From Keighley MRB, Williams NS. *Surgery of the anus, rectum, and colon.* Philadelphia: WB Saunders, 1993, with permission.)

Treatment of Perineal Fistulae

Perineal fistulae can be treated in a number of ways, depending on their location, the patient's condition, and previous surgical procedures undergone by the patient.

Mucosal Advancement

Mucosal advancement is the treatment of choice for postobstetric or cryptoglandular rectovaginal fistulae. The fistula track is first identified by careful probing. The vaginal side of the fistula is completely ignored unless there is sepsis, in which case it is cleared by local excision and curettage. An intra-anal retractor is inserted and, with the patient in the prone jackknife position, excellent exposure of the fistula is obtained. The mucosa surrounding the fistula is infiltrated with a weak adrenaline solution. The anterior aspect of the anal canal is also infiltrated in the submucosal and the intersphincteric plane. A transverse incision is made at the level of the fistula or just below it. The internal sphincter at this point is divided transversely, so upward dissection can proceed in the intersphincteric plane for a distance of approximately 4 to 5 cm. Lateral incisions are then made along the long axis of the anus on either side of the fistula opening but diverging from one another as they extend cranially. Thus, a flap of mucosa, submucosa, and internal sphincter is created, with a wide base and a tapering apex containing the fistula. The fistula is then excised by transverse exci-

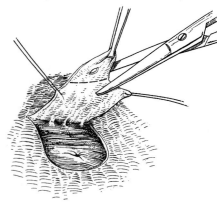

Fig. 28. Anal advancement flap. (From Keighley MRB, Williams NS. *Surgery of the anus, rectum, and colon.* Philadelphia: WB Saunders, 1993, with permission.)

sion of the lower part of the flap. Any infection in the intersphincteric plane is cleared by curettage. The mucosa and internal sphincter below the transverse incision of the anal canal are dissected free, and a direct anastomosis is made between the apex of the flap and the cut anal canal. The lateral margins are then secured with interrupted sutures (Fig. 28). It is rarely necessary to defunction a mucosal advancement flap unless there is underlying Crohn disease or severe perianal sepsis.

Transvaginal Mucosal Advancement

A vaginal mucosal advancement flap is an occasional alternative to anal advancement. The problem with vaginal advancements is that tissues are far less lax than tissues in the anal canal, and thus it is technically more difficult to bring down mucosa from above to close the defect. Nevertheless, for some postoperative fistulae, particularly after restorative proctocolectomy or a previous coloanal anastomosis, there is so much scarring in the anal canal that rectal advancement is impossible; under these circumstances, a vaginal advancement is a more satisfactory option. The technique is identical to that described for rectal mucosal advancement, and the operation may be performed with the patient in the prone jackknife or the lithotomy position.

Transsphincteric Mucosal Advancement

If the internal opening of the rectal component of a rectovaginal fistula is inaccessible through an anal speculum, access may be obtained using the transsphincteric approach or by a posterior rectotomy without division of the sphincters

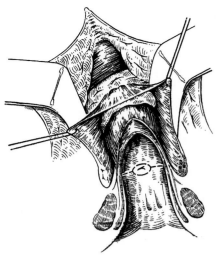

Fig. 29. Transsphincter repair. (From Keighley MRB, Williams NS. *Surgery of the anus, rectum, and colon.* Philadelphia: WB Saunders, 1993, with permission.)

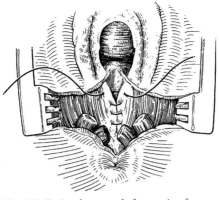

Fig. 30. Perineal approach for repair of a rectovaginal fistula. (From Keighley MRB, Williams NS. *Surgery of the anus, rectum, and colon.* Philadelphia: WB Saunders, 1993, with permission.)

The Gastrointestinal Tract

(Fig. 29). A posterior rectotomy is preferred to the transsphincteric approach, because it does not compromise sphincter function, but access is slightly more restricted. The patient is placed in the prone jackknife position, and a longitudinal incision is made slightly off the midline from the buttock down toward the anal margin. The upper part of the incision is deepened and, if necessary, the lower aspect of the coccyx is excised. If the sphincters are to be divided, they are carefully marked with sutures before division so that they can be reconstituted with ease at the close of the operation. The rectum is then opened between stay sutures or, in the case of the transsphincteric approach, the entire anorectum is opened to expose the fistula. A rectal mucosal advancement flap is created in the same manner as described previously. The only difference is that the internal sphincter is less well developed at this height, and the advancement involves the entire full thickness of the rectal wall. Once the advancement flap has been created and the defect closed, the anorectotomy is then closed in layers—first, the anorectal mucosa, then the internal sphincter, and, finally, the external sphincter, if divided. Closed-suction drainage is usually advisable.

Seton Fistulotomy
Seton fistulotomy is rarely indicated for the treatment of rectovaginal fistulae unless the fistulae complicate Crohn disease, in which case a loose seton provides an ideal method of draining pus. Occasionally, tight seton enclosure to provide delayed

division may be indicated in low perineal fistulae.

Opening and Sphincter Repair
A few perineal fistulae lie superficial to the sphincters. If this is the case, a superficial or intersphincteric fistula could be safely opened. Postobstetric fistulae may be treated by opening the fistula track and repairing the underlying defect in the sphincter. This method of treatment is particularly appropriate if a postobstetric rectovaginal fistula is complicated by a traumatic sphincter injury. (The technique of sphincter repair is described in another section.) If there is any evidence of sepsis, a proximal stoma might be advisable. In localized sepsis, the skin incisions may be left open to granulate (Fig. 30).

Special Considerations for Perianal Crohn Disease

 CLINICAL PRESENTATION

The following are the hallmarks of perianal Crohn disease:

1. Edematous skin tags
2. Painless fissures
3. Deep cavitating ulcers
4. Complex anorectal sepsis associated with complex anorectal fistulae
5. Rectal strictures

Approximately one third of all patients with perianal Crohn disease develop perianal disease before the macroscopic and symptomatic appearance of intestinal disease. Hence, in approximately one third of patients, perianal disease is the first mani-

festation and predates the label of Crohn disease. In 45% of patients, perianal Crohn disease appears at the same time as intestinal disease. In the remaining 25% of patients, perianal disease occurs subsequent to the established diagnosis.

CAUSES

Perianal Crohn disease is a further manifestation of a panmural granulomatous condition. In the anal region it is particularly prominent as a result of nonspecific cryptoglandular infection, as well as enormous lymphoid aggregates found in the anal region. It is thought that the primary process in the anal canal is a penetrating anal ulcer that causes lymphedema, fibrosis, and activation of cryptoglandular infection.

Perianal Crohn disease can be subclassified into benign or aggressive disease. Benign disease often pursues a low-grade course with remission and relapse. Indeed, complete resolution may occur without any specific treatment. Such remission often occurs after surgical treatment or successful medical treatment of the underlying intestinal disease. Benign anorectal disease consists of skin tags, fissures, simple anorectal sepsis, and fistulae. By contrast, certain manifestations of Crohn disease result in progressive anorectal destruction, sepsis, fibrosis, and eventual rectal excision. Aggressive forms of perianal Crohn disease include (a) deep penetrating anal ulcers, (b) complex anorectal fistulae, and (c) extensive perirectal fibrosis and stricture. The rectal excision rate in patients with aggressive disease during a period of 5 years exceeds 80%.

 DIAGNOSIS

Diagnosis of Crohn disease is by the typical clinical syndrome, in conjunction with typical radiology demonstrating intestinal ulceration, deep fissure, thickening of bowel wall, segmental disease, longitudinal ulcers, strictures, and cobblestoning of the mucosa. When possible, diagnosis should be supported by histopathologic evidence of noncaseating granulomas and deep fissured ulcers associated with transmural disease.

The typical appearances of perianal Crohn disease with skin tags, anal fissures and ulcers, complex anorectal fistulae, and anorectal strictures should be supported by biopsy, when possible, along with full intestinal radiology. The following conditions should also have been excluded: sexually transmitted disease, anorectal tuberculosis, anorectal and anogenital cancer, hidradenitis suppurativa, Behçet syndrome, and anorectal lymphoma.

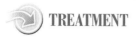 **TREATMENT**

Conservative Therapy

Conservative treatment is recommended for asymptomatic perianal Crohn disease. It is particularly appropriate for patients with minor skin tags, painless anal fissures, and simple anal fistulae (including simple, low rectovaginal fistulae), and in patients with other nonspecific anal disease, such as hemorrhoids. In some patients, surgical treatment may compromise continence. Perianal wounds tend to heal slowly. Hence, surgical treatment should be avoided when disease causes no symptoms or is likely to remit spontaneously.

Drainage of Pus

Perianal Crohn disease is likely to cause progressive fibrosis and anal destruction if sepsis is left without being adequately drained. Anorectal sepsis in Crohn disease is complex and should be carefully defined by imaging techniques and examination with the patient under anesthesia. The intersphincteric plane is a source of occult sepsis, and in patients with infective symptoms and in whom traditional drainage identified little pus, the intersphincteric plane should be explored to ensure that this is not the seat of sepsis. Anorectal sepsis is often associated with fistulae. Recurrent sepsis is common; we recommend the use of soft, loosely tied setons to establish prolonged drainage and subsequent resolution. Mushroom catheters can

also be used, particularly if irrigation is deemed necessary.

Defunction

In some patients, the progression of anorectal disease can be halted and even encouraged to completely resolve by diverting the fecal stream from the anorectal region. This method of treatment is particularly appropriate for severe anorectal sepsis and fistulae and in patients with anorectal strictures. Many patients undergoing loop ileostomy for fecal diversion in perianal disease eventually progress to proctocolectomy because, although fecal diversion switches off active disease, the chances of restoring intestinal continuity are less than 20%.

Selective Treatment

Certain forms of anorectal Crohn disease deserve specific treatment.

Steroid Injection

Local steroid injection may be useful as a means of healing penetrating ulcers complicating Crohn disease.

Dilation

Anorectal dilation may play a useful part in the management of patients with short diaphragmatic anorectal strictures.

Advancement Flaps

Mucosal advancement may play an important role in selected patients with anorectal and rectovaginal fistulae, but because of the risks of sepsis and the relatively poor healing in perianal Crohn disease, coexisting fecal diversion is often advised.

Seton Fistulotomy

Tight seton fistulotomy may be used in selected cases of anorectal fistulae. Each case must be judged on its own merit. Whenever anorectal fistulae are treated in Crohn disease, coexisting sepsis must be adequately drained, and fecal diversion may be necessary.

Proctocolectomy

Proctocolectomy is eventually required in many patients, particularly those with deep penetrating anal ulcers, complex anorectal fistulae, and progressive anorectal stenosis with sepsis. Proctocolectomy in these patients is difficult. An intersphincteric excision of the anorectum is impossible, and wide excision is often necessary to clear sepsis. These patients risk unhealed perineal wounds and persistent perineal sinus. Persistent perineal sinus in these patients may eventually require treatment by myocutaneous rectus abdominis flaps. Nevertheless, the quality of life in patients after proctocolectomy for anorectal Crohn disease is generally satisfactory, once patients have accepted that their lives are better with a permanent ileostomy.

SUGGESTED READING

Beck DE, Wexner SD. *Fundamentals of anorectal surgery.* New York: McGraw-Hill, 1992.

Corman ML. *Colon and rectal surgery,* 3rd ed. Philadelphia: Lippincott, 1993.

Fielding LP, Goldberg SM. *Surgery of the colon, rectum, and anus.* New York: Chapman and Hall.

Keighley MRB, Williams NS. *Surgery of the anus, rectum, and colon,* 2nd ed. Philadelphia: WB Saunders, 1999.

Phillips RKS. *Anal fistula.* New York: Chapman and Hall, 1995.

EDITOR'S COMMENT

We are indeed fortunate to have one of the most experienced and distinguished colorectal surgeons to provide commentary for anorectal disorders. In this complete and detailed chapter, Professor Keighley covers the extent of anorectal disease, including pilonidal disease, and sheds some light not often brought up in this country on the cause and some different treatments of this disorder.

This is appropriate because, as I stated in the commentary in the Fourth Edition, anorectal disorder is among the most poorly treated in the United States. "Most U.S. surgeons who are not specially trained in these areas consider anorectal disorders to be troublesome, and indeed they are—not to the surgeon but to the patient" (Baker RJ, Fischer JE, eds. *Mastery of surgery*, 4th ed. Philadelphia: Lippincott Williams & Wilkins, 2001:1656). However, it is clear that there is much

misery caused by anorectal disorders, and that probably more patients suffer for a longer period of time from something that surgeons and gastroenterologists consider an extraordinarily minor situation, and yet the amount of suffering, ounce for ounce, is, as it were, tremendous.

There are a number of pearls in this book that will help the surgeon who is not especially trained in colorectal disease in treating these patients. For example, the statement that 40% of anal fissures are anterior in women is not widely known, nor is it widely quoted. Presumably, at least theoretically, this is the result of tearing of the birth canal and, thus, the anterior stress on the rectal mucosa. This is extraordinarily helpful because most surgeons, when they examine the patient for anal fissures, feel posteriorly for the break in the mucosa and in the tenderness, so knowing that in women the defect in the

anal mucosa may be anterior will help in what to look for in the examination.

As to the cause of anal fissure, the mythology is that it results from increased resting anal canal pressures. However, as the author points out, motility studies reveal ultraslow waves indicative of increased internal anal sphincter activity. Other data suggest that anal fissure is associated with a local reduction in blood flow, which makes sense because it would probably impair healing. What is surprising is that healing of anal fissures is associated with a return of normal anal canal pressures and normal blood flow measurements. Theoretically, the increased anal sphincter pressures, with or without reduced blood flow, are chronically present and do not vary. Thus, the finding that the sphincter pressure is the result of, and not the cause of, the anal fissure should lead one to re-examine

(continued)

the entire concept of why anal fissures form. Whatever the cause, the relapse rate after medical treatment for chronic anal fissure is allegedly about 50%, which well agrees with my own personal experience. The question is, When does one undertake surgical therapy, whatever it is?

The simplest form of surgical therapy is anal dilation, usually accomplished under outpatient surgical conditions. Anal dilation works by tearing or disrupting the fibers of the internal sphincter and, inadvertently I suppose, causing damage to the external sphincter. It should not be carried out more than once because tears may occur in two different areas, in which case incontinence will result, and thus, the incontinence rate unfortunately is between 3% and 5%. It is usually transient, lasting only 2 or 3 months, but may be permanent.

The other alternative is lateral sphincterotomy. This can be done either open or closed. Happily, there is a Cochrane Collaboration, which, with its usual precision, analyzed 24 randomized clinical trials encompassing 3,475 patients who were included in the review (Nelson R. *The Cochrane Library* 2005; issue 3). In this review, the combined results for open versus closed partial lateral internal sphincterotomy showed little difference between the two procedures in both long- and short-term follow-up, both in fissure persistence and in the risk of incontinence. On the other hand, anal stretch and posterior midline internal sphincterotomy should probably be abandoned according to this review. The study concludes that more data are needed to assess the effectiveness of posterior internal sphincterotomy, anterior levatorplasty, wound suture, or papilla excision. Other proposed treatments include botulinum toxin injected into the sphincter. Arroyo et al. (*Am J Surg* 2005; 189:429), in a randomized prospective trial, compared the effectiveness and morbidity of surgical versus chemical sphincterotomy in the treatment of chronic anal fissure. There was a 3-year follow-up. While there was a 92% overall healing in the open sphincterotomy group, there was only 45% overall healing in the toxin botulinum group ($P <.001$). Higher recurrence seems to be associated with a sentinel pile before treatment and manometric criteria, such as persistently elevated mean resting pressure, slow wave time percentage, or the presence of ultraslow waves. After 3 years, incontinence was present, as with most other studies, in 5% of the open sphincterotomy group and in none of the botulinum toxin group. Because of the incidence of incontinence following sphincterotomy, the authors concluded that, despite the low healing, patients over 50 years of age who are at greater risk for incontinence should be treated with botulinum and patients under 50 should be treated with lateral sphincterotomy. All seem to agree, however, that posterior incision with or without open sphincterotomy runs the risk of a gutter deformity. In that case, perpetual soiling occurs. While some enclaves, such as The Cochrane Collaboration, believe that open posterior sphinc-

terotomy with excision of the ulcer should be tested further, most others disagree.

One of the wonderful points of this chapter is the necessity to culture a collection to see whether it will develop into a chronic fistula. Professor Keighley states that those that have coliform have a very good chance of developing into a fecal fistula, whereas those that are staphylococcal in origin by and large do not develop into fistulae.

I will not attempt to summarize the superb segment on hemorrhoidectomy with the various classifications, which are extremely important because the treatments are different. Not all cases require hemorrhoidectomy. The earlier stages of "piles," as they are called, require suture of the mucosa so that the piles no longer prolapse. However, for some of the advanced stages of piles, rubber-band treatment is probably most appropriate.

The discussion of pilonidal sinus and abscess is masterful. It is interesting how the concept and treatment of this annoyance—how it sometimes causes extreme discomfort, inability to hold a job, and repeated attempts at surgical cure—have changed over the years. Far from being congenital, with malunion of the bilateral plates of skin that come together in the midline, it does appear that the evidence for pilonidal sinus and abscess being acquired begins with pits and then hair inhabiting the pits, resulting in infection, abscesses, etc. It is probably appropriate to consider nonexcisional therapy as the initial step: Hair shaving, drainage of abscesses, trying to rid the central area of hair, laser hair ablation, and the insistence on excellent hygiene. However, if excision must be carried out, it seems likely that an off-midline incision is much more apt to heal than a midline incision.

Billingham et al. (*Curr Probl Surg* 2004;41[7]: 586) defined the ideal treatment of pilonidal sinus: It would be "easy to perform, require short or no hospitalization, have a low recurrence rate, have minimal pain and wound care, have a fast return to normal activity, and be cost effective. To date, no treatment, conservative or aggressive, meets all these criteria." After reviewing all the evidence, the authors stated that, "the best evidence that is available seems to favor flap or asymmetric closure over a simple incision in the midline, with or without primary closure of the wound." Armstrong and Barcia (*Arch Surg* 1994;129:914) carried out conservative treatment of pilonidal disease. They utilized conservative therapy with meticulous shaving and hair removal, but unfortunately the excisional group was not controlled for the type of operation performed. They then compared the number of occupied bed days and number of operations needed over 3 years in both groups, and found a highly significant difference in favor of conservative treatment. They did not, however, report on recurrence rates or healing. The criticism regarding this study is that the investigators knew nothing about what happened to the patients—whether they went to other hospitals for therapy or were still suffering from pilonidal disease.

There are, however, only four randomized prospective studies comparing midline incision with

or without primary closure. Fuzun et al. (*Dis Colon Rectum* 1994;37:1148) compared open excision with or without closure with follow-up to 3 years. Infections were present in 3.6% of the closed group and in 1.8% of the open group. There were no recurrences in the open group; the closed group had 4.4% recurrence ($P >0.01$). They did not, however, recommend open excision and leaving the wound open because, even though the rates of infection or recurrence are relatively low, there is much more discomfort and morbidity when leaving the wound open. Kronborg et al. (*Br J Surg* 1985;72:303) randomized 88 patients in one of three arms, thus inviting a type II error. They basically found no significant differences between excision with primary closure and excision with primary closure and the addition of clindamycin, including a 3-year follow-up. The time to healing, however, was significantly longer in the open group versus the primary closure group (64 vs. 15 days, $P >0.001$). There were no significant differences in the recurrence rate, but, then, I would not have expected that with groups so small. Sondenaa et al. (*Eur J Surg* 1996;162:237) found no difference in healing or recurrence in a study involving midline excision and primary closure, with or without cefoxitin prophylaxis. They did not recommend cefoxitin prophylaxis, which I find difficult to adhere to. The same authors randomized 60 patients in each group to excision with primary closure with a median follow-up of 4.2 years. There was no significant difference in recurrence between the groups. There were several trials concerning flap-based or asymmetrical closures off the midline, for example, the Limberg flap (Urhan et al. *Dis Colon Rectum* 2002;45:656) and several other flaps. The complications of the flaps seem to be higher, but in fact the long-term closure, in most studies, seems to be better. Thus, we are left with the dictum according to the current hypotheses that conservative treatment should be the cornerstone of the therapy, and includes meticulous shaving and hair removal by any means necessary, and general hygiene. Antibiotics, according to many authors, are not appropriate, although I continue to use them. Flap closures seem to work better for overall results, and midline excision does seem to work most of the time. Most authors believe that it is logical to reserve the more complex flap procedures for long-suffering patients with multiple recurrences or nonhealing wounds.

Finally, in the treatment of anorectal fistulae, the Kraske approach—splitting the rectum from behind in a parasacral incision—is something that is not often practiced, and requires a master surgeon to carry out a high rectal advancement flap in very high fistulae. I would add one additional matter to the perianal Crohn disease, and that is that usually, at least in my experience, the tags around the rectum, even in early disease, seem to indicate activity of Crohn disease.

Again, this is a masterful chapter, and we are very grateful to Professor Keighley for excellent effort.

J.E.F.

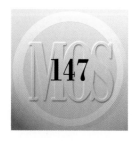

147 | Functional Bowel Disorders

MICHAEL R. B. KEIGHLEY

| Incontinence

Incontinence of feces is a demoralizing and psychologically devastating condition for the patient. It is far worse in terms of quality of life than incontinence of urine. So distressing is the condition that many patients afflicted by incontinence of feces never admit their problem to their families or closest medical attendants. Symptoms are therefore concealed, because patients feel ashamed that they are "dirty," with the inevitable consequence that they become social outcasts with loss of self-esteem, demoralization, and loss of confidence.

True fecal incontinence, or the loss of bowel contents without awareness, is the most distressing symptom, necessitating protective clothing and diapers. In many patients, there is loss of anorectal sensation and motor function. With urge incontinence, patients have to rush to the bathroom.

Hence, sensory awareness is retained, but motor control is only capable of preventing involuntary defecation for a short time. These patients fear traveling or moving out of social circumstances in which a bathroom is not available. Urgency is, of course, a common symptom in patients with rectal disease, particularly proctitis or a narrowed rectum, as well as after obstetric trauma.

Soiling is caused by the inability of the anal canal to close completely. Sensation is thus usually preserved, and there is a defect in the anal canal through which feces may seep.

Overflow incontinence is caused by fecal impaction. Liquid feces leak around a solid bolus of fecal material that occupies the entire lumen of the rectum. Overflow incontinence is often associated with the aging process; megacolon is associated with loss of sensory awareness in the rectum.

 CLINICAL PRESENTATION

Clinical presentation usually identifies the principal cause for incontinence. Women are affected far more commonly than men are, because obstetric injury is the most common cause of incontinence requiring surgical treatment. Some patients become incontinent after operations on the anal canal or on the rectum and colon. A further group includes patients who sustain trauma to the perineum. Any patient presenting with fecal incontinence should be closely questioned to exclude underlying neurologic disorders, particularly demyelinating disease in the young and cauda equina lesions at all ages. There is also a group of patients with congenital disease who present with incontinence. In such patients, there is usually a history of surgical treatment in the neonatal period for anorectal agenesis, Hirschsprung disease, meningocele, or other congenital lesions affecting the cauda equina or anorectum. Finally, 70% of patients with a rectal prolapse are incontinent; hence, prolapse must be excluded in all patients with symptoms of incontinence.

CAUSES

Factors Responsible for Normal Continence

Normal continence depends on a number of correlated factors that, in principle, include a reservoir, an anorectal junction that opens and closes at will, and a closed anal canal at rest.

The rectal reservoir may be compromised in patients with inflammatory disease affecting the rectal mucosa and the wall of the rectum, as in ulcerative colitis and Crohn disease. The rectal ampulla may be severely compromised in patients who have had previous radiation treatment or may have been surgically reduced in capacity among patients having ileoanal or coloanal anastomoses, particularly where no reservoir has been constructed. The voluntary control mechanism for opening and closing the anal canal consists of the pelvic diaphragm and puborectalis sling, particularly, as well as the striated external anal sphincter. These muscles may be damaged from trauma after obstructed vaginal deliveries. They may become neuropathic from prolonged second stage of labor, and they may be physically divided by the fetal head or by an obstetrician if an episiotomy extends through the sphincters. The striated muscle may fail to function if there has been severe infection resulting in fibrosis around the sphincters or pelvic floor, or the external sphincters may have been divided during anal operations, particularly fistulotomy, or by perineal trauma.

The phenomenon of the anal canal being closed at rest depends on the involuntary contraction of the circular smooth muscle around the anal canal. The internal sphincter is under autonomic control mediated through nitric oxide. The smooth muscle itself may be damaged by previous surgery, such as hemorrhoidectomy, anal dilation, or sphincterotomy. It may become neuropathic from operations that interrupt the normal intermyenteric fibers innervating the internal sphincter, and it may be defective in patients in whom normal chemical transmitters no longer function, as, for instance, in Hirschsprung disease.

The anorectum cannot function normally if it does not receive afferent signals. Thus, patients with impairment of rectal or anal sensation have compromised continence. The sensory fibers of the pudendal nerve supply the anorectum, and this nerve may be damaged after obstetric trauma and in cauda equina lesions. Cerebral degeneration from any cause may result in impaired rectal evacuation and incontinence.

Causes of Incontinence

Obstetric trauma may result in disruption of the fibers of the puborectalis and pelvic floor, a neuropathic injury affecting the pudendal nerve, which affects the motor and sensory components of the anorectum. Obstetric trauma may directly cause sphincter injury. Patients may have impairment of rectal evacuation and lack of control from sensory and motor deficiency.

Postoperative incontinence may be a result of damage to the internal or external anal sphincter after operations on the anus, such as hemorrhoidectomy, sphincterotomy, anal dilation, and anorectal fistula surgery. In some cases, the sphincter muscles may be divided. In others, a gutter deformity may develop in the anal canal, which prevents the anal canal from remaining closed at rest. Colorectal operations may also result in incontinence if they cause rectal strictures or fibrosis of the reservoir, which then is no longer compliant and is small in volume capacity. Incontinence may develop after transection of the low rectum or anal canal as a result of interruption of the intermyenteric autonomic nerve plexus. Thus, any operation on the colon and rectum, particularly if it involves a low anastomosis, may result in impaired continence.

Perineal trauma may result in damage to the sphincter, pelvic floor, anal canal, and rectum. There is often associated injury to the urethra, the bony pelvis, and the soft tissues of the buttocks.

Neurologic injury may involve upper motor neurons, which usually results in severe constipation, fecaloma, and soiling, or lower motor neurons, in which the anorectum is completely patulous and there is buttock anesthesia. More localized neurologic injury may involve the pudendal nerve in patients who strain or in whom there has been a prolonged second stage of labor. Diffuse neurologic abnormality may occur in demyelinating disease and in the neurologic degenerative process seen in the acquired immunodeficiency syndrome.

Sepsis around the anal canal may result in skeletal muscle destruction and fibrosis. This cause of incontinence may occur when inefficient or delayed drainage of anorectal sepsis has occurred and in patients with severe localized inflammatory disease of the anal canal, as may occur in Crohn disease or in deep penetrating ulcers associated with the acquired immunodeficiency syndrome.

Congenital causes of incontinence may be anorectal agenesis, Hirschsprung disease, rectal reduplication, and anorectal dermoids, or the congenital abnormality may affect the neural tube, as in patients with meningomyelocele or its variants.

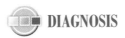

DIAGNOSIS

Clinical Examination

Clinical examination identifies the principal cause of incontinence in most patients, but in certain instances specialized anorectal physiology is required for diagnosis and as a means of recommending whether surgical treatment is indicated.

Inspection of the perineum can identify scars from previous anal surgery, episiotomy, or obstetric injury. Often, a defect in the sphincter ring is apparent. The site of the anus should be noted. Anterior displacement suggests an ectopic anus (minor variant of anorectal agenesis). The presence of skin tags, fistulae, or the presence of patulous anus should be recorded. Inspection should then include examination during straining to exclude a rectal prolapse and to assess the degree of perineal descent and vaginal descent, cystocele, and rectocele.

Rectal examination should attempt to assess resting tone and the contractile activity of the external anal sphincter and the puborectalis. Rectal examination should also identify any defect in the sphincter and any gutter deformity, in addition to any palpable pathologic abnormality in the rectum.

Proctosigmoidoscopy should be performed to exclude proctitis, polyps, or any other colorectal pathology.

Specialized Diagnostic Techniques

Anal manometry provides data on the maximum resting anal canal pressure and the maximum pressure generated during a maximum squeeze effort (Fig. 1). Manometry also helps to identify the length of the high-pressure zone, and vector manometry may be used to clarify areas of reduced anal pressure, signifying localized defects. In some circumstances, ambulatory manometry may be necessary. An inflatable balloon should then be inserted into the rectum and anal manometry performed during balloon distention to determine the presence or absence of the rectoanal inhibitory reflex. This reflex may be absent in Hirschsprung disease and in some patients with incontinence. Distention of a rectal balloon is a simple method of crudely assessing rectal capacity and rectal sensation. However, for compliance measurements of the rectum, integrated changes in intrarectal pressure are recorded with incremental volumes in the rectal balloon. Anal sensation should be measured using the technique of anal mucosal electrosensitivity in the lower, mid-, and upper anal canal.

Electromyography was formerly used for mapping the external anal sphincter in patients with sphincter defects and in assessing ectopic anus. However, the use of needle electrodes is painful and poorly tolerated by patients, particularly if there is scar tissue. Likewise, measurement of fiber density as an assessment of the degree of denervation may be performed by repeated sampling of the external sphincter and puborectalis by use of concentric needle electrodes. For the same reason, patients find this investigation difficult to tolerate and are not particularly compliant. By contrast, conduction studies are less invasive and give an assessment of pudendal neuropathy. Pudendal nerve terminal motor latency measurements can be made by stimulating the pudendal nerve as it winds around the ischial tuberosity and recording the evoked contraction in the external sphincter after stimulation (Fig. 2). Conduction delays are associated with pudendal neuropathy, but there is considerable observer variation with this measurement.

Ultrasound examination of the anal canal and rectum has superseded electromyography in the identification of sphincter defect. Anal ultrasonography can be used for dynamic assessment of contractility, as well as definition of anatomic defects (Fig. 3), morphology, and pathologic conditions (e.g., abscess and fistula). In the future, magnetic resonance imaging coils

The Gastrointestinal Tract

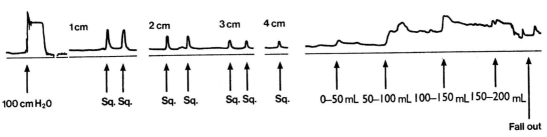

Fig. 1. A typical and pressure profile in fecal incontinence. (From Keighley MRB, Williams NS. *Surgery of the anus, rectum, and colon.* Philadelphia: WB Saunders, 1993, with permission.)

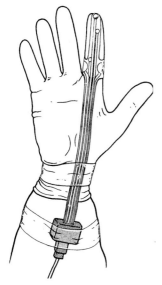

Fig. 2. Testing pudendal nerve latency. (From Keighley MRB, Williams NS. *Surgery of the anus, rectum, and colon.* Philadelphia: WB Saunders, 1993, with permission.)

placed within the lumen of the rectum may provide additional important information.

Many patients with fecal incontinence have some impairment of rectal evacuation. Thus, assessment of rectal emptying by isotopic techniques or during videoproctography is indicated for some patients. Videoproctography may also be needed to exclude coexisting abnormalities, such as

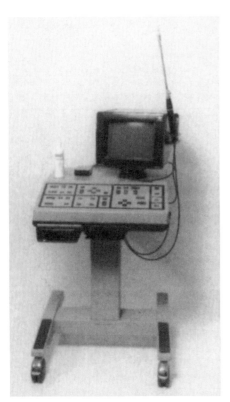

Fig. 3. Anal ultrasonography.

intussusception, perineal descent, and rectocele, as well as to provide playback images to record pelvic floor movements during contraction and attempted defecation.

In general, patients with low resting anal pressures or low squeeze pressures, patients with a short high-pressure zone, patients with gross perineal descent, and patients with anal anesthesia and gross prolongation of pudendal nerve terminal motor latency do badly after attempted reconstructive surgery. Thus, for such patients, counseling for a possible stoma might be a more appropriate policy than attempted reconstructions.

 TREATMENT

Conservative Therapy

Many patients with fecal incontinence have a history of diarrhea. Under these circumstances, particularly if the incontinence is relatively mild, control of the diarrhea may achieve sufficient improvement and further therapy becomes unnecessary. Use of codeine phosphate and loperamide can be important. In patients with rapid transit times, tablets or capsules may not be absorbed, but an elixir may be.

Physiotherapy and Biofeedback

Unquestionably, some patients can no longer contract the sphincter and pelvic floor complex appropriately in response to rectal distention. Others seem incapable of sphincter and pelvic floor contraction on command and tend to strain during attempted voluntary contraction. Another group finds it difficult to contract the sphincter and pelvic floor after recent injury because of pain and psychological trauma. Such patients may be improved dramatically by a series of pelvic floor exercises, faradism, electrical stimulation of the sphincter muscles, and biofeedback retraining. Biofeedback involves an afferent stimulus as a learning process to trigger pelvic floor and sphincter contraction. Biofeedback retraining may produce dramatic improvement in patients who have problems in learning the technique. Biofeedback may also heighten rectal sensory awareness. However, biofeedback requires complete cooperation by the patient. Hence, in motivated patients, this form of treatment is important, particularly for minor forms of incontinence. It may also be helpful as a preoperative conditioning process so that the discipline can be reinforced postoperatively.

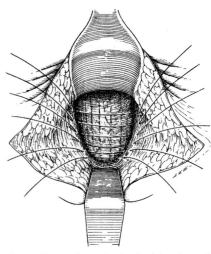

Fig. 4. Postanal repair. An incision is made posterior to the rectum and the anus retracted anteriorly (here depicted with the patient prone in the jackknife position). Prolene sutures are placed to bring the pubis rectalis together posterior to the rectum. (From Keighley MRB, Williams NS. *Surgery of the anus, rectum, and colon.* Philadelphia: WB Saunders, 1993, with permission.)

Postanal Repair

The aim of postanal repair is to restore the anorectal angle; this used to be considered essential for continence. The operation is performed with the patient in the lithotomy or prone jackknife position, and the patient is catheterized. A curved incision is made behind the anal canal, and a flap of skin is raised toward the anus. When the fibers of the external anal sphincter are reached, the intersphincteric plane is defined. The intersphincteric plane is then opened by retracting the external sphincter posteriorly to reach the retrorectal plane. At this point, Waldeyer fascia must be divided transversely so that the veins on the back of the rectum can be exposed (Fig. 4). By retracting the rectum anteriorly, one can display the striated muscle fibers of the puborectalis. Further upward dissection allows the retrorectal fat to be dissected from the pelvic floor. The operation involves closing the puborectalis in the midline behind the rectum with a series of interrupted Prolene sutures. The wound is closed over a suction drain.

Anterior Levatorplasty

Anterior levatorplasty is useful in patients with rectocele and in some patients requiring sphincter repair in whom there is a deficiency in the anterior aspect of the pelvic floor. The patient is placed in the prone jackknife or lithotomy position.

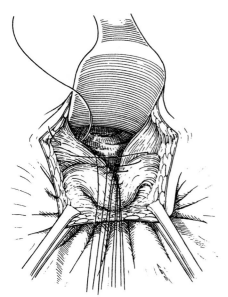

Fig. 5. Anterior levatorplasty. (From Keighley MRB, Williams NS. *Surgery of the anus, rectum, and colon.* Philadelphia: WB Saunders, 1993, with permission.)

Liberal infiltration of the rectovaginal septum with a weak adrenaline solution and a local anesthetic is necessary. A transverse incision is made across the perineum, between the rectum and the vagina, but in front of the anterior border of the anal sphincters. The external anal sphincter is identified posteriorly, and the entire rectovaginal septum is dissected free to the level of the pelvic peritoneum where the rectum and the vagina move away from one another at the rectovaginal cul-de-sac. The posterior vaginal wall is then dissected from the levator muscles, so that the anterior limbs of the puborectalis can be easily identified. Repair involves approximating the anterior aspect of the puborectalis in the midline between the rectum and the vagina. In some patients, the anterior aspect of the external anal sphincter is also plicated or repaired (Fig. 5).

Total Pelvic Floor Repair

Total pelvic floor repair is a combination of postanal repair with anterior levatorplasty. It must be performed through two separate incisions.

Sphincter Repair

Sphincter repairs are indicated for patients with a localized defect in the external anal sphincter. The operation may be needed for postobstetric injury, division of the sphincter after fistula surgery, or traumatic injuries of the perineum. In each of these

three situations, the specific method of repair may have to be modified according to the extent of damage.

The patient may be operated on in the prone jackknife or lithotomy position. Prior infiltration with a weak adrenaline solution and a local anesthetic is always advisable. In postobstetric sphincter injuries, a cruciate incision may be used to provide excellent access to the rectovaginal septum, the perineal body, and the sphincters (Fig. 6). The cruciate incision is usually closed as a Z-plasty, but there is a tendency for wounds to break down. Thus, a circumanal incision is preferred by most surgeons, leaving the center open for drainage. For a defect after previous fistulotomy, a circumanal incision is usually more appropriate. In traumatic perineal injuries, the incision depends on the precise site of the defect. The first task is to dissect the external anal sphincter on either side of the defect and preserve, where possible, the internal anal sphincter. Stay sutures are placed on either side of the sphincter defect, and the scar tissue is divided. In patients with postobstetric injuries, the entire rectovaginal septum is dissected free so that an anterior levatorplasty can be combined with sphincter repair. However, in the case of injury after sphincterotomy, levatorplasty is rarely necessary unless one is dealing with an anterior deficiency in a female patient. In patients with perineal trauma, it may be necessary to identify any defect that may be present in the rectum as well as any defect in the

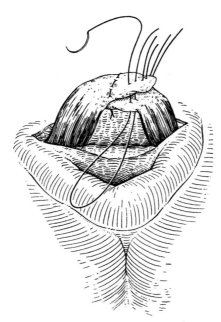

Fig. 6. Sphincter repair. (From Keighley MRB, Williams NS. *Surgery of the anus, rectum, and colon.* Philadelphia: WB Saunders, 1993, with permission.)

anal canal. In such cases, reconstitution of the anorectum by repair of its circular smooth-muscle fibers and mucosa may have to be combined with sphincter repair.

Sphincter repair itself involves a flap-over technique that takes one half of the divided sphincter muscle under the other, which thereby tightens the sphincter and eliminates the defect. It is wise to use a closed suction drain if there has been any difficulty with hemostasis. If the patient has a history of impaired rectal evacuation or gross constipation, it would be wise to consider a temporary covering loop colostomy.

Postoperative complications include sepsis, hematoma, stenosis with impairment of rectal emptying, and breakdown of the repair, which can lead to a supra-sphincteric fistula. Thus, it is essential that the patient be provided with perioperative antibiotic cover, mild laxatives, and careful attention to local dressings and hygiene. The overall success rate of sphincter repair is approximately 75% to 80%.

Rerouting of Ectopic Anus

The patient is catheterized and placed in the prone jackknife or the lithotomy position. Previous infiltration with a weak adrenaline solution in a local anesthetic is advised around the ectopic anus. The external anal sphincter should have been identified preoperatively by electromyography. A disk of skin is taken from the center of the defined external anal sphincter, and a plane of dissection is developed through the center of the sphincter ring. A gauze swab is placed in the future site of the anal canal.

The ectopic anus is then dissected from the back of the vagina or from the back of the prostate by use of a circumanal incision. The anus must be mobilized for at least 6 or 7 cm from the perineum above the levators before it is rerouted to its correct anatomic site. Stay sutures are placed on the lateral margins of the anus after it has been thoroughly mobilized, particularly anteriorly. The stay sutures are used to draw the anorectum through the center of the external anal sphincters to its correct anatomic position (Fig. 7). The mucosa is then sutured to the edges of the skin disk, and an anterior levatorplasty is performed to reconstitute the perineal body. The biggest hazard of rerouting the anal canal is fecal impaction. Many patients have chronic constipation and some impairment of evacuation. Thus, a regimen of postoperative laxatives is essential to achieve a satisfactory long-term outcome.

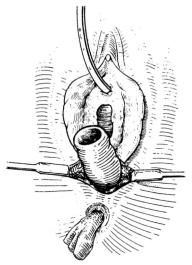

Fig. 7. Rerouting of the anal canal. (From Keighley MRB, Williams NS. *Surgery of the anus, rectum, and colon.* Philadelphia: WB Saunders, 1993, with permission.)

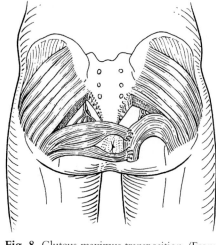

Fig. 8. Gluteus maximus transposition. (From Keighley MRB, Williams NS. *Surgery of the anus, rectum, and colon.* Philadelphia: WB Saunders, 1993, with permission.)

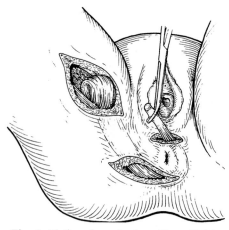

Fig. 9. Unilateral graciloplasty. (From Keighley MRB, Williams NS. *Surgery of the anus, rectum, and colon.* Philadelphia: WB Saunders, 1993, with permission.)

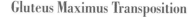

Gluteus Maximus Transposition

Gluteus maximus transposition is a relatively new operation that may prove extremely useful for patients with sphincter failure, particularly if the sphincters and puborectalis are neuropathic. The concept of taking normally innervated muscle, particularly from a muscle that is usually used to assist continence, is an attractive concept. Bilateral oblique gluteal incisions are made to expose the superficial fibers of the gluteus maximus on either side of the anus. The neurovascular bundle to the superficial fibers of the gluteus maximus is identified. The muscle insertion into the femur is detached or its origin from the ileum is detached. We prefer the former. Superficial fibers of the detached gluteus are then split. Subcutaneous tunnels are made anterior and posterior to the anus, so that the split muscle can be taken on either side of the anus and sutured to one another on the opposite side and to the opposite gluteus muscle itself (Fig. 8). Postoperative complications are hematoma and infection. Early results of this procedure are most encouraging.

Gracilis Muscle Transposition

A graciloplasty was introduced as a means of augmenting a damaged sphincter. The unique properties of the gracilis muscle are that it is long, has a strong tendinous insertion to the tibia, is not required for locomotor function, and has a proximal neurovascular supply. Hence, by detaching the distal tendon, two thirds of the distal

component of the muscle can be rerouted around the anus, and its tendon can be sutured to the opposite ischial tuberosity. The muscle may be rerouted clockwise or counterclockwise.

The patient is placed in the lithotomy position with the legs in stirrups. The gracilis muscle is mobilized through a single longitudinal incision or through multiple small incisions over the muscle. The mobilization of the muscle may also be performed laparoscopically, which improves cosmesis and reduces postoperative pain. We prefer a single longitudinal incision, because identification of the muscle can be difficult, and we do not think that morbidity is reduced by a series of small incisions. Tributaries of the long saphenous vein often require ligation. Great care must be taken to avoid injury to the saphenous nerve. The muscle is easily identified by its longitudinal muscle fibers, rounded belly, and long tendon. The tendon is detached from the medial border of the tibia as close to its insertion as possible. The distal two thirds of the muscle are delivered from its bed, but great care must be taken at the junction between the proximal third and the distal two thirds to identify the neurovascular bundle. The nerve is a branch of the anterior obturator nerve lying on adductor brevis. The blood supply is more variable, but the principal artery is nearly always just distal to the nerve, which splits into two branches before it reaches the muscle. If separate distal arteries are identified, they must be ligated. A separate incision is made over the buttocks, and a separate incision is made over the ischial tuberosity on the opposite buttock (Fig. 9). It may be possible to develop subcuta-

neous tunnels around the anus without making further incisions, but sometimes, additional anterior or posterior access is necessary. If this is the case, the anterior and posterior anal raphe should be preserved. After subcutaneous tunnels around the anus are developed and meticulous hemostasis is achieved, gauze swabs are left in each before muscle transposition.

We prefer to transpose the gracilis muscle by using an alpha loop, taking the muscle initially anterior to the anus around the right lateral margin of the anus underneath the posterior raphe and subsequently over itself, and then under the anterior raphe so that the tendon can be sutured to the opposite ischial tuberosity. It is crucial to obtain secure apposition between the periosteum of the ischial tuberosity and the tendon. We use three or four interrupted Prolene sutures on a heavy, round-bodied needle. The sutures are carefully positioned before they are tied. Closed suction drains are needed to evacuate hematoma, and the wounds are closed with Prolene sutures or staples.

A variant of unilateral nonstimulated graciloplasty is bilateral graciloplasty. This is a much more extensive operation, but the advantage is that a complete encircling sling of muscle, rather than tendon, is achieved around the anus, and each tendon is sutured to itself, thereby minimizing the consequences of local sepsis that causes disintegration of the sutures from the tendon to the ischial tuberosity (Fig. 10).

Complications of graciloplasty include pain, hematoma, infection, ischemic necrosis of tendon, and synergistic gangrene of the perineum. In view of these risks, some advocate a proximal colostomy until complete healing has been achieved.

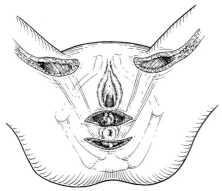

Fig. 10. Bilateral graciloplasty. (From Keighley MRB, Williams NS. *Surgery of the anus, rectum, and colon*. Philadelphia: WB Saunders, 1993, with permission.)

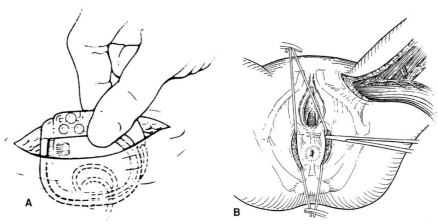

Fig. 11. Stimulated graciloplasty. **A:** The stimulator is placed in the pocket with the excess lead behind it. **B:** Gracilis muscle being rerouted around the anus. (From Keighley MRB, Williams NS. *Surgery of the anus, rectum, and colon*. Philadelphia: WB Saunders, 1993, with permission.)

The Gastrointestinal Tract

Graciloplasty seems to be effective for patients who are incontinent from anorectal trauma and in patients with Hirschsprung disease. It has been far less effective for patients with fecal incontinence in whom all other simpler methods of treatment have failed.

Gracilis Neosphincter

Gracilis neosphincter is a new and essentially experimental operation. The principle of the operation is to convert the gracilis muscle from a fast-twitch to a slow-twitch, continuously active muscle. Constant electrical stimulation of the nerve to the gracilis or to the muscle fibers themselves can convert the fast-twitch muscle of locomotor function to a slow-twitch, constantly active striated sphincter. Constant electrical stimulation is achieved by leads placed on the muscle itself or on the nerve to the gracilis muscle after the muscle has been transposed. Electrical stimulation is delivered through an implantable stimulator box placed in the subcutaneous tissues of the anterior abdominal wall, from which leads deliver the electrical stimulus to one or two gracilis muscles (Fig. 11). This operation can successfully replace a sphincter, but the device is expensive (at least $7,000), there is a risk of infection, and the battery life of the stimulator box is unknown. Furthermore, the operation must be selected only for patients who have a primary sphincter abnormality. Patients with incontinence often have coexisting impairment of rectal evacuation and impairment of anorectal sensation. Such patients are probably unsuitable for gracilis neosphincter. It is technically possible to perform a delayed implantation procedure. Thus, many advise unilateral or bilateral nonstimulated

graciloplasty in the first instance, with the placement of implantable electrodes, and placement of a stimulator box at a later stage if the nonstimulated muscle does not achieve continence. Currently, the three stages of the procedure are (a) delivery of a proximal stoma and mobilization of the gracilis muscle in situ; (b) rerouting of the gracilis muscle and placement of stimulator leads on the nerve or muscle, which is attached to an implantable stimulator box; and (c) reprogramming of muscle over a period of 6 months to convert the muscle from fast to slow twitch. At the end of the 6-month reprogramming period, the stoma is closed. Many surgeons now perform the operation as a single procedure without a stoma and continence stimulation after 6 to 8 weeks, provided there are no complications (Fig. 11A).

ABS Implantable Artificial Bowel Sphincter

An implantable device has been used for many years for treatment of urinary incontinence. A device using the same principle with a modified design has been made available for treatment of anal incontinence (Fig. 12). An inflatable cuff is placed around the anorectum through a single perineal or two para-anal incisions. The cuff is connected by a closed, water-filled system to a compliant reservoir placed in the retropubic space and is activated using a pump placed in the scrotum in the man or labia in the woman. Normally, the anorectal cuff is distended with fluid, which achieves continence. In the event of afferent signals from the rectum to initiate defecation, the patient squeezes the pump that deflates the cuff to allow stool to pass. This device has been im-

planted under controlled audit in North America and Europe. There is a risk of sepsis and extrusion of the implant in 10% to 20%. In those who have an intact device, continence is achieved in 80%.

Stoma Construction

For some patients, particularly the elderly and patients with severe neuropathy, the construction of a good stoma may be the best means of improving quality of life and restoring self-esteem to patients with fecal incontinence. The simplest stoma is an end colostomy, which can be constructed laparoscopically or through a small trephine in the abdominal wall. This stoma can be subsequently used for colostomy irrigation. Thus, patients are not necessarily committed to wearing a bag. Almost all patients with an improved quality of life with a colostomy eventually require rectal excision because they become incontinent of mucus from the defunctioned rectum.

For patients who are incontinent after extensive colorectal surgery, a covering ileostomy may be a better option than a colostomy. In a small number of patients, the option of a reservoir ileostomy should not be totally dismissed. Admittedly, this is an extensive operation, but patients do not have to wear an appliance. Furthermore, with stapling of the nipple valve, the proportion of patients requiring revision surgery after Kock reservoir ileostomy is not nearly as high as it used to be. For more information on stoma appliances, see Chapter 133. Finally, in some patients consideration should also be given to an appendicostomy or a continent colostomy irrigation device to facilitate antegrade colonic irrigation. Such techniques are particularly appropriate when impaired

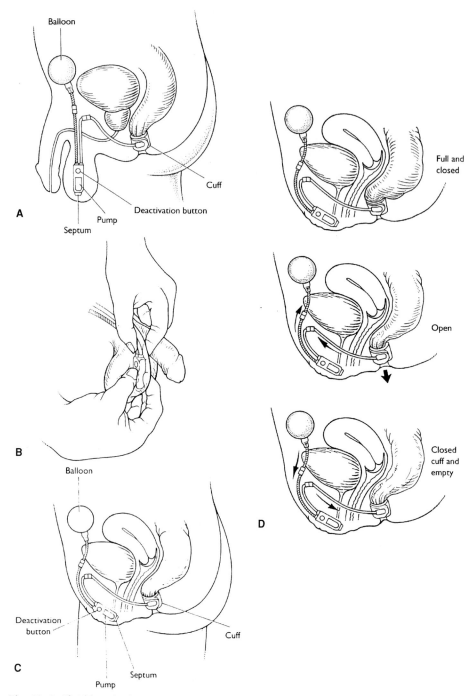

Fig. 12. Artificial bowel sphincter. **A:** A cuff is placed around the anal canal. An inflatable pump control assembly is placed in the scrotum and the balloon reservoir under the symphysis pubis. **B:** The pump in males is placed in the scrotum. To open the cuff to defecate, the pump must be squeezed and released several times. **C:** The same arrangement is used in women, but the pump is placed in the labia. **D:** When the cuff is closed, the stool stays in the rectum. When the pump is repeatedly squeezed (in the labia in women), the cuff opens, and the bowel can empty. Fluid then automatically returns to the cuff, which again closes around the anal canal.

rectal evacuation exists with the incontinence (Figs. 13 and 14).

Rectal Prolapse

Chapters 145A and B contain an account of the functional considerations of rectal prolapse.

 CLINICAL PRESENTATION

Rectal prolapse is a complete rectal intussusception. The prolapse appears on the perineum as a circumferential swelling that bleeds or becomes ulcerated. In 70% of patients, there is a history of incontinence. In 60% of patients presenting with

rectal prolapse who are younger than 40 years of age, there is an associated history of constipation.

CAUSES

Rectal prolapse, a complete intussusception of the rectum, results in attenuation of the lateral ligaments of the rectum.

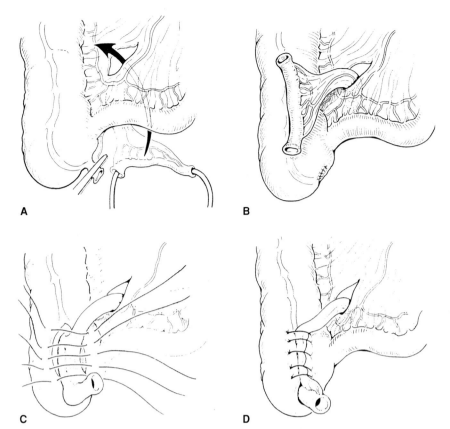

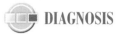

Fig. 13. Appendicostomy for antegrade colonic enema. **A:** The mesoappendix is preserved. **B:** The appendix is relocated through the mesentery along the cecum in an antiperistaltic fashion **(C)**. The appendix is laid within a submucosal space, its distal end is amputated, and this is then anastomosed to the cecum **(D)**. The seromuscular layer is closed over the enterocecostomy without compromising the mesenteric vascular pedicle. The proximal end of the appendix is exteriorized. (From Tsang TM, Dudley NE. *Pediatr Surg Int* 1995;10:33, with permission.)

There is often descent of the uterus associated with cystocele or rectocele. There is always a patulous anus and a weak pelvic floor associated with pudendal neuropathy. Rectal sensation is impaired because of the presence of the prolapse. Almost all patients with rectal prolapse give a history of discharge of mucus, which is commonly associated with pruritus ani.

DIAGNOSIS

A rectal prolapse is usually obvious on clinical examination during straining, but some patients are too embarrassed to strain and deliver the prolapse during clinical inspection. Bowel incontinence occurs in 70%. In such patients, videoproctography may be helpful, as may inspection of the perineum after defecation. It is important during clinical examination to assess whether uterine descent, cystocele, enterocele, or rectocele exists and to assess the tone of the anal sphincters at rest and during maximum voluntary contraction.

Physiologic study may be helpful to identify evidence of pudendal nerve delay, impairment of anorectal sensation, or extent of perineal descent. A videoproctogram may be helpful to identify a coexisting cystocele, rectocele, or enterocele.

TREATMENT

The treatment of rectal prolapse depends on the functional abnormality. In most young patients with rectal prolapse, there is coexisting straining, impaired rectal evacuation, and delayed colonic transit. In such patients, we believe that an abdominal rectopexy is advisable, with a variable colonic resection above the rectopexy (Fig. 15). If impaired rectal evacuation is a major feature and the prolapse is small, anterior resection might be a better option. By contrast, for elderly patients with rectal prolapse and associated co-morbidity, we believe that a perineal procedure is much

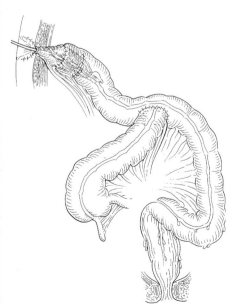

Fig. 14. Transverse colonic conduit.

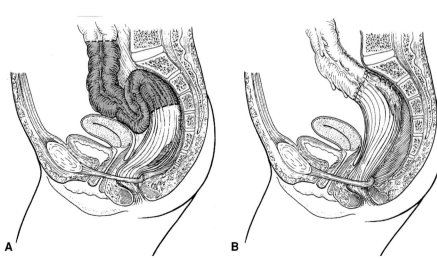

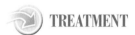

Fig. 15. Rectopexy **(A)** and sigmoidectomy **(B)**. (From Keighley MRB, Williams NS. *Surgery of the anus, rectum, and colon.* Philadelphia: WB Saunders, 1993, with permission.)

more appropriate and favor perineal rectosigmoidectomy with synchronous repair of the pelvic floor.

Megabowel

CLINICAL PRESENTATION

Megacolon or megarectum usually presents with severe constipation and soiling caused by a large fecaloma filling the rectum and around which liquid feces seep. Patients also frequently complain of abdominal discomfort and abdominal swelling, which is caused by gross fecal loading of the colon.

CAUSES

The cause of adult megacolon is not well understood. Some are almost certainly cases of adult Hirschsprung disease, usually with a short segment of aganglionosis. However, the majority of cases are acquired and associated with long-standing constipation or neurologic disease (e.g., hydrocephalus, epilepsy, or cerebral birth trauma), or result from degenerative disorders affecting the autonomic nervous system, as in Chagas disease.

There are four anatomic varieties: Megacolon alone, megarectum alone, megarectum and megasigmoid, and total megacolon with megarectum.

DIAGNOSIS

Megacolon may be suspected solely on clinical grounds. A huge fecal mass may be felt arising from the pelvis. Rectal examination may reveal an enormous fecaloma in a cavernous rectum with a patulous anus.

Plain abdominal radiographs may demonstrate gross dilation of the transverse diameter of the rectum filled with solid fecal material. In other cases, the diagnosis is less obvious, and a barium enema examination may be necessary. However, preparation for barium enema can prove difficult. Sometimes, patients require hospital admission for manual evacuation and repeated enemas to disimpact the fecaloma from the rectosigmoid region.

For the same reasons, anorectal physiology can prove extremely difficult in these patients and is virtually useless unless the fecaloma is disimpacted. If the rectal obstruction can be removed, resting and squeeze anal canal pressures are usually low, and the rectoanal inhibitory reflex is

usually absent. Rectal sensation is always impaired. Transit marker studies usually reveal some delay in colonic transit proximal to the dilated segment, but isotopic studies are much more useful in determining whether proximal colonic motility and transit are normal. Despite these theoretic considerations, the extent of resection is largely determined by the macroscopic appearance of the bowel at the time of laparotomy. The presence of normal ganglion cells in the anorectum may be verified by full-thickness rectal biopsy or anorectal myectomy. However, we would not advise anorectal myectomy in these patients, because it might compromise continence, and the histopathologic exclusion of Hirschsprung disease is really academic. In the presence of megarectum, these individuals do not have a normal lower rectum or upper anal canal, and full rectal excision is necessary.

TREATMENT

Conservative Therapy

There is no doubt that minor forms of megarectum may be controlled by keeping the rectum empty. Thus, a manual evacuation and thorough colon catharsis with purgatives and repeated enemas can be justified at first. Thereafter, the aim of conservative treatment is to keep the rectum empty by use of stimulant suppositories, enemas, and mild laxatives. This policy may be satisfactory, provided that anal sphincter function is sufficiently preserved for patients to be able to retain the enema and suppositories. This approach also needs a good deal of compliance by the patient, but sometimes, in mild disease and in patients who understand that surgical treatment is a major undertaking, these measures are successful.

Surgical Treatment

For most patients, surgical treatment is the only way to overcome overflow incontinence. Unlike the surgical treatment for pediatric Hirschsprung disease, the aim of surgical resection in the adult is to remove the dilated, nonfunctioning colonic and rectal segments. Thus, for megacolon alone, subtotal colectomy and ileorectal anastomosis are indicated (Fig. 16). For patients with megarectum or megarectum and megasigmoid, excision of the dilated nonfunctioning segment is undertaken, and

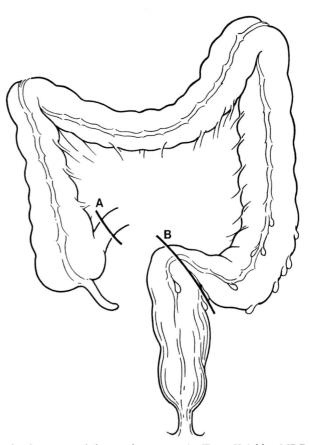

Fig. 16. Subtotal colectomy and ileorectal anastomosis. (From Keighley MRB, Williams NS. *Surgery of the anus, rectum, and colon,* 2nd ed. Philadelphia: WB Saunders, 1999, with permission.)

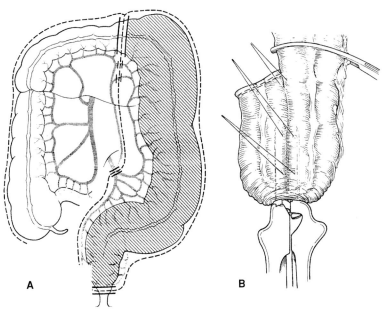

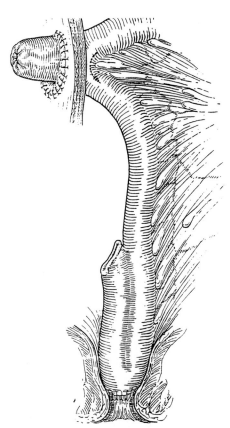

Fig. 17. Extended left colon resection **(A)** and coloanal anastomosis with pouch **(B).** (From Keighley MRB, Williams NS. *Surgery of the anus, rectum, and colon.* Philadelphia: WB Saunders, 1993, with permission.)

Fig. 18. Restorative proctocolectomy. (From Keighley MRB, Williams NS. *Surgery of the anus, rectum, and colon.* Philadelphia: WB Saunders, 1993, with permission.)

the normally innervated proximal colon of normal caliber is preserved with coloanal anastomosis (Fig. 17). Hence, operations described for the treatment of Hirschsprung disease, such as the Duhamel procedure, are inappropriate for adult megarectum. Also, for technical reasons, the Duhamel procedure is rarely possible in these patients, because the rectum completely fills the pelvis. In the small proportion of patients with gross megarectum and megacolon, total excision of the large bowel and rectum is indicated; if anal sphincter function is adequate, ileopouch–anal anastomosis is indicated (Fig. 18). One must admit, however, that there are some patients whose anal sphincter function is so badly compromised that no form of restorative resection is indicated. In such patients, proximal loop ileostomy alone may be used for treatment. If ablative surgery is indicated, conventional resection and a covering proximal stoma are advisable.

There are certain specific surgical strategies that have to be considered in patients with adult megarectum. These strategies are described below.

1. Preoperative mechanical bowel preparation may not be possible or desirable. Manual evacuation of a huge fecaloma before a reconstructive surgical procedure may cause iatrogenic damage to the sphincter and pelvic floor. Hence, we do not attempt mechanical bowel preparation preoperatively. We milk the

fecaloma from the anorectum during operation into the segment of bowel that is being resected.

2. Stapling procedures to perform a coloanal anastomosis are rarely possible in these patients. The dilated rectum imperceptibly continues downward into a dilated anus. Furthermore, the walls of the bowel are extremely thickened, which makes stapling transection almost impossible. Hence, for these patients, hand-sutured straight coloanal or ileoanal anastomosis is the only technique possible for restoring intestinal continuity. We do not advise constructing a colonic pouch.

3. Hemorrhage is a real problem in these patients. The pararectal veins are enormously enlarged. Hence, meticulous hemostasis is necessary at operation, and intense vigilance is needed postoperatively to detect blood loss and to assess transfusion requirements. In view of the risk of blood loss, it is often wise to retain the lower third of the rectum so that it can be transected at a site that can be easily controlled from above by the abdominal surgeon. In this manner, the proximal colon can be delivered through the anal stump without the necessity of a mucosectomy and a sleeve coloanal anastomosis at the dentate line (see Chapter 147). The same technique may be used for ileoanal anastomosis with pouch construction. In these complex surgical procedures, a covering ileostomy is always desirable

unless, of course, the dilated segment is confined to the colon, in which case an unprotected ileorectal anastomosis is an accepted option.

Slow Transit Constipation

 CLINICAL PRESENTATION

Slow transit constipation typically occurs in women between the ages of 20 and 35. There are often menstrual irregularities, which suggests abnormal ovulation and coexisting symptoms of nausea, backache, and abdominal distention. Many patients express evidence of psychological instability. Some may have a history of sexual abuse. Many patients are aggressive, and some are on psychotropic drugs for depressive illness. A few of these patients give a history of eating disorders. A few patients also experience intermittent diarrhea and constipation, and exhibit features of the irritable bowel syndrome.

CAUSES

There are a variety of organic disorders that may be associated with slow transit constipation. Endocrine causes include hypothyroidism, glucagonoma, hypercalcemia, pheochromocytoma, hypopituitarism, and pregnancy. Metabolic causes include amyloidosis, diabetes, systemic sclerosis, hypokalemia, porphyria, and uremia.

A variety of underlying neurologic disorders may be associated with slow transit constipation. They include demyelinating disease; neurologic ischemia; traumatic lesions of the brain and spinal cord, or tumors of the central nervous system; Parkinson disease; tabes dorsalis; autonomic neuropathy; von Recklinghausen disease; and multiple endocrine tumors.

A number of drugs may be associated with delay in the transit of fecal material through the colon. They include all analgesics (particularly opiates), anticholinergics, compounds formulated with calcium or aluminum, iron compounds, anticonvulsants, antidepressants, antihistamines, barium, bismuth, drugs for the treatment of Parkinson disease, ganglion-blocking drugs, long-standing laxatives, muscle relaxants, and psychotropic drugs.

There is also a large group of psychogenic disorders associated with slow transit constipation.

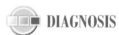 DIAGNOSIS

Constipation can be subclassified functionally into delayed colonic transit and impaired rectal evacuation. In practice, many patients exhibit both forms of motility disorder.

The history of prolonged incapacitating constipation given by many patients may be unreliable. Therefore, a variety of simple screening tests are needed to determine whether there is a physical problem and to ascertain whether the problem is one of impaired colonic transit or a disturbance of rectal evacuation. It is also important for clinicians to recognize that many in this group of patients are aggressive and expect instant attention for a long-standing problem. These patients must be counseled and told that a series of investigations is essential to unravel the source of the problem.

First, patients should be given the opportunity to carefully explain their normal dietary habits and their fluid intake. Definition of terms is important, because there is enormous variation in the understanding of the word "constipation." A careful drug history is essential. Some patients date the onset of symptoms to a previous operation; hysterectomy, oophorectomy, and other pelvic operations are predisposing factors to constipation. It is crucially important to exclude an eating disorder and to ascertain the patient's normal toilet practice: Many patients spend hours straining on the toilet.

A plain abdominal radiograph can help determine whether there is gross fecal loading in the colon. An inert marker study is also a useful method of screening for impaired colonic transit. However, it is not a sensitive test, and the results may vary markedly from week to week. Hence, the test may need to be repeated. The distribution of markers also gives some indication of the possible site of colonic delay. However, therapy should not be based on marker studies alone. Simple assessment of rectal emptying may be achieved by inserting a known volume of a semisolid inert physical substance into the rectum and asking the patient to attempt evacuation under normal circumstances in the bathroom for a specified period. This simple technique may give a rough guide as to whether there is impairment of rectal evacuation. For a more detailed study, colonic transit should be assessed by using an isotopically labeled meal, and rectal evacuation (Fig. 19) should be studied after inserting an isotopically labeled paste into the rectum. Further important information can be obtained by videoproctography, which can help to define any morphologic abnormality in the anorectum and the degree of pelvic floor movement during attempted contraction and evacuation. Incomplete intussusception can also be demonstrated, along with evidence of rectocele, cystocele, or entero-

cele. Definition of these abnormalities may involve placing contrast material in the vagina, bladder, peritoneal cavity, or the small bowel. Videoproctography also helps define the efficiency of rectal evacuation and the degree of perineal descent. Electromyography of the puborectalis can indicate whether there is failure of relaxation of the puborectalis during attempted defecation, but the technique is painful and has generally been superseded by other methods. Preoperative assessment is not complete without a detailed psychological evaluation. Previous physical and psychological trauma should be explored. Eating disorders should be identified, and sexual disturbance should be gently investigated.

A few physical disorders must be excluded in the patient with long-standing constipation. These disorders are sigmoid volvulus, cecal volvulus, and pseudo-obstruction. In addition, patients with constipation may have a disturbance of motility affecting the whole of the gastrointestinal tract. Hence, gastric emptying and small bowel transit should also be studied. Certainly, surgical treatment should not be undertaken without these investigations.

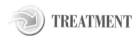 TREATMENT

Conservative Measures

Many patients pressure the surgeon to undertake something immediately to relieve pain and distress. However, it is essential to ensure that patients have an adequate fluid intake and a balanced diet. Excessive intake of fiber may be contraindicated in these patients, because it aggravates abdominal

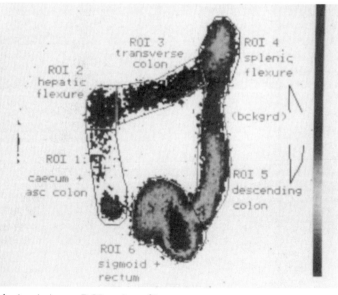

Fig. 19. Colonic scintigram. ROI, region of interest.

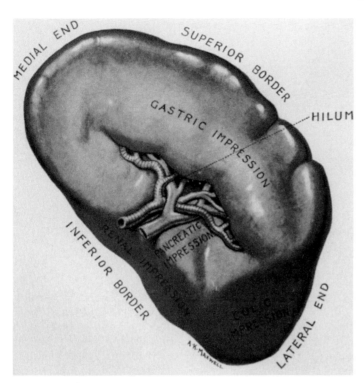

Fig. 1. Gross anatomy of the spleen.

capsulated organisms such as *Streptococcus pneumoniae*, *Neisseria meningitidis*, and *Haemophilus influenzae* is increased following splenectomy. In 1952, a postsplenectomy syndrome of severe, sometimes fatal meningitis and sepsis in four of five children splenectomized before the age of 6 months for congenital hemolytic anemia was reported, and the term *overwhelming postsplenectomy infection* (OPSI) was introduced in 1969. The true incidence of OPSI is not well defined, although a commonly used estimation of the incidence is 0.6% in children and 0.3% in adults. The risk of postsplenectomy septicemia, pneumonia, and meningitis was estimated to be 8.3% in trauma patients, or 166 times the 0.05% rate expected in the general population. OPSI is characterized by a sudden onset of symptoms and a rapid and fulminating course that often lasts only 12 to 18 hours. Common complaints include fever, nausea, vomiting, headache, and altered mental status. The disease is complicated by shock and disseminated intravascular coagulation and carries an overall mortality rate as high as 50% to 80%. Because of its severity, the use of polyvalent pneumococcal vaccine and close follow-up after splenectomy is routine. However, the effectiveness of the vaccine in splenectomized patients is unclear. The use of prophylactic antibiotics in asplenic patients is also controversial; however, minor infections in this group should be treated with antibiotics.

ligament, the splenorenal ligament, and the greater omentum. Accessory spleens have been noted in the pelvis, either in the presacral region or adjacent to the left ovary, and in the scrotum in juxtaposition to the left testicle (Fig. 5).

PHYSIOLOGY AND PATHOPHYSIOLOGY

During the early stages of fetal development, the spleen is responsible for red and white cell production, a function later assumed by the bone marrow. The most important functions of the spleen are those of a filter and an immune organ.

The spleen is responsible for the removal of old red cells, defective circulating cells, and circulating bacteria. In addition, normal erythrocyte morphology is maintained by the spleen as the spleen is able to process immature erythrocytes, removing their nuclei and changing the shape of the cellular membrane. The spleen is also responsible for the removal of the nuclear remnant of red cells (Howell-Jolly bodies), denatured hemoglobin (Heinz bodies), and iron granules (pappenheimer bodies). In disease states characterized by abnormal red cell morphology such as spherocytosis, thalassemia, and sickle cell anemia, the spleen is responsible for removal of these cells that are usually trapped in the splenic vasculature. To the

same extent, immune diseases affecting red cells, such as autoimmune hemolytic anemia, and macrophages in the spleen are responsible for red cell destruction.

The strongest evidence in favor of the important immune role of the spleen resides in the fact that the incidence of significant infection and sepsis caused by en-

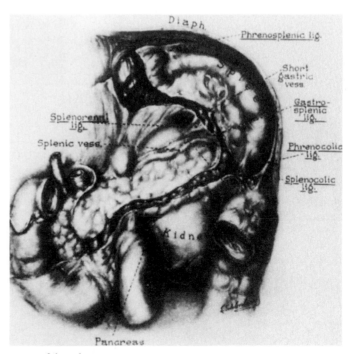

Fig. 2. Ligaments of the spleen.

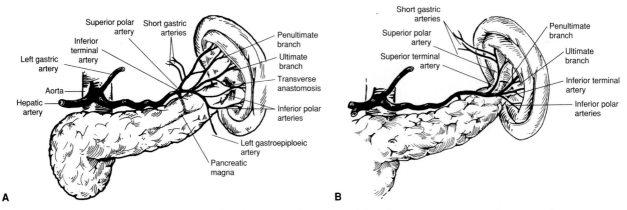

Fig. 3. A: Representation of the distributed anatomic formations of the splenic artery. **B:** magistral anatomic formations of the splenic artery.

Although the role of the spleen in the destruction of neutrophils under normal circumstances is not well defined, neutrophil removal may increase with splenic enlargement and in certain situations of autoimmune neutropenia. Normally, approximately one third of the platelet mass is pooled in the spleen, but in the presence of marked splenomegaly, up to 80% of the platelets can be sequestered in the organ. In thrombocytopenic states, platelet destruction in the spleen may be accelerated, or the spleen may mediate a moiety that causes widespread platelet destruction throughout the body. In addition to these cellular functions, the spleen has immunologic and secretory functions, being responsible for the synthesis of immunoglobulin M, tuftsin, opsonins, properdin, and interferon.

SPLENIC DISRUPTION

Splenic rupture is usually caused by blunt or penetrating trauma, although in rare instances spontaneous splenic rupture occurs. Rupture occurs at the moment of the injury but clinical manifestation (abdominal pain, hypotension, and tachycardia) may occur in a delayed fashion. A splenic injury scale has been developed to allow more precise therapeutic approaches (Table 1).

Hemodynamically stable patients undergo ultrasound examination. If the ultrasound is positive for free fluid and the patient remains stable, an abdominal computed tomographic (CT) scan is obtained to identify the source of bleeding and to evaluate for contrast extravasation and other intra-abdominal injuries that may require operative intervention. The CT appearance

will allow the treating physician to grade the injury (Fig. 6). Until recently, operative intervention was mandatory for the treatment of traumatic splenic rupture. At that time, surgical options included different techniques of splenic preservation or splenectomy. Currently, most hemodynamically stable patients without another indication for operative abdominal exploration are being treated by a nonoperative approach (bed rest, serial measurements of hematocrit and hemoglobin, serial abdominal examinations for 48 to 72 hours). The criteria for nonoperative management are depicted in Table 2.

A repeat CT scan before discharge is seldom necessary. Recent reports have shown that nonoperative management is safe. The current failure rate considering all injury grades varies from 3% to 20%.

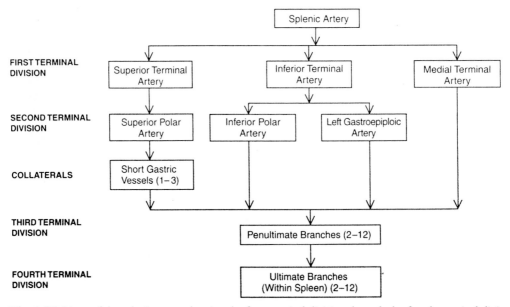

Fig. 4. Divisions of the splenic artery showing the first terminal division through the fourth terminal division, and origins of arteries including the short gastric and gastroepiploic vessels.

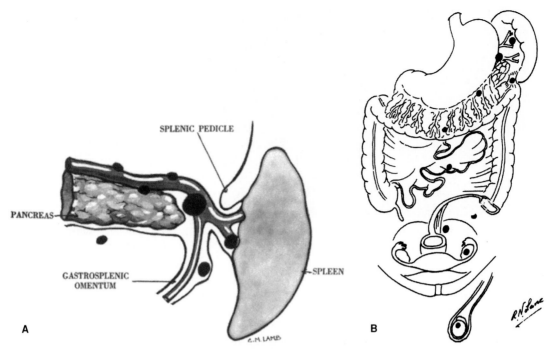

Fig. 5. Locations of accessory spleens. **A:** The more common locations of accessory spleens. Accessory spleens are also found in the left ovary, in the left testicle along the course of the left ureter, and in the lesser sac and greater omentum. **B:** Locations of accessory spleens. Note the positions of presacral and paraureteric spleniculi.

Surgical management is indicated in the presence of hemodynamic instability or shock on admission, associated injuries requiring operative intervention, and failure of nonoperative management (change in physical examination, decreased blood pressure, acidosis, tachycardia, and blood transfusion of more than 4 units in 24 to 48 hours). Angiographic embolization has also extended the percentage of patients that can avoid operative management.

smear demonstrating that more than 60% of the red cells are spherocytic, increased reticulocyte count, and a negative Coombs test. Splenectomy is the treatment of choice, decreasing the rate of hemolysis. Generally, the operation should be delayed until the 4th year of life. After removal of the spleen, the erythrocytes achieve a normal life span and jaundice, if present, disappears. The inherent membrane abnormality

persists. Hereditary elliptocytosis, pyropoikilocytosis, xerocytosis, and hydrocytosis represent variants of hereditary spherocytosis.

Hemolytic anemia is also associated with deficiency of glucose-6-phosphate dehydrogenase and pyruvate kinase. Glucose-6-phospate dehydrogenase deficiency is an X-linked hereditary disease and anemia occurs following exposure to drugs or

HEMATOLOGIC DISORDERS FOR WHICH SPLENECTOMY IS POTENTIALLY THERAPEUTIC

Anemias

Hereditary spherocytosis is transmitted as an autosomal dominant trait and is characterized by a defective erythrocyte membrane caused by the deficiency of a cytoskeletal protein named spectrin. This causes the cell to be smaller than normal, thick, rigid, and almost spherical. These cells have a tendency to be trapped and destroyed in the spleen. The salient features of the disease are anemia, reticulocytosis, jaundice, and splenomegaly. Cholelithiasis is reported in 30% to 60% of patients and ultrasound should be performed prior to operative intervention. The diagnosis is readily established by a peripheral blood

TABLE 1. AMERICAN ASSOCIATION FOR THE SURGERY OF TRAUMA— SPLEEN ORGAN INJURY SCALE

Class	Description
I	Nonexpanding subcapsular hematoma <10% of surface area
	Nonbleeding capsular laceration with parenchymal involvement <1 cm deep
II	Nonexpanding subcapsular hematoma 10%–50% of surface area
	Nonexpanding intraparenchymal hematoma <2 cm in diameter
	Bleeding capsular tear or parenchymal laceration 1–3 cm deep without trabecular vessel
III	Expanding subcapsular or intraparenchymal hematoma
	Bleeding subcapsular or subcapsular hematoma >50% of surface area
	Intraparenchymal hematoma >2 cm in diameter
	Parenchymal laceration >3 cm deep or involving trabecular vessels
IV	Ruptured intraparechymal hematoma with active bleeding
	Laceration involving segmental or hilar vessels producing major devasularization (>25% splenic volume)
V	Completely shattered or avulsed spleen
	Hilar laceration that devascularizes entire spleen

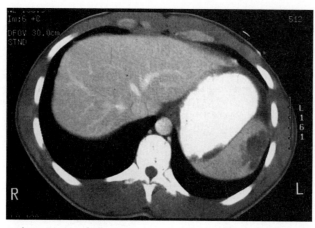

Fig. 6. Computed tomogram of splenic rupture secondary to blunt trauma.

certain chemicals. Splenectomy is seldom required to treat this condition.

Pyruvate kinase deficiency is an autosomal recessive disease characterized by increased red cell destruction caused by decreased red cell deformability and increased stiffness. Usually red cells are destroyed in the spleen. In addition to anemia, these patients often develop splenomegaly. Splenectomy may improve the anemia in patients with pyruvate kinase deficiency, but the procedure should be delayed, if possible, until after 4 years of age.

Thalassemia is transmitted as an autosomal dominant trait and is characterized by a defect in hemoglobin synthesis. In the United States, most patients are of southern European origin and suffer from β-thalassemia. Splenectomy is indicated only in those who have a marked increase in transfusion requirements, marked splenomegaly, hypersplenism, or repeated splenic infarctions.

Sickle cell anemia results from the homozygous inheritance of hemoglobin S. Sickle cell anemia is more frequently seen in African-Americans, as 0.5% of them are homozygous for hemoglobin S. Crystallization of hemoglobin S occurs under conditions of low oxygen tension, which leads to changes in red cell shape, splenic infarction, and, ultimately, autosplenectomy in some patients. Hypersplenism, a consequence of thalassemias and sickle cell anemia, is treated by splenectomy.

Idiopathic autoimmune hemolytic anemia is a disorder in which the life span of presumably normal erythrocytes is shortened when they are exposed to endogenous factors. Among patients in whom warm antibodies are detected and steroid therapy fails, splenectomy is successful in approximately 80%.

Thrombocytopenia

Thrombocytopenia from increased platelet dysfunction constitutes the most common indication for splenectomy for hematologic disease. Immune or idiopathic thrombocytopenic purpura (ITP) is an acquired autoimmune phenomenon resulting in the destruction of platelets. The spleen is likely the source of antiplatelet antibody production and the site of platelet destruction in most patients. The diagnosis is established by demonstrating normal or increased numbers of megakaryocytes accompanied by thrombocytopenia in the absence of any systemic disease or a history of ingestion of drugs capable of inducing thrombocytopenia. Adult female patients outnumber male patients. In children, it affects both sexes equally and spontaneous remissions are common. The most common presenting signs are petechiae and ecchymoses. The spleen is not enlarged. Characteristically, the platelet count is less than 50,000/mm³.

Acute ITP has an excellent prognosis in children younger than 16 years and rarely requires surgical intervention. Corticosteroids are the initial treatment. In adult patients, however, a long-term response to steroids, plasmapheresis, or immune globulin is uncommon. By contrast, 75% to 85% of patients who undergo splenectomy currently respond; their platelet counts generally rise above 100,000/mm³ within 7 days of splenectomy. Failure of splenectomy is usually associated with the presence of accessory spleens not identified and removed during the initial operation.

Refractory thrombocytopenia is associated with systemic lupus erythematosus and responds to splenectomy in a fashion similar to that of ITP. The same response has been noted in patients who have thrombocytopenia associated with the acquired immunodeficiency syndrome or positivity for the human immunodeficiency virus. Secondary hypersplenism with pancytopenia, thrombocytopenia, leukopenia, or anemia may occur whenever splenomegaly is present. In approximately 80% of patients, thrombocytopenia associated with splenomegaly is corrected by splenectomy. If, however, the splenomegaly is the consequence of portal hypertension, splenectomy alone is contraindicated.

Myeloproliferative Disorders

Hodgkin disease is a malignant form of lymphoma that usually affects young adults. Signs and symptoms include weight loss, night sweats, or asymptomatic lymphadenopathy. Hodgkin lymphoma is classified in four types: lymphocyte-predominant, nodular-sclerosing, mixed cellularity, or lymphocyte-depleted. The pathologic staging according to the Ann Arbor classification is depicted in Table 3.

Staging laparotomy with splenectomy was in integral part of the procedure for staging Hodgkin disease; it was generally reserved for patients with stage I or stage II disease to rule out subdiaphragmatic involvement. The procedure consists of celiotomy, splenectomy, liver biopsy, retroperitoneal node biopsy, and also biopsy of a hepatoduodenal node. This procedure has been largely supplanted by noninvasive studies and selected marrow and visceral biopsy.

Non-Hodgkin lymphoma is commonly accompanied by splenomegaly and hypersplenism. Splenectomy is indicated

TABLE 2. CRITERIA FOR NONOPERATIVE MANAGEMENT OF SPLENIC INJURIES

Hemodynamic stability
Negative abdominal examination
Absence of contrast extravasation on computed tomographic scan
Absence of other clear indications for exploratory laparotomy
Absence of associated health conditions that carry an increased risk of bleeding
  (coagulopathy, hepatic failure, use of anticoagulants, specific coagulation factor deficiency)

Stage	Description
1	Disease in a single lymphatic site
2	Disease in two or more lymphatic sites on the same side of the diaphragm
3	Lymphatic disease, including splenic involvement, on both sides of the diaphragm
4	Disseminated disease to extra lymphatic sites and organs

TABLE 3. ANN ARBOR STAGING CLASSIFICATION OF HODGKIN LYMPHOMA

in symptomatic splenomegaly and hypersplenism. Staging laparotomy and splenectomy is usually not indicated because of the systemic nature of the disease and its response to chemotherapy. In fact, only 1% of patients will present with disease confined to the spleen. Palliative splenectomy may be indicated in patients who are refractory to medical therapy to decrease pain, fullness, and hypersplenism.

Very large spleens are associated with myeloproliferative disorders. Splenectomy is indicated for symptomatic splenomegaly and for increasing transfusion requirements. If results are favorable, the patient can begin or continue chemotherapy. Splenectomy is a very effective therapy for hairy cell leukemia accompanied by neutropenia, thrombocytopenia, and anemia. Five-year survival in the range of 65% to 75% has been reported. Chemotherapy has been the mainstay of medical therapy for chronic lymphocytic leukemia. Splenectomy is used for palliation of symptomatic splenomegaly and hypersplenism. Chronic myelogenous leukemia is accompanied by progressive splenomegaly and splenic sequestration and leads to bleeding, anemia, and recurrent infections. The role of splenectomy in chronic myelogenous leukemia is controversial because no survival benefit has been observed following splenectomy performed during the early chronic phase or before allogeneic bone marrow transplantation.

Other Disorders

A variety of other disorders may benefit from splenectomy. These include Felty syndrome (rheumatoid arthritis, splenomegaly, and neutropenia), in which the symptomatic splenomegaly and neutropenia can be corrected but usually no change is seen in the rheumatoid arthritis. Sarcoidosis may be associated with an enlarged spleen, anemia, neutropenia, and pancytopenia, and is correctable by splenectomy. Gaucher disease is often characterized by splenomegaly and hypersplenism. In children with this disorder, partial splenectomy has been performed for symptomatic splenomegaly and hypersplenism to reduce the incidence of

overwhelming postsplenectomy infection. Cysts of the spleen are uncommon and may be nonparasitic (e.g., dermoid, epidermoid, epithelial, and pseudocyst) or parasitic (e.g., associated with echinococcal disease). Large, symptomatic, nonparasitic cysts can be widely unroofed and the spleen preserved; parasitic cysts are generally best managed by splenectomy. Splenic abscesses may be a consequence of infarction in patients with sickle cell anemia and are treated by drainage or splenectomy.

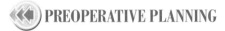 **PREOPERATIVE PLANNING**

In most instances, no specific treatment is required for the preoperative management of patients undergoing splenectomy. Vaccination against pneumococcus, meningococcosis, and *H. influenzae* should be administered preoperatively to reduce the risk of OPSI. Ideally, this should occur more than 10 days prior to splenectomy, but if not done preoperatively, this should be performed postoperatively approximately 1 week after surgery. Single-dose perioperative antibiotics are usually given and if a patient has had prolonged steroid treatment to treat this splenic disorder, then perioperative steroids with 100 mg of intravenous hydrocortisone should be given and tapered postoperatively.

Patients should be typed and crossed in advance of the operation as many patients are difficult to cross-match because of antibodies that have developed from many prior transfusions. All blood products should be warmed properly to avoid hemolysis by cold agglutinins found occasionally in patients with lymphoma.

In the case of an emergency splenectomy, pneumococcal vaccine should be administered in the early postoperative phase. The antibody response to pneumococcal polysaccharide antigen 6A and 19F has been shown not to be reduced after splenectomy.

A specific preoperative regimen is used in patients with myeloproliferative disorders who are prone to thrombosis of the splenic vein and superior mesenteric vein.

Medicating these patients with low-dose heparin (5,000 units subcutaneously twice daily) and an antiplatelet-aggregating drug such as aspirin or dipyridamole on the day before surgery is beneficial. This regimen is continued for 5 days postoperatively. In all patients, an orogastric tube is inserted into the stomach after endotracheal intubation to decompress the stomach and to facilitate ligation of the short gastric veins. The tube can be removed at the end of the procedure.

Platelets should not be administered preoperatively to those with ITP regardless of the extent of cytopenia because these cells will not survive. If thrombocytopenia is related to Marrow depression, preoperative administration of platelets is appropriate. Platelets should be available with thrombocytopenia (<50,000), and transfusion after splenic artery ligation is the best means to prevent splenic consumption of platelets. Preoperative embolization of the splenic artery can decrease operative blood loss and should be considered in patients with massive spleens.

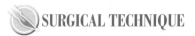 **SURGICAL TECHNIQUE**

Open Splenectomy

A variety of incisions can be used, depending on the nature of the disease and the surgeon's preference. For splenectomy related to blunt abdominal trauma, an upper midline incision is preferable because of the speed of performance and the accessibility of other potentially injured organs. Although uncommon today, this incision is also preferred when splenectomy is performed as part of the staging of Hodgkin disease to facilitate dissection of the lower periaortic and iliac nodes. In most patients in whom splenectomy is being carried out for hematologic disorder, a left oblique, subcostal incision beginning to the right of the midline and proceeding obliquely outward and downward approximately two fingerbreadths below the costal margin give excellent exposure. In patients with ITP and a small spleen, the oblique muscles do not have to be divided. With significant splenomegaly, the oblique muscles are divided laterally in the direction of their fibers.

In the case of marked splenomegaly with significant diaphragmatic adhesions, some surgeons advise a thoracoabdominal incision. Such an incision should be avoided because it is associated with a higher incidence of morbidity. Preoperative angiographic embolization can be considered to reduce bleeding in cases of massive splenography.

Splenectomy is performed with a technique of mobilization and dissection down to an ultimate pedicle of splenic artery and vein, keeping in mind the variable distribution of the splenic artery. With the surgeon positioned on the right side of the operating table, exploration with the right hand following the convex surface of the organ will define the ligamentous attachments posteriorly. In the case of splenic trauma, hematoma frequently has dissected these attachments, and rapid delivery into the wound is facilitated. In the case of elective splenectomy, the first step is transection of the ligamentous attachments, including the splenophrenic ligament at the superior pole and the splenocolic and splenorenal ligaments at the inferior pole (Fig. 7). This may be accomplished by blunt dissection or, if the ligaments are thickened, with scissors. These ligaments are avascular except when the patient has portal hypertension. Division of these ligaments will allow the spleen to be mobilized by continual retroperitoneal dissection. This allows better visualization of the short gastric vessels during ligation.

After the ligamentous attachments are transected, two to six gastric vessels that run from the spleen to the greater curvature of the stomach should be ligated in continuity and divided (Fig. 8). Often, this can best be performed before delivering

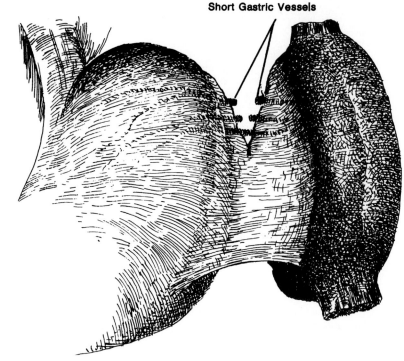

Short Gastric Vessels

Fig. 8. Ligation of short gastric vessels.

the spleen into the wound. If any question exists about ligation of these vessels, a Lembert suture should be placed in the gastric wall in a seromuscular fashion to avoid the complication of gastric fistulization.

After these maneuvers are completed, the spleen can be delivered into the wound

by blunt dissection of the posterior attachments (Fig. 9). Care should be taken not to divide the posterior attachments too far medially to avoid entering the splenic vein. One should also avoid axial rotation of the spleen because this may lead to disruption of the splenic artery or vein.

Dissection is carried out at the hilus as close to the spleen as possible to avoid injury to the pancreas. Individual ligation of the splenic artery or arterial branches and the splenic vein or venous branches is generally preferable. Splenic artery ligation is managed by double ligation and suture ligature, whereas the splenic vein can be doubly ligated and divided (Fig. 10). In the case of a markedly enlarged spleen, occasionally one must place a vascular clamp on the splenic vein and close the lumen with continuous vascular suture.

After removal of the spleen, hemostasis is checked in a specific fashion with observation of three major areas: (a) the inferior surface of the diaphragm, (b) the greater curvature of the stomach and the region of the short gastric vessels, and (c) the region of the hilus. This is readily accomplished by a rolled laparotomy pad into the left upper quadrant and unrolling it, exerting downward, with medial traction on the stomach and hilar region to permit visualization of the undersurface of the diaphragm. The pads are then rolled toward the midline to permit visualization of the greater curvature of the stomach and the

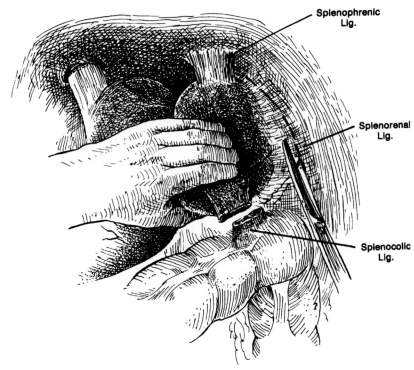

Splenophrenic Lig.

Splenorenal Lig.

Splenocolic Lig.

Fig. 7. Transection of ligamentous attachments.

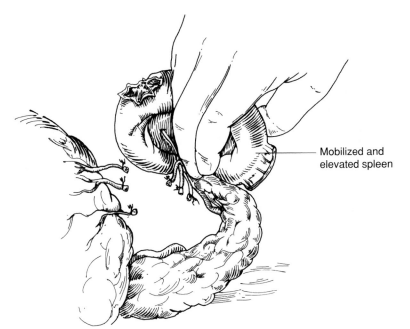

Mobilized and
elevated spleen

Fig. 9. Demonstration of the spleen mobilized and elevated into the wound following division of ligament attachments and posterior dissection.

short gastric vessels that have been divided. The final step is uncovering the hilar dissection. Direct visualization is facilitated using this technique, and hemostasis secured.

Initial ligation of the splenic artery and vein by entrance into the lesser sac is often done (Fig. 11). This maneuver rarely helps and, if the spleen is markedly enlarged, is difficult to perform. The only circumstance in which it is applied is a situation of marked lymphadenopathy in the hilar region of the spleen, which precludes safe dissection.

An integral part of splenectomy for hematologic disease is a thorough exploration to detect any accessory spleens. The more common locations of accessory spleens are the region of the hilus and the gastrosplenic ligament, the gastrocolic ligament and greater omentum, the mesentery, and the presacral space. It is very important to retrieve accessory spleens from patients with ITP. Failure to do so has been associated with recurrence of the disease.

Although the procedure is rarely performed now, when laparotomy was done for staging of Hodgkin disease, the first step was wedge biopsy of a portion of the right and left lobes of the liver. This was carried out early to avoid confusion in histologic evaluation; prolonged application of the retractors can result in leukocytic infiltration. Splenectomy was performed next, followed by biopsy of the

periaortic nodes and the hepatoduodenal nodes. The nodes were sent for pathologic study separately, with their locations mapped. Because the greatest yield was from the region of the 12th thoracic and first lumbar vertebrae, the colon was retracted craniad and the ligament of Treitz was resected to provide ready access to the upper retroperitoneum.

SPLENORRHAPHY AND AUTOTRANSPLANTATION

The techniques to preserve splenic tissue are dictated by the extent of damage. Small lacerations can be managed by compression and application of hemostatic agents such as oxidized cellulose or micronized collagen. Exposed areas of splenic parenchyma are readily controlled with an argon-beam coagulator. Bleeding associated with severe disruptions of the parenchyma can be managed with absorbable sutures that traverse the capsule and incorporate the parenchyma. Horizontal mattress sutures are advantageous because they minimize cutting through tissues (Fig. 12). These can be placed over pledgets to distribute the force and placed all the way through the spleen by threading sutures through spinal needles, which are then passed through the entire parenchymal surface.

If trauma is localized in one pole of the spleen, the area can be resected and edges approximated with a series of mattress sutures, or the omentum can be sutured over the raw surface of the spleen or into the defect (Fig.13). Autotransplantation of the spleen into the omental pockets has no place because, although the tissue survives, the vascularization is distinctly different from the normal splenic circulation and precludes adequate phagocytosis of encapsulated bacteria.

Partial splenectomy for Gaucher disease is best performed by isolating the vessels to

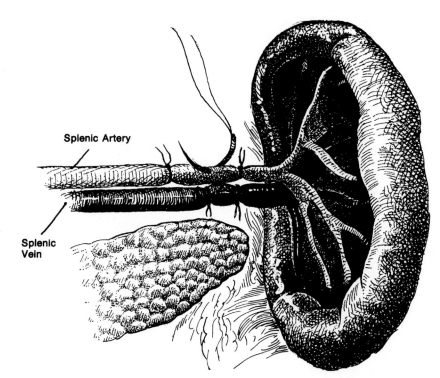

Splenic Artery

Splenic
Vein

Fig. 10. Ligation of the splenic artery and splenic vein in relation to the hilus.

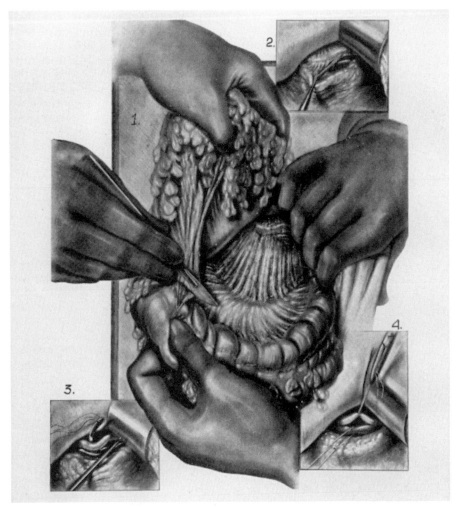

Fig. 11. Approach through the omental bursa to the splenic artery and vein (above the superior border of the pancreas). In some cases of splenomegaly in which the spleen is firmly attached to the diaphragm by numerous lesions, splenic artery ligation is sometimes selected. The splenic artery and vein should be cautiously dissected free from the back *(panel 1)* before silk ligatures are applied proximally *(panel 2)* and distally *(panel 3)* to them, and then each vessel is divided between the ligatures *(panel 4)*. After this procedure, the spleen is carefully mobilized from the diaphragm, tail of the pancreas, stomach, and colon before its pedicle is ligated once again and the organ is removed.

the segment of the spleen to be removed and ligating them in continuity and dividing them within the hilus, followed by transection of the parenchyma. The raw surface can then be coagulated with the argon-beam coagulator and an omental patch sewn over the surface of the spleen.

LAPAROSCOPIC SPLENECTOMY

Laparoscopic techniques have improved and most patients today are considered for elective laparoscopic splenectomy. The complicating factors are a large spleen (>500 g), suspected perisplenitis (most common in patients with previous infectious diseases of the spleen or portal hypertension), and previous gastric surgery. ITP patients are considered ideal for laparoscopic splenectomy, and staging laparotomy is suited ideally for laparoscopic approaches as well. The patient is positioned with the right side down (Fig. 14) and port sites are chosen with the first one placed near the midline and 4 cm below the spleen tip, the second is positioned near the tip of the 11th rib along the posterior axillary line, and a third is a middle port placed halfway between the other two, along the anterior axillary line. Occasionally, a fourth port may be required.

Laparoscopic splenectomy occurs in an order similar to the open technique, scissors with cautery, or preferably the harmonic Scalpel (Ethicon Endo-Surgery, Inc.) can be used to take down the lateral peritoneal attachments and can be used to ligate short gastric vessels. Endo stapling devices with vascular staples can be used to ligate and divide the short gastric vessels and used to ligate the splenic artery and vein.

Extraction of the spleen ordinarily involves morselization of the spleen in a bag, although occasionally the spleen is so large that commercially available bags may not contain the spleen adequately. A port site can be enlarged to facilitate removal; however, if the spleen is too large, a small incision can be made to remove the spleen. The use of a Pfannenstiel incision and removing the spleen through a suprapubic area may be more cosmetically satisfactory, particularly in women. Operative times for a splenectomy using a laparoscopic technique are longer, but laparoscopic splenectomy is associated with earlier return to diet, less ileus, less pain, less hospitalization, and less hospital expense.

Any serious bleeding or ineffectiveness of the usual maneuvers requires conversion to an open procedure. Laparoscopic splenectomy in children has increased with frequency and can be done for hematologic disease, hereditary spherocytosis,

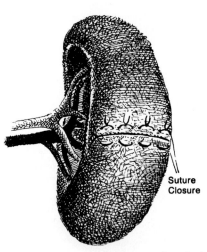

Fig. 12. Mattress suture closure of a splenic laceration.

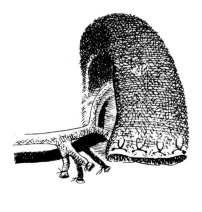

Fig. 13. Partial resection of the spleen following selected splenic artery ligation, parenchymal transection, and control of capsular bleeding.

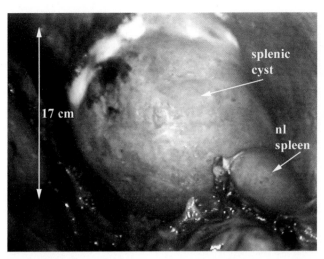

Fig. 4. Laparoscopic approach to splenic cyst.

tient. Creating the appropriate patient expectation preoperatively may avoid problems or unexpected disappointment from the patient postoperatively. Surgeons should give the patients a reasonable incidence of "conversion rates" to incisional surgery. While the surgical community does not view a "conversion" as a complication, the patient may have a different view unless properly educated. It is convenient to divide complications into four categories: those due to surgery, those due to laparoscopy, those due to operative splenectomy, and those due the nature of the treatment (Table 1). Surgeons will vary when advising prospective patients concerning the precise incidence of these events, but operators should be able to perform this procedure with less than 1% mortality and less than 4% incidence or pancreatic injury. Clearly splenectomy is not uniformly successful in all cases of ITP. Approximately 65% to 75% of patients will resolve their thrombocytopenia. Patients who are refractory to steroids and immune globulin therapy may have even less success with splenectomy. Patients need to be educated as to the risks that the asplenic patient engenders postoperatively in terms of infection. Overwhelming postsplenectomy sepsis (OPSS) is uncommon in adults; however, patients who consent to the procedure should be vaccinated against certain types of Gram-positive bacteria. Polyvalent pneumococcal vaccine should be administered at least 2 weeks prior to splenectomy. In addition, *Haemophilus influenza* type b (Hib) conjugate vaccine and meningococcal serogroup C conjugate vaccine should be administered as well. Even with vaccination, patients should be advised that should procedures associated with poten-

tial bacteremia be contemplated in the future, antibiotic prophylaxis is indicated. Patients should also be reminded about the need to communicate that a splenectomy has been performed in the past to health care providers taking a history. Patients often ask whether or not revaccination is needed. The answer to this is not clear. Some patients demonstrate low antibody level to capsular polysaccharide antigens after 5 to 10 years has lapsed postsplenectomy. When this occurs revaccination can be performed safely. Finally, to the extent that the risks and benefits

TABLE 1. POTENTIAL COMPLICATIONS OF LAPAROSCOPIC SPLENECTOMY THAT SHOULD BE REVIEWED IN THE PREOPERATIVE DISCUSSION

Surgical
  Anesthetic
  Deep venous thrombosis
  Intraoperative bleeding
  Infection
  Overall mortality
Laparoscopic
  Effect of pneumoperitoneum
  Entry injuries
  Trocar site hernia
Operative Splenectomy
  Increased risk of left-sided
    pulmonary complications
  Postoperative bleed from short
    gastric or splenic vessels
  Pancreatic fistula
  Left upper quadrant abscess
  Injury to adjacent organs
Treatment Related
  Failure to cure disease process
  Thrombocytosis

have been outlined and vaccinations administered, there is a need to document this and to make sure that the patient has this information as well, including which vaccines have been given and specific prophylactic antibiotic recommendations.

Splenic artery embolization has become less popular in the last decade. Despite this, some surgeons may find this useful when attempting to remove a very large spleen or as an adjunct to partial splenectomy. Care to preserve the blood to supply to the distal pancreas should be exercised by the angiographer (Fig. 5). Embolism can be performed at two levels along the splenic artery, and ideally the surgeon will conduct the dissection in between these sites for maximum hemostasis. When this adjunct is used it should be performed just prior to splenectomy, ideally on the same day. Infarction of the splenic mass can be extremely painful to the patient, and this should be anticipated in terms of counseling and the availability of pain medicine.

Just after entering the operating room, a single dose of antibiotic prophylaxis against Gram-positive organisms should be administered. Since many of these patients are on steroids, the plan for administering "stress doses" of steroids should be discussed with the anesthesia team. While the immediate availability of blood products and platelets must be assured prior to beginning the procedure, it is generally not necessary to actually administer platelets unless a bleeding diathesis is encountered. The old practice of "hanging platelets with the incision" does not appear to improve outcome or reduce blood loss in laparoscopic splenectomy. Sequential compression devices should be placed on the patient's lower extremities to minimize the risk of deep venous thrombosis. Urinary and (oro)nasogastric catheters are placed for decompression. Splenectomy is an advanced laparoscopic procedure requiring the dissection and control of several vascular structures. As such, the surgeon must have the appropriate tools immediately at his or her disposal. In addition to the usual array of graspers, I have found that a 10-mm right-angle dissector and a DeBakey-type noncrushing grasper are particularly useful while performing the dissection. Many surgeons control the main splenic vessels with linear endoscopic staplers. The surgeon should confirm the presence and number of "vascular loads" available for that device prior to initiating the procedure since halfway through the operation is the wrong time to find out that supplies might be short.

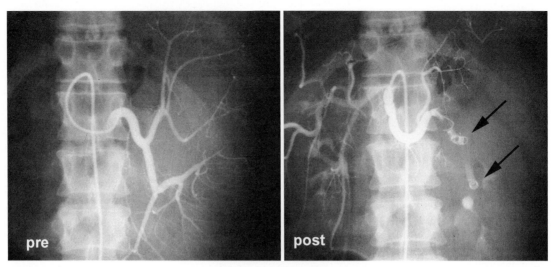

Fig. 5. Angiographic pre- (*left*) and postembolization (*right*) views of splenic artery with double coil technique (*arrows*).

Patient Positioning

Laparoscopic splenectomy was originally performed in the supine position with the surgeon standing between the legs or on the patient's right side. In 1995 Delaitre described the "hanged spleen" approach modeled after the lateral approach advocated for laparoscopic adrenalectomy described by Gagner et al. a few years earlier. The advantages of this become apparent when performing this procedure. The stomach falls away after the gastrosplenic ligament is divided, and the left lobe of the liver often does not require retraction (Fig. 6A). The spleen is then "hanging" on the peritoneal suspensory ligaments, facilitating the dissection of the hilum. Performance of concomitant surgical procedures (such as cholecystectomy) is more difficult through a lateral approach and may require repositioning. In addition, the search for accessory spleens may be more difficult in the lateral position; however, more than 80% of these accessory spleens can be reached in the lateral position. The advantages of the lateral technique probably outweigh this mild difficulty. Furthermore, when the patient is in the supine position, blood pools right into the hilum, obscuring vision. In general,

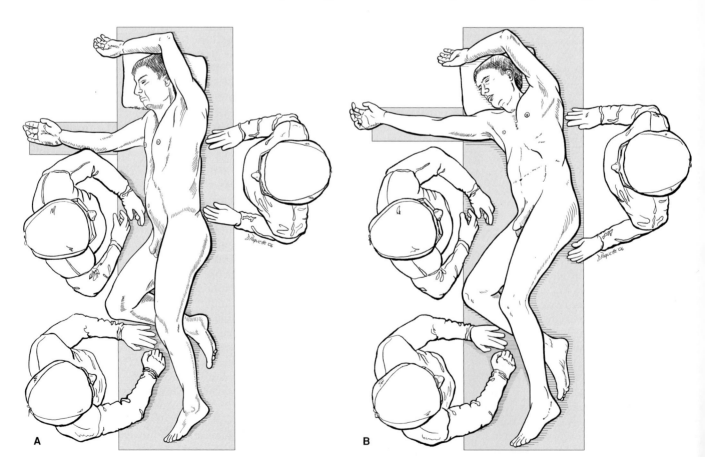

Fig. 6. A: Demonstration of lateral decubitus position. **B:** Demonstration of semi-lateral decubitus position.

there is almost no reason to remove a reasonably sized spleen from supine position. If the operator would prefer to cannulate the umbilicus for initial entry as might be the case in a smaller-sized patient, then reducing the amount of patient rotation from 90 degrees to 45 to 60 degrees is useful to clear the abdominal contents from the underside of the umbilicus (Fig. 6B). This facilitates entry and maintains a clear view to the spleen.

The lateral approach is executed by placing the patient in the right lateral decubitus position (left side up) with the abdominal side closest to the edge of the operating table, either utilizing a vacuum-stabilized beanbag or tape to secure the patient. The right arm is placed on an arm board and the left arm is supported in a sling or tray as for thoracotomy. The "kidney bar" is raised and the bed is flexed. This requires the surgeon to be precise in the patient's alignment on the operating table to take advantage of these maneuvers that spread the distance between the ribs and the iliac crest. Using somewhat less than the full lateral position allows a greater degree of freedom of the instruments along the costal margin, especially when moving the tips anteriorly. A reversed Trendelenburg position allows shifting the visceral contents in a caudad direction, bringing the spleen off the diaphragm. With the patient in the lateral or semi-lateral position, an urgent entry into the abdomen or even one made for futility would almost certainly be made through a flank incision. It is prudent to mark out such an incision prior to initiation of pneumoperitoneum, since this is ideally the line upon which the subcostal trocars should be placed.

SURGICAL TECHNIQUE

If the umbilicus is not used for the initial entry, then three trocar sites are marked along the anterior costal margin. While a Veress needle entry and blind initial puncture have been used by some, I prefer to make a small incision where the middle trocar site is anticipated and dissect down to the anterior fascia, which is incised under direct visualization, and then spread the underlying muscles bluntly, revealing the endoabdominal fascia and peritoneum. These layers can be incised or bluntly traversed, allowing access to the abdominal cavity. If this entry is made too far laterally then one encounters a thicker musculature and runs a small risk of landing in the retroperitoneum upon entry. Once entry into the peritoneal cavity is established,

we use a blunt balloon-tipped 12-mm trocar to minimize CO_2 leak. Later when this site is expanded somewhat during spleen extraction, a good seal can be easily maintained using this device for the final inspection. The other cannulae are placed under direct visualization.

Alternatively, an optical trocar can be used, which allows visualization of the abdominal wall layers during trocar insertion. Experience with this device is recommended prior to using it in the left upper quadrant. A fourth and more lateral trocar can be placed after the splenic flexure is mobilized. When the patients are not too large, the umbilicus trocar and just three subcostal trocars can be used. The exact location of these ports is driven by the size of the spleen and configuration of the patient's chest wall relative to the spleen. Early in one's operative experience, it is convenient to place 12-mm trocars along the costal margin for maximum flexibility in passing staplers, camera, and clip appliers. Over time even "needlescopic" laparoscopic splenectomy can be performed.

The procedure is initiated by mobilizing the splenic flexure of the colon with ultrasonic dissectors or cautery. This allows placement of a posterior cannula if needed. The gastrosplenic ligament containing the short gastric vessels is then opened. At this point some operators will dissect the hilum, transect the splenic artery(s) and vein(s), and divide the remainder of the short gastric vessels later. Other surgeons will first complete the division of all of the short gastric vessels immediately. This has a few advantages. The division of the short gastric vessels will allow the stomach to fall away to the right, exposing the distal pancreas and splenic hilum completely. Since many surgeons who undertake splenectomy are familiar with short gastric mobilization for fundoplication, this task is readily accomplished. If perchance immediate abdominal entry is needed later due to significant hemorrhage of the hilar vessels or spleen, then mobilizing the spleen quickly is quite easy without fear of additional problems from torn short gastric vessels. The short gastric vessels can be transected in a number of ways. Clips, vascular staples, ultrasonic shears, bipolar cautery, and thermal cautery have all been used to divide these vessels with good effect (Fig. 7). Occasionally a suture might be needed to control a recalcitrant short gastric vessel. The choice will ultimately depend on surgeon preference and operating room availability. Once the first short gastric (the most cephalad) has been transected, it is convenient to divide the uppermost part of the phrenocolic ligament at the superior pole of the spleen for a short distance to facilitate removal later. A careful search for accessory spleen should be undertaken at this point. The majority of accessory spleens will be found adjacent to the spleen, in the hilum, in the region of the pancreatic tail, or near the splenic flexure (Fig. 4). Less often they can be found remotely in the greater omentum, intestinal mesentery, or even the pelvis. Next, incising the remainder of splenocolic ligament and then the lower portion of the phrenocolic ligament allows elevation of the spleen to

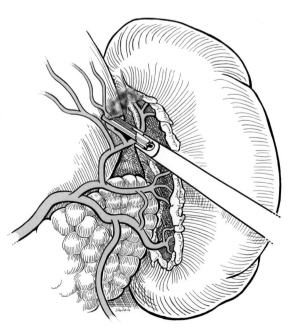

Fig. 7. Division of short gastric arteries using ultrasonic dissector.

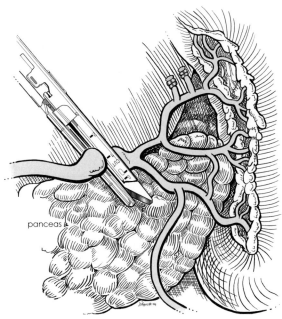

Fig. 8. Division of splenic artery using laparoscopic linear cutting device placed from cephalad port.

facilitate identification of the tail of the pancreas and begin the hilar dissection. If one leaves a 1- to 2-cm segment of the phrenocolic peritoneum attached to the spleen, then this can be used as a handle to elevate the lower pole of the spleen and separate it from the pancreas by dissection of the filmy avascular tissue in the retroperitoneum. Since almost one third of patients have a pancreatic tail that abuts the spleen, it is essential that this anatomy be delineated prior to transection of the splenic vessels.

As in open surgery, some surgeons prefer ligating the splenic artery with a clip or suture prior to dissecting the hilum. This is performed by identifying it at the superior border of the pancreas, carefully dissecting it with a right-angled instrument, passing a ligature (or using a hemoclip), and securing with an intra- or extracorporeal tie. The splenic vein will be just beneath the artery. Depending on the actual arrangement of the blood supply, this will devascularize most or all of the spleen. The splenic size will shrink somewhat. This is helpful when there are many branches in the hilum that require an extensive dissection. When the blood supply is in a bundled configuration, a single vascular staple load may be sufficient to divide the splenic artery and vein located along the superior border of the spleen in the lienorenal ligament (Fig. 8). When the blood supply is distributed the vessels can either be individually ligated or divided with multiple firings of the stapler. It is hazardous to simply elevate the spleen and apply the stapler close to parenchyma, as this method can

result in significant hemorrhage, splenosis, and pancreatic injury. In order to create the proper viewing angles to perform these maneuvers, it is often necessary to move the camera to different positions. Often the most advantageous stapling angle to divide the hilar vessels is achieved from the most anterior cannula. Once the hilar vessels are divided, short gastric vessels are transected (if not already) and the spleen is "hanging" and is elevated, exposing the remaining peritoneal attachment of the phrenocolic ligament and the areolar tissue of the retroperitoneum. A large extraction bag is then introduced into the abdomen (Fig. 9A,B). There are several choices including sterilizing supermarket freezer bags, but the material must be heavy to avoid rupture during splenic morsellation. By placing the bag medial to the spleen, unfolding it completely, and holding the mouth open with two grasping forceps, the spleen can then be rolled, pushed, or flipped from lateral to medial into the bag without actually grasping the parenchyma and risking splenosis. The edges of the bag are then brought out through the wound. It is helpful to enlarge the incision just a bit but usually to no more than 2 to 3 cm to facilitate spleen removal (Fig. 10). By elevating the extraction bag the spleen is brought closer to the surgeon and the spleen is first finger-fractured and then morsellated with ring forceps to create pieces small enough to fit through the wound. Commercial "morsellation" devices are available as well. Sharp instruments should not be placed into the bag since perforation would lead to splenosis. With patience, even a relatively large spleen can be removed through a small incision. Alternatively, a small Pfannenstiel incision can be made to remove very large spleens.

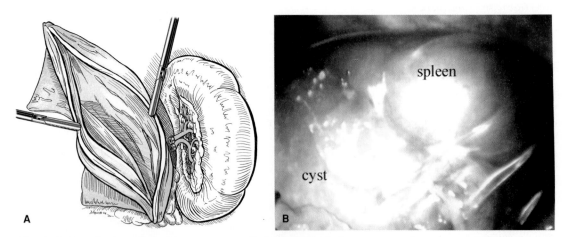

Fig. 9. A: Introduction of splenic entrapment sac. **B:** Spleen and splenic cyst as seen through entrapment sac.

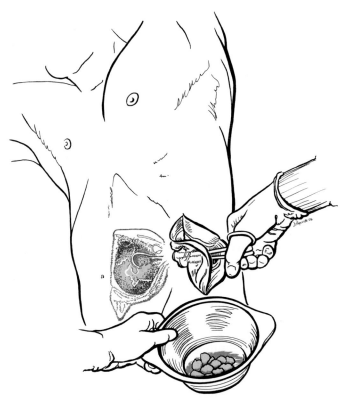

Fig. 10. Morsellation and removal of spleen in entrapment sac.

Once the spleen has been removed, the balloon-tipped trocar is reinflated, creating an adequate seal, and the abdomen is inspected. Unless there is specific concern about the integrity of the tail of the pancreas, there is no specific indication for a drain (closed suction type) to be placed. Ports 12 mm (or larger) are closed with fascial sutures and the skin is closed with subcuticular absorbable suture and reinforced with adhesive strips on skin prepared with tincture of benzoin.

Hand-assisted Laparoscopic Splenectomy

Hand-assisted laparoscopic splenectomy (HALS) was described by Kusminsky et al. in 1995. The technique involves making an incision usually either in the upper midline or in the Pfannenstiel position that allows the surgeon or assistant to place a hand into the abdomen to facilitate splenic retraction and dissection. There are a host of variations on this theme. Generally the surgeon stands on the patient's right side and retracts the spleen with the nondominant hand. Initial techniques and devices were cumbersome in terms of how the operator would insert or remove his or her hand into the abdomen. Recent modifications to these various devices have made this a much

more straightforward affair. A disc-shaped device is inserted through a 7- to 10-cm incision, creating a seal that can be traversed by the operator's hand without losing the pneumoperitoneum (Fig. 11). Although the creation of an incision would seem to negate the benefits of the minimally invasive approach, results appear comparable. Certainly, the size of the spleen range approachable by minimally invasive splenectomy techniques is extended by this methodology. Some authors have advocated this approach for all splenectomies, citing that it can be performed more quickly than a purely laparoscopic approach.

Partial Splenectomy

While the specific indications for such a splenectomy can be debated for hamartomas, cysts, and some storage diseases, this technique has been described and can be performed successfully by sufficiently experienced splenic operators. The patient is placed in the lateral or semi-lateral position as before. The keys to this procedure are opening the gastrosplenic, splenocolic, and phrenocolic ligaments and fully mobilizing the spleen so that the lesion and the associated blood supply can be identified. This requires a tedious dissection of the blood supply of the involved segment of spleen and confirming that adequate devascularization has been achieved by individually ligating the arterial branches. I have found that a preoperative angiogram is helpful when planning a partial splenectomy. The extent of the vessels to be ligated can also

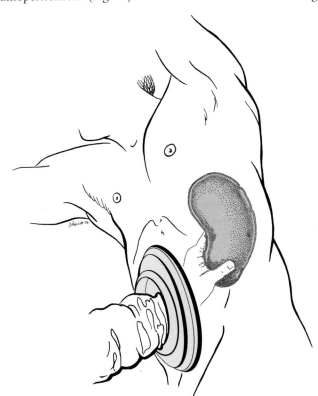

Fig. 11. Hand-assisted splenectomy.

be somewhat predicted by the number and placement of lobes and notches seen on the splenic surface. After the relevant arterial supply is divided, the venous supply is similarly treated. The planned transection margin of the spleen should be at least 5 to 10 mm from the line of demarcation; otherwise, breakthrough bleeding may ensue. Splenic division using linear staplers has been demonstrated in the veterinary/laboratory setting, but the thicker configuration of the human splenic has made this impractical clinically. If an adequate devascularized margin is achieved, then any resultant bleeding can usually be managed with cautery. When performing a partial splenectomy, special consideration needs to be given to the specimen extraction since morselation may not be appropriate depending on the indication for the procedure. In that case a small incision will be required for extraction.

Robotically Assisted Splenectomy

The introduction of approved robotic devices for general surgery has resulted in a number of procedures being performed using this technique. The presence of the robotic "wrist" with the multiple degrees of freedom gained could in theory allow for certain precisions of dissection not achievable using conventional laparoscopic techniques. Specific advantages remain unproven at the time of this writing.

Conversion to Incisional Surgery

Conversion of any laparoscopic procedure to an incisional one is the culmination of a complex decision-making process. Splenectomy in particular is subject to conversion issues since the procedure involves the manipulation and transaction of a significant number of arteries and veins. The ability of any one surgeon to control a significant bleeding situation is a matter of three factors: skill set, experience, and available necessary tools. If any of these are lacking, then early conversion is preferable to later incision; the surgeon should not let pride get in the way of a good decision. The need for conversion is also based on the patient's hemodynamic status. Pneumoperitoneum in the face of hypovolemia can potentiate hypotension significantly. Ideally direct compression of the offending vessel should be achieved while the incision is made. A non-crushing clamp can be applied or a gauze sponge can be introduced through the largest trocar and held in place. If the patient is in the lateral position, an incision

along the costal margin is then made and is quite satisfactory for attaining vascular control and finishing the splenectomy. The dictum *primum no nocere* truly applies when significant hemorrhage is encountered during laparoscopic splenectomy.

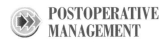

POSTOPERATIVE MANAGEMENT

Empiric observations after laparoscopic fundoplication have demonstrated that long periods of gastric decompression to prevent rupture of the short gastric vessel ligatures previously thought essential are not necessary unless unusual circumstances were encountered. The nasogastric and urinary catheters can be removed prior to discharge from the postanesthesia care unit. Early ambulation and oral intake are encouraged. Deep venous thrombosis prophylaxis is indicated. Patient-controlled analgesia (PCA) is used for the first 36 hours and the patient is transitioned to a combination of oral narcotics plus nonsteroidal anti-inflammatory (unless contraindicated by a persistently low platelet count) medication. Patients are allowed to shower on the second postoperative day. Most patients are discharged by day 3. Platelet counts often rise promptly and should be monitored for a successful therapeutic result or thrombocytosis. As many as one half of patients postsplenectomy may experience thrombocytosis. Severe thrombocytosis can be associated with both hemorrhage and thromboembolic phenomena. Many surgeons prophylactically treat platelet counts in excess of $750,000$ mm^3 with aspirin, or "minidose" heparin, but this is becoming less common. Platelet counts in excess of 1 million mm^3 can be considered for hydroxyurea therapy if symptomatic.

Postoperative Complications

There are specific complications of laparoscopy, such as CO_2 embolism, trocar site bleeding, or hernia, that apply to all such procedures. The postoperative complications of splenectomy are the same regardless of the method of access. Foremost is hemorrhage, which is usually recognized intraoperatively and treated, but can occur postoperatively as well. The two obvious sites are the splenic vessels at the tail of the spleen and the short gastric vessels along the greater curvature of the stomach. This is manifested by a falling hemoglobin level and a systemic reaction to hemorrhage. Kehr sign of left shoulder pain could tip the surgeon to a subdi-

aphragmatic event but could also be a normal consequence of irritation of the diaphragm in a perfectly executed procedure. Hemodynamically unstable patients should be simultaneously resuscitated and moved to the operating room for exploration generally performed via an incisional approach. Re-exploration may be performed laparoscopically in a stable patient since the problem could be a technically simple problem to correct, such as bleeding from a short gastric vessel or trocar site. Patients must be adequately resuscitated prior to the initiation of pneumoperitoneum to avoid hemodynamic compromise from the effects of increased intra-abdominal pressure in the hypovolemic patient. Intraoperative conversion to incisional surgery is warranted for severe hemorrhage or persistent bleeding from a site not controlled or identified laparoscopically.

Structures adjacent to the spleen (i.e., the colon, stomach, diaphragm, and pancreas) can be injured in the course of laparoscopic splenectomy. Injury to the tail of the pancreas occurs in 1% to 2% of cases and can occur from direct trauma to the organ or from devascularization of the blood supply to the tail of the pancreas. Direct trauma most often occurs from en mass stapling across the hilum of the spleen during which pancreatic tissue is included in the staple line. If leakage from the pancreatic duct ensues, this will often manifest as left upper quadrant pain, fever, pleural effusion, and elevated white blood cell count. Hyperamylasemia may be present as well. Computed tomography–guided catheter placement is usually sufficient to drain and control the fistula until it closes, but operative intervention may be required. Left lower lobe pulmonary complications such as pleural effusion, atelectasis, or pneumonia are seen more frequently after splenectomy than other upper abdominal procedures not directly under the left diaphragm. These are minimized by aggressive attention to pulmonary care in the immediate postoperative period. Postoperative thrombosis of the splenic vein can occur following splenectomy. This may occur more frequently than previously recognized. Up to 20% of patients may experience thrombosis of their splenic vein. This condition may be asymptomatic but could be associated with a vague abdominal pain, suggesting that performing routine postoperative Doppler ultrasound to assess for this condition may be warranted to detect those patients who may benefit from anticoagulation to avoid portal vein involvement or cavernous transformation of the portal vein.

The most frustrating complication of laparoscopic or open splenectomy is recurrent or persistent thrombocytopenia. The retention of even a small amount of splenic tissue can result in recurrent ITP. Modalities such as computed tomography, magnetic resonance imaging, or nuclear imaging with indium-111–labeled autologous platelets might localize suspicious tissue for subsequent resection. This exploration can be conducted laparoscopically by experienced operators or through an open approach. Intraoperative gamma probe scanning may be useful in locating small foci of splenic tissue. Despite successful resection of persistent splenic tissue, durable remission still might not be achievable.

SUMMARY

Laparoscopic splenectomy is an advanced minimally invasive procedure that can be performed with a similar therapeutic success and technical complication rate as compared with the incisional counterpart. As the operator gains experience with this procedure, progressively larger spleens can be removed using these techniques.

SUGGESTED READING

Delaitre B. Laparoscopic splenectomy. The "hanged spleen" technique. *Surg Endosc* 1995;9(5):528.

Gagner M, Lacroix A, et al. Early experience with laparoscopic approach for adrenalectomy. *Surgery* 1993;114(6):1120, discussion 1124.

Kusminsky RE, Boland JP, et al. Hand-assisted laparoscopic splenectomy. *Surg Laparosc Endosc* 1995;5(6):463.

Landgren O, Bjorkholm M, et al. A prospective study on antibody response to repeated vaccinations with pneumococcal capsular polysaccharide in splenectomized individuals with special reference to Hodgkin's lymphoma. *J Intern Med* 2004;255(6):664.

Pietrabissa A, Moretto C, et al. Thrombosis in the portal venous system after elective laparoscopic splenectomy. *Surg Endosc* 2004; 18(7):1140.

Poulin EC, Thibault C. The anatomical basis for laparoscopic splenectomy. *Can J Surg* 1993;37(5):484.

Nongastrointestinal Transabdominal

EDITOR'S COMMENT

For the small or normal-sized spleen, the laparoscopic splenectomy is the preferred approach to remove the spleen of many patients for most referring physicians. ITP is an ideal disease for laparoscopic splenectomy. The minimal-access technique makes it easier for patients to choose splenectomy without the fear of a major laparotomy. Many patients recuperate quickly through three to four small ports in just a couple of days.

The key to laparoscopic splenectomy as Dr. Schwaitzberg emphasizes is attention to patient positioning and the surgeon's knowledge of anatomy. I place the patient right side down, and the patient is rotated about 45 degrees with a roll supporting the back. The left arm crosses the chest and is supported on a pillow or arm holder. All pressure points are well padded to avoid neuropathy. The operating table is cracked with the kidney rest lifted, and the 12th rib and iliac crest is separated for optimal placement of the fourth port. This patient position will displace the intestine and colon by gravity, better exposing the spleen. I gain access with a Veress needle in the mid–left subcostal site, and enter the abdomen with an optical trocar. The 15-mm port is placed at this site and at the conclusion of the operation will be used for specimen extraction. The larger port allows a large 15-mm entrapment sac (USSC, Norwalk, CT).

Mobilization of the spleen begins by dividing the splenocolic ligament with harmonic shears.

Medial and lateral division of the gastrosplenic and phrenocolic ligaments further mobilizes the spleen from the tail of the pancreas. As the hilum is dissected, the surgeon needs to appreciate the distributed and magistral vascular arrangement and possible need for multiple staplers to get all vascular branches. Rather than bring the linear stapler from above, I introduce the endoscopic linear stapler from below. The inferior approach allows the linear endoscopic vascular stapler to hug the hilum and avoid pancreatic tissue.

Usually excellent hemostasis is achieved with stapler devices. Bleeding when it occurs can usually be well controlled with direct pressure between two instruments or with gauze until a clip can be applied. Occasionally fibrin glue may be used for more diffuse ooze. I will leave a drain if I have any concern about pancreatic disruption. While conversion to open splenectomy is very rare, nevertheless, an open laparotomy tray should be open and readily available. Postoperative hemorrhage should signal immediate return to the operating room to exclude surgical bleeding.

Prior to elective splenectomy, vaccination is important. While overwhelming sepsis is very rare, patients should be counseled as to the risks of postoperative infection. While most operations are completed laparoscopically, patients should appreciate that conversion to an open operation may be necessary.

Accessory splenic tissue should be routinely sought at time of splenectomy. Even though accessory splenic tissue is rarely identified during splenectomy, the hilum and mesentery should be inspected. Patients who fail to respond after splenectomy for ITP should be imaged to locate any retained splenic tissue.

Dr. Schwaitzberg describes the hand-assisted approach for splenectomy. While this technique may have value with larger spleens, I find that my hand only gets in my line of vision. Advocates of the hand-assisted approach note ease of specimen retrieval. Yet, with a little patience the spleen is easily morcellated with a ring forceps. The hand assist may have a role for surgeons very early in their laparoscopic splenectomy learning curve who already have hand port experience.

The robotic approach to splenectomy is over the top. Why the surgeon would want to use this technology for a splenectomy is unclear to me. One adds operative time and costs and is unlikely to simplify the procedure. Robotic splenectomy is interesting but is best avoided by the surgeon skilled in laparoscopy.

Trauma splenectomy is reserved for the "open" general surgeon. All surgeons performing laparoscopic splenectomy should be prepared to convert urgently to open surgery if necessary.

D.B.J.

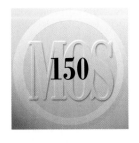

Splenic Preservation

CHARLES E. LUCAS AND ANNA M. LEDGERWOOD

HISTORICAL VIGNETTES

Roger Sherman, in 1979, provided a detailed historical perspective of splenic physiology and splenic injury in his presidential address to the American Association for the Surgery of Trauma. Although a number of so-called splenectomies were reported prior to the 19th century, Riegner, in 1892, introduced the modern era of splenic surgery when he performed a successful splenectomy following a blunt injury in a 14-year-old construction worker who fell from a scaffold. This young man had grade V splenic injury (Table 1) with portions of the spleen lying free in the peritoneal cavity. This operation helped establish two principles. First, laparotomy

with definitive control of bleeding, rather than extra-abdominal compression for refractory intra-abdominal bleeding, leads to a better outcome. Second, splenectomy is safe and well tolerated, thus laying to rest the 19th century concept that the spleen was necessary for life.

DANGERS OF THE ASPLENIC STATE

Throughout the past millennium, knowledge of splenic function has been elusive. The spleen has been portrayed as a vestigial organ without function; many senior surgeons still practicing were thus taught during their residency years. In contrast, the spleen has been considered essential for such diverse functions as laughter, humor, purification of the blood, and the maintenance of life. Scientific reconciliation of these conflicting opinions awaited 20th century investigations. During most of the 19th century, the pendulum had swung to the extreme concept that the spleen was not an important organ. Early 20th century reports drew the same conclusions, despite data suggesting the contrary. For example, Pearce, in 1918, noted that 25% of animals undergoing splenectomy died from either peritonitis or pneumonitis; unfortunately, these deaths were thought to be unrelated to the asplenic state, as reflected in the conclusion that animals survived splenectomy with "relative impunity." Pearce also noted that splenectomy leads to eosinophilia and leukocytosis, which were of unknown significance. Shortly thereafter, Morris and Bullock documented the importance of the spleen as an immune organ. Asplenic rats, subjected to a *Pasteurella* bacterial challenge, did poorly when compared with their normal controls; they suggested that the spleen was important for immunity. The surgical leadership in the Western world, however, rejected these findings by concluding that fears of infection after splenectomy were poppycock; thus, routine splenectomy for even the smallest of injuries became the norm for the ensuing generation.

The seed that gave rise to our current appreciation of splenic function was planted

when King and Shumacker reported two deaths in five children who died of an overwhelming postsplenectomy infection (OPSI) after splenectomy for spherocytosis. Smith, in 1957, reported the first death from OPSI following splenectomy in an injured patient without preexisting co-morbidities. Subsequent studies demonstrated that OPSI occurs in approximately 2% of children and 1% of adults; the mortality rate of OPSI in the nonvaccinated patient is approximately 50%. These findings led to a reassessment of splenic function.

SPLENIC FUNCTION

The spleen at birth is small and remains immature throughout the neonatal period. During this phase, there are few lymphoid follicles and a relative absence of germ centers. Throughout childhood, the spleen slowly increases in size and reaches its maximal weight during puberty when it represents approximately 25% of the total body lymphoid mass. Perfusion through the mature spleen facilitates leukocyte sequestration and the production of both immunoglobulins and antibodies to circulating antigens. This immunologic protection is thought to be mediated through the perifollicular cells. The result is enhanced opsonization and phagocytosis of bacteria. The resultant enhancement of bacterial clearance is directed primarily toward the encapsulated Gram-positive bacteria but also affects Gram-negative bacteria. These protective responses may also affect bacteria accessing the body by way of the respiratory route.

Immunologic Efficiency

The immune protection appears to correlate with the amount of spleen that is present; animals with hemisplenectomy do far better than their asplenic controls. The common organisms responsible for OPSI are the Gram-positive–encapsulated bacteria, namely, *Pneumococcus, Meningococcus, Staphylococcus*, and *Streptococcus*; however, *Escherichia coli, Haemophilus influenzae*, and other coliform organisms may lead to this syndrome. Furthermore, the volume of the remaining

TABLE 1. SEVERITY OF SPLENIC INJURY	
Grade	**Injury Description**[a]
I	Small subcapsular hematoma (<10% surface area)
	Small laceration (<1 cm deep)
II	Medium subcapsular hematoma (10% to 50% surface area)
	Intraparenchymal hematoma (<5 cm in diameter)
	Medium laceration (1 to 3 cm deep)
III	Large subcapsular hematoma (>50% surface area)
	Intraparenchymal hematoma (>5 cm in diameter)
	Expanding hematoma
	Large laceration (>3 cm deep or involving trabecular vessels)
IV	Laceration involving hilar vessels
V	Shattered or devascularized spleen

[a]Condensed from Organ Injury Scaling Committee for the American Association for the Surgery of Trauma (1994 revision).

spleen following partial splenectomy correlates directly with the antigenic response. Thus, preservation of the maximal amount of splenic tissue affords the best protection against OPSI. The intact spleen participates in the normal response to the polyvalent pneumococcal vaccine. Thus, vaccination is best administered before splenectomy.

OPERATIVE SPLENIC SALVAGE AFTER INJURY

Once the spleen became recognized as a vital link in the immune response to infection, operative attempts at splenic salvage became fashionable. A few far-sighted surgeons, however, practiced splenic salvage before their less prescient colleagues. Zikoff, in 1897, may have performed the first splenorrhaphy; Dretzka, in 1930, published a report of the first splenorrhaphy performed on a child. This early report by Dretzka and the subsequent report by Morgenstern and Shapiro highlight the technical factors involved with achieving successful splenorrhaphy. These authors emphasized the importance of a generous incision, which is necessary to provide good exposure.

Typically, in the injured patient, this is a midline incision, although a left subcostal incision provides excellent exposure in patients who are known to have injury limited to the left upper quadrant. The actively bleeding spleen should be packed in order to obtain temporary hemostasis while full splenic exposure is accomplished. The lesser sac is entered through the greater omentum outside the arcades of the gastroepiploic vessels (Fig. 1). As this dissection is carried superiorly along the greater curvature of the stomach, the proximal branches of the left gastroepiploic vessels may need to be divided; this facilitates the dissection near the apical fat pad and the cardiophrenic ligament. Mobilization of the proximal stomach anteriorly and medially allows one to visualize the short gastric vessels coming from the superior branches of the splenic artery as these branches enter into the superior segment of the spleen. Careful dissection of these vessels permits safe division. The splenic flexure of the colon is then mobilized. Typically, there will be two (sometimes one) short vessels extending from the colonic mesentery to the inferior pole of the spleen. These are the same "aberrant" vessels that are notoriously avulsed from the splenic capsule when too much anterior and medial pressure is placed on the omentum during gastric mobilization for

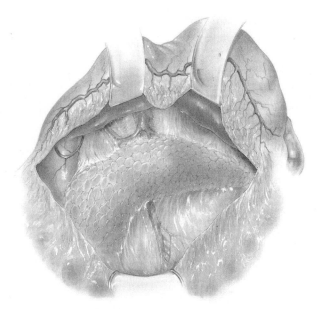

Fig. 1. When splenic exposure is not hurried, access to the lesser sac is achieved through the greater omentum outside the arcades of the gastroepiploic vessels. Proximal dissection exposes the short gastric vessels near the apical fat pad of the stomach, whereas lateral dissection exposes the splenic hilar vessels.

truncal vagotomy. These vessels are always present; they should be identified and made hemostatic by coagulation or individually tied prior to division.

The spleen can then be detached from its "avascular" diaphragmatic and retroperitoneal attachments, remembering that small vessels are often present in these attachments; they can be controlled by electrocoagulation. When bleeding occurs, placement of packs posterior to the area of digital dissection controls bleeding and allows the operation to proceed. The plane posterior to the spleen and both the body and tail of the pancreas are then bluntly dissected, taking care to remain within the plane and not extend posteriorly, where one might injure the adrenal vessels or renal vessels. The pancreas with spleen is then gently pushed anteriorly and medially; one must never pull on the spleen in an effort to lift the pancreas (Fig. 2). When the injured

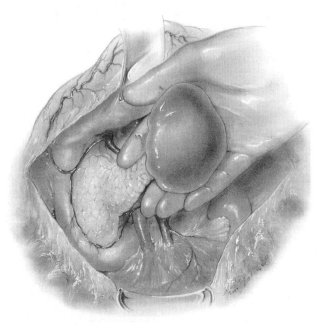

Fig. 2. After dividing the posterior and lateral splenic attachments to the diaphragm, the plane posterior to the spleen and pancreas is digitally dissected so that the pancreas with spleen can be gently rotated anteriorly and medially. Pulling on the injured spleen will inevitably aggravate the injury, necessitating total splenectomy.

spleen is actively bleeding, control of hemorrhage can be achieved by compressing the splenic hilum with the fingers and thumb of the left hand while the right hand is used to continue the anterior and medial mobilization of both the pancreatic body with tail and the spleen. Again, packs can be placed posteriorly in the plane that was previously occupied by these organs. When digital pressure does not control splenic bleeding, the operation will likely be hurried; this almost certainly will result in the patient requiring a total splenectomy. Therefore, this tedious and compulsive mobilization with digital hemostasis should be continued until the spleen has been fully delivered to the wound (Fig. 2).

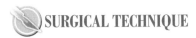

SURGICAL TECHNIQUE

Splenorrhaphy

Once fully mobilized, there are a variety of suture techniques for obtaining splenic hemostasis. For large, deep injuries, the authors prefer the placement of 2-0 chronic sutures swedged on a 2-inch blunt-tip needle; these are placed approximately 1 to 2 cm away from the torn margin and passed deep into the wound crevice; the suture exit tract should be a mirror image of the entrance placement (Fig. 3). Often, two of these sutures are placed sequentially so that the surgeon can tie one while the other suture is held by the assistant with the exact tension to achieve gentle compression of the spleen without tearing the parenchyma or causing tissue necrosis. Equal tension on both sides of the crevice is best obtained with two-handed ties, with each hand being close to the splenic surface. Displays of virtuosity by immature residents using fancy one-handed ties should be discouraged; these cause uneven tension, which promotes parenchymal injury with additional bleeding. Once apposed, most bleeding will rapidly subside; minor oozing through the needle holes is best treated by placing a dry sponge over the spleen and returning the spleen to the left upper quadrant for approximately 10 minutes while other organs are assessed. If hemostasis appears good when the pack or sponge is removed, the "no-touch" technique applies; the surgeon should leave it alone

Partial Splenectomy

When performing a partial splenectomy for extensive injury to the splenic segment or for splenic ischemia distal to transected hilar

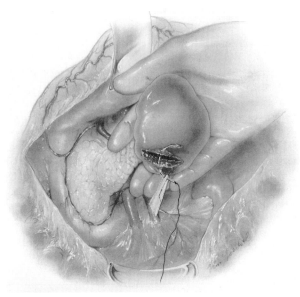

Fig. 3. Deep splenic lacerations can be sutured with the blunt-tipped, swedged-on, 2-0 chromic suture, which is placed 1 to 2 cm away from the tear and passed deeply into the wound crevice. When two sutures are placed, one can be held at the desired apposition while the other is gently tied.

segmental vessels, transverse intraparenchymal arteries may continue to bleed. Sometimes these transverse spurting vessels can be made hemostatic by electrocoagulation applied to an occlusive clamp, whereas other bleeding vessels require suture ligatures (Fig. 4). The authors prefer to use the 4 "0" silk sutures placed in a figure-of-eight manner to best avoid tearing of the adjacent splenic tissue while getting hemostatic occlusion of the pumper (Fig. 4). The same principles of gentleness apply when suturing the splenic parenchyma surrounding a

spurting vessel; a two-handed tie with equal tension reduces the chance for added parenchymal injury.

Following partial splenectomy, the splenic capsule may be approximated, especially if the crevice angles towards a central valley. This approximation should be done with fine sutures, such as 4-0 silk, and they should be tied quite gently. Bleeding through the needle holes is best contained by placing a pack over the repair and returning the spleen to the left upper quadrant, as previously indicated.

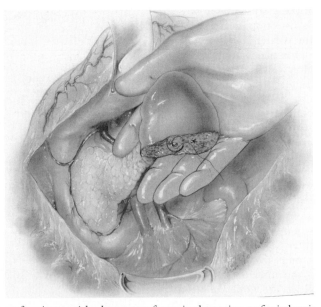

Fig. 4. When performing partial splenectomy for major laceration or for ischemia caused by hilar segmental vessel disruption, the trabecular vessels may be made hemostatic by electrocoagulation or suture ligation. Carefully placed figure-of-eight sutures followed by gentle tying give good hemostasis without excessive injury to the adjacent parenchyma.

When the injury causes disruption of hilar vessels, identification and ligation provide good hemostasis, whereas an obviously ischemic splenic segment distal to the ligation is best resected using the techniques described previously. There are many adjuncts of these techniques. These include the use of a variety of hemostatic agents to augment the hemostatic effect afforded by temporary packs; the argon laser may be more effective than simple electrocoagulation for larger splenic tears; the use of stapling devices gives quicker control but may cause ischemia or tearing; the placement of absorbable meshes around the badly injured spleen, which is then restored to the left upper quadrant and covered, may provide salvage of grade V injuries. In general, the authors advocate simplicity in providing splenic preservation; when complicated techniques must be used, the surgeon must ask the question whether the added efforts are conducive to an enhanced risk-to-benefit ratio in the patient with ongoing bleeding.

Using these techniques, the success of operative splenic salvage is 50%. The best results have been obtained in patients with blunt injury. The same techniques apply, though, for penetrating wounds. However, such efforts should not be made in the unstable patient with active bleeding from the spleen and/or from other organs; the extra time required for splenic preservation will increase the need for blood transfusion and compromise the patient's overall well-being.

Splenectomy with Splenic Replantation

Splenosis is a condition whereby patients with shattered spleens will sometimes develop islets of splenic growth following splenectomy when not all of the splenic fragments are identified and removed. Stimulated by this unusual event, the use of splenic preservation, by placing small fragments of splenic tissue with the omentum, has been promulgated. This "omental omelet" of multiple splenic fragments measuring no more than 1 cm in size is constructed. This technique has often been used in patients requiring rapid splenectomy for bleeding after penetrating wounds. Large clinical series have demonstrated that the splenic fragments remain viable and will concentrate isotope. The clinical protection against OPSI afforded by this omelet, however, has not lived up to expectations. Like-

wise, the patients with splenic replantation do not respond in the same way as patients with splenic salvage in the normal position with maintained splenic blood flow or in patients with splenic injury. The longest animal study, using a canine replantation model of splenic replantation in an omental omelet, followed these animals for 18 months; the results of this study explain why the omental omelet does not provide full immunologic protection. The splenic omelets uniformly survive and take up isotope, but the histology of these surviving segments shows that the perifollicular lymphoid tissue is absent. This is the tissue thought by most researchers to be the source of the protective immune response. Based on these animal studies and on bad clinical observations, the authors no longer recommend this technique.

Nonoperative Splenic Preservation after Injury

Billroth, in the 1870s, suggested that the injured spleen could be treated nonoperatively. He reported on a patient who sustained a lethal closed-head injury and died on postinjury day 5; the autopsy revealed a splenic rupture that had completely coagulated. Despite this early prophetic observation, nonoperative treatment of splenic injury, for all practical purposes, was avoided until the 1950s in children and the 1970s in adults. During the past 25 years, nonoperative splenic preservation has become the norm; successful observation in both children and adults approaches 90% after blunt injury. Success with this regimen correlates with a number of factors, with the grade of splenic injury and presence of associated injuries requiring laparotomy being high on the list (Table 1).

Many important advances in the successful nonoperative splenic preservation have been made in the past few years. The clinical presentation is now recognized as the single most important factor in deciding on nonoperative therapy; age and grade of splenic injury are less important in the clinically stable patient. A vital clinical decision about aborting the nonoperative approach relates to the need for blood transfusion during the period of observation. When the patient requires more blood transfusions than would be predicted on the basis of associated injuries, especially to bones, or when the patient with an isolated splenic injury requires any blood transfusion because the hemoglobin has drifted below

a critical range of 8 to 10 g, the authors recommend immediate operative intervention for a recently ruptured spleen. Like any clinical decision, the risk-to-benefit ratio must be assessed and comorbidities must be taken into consideration. As long as one does not endanger the patient with the risk of multiple blood transfusions, which could be avoided with splenectomy, the main complication of nonoperative therapy for splenic injury is the need to do a later exploration.

When nonoperative therapy fails and the patient requires exploration, the same principles of splenic preservation by the techniques described previously apply; the likelihood of successful operative splenic salvage, however, is much lower after unsuccessful observation. In retrospect, it appears that patients who had injuries that could be successfully treated with splenorrhaphy or partial splenectomy are now being treated successfully by nonoperative therapy. Thus, the 50% success rate for operative splenorraphy, when exploration is used as the primary treatment modality falls to approximately 10% in patients who fail nonoperative therapy and require operation.

One of the important subgroups, for patients being observed nonoperatively for splenic injury, includes those patients who have evidence of a splenic blush on computed tomography. This includes active bleeding. The stable patient with a splenic blush is a candidate for angiography and embolization of the intrasplenic vessel. This has an excellent success rate of providing hemostasis with a significant but acceptable incidence of long-term pain from segmental splenic infarction or of rebleeding requiring operative intervention.

Distal Pancreatectomy with Splenic Salvage

The use of splenic preservation while performing distal pancreatectomy for grade II pancreatic injury was promulgated by Pachter (Fig. 5), with ductal disruption to the left of the superior mesenteric vein. This distal pancreatectomy is performed by ligating each branch of the splenic artery and splenic vein as they enter into the pancreas, while at the same time protecting their terminal branches at the splenic hilum in order to maintain splenic perfusion. This technique has subsequently been applied to localized pancreatic tumors that are benign, cystic in nature, or have low potential for malignancy, such as the papillary tumors. Most reports describe the open laparotomy approach.

Access to the pancreas and spleen may be achieved through a midline incision, although the authors prefer a left subcostal incision, which may be extended as needed into the right subcostal area to give good exposure to all of the pancreas and the splenic hilum. The omentum is divided as previously described and the splenic flexure is mobilized to fully expose the retroperitoneal tissues (Fig. 6). The posterior leaf of the lesser omentum attaches to the superior border of the pancreas. These attachments, likewise, should be severed through the avascular plane, which is quite close to the pancreas. There will also be some avascular attachments between the posterior greater curvature of the stomach and the tail of the pancreas; these should also be divided close to the pancreas. These techniques leave the pancreas fully exposed on the anterior, superior, and inferior surfaces.

The splenic vein and its branches should be approached first. This is best achieved by rotating or lifting the inferior border of the pancreas superiorly and anteriorly, thus exposing the posterior surface (Fig. 7). Careful dissection in this area will identify the short branches of the splenic vein as they enter into the pancreatic parenchyma (Fig. 7). These short veins should be carefully freed, divided, and ligated. This ligation can be achieved with fine 4-0 silk ties with small hemoclips; the authors prefer the fine silk ties, which do not get caught by sponges, as may happen when staples come in proximity to sponges. The sequential division of the venous branches is more easily accomplished by moving from the superior mesenteric area toward the inferior mesenteric vein and, finally, to the splenic hilum.

Once the hilum is identified, the small terminal arterial branches of the splenic artery can be identified and controlled in the same manner prior to moving from the splenic hilum back to the splenic artery as it descends from the celiac axis. Once all of these branches have been divided, while at the same time preserving terminal branches of the splenic artery and vein within the hilum, the pancreas can be removed. The division of the pancreas would be at the point of transaction in injured patients or to the right of the neoplastic lesion in patients with tumor or cysts. The pancreatic division can be performed by electrocoagulation followed by suture ligation of small parenchymal vessels that exhibit refractory bleeding; the pancreatic duct, if it

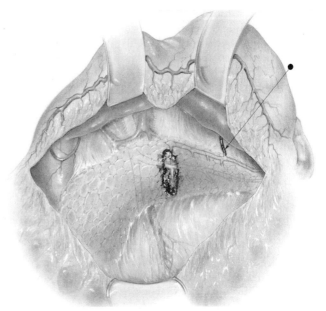

Fig. 5. A grade II pancreatic injury, typical for what is seen after blunt trauma, is depicted. The pancreatic transection is to the left of the superior mesenteric vein and is associated with ductal disruption. The dot indicates the posterior gastric artery, which arises from the splenic artery approximately 3 to 4 cm proximal to the splenic hilum, and enters into the stomach posteriorly and slightly inferior to the short gastric vessels.

can be identified, should be suture-ligated. The remaining pancreatic stump is then approximated with fine "capsular" sutures to decrease the likelihood of later bleeding or fistulization. When this technique of splenic preservation is performed, the spleen does not have to be fully mobilized from its retroperitoneal attachments. When

dissection is difficult, however, mobilization is recommended.

Warshaw described an alternate technique for splenic preservation while doing distal pancreatectomy for small, localized neoplasms (Fig. 8). This consists of dividing the pancreas with the splenic artery and splenic vein at the site of division but pre-

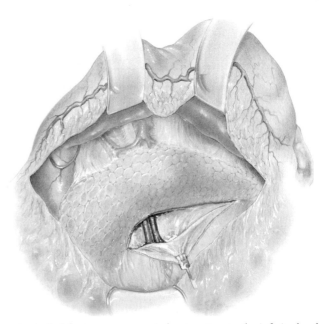

Fig. 6. The anterior leaf of the transverse mesocolon inserts onto the inferior border of the pancreas. Division of this mesenteric leaf is best performed immediately adjacent to the pancreas, where there are no collateral vessels. This schematic highlights how the underlying mesenteric vessels are exposed after separation of this anterior leaf from the pancreas.

serving the splenic hilar branches so that perfusion of the spleen is maintained by means of backflow through the short gastric vessels and posterior gastric artery (Fig. 5). The short gastric vessels arise from the superior segmental branches of the splenic vessels and enter into the greater curvature of the stomach just below the apical fat pad. The posterior gastric artery arises from the splenic artery approximately 3 or 4 cm inferior and medial to the short gastric vessels (Fig. 5). When using this technique for splenic salvage, one has a better chance for maintaining retrograde flow to the spleen if both the short gastric vessels and the posterior gastric vessels are protected. One of the complications of this technique for splenic preservation is partial splenic infarction of the inferior pole, which was documented in the Warshaw report of distal pancreatectomy for small tumors and has been observed by the authors following distal pancreatectomy with splenic preservation after injury.

Distal pancreatectomy with splenic preservation in patients with gunshot wounds or stab wounds involving the distal pancreas is more likely to be accomplished by the technique of dividing the splenic artery and the splenic vein at the site of pancreatic injury because ongoing bleeding or significant hematoma following penetrating wounds in this area is more common. Blunt rupture of the pancreas is seldom associated with major bleeding, which compromises active exposure. When splenic preservation with distal pancreatectomy is performed after penetrating injury, the surgeon must be sure that the patient is stable and that there is no persistent bleeding from other sites (Fig. 9). The risk of spending extra time preserving the spleen in a patient with marginal stability or ongoing bleeding outweighs the risk of OPSI following rapid distal pancreatectomy with splenectomy.

Treatment of Pancreatic Head Lesions/Tumors with Splenic Preservation

Some patients with blunt abdominal injury will present with a stellate laceration in the head of the pancreas anterior to the intrapancreatic portion of the distal common bile duct (Fig. 10). Although superficial lacerations in this area after blunt injury can be treated with wide drainage, the deep lesion requires careful assessment for complete transection and for involvement of the bile duct. When

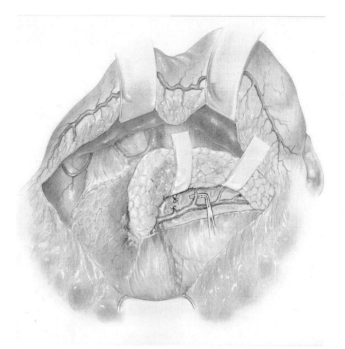

Fig. 7. By gently rotating the inferior border of the pancreas anteriorly and superiorly, the splenic vein, with its branches into the pancreatic parenchyma, is identified. These branches, which are much shorter than those depicted in this schematic, are individually divided and hemostasis is obtained by means of small clips or ligatures.

complete transection occurs, preservation of the lateral portion of the head of the pancreas, the pancreatic neck, and the distal pancreas with spleen preservation can be achieved by creating a Roux-en-Y jejunal limb, which is anastomosed to the distal pancreas in an end-to-end or, in the authors' preference, an end-to-side pancreaticojejunostomy (Fig. 11). The residual pancreatic rim along the duodenal sweep is made hemostatic followed by "capsular" approximation

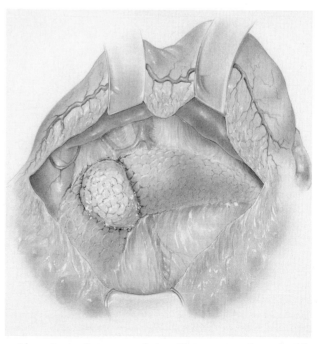

Fig. 8. Patients with cystic neoplasms or atypical papillary masses at the neck of the pancreas may be treated by local resection of the neoplasm followed by closure of the duodenal segment of remaining pancreas and decompression of the distal pancreas into a Roux-en-Y jejunal limb.

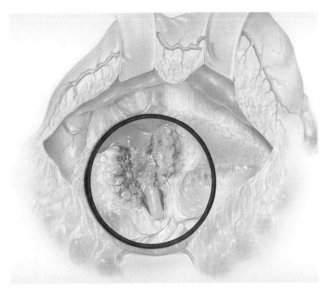

Fig. 9. Major gunshot wounds to the neck of the pancreas seldom lend themselves to splenic preservation when performing distal pancreatectomy. The associated bleeding from adjacent vessels and the surrounding hematoma impairs the type of delicate dissection that is required when performing distal pancreatectomy with splenic salvage.

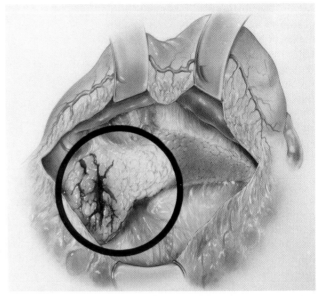

Fig. 10. Patients with blunt abdominal injury may sustain a stellate fracture of the head of the pancreas in the vicinity of the intrapancreatic portion of the common bile duct. Patients with large gunshot wounds to this area usually die on the operating table.

(Fig. 11). When this injury occurs following a gunshot wound, the associated bleeding from injuries to adjacent vessels usually makes this approach impractical and unsafe. Occasional cystic tumors or benign pancreatic tumors lying between the superior mesenteric vein and the intrapancreatic portion of the bile duct can be treated in the same manner with local resection of the tumor, closure of the residual pancreas along the duodenal sweep, and Roux-en-Y pancreaticojejunostomy.

Laparoscopic Approach to Splenic Preservation

The rising trend toward laparoscopic surgery has expanded into the domain of splenic preservation. Removal of a benign pancreatic cyst with distal pancreatectomy and splenic preservation has been described using a three-port technique. The laparoscopic approach follows the same steps summarized previously with the open approach; each step is followed sequentially. The authors have no experience with this technique.

Distal pancreatectomy with splenic preservation has also been described in patients with pancreatitis requiring distal resection for ductal ectasia. This approach, however, must be scrutinized carefully; the authors have had extensive experience with surgery of the inflamed pancreas, which can be quite tedious. Dissection of the severely inflamed pancreas is most difficult using the open approach. The authors question the severity of pancreatitis that would need pancreatectomy in a setting in which this could be accomplished laparoscopically. Furthermore, most patients with benign pancreatic ductal obstruction are best treated with Roux-en-Y pancreaticojejunostomy rather than distal pancreatectomy, thus preserving both endocrine and exocrine functions.

The use of the laparoscopic approach has also been used for the resection of simple splenic cysts, thus providing for splenic preservation. These are true cysts of the spleen. The results of these studies have not been uniformly good. These techniques can be facilitated by radiofrequency

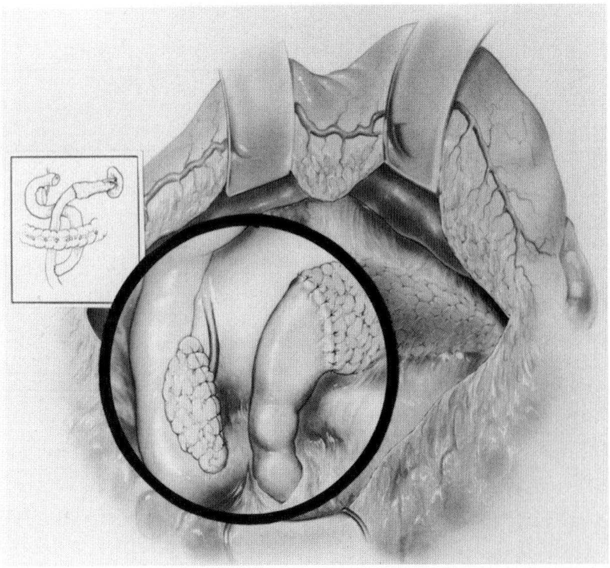

Fig. 11. When extensive injury to the head of the pancreas occurs anterior and to the left of the intrapancreatic portion of the common bile duct, the transection can be completed and followed by end-to-side Roux-en-Y pancreaticojejunostomy and oversewing of the residual pancreatic remnant adjacent to the duodenum.

control of bleeding. The true role of such techniques needs to be determined by future experience.

Finally, the need for splenectomy as part of the devascularization procedure for bleeding esophageal varices has been challenged; the authors have used the devascularization procedure for refractory bleeding varices in patients with cirrhosis, and continue to recommend splenectomy because of the significant portal inflow by way of the splenic artery.

SUGGESTED READING

Lillemore KD, Kaushal S, Cameron JL, et al. Distal pancreatectomy: indications and outcomes in 235 patients. *Ann Surg* 1999;229:693.

Lucas CE. Splenic trauma: choice of management. *Ann Surg* 1991;213:98.

Pachter HL, Grau J. The current status of splenic preservation. *Adv Surg* 2000;34:137.

Saxe JM, Hayward SR, Lucas CE, et al. Splenic reimplantation does not affect outcome in chronic canine model. *Am Surg* 1994;60:674.

Sherman R. Prospectives in management of trauma to the spleen: 1979 presidential address. American Association for the Surgery of Trauma. *J Trauma* 1980;20:1.

Warshaw AL. Conservation of the spleen with distal pancreatectomy. *Arch Surg* 1988;123:550.

EDITOR'S COMMENT

In this excellent chapter, Drs. Lucas and Ledgerwood, acknowledged experts in the treatment of trauma, have given us a very good history of splenic preservation starting in the 19th century and indicating how the pronouncements of great yet uninformed surgeons delayed the acceptance of overwhelming postsplenectomy infection. For those who have seen overwhelming postsplenectomy infection, it is dramatic. The patient enters the hospital within 24 hours of the onset of a seemingly trivial, usually respiratory, infection. In extremis with a white count less than 1,000, bacteria growing in the bloodstream, and, despite all efforts, the patient is generally lost.

It took a while for the existence of the syndrome of overwhelming postsplenectomy infection to be recognized. In the pediatric surgical literature, children with blood diseases, such as thalassemia and other hematologic diseases necessitating splenectomy, seemed to have a larger incidence of overwhelming postsplenectomy infection, perhaps as high as 13% or 14%.

I first became aware of the postsplenectomy syndrome as a junior resident, perhaps in the early 1960s. When I was a senior resident, after returning from the National Institutes of Health in the late 1960s, I tried to analyze the incidence of postsplenectomy infection at Massachusetts General Hospital. I selected 800 patients who had undergone splenectomy because of trauma without any evidence of hematologic disease. I could not complete the chart review as I was trying to do this without help, but found that after going through several hundred charts I had still not encountered a single case of postsplenectomy infection. The exact incidence did, therefore, seem to be very low in these patients who were normal prior to splenectomy, and I would accept the incidence of 1%, especially in adults.

By the time the late 1970s arrived, this was generally accepted by most general surgeons, even those who were not dealing with trauma, and led, at least in one case that I am familiar with, to the death of a patient who probably would have survived if splenic preservation had not been attempted. This remains a danger to patients even without associated injuries, and I accept entirely the repeated dictum mentioned by the authors that a poorly conceived attempt at splenic salvage in a situation in which an expeditious splenectomy would probably have salvaged the patient without the need for major transfusion and some of the complications of prolonged hemorrhage and prolonged transfusion.

The technique is very well described in a series of very nice illustrations. I tend to approach this operation differently, perhaps influenced by my experience with central splenorenal shunt and doing the splenectomy initially by mobilizing the spleen later-ally. In the case of portal hypertension, as I state in my chapter on the central splenorenal shunt (Chapter 120), I generally start the dissection approximately 2 cm lateral to the spleen and control the collaterals in the retroperineum with mattress sutures, which are later oversewn with a running suture to prevent oozing from the lateral edge of the cut retroperineum. However, once the branches to the colon are tied in continuity and divided, mobilizing the inferior border of the spleen, one then proceeds to ligating the short gastric vessels in continuity and later oversewing the greater curvature of the stomach to prevent the occasional case of gastric perforation along the greater curvature. The authors are correct in that dividing the highest short gastric can sometimes be technically challenging and one must take great care, including mobilization of the stomach at the hiatus, in order to avoid an injury to the spleen in so doing. Once the injury is identified, one can then bring the spleen and the tail of the pancreas down and forward by careful and gentle retroperitoneal dissection, staying in the appropriate plane until the entire spleen and the accompanying tail of the pancreas are elevated into the wound, so one can clearly see what one is doing. Whatever hilar vessels are avulsed are then doubly ligated and oversewn so as to prevent subsequent bleeding. If a portion of the spleen is devascularized, I prefer a chromic suture No. 127 for mattress sutures in which one ties the cut edge of the spleen anteriorly with two-handed ties. If the spleen is especially soft, small Teflon pledgets may be attached to the chromic suture in order to avoid tearing the spleen. The reason I like that particular suture, which I also use to a cut edge of the liver, is that the needle and the suture are essentially of the same diameter so that the needle holes do not bleed excessively. The insistence on two-handed ties to equally maintain tension is essential if one is to avoid tearing a soft splenic capsule. If the operation lends itself, one can then do a fish-mouth type of excision of the devascularized splenic parenchyma, as in a V, ligating the vessels with fine silk suture at the base of the V, and then using mattress sutures to close the capsule. An argon beam coagulator is excellent for completing the hemostatic process.

With respect to pancreatic tail resection, I have on occasion maintained the function of the spleen. Here the splenic vein may be more adherent to the tail of the pancreas, especially if there has been chronic pancreatitis because of a lesion and because of the obstruction of the distal pancreatic duct. The degree of separation of the splenic vein and the pancreas is often considerably less than is pictured in Figure 7; however, the technique I use is the same except I use a right-angled Jacobsen clamp, passing two 4-0 silk sutures separately around the splenic vein branches and dividing them either with a No. 15 scalpel blade or Potts scissors, which come in very useful here. When the pancreas is transected, I again use a fish-mouth type of approach identifying the pancreatic duct and oversewing it with a purse-string suture of 5-0 prolene. The V shaped pancreatic parenchyma is then approximated after hemostasis is secured with a 2-0 silk suture again tied in mattress fashion.

I agree with all of the various combinations and permutations of splenic preservation put forth by the authors. The spleen only functions when the splenic artery and splenic vein are intact, at least with a few hilar branches. Recently, Buffett et al. (*Blood* 2006;107:3745; epub Dec 29, 2005), writing from the Hospital Necker in Paris, took advantage of the occasion of distal pancreatectomy and splenectomy to perform ex vivo perfusion of retrieved intact spleens using labeled red cells with *Plasmodium falciparum*-infected erythrocytes pre-exposed to the antimalarial drug artesunate. They found that, in three spleens, more than 95% of the artensunate (ART)–red blood cells were cleared from the perfusate in 2 hours, and that each transit through the isolated perfuse spleens parasitic remnants removed from 0.2 to 0.23 of ART, infected red blood cells (IRBCs), which was consistent with what had been estimated in vivo.

The change in the management of adult splenic injury was reviewed by Hartnett. et al. (*Am Surg* 2003;69:608). They reviewed 20 years of experience with patients from the Maine Medical Center discharged between January 1, 1981, and December 31, 2000, using the *International Classification of Disease,* 9th Revision, codes indicating splenic injury. They found that the number of splenic injuries increased from 75 per year for the first 15 years to 96 per year in the last 5-year period. In keeping with the emphasis of splenic preservation and observation in both adults and children, operative intervention decreased from 71% to 41% and was lower at various trauma hospitals with which these results were compared. After 24 hours of successful intervention, the rate of operative intervention, at times greater than 24 hours, was 2.2% in the last 10 years of study. The rate of splenorrhaphy remains stable at approximately 12%. Mortality rates were greater in patients with an injury severity score of greater than 25. They found that the frequency of delayed intervention was low and did not increase during the period of the lower intervention rate. This suggests that an experienced team that did not attempt to use nonoperative intervention in patients who should not have been subjected to observation can be carried out in a large number of patients without an increased mortality.

If one gets into difficulty with an isolated splenic injury and cannot achieve hemostasis with suture alone, the use of mesh has come into use. Reddy et al. (*ANZ J Surg* 2004;74:596) used a two-layer mesh plenorhaphy in which oxycel is sutured

(continued)

Nongastrointestinal Transabdominal

to the inside of the Dexon mesh (Syneture, Mansfield, MA) and used to wrap the spleen. They claim that the use of the double-layer mesh, one hemostatic (oxycel), and the Dexon mesh enabled one to get a greater security in suturing the spleen.

Finally, I. Kolar (*Eur J Pediatr Surg* 2005;15:132) reported four children treated with early and delayed distal pancreatectomies without splenectomy and with preservation with the splenic vessels after traumatic transection of the distal pancreas. In this brief case report of four patients, one was operated on early because of a concomitant gastric perforation. The other three cases were operated on after delays of between 24 and 38 hours because of spreading peritonitis secondary to the pancreatic injury. The distal pancreas was resected, although the author comments that it was technically much more demanding. However, the surgical team managed to retain splenic function and, although two children were reoperated because of abdominal abscess, all survived.

As this nice chapter indicates, the care of patients with splenic injuries has changed dramatically during the past 30 years, especially as the importance of the spleen to immunologic function and the phagocytosis of encapsulated organisms has been elucidated. The technique is somewhat demanding and should not be used in the event of other complicated injuries at which time an expeditious splenectomy will save the life of the individual. However, the extension of observation from children to adults seems to have caught on and is being practiced without additional mortality.

J.E.F.

Surgery of the Urinary Tract and Bladder

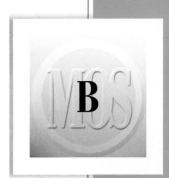

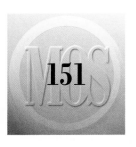

151   Anatomy of the Kidneys, Ureter, and Bladder

RICHARD L. DRAKE

KIDNEYS

The kidneys are located in the retroperitoneal connective tissue of the posterior abdominal wall. They develop as pelvic organs that ascend into their final position in the abdomen. The kidneys are bean-shaped structures with a reddish-brown coloration and are approximately 11 to 12 cm long, 5.0 to 7.5 cm wide, and 2.5 to 3.0 cm thick. The left kidney is usually somewhat longer and narrower than the right kidney. Their location in the posterior abdominal wall is usually between the upper border of T-12 and L-2. However, the right kidney is usually slightly lower than the left kidney because of the presence of the liver.

Relationships and Fascias

The location of the kidneys against the posterior abdominal wall provides development of unique relationships with numerous other structures. Structures anterior to the right kidney are the suprarenal gland, the liver, the second part of the duodenum, the right colic flexure, and the small intestine (Fig. 1A). Structures posterior to the right kidney include the diaphragm; the costodiaphragmatic recess; the 12th rib; the psoas major muscle; the quadratus lumborum muscle; the transversus abdominis muscle; and the subcostal, iliohypogastric, and ilioinguinal nerves (Fig. 1B). Structures anterior to the left kidney include the suprarenal gland, the spleen, the stomach, the body (or tail) of the pancreas, the left colic flexure, and

the small intestine (Fig. 1A). The listed structures lie directly against the fascias covering the kidney without any intervening tissues except for the liver, the stomach, the spleen, and the small intestine, which are covered with peritoneum. The structures listed as posterior to the right kidney are also posterior to the left kidney, with the addition of the 11th rib because of the higher position of the left kidney (Fig. 1B). Thus, numerous structures must be considered in any surgical approach to the kidneys.

The fascias covering the kidneys are unique. Enclosing the renal parenchyma is a fibrous tissue called the *renal capsule*. This layer of tissue is lightly bound to the kidneys and can be removed easily except in certain disease processes. Immediately adjacent to the renal capsule is the perinephric (perirenal) layer of fat (Fig. 2). This layer covers the kidneys and the ureter and is called the *adipose capsule*. Continuing outward is a membranous condensation of the extraperitoneal connective tissue called the *renal (Gerota) fascia* (Fig. 2). This specialized membrane separates the perirenal fat from the adipose tissue covering the posterior abdominal wall and must be incised in any operation, whether an anterior or posterior approach is used. The renal fascia consists of anterior and posterior layers that surround the kidneys and the suprarenal gland, usually sending an intervening septum between the two structures. Moving laterally, the anterior and posterior layers may fuse and become continuous with the transversalis fascia. Medially, the posterior layer fuses

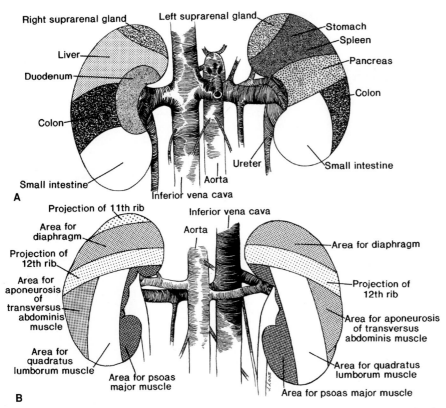

Fig. 1. A: Anterior relations of the right and left kidneys. All of the structures lie against the fascias covering the kidneys, except for the liver and the small intestine on the right and the stomach, the spleen, and the small intestine on the left, which are covered with peritoneum. **B:** Posterior relations of the right and left kidneys.

with the fascia covering the psoas muscle, and the anterior layer may fuse with the sheaths of the blood vessels in the area or cross to the opposite side and fuse with the anterior layer from that side (Fig. 2). Superiorly, the anterior and posterior layers fuse after passing over the suprarenal gland and, inferiorly, the layers also fuse, except where the ureter passes through these tissues. Because of the opening around the ureter, infections around the kidneys may descend into the pelvis and vice versa. Finally, outside the renal fascia is the paranephric (pararenal) fat (Fig. 2). This is a layer of adipose tissue on the pos-

terior abdominal wall and is usually in a posterolateral position.

Structure

The renal parenchyma consists of the outer cortex and the inner medulla (Fig. 3). The cortex is an outer, pale, continuous broad band of tissue. It is dense, homogeneous tissue and consists of renal corpuscles and convoluted portions of renal tubules. The medulla is an inner layer of discontinuous tissue caused by the inward projections of cortical tissue called the *renal columns*. The medulla is darker brown

than the cortex and is composed of the renal pyramids. The renal pyramids appear to have longitudinal striations, which extend into the cortex as medullary rays. Each pyramid contains the descending and ascending limbs of the renal tubules and the collecting tubules. The apex of each pyramid is called a *renal papilla*, and it projects into a minor calyx, which is a subdivision of the renal pelvis.

The medial margin of each kidney is occupied by the hilum. The hilum expands into a central cavity called the *renal sinus* and is the site of entrance or exit for blood vessels, lymphatics, and nerves. It transmits, from anterior to posterior, the renal vein, the anterior branch of the renal artery, the ureter, and the posterior branch of the renal artery. It also contains fat and the renal pelvis. The renal pelvis is the expanded upper end of the ureter. It divides into two or three major calyces that further subdivide into many minor calyces. Each minor calyx is indented by a renal papilla. The renal pelvis continues inferiorly and tapers to a narrow tube that becomes the ureter. The ureteropelvic junction is rather indefinite but is usually referred to as located opposite the lower pole of the kidneys.

Vascular Supply and Lymphatics

The kidneys are supplied by the renal arteries, which arise from the lateral aspect of the aorta just inferior to the origin of the superior mesenteric artery (usually between L-1 and L-2). On occasion, the right renal artery may arise a little higher than the left and has a unique pathway to the right kidney in that it passes posterior to the inferior vena cava as it crosses the posterior abdominal wall. As each renal artery approaches the renal pelvis, it divides into anterior and posterior branches that pass on either side of the renal pelvis and major calyces. This provides a somewhat bloodless horizontal plane through the kidney because the anterior branch supplies the anterior half of the organ, and the posterior branch supplies the posterior half of the organ. Additional accessory renal arteries may be found entering the hilum or extrahilar regions. Generally, the accessory arteries do not anastomose with the major renal arteries and may arise from the aorta, the renal artery, or from a different vessel.

The venous drainage of the kidneys consists of anastomosing channels forming a single renal vein that exits at the hilum. Most tributaries of the renal vein

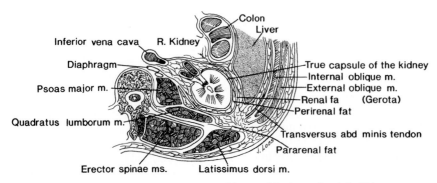

Fig. 2. Transverse section showing the relation of the renal fascias to the right kidney.

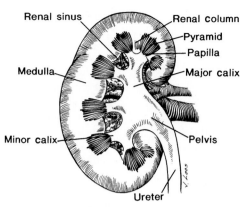

Fig. 3. Longitudinal section showing the internal structure of the kidney, which consists of an outer cortex and inner medulla. Note that each renal pyramid ends as a renal papilla that projects into a minor calix.

pass anterior to the renal pelvis, but on occasion one may pass posterior to this structure. After exiting the hilum, the left renal vein passes anterior to the aorta and posterior to the superior mesenteric artery as it approaches the inferior vena cava. The right renal vein has a short, direct path to the inferior vena cava and enters this vessel at approximately the same level as the left renal vein.

The lymphatic drainage of each kidney is to the lateral aortic group of lumbar nodes around the origin of the renal artery.

URETER

The ureters are muscular tubes that extend approximately 25 cm from the kidneys to the posterior surface of the bladder. Each ureter has an upper expanded end called the *renal pelvis*. Of clinical relevance is the fact that three constrictions are present as the ureter descends from the kidney to the bladder. These constrictions occur at the ureteropelvic junction, where the ureter crosses the pelvic brim and where the ureter enters the bladder wall. In addition, obstruction of the ureter may be caused by stenosis of the ureteropelvic junction, compression of the ureter, a urinary calculus lodged anywhere along the ureter, or from abnormalities at the junction of the ureter with the bladder.

Pathway

Inferior to the ureteropelvic junction, the ureter descends more or less vertically in the extraperitoneal connective tissue of the posterior abdominal wall on the psoas major muscle (Fig. 4). In this retroperitoneal position, the proximal ureter is lateral to the testicular/ovarian vessels before being crossed by these vessels and continuing distally on their medial side. Additionally, in

this retroperitoneal position, the left ureter travels for a considerable distance along the lateral border of the inferior mesenteric vein. It should also be mentioned that as the left ureter nears the common iliac vessels, it lies lateral to the superior rectal (hemorrhoidal) artery. As the left ureter approaches the pelvic brim, it lies in the base of the sigmoid mesocolon. This is a unique relationship that exists only on the left side. At the pelvic brim, the ureters cross the common iliac vessels, usually at the level of the bifurcation of these vessels into the external and internal iliacs. From this point to their en-

trance into the bladder, the pathway is somewhat variable in the man and woman. Each one is discussed here separately.

The Female Pathway
At the pelvic brim in the female, the ureters are closely related to the ovarian vessels (Fig. 4). The ureters cross the pelvic brim just medial to these vessels. During surgical procedures involving the ovaries, the ureters may be damaged when the ovarian vessels are secured. Continuing inferiorly, the ureters lie deep to the peritoneum and are located near the internal iliac vessels as they pass down the lateral pelvic wall. The ureters pass posterior to the ovaries and enter the uterosacral folds toward the floor of the pelvis. They continue in a medial and anterior direction in these folds along with numerous vessels and nerves. At the base of the broad ligament, associated with the lateral cervical or cardinal ligament, the ureters are located inferior to the uterine artery as this vessel passes in a transverse direction toward the uterus (Fig. 5). Crossing of the ureters by the uterine artery occurs just lateral to the uterus and is a possible site of surgical injury to the ureter. After crossing inferior to the uterine arteries, the ureters continue in their anterior and medial pathway, passing just lateral to the lateral

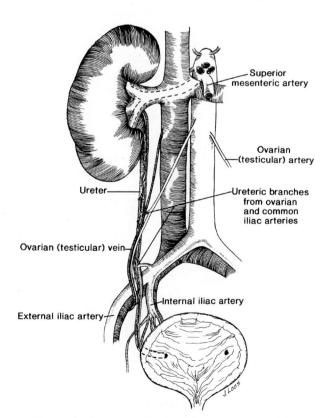

Fig. 4. The path of the ureter, showing its blood supply as it passes down the posterior abdominal wall toward the bladder. The ureter receives arterial branches from the renal, ovarian (testicular), and common iliac arteries.

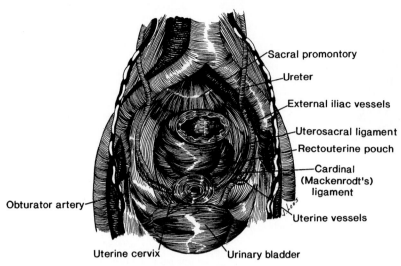

Fig. 5. Superior view looking into the pelvis with the peritoneum removed. As the ureters move toward the bladder, they are located inferior to the uterine artery as this vessel passes in a transverse direction to supply the uterus.

fornix of the vagina before entering the posterolateral aspect of the bladder (Fig. 6).

The Male Pathway

Near the pelvic brim in the male, the ureters and the testicular vessels separate and the testicular vessels follow the external iliac vessels. The ureters cross the pelvic brim and continue to descend in a slightly medial direction as they continue their intrapelvic course to the bladder. As in the woman, they lie deep to the peritoneum and near the internal iliac arteries as they pass down the lateral pelvic wall. Toward the floor of the pelvis, the ureters enter the sacrogenital folds along with several vessels and nerves. As they continue anteriorly and medially in these

folds, the ureters pass inferior to the ductus deferens and anterior to the seminal vesicles before entering the posterolateral aspect of the bladder (Fig. 7).

Vascular Supply and Lymphatics

The ureters receive arterial branches from adjacent vessels as they move toward the bladder (Fig. 4). The renal arteries supply the upper end, and the middle portion may receive branches from the aorta, the testicular or ovarian arteries, and the iliac arteries. In the pelvis, the ureters are supplied by one or more arteries from branches of the internal iliac arteries. In all cases, arteries reaching the ureters divide into ascending and descending

branches that form a longitudinal anastomosis.

Lymphatic drainage of the ureters follows a pattern similar to that of the arterial supply. Lymph from the upper portion of each ureter drains to the lateral aortic group of lumbar nodes, from the middle portion drains to lymph nodes associated with the common iliac vessels, and from the inferior portion drains to lymph nodes associated with the external and internal iliac vessels.

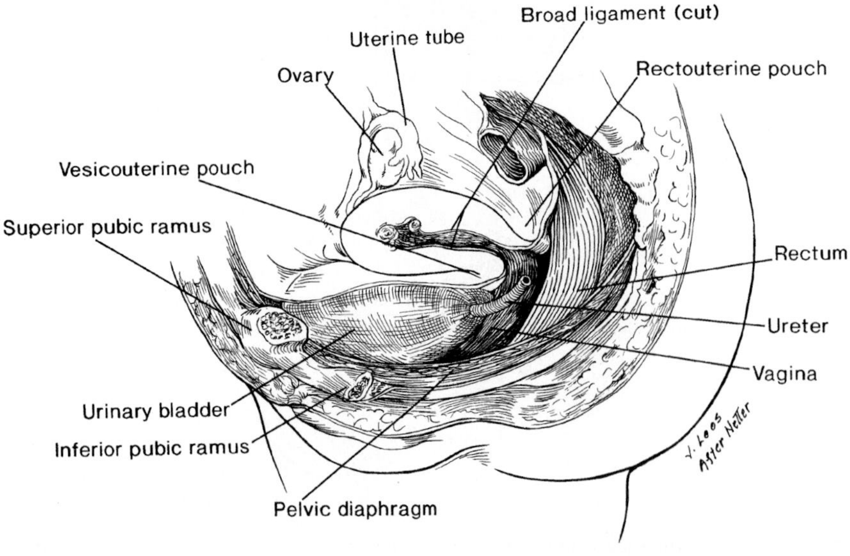

BLADDER

The bladder is a musculomembranous sac located behind the pubic bones and the pubic symphysis. The empty bladder has a pyramidal shape with an apex, a base, and a superior and two inferolateral surfaces. It also has a neck that extends inferiorly. The empty bladder is within the pelvic cavity. As it fills, it rises above the pelvic brim, contacting the posterior surface of the anterior abdominal wall.

Structure

As mentioned, the bladder, when empty, has a pyramidal shape (Fig. 8A). The apex (or vertex) of the bladder points anteriorly and is connected to the umbilicus by the median umbilical ligament (a remnant of the allantois). The base (or fundus) of the bladder is the area between the two ureteric openings and the internal urethral orifice. It is triangular and points posteriorly. Internally, the smooth triangular area outlined by the three openings is called the *trigone* (Fig. 8A). This area is smooth compared with the rest of the internal surface of the bladder because here the mucous membrane is firmly bound to the underlying muscular coat.

There are two additional internal structures. One is found in men and women, and the other is found only in men. In men and women, there is a ridge between the two ureteric openings called the *interureteric crest* (Fig. 8). The second structure, observed in men only, is the uvula vesicae. This is a small swelling produced by bulging of the prostate's median lobe into the bladder at the inferior corner (apex) of the trigone, just above the internal urethral orifice.

The musculature in the wall of the bladder (tunica muscularis) is called the *detrusor muscle*. It consists of three layers of smooth-muscle fibers arranged as an outer longitudinal layer, a middle circular layer, and an inner longitudinal layer. At the neck of the bladder, the middle circular layer forms the sphincter vesicae muscle.

Fig. 6. Parasagittal section of the female pelvis showing the ureter passing just lateral to the lateral fornix of the vagina before entering the posterolateral aspect of the bladder.

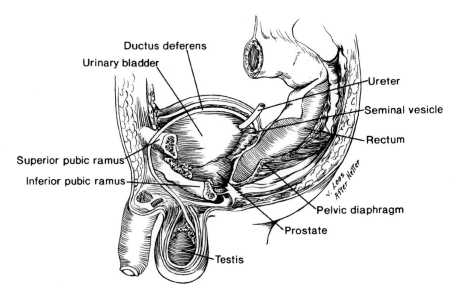

Fig. 7. Parasagittal section of the male pelvis showing the ureter passing inferior to the ductus deferens and anterior to the seminal vesicle before entering the posterolateral aspect of the bladder.

Relationships and Fascias

Peritoneum covers the bladder on its superior surface and is continuous anteriorly with the median and medial umbilical folds and with the parietal peritoneum of the supravesical fossa. Posteriorly, the peritoneal reflections differ between men and women. In the man, the peritoneum descends to the base of the bladder, lines the rectovesical pouch, and continues posterolaterally as the sacrogenital folds. In the woman, the peritoneum reflects onto the uterus without covering the base of the bladder and lines the shallow vesicouterine pouch.

Numerous structures are directly related to the bladder because of its location in the pelvic cavity. In the man, the neck of the bladder rests on the upper surface of the prostate gland. Anterior to the bladder are the pubic symphysis, the retropubic pad of fat, and the anterior abdominal wall. Posterior to the bladder are the rectovesical pouch, ductus deferens, seminal vesicles, rectovesical fascia, and the rectum. Lateral to the bladder are the obturator internus muscle above and the levator ani muscle below. Superior to the bladder are the peritoneal cavity, coils of the ileum, and the sigmoid colon. Inferior to the bladder is the prostate gland. In the woman, the bladder lies at a lower level than it does in the man, and the neck of the bladder lies directly on the deep perineal pouch. Anterior to the bladder are the pubic symphysis, the retropubic pad of fat, and the anterior abdominal wall. Posteriorly, the bladder is separated from the rectum by the vagina. Lateral to the bladder are the obturator internus muscle above and the levator ani muscle below. Superior to the bladder are the vesicouterine pouch of the peritoneal cavity and the body of the uterus. Inferior to the bladder is the deep perineal pouch.

The bladder is held in position by ligaments attached to the base of the bladder near the exit of the urethra and the apex of the bladder. In the man, because the prostate is attached to the bladder in this region, the ligaments pass between the prostate gland and pubic bone. These ligaments are called the *medial* and *lateral puboprostatic ligaments*. In the woman, the ligaments attach directly between the bladder and the pubic bone. These ligaments are called the *pubovesical ligaments*. The base of the bladder is also attached posteriorly to the sides of the rectum and the sacrum by the rectovesical ligaments in the man and by the uterovesical and uterosacral ligaments in the woman. Finally, the apex of the bladder is attached anteriorly by the median umbilical ligament, which is a fibrous cord extending from the bladder to the umbilicus.

Vascular Supply and Lymphatics

There are usually two, and sometimes three, arteries that supply the bladder (Fig. 4). The superior vesical arteries are present in men and women. They arise from the paired umbilical arteries and are distributed to the apex and body of the bladder. The other constant arterial supply to the bladder is through the inferior vesical arteries. These arteries are variable in their origin and

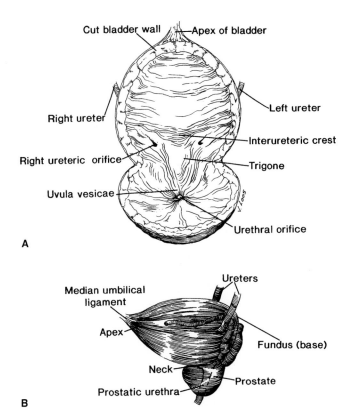

A

B

Fig. 8. A: The interior of the male urinary bladder from the front. The median lobe of the prostate bulging into the bladder at the inferior corner of the trigone produces the small swelling called the *uvula vesicae*. **B:** The urinary bladder showing the general shape, surfaces, and relation to nearby structures.

Nongastrointestinal Transabdominal

supply the inferolateral region of the anterior surface of the bladder. In the woman, a vaginal artery is usually identified as having a distribution pattern similar to that on the bladder. In men, a third artery has been described as supplying approximately one third of the posterior surface of the bladder. This artery is usually a branch of the artery of the ductus deferens. The venous drainage of the bladder is through a network of veins that drain down toward the neck of the bladder to form the vesical venous plexus. From this point, the plexus receives drainage from other nearby structures before draining laterally to the internal iliac vein. Lymphatic drainage is through lymph nodes associated with the common, internal, and external iliac arteries.

EDITOR'S COMMENT

Despite the fact that this is intended as an introduction to the area that is most usually populated by urologists, general surgeons do need to have a working knowledge of the urinary system, starting with the kidneys, which are relatively straightforward except for the vasculature, and going to the ureter, and especially the ureters in the male and how they course down and into the bladder. There are three areas in which the ureter could be injured during the course of operations in the pelvis. The first is where the left ureter runs very close to the superior hemorrhoidal vessels. I do not have the ureter cannulated when I expect a difficult time with the ureter in a procedure in which there is a substantial amount of inflammation in the sigmoid area. For one thing, a stent makes the ureters much more rigid and, at least to my thinking, they are much more likely to be damaged. Better to find the ureters as high as one can as they come off the kidney and trace it down. I put a vessel loop around the ureter and then as I free it up I stay a respectful distance away from the ureter so as not to interfere with the vasculature. Where the ureter crosses the iliac vessels tends to be, at least in my experience, quite variable, variable as to 2 or 3 cm difference. This is particularly true in situations in which there is some inflammation in the area. A vessel loop around the ureter, which is left in place loosely so that there is no obstructing the ureter with a Kelly clamp attached to it and long enough to be out of the field but easily accessible, will enable one to continually refer it to the presence of the ureter and where it is without losing too much time. I always point out to residents, when doing a high ligation of the sigmoid vasculature for carcinoma, how close the superior hemorrhoidal vessels and the inferior mesenteric artery the ureter travel in some pa-

tients. The right ureter also should be identified but this does not have to be freed up to do so. The right ureter tends to be somewhat higher along the pelvis and, except in patients in whom there is a lot of fat in the retroperitoneum, the ureter is usually seen easily and can be identified without freeing it up.

The second area in which the ureter is vulnerable is where it crosses adjacent to the ovarian veins. In most oncologic procedures involving removal of the ovaries, be they ovaries that contain metastatic deposits from carcinoma of the colon or the occasional patient whom a general surgeon stumbles onto in carcinoma of the ovary, the ovarian vessels should be taken fairly high. Dissecting out the ovarian vessels when one may cause inadvertent injury to the ureter.

The third area in which the ureter can be injured is where it passes along adjacent to the uterine artery or passes close to the uteralsacral ligaments. On the occasion of having to do a hysterectomy for malignant disease, which basically is a posterior exenteration, if one is not careful, one can take the two uterosacral ligaments too far away from the uterus and thus inadvertently injure the ureter. The second place is at the base of the bladder close to the uterine artery. If one injures the uterine artery and gets into bleeding, one must be very careful not to clamp the ureter inadvertently when trying to control the bleeding.

As laparoscopic harvesting usually is hand-assisted for renal transplantation it has become more common and laparoscopic donor nephrectomy has become the standard method of voluntary donor harvest in most transplant programs. Most programs will prefer to do the left side because the vasculature tends more often to be single and is easier to harvest with the longer length of vessels that can be plugged into the iliac vessels. On the right side there is a

considerably shorter renal vein, which has significant implications to resection of the donor kidney and reimplantation. The observation of Satyapal (*Anat Rec* 1999;256:202) concerning the entry angle and height of the renal veins is that the left renal vein enters the inferior vena cava higher than the right renal vein in 54% of the cases, lower in 36% of the cases, and directly opposite in only 10%. The vertical distance between the lower borders of the veins was approximately 1 cm. Veins enter at a vertebral level between T-12 and L-2.

A very important aspect of anatomy of the kidneys and bladder is the place of the nerves that control both sexual and bladder function, especially after urologic oncologic surgery. As one will see repeatedly in the chapters in this section, particularly in radical prostatectomy and in radical cystectomy, knowledge of these nerves is paramount. In Chapter 140 by Professor Heald, total mesenteric excision, which has become the sine qua non of low anterior resection of the rectum, even the lower rectum, the place of the nerves is very carefully catalogued.

Finally, one needs to call attention to the segmental vascular supply of the ureter, enabling sections of the ureter to survive if others have been taken inadvertently or injured. The fact that one can split the kidney, the anterior and posterior halves work on each, in turn sometimes with bench surgery, is of importance, particularly in patients who have a single kidney.

In short, as urology has become more differentiated and more adventuresome, the knowledge of anatomy of these important urologic vessels is essential.

J.E.F

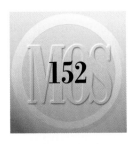

152

Calculous Disease of the Urinary Tract: Endourinary Procedures

MICHAEL P. O'LEARY AND GLEN W. BARRISFORD

INTRODUCTION

Calculous disease of the urinary system has been recognized panculturally for thousands of years. The earliest recorded urinary calculous was obtained from the grave site of a 16-year-old Egyptian boy. It was dated to approximately 4800 BC and was likely a complication of schistosomal disease.

Included among the earliest surgical therapies for urolithiasis were perineal and endourethral lithotomy. These procedures were invasive and carried such a high complication rate that physicians were encouraged by the Hippocratic Oath to "not use the knife on sufferers from the stone" in favor of more highly specialized men. However, during the era of "open" surgery,

invasive procedures offered greater therapeutic value with a reduced morbidity.

During the past several decades, the treatment for urinary stone disease has changed dramatically. Improvements in endoscopic instrumentation and techniques have allowed access to virtually all aspects of the urinary system. Improved modalities have offered a greater reduction of stone burden while providing effective treatment for all stone compositions.

CLINICAL ASPECTS

Urinary calculi represent the third most common affliction of the urinary system (the first being infection; the second, prostatic pathology). The lifetime risk for developing urolithiasis in industrialized countries approximates 1% to 5%. The most commonly affected age group ranges from 20 to 50 years, with men three times more likely than women to develop urinary calculi. Individuals of Caucasian/Asian descent are at increased risk, while those of Native/African-American ancestry are at reduced risk. The risk of recurrent disease within 5 years approximates 50%. A variety of hereditary calculous-forming syndromes have been described.

The typical clinical presentation of urinary calculi is intermittent unilateral flank pain that radiates to the inguinal/genital region. Hematuria is common, but not universally present. Other typical signs and symptoms include leucocytosis, pyuria, fever, and an inability to obtain a position of comfort.

Workup typically begins with history, physical examination, urinalysis, complete blood count, and electrolytes. Imaging with noncontrast spiral computed tomography (CT) remains the diagnostic study of choice (sensitivity 96%, specificity 100%). CT offers the most precise imaging while providing an evaluation of multiple potential sources of flank and abdominal discomfort. When appropriate CT imaging is unavailable, intravenous urogram (IVU) is an acceptable alternative (sensitivity 87%, specificity 94%). IVU provides detailed anatomic and functional information; however, it is more labor intensive and time-consuming. Renal ultrasound is specifically indicated for the evaluation of hydronephrosis, for renal pelvis/ureteropelvic junction calculi, and in gravid patients (sensitivity 11% to 24%, specificity 90%).

Indications for the treatment of urinary calculi are largely dependent upon the size and location of the calculus, with a consideration for the likelihood of spontaneous passage. Individuals who are immunocompromised or who have solitary/transplanted kidneys, intractable pain, obstruction, infection, or staghorn calculi are candidates for early intervention. Additionally, patients in occupations unable to tolerate renal colic while "on the job" warrant aggressive treatment (i.e., airline pilots).

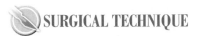 ## SURGICAL TECHNIQUE

Approximately 10% to 20% of urinary calculi will eventually require surgical management. The treatment modality of choice largely depends upon several properties intrinsic to the calculus including size, location, composition, and configuration. Additionally, an overall assessment of the patient's co-morbidities and anatomy assist in treatment planning. A variety of therapeutic approaches exist for the treatment of urinary stone disease. Each technique will be discussed briefly, but the emphasis of this chapter will be upon ureteroscopic stone manipulation.

Noninvasive treatment includes medical therapy and extracorporeal shock wave lithotripsy (ESWL). Unfortunately, the available medical therapies have had marginal success in only a small percentage of urinary calculi. Conversely, since the introduction of shock wave lithotripsy in the early 1980s, it has taken on a role for the initial treatment of renal pelvis and proximal ureteral calculi that are less than 2.0 cm. ESWL is considered suboptimal for cysteine stones and distal ureteral or impacted calculi. The most commonly associated complications of therapy include intrarenal hemorrhage, perinephric hematoma, and cortical fibrosis. In rare instances when treating patients with large stone burdens, fragments can accumulate and obstruct the ureter, resulting in steinstrasse ("stone street").

Ureteroscopy represents the next least invasive level of therapy for urinary calculi. It is ideally suited for large or impacted calculi below the pelvic brim. It is optimally performed under general anesthesia, providing a reduction in abdominal and lower extremity movement. Although laryngeal mask airways (LMAs) are commonly used in our institution, airway management with an endotracheal tube (ETT) allows for optimum control of the respiratory variability/movement throughout challenging procedures and can minimize ureteral injuries. Epidural analgesia with adequate sedation can provide an acceptable alternative. Appropriate patient positioning is of paramount importance in order to obtain proper access. Typically, the contralateral lower extremity is widely extended, providing significantly improved access to the affected side. This maneuver is performed with great care to prevent hyperextension of the hip. Plain radiographic imaging can be utilized with adequate results. However, optimum imaging and improved operative efficiency are provided in the presence of fluoroscopic guidance.

Evaluation of the upper urinary system begins with a gentle ureteropyelogram utilizing dilute contrast material allowing for precise calculus localization. A 0.038-mm flexible-tipped guidewire is used to initiate endoscopic access to the upper urinary tract. With the assistance of an open-ended ureteral catheter, a guidewire is inserted into the ureteral orifice and carefully negotiated past the calculus. Occasionally the initial guidewire is unable to pass an impacted or obstructing stone. In this case one may choose a guidewire with a specialized hydrophilic coating or an angled tip in order to obtain access. Several distinct guidewires are commercially available, each possessing unique properties designed to overcome troublesome upper tract access. Once a guidewire is safely placed in the ureter proximal to the calculus, balloon dilation of the ureteral orifice can be performed. A balloon-tipped catheter slides over the previously placed guidewire and the balloon is inflated to 3 to 10 atmospheres of pressure, then held in place for approximately 3 minutes. Alternatively, access can be obtained with the use of a ureteral access sheath. This is a tapered, firm, soft plastic device that provides access to the ureter and eliminates the need for dilation of the orifice. At this point, either a semirigid or flexible ureteroscope can be used to access the ureter. These instruments range on the order of 3 to 10 French and have working and irrigating ports that range from 2 to 6 French. The distal ureter is easily accessed with a semirigid ureteroscope, while the renal pelvis and proximal ureter are more safely accessed using a flexible scope. It is essential to keep the guidewire under vision while passing instruments retrograde through the ureter. Using the wire as a guide allows the surgeon to maintain orientation and prevents unnecessary ureteral injuries (false passages/perforation/disruption). Saline irrigation is used with pressure infusion devices to maintain adequate visibility. In order to prevent loss of access, additional guidewires known as "safety wires" are occasionally placed. In the event that the ureteroscope is inadvertently removed from the ureter, a safety wire provides access to a previously instrumented upper tract. This is particularly important in the case of flexible ureteroscopy. Ureteroscopy remains the treatment of choice for ureteral calculi and has a greater than 90% success rate when treating distal ureteral calculi.

When calculi are over 2.5 cm, percutaneous lithotripsy (PL) becomes the method of choice. In comparison to ESWL, PL is more successful in reducing stone volume.

The experienced urologic surgeon may obtain percutaneous access on his or her own. However, in our institution we work in conjunction with the interventional radiologist, who safely establishes access to the renal pelvis under fluoroscopic guidance. Once in the operating suite, the tract is dilated prior to the procedure. When percutaneous therapy is unsuccessful open surgery becomes the treatment of choice. However, less than 1% of all urinary calculi require nephrolithotomy. Indications for open surgery include failed ESWL/PL, morbid obesity, distal obstruction, stenotic calyceal infundibula, large or complex renal calculi, or co-morbidities preventing long endourologic procedures.

TREATMENT MODALITIES

Urinary calculi can be treated with a varied level of invasiveness using an array of modalities. Thus far we have considered different surgical approaches without consideration of the modality used for calculus destruction/extraction. Electrohydraulic, ultrasonic, and laser lithotripsy and basket extraction of urinary calculi will be briefly described.

Electrohydraulic lithotripsy (EHL) was first utilized for the treatment of bladder calculi in 1950. An electrical charge is generated at the tip of the EHL probe. A spark is created and results in intense heat. Subsequently, a cavitation bubble is formed, which gives rise to a multidirectional shock wave. Following this, the bubble collapses, initiating a second shock wave. Approximately 50 to 100 waves per second are generated, resulting in effective stone fragmentation of even the hardest calculi. Unfortunately, EHL is highly injurious to the tissue and can result in significant ureteral damage. Although it has been used in renal and ureteral calculi since 1975, it is presently primarily indicated for bladder calculi.

Ultrasonic lithotripsy, originally described in 1979, is a modality that converts electrical energy into ultrasonic waves. These waves are transmitted through a hollow metal probe and result in vibration at the tip. The vibration is used to fracture the calculi. As previously mentioned, it is most commonly used in percutaneous lithotripsy and is the modality of choice for large calculi. However, it is not useful for very hard calculi (uric acid, cysteine, calcium oxalate/monohydrate). Additionally, therapy is required in 3% to 35% of cases due to retained stone fragments.

Laser lithotripsy has been utilized in a variety of forms since 1968. Initial attempts required a ruby-based beam with energy on the order of 50 to 300 J. Greatest success was achieved against struvite stones, but calcium-based stones were resistant to therapy. Over the subsequent 30 years, a variety of laser types gained and lost favor for a variety of reasons. Currently, the holmium laser is the most widely used for urinary lithotripsy. It is the newest modality and fragments calculi by vaporizing the surface, resulting in a crater and eventually cracking the stone. Temperatures in excess of 4,000° C are required. Tissue damage is minimized by the pulsatile nature of the laser combined with cooling irrigant and direct contact with the stone surface. The holmium laser will eventually fragment any stone of any composition, giving it a decided advantage over other laser types. The holmium laser can be delivered through a flexible ureteroscope with varied laser fiber sizes. Generally the fibers are 200, 400, 600, or 1,000 micrometers. The larger fiber provides greater surface area to fragment the stone in a more rapid manner. However, with increasing fiber size a limitation in the ureteroscopic flexion develops. Therefore, smaller fibers are required for calculi that are in positions requiring great flexibility to visualize. The holmium laser is primarily indicated for ureteral and renal calculi of any composition.

Prior to the widespread use of laser lithotripsy, basket extraction of calculi held a more prominent position in the treatment algorithm. However, most calculi can be fractured to spontaneously passable fragment sizes. In certain cases basket extraction can serve as an adjunct to laser therapy in order to reduce the operative time or to obtain a specimen for analysis. However, basket extraction of fragments larger than 5 to 7 mm is ill advised as the risk for a retained stone basket increases greatly. This complication can be averted with patience and adequate laser time.

Urinary stone disease and management will likely affect a variety of patients under the care of a wide range of surgical and medical specialists. A basic understanding of the available treatments/modalities and indications for each will enhance the armamentarium of the practitioner and will expedite and improve the evaluation and care of the many patients affected.

SUGGESTED READING

Bagley DH. Ureteroscopic lithotripsy. *Diagn Therap Endosc* 1997;4(1):1.

Clayman M, Uribe CA, Eichel L, et al. Comparison of guide wires in urology. Which, when, and why. *J Urol* 2004;171:2146.

Dretler SP. An evaluation of ureteral laser lithotripsy: 225 consecutive patients. *J Urol* 1990;143:267.

Ehreth JT, Drach GW, Arnett ML, et al. Extracorporeal shock wave lithotripsy: multicenter study of kidney and upper ureter versus middle and lower ureter treatments. *J Urol* 1994;152:1379.

Francesca F, Grasso M, Lucchelli M, et al. Cost-efficiency comparison of extracorporeal shock wave lithotripsy and endoscopic laser lithotripsy in distal ureteral stones. *J Endourol* 1993;7(4):289.

Huffman J, Bagley D, Lyon E. *Ureteroscopy.* Philadelphia: WB Saunders, 1995.

Miller OF, Rineer SK, Reichard SR, et al. Prospective comparison of unenhanced spiral computed tomography and intravenous urogram in the evaluation of acute flank pain. *Urology* 1998;52:982.

Mulvaney WP, Beck CW. The laser beam in urology. *J Urol* 1968;99:112.

Shokeir AA, Mahran MR, Abdulmaaboud M. Renal colic in pregnant women: role of renal resistive index. *Urology* 2000;55:344.

Sosa E, Jenkins A, Albala D, et al., eds. *Textbook of endourology.* Philadelphia: WB Saunders, 1995.

Teichman J. Acute renal colic from ureteral calculus. *N Engl J Med* 2004;350:684.

Vieweg J, Teh C, Freed K, et al. Unenhanced helical computerized tomography for the evaluation of patients with acute flank pain. *J Urol* 1998;160:679.

Weiss RM, George NJR, O'Reilly PH. *Comprehensive urology.* Mosby International, 2001:1, 313, 326, 651.

⑂⑂⑂ EDITOR'S COMMENT ⑂⑂⑂

In this brief but cogent chapter, the authors give an excellent review of various endourinary procedures. There is also a very good biophysical exposition on the various types of lasers and endourinary procedures as well as the types of stones for which they are, and are not, useful.

These procedures are, after all, blind procedures. Although one can argue that the various uteroscopes, guidewires, and different technological innovations have enabled a degree of safety for these procedures, there nonetheless remains a basic problem of the inability to see what is going on. The copious use of irrigation helps, but in the final analysis, as the authors say, depending on the stone and depending on the type of laser or ultrasonic technique used, between 3% and 35% of patients require further procedures.

Because urology staff in our institution participate in the mortality and morbidity conferences

(continued)

on a regular basis, I have had the opportunity to view in this referral center a number of complications in the endourinary procedures that have been carried out elsewhere. The most recent complication that was presented was not a complication that occurred here, but it was presented at the conference because it was a case of failure of imaging that the patient had initially had done here, and a lot of different images done elsewhere, of a somewhat large stone that was, in fact, extraureteral. The patient had undergone ultrasonic lithotripsy, perhaps ill-advised in view of the size of the stone and/or perhaps its composition, and had a double ureter. This, too, was not appreciated in the previous institution; it finally turned up when both orifices were identified and the appropriate dye studies were obtained. The logical question that could be asked is, how is it possible that this extraureteral stone remained in place for months, although the patient was asymptomatic? This is difficult to comprehend, but one must fault previous procedures.

In addition, the widespread presence of spicules following ultrasonic percutaneous lithotripsy re-mains a cause of concern. This again is an instance of one being unable to see. Most of the time, the spicules are too small to be visualized by whatever imaging techniques are used at that particular time. There is ample evidence that the presence of spicules in the wall of a ureter may actually pass through, or worse, do not pass through and form a locus of fibrosis.

These particular findings carry with them a theme that I have used previously in this volume: that is, in our rush to not injure the patient with an incision, we sometimes take risks that are not only inappropriate but end up being harmful. In a society in which minimally invasive surgery has gotten the hype that it has, it is difficult for a practitioner to simply say to a patient, "Look, it is not in your best interest to carry this out in a minimally invasive manner." In this situation, no number of statistics may suffice for certain patients and families who simply say, "Well, if you can't do it this way, I will find someone who does," and, in fact, one can always find someone who does. This is true not only of urologic procedures, but of other procedures as well. It is clear, for example, in the presence of coronary disease, if one were to compare the ever-shrinking results of open coronary bypass artery graft and what the indications are versus either drug-eluding stents and other types of stents, that there are more procedures necessary in the posttherapeutic period, and the cost is greater following stenting as well as earlier occlusion and the requirement for further procedures. How does one explain this and justify it in an era in which all aspects of medical costs are being carefully evaluated? The only way to explain this is that patients are so fearful of an open procedure including, in this case, for the most part, median stenotomy, that they—and society—will tolerate increased numbers of procedures and the increased expense in an effort to avoid an incision. Unless and until society is able to deal with this issue, it is likely that patients will undergo, not only in urinary calculous disease but in other diseases such as those enumerated, procedures that are less likely to be as efficient or as inexpensive in the long run as the procedures they finally do undergo. I believe this will turn out to be a societal problem that will have to be dealt with at some time and, one hopes, not by health economists.

J.E.F.

Chapters 152a and 153, see www.masteryofsurgery.com

Nongastrointestinal Transabdominal

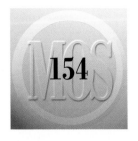

Radical Nephrectomy for Renal Cell Carcinoma

WILLIAM C. DEWOLF AND JAMES C. HU

INTRODUCTION

Renal cell carcinoma (RCC) is the most common malignancy of the kidney and accounts for about 3% of all adult neoplasms. The estimated number of new cases per year in the United States is 35,000, with almost 12,500 deaths per year. Interestingly, the term "hypernephroma" is commonly used in the literature to refer to parenchymal tumors of renal origin. This somewhat mistakenly used term derived from an antiquated misconception that renal tumors arose from adrenal rests within the kidney as proposed by Grawitz in 1883. Surgery has a special place in the treatment of renal cell carcinoma for three reasons. First, renal cell carcinoma is, in general, refractory to chemotherapy and radiation and therefore surgery is the primary mode of therapy. Second, as in most other surgical disciplines, technology has significantly advanced such that newer techniques and approaches are being introduced so that past habits and customs are being challenged. Hence, a new chapter involving the basic goals of treatment as well as technique of treating renal cell carcinoma is important. Third, the incidence of treatment of renal cell carcinoma is increasing; this is not so much due to an actual increase in prevalence but rather to expanded and more sensitive use of imaging studies with the resultant "incidental" discovery of renal masses. In addition, it is now not uncommon to perform "debulking nephrectomies" in preparation for immune/biologic treatment for metastatic disease. Hence, the increase in demand for nephrectomy is for both low- and high-stage disease.

PATHOLOGY

Most examples of renal cell carcinoma arise from the proximal tubular epithelial cells. Because of numerous scientific advances, it now seems clear that a number of distinct entities exist under this heading including clear cell (the most common type), papillary, chromophobe, and the much less common collecting duct tumor as well as the sarcomatoid variant. Differentiating between these tumors can be important for many practical reasons. For example, papillary tumors tend to be more multifocal (i.e., 7% to 20 %) and therefore wider margins may be desirable. If a partial nephrectomy is done, then follow-up should be longer compared to other variants because of the possibility of smaller undiagnosed microscopic tumors that may exist in the remaining "normal" kidney (either ipsilateral or contralateral kidney), which may present at a later time. On the other hand, clear cell carcinoma tends to respond better than other subtypes to immunotherapy and some interleukin (IL)-2 based protocols will address only clear cell carcinoma. Finally, sarcomatoid or spindle cell variety tends to be more locally invasive than pathologic variants.

RCC is also associated with cysts, both acquired and hereditary (such as the polycystic variety). There is an estimated 10- to 50-fold increase in the risk of RCC for patients with chronic renal failure and associated acquired cystic disease. This type of tumor varies according to length of time on dialysis and number of cysts and has even been reported in a transplanted kidney in a patient on hemodialysis after failure of the transplant. The most important risk factor is chronic renal failure and not dialysis. The cause is unknown.

About 10% to 15 % of renal tumors are benign and usually are either oncocytomas or angiomyolipomas, although other more rare tumors help make up this list. Quite often it is difficult to identify such tumors by preoperative needle biopsy for many technical reasons and therefore partial nephrectomy often "saves" a patient an unnecessary nephrectomy.

The grading of RCC is one of the most important prognostic indices of the final pathologic specimen and this includes ploidy. The most commonly used system is that of Fuhrman. The characteristics of the four groups of the Fuhrman grading system are detailed in Table 1. Practically speaking, most pathologists rely on presence and relative size of nucleoli to assess grade. This means that the quality of fixation is unusually important because nucleoli identification is easily disrupted by poor fixation. Another caveat in the use of Fuhrman grading involves heterogeneity of grade within a single tumor. This has not been totally worked out, but most pathologists use the "worst grade approach."

ETIOLOGY/GENETICS

Numerous etiologic factors have been investigated including viruses, lead compounds, x-rays, and over 100 chemicals including aromatic hydrocarbons. Many have been important in experimental induction of malignancy, but none has been found to play a role in human renal cancer. However, certain risk factors exist; most important includes tobacco, which produces a 2- to 2.5-fold increased risk for smokers compared with nonsmokers. Hypertension and obesity have also been linked. Over the past two decades the specific genetic abnormalities associated with most forms of RCC have been worked out so that most common tumors of the kidney can be traced to known genetic abnormalities. This makes RCC a genetic prototype similar to colon cancer. As with many malignant disorders, the genetics of RCC was worked out through familial RCC and associated pedigrees. For example, to identify the gene for sporadic clear cell carcinoma, patients with hereditary von Hippel-Lindau disease (VHL) were studied. Such patients are generally at risk for (a) bilateral clear cell RCC, (b) pheochromocytoma, (c) malignant neuroendocrine tumors of the pancreas, and (d) cerebellar and spinal hemangiomas and others. It is now known that VHL disease is inherited in an autosomal dominant fashion and results from a genetic defect of the VHL gene located on chromosome 3p25. The function of the gene is to act as a ubiquitin ligase and target hypoxia inducible factor 1-alpha (HIF 1-α) for ubiquitin-mediated destruction. If HIF 1-α is overproduced, it will stimulate production of several growth factors, such as vascular endothelial growth factor (VEGF), that are important for malignant transformation. This same gene is responsible for nonhereditary sporadic RCC. Similar studies were performed with hereditary papillary renal cell carcinoma

TABLE 1. FUHRMAN NUCLEAR GRADING SYSTEM

Grade	Nuclear size	Shape	Chromatin	Nucleoli
1	<10 μm	Round	Dense	Inconspicuous
2	15 μm	Round	Finely granular	Small, not visible with 10x objective
3	20 μm	Round/oval	Coursely granular	Prominent
4	>20 μm	Pleomorphic Multilobulated	Open, hyperchromatic	Macronucleoli

(type I) and the affected gene was identified as c-MET. The mutations are known to be missense and tend to "activate" the gene. The gene for papillary RCC type II was found to be the fumarate hydrolysate gene (a Krebs cycle enzyme). The gene for oncocytoma and chromophobe RCC has been found but not characterized; it is located on l7p and was identified through studies of patients with Birt-Hogg-Dube syndrome, who are at risk for cutaneous fibrofollicular lesions, lung cysts, and renal tumors (in this case oncocytoma and/or chromophobe RCC). The function of the gene is not yet known.

 DIAGNOSIS

As with other malignancies, the diagnosis of RCC is really divided into two parts: Clinical presentation (which includes paraneoplastic syndromes) and diagnostic testing. Because of the rather remote location of the kidneys, RCC may remain clinically occult for long periods of time. Patients manifesting the classical "triad" of hematuria, flank pain, and flank mass would therefore have advanced disease. Such clinical presentation now occurs relatively infrequently. Other more nonspecific symptoms such as fever, weight loss, fatigue, and nausea are more common. Perhaps more interesting, however, is the paraneoplastic syndromes that have been described in association with RCC, which can be considered the prototype malignancy for ectopic hormone production (which is considered the primary cause of paraneoplastic syndrome). For example, RCC has been described to produce parathormone, erythropoietin, gonadotropins, placental lactogen, enteroglucagon, insulin-like substances, prostaglandin A, and prolactin. Related to that is a peculiar "idiopathic" liver dysfunction associated with increased alkaline phosphatase, indirect bilirubin, and altered international normalized ratio (INR) that is reversible after removing the tumor.

An increasing number of newly diagnosed cases are taking the form of inciden-

tal findings during unrelated imaging exams. Contrast enhanced studies are most commonly used, either computed tomography (CT) or magnetic resonance (MR), with about equal results. MR, however, is becoming more popular because resolution continues to improve and it can be used in people with history of iodinated contrast allergy, renal insufficiency, or suspected venacaval thrombus. In addition, MR is especially good for diagnosing *malignancy* in the complex renal cyst; nodular enhancement will predict RCC with 95% positive predictive value. From these studies the patient should be evaluated for tumor size, lymphadenopathy, metastasis, status of adrenals, and contralateral "good" kidney. Ultrasound may be used to diagnose solid lesions, but it is poor for other staging information that is offered by CT or MR. And, finally, arteriography, once a major diagnostic tool for RCC, is rarely used and reserved for very individualized special circumstances. Needle biopsy may be difficult and somewhat inaccurate and is generally reserved for diagnosing non-

RCC histology such as lymphoma; differentiating oncocytoma from RCC may be extremely difficult and the absence of malignant cells on biopsy does not rule out the possibility of a neoplasm. There appears to be little risk of seeding the needle tract.

STAGING

Although several schemes have been reported to correlate extent of tumor and its prognosis, the TNM staging system of the American Joint Committee on Cancer (AJCC) is still the most universally used and best understood (Table 2). For example, the 10-year cancer-specific survival rates for stage T1a and T1b groups are 98% and 81%, respectively. Systematic lymphadenectomy may be valuable for staging RCC, but there is decreasing enthusiasm for this procedure in the surgical community because of a low positive rate in patients with negative preoperative staging studies (3% to 8%). In addition, the increasing use of minimally invasive procedures do not adapt themselves well to lymphadenectomy. The proponents of lymphadenectomy argue that removal of nodes for pathologic evaluation will provide important staging information and have prognostic implications. In addition, it is possible that removal of positive nodes, especially in situations of limited nodal involvement, may be curative as noted with bladder and breast cancer. Those arguing against the chance of finding positive nodes in the face of negative imaging point out that the odds are exceedingly small, especially considering the increasing

TABLE 2. AMERICAN JOINT COMMITTEE ON CANCER TNM STAGING OF RENAL CELL CARCINOMA (2002)

Primary tumor (T)		
	TX	Primary tumor cannot be assessed
	T0	No evidence of primary tumor
	T1a	Confined to kidney, ≤4.0 cm
	T1b	Confined to kidney, >4.0 cm and ≤7.0 cm
	T2	Confined to kidney, >7.0 cm
	T3a	Tumor invades the perinephric fat or the adrenal gland but not beyond Gerota's fascia
	T3b	Tumor grossly extends into the renal vein(s) or vena cava below the diaphragm
	T3c	Tumor grossly extends into the renal vein(s) or vena cava above the diaphragm
	T4	Tumor invades beyond Gerota's fascia
Regional lymph nodes (N)		
	NX	Regional lymph nodes cannot be assessed
	N0	No regional lymph node metastasis
	N1	Metastasis in a single regional lymph node
	N2	Metastasis in more than one regional lymph node
Distant metastasis		
	MX	Distant metastasis cannot be assessed
	M0	No distant metastasis
	M1	Distant metastasis

Nongastrointestinal Transabdominal

low-stage low-grade tumors that we are now finding with the increasing use of abdominal imaging for miscellaneous reasons and discovery of smaller tumors. Lymphadenectomy would interfere with the current wave of enthusiasm for minimally invasive approaches for nephrectomy. The true answer is still unknown.

PRINCIPLES OF MANAGEMENT

Preoperative Evaluation

Preoperative evaluation includes a complete metabolic panel including serum creatinine, calcium, and liver function studies. If the creatinine is abnormal, then every effort should be made to do a partial nephrectomy, which, when done correctly, yields results as good as total radical nephrectomy with regard to tumor control for malignancies less than 4 cm in diameter. If the calcium or alkaline phosphatase are up, then a bone scan and possibly long bone radiographs should be done to rule out metastatic disease; if no metastases are found, then every effort should be made to rule out hyperparathyroidism versus paraneoplastic syndrome. Chest radiography is always required and a brain scan only for stage T2 or greater. Hemoglobin and hematocrit are evaluated to rule out erythropoietin-producing tumors with polycythemia or lactoferrin-producing tumors with anemia. If venacaval thrombus is suspected, then an MR scan is probably optimal for staging. Preoperative renal infarction is rarely indicated in today's surgical approach to the treatment of RCC. There are two circumstances, however, in which it may be helpful: First, when dealing with an inferior venacaval thrombus that is vascularized, preinfarction often shrinks the thrombus, making it easier to remove. The second indication may occur in planning a debulking operation in which the renal vasculature is completely encased in nodal disease and the surgeon anticipates difficulty in finding the major vessels. In both cases it is probably better to infarct 24 hours in advance to allow clot to develop and mature.

Status of Adrenal and Its Role in Choice of Operation

Special attention must be paid to the status of the adrenal gland in the preoperative imaging assessment of the kidney. Preoperative CT or MR is almost 100% sensitive in predicting metastatic disease to the adrenal; therefore, if the CT or MR shows a normal adrenal, the surgeon has the option of simply leaving the adrenal in place at the time of nephrectomy. This decision is especially important when dealing with partial nephrectomy where the adrenal is preferentially left in situ. Adrenal mets are just as likely to occur with lower pole lesions as they are with upper pole lesions.

Compensatory Hypertrophy

Renal counterbalance and hypertrophy theory was first introduced by Himnan in 1926. The theory is based on the premise that there is a mechanism to monitor total renal function and that the function of each kidney can be modulated up or down as appropriate. Thus, if one kidney is removed or rendered nonfunctioning by whatever means, the opposite kidney would undergo compensatory hypertrophy. The growth involves both hypertrophy and hyperplasia and apparently the process slows down with age. Unfortunately, our understanding of the exact mechanism and especially how the effect interacts with any comorbid disease that affects renal function (such as diabetes or hypertension) is not enough to make useful clinical predictions. Therefore, anticipated nephrectomy in the face of already compromised renal function is still problematic with regard to estimating postoperative renal function, which may be significantly reduced.

Surgery vs. Surveillance: The Natural History of Small Renal Cell Carcinoma

It is sometimes harder not to operate rather than follow the natural surgical reflex to take out a mass, especially if the mass is small. Such decisions, however, are becoming clinically important considering that during the past 20 years the discovery of less than 3-cm incidental renal tumors has significantly increased due to the widespread use of sonography and CT for evaluation of various abdominal complaints.

Our understanding of how these small renal masses grow is still rudimentary, but nonetheless there are two important observations that must be kept in mind when dealing with the disposition of renal masses. First, in general, renal masses seemingly grow slowly. There is now an increasing number of publications tracing the natural history of growth of RCC. In general, they report that tumor growth is between 0.1 and 1.5 cm per year. Collectively, reports indicate that it is rare for a patient to develop metastases with a combined median follow-up of about 36 months. Indeed, on those patients who do receive surgery, there even seems to be a higher incidence of benign tumors approaching 25%.

The second observation to keep in mind is that the potential of metastatic spread seems to be size dependent. This is actually an old and perhaps historic observation by Bell, who in 1938 reported an autopsy series and found only 1 in 38 renal cortical tumors less than 3 cm in diameter to be associated with metastasis. In contrast, 70 of 106 tumors larger than 3 cm revealed metastasis. Interestingly, more than a half century later, the National Institutes of Health confirmed this with a kindred analysis of 181 patients with von Hippel-Lindau disease (who are at risk for renal cell carcinoma). In that series none of the 108 patients with tumors less than 3 cm followed prospectively for 5 years developed metastasis. The incidence then increased according to tumor size.

Debulking Nephrectomy

The concept of cytoreductive surgery is very appealing in the treatment of renal cell carcinoma for several reasons. First, it is well known that spontaneous regression of pulmonary nodules may occur following excision of primary tumor. Second, it is known that cancer patients and tumor-bearing mouse models have been shown to have impaired immune responses by several criteria. Therefore, removing the primary should improve immune-enhancing therapy. Third, metastatic RCC has a poor prognosis and resists conventional chemotherapy and radiation. Several studies have now shown improved survival with biologic response modifier therapy in combination with debulking cytoreductive surgery prior to therapy.

Intraoperative Renal Ischemia

Often temporary occlusion of the renal artery is necessary for a variety of operations on the kidney. This diminishes intraoperative blood loss and improves access to intrarenal structures through improved visibility and decrease in tissue turgor.

Prevention of ischemic damage first requires an appreciation of the sensitivity of the kidney to warm ischemia, which is mainly derived from the fact that the kidney has several complex metabolic requirements, which are predominantly aerobic. The extent of damage after normothermic arterial occlusion depends on the duration of occlusion. Canine studies have shown that warm ischemic intervals of up to 30 minutes can be sustained with full recovery. Ischemia beyond 30 minutes results in permanent damage to the nephron, with the tubules more sensitive than the glomeruli. Interestingly, it is thought that the solitary kidney is more resistant to ischemic damage than the paired kidney. Likewise, animal studies have shown that renal damage is less when the renal artery alone is occluded in contrast to occlusion of both the renal artery and the renal vein. This is thought to be due to factors relating to retrograde venous perfusion and also venous congestion of the kidney. Other important points of technique include lessons from animal studies that show that intermittent occlusion of the renal artery with short periods of recirculation is more damaging than continuous occlusion (probably due to recirculation injury) and that manual compression to control intraoperative hemorrhage is more deleterious than simple arterial occlusion.

The prevention of damage during and after renal ischemia therefore requires observance of a few basic rules:

1. Preoperative and intraoperative hydration should be adequate.
2. Avoid intraoperative hypotension.
3. Avoid traction on the renal artery.
4. Clamp only the artery, not the vein.
5. Use intraoperative mannitol immediately prior to clamping the renal artery.
6. Use hypothermia (crushed ice), especially if clamp time will be longer than 30 minutes.
7. The systemic use of heparin is not necessary.

The use of mannitol is beneficial because it increases renal plasma flow, decreases intrarenal vascular resistance, minimizes intracellular edema, promotes an osmotic diuresis when renal circulation is restored, and acts as a free radical scavenger. It basically prevents proximal tubular damage.

Several methods for hypothermia induction have been described, but the easiest is simply to use chopped ice. The kidney is surrounded by a plastic bag (like an intestinal bag) after the artery is clamped. The vein is not clamped. The chopped ice is then placed into the intestinal bag around the kidney; it takes about 10 minutes for the core temperature of the kidney to cool. This method will allow safe cold ischemic times of up to 4 hours.

INCISIONS

Exposure of the kidney in radical nephrectomy is particularly important aside from the usual reasons because (a) many *potential* routes exist, so there will be a process of selection, and (b) the kidney, especially in males, is deeply placed with numerous surrounding vital structures that can easily be avoided with proper exposure and knowledge of where they are. Furthermore, if unexpected injuries and problems occur, proper visibility and access are important to

avoid catastrophes. For example, in cases where visibility to the hilum of the left kidney is compromised by nodal involvement, difficult dissection may lead the surgeon to wrongly ligate the superior mesenteric artery that is mistaken for the left renal artery. Better exposure will, in part, avoid such complications. Therefore, to be considered in selection of incision are (a) kidney location, (b) size of tumor, and (c) associated pathology (such as colon involvement, increased or altered vascularity, previous operations, and body habitus). Although there are several classic incision types and names that are mentioned in each reference text, there are really only two basic approaches for cancer of the kidney that can be used for either partial nephrectomy or total radical nephrectomy. The first is flank and the second is anterior (minimally invasive is discussed separately at the end of the chapter). For cancer both are best done as a transperitoneal procedure (Fig. 1).

Flank/Thoracoabdominal Approach

The renal arteries usually arise between the L1 and L2 vertebrae, and the umbilicus is approximately at L4 (Fig. 2). This means that a "flank" incision beginning at the anterior axillary line in the interspace between the 10th and 11th ribs and that is aimed at an area about 1 cm above the umbilicus should have its midpoint right at the renal hilum (Figs. 1 to 3). The incision can be moved inferiorly (i.e., 12th rib, etc.), but the exposure to the adrenal and renal hilum will decrease accordingly. Keep in mind that it is also important to have clear visualization to the upper pole for both partial nephrectomy (for placement of intestinal bag for ice slush and dissection of adrenal off of the kidney) and total nephrectomy (to include or exclude the adrenal). For the average nephrectomy, the easiest placement of the patient is up at "full flank" or at near 90 degrees to the table. This allows an approach to hilum and kidney from virtually any direction, which is particularly helpful on tougher cases. However, if central abdominal exposure is more important than lateral kidney exposure (as, for example, for node dissection), then the patient can be rotated to a more flat position with the pelvis and shoulder resting on a rolled towel to provide a 30-degree tilt-up position (Figs. 1 and 3). This can be further modified by simply tilting the table sideways in either direction during the operation for anterior (i.e., to view the great vessels) or posterior (i.e., for renal artery control) view.

To begin, the patient is placed in the lateral position after anesthesia induction. It is also advantageous to have a nasogastric

tube in place, which can be either left in place or removed at the end of the case depending on the surgeon's preference. The surgeon, however, should check the position of the nasogastric tube in the stomach after the incision is made. In the lateral position, the tip of the 12th rib should be over the kidney rest. The bottom leg should be flexed to 90 degrees with the top leg straight to maintain stability. An axillary roll (usually a rolled small towel) is placed under the axilla to prevent compression of the axillary vessels and nerves. The patient is secured in this position with a 2- or 3-inch adhesive tape passed over the greater trochanter and attached to the edge of the table (Fig. 3). The patient's ipsilateral shoulder is rotated approximately the same degree as the pelvis and the arm extended over the bed and supported on a padded arm rest. The table should be flexed before the arm is positioned and axillary roll placed because flexion changes body position. Flexion also increases the space between the costal margin and the iliac crest and puts the flank muscles and skin on tension, making the incision and exposure easier and better. This effect may be accentuated by raising the kidney rest. These maneuvers, of course, must be done with care in older patients with a deformed spine or any patient with scoliosis.

The best "universal" flank incision for surgery of malignancy of the kidney is made between the 10th and 11th ribs (supra 11th) and extended toward a point about 1 cm above the umbilicus and extending to but not beyond the edge of the rectus muscle. The posterior extent of the incision should not go beyond the latissimus dorsi muscle, although the extent of each end may vary depending on the conditions. Resection of the rib is not necessary and may even cause some wound instability and pain after closure. After the intercostal muscles have been cut and the flank muscles incised down to the transversalis muscle, attention must be directed at the pleural reflection, which generally crosses the ribs at the area of the junction of the anterior and middle third of the ribs (Fig. 3). The pleura may be reflected upward by simply dividing the fascial attachment to the diaphragm. Alternatively, the lower fibers of the diaphragm can be detached from the insertion into the posterior inner aspect of the 12th and 11th ribs. This allows the lower diaphragm and pleura to be retracted upward out of the wound. On the other hand, if the pleural space is low, as is usually the case, the incision can be carried into the pleural space, with care taken not to injure the lung. A small incision is then made into the lumbodorsal fascia to expose peritoneum. On the right side this is usually

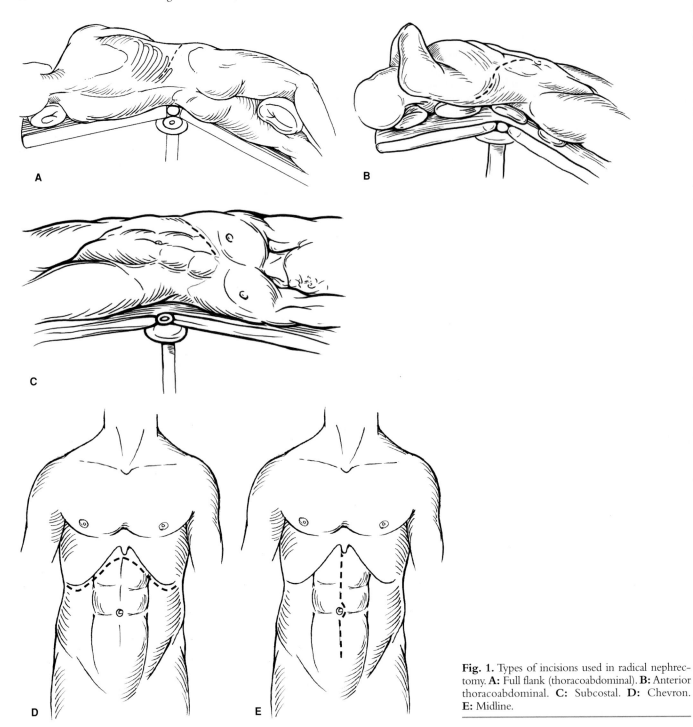

Fig. 1. Types of incisions used in radical nephrectomy. **A:** Full flank (thoracoabdominal). **B:** Anterior thoracoabdominal. **C:** Subcostal. **D:** Chevron. **E:** Midline.

over the liver, and after the fat is pushed away and the peritoneum is found, the peritoneal cavity is then entered. On the left, care must be taken not to dissect too deep to avoid injury to the colon or spleen. The peritoneal cavity is more easily found anteriorly toward the rectus. A Bookwalter retractor is placed, which allows constant changing of retractor blades depending on exposure and the progress of the operation. With the lung protected, the diaphragm is divided for a few centimeters in the direction of the muscle fibers.

After the nephrectomy (or partial nephrectomy) is completed, the kidney bar is lowered and the table slowly taken out of flexion during various phases of the closure. A 24 French chest tube is inserted through a separate stab wound, usually cephalad of the ninth rib at the midaxillary line, and aimed at the apex of the chest cavity. The diaphragm is closed with interrupted zero silk with the knots aimed toward the abdominal cavity and away from the chest. The ribs need not be approximated with separate sutures, although the lumbodorsal fascia should be

reapproximated with zero nonabsorbable suture for stability. If possible, intercostal muscles are closed with running zero absorbable suture, which will facilitate removing the chest tube within 24 hours. The various layers of the abdominal cavity are all closed separately with running zero absorbable suture, such as Vicryl. Care should be taken not to injure intercostal nerves that run between the transversalis and internal oblique layers. The external oblique is closed with heavy absorbable or nonabsorbable suture. I prefer interrupted zero Ethibond sutures to

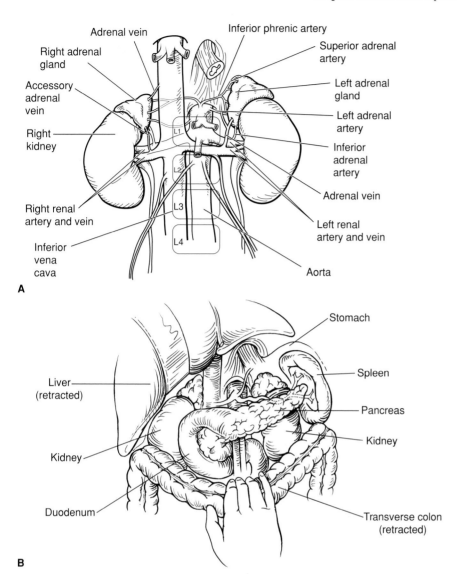

A

B

Fig. 2. A: Vascular anatomy of the kidney and adrenal glands. **B:** Vascular anatomy of associated organs.

the falciform ligament is divided between Kelly clamps and suture-ligated with 2-0 silk suture. A self-retaining retractor is then placed for the nephrectomy.

Total Radical Nephrectomy

Total radical nephrectomy, in contrast to partial nephrectomy, is indicated when the tumor is compressing any portion of the primary renal vasculature or true renal pelvis, or if it is known to be invading the capsule. In addition, the contralateral kidney should be normal. The basic goal is to remove the tumor-containing kidney and the perirenal fat within Gerota's fascia. Theoretically, this encompasses the ipsilateral adrenal gland, although it is now becoming more accepted to leave the adrenal gland if it appears normal on the preoperative imaging studies. The question of performing a paracaval or para-aortic node dissection is controversial, especially with clinical T1 N0 MX lesions (which are the most common). I personally perform a node dissection on all radical nephrectomy patients because it provides patients with prognostic information that significantly impacts personal lives. In addition, there may be a subset of patients with micrometastatic lymph node involvement who benefit from the lymphadenectomy.

Irrespective of the choice of incision or side, the basic steps are about the same. After entering the peritoneal cavity, the colon is reflected medially (Fig. 5). This is initiated by incising the posterior peritoneum lateral to the colon along the length of the descending colon (left side) or ascending colon (right side). For left-sided exposure the lienorenal ligament is incised to mobilize the spleen cephalad and medial. On the right side the hepatic flexure of the colon is mobilized. It is important to avoid injury to the mesocolon. Dissection of the mesocolon off of Gerota's fascia on either side should be done carefully and if done properly should be bloodless and will lead the surgeon down to the duodenum, thence the renal vein on both sides and the IVC on the right side. The maneuver is facilitated by holding the colon/mesocolon at 90 degrees to Gerota's fascia (i.e., "tenting" up the colon) and the Gerota fascia–mesocolon bloodless plane should define itself nicely. On the left side special care should be used sweeping the mesocolon off Gerota's fascia when moving in the cephalad direction because the superior limit of Gerota's fascia borders the splenic vessels and the pancreas. In some obese patients, or in patients with scarring in the area from infection or malignancy, it is easy for the pancreas to inadvertently enter the

accommodate the "shearing" effect of the wound and its inherent ability to slowly shift over time. If the incision is used for a partial nephrectomy, then a Jackson-Pratt or other similar drain should be brought out through another stab wound exiting below the wound to avoid the chest cavity.

Anterior Transabdominal Incisions (Chevron or Subcostal)

The principal advantage to the anterior transabdominal approach is that the surgeon has access to the origin of the renal vessels on both sides (right and left) simultaneously. In addition, other intra-abdominal contents can be surveyed or approached for other procedures. The most commonly used modification is the chevron or subcostal approach; however, in some cases, especially thin people, this can be done through a midline or paramedian approach. This approach is espe-

cially appropriate with patients who have spinal deformities in which the flank approach represents a hazard or in those cases where a laparoscopic nephrectomy needs to be emergently converted to an "open" case. It is often helpful to place a rolled sheet under the lumbar area on the side of the nephrectomy (Fig. 4). The chevron incision begins at the tip of the ipsilateral 11th rib and stays two fingerbreadths below the costal margin and extends medially to the midline near the xiphoid process; the incision can then be extended across in either direction as far as necessary for other parts of the operation. The incision is then carried down to the anterior rectus fascia, which is the divided. Along with this, the incision is extended laterally to divide the external and internal oblique muscles, and finally the fibers of the transversus muscle are split. When encountered, the superior epigastric artery is ligated with 2-0 silk and divided. Likewise,

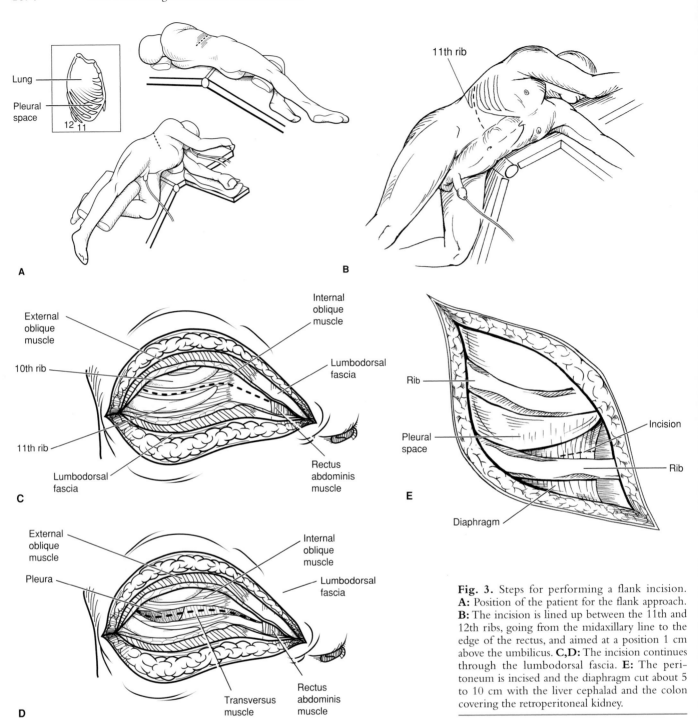

Fig. 3. Steps for performing a flank incision. **A:** Position of the patient for the flank approach. **B:** The incision is lined up between the 11th and 12th ribs, going from the midaxillary line to the edge of the rectus, and aimed at a position 1 cm above the umbilicus. **C,D:** The incision continues through the lumbodorsal fascia. **E:** The peritoneum is incised and the diaphragm cut about 5 to 10 cm with the liver cephalad and the colon covering the retroperitoneal kidney.

field of surgery. On the right side kocherizing the duodenum exposes the vena cava and the renal vein.

One of the advantages of the thoracoabdominal transperitoneal approach is that the kidney, at this point, can be approached from four directions: inferior, superior, lateral, and medial. It is usually easiest to begin dissection laterally and dissect in a medial direction staying close to posterior wall. This leads to the hilum but also clears the way to the inferior portion, where the ureter and gonadal vessels may be approached and ligated. This can be aided by moving the kidney cephalad

with the finger behind the "packet" containing the ureter (Fig. 6). The dissection may then proceed in any of the major directions as allowable as already noted above; that is, the surgeon may continue in the cephalad direction along the paracaval area (right side) or para-aortic area (left side), leaving the nodal tissue around the great vessels for later dissection. On the other hand, dissection from the lateral approach may continue until the renal artery is encountered posterior to the kidney. Interestingly, there seems to be a plane between the perinephric fat and the perihilar fat that signals the presence of the

renal artery (Fig. 7). Finally, dissection may be directed superiorly in which the attachments between Gerota's fascia and the liver (right side) and spleen (left side) are divided with electrocautery or hemoclips. This maneuver is aided by pulling down the upper pole of the kidney with progressive exposure as the avascular connective tissue and peritoneal attachment are progressively divided (Fig. 7B). Dissection is usually easier lateral to medial and care must be exercised to divide all vessels step by step. If the adrenal is to be spared, a plane between the upper pole of the kidney and adrenal is followed and hemoclips

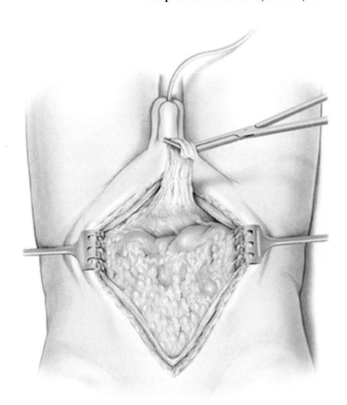

Fig. 2. Wide excision of the urachal remnant en bloc with the cystectomy specimen. (From Stein JP, Skinner DG. Surgical atlas–radical cystectomy. *Br J Urol Int* 2004;94:197.)

Following mobilization of the bowel, a self-retaining retractor is placed. The right colon and small intestine are carefully packed into the epigastrium with three moist lap pads, followed by a moistened towel rolled to the width of the abdomen. The descending and sigmoid colon are not packed and are left as free as possible, providing the necessary mobility required for the ureteral and pelvic lymph node dissection.

Successful packing of the intestinal contents is an art and prevents their annoying spillage into the operative field. Packing begins by sweeping the right colon and small bowel under the surgeon's left hand along the right sidewall gutter. A moist open lap pad is then swept with the right hand along the palm of the left hand, under the viscera along the retroperitoneum and sidewall gutter. In similar fashion, the left sidewall gutter is packed, ensuring not to incorporate the descending or sigmoid colon. The central portion of the small bowel is packed with a third lap pad. A moist rolled towel is then positioned horizontally below the lap pads, but cephalad to the bifurcation of the aorta. Occasionally, prior to placement

right triangle, the base formed by the third and fourth portions of the duodenum, the right edge represented by the white line of Toldt along the ascending colon, the left edge represented by the medial portion of the sigmoid and descending colonic mesentery, and the apex represented by the ileocecal region (Fig. 3). This mobilization is critical in setting up the operative field and facilitates proper packing of the intra-abdominal contents into the epigastrium.

The left colon and sigmoid mesentery are then mobilized to the region of the lower pole of the left kidney by incising the peritoneum lateral to the colon along the avascular/white line of Toldt. The sigmoid mesentery is then elevated off the sacrum, iliac vessels, and distal aorta cephalad to the origin of the inferior mesenteric artery. This maneuver provides a mesenteric window through which the left ureter will pass (without angulation or tension) for the ureteroenteric anastomosis to the urinary reservoir at the terminal portions of the operation, and also facilitates retraction of the sigmoid mesentery while performing the lymph node dissection—particularly the superior limits (Fig. 4). Care should be taken to dissect along the base of the mesentery and avoid injury to the inferior mesenteric artery and blood supply to the sigmoid colon.

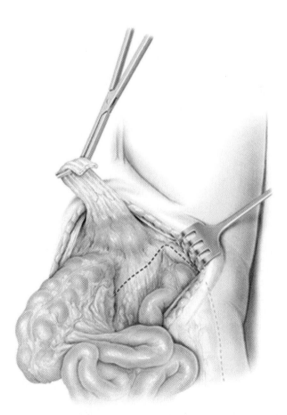

Fig. 3. View of the pelvis from overhead. Note that the ascending colon and peritoneal attachments of the small bowel mesentery (*dotted line*) are mobilized up to the level of the duodenum. This mobilization allows the bowel to be properly packed in the epigastrium and exposes the area of the inferior mesenteric artery, which is the superior limits of the lymph node dissection. (From Stein JP, Skinner DG. Surgical atlas–radical cystectomy. *Br J Urol Int* 2004;94:197.)

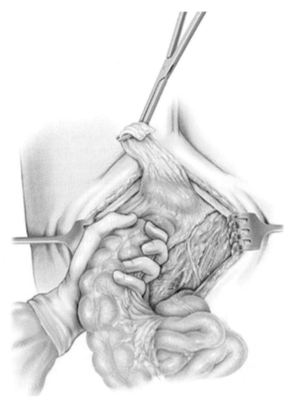

Fig. 4. View of the pelvis from overhead. Note that the sigmoid mesentery is mobilized off the sacral promontory, common iliac vessels, and distal aorta up to the origin of the inferior mesenteric artery. (From Stein JP, Skinner DG. Surgical atlas-radical cystectomy. *Br J Urol Int* 2004;94:197.)

of the first moist lap pad, a mobile greater omental apron can be used to facilitate packing of the intestinal viscera in a similar fashion to the lap pad. After the bowel has been packed, a wide Deaver retractor is placed with gentle traction on the rolled towel to provide cephalad exposure.

Ureteral Dissection

The ureters are most easily identified in the retroperitoneum just cephalad to the common iliac vessels. They are dissected into the deep pelvis (several centimeters beyond the iliac vessels) and divided between two large hemoclips. A section of the proximal cut ureteral segment (distal to the proximal hemoclip) is then sent for frozen section analysis to ensure the absence of carcinoma in situ or overt tumor. The ureter is then mobilized cephalad and tucked under the rolled towel to prevent inadvertent injury. Frequently, an arterial branch from the common iliac artery or the aorta needs to be divided to provide adequate ureteral mobilization. In addition, the rich vascular supply emanating from the gonadal vessels should remain intact and undisturbed. These attachments are an important blood supply to the

ureter and ensure an adequate vascular supply for the ureteroenteric anastomosis at the time of diversion. This is particularly important in irradiated patients. Leaving the proximal hemoclip on the divided ureter during the exenteration allows for hydrostatic ureteral dilation and facilitates the ureteroenteric anastomosis. In women, the infundibulopelvic ligaments are ligated and divided at the level of the common iliac vessels.

Distal Retroperitoneal and Pelvic Lymphadenectomy

A meticulous pelvic lymph node dissection is routinely performed with radical cystectomy. The extent of the lymphadenectomy may vary depending on the patient and surgeon preference. As mentioned, an accumulating body of evidence strongly suggests that a more extended lymphadenectomy may be beneficial in patients undergoing cystectomy for high-grade, invasive bladder cancer. When performing a salvage procedure following definitive radiation treatment (greater then 5,000 rads), a pelvic lymphadenectomy is usually not performed because of the significant risk of iliac vessel and obturator nerve injury.

For a combined lower retroperitoneal, common, and pelvic–iliac lymphadenectomy, the lymph node dissection is initiated at the inferior mesenteric artery (superior limits of dissection) and extends laterally over the inferior vena cava to the genitofemoral nerve, representing the lateral limits of dissection. Distally, the lymph node dissection extends to the lymph node of Cloquet medially (on the Cooper ligament) and the circumflex iliac vein laterally. The cephalad portion of the lymphatics at the level of the inferior mesenteric artery are ligated with hemoclips to prevent lymphatic leak, while the caudal (specimen) side is ligated only when a blood vessel is encountered. Frequently, small anterior tributary veins originate from the vena cava just above the bifurcation, which should be clipped and divided. In men, the spermatic vessels are retracted laterally and spared. In women, the infundibulopelvic ligament along with the corresponding ovarian vessels are ligated and divided at the pelvic brim as previously described.

All fibroareolar and lymphatic tissue are dissected caudally off the aorta, vena cava, and common iliac vessels over the sacral promontory into the deep pelvis. The initial dissection along the common iliac vessels is performed over the arteries, skeletonizing them. As the common iliac veins are dissected medially, care is taken to control small arterial and venous branches coursing along the anterior surface of the sacrum. Electrocautery is helpful at this location and allows the adherent fibroareolar tissue to be swept off the sacral promontory down into the deep pelvis with the use of a small gauze sponge. Significant bleeding from these presacral vessels can occur if not properly controlled. Hemoclips are discouraged in this location as they can be easily dislodged from the anterior surface of the sacrum, resulting in troublesome bleeding.

Once the proximal portion of the lymph node dissection is completed, a finger is passed from the proximal aspect of dissection under the pelvic peritoneum (anterior to the iliac vessels), distally toward the femoral canal. The opposite hand can be used to strip the peritoneum from the undersurface of the transversalis fascia, and connects with the proximal dissection from above. This maneuver elevates the peritoneum and defines the lateral limit of peritoneum to be incised and removed with the specimen. In men, the peritoneum is divided medial to the spermatic vessels, and lateral to the infundibulopelvic ligament in female patients. The only structure encountered is the vas deferens in the

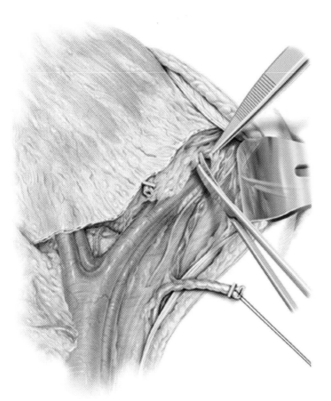

Fig. 5. Technique of skeletonizing the external iliac artery and vein. (From Stein JP, Skinner DG. Surgical atlas–radical cystectomy. *Br J Urol Int* 2004;94:197.)

male or round ligament in the female; these structures are clipped and divided.

A large right-angled rake retractor (Israel) is used to elevate the lower abdominal wall, including the spermatic cord or remnant of the round ligament, to provide distal exposure in the area of the femoral canal. Tension on the retractor is directed vertically toward the ceiling, with care taken to avoid injury to the inferior epigastric vessels. This provides excellent exposure to the distal external iliac vessels. The distal limits of the dissection are then identified: the circumflex iliac vein crossing anterior to the external iliac artery distally, the genitofemoral nerve laterally, and the lymph node of Coquet sitting on the Cooper ligament medially. The lymphatics draining the ipsilateral leg, particularly medial to the external iliac vein, are carefully clipped and divided to prevent lymphatic leakage. This includes the lymph node of Cloquet (also known as Rosenmüller), which represents the distal limit of the lymphatic dissection at this location. The distal external iliac artery and vein are then circumferentially dissected and skeletonized, with care taken to ligate an accessory obturator vein (present in 40% of patients) originating from the inferomedial aspect of the external iliac vein.

Following completion of the distal limits of dissection, the proximal and distal

dissections are joined. The proximal external iliac artery and vein are skeletonized circumferentially to the origin of the hypogastric artery (Fig. 5). Care should be taken to clip and divide a commonly encountered vessel arising from the lateral aspect of the proximal external iliac vessels coursing to the psoas muscle. The external iliac vessels are then retracted medially, and the fascia overlying the psoas muscle is incised medial to the genitofemoral nerve. On the left side, branches of the genitofemoral nerve often pursue a more medial course and may be intimately related to the iliac vessels, in which case they are excised.

At this point, the lymphatic tissue surrounding the iliac vessels are composed of a medial and lateral component attached only at the base within the obturator fossa. The lateral lymphatic compartment (freed medially from the vessels and laterally from the psoas) is bluntly swept into the obturator fossa by retracting the iliac vessels medially, and passing a small gauze sponge lateral to the vessels along the psoas and pelvic sidewall (Fig. 6). This sponge should be passed anterior and distal to the hypogastric vein, directed caudally into the obturator fossa. The external iliac vessels are then elevated and retracted laterally while the gauze sponge is carefully withdrawn from the obturator fossa with gentle traction using the

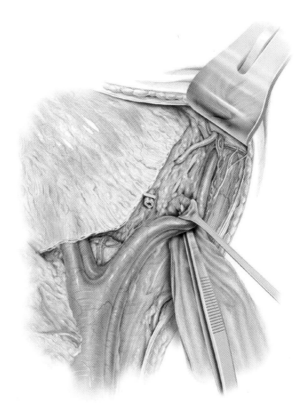

Fig. 6. Technique of passing a small gauze sponge lateral to the external iliac vessels and medial to the psoas muscle. (From Stein JP, Skinner DG. Surgical atlas–radical cystectomy. *Br J Urol Int* 2004;94:197.)

Nongastrointestinal Transabdominal

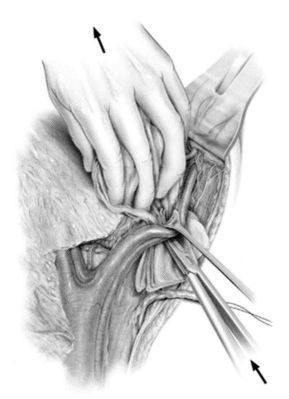

Fig. 7. Technique of withdrawing the gauze sponge with the left hand. Note that this will aid in dissecting the obturator fossa, sweeping all fibroareolar and lymphatic tissue toward the bladder. (From Stein JP, Skinner DG. Surgical atlas-radical cystectomy. *Br J Urol Int* 2004;94:197.)

a safe cystectomy with proper vascular control. Isolation of the lateral vascular pedicle is performed with the left hand. The bladder is retracted toward the pelvis, placing traction and isolating the anterior branches of the hypogastric artery. The left index finger is passed medial to the hypogastric artery and posterior to the anterior visceral branches. The index finger is directed caudally toward the endopelvic fascia, parallel to the sweep of the sacrum. This maneuver defines the two major vascular pedicles to the anterior pelvic organs: the lateral pedicle, anterior to the index finger, composed of the visceral branches of the anterior hypogastric vessel; and the posterior pedicle, posterior to the index finger, composed of the visceral branches between the bladder and rectum.

With the lateral pedicle entrapped between the left index and middle fingers, firm traction is applied vertically and caudally. This facilitates identification and allows for the individual branches off the anterior portion of the hypogastric artery to be isolated (Fig. 9). The posterior division of the hypogastric artery including the superior gluteal, iliolumbar, and lateral sacral arteries are preserved to avoid gluteal claudication. Distal to this posterior division, the hypogastric artery may be ligated for vascular control, but should

left hand (Fig. 7). This maneuver effectively sweeps all lymphatic tissue into the obturator fossa and facilitates identification of the obturator nerve deep to the external iliac vein. The obturator nerve is best identified proximally and carefully dissected free from all lymphatics. The obturator nerve is then retracted laterally along with the iliac vessels (Fig. 8). At this point, the obturator artery and vein are entrapped between the index finger (medial to the obturator nerve) laterally and the middle finger medially with the left hand. This isolates the obturator vessels exiting the obturator canal along the pelvic floor. These vessels are then carefully clipped and divided, ensuring to stay medial to the obturator nerve. The obturator lymph node packet is then swept medially toward the sidewall of the bladder, ligating small tributary vessels and lymphatics from the pelvic sidewall, and removed.

Ligation of the Lateral Vascular Pedicle to the Bladder

Following dissection of the obturator fossa and dividing the obturator vessels, the lateral vascular pedicle to the bladder is isolated and divided. Developing this plane isolates the lateral vascular pedicle to the bladder, a critical maneuver in performing

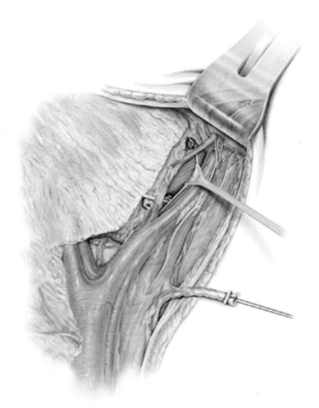

Fig. 8. Obturator fossa cleaned. This allows proper identification of the obturator nerve passing deep/posterior to the external iliac vein. Note that this nerve is retracted with the external iliac vessels. (From Stein JP, Skinner DG. Surgical atlas-radical cystectomy. *Br J Urol Int* 2004;94:197.)

TABLE 2. THE PERIOPERATIVE MORTALITY AND EARLY COMPLICATION RATES IN 1,054 PATIENTS WHO UNDERWENT RADICAL CYSTECTOMY FOR TRANSITIONAL CELL CARCINOMA OF THE BLADDER

	Number of Patients	Perioperative Mortality[a]	Early Complication[b]
Form of urinary diversion			
Coundit[c]	278 (26%)	8 (3%)	83 (30%)
Continent[d]	776 (74%)	19 (2%)	209 (27%)
Perioperative adjuvant therapy			
None	884 (84%)	26 (3%)	247 (28%)
Radiation only	108 (10%)	1 (1%)	30 (30%)
Chemotherapy only	49 (5%)	0	12 (25%)
Radiation and chemotherapy	13 (1%)	0	3 (23%)
Totals	1,054	27 (3%)	292 (28%)

[a]Any death occurring within 30 days of surgery or before discharge.
[b]Any complication occurring within the first 4 months postoperative.
[c]Including ileal conduits and colon conduits.
[d]Including continent cutaneous, orthotopic, and rectal reservoirs.
From Stein JP, Lieskovsky G, Cote R, et al. Radical cystectomy in the treatment of invasive bladder cancer: long-term results in 1054 patients. *J Clin Oncol* 2001;19:666, with permission.

that the ideal outcome for patients with high-grade, invasive bladder cancer is when the primary bladder tumor is confined to the bladder, without evidence of extravesical extension or lymph node metastases. Significant delays in patients with invasive bladder cancer should obviously be avoided. There is evidence to suggest that prolonged delays may lead to more advanced pathologic stages and decreased survival in patients with muscle-invasive bladder cancer. Furthermore, it should be emphasized that care should taken in delaying a more definitive therapy in patients with high-risk superficial bladder tumors, or those tumors that are superficial that have not appropriately responded to conservative forms of therapy.

Extravesical, Lymph Node–negative Tumors

Non–organ-confined (extravesical), lymph node–negative tumors were found in approximately 20% of our patients undergoing cystectomy (Table 3). In this pathologic subgroup, no obvious survival differences between extravesical P3 and P4 tumors were observed. The recurrence-free survival in this pathologic subgroup of extravesical, non–organ-confined, lymph node–negative tumors was 58% at 5 years and 55% at 10 years. It is clear that patients with these locally advanced tumors have higher recurrence rates and decreased survival compared to the subgroup of patients with organ–confined, lymph node–negative tumors. In view of this, one may consider adjuvant treatment strategies for this pathologic subgroup of patients.

In 1997, the TNM (tumor, node, metastases) staging system for bladder cancer was modified by the American Joint Committee on Cancer (AJCC) and the International Union against Cancer (UICC). The revised TNM classification stratifies extravesical tumor involvement (previously defined as pT3b) into microscopic (pT3a) and gross (pT3b) extravesical tumor extension. In order to determine the clinical significance of this new pathologic subgrouping, we evaluated the clinical outcomes in our group of patients following radical cystectomy with pathologic pT3 disease stratified by microscopic and gross extravesical tumor involvement. We found no significant difference in the recurrence-free and overall survival in patients when evaluating for pT3a and pT3b extravesical tumor extension. The incidence of lymph node involvement was not different (approximately 45%) between the

TABLE 3. PATHOLOGIC STAGING OF PATIENTS AND RECURRENCE-FREE AND OVERALL SURVIVAL RATES

Variable		Number of Patients	Recurrence-Free Survival (%) 5 yr	Recurrence-Free Survival (%) 10 yr	Overall Survival (%) 5 yr	Overall Survival (%) 10 yr
Pathologic stage[80]	P0	66 (6%)	92	86	84	67
	Pis	100 (9%)	91	89	89	72
	Pa	42 (4%)	79	74	80	56
	P1	194 (19%)	83	78	76	52
	P2a (superficial muscle)	94 (9%)	89	87	78	57
	P2b (deep muscle)	98 (9%)	78	76	64	44
	P3 (extravesical extension)	135 (13%)	62	61	49	29
	P4	79 (7%)	50	45	44	23
Lymph node negative	All patients	808 (76%)	78	75	69	49
Lymph node positive	All patients	246 (24%)	35	34	31	23
	1–4 nodes	160	41	40	39	32
	≥5 nodes	86	24	24	17	8
	Organ confined (P-stage)	75	46	44	47	41
	Extravesical (P-stage)	171	30	30	24	19
Pathologic subgroups	Organ confined[a]	594 (56%)	85	82	78	56
	Extravesical[b]	214 (20%)	58	55	47	27
Entire group		1,054	68	66	60	43

[a]Including P0 and Pa, Pis, P1, P2a and P2b (lymph node negative).
[b]Including P3 and P4 (lymph node negative).
Note: P-stage reflects 1997 TNM staging system.
From Stein JP, Lieskovsky G, Cote R, et al. Radical cystectomy in the treatment of invasive bladder cancer: long-term results in 1054 patients. *J Clin Oncol* 2001;19:666, with permission.

Nongastrointestinal Transabdominal

TABLE 4. INCIDENCE OF LYMPH NODE INVOLVEMENT WITH PRIMARY BLADDER TUMORS

Primary Bladder Tumor (P-Stage)	Number of Patients	Lymph Node Involvement	
		Positive	Negative
P0, Pis, Pa, P1[a]	421 (40%)	19 (5%)	402 (95%)
P2a (superficial muscle)	115 (11%)	21 (18%)	94 (82%)
P2b (deep muscle)	133 (13%)	35 (27%)	98 (73%)
P3 (extravesical extension)	248 (23%)	113 (45%)	135 (55%)
P4	137 (13%)	58 (43%)	79 (57%)
Entire group	1,054	246 (24%)	808 (76%)

[a]Superficial (nonmuscle) tumors.
Note, the P-stage reflects the 1997 TNM staging system.
From Stein JP, Lieskovsky G, Cote R, et al. Radical cystectomy in the treatment of invasive bladder cancer: long-term results in 1054 patients. *J Clin Oncol* 2001;19:666, with permission.

groups; however, as one would expect, the presence of lymph node involvement was associated with a higher risk of recurrence and worse overall survival. Because no differences were observed between the clinical outcomes for patients with pT3a and pT3b disease, we believe they should be treated similarly. Furthermore, future staging systems may consider classifying these tumors collectively, which may also facilitate comparisons with historical cystectomy series.

Lymph Node–positive Disease

Despite an aggressive treatment philosophy and approach to bladder cancer, 24% of our patients demonstrated lymph node–positive disease at the time of cystectomy (Table 3). This underscores the virulent and metastatic capabilities of high-grade, invasive bladder cancer. Although patients with lymph node tumor involvement are a high-risk group of patients, nearly one third of these patients in our series were alive at 5 years, and 23% were alive at 10 years. It is possible that the surgical approach (with an extended pelvic–iliac lymph node dissection) may provide some advantage with long-term survival in selected individual with lymph node–positive disease. The impact of adjuvant therapy in this group of patients, although difficult to assess and subject to selection bias, may also play a role in the outcomes of patients with lymph node–positive disease. In fact, in a separate analysis of lymph node–positive patients, we found that the administration of adjuvant chemotherapy was a significant and independent predictor for recurrence and overall survival in these patients.

The prognosis in patients with lymph node–positive disease can be stratified by the number of lymph nodes involved (tumor burden), and by the P stage of the primary bladder tumor (Table 3). In our cystectomy series, patients with fewer than five positive lymph nodes had improved survival rates compared to patients with five or more lymph nodes involved. A significant difference was also observed when stratifying patients by their primary bladder stage. Patients with lymph node–positive disease and organ-confined bladder tumors had a significant improved recurrence-free survival compared to those with non–organ-confined, lymph node–positive tumors. Similar results with lymph node–positive tumors following cystectomy have been previously reported.

We believe that the number of lymph nodes involved with tumor and the extent of the lymph node dissection are both important variables for patients undergoing cystectomy for bladder cancer. We have re-examined our 246 patients with lymph node tumor involvement following radical cystectomy to evaluate other prognostic factors in this high-risk group of patients. This re-evaluation subsequently stimulated the concept of *lymph node density*—an important prognostic factor that better stratifies lymph node–positive patients following radical cystectomy. Lymph node density (defined as the total number of positive lymph nodes divided by the total number of lymph nodes removed) accounts for the extent of the lymph node dissection (number of lymph nodes removed) and the tumor burden (number of positive lymph nodes) following radical cystectomy for patients with lymph node–positive disease. Therefore, lymph node density incorporates these concepts simultaneously.

If lymph tumor burden and the extent of the lymphadenectomy are important variables in patients with lymph node–positive disease, it is only logical that lymph node density is also important. In fact, we found lymph node density to be a significant and independent prognostic variable in patients

with lymph node metastases, which may best stratify this high-risk group of patients. It is possible that future staging systems and the application of adjuvant therapies in clinical trials should consider applying these concepts to help better stratify this high-risk group of patients following radical cystectomy. Regardless, patients with any lymph node involvement remain at high risk for disease recurrence and should be considered for adjuvant treatment strategies.

RECURRENCE FOLLOWING CYSTECTOMY

Recurrence following radical cystectomy for bladder cancer is not unusual and correlates directly to the pathologic stage and subgroup. In our report of 1,054 patients with long-term follow-up (median 10 years), recurrences were classified as local (pelvic), distant, and urethral. Local recurrences by definition are those tumor recurrences that occur within the soft tissue field of exenteration. Distant recurrences are defined as those that occur outside the pelvis, while urethral tumors are classified as a new primary tumor that occurs in the retained urethra. Overall, 30% of the 1,054 patients experienced a local or distant tumor recurrence (Table 5). The median time to any recurrence was 12 months, with 86% of all patients developing their recurrence with the first 3 years postoperatively. Of the 311 patients in our series who developed a recurrence, 75% were distant (median time to distant recurrence, 12 months) and 25% local (median time to local recurrence, 18 months).

Pelvic (Local) Recurrence

Radical cystectomy clearly provides the best local (pelvic) control of the disease (Table 5). An overall local pelvic recurrence rate of 7% was observed in the USC cystectomy series. Patients with organ-confined, lymph node–negative tumors demonstrated only a 6% local recurrence rate, compared to a 13% local recurrence rate in those with non–organ-confined, lymph node–negative tumors. Even those at highest risk of a local recurrence (lymph node–positive disease) had only a 13% local recurrence rate following cystectomy. The use of a high-dose, short course of preoperative radiation therapy does not reduce the risk of pelvic recurrence. Nearly all patients suffering a pelvic recurrence following cystectomy will die of their disease despite additional and even aggressive therapeutic efforts.

TABLE 5. BLADDER CANCER RECURRENCE BY PATHOLOGIC SUBGROUPS

Pathologic Groups	Total Number of Patients	Recurrence Site	
		Local	Distant
Organ confined[a]	594 (56%)	27 (6%)	62 (13%)
Extravesical disease[b]	214 (20%)	22 (13%)	59 (32%)
Lymph node positive	246 (24%)	28 (13%)	113 (52%)
Totals	1,054	77 (7%)	234 (23%)

[a]Including P0, Pa, Pis, P1, P2a, and P2b.
[b]Including P3 and P4.
Note: P stage reflects 1997 TNM staging system.
From Stein JP, Lieskovsky G, Cote R, et al. Radical cystectomy in the treatment of invasive bladder cancer: long-term results in 1054 patients. *J Clin Oncol* 2001;19:666, with permission.

Metastatic (Distant) Recurrence

Recurrences following radical cystectomy are most commonly found at distant sites (Table 5). Distant recurrences can also be stratified by pathologic subgroups. In our series, patients with organ-confined lymph node–negative tumors demonstrated a 13% recurrence rate, which increased to 32% for those with extravesical lymph node–negative and 52% for those with lymph node–positive tumors. Patients at high risk for tumor recurrence should clearly be considered for adjuvant chemotherapy protocols.

Urethral Recurrence

It is generally believed that urethral tumors in patients with a history of bladder cancer following radical cystectomy represent a second manifestation of the multicentric defect of the primary transitional cell mucosa that led to the original bladder tumor. The term "urethral recurrence" may therefore be somewhat misleading, suggesting a failure of definitive treatment of the bladder cancer as the cause of the urethral lesion. Rather, most urethral tumors probably represent simply another occurrence of the transitional cell carcinoma in the remaining urothelium. As radical cystectomy has emerged as the most effective therapy for invasive bladder cancer and as orthotopic diversion to the native intact urethra has increasingly been performed, the fate of the retained urethra has become an increasingly important oncologic issue.

The advent of orthotopic lower urinary tract reconstruction has arguably improved the quality of life in patients following radical cystectomy for bladder cancer. Approximately 90% of all patients undergoing cystectomy for bladder cancer at our institution receive an orthotopic neobladder substitute. From an oncologic perspective, only those patients found to have a positive margin at the proximal urethra (distal to the apex of the prostate in men and just distal to the bladder neck in women) on intraoperative frozen section are absolutely excluded from orthotopic reconstruction. This enthusiasm to preserve the native urethra following radical cystectomy and allow for orthotopic reconstruction has rightfully increased concerns for the potential for urethral recurrence in these patients.

Prior to the orthotopic era in women, urethral tumor recurrence was not considered an important oncologic issue, as the entire urethra was routinely removed at the time of cystectomy. With a better understanding of female pelvic anatomy and the innervation of the rhabdosphincter and continence mechanism in women, along with the identification of various pathologic risk factors for urethral tumor involvement in these patients, orthotopic diversion has now become a commonly performed form of urinary diversion in women following cystectomy. We have demonstrated that tumor involving the bladder neck is the most important risk factor for urethral tumor involvement in women. Although bladder neck involvement is a significant risk factor for urethral tumors, not all women with tumor involving the bladder neck will have urethral tumors. Approximately 50% of women with tumor at the bladder neck will have a urethra free of tumor. In this situation, the patient may potentially be considered an appropriate candidate for orthotopic diversion. Furthermore, we have shown that intraoperative frozen section analysis of the distal surgical margin provides an accurate and reliable means to evaluate the proximal urethra, and currently is the primary pathologic factor that determines appropriate candidacy for orthotopic diversion. With this selection process, to date, we have not had a female urethral recurrence.

A growing number of male patients reconstructed to the urethra following cystectomy exist today, and with longer follow-up will expose them to a greater risk for a urethral recurrence. The historical incidence of urethral recurrence in the retained urethra following cystectomy for bladder cancer ranges from 6% to 10%. Specific clinical and pathologic risk factors that have been studied and may provide some risk assessment for urethral recurrence include multifocal tumors, carcinoma in situ, tumor involvement of the prostate (particularly invasion of the prostatic stroma), and the form of urinary diversion (orthotopic or cutaneous) performed.

We recently evaluated our clinical experience regarding the incidence and associated risk factors for urethral recurrence in a large group of male patients undergoing radical cystectomy and urinary diversion for transitional cell carcinoma of the bladder with long-term follow-up. We analyzed the clinical and pathologic results of 768 consecutive male patients undergoing radical cystectomy with the intent to cure for high-grade, invasive bladder cancer (median follow-up 13 years); 397 men (51%) underwent an orthotopic urinary diversion (median follow-up 10 years) and 371 men (49%) underwent a cutaneous urinary diversion (median follow-up 19 years). Overall, a total of 45 patients (7%) developed a urethral recurrence, with an overall median time to recurrence of 2 years (range 0.2 to 13.6 years): 16 men (5%) with an orthotopic and 29 men (9%) with a cutaneous form of urinary diversion.

In this cohort of male patients, multiple risk factors were analyzed with regard to urethral recurrence. In a multivariable analysis, two important variables were identified that significantly increased the risk of a urethral tumor recurrence following cystectomy: Any prostate tumor involvement and the form of urinary diversion. The estimated 5-year probability of a urethra recurrence was 5% without any prostate involvement, and increased to 12% and 18% with superficial (prostatic urethra and ducts) and invasive (stroma) prostate involvement, respectively. Furthermore, patients undergoing an orthotopic diversion demonstrated a significantly lower risk of urethral recurrence compared to those undergoing a cutaneous form of urinary diversion.

The overall management of the urethra in male patients treated for high-grade invasive bladder cancer is an important issue. This concern has become even more critical from an oncologic perspective since the advent of orthotopic diversion. The indications and timing of a prophylactic urethrectomy in those undergoing cystectomy and a cutaneous diversion is debatable. This may include urethrectomy at the time of cystectomy based on preoperative clinical parameters or on the intraoperative frozen section analysis of the urethral margin, or a delayed urethrectomy based on final pathologic evaluation of the cystectomy specimen.

Our long-term findings provide some insight regarding the issues and management of the retained urethra in both men and women following cystectomy for bladder cancer. We believe that intraoperative frozen section analysis of the proximal urethra by an experience pathologist is a reliable and accurate means to determine candidacy for orthotopic diversion in all patients. It has been our practice to perform an orthotopic neobladder in men and women whose intraoperative frozen section of the proximal urethra is without tumor. Our data suggest that this approach does not appear to increase the risk of a urethral recurrence in these patients. Male patients with known prostatic tumor involvement should not necessarily be excluded from an orthotopic substitute if the intraoperative biopsy is normal. Similarly, female patients with bladder neck involvement should not necessarily be excluded from an orthotopic neobladder if the intraoperative biopsy is also normal. All patients should be carefully counseled regarding the careful follow-up, the long-term risks of a urethral recurrence, and the possible need for urethrectomy following cystectomy for transitional cell carcinoma of the bladder.

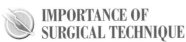

IMPORTANCE OF SURGICAL TECHNIQUE

The dedication of the surgeon and technical commitment to a properly performed cystectomy and adequate lymphadenectomy is important to the success and clinical outcomes in patients with high-grade bladder cancer. The importance of surgical technique is well illustrated in the role this may have played in a recently reported randomized multi-institutional cooperative group trial. In this prospective study, 270 patients underwent cystectomy with half of the patients receiving neoadjuvant chemotherapy. In a separate analysis of this trial, various surgical factors were subsequently analyzed. In these 270 patients, 24 had no lymph node dissection, 98 had a limited dissection of the obturator lymph nodes only, and 146 patients had a so-called standard (not extended) pelvic lymph node dissection. The 5-year survival rates for these groups were 33%, 46%, and 60% respectively. The median number of lymph

nodes removed for the entire cohort was ten. As expected, the survival rate for patients with less than ten lymph nodes removed was significantly lower compared to patients with more than ten lymph nodes removed: 44% versus 61%, respectively. In a multivariate analysis, the extent of the lymph node dissection, number of lymph nodes removed, and number of cases performed by the individual surgeon were the most significant factors influencing survival in patients undergoing cystectomy for bladder cancer. It is emphasized that, although this well-publicized study was not intended to analyze the surgical approach and/or technical differences in the treatment of bladder cancer, it was the surgical factors and not neoadjuvant chemotherapy that were most critical as predictors in the outcomes of these patients.

CONCLUSIONS

Unlike other therapies, radical cystectomy pathologically stages the primary bladder tumor and regional lymph nodes. This histologic evaluation provides important prognostic information and identifies high-risk patients who may benefit from adjuvant therapy. Our data suggest that patients with extravesical tumor extension or with lymph node–positive disease appear to be at increased risk for recurrence and may be considered for adjuvant chemotherapy strategies. Additionally, the recent application of molecular markers based on pathologic staging and analysis may also serve to identify patients at risk for tumor recurrence who may benefit from adjuvant forms of therapy.

The clinical results and outcomes following radical cystectomy demonstrate good survival, with excellent local recurrence rates for high-grade, invasive bladder cancer. These results provide sound data and a standard to which other forms of therapy for invasive bladder cancer can be compared. Furthermore, improvements in orthotopic urinary diversion have improved the quality of life in patients following cystectomy. Continence rates following orthotopic diversion are good and provide patients a more natural voiding pattern per urethra. Contraindication to orthotopic urinary diversion is the presence of tumor within the urethra or extending to the urethral margin as determined by frozen section analysis of the distal surgical margin at the time of cystectomy, compromised renal function (creatinine >2.5 ng/mL), or the presence of inflammatory bowel disease. Even in patients with locally advanced disease, or-

thotopic diversion can be employed without concern over subsequent tumor-related reservoir complications.

The question whether patients have a better quality of life following cystectomy or following bladder-sparing protocols, which require significant and prolonged treatment to the bladder with the potential for tumor recurrence, has not been elucidated. Currently, orthotopic diversion should be considered the diversion of choice in all cystectomy patients and the urologist should have a specific reason why an orthotopic diversion is *not* performed. Patient factors such as frail general health, motivation, or co-morbidity and the cancer factor of a positive urethral margin may disqualify some patients. Nevertheless, the option of lower urinary tract reconstruction to the intact urethra has been shown to decrease physician reluctance and increase patient acceptance to undergo earlier cystectomy when the disease may be at a more curable stage.

In conclusion, a properly performed radical cystectomy with an appropriate and extended lymphadenectomy provides the best survival rates, with the lowest reported local recurrence rates for high-grade invasive bladder cancer. The surgical technique is critical to optimize the best clinical and technical outcomes in patients with this procedure. Advances in lower urinary tract reconstruction provide a reasonable alternative for patients undergoing cystectomy and have improved the quality of life of these patients requiring removal of their bladder.

SUGGESTED READING

Grossman HB, Natale RB, Tangen CM, et al. Neoadjuvant chemotherapy plus cystectomy compared with cystectomy alone for locally advanced bladder cancer. *N Engl J Med* 2003;349:859.

Hautmann RE, Paiss T. Does the option of the ileal neobladder stimulate patient and physician decision towards earlier cystectomy? *J Urol* 1998;159:1845.

Herr HW. Surgical factors in bladder cancer: more (nodes) + more (pathology) = less (mortality). *B J U Int* 2003;92:187.

Herr HW, Bochner BH, Dalbagni G, et al. Impact of the number of lymph nodes retrieved on outcome in patients with muscle invasive bladder cancer. *J Urol* 2002;167:1295.

Jemal A, Tiwari RC, Murray T, et al. Cancer statistics, 2004. *CA Cancer J Clin* 2004;54:8.

Leissner J, Ghoneim MA, Abol-Enein H, et al. Extended radical lymphadenectomy in patients with urothelial bladder cancer: results of a prospective multicenter study. *J Urol* 2004;171:139.

Leissner J, Hohenfellner R, Thuroff JW, et al. Lymphadenectomy in patients with transitional cell carcinoma of the urinary bladder; significance for staging and prognosis. *Br J Urol Int* 2000;85:817.

Poulsen AL, Horn T, Steven K. Radical cystectomy; extending limits of pelvic lymph node dissection improves survival for patients with bladder cancer confined to the bladder wall. *J Urol* 1998;160:2015.

Quek ML, Stein JP, Clark PE, et al. Microscopic and gross extravesical extension in pathologic staging of bladder cancer. *J Urol* 2004;171:640.

Sanchez-Ortiz RF, Huang WC, Mick R, et al. An interval longer than 12 weeks between the diagnosis of muscle invasion and cystectomy is associated with worse outcome in bladder carcinoma. *J Urol* 2003;169:110.

Skinner DG, Daniels JA, Russell CA, et al. The role of adjuvant chemotherapy following cystectomy for invasive bladder cancer: a prospective comparative trial. *J Urol* 1991;145:459.

Stein JP. Indications for early cystectomy. *Urology* 2003;62:591.

Stein JP. The role of lymphadenectomy in bladder cancer. *Am J Urol Rev* 2003;1:146.

Stein JP, Cai J, Groshen S, et al. Risk factors for patients with pelvic lymph node metastases following radical cystectomy with en bloc cystectomy: the concept of lymph node density. *J Urol* 2003;170:35.

Stein JP, Clark P, Miranda G, et al. Urethral tumor recurrence following cystectomy and urinary diversion: clinical and pathologic characteristics in 768 patients. *J Urol* [Submitted for publication].

Stein JP, Cote RJ, Freeman JA, et al. Indications for lower urinary tract reconstruction in women after cystectomy for bladder cancer: a pathological review of female cystectomy specimens. *J Urol* 1995;154:1329.

Stein JP, Esrig D, Freeman JA, et al. Prospective pathologic analysis of female cystectomy specimens: risk factors for orthotopic diversion in women. *Urology* 1998;51:951.

Stein JP, Grossfeld G, Freeman JA, et al. Orthotopic lower urinary tract reconstruction in women using the Kock ileal neobladder: updated experience in 27 patients. *J Urol* 1997;158:400.

Stein JP, Lieskovsky G, Cote R, et al. Radical cystectomy in the treatment of invasive bladder cancer: long-term results in 1054 patients. *J Clin Oncol* 2001;19:666.

Stein JP, Lieskovsky G, Ginsberg DA, et al. The T-pouch: an orthotopic ileal neobladder incorporating a serosal lined ileal antireflux technique. *J Urol* 1998;159:1836.

Stein JP, Quek MD, Skinner DG. Contemporary surgical techniques for continent urinary diversion: continence and potency preservation. In: Libertino JA, Zinman LN, eds. *Atlas of urologic clinics of North America.* Philadelphia: W. B. Saunders, 2001:147.

Stein JP, Skinner DG. Orthotopic bladder replacement. In: Walsh PC, Retik AB, Vaughan ED, et al., eds. *Campbell's urology,* 8th ed. Philadelphia: W. B. Saunders, 2002:3835.

Stein JP, Skinner DG. Radical cystectomy in the female. In: Montie, JA, ed. *Atlas of urologic clinics of North America.* Philadelphia: W. B. Saunders, 1997:37.

Stein JP, Stenzl A, Esrig D, et al. Lower urinary tract reconstruction following cystectomy in women using the Kock ileal reservoir with bilateral ureteroileal urethrostomy: initial clinical experience. *J Urol* 1994;152:1404.

Vazina A, Dugi D, Shariat SF, et al. Stage specific lymph node metastasis mapping in radical cystectomy specimens. *J Urol* 2004;171:1830.

Vieweg J, Gschwend JE, Herr HW, et al. The impact of primary stage on survival in patients with lymph node positive bladder cancer. *J Urol* 1999;161:72.

EDITOR'S COMMENT

This chapter is in keeping with the theme in other areas of the book such as rectal cancer, in which restorative function has advanced in the past decade to the point that what was previously a very destructive operative procedure with a conduit that ends on the abdominal wall is now being replaced by orthotopic reconstruction of the bladder for bladder cancer. The chapter also argues for an aggressive approach for organ-confined, lymph node–negative carcinoma of the bladder, including muscle-invasive p2A and p2B, in which their own results show 85%, 5-year disease-free survival and 82% 10-year disease-free recurrence. It also argues for early, aggressive cystectomy for superficial tumors limited to the lamina propria that have not responded to therapy (Stein JP. *Urology* 2003;62:591). Also, other evidence (Sanchez-Ortiz RF. *J Urol* 2003;169:110) is seen that indicates that delay in definitive therapy for more than 12 weeks following bladder invasion leads to a poorer outcome.

In view of these data, the report of Prout Jr et al. (*Cancer* 2005;104:1638) based on 820 patients from the National Cancer Institute's Surveillance, Epidemiology, and End Results program diagnosed in 1992, at age 55 years, borders on the shocking. "Among the patients with muscle invasion, those age 75 years and older were less likely to undergo radical cystectomy (14%) compared with patients ages 55-64 years (48%) and those ages 65-74 years (43%)." One hopes that the percentages undergoing radical cystectomy since that time have increased because the patients, certainly those under the age of 75, are exquisitely amenable to improvement in survival as the authors argue for cogently.

Unfortunately, there is no level I evidence of quality of life and the reconstruction. Gerharz et al. (*J Urol* 2005;174:1729) failed to find any report rising above level III concerning the quality of life depending on reconstruction following radical cystectomy. They pointed out that even patients who are in hospice may have a reasonable quality of life. They called for randomized prospective trials. Many of the centers with excellent volumes could pool their patients and come up with a randomized prospective trial, which would answer these questions. However, unless individuals who are so convinced of the superiority of their method will do a randomized prospective trial between ileal conduits, for example, ending on the abdominal wall and orthotopic reconstruction, participation is unlikely.

Despite these difficulties, this is a difficult and lethal lesion and needs therapy in a timely fashion. The reason more patients did not undergo radical cystectomy, I believe, is that this is a tedious and difficult operation, which should not be performed outside of centers experienced in this procedure. This statement is not easy for me to make. The demographics of patients throughout this country are such that a number of patients with this quite common disease are reluctant to travel to other institutions distant from where they are, and will be treated in areas in which this expertise is not available. Nonetheless, it appears that this is worthwhile. In addition, as I found in Cincinnati working with Lester Martin on the S-pouch ileal pouch–anal anastomosis, which we began to perform together in 1979, once it was clear that one could restore transrectal function in moving one's bowels, the referrals from gastroenterologists took place at an earlier time in the disease. Hopefully, as Prout said in his article (previously cited), the interval between 1992 and the present has spread the ability to perform this operation, which, indeed, does seem to offer a great deal more than radiation and chemotherapy for a disease that has invaded the muscle.

A few technical details. Were I doing an operation of this magnitude in a patient with impaired cardiac disease, I probably would not digitalize them preoperatively but monitor their fluid status with a central venous pressure (CVP) monitor. We are currently treating patients in the elderly group, and in general, with Kehlet's Fast Track surgery, which minimizes crystalloid therapy during the operation and following the operation minimizes opiates with epidurals. Thus, the mobilization of intraoperative fluid is less pronounced and occurs earlier in the second or third postoperative day. If one is concerned about the failure, one should probably use the CVP to monitor fluid status. As far as antibiotics in the postoperative period, my own practice is to use only a single dose of perioperative antibiotics in patients in whom there is not widespread contamination and the operation lasts 3.5 hours or less. In excess of this time period, a second dose is given of short-acting antibiotics. At the most, I may give a single additional dose in the recovery room. It does not seem to me that there is any evidence that treating patients such as this, just because the small bowel was violated, offers any improvement in outcome.

What is the nature of the extensive lymph node dissection? Is this for staging or is it for cure? In many diseases, including breast cancer, the predominance of opinion has shifted from that of excision of lymph nodes not related to an attempted cure, but at staging. However, it is my belief, as well as many others dealing with carcinoma of the breast, that this is a systemic disease when it is initially discovered. This seems to be different. The extent of dissection and the median number of lymph nodes appears to correlate with long-term survival as the authors argue the number of lymph nodes removed seems to correlate with survival. Is this a question of experience in carrying out the cystectomy or is this a question of surgical skill? It is interesting that in the multidisciplinary study referred to (Grossman HB, et al. *N Engl J Med* 2003;349:859; Herr HW. *Br J Urol Int* 2003;92:187), 14% of the patients undergoing cystectomy had no lymph node dissection at all. Thus, if this disease is not systemic at the time of discovery, patients may have a better chance the more lymph

(continued)

nodes are resected, especially if there are some positives.

What about chemotherapy postoperatively? Lehmann et al. (*Br J Urol Int* 2006;97:42), from Mainz, Germany, in a center for bladder carcinoma began a randomized prospective trial in postoperative chemotherapy for observation only or systemic chemotherapy with methotrexate, vinblastine, and doxorubicin. They initially intended to randomize 100 patients, 50 to each group. When analyzing the results at the midway point, they noted that the differences between survival were so striking, with 10-year reoccurrence-free survival of 47% estimated and 13% in the control group, that the trial was stopped. The authors of the chapter are vigorous proponents of aggressive chemotherapy postoperatively.

Who are candidates for this type of therapy? Women, of course. Nesrallah et al. (*Br J Urol Int* 2005;95:1045) reported on 29 women who underwent orthotopic ileal neobladder (without the

p-piece). Sixty-five percent of their patients, 1,929, were alive and disease free with a mean follow-up of 35 months. Age is also an issue. Zebic et al. (*Br J Urol Int* 2005;95:1211), writing from Essen, Germany, analyzed 53 patients between the ages of 75 and 90 undergoing radical cystectomy between 1994 and 2002. Forty-six patients were treated with curative intent and seven with palliative intent for severe irritative voiding symptoms, severe pain, and recurrent macrohematuria requiring blood transfusions. The mortality was 4% in the curative group and two of the seven died after palliative surgery with prolonged complications. This is consistent with the experience of most other patients with advanced disease undergoing palliative care. Patients who undergo renal transplantation also developed bladder cancer and they, according to Lang et al. (*J Urol* 2005; 173:881), should be offered radical cystectomy and orthotopic reconstruction. Four patients were reported: Two patients died at 11 and 15 months of tumor progression and a pulmonary embolus, whereas two were alive with no evident disease at 90

months. Thus, at least in two patients the specter of tumor progression with immunosuppression did not appear to be a factor.

Finally, and inevitably, there is evidence of a laparoscopic approach to this operation. Turk et al. (*J Urol* 2001;165:1863) and Gill et al. (*J Urol* 2002; 168:13) reported the totally intracorporeal laparoscopic approach to radical cystectomy. While this can be done, the operation may be slightly different. I would think that trying to do a T-valve orthotopic neobladder would probably be extraordinarily difficult. Finally, given the data of the number of lymph nodes excised and the more favorable outcome with a more aggressive lymph node dissection, one wonders whether an operation that takes 9 or 10 hours, at least with initial experience, will give us good results when the lymph node dissection will probably be more difficult carried out closed then open. However, with increased experience it may prove to be as effective.

J.E.F.

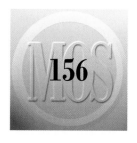

Laparoscopic Pelvic and Retroperitoneal Lymph Node Dissection

GUILHERME LIMA, MARK NOGUEIRA, AND LOUIS R. KAVOUSSI

Regional lymphadenectomy is an important part in the management of genitourinary malignancies. In an effort to minimize the morbidity of lymph node dissection, laparoscopic techniques have been applied to perform these procedures. The principal types of urologic laparoscopic lymph node dissection are pelvic lymphadenectomy for prostate, bladder, and penile cancer and retroperitoneal lymphadenectomy for testis cancer.

Laparoscopic Pelvic Lymphadenectomy

Prostate cancer is the most common noncutaneous malignancy in men. In 2003, approximately 220,900 cases were diagnosed and 28,900 died of prostate cancer in the United States. Curative therapy for prostate cancer is either surgical removal via the retropubic, laparoscopic, or perineal approaches as well as radiation therapy delivered by external beam or placement of interstitial implants. Pelvic lymphadenectomy has been performed to identify patients with lymphatogenous metastasis who would not be cured by localized therapy and, as such, is performed purely for staging purposes.

Open pelvic lymph node dissection (PLND) at the time of prostatectomy remains the most common method for detecting lymphatogenous metastasis. Imaging modalities such as computed tomography (CT) and magnetic resonance imaging (MRI) evaluate lymph node size rather than the presence of tumor within the nodes, which results in a high false-positive rate. Other diagnostic modalities such as fine needle aspiration cytology and immunoscintigraphy are also not very accurate.

In order to obtain accurate staging in men with prostate cancer, laparoscopic pelvic lymph node dissection (LPLND) was introduced by Schuessler in 1991. Subsequent studies have demonstrated that the LPLND and open PLND are equivalent with respect to nodal yield. Many studies confirmed that analgesic use, length of hospital stay, and duration of convalescence are less with LPLND than with standard open PLND.

CLINICAL PRESENTATION

Owing to increased public awareness and the use of prostatic-specific antigen (PSA) screening, most men with prostate cancer

present with low-stage organ-confined disease. In fact, only 5% of individuals with prostate cancer have lymph node metastasis at time of diagnosis. With the advent of reliable nomograms, based on patient clinical stage, PSA level, and histologic Gleason score, PLND for prostate cancer is no longer universally required.

Recognizing that only patients at risk require lymphadenectomy, what clinical situations warrant LPLND? Low-risk patients electing to undergo radical retropubic prostatectomy would not benefit from LPLND, because open PLND is performed through the same incision as prostatectomy. Specific clinical situations that would require LPLND include high-risk patients considering perineal prostatectomy and those that need nodal staging before initiating radiation therapy.

LPLND has also been applied to other nonprostatic genitourinary malignancies. Select patients with carcinomas of the bladder, penis, or urethra may require a LPLND. In cases of transitional cell carcinoma of the bladder, PLND offers both prognostic and potentially therapeutic benefits. The number of lymph nodes removed during cystectomy has been shown to correlate with survival, and it is currently recommended that a minimum

Nongastrointestinal Transabdominal

of 10 to 14 nodes be removed. With respect to penile carcinoma, radical ilioinguinal lymph node dissection is associated with a potential for high morbidity. In patients with positive pelvic lymph nodes, excision of ilioinguinal lymph nodes is not curative. As such, PLND may obviate the need for ilioinguinal dissection, thereby sparing the patient additional morbidity. PLND is indicated in patients with penile cancer who have enlarged pelvic lymph nodes on CT (>2 cm) and/or more than two positive nodes involved with disease at the time of inguinal lymphadenectomy. Urethral carcinoma is relatively rare, and therefore the role of lymphadenectomy is not clearly outlined in most treatment strategies. Positive lymph nodes in this setting, however, are believed to portend a poor prognosis and would likely preclude aggressive surgical management. Differences in technique for each of these disease processes will be discussed in the technical portion of the chapter.

 PREOPERATIVE PLANNING

For those patients at high risk of lymphatic metastasis, radiographic studies, such as CT of the abdomen and pelvis, should be obtained before surgery to detect gross nodal disease. Diagnostic biopsy in patients with adenopathy may preclude the need for surgical intervention. Bone scan should be reserved for those patients who have PSA of or above 20, who have an elevated alkaline phosphatase, or who are symptomatic with bone pain.

Patients should receive appropriate preoperative antibiotic coverage, typically a first-generation cephalosporin. A type and screen for blood products is appropriate. In addition, patients who are scheduled to undergo concurrent prostatectomy should receive a mechanical bowel prep. A full bowel prep may be helpful in patients who are expected to have extensive intra-abdominal adhesions.

Positioning and Setup

A general anesthesia is utilized and an orogastric tube is placed to empty the stomach. A Foley catheter is inserted to decompress the bladder. The scrotum and penis are wrapped with a compressive gauze to prevent pneumoscrotum/penis. The scrotum represents a potential space into which gas can track during the procedure. The patient is placed supine with both arms secured at the side (Fig. 1).

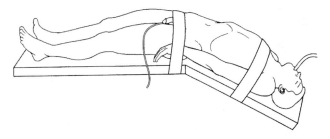

Fig. 1. The patient is positioned supine, and, after trocar placement, the table is flexed to move the bowel after the pelvis. A bladder catheter and orogastric tube are placed. The patient is secured to permit maximal table rotation.

The positioning of the surgical team is represented in Figure 2. The anesthesiologist is at the head of the table. The operating surgeon is on the contralateral side of the table from the lymph node packet to be excised. The assistant is opposite the surgeon while the scrub nurse and Mayo stand are placed adjacent and superior to the operating surgeon. The video equipment is placed at the foot of the table such that the surgeon is facing the same direction as he or she is operating.

Port Placement

Pneumoperitoneum is initiated by the placement of a Veress needle into the base

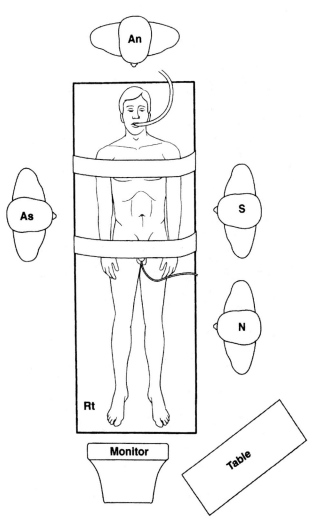

Fig. 2. Surgical team is positioned as depicted for laparoscopic pelvic lymph node dissection. An, anesthesiologist; As, assistant surgeon; N, scrub technician or nurse; S, surgeon.

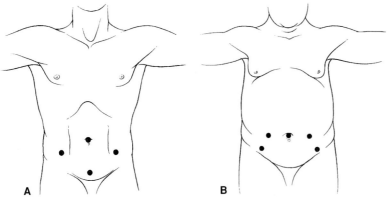

Fig. 3. A: "Diamond" configuration for laparoscopic pelvic lymph node dissection port placement. **B:** "Fan" configuration for port placement in obese patient.

of the umbilicus. The surgeon's hand or towel clamp is used to elevate the abdominal wall during placement of the Veress needle. Proper placement is confirmed by the observation that intraabdominal pressure remains low during low-flow gas insufflation and by the saline "drop test." The abdomen can then be insufflated to a pressure of 15 to 20 mm Hg. A 1-cm incision is made at the umbilicus. A hemostat is used to dissect the subcutaneous fat down to the fascia. A laparoscope with a 0-degree lens is placed within the 10-mm Visiport (U.S. Surgical, Norwalk, CT) or Optiview (Ethicon Endosurgical, Cincinati, OH) incising visual obturator. The camera is focused on the tip of the obturator. The camera and trocar can then be advanced under direct vision into the peritoneal cavity. After removal of the obturator, the 30-degree camera lens is placed through the umbilical trocar. After inspection of the abdominal cavity to rule out viscus or vascular injury and adhesions, additional working trocars are placed.

The typical port site pattern is illustrated in Figure 3A. A "diamond" configuration is most commonly used. The camera is typically situated at the umbilical port. A trocar is placed approximately four fingerbreadths above the pubic bone. The lateral trocars are placed one third of the way from the umbilicus to the anterior superior iliac spine on each side. In obese patients, a "fan" configuration facilitates retraction and dissection (Fig. 3B). For the nonumbilical ports, any combination of 5- and 10-mm ports is acceptable, depending on the surgeon's preference. After trocar placement, the patient is put in the Trendelenburg position, which allows gravity to keep the intestines out of the pelvis during dissection.

SURGICAL TECHNIQUE

The anatomic landmarks are illustrated in Figure 4. The limits of resection are the pubic bone distally, the bifurcation of the common iliac vessels proximally, the external iliac vein anteriorly, the obturator nerve posteriorly, the medial umbilical ligament medially, and the pelvic sidewall laterally. Note that during dissection, metal clips should be judiciously used on the lymphatic tissue to decrease risk of lymphocele formation.

A longitudinal incision is made in the peritoneum lateral to the medial umbilical ligament (Fig. 5). This extends from the pubic symphysis to just proximal to the iliac vessels. On the left side, it is quite common to encounter adhesions to the sigmoid colon that need to be incised first. Once the peritoneum is opened, the vas deferens is identified and divided (Fig. 6). Next, the medial edge of the iliac vein is identified and, by retracting the nodal tissue medially, the node tissue is freed from the pubic bone to the bifurcation of the common iliac vessels (Fig. 7). This defines the lateral border of the nodal packet. The nodal packet is then dissected free posteriorly from the obturator internus muscle. The dissection proceeds proximally toward the junction of the medial umbilical ligament and the bifurcation of the iliac vessels (Fig. 8). This maneuver exposes the obturator nerve and vessels (Fig. 9). Care must be taken to avoid injury to the ureter, which lies medial at this point.

The medial edge of the dissection is defined by retracting the medial umbilical ligament medially while pulling the nodal packet laterally. Blunt dissection at this point frees nodal tissue. Distal attachments beneath the pubis are clipped and transected. The entire packet is pulled cranially, and final attachments at the junction of the medial umbilical ligament and the hypogastric artery are clipped and divided.

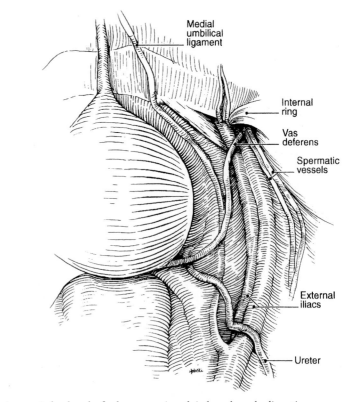

Fig. 4. Anatomic landmarks for laparoscopic pelvic lymph node dissection.

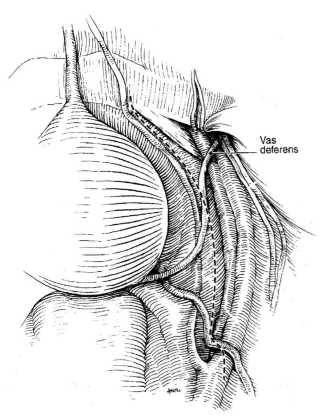

Fig. 5. An incision is made lateral to the medial umbilical ligament. This is extended from the pubic bone to the bifurcation of the common iliac vessels.

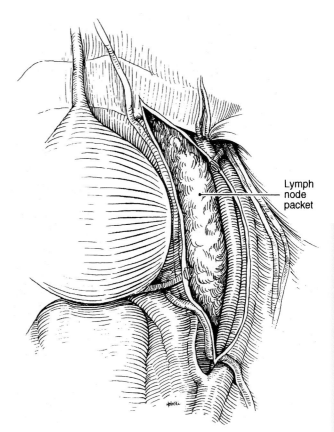

Fig. 7. The lateral edge of the lymph node packet is developed. The medial edge of the iliac vein and the nodal tissue are identified.

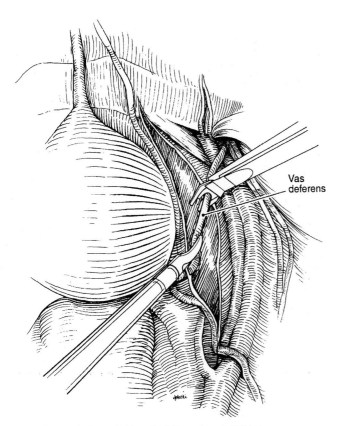

Fig. 6. The vas deferens is identified, ligated, and divided.

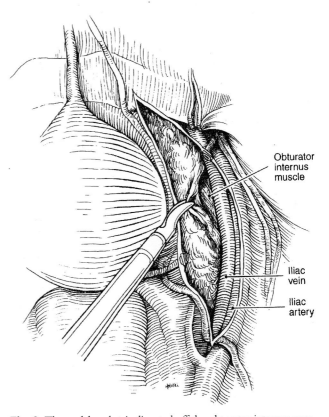

Fig. 8. The nodal packet is dissected off the obturator internus muscle, and the dissection proceeds proximally toward the junctions of the medial umbilical ligament and the bifurcation of the iliac vessels.

Nongastrointestinal Transabdominal

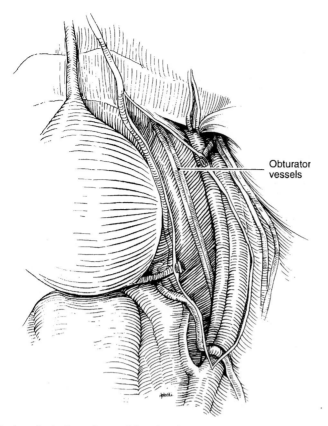

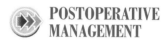

Fig. 9. With the lymphatic tissue dissected free, the obturator nerve vessels should be visible.

The specimen can then be extracted from the body using an Endocatch bag (U.S. Surgical, Norwalk, CT) or a laparoscopic spoon forceps (Fig. 10). The contralateral side is addressed in a similar fashion.

After completing the lymph node dissection, it is imperative to examine the operative site under low insufflation pressure to ensure hemostasis. Hemostasis is achieved using cautery and surgical clip

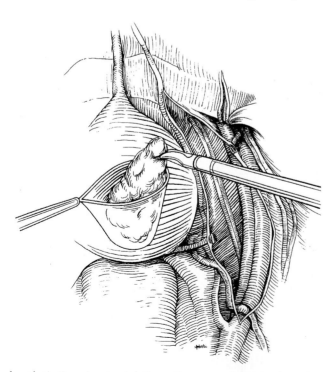

Fig. 10. The lymphatic tissue is extracted. Depending on specimen size, it can be extracted with an Endocatch bag.

placement. A final survey of the peritoneal cavity is performed to rule out visceral injury. Closure of trocar entry sites is achieved under direct vision. Before securing the last trocar site, an effort is made to expel all CO_2 from the peritoneum. The port site incisions are closed with absorbable sutures in a subcuticular fashion or with skin glue.

Modification of the dissection template is necessary when performing lymphadenectomy for other genitourinary malignancies. Carcinomas of the penis, bladder, and urethra require an extended version of the pelvic lymphadenectomy. The margins of the resection are extended to the genitofemoral nerve laterally and the common iliac artery proximally.

POSTOPERATIVE MANAGEMENT

The orogastric tube is removed at the end of the procedure. The Foley catheter is removed when the patient is ambulatory. Oral intake can begin the evening of the surgery. Typically hospitalization is less than 24 hours.

COMPLICATIONS

General complications of LPLND are similar to those seen in all laparoscopic surgery and include ileus, deep vein thrombosis, or urinary retention. Vascular injuries can occur during trocar placement or nodal dissection. Most commonly, the inferior epigastric vessels are injured during lateral trocar placement. The external iliac and obturator vessels can also be injured during nodal dissection. Despite the close proximity of these vessels, vascular injury is rare, occurring in approximately 2% to 3% of cases.

Care must be taken to identify and avoid clipping or transecting the obturator nerve. Also, cases of transection or occlusion of the ureter have been reported. Identification of these structures will minimize this risk.

Viscus injuries are also rare; most of these are bowel and bladder injuries. These injuries can occur during trocar placement or dissection. Decompression of viscus by orogastric tubes or Foley catheters can minimize the potential for these injuries. Injuries that are recognized intraoperatively can be repaired at the same time as surgery. Unrecognized bowel injury can present postoperatively as fever, abdominal pain, ileus, or diarrhea. Prompt imaging of

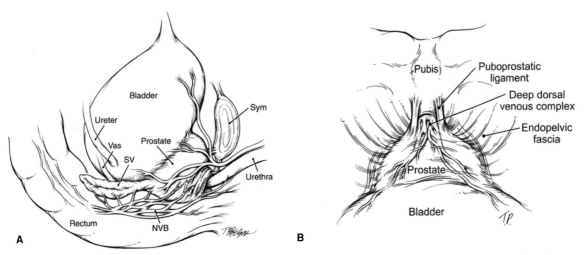

Fig. 1. Details of male retropubic anatomy that are relevant to radical prostatectomy. **A:** Sagittal view. **B:** View from surgeon's perspective. (Copyright 2005 Johns Hopkins University.)

Though historically performed routinely during radical prostatectomy, lymphadenectomy can also be performed selectively in just those cases with risk factors for extraprostatic extension (such as serum prostate-specific antigen [PSA] level >10 ng/mL or Gleason score >6). The purpose of the lymphadenectomy in radical prostatectomy is purely diagnostic, with the results possibly influencing use of adjuvant therapies or frequency of follow-up. However, the use of frozen section at the time of radical prostatectomy as a decision point for determining whether or not to proceed with prostatectomy has largely been abandoned, in part because it is recognized that prostatectomy can provide effective local control that may have benefits even in the setting of lymph node metastases. For pelvic lymphadenectomy, borders include the external iliac vein anteriorly, the obturator nerve posteriorly, the bifurcation of the iliac vein as the cephalad extent, and the pelvic side wall as the caudal extent of the removed lymph node specimen. One or two clips placed at the proximal and distal border of the nodal packet are usually sufficient to prevent significant lymphatic leak.

The Deep Dorsal Vein and Anterior Prostatic Apex

Many components of the dissection of the prostate, nerve-sparing, and subsequent vesicourethral anastomosis are performed using modifications of technique first described by Walsh. To expose the deep dorsal vein and anterior prostatic apex (Fig. 1B), a notched retractor blade is used to retract the bladder superiorly by traction on the Foley catheter and balloon within the bladder dome. The endopelvic fascia is incised, the puboprostatic ligaments are divided with scissors, and the superficial dorsal vein is cauterized and divided. Excessive use of electrocautery beyond the prostatic apex should be avoided, as it can injure sphincteric nerves. Cephalad retraction of the prostatic apex by a sponge stick improves retropubic exposure of the deep dorsal vein. For hemostasis before dividing the deep dorsal vein, two figure-of-eight suture ligatures (0-chromic on a CT-1 needle) are placed to secure the deep dorsal vein proximally and distally (Fig. 2). These suture ligatures can control the anterior component of the dorsal venous complex, but in many cases may not control the posterolateral extensions of the deep dorsal vein. A harmonic scalpel or ultrasonic shears are advantageous for division of the deep dorsal venous complex as these provide improved hemostasis during division of the dorsal vein, particularly in the posterolateral extension of this venous complex as it drapes around the membranous urethra. Care again should be taken to avoid excessive use of ultrasonic or harmonic scissors, as these can generate significant heat that can cause thermal injury to adjacent nerves. The cavernous nerves and sphincteric nerves course posterolateral to the membranous urethra (Fig. 3), so use of the harmonic scalpel posterior to the urethra should be avoided. In cases when hemostasis is not adequate following division of the deep dorsal vein, the distal venous complex can be oversewn with a running 2-0 chromic suture on a UR-6 needle (the UR-6 nee-dle size facilitates effective hemostasis suturing of the deep dorsal vein while avoiding both the levator ani and the urethra within the narrow confines of the male pelvis).

Dissecting the Membranous Urethra and Prostatic Apex

Division of the deep dorsal vein exposes the urethra below. After incision of the anterior and lateral urethral wall with scissors, sutures for the eventual vesicourethral anastomosis (2-0 Monocryl) are anchored in the urethra at the 12 o'-clock, 3 o'clock, and 9 o'clock positions. The Foley catheter is then divided at the urethral meatus, the cut end withdrawn into the pelvis and there secured with a cocker clamp to keep the balloon inflated in the bladder, to later serve for traction and as a guide for bladder neck transection. The fourth anastomotic suture is placed at the 6 o'clock position, and the posterior urethra is then cut to complete transection of the urethra at the prostatic apex. The posterior striated sphincter, or rectourethralis muscle, is then divided sharply to reveal Denonvilliers fascia beyond the edge of the posterior prostatic apex below (Fig. 4).

Posterolateral Dissection of the Cavernous Nerves and Prostatic Pedicles

Denonvilliers fascia is divided sharply in the midline, beyond the prostatic apex and between the laterally positioned neurovascular bundles (composed of cavernous

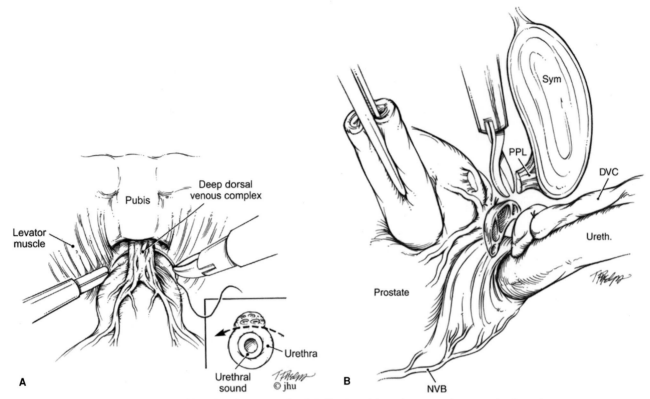

Fig. 2. A: Suture ligation of deep dorsal vein complex (DVC), viewed from the surgeon's perspective. Inset shows proper plane of needle passage between DVC and urethra. **B:** Division of the deep dorsal vein accomplished by harmonic scalpel after placement proximal and distal suture ligature, sagittal view. (Copyright 2005 Johns Hopkins University.)

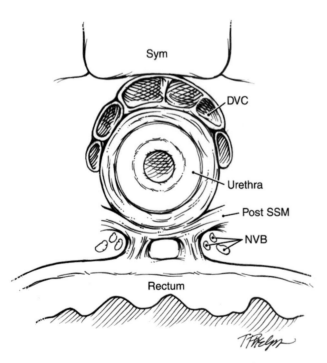

Fig. 3. Transverse view at the distal urethral margin of prostatic apical dissection, demonstrating the deep dorsal vein draped over the urethra anterolaterally, striated sphincteric fibers posteriorly, and neurovascular bundles just posterolateral to the striated urinary sphincter/rectourethralis muscle. Note the course of the neurovascular bundles at the 5 and 7 o'clock position along the urethra.

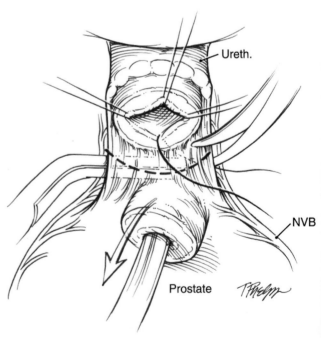

Fig. 4. Positioning of the urethral anastomotic sutures followed by division of the posterior striated sphincter/rectourethralis muscle just anterior to the neurovascular bundle.

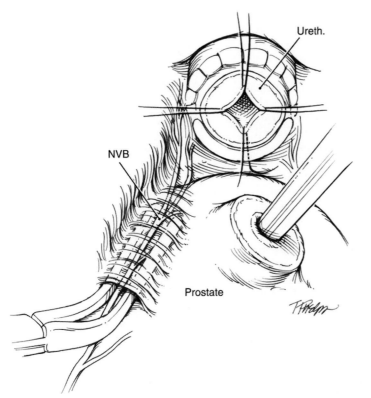

Fig. 5. Elevating the lateral pelvic fascia off the lateral prostate to facilitate preservation of the cavernous nerves (neurovascular bundle, NVB).

Wide Excision of the Neurovascular Bundle

If preoperative studies (e.g., findings on rectal examination or endorectal, contrast-enhanced magnetic resonance imaging [MRI] scan) or intraoperative findings indicate presence of tumor close enough to the neurovascular bundle that sparing of the cavernous nerves would jeopardize surgical margins, then the neurovascular bundle on the affected side should be widely excised. Wide excision is accomplished by retrograde dissection identical to that described above, except that the lateral pelvic fascia is not incised, and hence the neurovascular bundle and any associated extraprostatic tumor remains closely attached to the posterolateral border of the prostate. The dissection proceeds laterally across the neurovascular bundle beyond the prostatic apex, clipping and dividing the bundle immediately after it is exposed following division of the rectourethralis muscle and incision of Denonvilliers fascia beyond the prostatic apex. The retrograde dissection separating the prostate from rectum proceeds superiorly and laterally beyond the neurovascular bundle, and generally little need for hemostatic clips is encountered until the dissection reaches the seminal vesicles, where the posterolateral pedicles to the prostate are encountered and managed as described above.

Transection of the Bladder Neck and Vasa Deferentia; Dissection of the Seminal Vesicle

After completing retrograde dissection of the prostate, the Foley balloon is released

nerves that mediate erectile function and sphincteric nerves that mediate urethral sphincter tone). For nerve-sparing dissection, the lateral pelvic fascia (that covers the lateral prostate and cavernous neurovascular bundle) is elevated from the prostate and nerves below with a sharp right-angle clamp and is divided sharply from prostatic apex to the bladder neck. This maneuver exposes the prostatic border and neurovascular bundle, and also releases the neurovascular bundle laterally, facilitating its subsequent preservation (Fig. 5). A fine-tipped right-angle clamp is then used to sequentially separate the remaining attachments of the neurovascular bundle from the lateral border of the prostate, with vascular branches clipped for hemostasis, while minimizing traumatic traction to the neurovascular bundle by minimizing cephalad traction on the prostate. During the retrograde dissection (Fig. 6), the midposterior prostate capsule and Denonvilliers fascia are separated with ease from the prerectal fat in the midline, although fibrous remnants from prostate biopsies can be encountered, and these are best divided sharply with scissors. At the level of the seminal vesicles, Denonvilliers fascia is again incised sharply, and posterolateral vascular pedicles to the prostate are clipped and divided to reveal the border

between the seminal vesicle and posterior bladder neck. The space between the seminal vesicle and bladder neck is developed with a blunt right-angle clamp that can be passed entirely though the space from right to left; this maneuver, mobilizing the seminal vesicles away from the posterior bladder neck, facilitates subsequent transection of the posterior bladder neck.

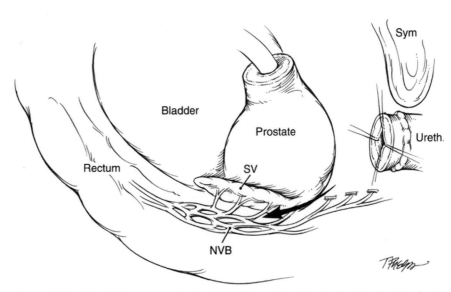

Fig. 6. Relationship of the neurovascular bundle, bladder neck, and seminal vesicles: Sparing the tips of large seminal vesicles can reduce dissection and traction injury to the cavernous neural plexus.

from under the cephalad retractor and is placed on caudal traction to define the border between the bladder neck and anterolateral prostate. Indigo carmine is administered intravenously to subsequently facilitate identifying the ureteral orifices. Vascular pedicles coursing from the inferior vesicle pedicle to the prostate are isolated, clipped, and divided. Electrocautery is used to incise the anterior bladder neck 1 to 2 cm above the prostate, and a gooseneck clamp (e.g., Semb clamp) is passed between the seminal vesicles and posterior bladder neck to elevate the posterior bladder neck and to clearly define the border between the posterior bladder neck and prostate, where the bladder neck is then transected. Some surgeons have espoused bladder neck "preservation" for optimizing functional recovery (efforts to preserve circular muscle fibers at the junction of the prostate and bladder). However, outcomes studies showed no such benefit when bladder neck sparing was evaluated, whereas higher rates of cancer present at the surgical margins were encountered.

After transection of the bladder neck (Fig. 7), the vasa deferentia are clipped and divided, and seminal vesicles are freed from investing neurovascular attachments (which are clipped and divided), thereby completing the detachment of the entire prostate, seminal vesicles, and ampullae of the vasa en bloc. The close proximity of the tips of the seminal vesicles to the plexus of the cavernous nerves, however, has prompted some to consider sparing of the seminal vesicle tips as a means of further reducing traumatic traction and unintended injury to the cavernous nerves. This refined excision plan should be reserved only for cases that have a favorable cancer severity profile (clinical stage = T1, or Gleason pattern <7, PSA <10, and cancer involving <50% of any biopsy core) wherein seminal vesicle involvement by the cancer is unlikely.

Interposition Nerve Grafts for Replacing Widely Excised Cavernous Nerves

Interposition nerve grafts can be placed to span the excised course of the cavernous nerves. The graft is typically harvested from the sural nerve, though use of genitofemoral nerves has also been described. The nerve for grafting can be harvested by a plastic surgery team operating in tandem on the sural nerve during the latter phases of retrograde dissection of the prostate. A graft length of 7 to 10 cm is generally required, and the anastomosis is completed after using interrupted 6-0 suture after removal of the prostate and before completion of the vesicourethral anastomosis. The distal anastomosis is readily accomplished as the cavernous nerves are coalesced in the distal stump. However, the cavernous nerve plexus has a propensity to fan out into multiple smaller branches more proximally, often leaving smaller-caliber recipient ends for the proximal graft anastomosis. It has been proposed that such interposition grafts may benefit urinary or erection recovery; however, in our experience grafts were associated with recovery benefit only when the contralateral neurovascular bundle was able to be spared, leaving some uncertainty as to whether recovery was consequent to the interposition graft or due to unintentional bias toward more meticulous technique on the side of the preserved cavernous nerves.

Vesicourethral Anastomosis and Closure

After hemostasis is secured following removal of the prostate and seminal vesicles, the caliber of the transected bladder neck opening is reduced by placement of interrupted 2-0 chromic sutures with care taken to avoid ureteral orifices that are visualized by their excretion of indigo carmine. The mucosa is everted using 4-0 chromic suture placed at the lateral and anterior aspect of the bladder neck; mucosa at the posterior edge of the reconstructed bladder neck is everted by placement of a full-thickness, mucosa-muscularis-mucosa vesical stitch of 2-0 chromic on a UR-6 needle. Maintaining a 22 French caliber opening in the reconstructed bladder neck can help prevent later urethral strictures. Although use of a variety of anterior bladder "tubes" fashioned to reduce early incontinence can lead to marginally earlier continence recovery, such reconstructive maneuvers have also been associated with a significantly increased rate of later urethral strictures, the adverse consequences of which outweigh the marginally earlier continence benefits. After the bladder neck is calibrated to 22 French and mucosa everted, the previously placed 2-0 Monocryl sutures in the urethral stump are brought to their corresponding position on the bladder neck with a French eye needle, and a clear 20 French Foley catheter is positioned into the bladder and balloon filled with 5 mL of saline. Retaining the hyperextended position improves access to and visibility of the vesicourethral anastomosis, and thereby facilitates tying of the anastomotic sutures in place as the bladder is reapproximated to the urethral stump (Fig. 8). The catheter is irrigated; a watertight anastomosis is the goal. Minor leaks can be expected to resolve with drainage, whereas copious leaks warrant closer inspection to ascertain integrity of the vesicourethral anastomosis. A closed suction drain is placed in the space of Retzius through a lateral stab incision, the midline fascia is closed with running monofilament suture, and the skin is closed with running subcuticular suture.

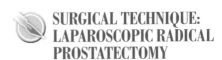

SURGICAL TECHNIQUE: LAPAROSCOPIC RADICAL PROSTATECTOMY

LRP can be performed by either a transperitoneal or extraperitoneal approach. In this section we will describe the transperitoneal

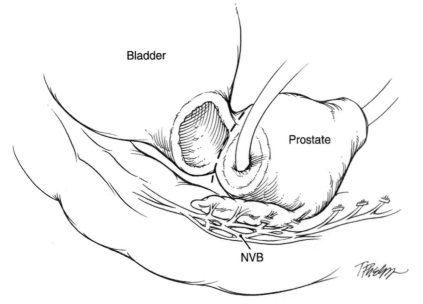

Fig. 7. Transection of the bladder neck.

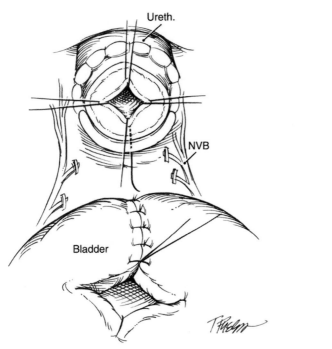

Fig. 8. Reapproximating the reconstructed bladder neck to the membranous urethra.

laparoscopic approach and highlight minor differences in the extraperitoneal technique and RAP technique. For preoperative preparation, patients are advised to remain on clear liquids 24 hours prior to surgery and to administer one bottle of citrate of magnesium as a bowel preparation, as well as to self-administer a Fleets enema the evening prior to laparoscopic prostatectomy.

Patient Positioning

After induction of general endotracheal anesthesia, the patient is placed in the supine position with arms tucked and padded at the sides. The legs are spread as far as possible to allow for access to the rectum and perineum. An AESOP robotic arm (Intuitive Surgical, Sunnyvale, CA) is attached to the operative table at the level of the patient's right shoulder and can be controlled either by voice activation or by the assistant using a handheld remote control device. The patient is secured to the table at the level of the shoulders and thighs with cloth tape. The table is then placed in a steep Trendelenburg position. An orogastric tube and urethral catheter are placed to decompress the stomach and bladder respectively. In the RAP technique, the patient's legs are placed in stirrups in the low lithotomy position and spread widely to allow the daVinci robot to be "docked" to the operating table between the patient's legs.

Abdominal Access

For a transperitoneal LRP approach, a Veress needle is inserted at the umbilicus and abdominal insufflation is achieved. The abdominal insufflation pressure is maintained at 15 mm Hg. Primary trocar placement is accomplished using a Visiport device (United States Surgical Corporation, Norwalk, CT) inserted through a 1.5-cm horizontal incision at the base of the umbilicus. Alternatively, an open or Hasson technique may be used to place the primary trocar. Secondary trocars are then placed under laparoscopic view including a 12-mm right pararectus trocar, a 5-mm left pararectus trocar, and two 5-mm trocars placed halfway between the anterior superior iliac crest and pararectus trocar on the right and left sides (Fig. 9). The surgeon operates primarily through the two pararectus ports and the assistant through the 5-mm trocar in the right lower quadrant. The left lower quadrant 5-mm trocar is used for retraction purposes and can be manipulated by a second assistant or endoscopic instrument holder.

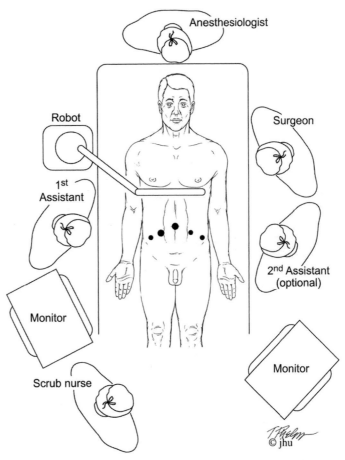

Fig. 9. Trocar configuration for laparoscopic radical prostatectomy. (Copyright 2005 Johns Hopkins University.)

Nongastrointestinal Transabdominal

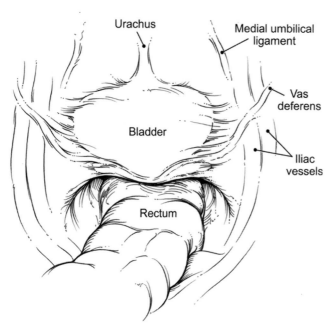

Fig. 10. Initial view of the pelvis following trocar placement. Relevant landmarks include the bladder, rectum, vas deferentia, and median umbilical ligaments (Copyright 2005 Johns Hopkins University.)

The robotic-assisted approach is similar to the transperitoneal approach described above with the exception of trocar configuration. After Veress needle insufflation, a 12-mm trocar is introduced immediately above the umbilicus and is used for introduction of the three-dimensional laparoscope lens. Two 8-mm daVinci metal trocars are placed bilaterally in the pararectus location, approximately 2.5 cm below the level of the umbilicus, and serve as the primary trocars for insertion of the two robotic arms and instruments. A 5-mm trocar is placed between the umbilicus and the 8-mm port on the right side of the abdomen. A 12-mm trocar is placed in the midaxillary line and 2.5 cm above the iliac crest on the right side for use by the first assistant. An optional 5-mm trocar is placed to mirror the 12-mm trocar 2.5 cm above the left iliac crest for use by a second assistant if available. The surgeon is seated at the operating console and conducts the operation by controlling two micromanipulators affixed to the surgeon's thumb and index finger. At the bedside, the surgeon's hand and wrist movements are replicated in real time by the daVinci robot using specially designed, wristed instrumentation with 7 degrees of freedom. The steps of RAP are accomplished similar to that of the transperitoneal LRP approach.

Seminal Vesical and Vas Deferens Dissection

Upon initial inspection of the operative field, the relevant landmarks include the bladder, median (urachus) and medial umbilical ligaments, vas deferentia, iliac vessels, and rectum (Fig. 10). Dissection is carried out using bipolar forceps in the surgeon's left hand and monopolar electrocautery shears in the right hand.

During the transperitoneal LRP approach, the initial step is the retrovesical dissection of the vas deferentia and seminal vesicles. The peritoneum overlying the vas and seminal vesicles is incised sharply. The vas is clipped and divided and traced distally toward the ipsilateral seminal vesicle. Hemoclips are placed hugging the lateral surface of the seminal vesicle to control tiny vascular branches feeding the lateral aspect of the seminal vesicle. "Cold" transection is

used to divide these branches, thus avoiding thermal injury to the cavernous nerves lying in close proximity to the seminal vesicle (Fig. 11). By lifting both seminal vesicles and vasa anteriorly, a 2- to 3-cm horizontal incision is made approximately 0.5 cm below the base of the seminal vesicles and blunt dissection is carried out between Denonvilliers fascia and the rectum distally toward the prostatic apex (Fig. 12).

Developing the Space of Retzius

The bladder is dissected from the anterior abdominal wall by dividing the urachus and incising the peritoneum bilaterally just medial to the medial umbilical ligaments. Applying cephalad traction on the urachus, the prevesical fat is incised with a monopolar electrocautery hook device, thus entering the space of Retzius (Fig. 13). The fat overlying the anterior prostate is dissected free exposing the periprostatic fascia, puboprostatic ligaments, and pubis (as in Fig. 1A). The endopelvic fascia and puboprostatic ligaments are sharply divided, exposing levator muscle fibers attached to the lateral and apical portions of the prostate. These fibers are meticulously and bluntly dissected from the surface of the prostate exposing the prostatourethral junction.

Ligation of the Dorsal Venous Complex

The deep dorsal venous complex (DVC) is a potential source of bleeding and must be controlled prior to transection. Using a 0-Polyglactin GS21 needle, the dorsal vein complex is suture-ligated using a figure-of-eight suture (as depicted in Fig. 2A). The needle is passed beneath the

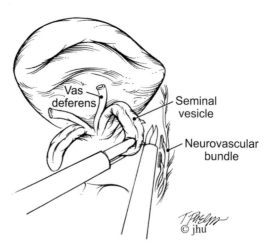

Fig. 11. Dissection of seminal vesicle. Hemoclips and "cold" transection of vascular branches to the seminal vesicle are utilized in lieu of electrocautery in order to minimize damage to nearby neurovascular bundle. (Copyright 2005 Johns Hopkins University.)

Nongastrointestinal Transabdominal

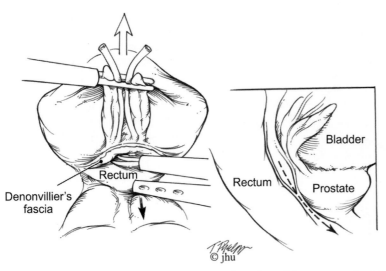

Fig. 12. Incision of Denonvilliers fascia and posterior dissection of the prostate gland. Sagittal view shows proper plane of dissection posterior to the prostate. (Copyright 2005 Johns Hopkins University.)

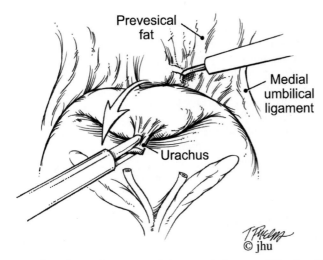

Fig. 13. Division of urachus and exposure of the prevesical space of Retzius. (Copyright 2005 Johns Hopkins University.)

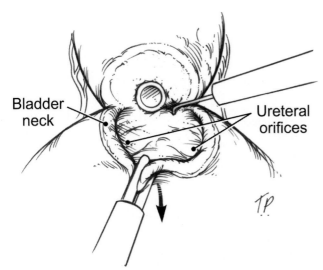

Fig. 14. Bladder neck transection. A curved 20 French van Buren urethral sound is useful in delineating the precise border between the bladder neck and prostate. (Copyright 2005 Johns Hopkins University.)

DVC but anterior to the urethra. The DVC is not divided until later in the operation during the apical dissection of the prostate.

Lateral Release of the Neurovascular Bundles

The cavernous nerves to the penis course as two separate bundles along the posterolateral surface of the prostate intertwined with blood vessels (a.k.a. neurovascular bundles [NVBs]). The NVB lies between two distinct fascial planes that surround the prostate, namely the lateral prostatic fascia and levator fascia. The plane between the levator and prostatic fascia is developed gently using blunt dissection with a fine curved dissector and working in a posterolateral direction until a groove between the NVB and prostate is achieved (i.e., lateral NVB groove). Electrocautery should be avoided if possible during dissection near the NVBs in order to minimize potential thermal injury to the delicate cavernous nerves.

Bladder Neck Transection and Prostatic Pedicle Ligation

A 20 French metal Van Buren urethral sound is introduced to help delineate the proper plane of dissection between the bladder neck and prostate. The anterior bladder is divided using ultrasonic shears followed by the posterior bladder neck, which is divided using a hook monopolar electrocautery device (Fig. 14). During a transperitoneal LRP approach, the previously dissected seminal vesicles and vas deferentia are grasped and brought through the opening created between the bladder neck and prostate. During an extraperitoneal LRP approach, the seminal vesicles and vasa are identified and dissected at this time. In both techniques, the seminal vesicles are lifted anteriorly, placing the prostatic pedicles on slight traction. The prostatic pedicles are secured with large hemoclips and sharply divided without electrocautery in order to avoid thermal injury to the nearby NVBs (Fig. 15).

Antegrade Neurovascular Bundle Preservation

After division of the prostatic pedicles, dissection is carried out toward the previously defined lateral NVB groove (Fig. 15). The remaining attachments between the nerve bundles and prostate are gently teased off of the posterolateral surface of

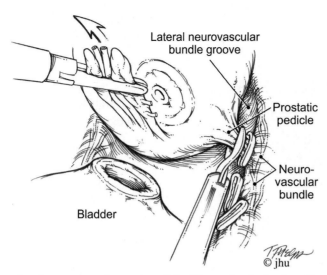

Fig. 15. Control and transection of prostatic pedicles. The previously developed lateral neurovascular bundle groove serves as a landmark for antegrade dissection and release of the neurovascular bundle from the prostate gland. (Copyright 2005 Johns Hopkins University.)

the prostate using a series of blunt and sharp dissection maneuvers as far distally toward the apex as possible. The use of electrocautery and direct manipulation of the NVB is avoided to minimize injury to the cavernous nerves.

Division of Dorsal Venous Complex and Prostatic Apex

The DVC is divided just proximal to the previously placed DVC stitch. Great care must be taken to avoid inadvertent entry into the prostatic apex, resulting in an iatrogenic positive apical margin. The anterior and posterior urethra is divided by sharp dissection, taking care to avoid transecting the NVBs coursing along the 5 and 7 o'clock position along the urethra (Fig. 16). The remaining attachments between the NVB and prostatic apex are dissected free using sharp dissection. Once the prostate specimen is released completely, it is closely inspected and stored in the right lower quadrant of the abdomen until the end of the procedure.

Pelvic Lymphadenectomy

Laparoscopic bilateral pelvic lymphadenectomy is performed (when indicated, e.g., Gleason score ≥7 or PSA >10 ng/mL)

removing all lymphatic tissue bordered by the external iliac vein anteriorly, obturator nerve posteriorly, Cooper ligament distally, bifurcation of the iliac vessels proximally, medial umbilical ligament medially, and pelvic side wall laterally. Sharp dissection and electrocautery should be avoided if possible to avoid iatrogenic injury to the iliac vessels and obturator nerve. Hemoclips are used to secure the small vascular and lymphatic branches traveling to the lymph node packet (Fig. 17). The lymph nodes and prostate specimen are placed together in an entrapment sac and stored in the right lower quadrant of the abdomen until completion of the anastomosis.

Vesicourethral Anastomosis

Either a running or interrupted vesicourethral anastomosis is accomplished with 2-0 polyglactin suture on a UR-6 needle. Our preference is the interrupted closure starting at the 6 o'clock position and continuing in both the clockwise and counterclockwise direction up to the 12 o'clock position (Fig. 18). Approximately six to eight sutures are required to complete the anastomosis. Great care must be taken so as to avoid damaging the ureteral orifices when taking the bladder bites and the NVBs when taking the urethral bites. Either an anterior or posterior tennis racquet closure of the bladder neck may be required if there is significant discrepancy between the bladder neck opening and urethra. An 18 French silicone urethral catheter is placed prior to completion of the anastomosis and the anastomosis tested by filling the bladder with 100 to 150 mL saline. Visible leaks at the anastomosis may be repaired with additional sutures as necessary. A closed suction drain is left in the prevesical space, exiting the 5-mm right lower quadrant trocar site at the end of the operation.

Extraperitoneal Approach to Laparoscopic Prostatectomy

In an effort to avoid possible ileus or other bowel complications that can be encountered when LRP is conducted transperitoneally, and to avoid adhesions that could be encountered in a previously operated abdomen, an extraperitoneal approach to LRP has been developed. For the extraperitoneal LRP approach, a 1.5-cm incision is made at the base of the umbilicus and dissection is carried out down to the peritoneum. Using blunt finger dissection,

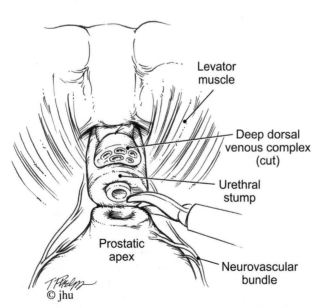

Fig. 16. Division of the previously ligated dorsal venous pedicle and urethra. (Copyright 2005 Johns Hopkins University.)

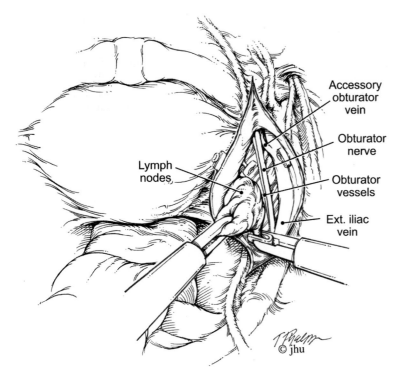

Fig. 17. Laparoscopic dissection of right obturator lymph node packet. Hemoclips are used to avoid electrocautery damage to the iliac vessels and obturator nerve. (Copyright 2005 Johns Hopkins University.)

a space is created anterior to the peritoneum. A trocar-mounted kidney-shaped balloon dilator device (U.S. Surgical, Autosuture, PDB Balloon, Norwalk, CT) is inserted into the preperitoneal space and 500 to 700 mL of air inflated (40 to 50 pumps) to develop the space of Retzius immediately anterior to the bladder and prostate (Fig. 19). Secondary trocars are then inserted as described previously. This approach leads to the preperitoneal view of the space of Retzius as shown in Figure 1B, and dissection proceeds from the dorsal venous ligation as described in the transperitoneal approach above. In the extraperitoneal LRP approach, dissection of the seminal vesicles, vas deferentia, and Denonvilliers fascia is performed late in the procedure after the bladder neck has been completely divided from the prostate. With cephalad traction on the bladder, each vas and seminal vesicle is identified, dissected, and lifted anteriorly, and Denonvilliers fascia dissected as described previously. Other aspects of the extraperitoneal dissection are conducted as described in the transperitoneal technique.

Exiting the Abdomen

The entrapment sac containing the prostate and lymph node specimens is delivered via extension of the infraumbilical incision and fascia. The fascia of the infraumbilical and 12-mm trocar sites is closed primarily to prevent incisional hernia. Skin edges are closed using 4-0 polyglactin subcuticular stitches.

MANAGEMENT AND OUTCOMES AFTER RETROPUBIC OR LAPAROSCOPIC PROSTATECTOMY

Postoperative Care

Patients are given intravenous ketorolac (15 mg IV every 6 hours) with parenteral narcotics for postoperative pain on the night of surgery, changed to an oral pain medication on the first postoperative day. The use of ketorolac has been a major advance in reducing narcotic requirements and avoiding narcotic-associated ileus. To avoid nephrotoxicity, however, it is prudent to reserve ketorolac initiation until after the patient has shown sufficient hemodynamic stability for transfer from the monitored recovery room setting, and should be withheld or discontinued if persistent hematuria develops. Sequential compression devices for the prevention of deep venous thrombosis should be continued until the patient is fully ambulatory. Clear liquids are initiated on the morning of the first postoperative day, and patients are advanced to a regular diet for lunch as tolerated. The closed suction drain is removed when the output is minimal (<50 mL in 8 hours), and the patient can be discharged home on the first or second postoperative day with the urethral catheter to straight drainage. Discharge medications may include ibuprofen 600 mg orally every 6 hours to prevent bladder spasms and incisional pain, stool softener daily, narcotic pain medication as needed, and a 2- to 3-day course of antibiotics to be initiated prior to catheter removal. The Foley catheter can be

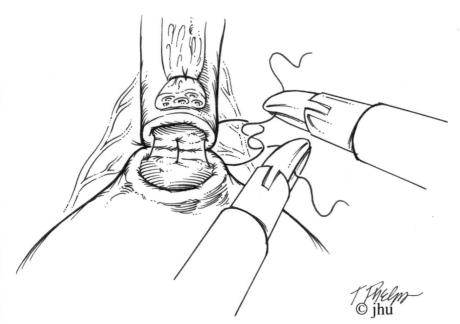

Fig. 18. Interrupted vesicourethral anastomosis using 2-0 polyglactin sutures. (Copyright 2005 Johns Hopkins University.)

Nongastrointestinal Transabdominal

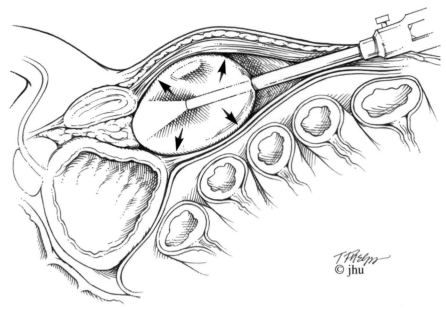

Fig. 19. Creation of working space for extraperitoneal laparoscopic radical prostatectomy. A trocar-mounted balloon dilator device is used to create the preperitoneal working space. (Copyright 2005 Johns Hopkins University.)

removed any time in the second week postoperatively; for early removal (before postoperative day 8), a gravity cystogram is advised as 10% to 20% of vesicourethral anastomoses may show extravasation at that time. After day 10, extravasation is rare and a cystogram is ordered for cases entailing mitigating circumstances.

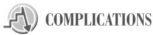 COMPLICATIONS

The most common acute complications following either RRP or LRP include bleeding requiring transfusion (3% to 20%), bladder neck contracture (2% to 10%), or anastomotic leak requiring extended period of catheter or pelvic drain. Blood loss requiring transfusion may be more consistently lower for LRP or RAP series than among RRP series, though some surgeons have reported refined RRP techniques reducing transfusion rates to minimal levels such as those observed with laparoscopic approaches. Complications that are more common after LRP than RRP include ileus (3%) and conversion to conventional RRP (1% to 2%). In contrast, wound infection has been reported more commonly after RRP (5%) than LRP. The learning curve for these procedures is substantial, with declines in complication rates evident after a case experience of over 50 cases ($P = 0.019$). Annual prostatectomy case volume was also found to be associated with complication rates, as urologists

who performed more than 15 radical prostatectomies annually (the highest quartile of annual prostatectomy volume) had urinary complications (predominantly urethral strictures) less commonly than those who performed fewer than five radical prostatectomies annually (the lowest quartile of annual prostatectomy volume). Less common are deep venous thromboses (2%), whereas pulmonary embolus, myocardial infarction, or other cardiopulmonary events are rare (<1%).

Long-term complications of both RRP and LRP include urinary incontinence, urethral strictures, and erectile dysfunction. Urinary incontinence is commonplace in the first several months following prostatectomy, with median time to recovery of urinary control of 2 to 3 months. Depending on how urinary continence is defined and on the age of patients selected for RRP or LRP, long-term stress urinary incontinence persists as a moderate or major urinary problem in 6% to 15% of patients more than 1 year after radical prostatectomy. Ultimately, 2% to 3% of patients opt for placement of an artificial urinary sphincter to restore urinary continence. Erectile dysfunction is even more pervasive than urinary incontinence after RRP or LRP, and the recovery of erections adequate for intercourse can take 1 to 2 years after surgery. Key factors influencing recovery of erections after RRP or LRP include patient age and quality of erectile function prior to prostatectomy. Whereas prospects for erec-

tion recovery among men older than 70 years of age or among those who have some degree of erectile dysfunction prior to prostatectomy are dim, the prospects of erection recovery among men in their 40s or 50s are favorable, with a majority of men in this age group expected to recover adequate erections if a nerve-sparing surgical technique is employed.

CANCER CONTROL

Prostate cancer–specific survival following radical retropubic prostatectomy has been consistently observed to be higher than 95% at 5 to 10 years or longer follow-up by many case series as well as in multi-institutional studies. Although laparoscopic prostatectomy lacks sufficiently long follow-up to comment regarding cancer-specific survival after LRP, data regarding positive surgical margins after RRP or LRP provide a glimpse of one surrogate measure of cancer control efficacy. Whereas overall positive surgical margin rates of 11% to 26% have been reported in the literature, with 7.8% to 16.8% for those patients with organ-confined disease, we observed overall and pT2 positive margin rates of 11.3% and 4.7%, respectively, after LRP. Recurrence-free survival rates in the first 3 years after LRP also appear to exceed 90% (as do similar RRP series), providing additional evidence that, at least in early follow-up, LRP appears to provide acceptable cancer control as compared to RRP. Multi-institutional, prospective studies directly comparing LRP and RRP outcomes, however, have not yet been reported, though several are under way.

SUGGESTED READING

Abbou CC, Salomon L, Hoznek A, et al. Laparoscopic radical prostatectomy: preliminary results. *Urology* 2000;55(5):630.

Bill-Axelson A, Holmberg L, Ruutu M, et al. Scandinavian Prostate Cancer Study No. 4. Radical prostatectomy versus watchful waiting in early prostate cancer. *N Engl J Med* 2005;352(19):1977.

Guillonneau B, El-Fettouh H, Baumert H, et al. Laparoscopic radical prostatectomy: oncological evaluation after 1000 cases at Montsouris institute. *J Urol* 2003;169:1261.

Guillonneau B, Rozet F, Cathelineau X, et al. Perioperative complications of laparoscopic radical prostatectomy: the Montsouris 3-year experience. *J Urol* 2002;167:51.

Guillonneau B, Vallancien G. Laparoscopic radical prostatectomy: the Montsouris experience. *J Urol* 2000;163:418.

Hollenbeck BK, Dunn RL, Wei JT, et al. Determinants of long-term sexual HRQOL after radical prostatectomy measured by a validated instrument. *J Urol* 2003;169(4):1453.

Johansson JE, Andren O, Andersson SO, et al. Natural history of early, localized prostate cancer. *JAMA* 2004;291(22):2713.

Katz R, Salomon L, Hoznek A, et al. Patient reported sexual function following laparoscopic radical prostatectomy. *J Urol* 2002; 168:2078.

Kim ED, Scardino PT, Hampel O, et al. Interposition of sural nerve restores function of cavernous nerves resected during radical prostatectomy. *J Urol* 1999;161(1):188.

Lepor H, Nieder AM, Ferrandino MN. Intraoperative and postoperative complications of radical retropubic prostatectomy in a consecutive series of 1,000 cases. *J Urol* 2001; 166(5):1729.

Menon M, Tewari A, Baize B, et al. Prospective comparison of radical retropubic prostatectomy and robot-assisted anatomic prostatectomy: the Vattikuti urology institute experience. *Urology* 2002;60(5):864.

Rassweiler J, Sentker L, Seemann O, et al. Laparoscopic radical prostatectomy with the Heilbronn technique: an analysis of the first 180 cases. *J Urol* 2001;166:2101.

Su LM. Laparoscopic and robotic-assisted radical prostatectomy. *Campbell Urol Updates* 2003;1(4):1.

Su L, Link RE, Bhayani SB, et al. Nerve-sparing laparoscopic radical prostatectomy: replicating the open surgical technique. *Urology* 2004; 64:123.

Walsh PC. Anatomic radical retropubic prostatectomy. In: Walsh PC, Retick AB, Vaughn ED, et al., eds. *Campbell's urology,* 8th ed., volume IV. Philadelphia: Saunders, 2002.

Wei JT, Dunn RL, Marcovich R, et al. Prospective assessment of patient-reported urinary continence following radical prostatectomy. *J Urol* 2000;164:744.

EDITOR'S COMMENT

This chapter comes at a very good time for discussing transitions in radical retropubic prostatectomy in the treatment of both of organ-confined prostatic cancer and of patients in which extension of cancer outside the prostate has occurred. Since the description in 1983 by Walsh of the nerve-sparing radical retropubic prostatectomy as described by the authors, there have been numerous technical advances that have resulted in some better outcomes. However, to say that continence is universal is probably not correct, and as the authors detail, the results are someplace above 80% for relative continence, with a small percentage requiring or desiring the insertion of a prosthesis in order to achieve continence when leakage is to the extent that it is socially embarrassing. The aspect of sexual function and erection seems somewhat more guarded (Rassweiler J, et al. *Eur Urol* 2006;49:113), reporting 85% continence after 12 months; 53% of those patients who engaged in intercourse preoperatively and underwent bilateral nerve preservation reported the ability to engage in sexual intercourse, but this included the use of phosphodiesterase-type 5 inhibitors. The authors in this chapter are more guarded, which is appropriate.

What is desired is a cancer-specific survival of 90% or more. In this chapter, 95% cancer-specific survival occurring 5 to 10 years after the procedure is described. Nelson and Lepor (*Urol Clin N Am* 2003;30:703) reported cancer-specific survival of up to 90% 10 years and metastatic-free survival of 76% to 82% 15 years after radical retropubic prostatectomy.

Whether or not one can achieve a similar degree of freedom from the disease laparoscopically is questionable in the minds of Toujier and Guillonneau, writing for Memorial Sloan-Kettering Cancer Center (*Eur Urol* in press), in which they questioned radical laparoscopic prostatectomy and pointed out that positive margins range from 11% to 26%, which includes the organ-confined disease (6% or 8%) and extraprostatic extension (35% to 60%). They logically argued that this cannot result in anything else but earlier recurrence.

Morrell and Smith Jr. (*J Urol* 2005;66[Suppl 5A]:105) argued that the results obtained with robotic-assisted radical retropubic prostatectomy carried out can only be achieved, in the senior author's opinion, after 150 procedures and that surgeon comfort and confidence compared to what was achieved with open radical retropubic prostatectomy did not occur until after 250 robotic-assisted laparoscopic prostatectomies. This gives one pause since advertising about various hospitals with the occasional practitioner using the robot carrying out 5 to 15 procedures a year are unlikely to achieve the degree of comfort that these authors feel necessary in order to achieve comparable results to open radical retropubic prostatectomy. This is discouraging, but then advertising is the American way.

From the same institution, Webster et al. (*J Urol* 2005;174:912) compared the requirement for pain medication in robotic-assisted laparoscopic prostatectomy with open radical retropubic prostatectomy and found no difference. Of course, both of these operations are lower abdominal procedures and are reported to have no excessive pain medication requirements.

A large German laparoscopic working group reported their results (Rassweiler J, et al. *Eur Urol* 2006;49:113). Almost 6,000 patients were accumulated in 18 centers with laparoscopic radical prostatectomy performed by 50 individual urologists between March 1999 and August 2004. Three centers performed more than 500 and six more than 250 cases. Conversion rates to open surgery averaged 2.4%. The rate of positive margins was 10.6% for pT2 and 32.7% for pT3A tumors. As stated previously, continence was 85%, and seven centers reported potency with bilateral nerve preservation as stated previously at 53%, including Viagra-type drugs. Of concern is a 5-year PSA recurrence rate in three centers of 8.6% (4% to 15.3%) for pT2 tumors and 17.5% (15% to 20.6%) for pT3A stages, thus confirming the concerns of the previously quoted Memorial-based group.

Tewari et al. (*Future Drugs* 2006;6[1]:11) analyzed a pooled analysis of the published literature on robotic prostatectomy and believe that at short-term follow-up the continence and potency results appear to be the equivalent of radical retropubic prostatectomy and laparoscopic prostatectomy. They also claim that the learning curve for robotic prostatectomy is faster than that of laparoscopic prostatectomy. However, they do not mention outcomes. It does appear that other authorities disagree with this point of view and have concerns about the long-term outcome and long-term cure rate, which these authors seem to have rose-colored glasses in discussing. They do raise cost factors.

Finally, Scales et al. (*J Urol* 2005;174:2323) discussed the costs of robotic-assisted prostatectomy versus radical retropubic prostatectomy. At the base analysis, the cost of robotic-assisted prostatectomy (not including the $2 million investment for two robots, one in the laboratory and one in the operating room) of $783 and $195 in the specialist and generalist setting, respectively. They do say that the robotic approach could achieve cost equivalence with a surgical volume of 10 cases weekly, and if the case volume was increased to 14 cases weekly, the robotic approach would be less expensive in some practice settings if the length of stay was less than 1.5 days. I do not know whether or not the latter is achievable.

In any event, whatever the cost, it does appear as if the advertising for the robot, which will catch many potential customers' eyes, is upon us. Whether or not this is ethical, whether or not the results are good, and whether or not the patient is being fully informed I cannot comment on, but I have grave concerns.

J.E.F.

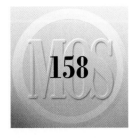

158   Laparoscopic Radical Prostatectomy

JEFFREY A. CADEDDU AND J. KYLE ANDERSON

Prostate cancer is the most common non-skin cancer and the second largest killer of men among all malignancies. In 2004 there were 230,110 new cases diagnosed and 29,500 men died from prostate cancer. Given the scope of prostate cancer, it is little surprise that multiple treatment options exist. Currently, these include watchful waiting, hormone therapy (gonadotropin-releasing hormone agonists or orchiectomy), ablative technologies (cryotherapy or high-intensity focused ultrasound), brachytherapy, external beam radiation therapy, open radical perineal prostatectomy, open radical retropubic prostatectomy (RRP), and laparoscopic radical prostatectomy (LRP). Of these options, the various techniques for prostatectomy provide the most definitive treatment. Not only is the entire gland removed but surrounding lymph nodes are obtained in select cases. In addition to providing both pathologic staging and prognostic information, open prostatectomy has a long track record as an unsurpassed treatment for localized prostate cancer.

Radical prostatectomy was first reported as a treatment for prostate cancer in 1905 by Hugh Hampton Young. Initial technique was perineal, with incision anterior to the anus and dissection retrograde toward the bladder neck. A major innovation came with the anatomic retropubic approach pioneered by Walsh in the 1970s. This technique provided much improved vascular control of the dorsal venous complex, superior dissection of the prostatic apex, and preservation of the neurovascular bundles responsible for erections. Postoperative incontinence and impotence had always been the major deterrents to radical prostatectomy, but with preservation of the external urethral sphincter and neurovascular bundles these complications were greatly reduced. The most recent improvement in prostatectomy technique has been laparoscopic radical prostatectomy. Schuessler et al. performed the first LRP in 1991. The technique was further described by two French groups: Guillonneau and Vallancien at Mountsouris Hospital and Abbou et al. at Henri Mondor Hospital. With their work, LRP allows removal of the prostate with less blood loss, shorter postoperative conva-

lescence, and comparable oncologic efficacy when compared with open surgical approaches. In this chapter, we will cover the important technical points of LRP and briefly discuss surgical outcomes relative to open radical retropubic prostatectomy.

PATIENT SELECTION

Prostatectomy is suitable for patients with at least 10 years of life expectancy and medical condition suitable for a major operative procedure. Diagnosis of prostate cancer should be documented with appropriate biopsies, and preoperative clinical staging workup (digital rectal examination and prostatic-specific antigen [PSA] level) should demonstrate organ-confined disease. Additionally, bone scan and abdominal computed tomography scan for patients with Gleason score of 8 or above or PSA more than 20 should be obtained. Although prostate size on either extreme (below 20 g or above 80 g) can increase the difficulty of the procedure, there is no absolute limit on gland size that can be removed. Neoadjuvant hormone ablation does not improve survival and can increase periprostatic adherence of tissues, and thus it should be avoided if possible. LRP following previous radiation treatment to the pelvis has not been described and is not recommended. Finally, the question of nerve-sparing prostatectomy to preserve potency must be addressed with the patient preoperatively. Relative contraindications to nerve sparing are impotence, large nodule palpable at the prostatic apex, locally advanced disease, and PSA more than 20 ng/mL. Intraoperatively, adherence of the neurovascular bundles to the prostate or unusual thickness of the bundles would be additional contraindications to nerve-sparing technique.

Additional contraindications specific to LRP are few. Patients with previous extensive intra-abdominal surgery or history of peritonitis are better served by alternative modalities. Additionally, a history of cerebral vascular abnormalities (aneurysms, arteriovenous malformations, or cerebral vascular accidents) may increase the risk of complication given the extreme Trendelenburg position needed for this procedure.

Obesity is a relative contraindication as a large pannus can markedly change instrument angle of entry into the abdomen and make intra-abdominal manipulation much more difficult. Finally, pelvic lipomatosis or previous open bladder or prostate surgery are contraindications to this procedure.

SURGICAL TECHNIQUE

There are two described approaches to laparoscopic prostatectomy: intraperitoneal and extraperitoneal. Choice of approach should be surgeon preference, as outcomes following these techniques have not been shown to be significantly different. Of the two, the intraperitoneal approach is more commonly described and is probably easier to master given the larger working space and easy access to the seminal vesicles. Thus, it is the intraperitoneal procedure that we will describe first. The intraperitoneal LRP with nerve sparing can be broken down into a number of steps including placement of trocars, dissection of the vas and seminal vesicles, mobilization of the bladder, opening of the endopelvic fascia, ligation of the dorsal venous complex, bladder neck dissection, preservation of the nerves, division of the prostatic pedicle, dissection of the prostatic apex, removal of the prostate, and urethrovesicle anastomosis. Minor deviations from this approach have been reported and will be mentioned where appropriate. Differences between the intraperitoneal and extraperitoneal approach will be highlighted as well, although once the respective space has been accessed, the two procedures are quite similar.

Surgical preparation begins the day before surgery with a magnesium citrate bowel preparation. This decompresses the colon (as colonic or rectal distention can greatly hinder exposure) and allows primary repair in the unlikely event that a rectal injury occurs. On the day of surgery, an intravenous first-generation cephalosporin antibiotic is administered preoperatively, two or more intravenous access points are obtained, and sequential compression devices are applied to the lower extremities.

On entering the operating room, general anesthesia is induced and the patient

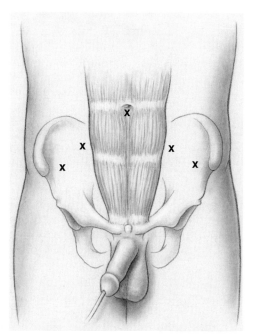

Fig. 1. Placement of ports.

is positioned with the umbilicus over the kidney rest. We prefer straps or tape placed in an "X" over the patient's shoulders and chest in order to prevent patient movement when the bed is placed in deep Trendelenburg position later in the procedure. An oral or nasal gastric tube is used to decompress the stomach, and as always during laparoscopy, nitrous oxide inhalation gas should be avoided. A rectal bougie may be placed at this time for later manipulation of the rectum, but we have not found this necessary. We do, however, spread the legs to allow access to the perineum later in the procedure. Finally, an important goal for the anesthesiologist is to minimize intravenous fluids. With the steep Trendelenburg position required for this procedure, facial and laryngeal edema and subsequent difficulty removing the endotracheal tube is a significant risk.

With sterile preparation and draping complete, a No. 18 French foley catheter is inserted into the bladder. A transverse incision is made immediately cranial to the umbilicus and the intraperitoneal space is inflated to a pressure of 15 mm Hg. A 12-mm trocar is placed at this site and a 0-degree telescope is inserted. This is the only lens necessary for the surgery. Four more trocars are placed as shown in Figure 1. The medial two ports are 12 mm in size and are located 4 to 5 cm laterally and caudally to the umbilical trocar. The two lateral ports are 5 mm in size and are placed 4 to 5 cm laterally and slightly caudally from the 12-mm trocars. Once the

trocars are in position, the bed is placed in maximal Trendelenburg position (approximately 30 degrees, head down).

These trocar locations allow the operating surgeon to work through the two ports on the left side, and the assistant to function autonomously via the two right-side trocars. Visualization is provided almost exclusively through the umbilical port with a 0-degree telescope. A second assistant can operate the camera from a position at the head of the bed, or alternatively a robotic

arm or other positioning device can be mounted on the right bed rail and used for camera control. Monitors are positioned at the foot of the bed with one monitor per side. Cautery and ultrasonic shears are placed at the foot of the bed as well. Instrumentation used during LRP includes monopolar scissors, bipolar graspers, tissue graspers, suction irrigation device, needle drivers, and ultrasonic shears.

The surgeon begins the procedure with grasper and monopolar scissors in the left-sided ports. The assistant uses a blunt-tip grasper in the medial port and suction irrigator in the lateral port. Frequently on entering the pelvis, adhesions of the sigmoid colon are encountered. These are easily taken down and the rectovesical pouch is well visualized. A thorough anatomic understanding of the posterior aspect of the prostate and seminal vesicles is important given that structures to be avoided (namely rectum and ureters) are in close proximity. Figure 2 shows the initial peritoneal incision over the seminal vesicles and vas deferens. With the assistant applying upward retraction with the suction irrigator and sigmoid colon retraction with the grasper, the peritoneum overlying the seminal vesicles and vas deferens is opened. The vas are the most easily identified structure and can be traced medially from the internal ring. Awareness of the ureters, which lie anterior and lateral from the vas, is important as the potential for ureteral injury exists. The peritoneum over the vas is opened, the vas are dissected free for 3 to 4 cm, and each is divided. Dissection of the seminal vesicles is

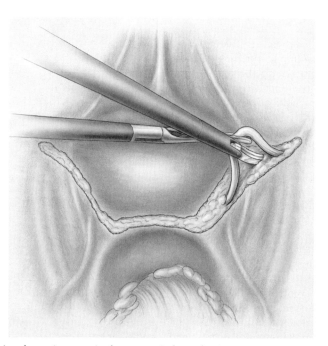

Fig. 2. Opening the peritoneum in the rectovesical pouch.

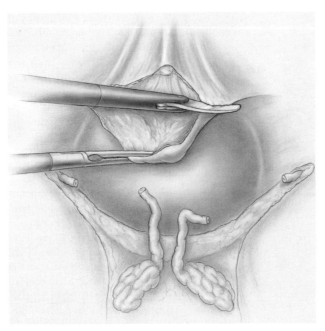

Fig. 3. Mobilization of the bladder.

undertaken with the assistant providing anterior and posterior retraction at the respective peritoneal edges. Progress is made toward the tip of the seminal vesicle where the vascular supply is encountered and controlled, generally with clips. During a nerve-sparing procedure, care must be taken when approaching the tips of the seminal vesicles as the neurovascular bundle is in close proximity and use of cautery can have a deleterious effect on the nerves. Once both seminal vesicles and vas are free, these structures are retracted anteriorly and Denonvillier fascia is opened. The space between the prostate and anterior rectal wall is developed, as this will greatly simplify later dissection of the prostatic pedicles.

The next component of the procedure is the mobilization of the bladder and opening of the endopelvic fascia (Fig. 3). To begin, the bladder is filled with 200 mL of saline to aid in identification and dissection of the bladder from the anterior abdominal wall. Initial incision can be medial or lateral to the medial umbilical ligament, but regardless, awareness of the external iliac vein location is important as it is frequently in close proximity. The most important landmark is the pubic bone. Once this is identified, the space of Retzius is entered and the bladder is mobilized posteriorly.

With the bladder dropped posteriorly, adipose tissue overlying the endopelvic fascia and prostate is removed. The endopelvic fascia is easily opened, and with sharp and blunt dissection, levator muscle fibers should be separated from the prostate. Dissection is

continued to the prostatic apex and when the superficial dorsal vein and puboprostatic ligaments are encountered, these structures are cauterized and divided. Control of the dorsal venous complex at the prostatic apex is next accomplished with intracorporeal stitch placement and knot tying using a figure of eight 0-vicryl stitch on a

CT-1 needle (Fig. 4). This stitch should be deep enough to encompass the complex but should not enter into the urethra. Division of the dorsal venous complex is delayed until later in the procedure, as division at this time results in increased blood loss.

The next important maneuver is the separation of the base of the prostate from the bladder neck (Fig. 5). Correct identification of the plane of dissection is critical to achieve a satisfactory bladder neck; however, this plane is not always obvious. Thus, a number of techniques have been developed to identify the junction between the prostate and bladder. First, the adipose tissue is generally easily removed from the prostate using blunt dissection. This is not the case with the bladder, and thus this change in adipose tissue adherence marks the vesicoprostatic junction. Next, the Foley catheter may be exchanged for a Van Buren sound. By angling the tip of the sound anteriorly while moving through the area of the bladder neck, the junction between bladder and prostate becomes quite obvious. Alternatively, movement of the Foley catheter balloon against the bladder neck highlights the junction. Additional information about the presence of a median lobe is also gleaned from this final maneuver, as a large median lobe will often cause the balloon to deviate to one side. Once the

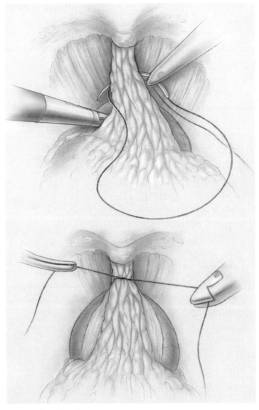

Fig. 4. Dorsal venous complex ligation.

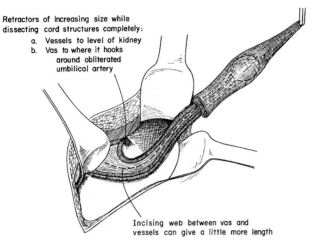

Retractors of increasing size while dissecting cord structures completely:
a. Vessels to level of kidney
b. Vas to where it hooks around obliterated umbilical artery

Incising web between vas and vessels can give a little more length

Fig. 8. Continued mobilization into retroperitoneal space.

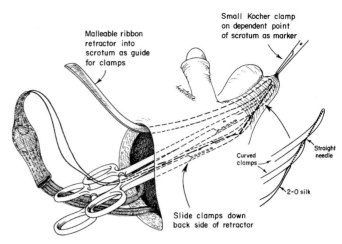

Malleable ribbon retractor into scrotum as guide for clamps

Small Kocher clamp on dependent point of scrotum as marker

Curved clamps

Straight needle

2-0 silk

Slide clamps down back side of retractor

Fig. 11. Passing suture to scrotum.

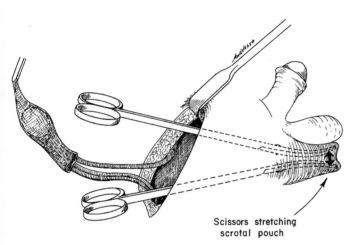

Scissors stretching scrotal pouch

Fig. 9. Preparing scrotum.

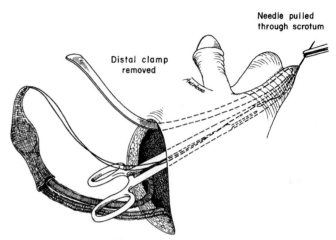

Distal clamp removed

Needle pulled through scrotum

Fig. 12. Pulling fixation suture through scrotum.

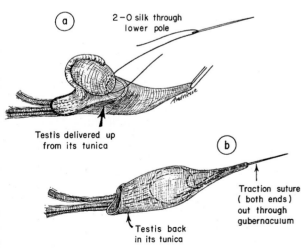

(a)

2-0 silk through lower pole

Testis delivered up from its tunica

(b)

Testis back in its tunica

Traction suture (both ends) out through gubernaculum

Fig. 10. Placing fixation suture in testis.

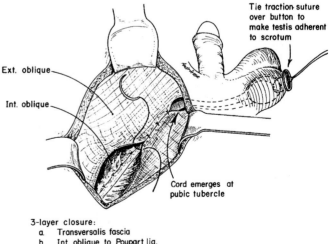

Tie traction suture over button to make testis adherent to scrotum

Ext. oblique

Int. oblique

Cord emerges at pubic tubercle

3-layer closure:
a. Transversalis fascia
b. Int. oblique to Poupart lig.
c. Ext. oblique

Fig. 13. Testis fixation.

Nongastrointestinal Transabdominal

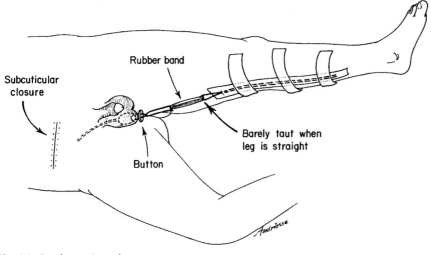

Fig. 14. Gentle traction when necessary.

The limiting factor in bringing a high testicle down is always the spermatic vessels, not the length of the vas deferens. When a testis is high in the abdomen, even a wide mobilization of the spermatic vessels may not gain enough length to bring the testis into the scrotum. Autotransplantation with anastomosis of the spermatic vessels to the deep inferior epigastric vessels has been shown to be possible with microvascular technique. However, we doubt the practicality of this approach. First, the very high testis is often abnormal initially. Second, if its histologic features are favorable, the operation would require performance at a very early age. Both of these factors lead us to question the use of testicular autotransplantation, particularly if the other side appears normal.

It has been shown that the spermatic vessels are not end vessels but have extensive collateral with the adjacent blood vessels that accompany the vas deferens. Thus, spermatic vessels can be ligated and divided high, with survival of the testis based on its blood supply with the vas deferens. Therefore, if the decision is made *early in the operation,* before the cord structures are skeletonized, the spermatic vessels can be ligated high. Then the vas is mobilized, maintaining with it all of the surrounding tissue, including a wide strip of peritoneum. The testis and its pedicle are then brought through the abdominal wall near the pubic tubercle, the shortest distance down to the scrotum. In the prune belly syndrome, there is a particularly rich vascular plexus in the tissues surrounding the vas. The vas itself is often abnormal. The degree of success with this type of orchidopexy, in which the vessels are divided, is proportional to the degree

of care of maintaining the tissues around the vas. If the vas is skeletonized, the testis will become infarcted.

Two other approaches have been used when it is evident early in the operation that the vessels are too short to allow successful orchidopexy. One is to perform a staged orchidopexy, bringing the testis as low as it will come and suturing it there. Reoperation is carried out a year later, with remobilization of the testicle to bring it lower. The testis can be wrapped, meanwhile, with a thin sheet of Silastic. In our experience, the reaction despite the use of Silastic is so great that the staged approach is not a very practical one. Another procedure used recently is preliminary ligation of the short spermatic vessels—either at open operation or laparoscopically—to allow enlargement of the collateral supply to the testicle via the vas deferens, with the orchidopexy performed at a later date.

Orchiectomy is a reasonable option for a high intra-abdominal testis when it is obvious that the testis is poorly developed.

REOPERATION FOR FAILED ORCHIDOPEXY

The most common cause of failure of orchidopexy is inadequate mobilization. Usually, reoperation is successful in such cases. In most cases, the surgeon finds that the previous operation did not extend above the level of the internal ring. Therefore, the reoperation should start in virgin territory higher than the inguinal canal, opening the internal oblique and transversalis fasciae to visualize the spermatic cord structures behind the peritoneum. Once they are identified, they can be followed downward, into the scar secondary

to the previous orchidopexy. To begin the dissection lower, at the level of the testis, and proceed upward is dangerous because the spermatic vessels and vas are not easily identified in scar tissue. During orchidopexy, the assistant should be warned to be very gentle when keeping traction on the spermatic vessels. We have seen these vessels avulsed by heavy-handed traction in two cases: In one the testis survived; in the other it did not.

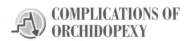

COMPLICATIONS OF ORCHIDOPEXY

The most common complication of orchidopexy is failure to place the testis into the scrotum because an *inadequate operation* was performed. *Atrophy of the testis* results from rough handling or excessive traction on the vessels. *Inadvertent injury to the vessels and vas* can occur during orchidopexy, just as in herniorrhaphy. Massive *retroperitoneal hemorrhage* can be caused by inadequate ligation of deep inferior epigastric vessels. We saw such a case many years ago. *Late malignancy* can develop in a testis despite orchidopexy. Orchidopexy does not seem to decrease the incidence of cancer, but it does put the testis in a position where it can be readily examined by the patient, which is not possible with an intra-abdominal testis. We routinely advise all of these patients to examine themselves for the rest of their lives as a precaution. *Postoperative wound infection* should be extremely rare with good surgical technique. We no longer use nonabsorbable suture material in children undergoing this type of surgery, because if a wound infection does occur, it cannot be eradicated unless all of the infected suture material is removed, especially if it is silk or a braided nonabsorbable material. Orchidopexy is a beneficial operation in most patients if performed correctly.

Hutson and Hasthorpe have recently related a fascinating account of the importance of normally descended testes. It is an anecdote to be enjoyed by all surgeons: "In the middle ages a female pope was elected, leading to a scandal when she gave birth to a baby during a papal procession through Rome. Following this episode, the porphyry chair was produced as a way of determining definitively whether any future pope was a man and hence could become the Holy Father. The chair has a cut out in the seat such that the elected cardinal could sit on the chair, suitably robed, but a junior cardinal could reach in from behind and palpate the scrotum. If the scrotum contained 2 testes, they would chant '*duo testes bene pendulum*' (he has 2 testes and they hang well), confirming masculinity and eligibility for the papacy."

SUGGESTED READING

Bailey RW, Flowers JL. *Complications of laparoscopic surgery*. St. Louis: Quality Medical Publishing, 1994.

Colodny AH. Laparoscopy in pediatric urology: too much of a good thing? *Semin Pediatr Surg* 1996;5(1):23.

Fischer MC, Milen MT, Bloom DA. Thomas Annandale and the first report of successful orchiopexy. *J Urol* 2005;174(1):37.

Grosfeld JL, Hendren WH, eds. *Seminars in pediatric surgery*, vol 5. Philadelphia: WB Saunders, 1996

Huff DS, Hadziselimovic F, Snyder HM III, et al. Histologic maldevelopment of unilaterally cryptorchid testes and their descended partners. *Eur J Pediatr* 1993;152(Suppl 2): S11.

Hutson JM, Hasthorpe S. Testicular descent and cryptorchidism: the state of the art in 2004. *J Pediatr Surg* 2005;40(2):297.

Ivell R, Hartung S. The molecular basis of cryptorchidism. *Mol Hum Reprod* 2003;9(4): 175.

Lee PA. Fertility after cryptorchidism: epidemiology and other outcome studies. *Urology* 2005;66(2):427.

Misra M, MacLaughlin DT, Donahoe PK, et al. Measurement of Mullerian inhibiting substance facilitates management of boys with microphallus and cryptorchidism. *J Clin Endocrinol Metab* 2002;87(8):3598.

Moore RG, Peters CA, Bauer SB, et al. Laparoscopic evaluation of the nonpalpable testis: a prospective assessment of accuracy. *J Urol* 1994;151:728.

Oh J, Landman J, Evers A, et al. Management of the postpubertal patient with cryptorchidism: an updated analysis. *J Urol* 2002; 167(3):1329.

Peters CA. Laparoscopic and robotic approach to genitourinary anomalies in children. *Urol Clin North Am* 2004;31(3):595.

Peters CA. Laparoscopy in pediatric urology: challenge and opportunity. *Semin Pediatr Surg* 1996;5(1):16.

Raman JD, Schlegel PN. Testicular sperm extraction with intracytoplasmic sperm injection is successful for the treatment of nonobstructive azoospermia associated with cryptorchidism. *J Urol* 2003;170(4 Pt 1):1287.

Wenzler DL, Bloom DA, Park JM. What is the rate of spontaneous testicular descent in infants with cryptorchidism? *J Urol* 2004;171 (2 Pt 1):849.

EDITOR'S COMMENT

The undescended testicle is a very common situation, usually requiring surgery. Historically, the scholarly activity dates back to Thomas B. Curling, who in 1866 summarized what was known at that time regarding undescended testicle in his book, *A Practical Treatise on the Diseases of the Testis* (London: J Churchill, 1866:12). A number of observations made by Curling hold true today, although it is not known exactly how these conclusions were reached. For example, his statements, "A retained testicle only imperfectly executes its function" and "If the evolution does not take place within a twelvemonth after birth, it is rarely fully and perfectly complete afterwards," as reported by Fischer et al. (*J Urol* 2005; 174:37), in fact, are correct. Most of Curling's other observations are also correct, as Kollin et al. (*Acta Paediatr* 2006;95[3]:318) demonstrated in a randomized controlled trial of the effect of orchidopexy at age 9 months on testicular growth. Seventy boys with cryptorchidism were randomized to surgical treatment at 9 months, and 79 boys to treatment at 3 years of age. The boys were then followed at 12 and 24 months. Ultrasonography was used to determine testicular volume. After orchidopexy, the previously retained testes resumed growth and were significantly larger than the nonoperated testes at 2 years (0.49 mL vs. 0.36 mL, $P < 0.001$). Testicular growth after orchidopexy also increased the ratio between the operated testes and the previously normal scrotal testes to 0.84 for the surgically treated group, compared to 0.63 for the untreated group. The authors concluded that there is a beneficial effect on testicular growth of the previously undescended testicle. Thomas Annandale, chair of surgery at the Edinburgh Royal Infirmary, succeeded Joseph Lister as the Regius professor, and was fully cognizant of the principles of antisepsis. He performed the first successful orchidopexy in 1877 (*Br Med J* 1879;I:7), in which he treated the operative field with carbolic acid dressings. Previous unsuccessful attempts at orchidopexies were reported by James Adams (*Lancet* 1871:710). One of the procedures failed because his patient died of peritonitis following development of erysipelas at home, after an outpatient attempt to replace a perineal testis in an 11-month-old into an empty left scrotum. The testis, in fact, was replaced normally into the scrotum, and anchored by a suture of catgut. At autopsy, a patent processus vaginalis allowed the infection in the local operative site to spread into the peritoneum, and the ensuing peritonitis was responsible for the death of this child, as well as of a number of others. It is interesting that in the early history of orchidopexy, there seemed to be a relatively large number of peritoneal testes, suggesting that perhaps mixed male-female gender difficulties were present in these children.

The cause of cryptorchidism has long been assumed to be accounted for by abnormalities in hormonal development. In a very nice review by Hutson and Hasthorpe (*Cell Tissue Res* 2005;322:155), the process of downward migration is well described. At 7 to 8 weeks of development, the ambisexual gonad begins to develop into either a testis or an ovary (Hutson JM, et al. *Endocrinol Rev* 1996; 18:259). If the genome contains a Y chromosome, the SRY gene begins to trigger a complex sequence of events, which results in a testicle. The developing Sertoli cells will then begin to produce Müllerian-inhibiting substance/anti-Müllerian hormone (MIS/AMH). Testosterone production is begun by the Leydig cells. The testis in the developing urogenital ridge has two ligaments as its anchor, the cranial suspensory ligament and the caudal genitoinguinal ligament, or gubernaculum, which was first described by John Hunter (Hunter J (1786) Observations on certain parts of the animal Oeconomy. 13 Castle St., London, pp 1–26; 1786:1). The initial intra-abdominal position of the testicle is at the same level of the ovary. But testicular descent is now identified as occurring in two phases. The first or transabdominal phase is more mechanical, and the hormonally controlled elements apparently have less that can possibly go wrong with them. The mechanical aspect of this is a hormonally controlled enlargement of the distal gubernaculum, so that it becomes a more powerful anchoring ligament for the testis. The cranial suspensory ligament regresses. It was thought that this regression is under the control of testosterone. However, the hormone controlling the enlargement of the gubernaculum, which is critical to this process, has recently been determined, and is a newly described insulin-like hormone 3 (Insl3), which is made by the Leydig cells. The swelling reaction of the distal gubernaculum then draws the testis down toward the inguinal ring. In contrast, in the female fetus, the gubernaculum does not undergo a swelling reaction. It develops into the round ligament, and the ligament of the ovary. As the embryo enlarges, the ovary is not held close to the inguinal region, because the gubernaculum enlarges only in proportion to the overall embryo and fetus. This phase of descent takes place between 7 and 8 weeks, and is complete by 15 weeks.

The second phase of descent occurs between 25 and 35 weeks of gestation. The reason for the pause between phases is not known. What transpires next is that the gubernaculum grows out from the inguinal abdominal wall, and physically migrates across the pubic region into the scrotum. Inside the gubernaculum, the processus vaginalis enlarges to create an extension of the abdominal cavity into the scrotum. The direction of migration appears to be controlled by the genitofemoral nerve and the release of neurotransmitters, notably calcitonin gene-related peptide (Hutson JM, et al. *Turk J Pediatr* 2004;46(Suppl):3).

The descent of the testis into the scrotum allows a neonatal gonocyte to transform into a type A spermatogonia at 3 to 12 months of age. This is absolutely crucial to the development of subsequent fertility, as the stem cells for spermatogenesis are created in this structure. In the undescended testis, this step is blocked, and is the origin of the current thinking that orchidopexy is recommended at 6 to 12 months of age. In addition, Hadziselimovic and Herzog (*Hormonal Res* 2001;55:6) have shown that the inadequate development of the type A spermatogonia results in a low sperm count after puberty. Moreover, congenitally abnormal gonocytes may subsequently turn into carcinoma in situ (CIS) cells, or gonocytes that fail to transform into type A spermatogonia may subsequently be mutated into CIS cells. These CIS cells, in the high-temperature environment associated with undescended testicle, then predispose to the well-known risk of cancer after puberty.

In further pursuit of the normal or abnormal function of the hypothalamic-pituitary-gonadal axis, Suomi et al. ((c) The Endocrine Society, 2006, first published online Jan. 4, 2006, by the *Journal of Clinical Endocrinology and Metabolism*, as doi:10.1210/jc.2004-2318) studied 388 Finnish

(continued)

Nongastrointestinal Transabdominal

boys and 433 Danish boys (88 and 34 with cryptorchidism, respectively). Clinical examinations were carried out at 0 and 3 months, and blood samples at 3 months. There was significantly higher follicle-stimulating hormone (FSH) in Finnish boys, and lower inhibin B than Finnish control boys. Danish cryptorchid boys had higher FSH levels than controls, and healthy Danish boys had lower inhibin B levels than Finnish boys. Inhibin B was normal in Danish cryptorchid boys. Changes in the hormone levels apparently were most striking in boys with severe, persistent cryptorchidism, but also detectable in milder cases. Effects on Leydig cell function, however, were subtle in Finnish but not Danish boys, but testosterone levels remained in normal range. These findings suggest that gonadotropins and androgens may play a role in what is seen to be a primary testicular disorder, but they may be secondary to the cryptorchidism itself. Other data will need to be brought to bear in order to ascertain which comes first.

Since hormonal abnormalities are thought to be important in the cause of cryptorchidism, it would not be surprising if gonadotropins were used in an effort to have the testis moved down into proper scrotal position. However, tests of gonadotropin administration in primary cryptorchidism have not been successful (Rajfer J, et al. *N Engl J Med* 1986; 314:466; DeMuink KS, et al. *Lancet* 1986;1:876).

The question of laparoscopic mobilization and its role in the therapy of cryptorchidism remains unanswered. The open procedure itself is carried out as an outpatient one, and thus, there is no length of stay. The approach is carried out retroperitoneally.

The technique described so well in this chapter by Dr. Hendren has worked well in excellent hands, and is quite adequate for exploring the retroperitoneum. Thus, individuals still struggle with determining the role of laparoscopic mobilization. It should be something other than, "I can do this," because there is the possibility of injury to the bowel, bleeding, etc., in a procedure that really has a very low morbidity when done open, especially as Dr. Hendren describes it. Leung et al. (*Pediatr Surg Int* 2005;21:767) reported 15 cases, of which 13 were "peeping" (i.e., within 2 cm of the internal inguinal ring), and two were canalicular testes. Three were redo's, because of unfavorable testicular position following previous surgery. I am concerned about the need to do laparoscopic mobilization, including all of the inherent risks, because if the testes were within 2 cm of the inguinal canal, it should be entirely possible to carry these down to the scrotum by employing the technique described in this chapter. In the previous comment, in the fourth edition, I stated that the role of laparoscopy was still not entirely decided. The one goal in which I think it might be useful is to see whether or not there really is a testis, or whether it is a nubbin, in which case it needs to be removed. I am not certain that using the laparoscope to ligate the vessels is reason enough to deviate from a tried-and-true procedure. It may be that laparoscopic division of the testicular vessels, the first stage of the Fowler-Stephens procedure, could be one area where laparoscopy may be useful. On the other hand, in good hands this can be carried out as part of the open procedure, and as part of a first stage. In the previous commentary, I also indicated that perhaps some type of magnetic resonance angiography or other gadolinium-assisted magnetic res-

onance imaging might yield information as to where the testis really is.

Finally, there is the acquired or secondary cryptorchidism. This is a situation in which a testis previously well seated in the scrotum rides higher in boys aged 5 to 10 years. Here there seems to be a difference of opinion on how these patients should be treated. While Hutson and Hasthorpe (previously cited) believe that the primary treatment of this is surgical, Mack et al. (*Br J Surg* 2003;90:728) believe that with puberty the majority of these testes will move down, and in the majority of cases, treatment with human chorionic gonadotrophin (HCG) is effective in achieving full scrotal descent. The mechanism appears to be, according to the authors, that HCG stimulates the Leydig cells to produce testosterone, resulting in high local levels. Secondly, it does not appear as if, in the high-riding testes in the scrotum, or even in the inguinal canal, failure to operate early results in decreasing fertility.

Lastly, Yonkov and Chatalbashev (*Folia Med* 2004;46[4]:27) reviewed 1,466 patients aged 1 to 16 years who were operated on between 1979 and 2003 in a Bulgarian children's clinic. Success rates were variable, with the early results successful in 42% of all patients with intra-abdominal testes, in 74% with testes high in the inguinal canal, in 87% with testes low in the canal, and in 98% with ectopic testes. I am not certain how these results compare with the results in this country, but it seems that they are somewhat lower than the success rates that Dr. Hendren and his colleagues have achieved.

J.E.F.

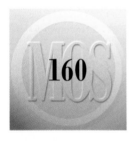

Surgical Management of Wilms Tumor

PETER F. EHRICH

INTRODUCTION

Wilms tumor (WT) is the most common tumor of renal origin found in children. It accounts for 6% of all pediatric tumors and is the second most frequent intra-abdominal solid organ tumor found in children. The annual incidence is 8.1 per million children. This results in about 650 new cases each year in North America. Initial survival rates in the early part of the last century were only 30%, but now long-term survival in both North America and European trials is approaching 85%, with many low-stage tumors significantly higher (Table 1). This remarkable progress in the treatment and understanding of children with Wilms tumor is the result of many factors. These include the development of multiagent chemotherapy, cooperative pediatric in-

terdisciplinary groups conducting large randomized controlled clinical trials, new diagnostic modalities, and radiation therapy. Treatment is now progressing toward "risk-based management"—based not only on stage and histology but also on incorporating genetic markers. Therapy has been refined so that children with low-risk tumors can be spared intensive chemotherapy and radiation with their long-term side effects without sacrificing excellent outcomes. Alternatively, research continues to look for novel strategies in children, including treatment intensification, with high-risk tumors for improved survival. Within the multidisciplinary treatment team, the surgeon plays a critical role in the diagnosis and staging and the surgeon's technical skills and judgment direct therapy and impact outcome.

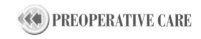

PREOPERATIVE CARE

Clinical Presentation

A typical child with WT presents with a large, smooth, round, nontender abdominal flank mass. The mean age at diagnosis is 3 years with most children between the ages of 1 and 4 years. Wilms tumor is rare over 10 years and under 6 months of age. A functional review of patients with Wilms tumor does not show any tumor-specific symptoms. Typically the mass is asymptomatic and discovered either by a parent or a physician. Twenty percent of children with WT have hematuria, 10% have coagulopathy, and 20% to 25% present with hypertension due to activation of the renin-angiotensin system. Fever, anorexia, and weight loss occurs in 10%. In rare instances tumor rupture and

TABLE 1. WILMS TUMOR STAGING

Stage	NWTSG	SIOP
I	Tumor limited to the kidney, completely resected Capsule not ruptured No renal vessels involved	Same
II	Tumor extends outside of renal capsule, direct extension but completely resected Invasion of renal vessels Tumor spillage but confined to the flank not involving the peritoneal surface	Extrarenal tumor extension by extracapsular invasion Regional lymph node invasion Vascular or ureteral invasion Tumor completely excised
III	Incomplete tumor resection with any of the following: Lymph node metastases Tumor penetrating peritoneal surface Infiltrating vital structures Tumor spill not confined to the flank occurred before or during surgery	Incomplete surgical resection of extracapsular invasion including: Preoperative biopsy Preoperative rupture Peritoneal implants or nodal metastasis beyond regional lymph nodes
IV	Hematogenous metastasis of lymph node metastasis outside the abdomen or pelvis	Same
V	Bilateral tumors at presentation	Same

NWTSG, National Wilms Tumor Study Group; SIOP, The International Society of Pediatric Oncology.
NWTSG: The tumor is staged at surgery and before the initiation of chemotherapy.
SIOP: Chemotherapy is given prior to surgery; staging is based on imaging studies initially and then the tumor is restaged after surgery.

bleeding can cause an acute abdomen. Between 5% and 10% of tumors are bilateral, and bilateral tumors can either be synchronous or metachronous. Bilateral tumors are more commonly found in children with syndromes such as Beckwith-Wiedemann syndrome. The incidence of bilateral WT in sporadic cases is less then 4%.

Physical examination reveals congenital anomalies (aniridia, genitourinary malformations, hemihypertrophy, or signs of overgrowth) in 13% to 28% of children. The syndromes associated with the highest risk of developing Wilms tumor include the syndrome of aniridia, genitourinary malformation, and mental retardation (generally referred to as WAGR syndrome); the Beckwith-Wiedemann syndrome (visceromegaly, macroglossia, omphalocele, and hyperinsulinemic hypoglycemia), and the Denys-Drash syndrome (nephropathy, renal failure, male pseudohermaphroditism, and Wilms tumor). Other syndromes that have been associated with Wilms tumor include hemihypertrophy, Klippel-Trenaunay-Weber syndrome, Perlman syndrome, and genitourinary malformations.

Diagnostic Imaging

A child with an abdominal mass requires diagnostic imaging in order to establish the nature and origin of the mass. The differential diagnosis of an abdominal mass is extensive and includes other solid organ tumors such as hepatoblastoma, neuroblastoma, germ cell tumors, and rhabdomyosarcoma. Abdominal ultrasound with vascular assessment of the renal vein and cava should be the initial study. A computed tomography (CT) scan of the abdomen with oral and intravenous contrast typically demonstrates an intrarenal neoplasm that displaces the collecting system medially. It is critical to imaging both kidneys because of bilateral tumors. Radiographic imaging of the chest by CT scan is mandated. WT can spread via the vascular system to the renal vein, inferior vena cava (IVC), and atrium as well as invade the vessel walls. B-mode ultrasound and echocardiography are the best methods to imaging these areas. About 4% of WTs present with IVC or atria involvement and 11% with renal vein involvement.

Magnetic resonance imaging (MRI) scanning is helpful, but to date has not been shown superior to CT scanning in standard assessments. The value of MRI is that it can help to distinguish between nephrogenic rests (discussed later) and Wilms tumor. Positron emission tomography (PET) scanning is a new modality to cancer imaging. It appears to be useful in some malignancies. In a variety of tumors PET scanning has been helpful because of uptake of 2-(fluorine-18)-fluoro-2-deoxy-D-glucose (FDG), which helps distinguish normal and malignant tissue. In WT there have been a few case reports, but its role has not yet been defined.

Preoperative Preparation

After completing the imaging assessment the child should be prepared for the operating room. The child must be properly hydrated with an intravenous line and have nothing to eat for at least 6 hours prior to surgery. Preoperative blood tests prior to surgery should include a complete blood count, a cross and type for at least 10 mL/kg, and coagulation studies. Although rare, the blood pressure may be significantly elevated requiring pharmacologic control. Standard monitoring in the operating room should include continuous electrocardiographic, blood pressure, temperature, and pulse oximetry monitoring. An arterial catheter is rarely required but in hypertensive or pulmonary compromised patients it may be value. Urine output is monitored through an indwelling Foley catheter. Two large-bore intravenous lines placed in the upper limbs are recommended. A long-term central catheter is often placed in these children for postoperative chemotherapy under the same anesthetic. If placed prior to the abdominal operation, it can function as one of the large-bore intravenous lines. Lower limb lines should be avoided if possible.

UNRESECTABLE TUMORS

In European studies through the International Society of Pediatric Oncology (SIOPEL), preoperative chemotherapy is used routinely. In the National Wilms Tumor Study Group (NWTSG) and Children's Oncology Group (COG) studies, confirmation of pathology and nephrectomy is preferred. Survival rates are similar in both protocols. In the North American studies, preoperative chemotherapy is used only for unresectable tumors. There are four main reasons a tumor maybe classified as initially unresectable. *First,* patients with extension of tumor thrombus above the level of the hepatic veins should be managed with preoperative chemotherapy. *Second,* tumors that involve contiguous structures whereby the only means of removing the kidney tumor requires removal of the other structure (excluding the adrenal gland) should be biopsied and the tumor assigned a surgical stage. The majority of these tumors will compress and adhere to the adjacent organ without actual invasion. These patients can be treated with chemotherapy to shrink the tumor, thereby allowing nephrectomy with preservation of the contiguous organs. A *third* indication for an unresectable tumor is if in the surgeon's judgment a nephrectomy would result in significant or unnecessary morbidity/mortality, diffuse tumor spill, or residual tumor. In this clinical scenario the tumor should be biopsied and the patient given preoperative chemotherapy. *Fourth,* patients with pulmonary compromise due to extensive pulmonary metastases should receive chemotherapy prior to surgery to decrease the operative risk.

Past experience in the NWTSG and SIOPEL studies have shown that pretreatment with chemotherapy almost always reduces the bulk of the tumor and renders it resectable. However, this method does not result in improved survival rates, and does result in the loss of important staging information. It is recommended that all patients undergo initial exploration to assess operability. It is only then that a tumor biopsy should be considered. Patients who are staged by imaging studies alone are at risk for understaging and overstaging. If one chooses to give preoperative therapy based on imaging alone, with or without a needle biopsy, the local tumor should be considered to be stage III, and treatment for patients with favorable or focal anaplasia histology or unknown histology and for patients with diffuse anaplasia histology should be with given. Once there is an adequate reduction in the size of the tumor, nephrectomy is performed following the guidelines described below. For the unresectable patients, radiographic re-evaluation should be performed at week 6. The operative procedure can be performed shortly thereafter if sufficient tumor shrinkage has occurred.

Patients with invasion of the vena cava should be considered for tumor resection when there is evidence of regression of the vena caval thrombus regardless of the degree of response of the primary tumor. Serial imaging evaluation is helpful to assess response, but radiographic evidence of persistent disease can occasionally be misleading

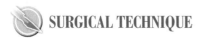 **SURGICAL TECHNIQUE**

Positioning

This procedure is performed under general endotracheal anesthesia. The patient

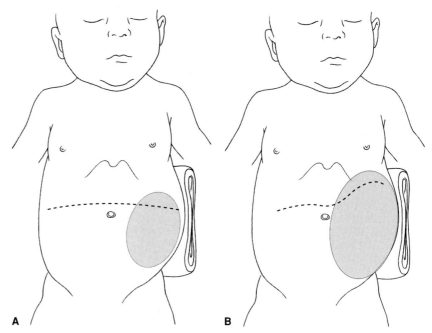

Fig. 1. A: This figure demonstrates the recommended positioning and incision for a Wilms tumor. The child should be slightly elevated on the side of the tumor. A transverse supraumbilical incision is made extending from the midaxillary line on the side of the tumor to the anterior axillary line on the opposite side. **B:** When the tumor is large enough to push up the diaphragm, a thoracoabdominal incision can be very helpful for exposure.

should be positioned supine with the side of the tumor elevated slightly (Fig. 1A,B). In a child a 500-mL intravenous bag or a couple of sterile cloth towels rolled together is usually sufficient. The abdomen and the lower portion of the chest should be prepped and draped appropriately.

Incision and Exposure

A generous transabdominal, transperitoneal, or thoracoabdominal incision is recommended for adequate exposure. The abdominal incision should be one to two fingerbreadths above the umbilicus (Fig. 1A). The incision should extend from the midaxillary line on the side of the tumor to the anterior axillary line on the contralateral side. For very large tumors or those that come off the superior pole and extend up to the diaphragm, a thoracic extension of the incision through the eighth or ninth rib helps with exposure (Fig. 1B). Electrocautery will help control the subcutaneous bleeding. The anterior rectus muscle should be opened on both sides of the abdomen and extended laterally to the external oblique fascia. The posterior rectus and internal and oblique muscles should be opened in a similar fashion. The peritoneum is then incised at a safe free spot within the incision. A moist lap pad should be gently placed over the tumor. A pediatric retractor such as the "Omni tract"

helps facilitate exposure. Complete exploration of the abdomen should be performed. Typically WT can be quite large and will displace other organs and the intestine. Invasion of the other organs, however, is rare. Alternately, the colon is frequently adherent to the tumor but can be easily dissected off. Thorough exploration of the abdomen is necessary to detect evidence of extrarenal extension of tumor. If suspicious lymph nodes or other metastatic deposits are found, these should be biopsied to document tumor involvement. Routine exploration of the contralateral kidney is not necessary if imaging is satisfactory and does not suggest a bilateral process. If the initial imaging studies were suggestive of a possible lesion on the contralateral kidney, the contralateral kidney should be formally explored to rule out bilateral involvement. This should be done prior to nephrectomy to exclude bilateral Wilms tumor. To do this exploration adequately, the colon and its mesentery should be mobilized from the anterior surface of the contralateral kidney, Gerota fascia incised, and the kidney turned forward to palpate and visualize both its anterior and posterior surfaces. Any areas suggestive of bilateral involvement should be biopsied. If positive, a nephrectomy should not be performed (see bilateral section below). In addition, any evidence of a preoperative tumor rupture should clearly be documented in the operative report.

Resection

A radical nephrectomy is performed with the ureter divided as distally as possible. Initial recommendations included an attempt to dissect, expose, and ligate the renal vessels to lessen the chance of hematogenous spread of tumor cells while removing the tumor; also, vascular control prior to nephrectomy will lessen the risk of bleeding prior to mobilizing the primary tumor. However, in many instances the tumor size may make it difficult and unsafe to do this initially. Furthermore, WT studies have not demonstrated any adverse patient outcomes based on when the renal vessels were ligated. Therefore, preliminary ligation should not be pursued if technically difficult or dangerous. In large tumors, the kidney and tumor should be mobilized laterally followed by the inferior and superior poles. Thus, the kidney will be free on its vascular pedicle and ligation of the vessels is technically easier.

When the renal vein is exposed and controlled, the vein and inferior vena cava should be palpated carefully before ligation to rule out extension of the tumor into the wall or the lumen of the vein. If tumor extension is present, this should be removed en bloc with the kidney, if possible, prior to ligation of the vein. Note should be made of whether the tumor penetrates the vessel wall or is attached to the intima. Patients with extension of tumor thrombus above the level of the hepatic veins should be biopsied and managed with preoperative chemotherapy. The majority of these cases should be on preoperative imaging. This approach will often achieve significant shrinkage of the intravascular thrombus facilitating subsequent surgical removal. Both the renal vein and artery should be double-ligated with 00 silk ties and/or a 000 silk suture ligature on the aortic or caval side. To mobilize the kidney, the lateral peritoneal reflection is opened, and the colon is reflected medially. A plane is established outside of Gerota fascia by sharp and blunt dissection. Retroperitoneal perforating vessels should be tied with 000 silk or polyglactin. The adrenal gland may be left in place if it is not abutting the tumor; however, if the mass arises in the upper pole of the kidney, the adrenal gland should be removed with the neoplasm. The lateral and posterior portion of the kidney is mobilized through freeing the retroperitoneal attachments. The ureter is ligated and divided as low as conveniently possible, but it is not necessary to remove the ureter completely. There is a potential for urothelial spread of the tumor cells arising from a lesion that extends into the collecting system. The tumor and the uninvolved portion of the kidney are mobilized and removed intact. Any enlarged or suspicious lymph nodes should be included with the specimen. Any suspicious areas that represent metastases should be biopsied, specifically identified as to the site from which it was removed, and the site(s) identified with small titanium clips so that the locations can be determined later by roentgenograms.

Side-Specific Considerations

Tumors on the right present unique problems for the surgeon (Fig. 2A–D). The

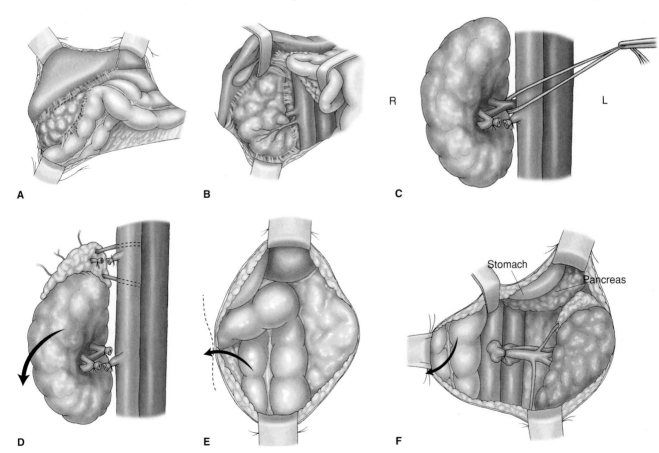

Fig. 2. Anatomic consideration for a right Wilms tumor resection. **A:** The ascending colon and hepatic flexure need to be mobilized. A plane of dissection needs to be established between the tumor and the liver. The dashed lines mark the locations at where the dissection should begin. **B:** The right renal vein is significantly shorter than the left. **C:** Careful dissection will allow for safe ligation of the renal vessels. **D:** On the right side the adrenal vein can be closely adherent or displaced by the tumor mass. **E:** A left Wilms tumor tends to displace the colon medially and anterior. The white line of Toldt guides the dissection plane. **F:** The renal vessel for a left-sided tumor is longer and easier to identify compared to a right-sided tumor. Exposure is facilitated by mobilizing the colon medially and the pancreas superiorly.

right main renal vein is short and easier to tear during dissection. In addition, the right adrenal vein may be adherent to the tumor mass. To help with exposing the vein and the vena cava, the hepatic flexure and transverse colon must be mobilized off the liver and retracted medially. In addition, the duodenum must also be mobilized and retracted medially. A partial Kocher maneuver is helpful. Anatomic considerations for a left nephrectomy include remembering that the left renal vein crosses over the aorta and that the left gonadal (testicular or ovarian vein) and the left adrenal vein enter the left renal vein directly (Fig. 2E,F). Elevating the spleen and pancreas superior and medially to the tumor will facilitate exposure for left-sided tumors.

Lymph Node Documentation

The presence or absence of disease in hilar and regional lymph nodes is an extremely important factor in accurate staging and therefore appropriate treatment. Routine lymph node sampling from the renal hilum and the pericaval or para-aortic areas must be done for accurate staging (Fig. 3). Involved or suspicious lymph nodes should be excised. Formal lymph node dissection is not recommended. The nodes should be carefully separated for microscopic examination. Failure to sample lymph nodes is one of the major technical errors noted in Wilms tumor surgery. Children with positive lymph nodes are classified as stage III. Studies have demonstrated a higher risk of recurrence in children who did not have the lymph node status documented at the time of nephrectomy.

Contiguous Organs

Wilms tumors are frequently adherent to adjacent organs. In the majority of cases, there is not frank invasion by the tumor and the organs can be dissected freely from the tumor. Radical en bloc resection (e.g., partial hepatectomy) is not generally warranted. Extensive resection including multiple organs (e.g., spleen, pancreas, and colon) is also not advised as this is associated with an increased frequency of complications. Furthermore, WTs are very chemosensitive and in these situations a biopsy followed by chemotherapy will allow for a safer resection. If removal of a small section of diaphragm, psoas muscle, or tip of the pancreas allows the tumor to be removed intact, then proceed.

Tumor Spills and Ruptures

The local stage of the tumor and the operation play an important role in directing adjuvant therapy. Studies have shown a higher risk of recurrence in patients who had tumor spills or ruptures irrespective of the cause or extent of the soiling. These events resulted in an increased risk of local recurrence and increased adjuvant therapy with the attendant risks. "Spillage" refers to transgression of the tumor capsule during operative removal, whether accidental, unavoidable, or by design. Spill would occur if the surgeon transected the renal vein or ureter at the site of tumor extension. When the tumor extends into the renal vein or inferior vena cava, a precise description of the technique of removal should be given in the operative note. It must be stated in the operative report if the intravascular tumor extension was removed en bloc or if

the tumor was transected, as well as if the tumor thrombus was removed completely and if there was evidence of either adherence or invasion of the vein wall. Preoperative percutaneous needle biopsy from the anterior or posterior approach is also considered "local spillage." Open incisional biopsy prior to nephrectomy is considered a local spill unless, in the surgeon's judgment, the whole peritoneal cavity has been soiled in the process

"Rupture" refers to either the spontaneous or posttraumatic rupture of the tumor preoperatively with the result that tumor cells are disseminated throughout the peritoneal cavity. Bloody peritoneal fluid shall be considered a sign of major soilage, whether or not gross or microscopic tumor is identified in the fluid. There are times when the tumor may rupture posteriorly and the perforation is confined to the retroperitoneal space, thus qualifying as local soilage. When a hematoma is present, it is assumed that tumor cells will spread with the blood. If primary nephrectomy is undertaken, this increases the risk of contamination of the peritoneal space. The superior, inferior, medial, and lateral margins of the associated hematoma should be described fully in the operative note, and the margins marked with titanium clips. Tumor may penetrate the kidney capsule and the overlying peritoneum, the raw neoplastic tissue surface being in free communication with the peritoneal cavity. This is considered major soilage. Separate, distinct nodules of tumor on the peritoneal or serosal surfaces at a distance from the primary neoplasm ("satellite implants") are considered a sign of major soilage.

Closure

After the tumor resection is complete, the tumor bed should be irrigated with saline/Ringers solution and inspected for bleeding. If during the operation any soilage was noted, the tumor bed should be outlined with a titanium clip and it should be clearly documented in the operative dictation. The colon is then laid over the tumor bed and all structures placed back into their normal anatomic position. The peritoneum, transversalis fascia, and posterior rectus should be closed as the first inner layer with 00 or 0 polypropylene with a tapered needle. Next, the internal and external oblique fascia and the anterior rectus are closed in a similar fashion. The subcutaneous portion of the wound should be irrigated and assessed for bleeding. Scarpa fascia in a child is a delineable layer and can be closed with interrupted or continuous

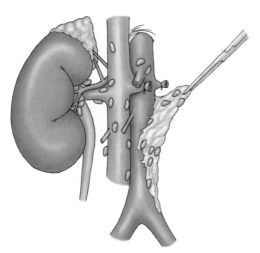

Fig. 3. Lymph node sampling is a critical staging and prognostic consideration for children with Wilms tumor.

4-0 polyglactin suture. Suture removal in children is very frightening and painful; therefore, skin staples should be avoided. The skin should be closed using a dermal continuous 4-0 polyglactin suture. Sterile strips are used to coapt the skin.

Insertion of a central venous catheter at the time of nephrectomy has become routine for these operations. The child will require adjuvant chemotherapy to effect a cure for this neoplasm. The surgeon should consider placing a central venous catheter under the same anesthetic to avoid a second operation or a delay in therapy. A subcutaneous port is the best choice for the child, or an external line if the child is too small for a port placement.

SPECIAL CONSIDERATIONS

Horseshoe Kidney

There are several conditions in children that have a predisposition to developing WT. These include children with horseshoe kidneys, sporadic aniridia, hemihypertrophy, Beckwith-Wiedemann syndrome, and nephroblastomatosis. Children with these conditions need to be monitored carefully with renal ultrasound every 3 to 6 months until they are at least 10 years of age. Resection of a WT in a child with a horseshoe kidney presents unique challenges (Fig. 4). Children with horseshoe

kidneys and WT must be carefully imaged prior to any surgery. The blood supply to the kidney as well as the ureters must be identified and isolated. Exposure and mobilization of the kidney on the side of the tumor is carried out as if one is performing a unilateral resection. The side of the kidney containing the tumor, the isthmus, and the ipsilateral ureter are resected. The lower end of the remaining kidney is oversewn with 00 polyglactin mattress sutures. As with other unilateral procedures, the lymph node groups are sampled for staging purposes.

Synchronous Bilateral Wilms Tumor (BWT)

Survival in patients with bilateral synchronous tumor has improved dramatically with the approach to therapy becoming evidence based and standardized. Therapy for patients with BWT is focused on sparing renal parenchyma. Review of National Wilms Tumor Study Group/Children's Oncology Group (NWTSG/COG) patients found that 9.1% of those with synchronous BWT developed renal failure. The cause of renal failure in 74% of the patients was bilateral nephrectomy for persistent or recurrent tumor in the remaining kidney after initial nephrectomy. Therefore, avoiding total nephrectomy at initial surgery is advised. For a child with

suspected BWT, initial surgical therapy is directed to establishing the pathologic diagnosis in each kidney through biopsy of each kidney. The COG has recommended that all children with BWT receive chemotherapy prior to surgical resection. Extensive algorithms have been developed to help direct therapy in these patients and can be found on the COG Web site at www.childrensoncologygroup.org (surgical discipline). It is strongly recommended that when one encounters a BWT, he or she review the therapy guidelines as they are regularly revised. Primary excision of large tumor masses should not be attempted. When biopsies are obtained, a posterior approach is advised to limit contamination of the peritoneal cavity. Solitary peripheral renal lesions less than 2 cm in diameter can be completely excised at diagnosis.

After initial chemotherapy, the patient is evaluated by repeat imaging at 6 weeks. If imaging suggests the viability of a partial resection, a second-look procedure is carried out and surgery should be performed. The goal of second-look surgery, whether at week 6 or 12, is to achieve complete resection of tumor with negative margins while preserving the greatest amount of viable kidney. All steps are taken to avoid bilateral nephrectomy. If the response to therapy does not allow for a partial nephrectomy, further treatment is used to attempt to shrink the tumor. It may be necessary to do third- and fourth-look procedures prior to bilateral nephrectomy.

Biopsies are essential in patients who are not responding to chemotherapy, since tumors with complete necrosis and predominantly regressive changes can increase in size during therapy. A clinically good response (by imaging) is usually associated with a pathologically good response in terms of regressive histologic changes. The converse is not always true. Tumors with complete necrosis and predominantly regressive changes can increase in size during therapy. Differentiation of the tumor after chemotherapy has been noted. Stromal and epithelial predominant tumors are found more often after chemotherapy. These histologic subtypes may demonstrate a poor clinical response to therapy but have an excellent prognosis if the tumor is completely excised.

Biopsies of nonresponding tumors are also needed to exclude anaplasia, which occurs in 10% of BWTs. Anaplastic tumors have been noted to be resistant to chemotherapy. Any surgical procedure in patients with anaplasia must ensure complete resection of the tumor. Complete

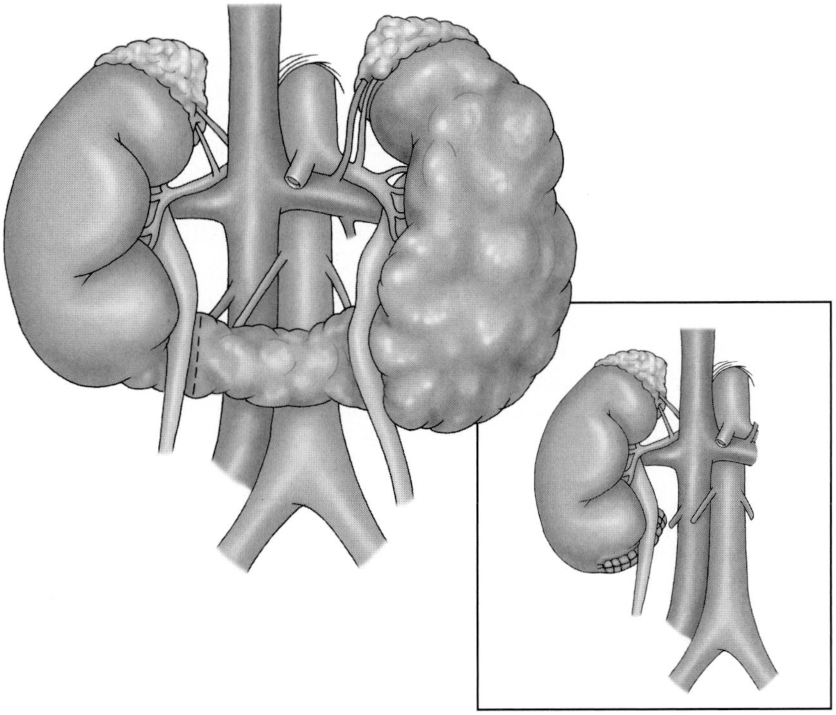

Fig. 4. This diagram represents a horseshoe kidney with a Wilms tumor. The tumor and the isthmus must be resected. The dashed line shows the line of resection. The insert demonstrates anatomy postresection.

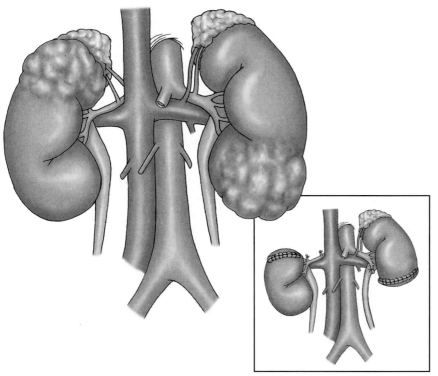

Fig. 5. Children with bilateral tumors present unique challenges. Chemotherapy is used as the first line of therapy. When the tumor becomes amenable to a partial nephrectomy, surgery should be performed.

excision of anaplastic tumors can improve survival. For patients with unilateral tumors with less than 50% reduction in the size of the tumor, nephrectomy should be performed if partial resection is not feasible. In BWT, nonresponders undergo open biopsy of the tumor(s) to guide subsequent chemotherapy decisions. Needle biopsy of the tumors is not sufficient at this time. Tumors judged to be amenable to resection are removed by partial nephrectomy or wedge excision (Fig. 5). The surgeon should always attempt to achieve negative surgical margins. Enucleation of the tumor should only be considered for patients with favorable histologic BWT if removing a margin of renal tissue would compromise the vascular supply to the kidney (e.g., a centrally located tumor encroaching on the renal hilum). Biopsy of the tumor should be done before considering enucleation. If anaplasia is found on the biopsy, enucleation should not be performed.

Other groups of children that could benefit from renal parenchymal–sparing surgery are those known to be at increased risk for development of metachronous Wilms tumor. Patients with aniridia and a number of overgrowth syndromes (e.g., Beckwith-Wiedemann syndrome and idiopathic hemihypertrophy) have an increased incidence of nephrogenic rests (a premalignant lesion) in comparison to patients with unilateral Wilms tumor not associated with congenital anomalies.

In a few cases a bench operation (after the kidney is perfused with iced Ringers saline solution and perfusate similar to that used for renal transplantation) to dissect the neoplasm from the kidney and autoimplant the residual renal tissue in the pelvis has been described. A large experience with these cases has not been reported and should only be used in experienced hands in rare circumstances. Children with BWT who require bilateral nephrectomies can be considered for renal transplantation after therapy is completed but will be at risk due to immunosuppression of tumor reactivation and other associated risks of renal transplantation.

Intravascular Extension

Vascular invasion of the renal vein, cava, and atrium presents special surgical challenges. These tumors will often respond to preoperative therapy. Renal vein involvement has been noted in 11% of cases (most often detected at operation) and caval and atria involvement in 5% of cases. Tumor extension into the renal vein and proximate inferior vena cava can in most cases be removed en bloc with the kidney (Fig. 6A,B). However, primary resection of extension into the inferior vena cava to the hepatic level or into the atrium is associated with higher operative morbidity. In these circumstances, preoperative chemotherapy decreases the size and extent of the tumor thrombus without increasing its adherence to the vascular wall, thereby facilitating subsequent excision. Ultrasonographic studies are essential to identify vascular extent of the tumor. The tumor that extends into the renal vein and cava may simply extend as a floating attachment and can then be "fished out." Control of the renal vein and cava above and below the tumor with vessel loops is necessary. The tumor should not be transected. Silk 2-0 stitches can then be placed on either side of the renal vein. This will help with vascular control and limit bleeding. The tumor and kidney should be completely mobilized prior to removing vascular thrombus. A venotomy is then done and the tumor pulled out of the vein. A Foley balloon technique can also be used to pull out the tumor. In other instances the tumor may be fixed to the vascular lumen. Extraction is more difficult and a larger venotomy may be required. A similar technique used for removing plaque for a carotid endarterectomy is helpful to lift the tumor off the vein wall. If after preoperative chemotherapy the tumor still extends above the hepatic veins, cardiopulmonary bypass is needed to remove the vascular extent of the tumor. The abdominal tumor is mobilized and removed first, prior to administration of heparin. After placing the child on bypass, the right atrium is opened and the tricuspid valve inspected. The tumor is removed from the heart above and the below at the same time to prevent tumor emboli. This aggressive approach is similar to that used in those children with stage II tumors.

Nephroblastomatosis

Nephroblastomatosis or nephrogenic rests (NRs) are defined as "persistent metanephretic tissue after the 36th week of life." It is considered a premalignant lesion. There are two clinical situations when a surgeon may encounter NRs. The first is within a WT specimen. NRs within a kidney that contains a WT result in an increased risk of that child developing a metachronous tumor in the other kidney. The second is as an independent lesion. These children can also develop de novo Wilms tumors within the NRs and must be followed carefully. NRs can be subclassified according to the rest category present (e.g., diffuse hyperplastic perilobar

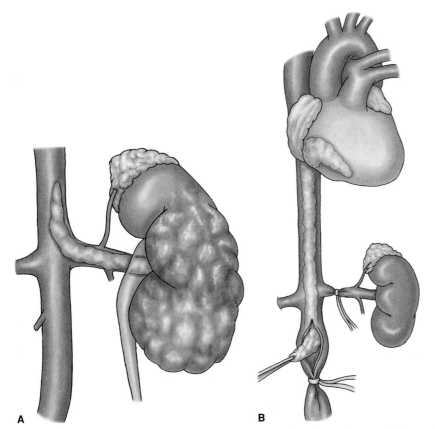

Fig. 6. A: Intravascular extension of a left Wilms tumor. Note the "floating" tumor in the caval. **B:** Tumor extending to the atrium. Cardiopulmonary bypass plus complete vascular controlled is needed to safely remove these tumors.

nephrogenic rests [DHPLNRs]). NRs are also categorized based on their growth phase. These include incipient or dormant nephrogenic rests, hyperplastic nephrogenic rests, and regressing or sclerosing nephrogenic rests. Those that form a thick rind around the kidney, DHPLNRs, are the least difficult to identify. The NRs that cause the greatest diagnostic difficulty are those that are actively proliferating or hyperplastic, as these are often mistaken for WT. Hyperplastic NRs can produce masses as large as conventional Wilms tumor. Neoplastic induction of NRs can occur and is the biggest challenge for the surgeon managing these patients. Pathologic distinction between NR and WT is difficult. Incisional biopsies are of no value. One needs to examine the juncture between the lesion and the surrounding renal parenchyma to be able to distinguish between the two entities. Most hyperplastic NRs lack a pseudocapsule at the periphery, while most Wilms tumors will have this feature.

In DHPLNRs, the cortical surface of the kidney is composed of hyperplastic NRs. The entire nephrogenic zone is involved with a thick rind capping the entire kidney. Cut sections reveal a rind of pale tissue encasing the kidney. This extends from the capsule into the upper cortex. It is well delineated from the normal renal parenchyma. Histologically, the lesion consists of predominantly blastemal cells, but a significant epithelial component can be present. With multicentric NRs, the lesions are separated by recognizable renal parenchyma. These patients are prone to WT development and bilateral lesions are common.

Radiology of Nephrogenic Rests

Radiologic studies may be helpful to help distinguish NR from Wilms tumor. A few studies suggest the utility of MRI in detecting NRs, but each of these series is small and retrospective. In patients with multicentric or bilateral tumors, it has become apparent that many lesions previously thought to be Wilms tumor are indeed hyperplastic NR. Nephroblastomatosis appears homogenous on CT compared to the cortex after contrast injection. On MRI, nephroblastomatosis is isointense or slightly hypointense to the cortex on T1-weighted images. They remain hypointense after gadolinium injection. Wilms tumor can be distinguished due to

mixed echogenicity and inhomogeneity. Some have suggested that imaging appearance is more useful than biopsy in the diagnosis and follow-up of nephroblastomatosis. Hyperplastic NRs are also suspected if the lesions retain the shape of the NR, ovoid, lenticular, or band-like.

The technology of MRI and CT is quickly advancing. MRI used to have the advantage by displaying the images in multiple planes, thus guiding the surgeon for the nephron-sparing surgery. With multislice technique, CT now can be reconstructed into multiple planes. CT, however, accounts for the majority of diagnostic ionizing radiation exposure these patients receive. There is still no consensus about which modality is best to detect the rests. However, MRI may have an additional advantage of distinguishing the sclerotic NR (dark on T2-weighted or short tau inversion recovery [STIR] sequences) from hyperplastic or dysplastic rests and Wilms tumor.

In addition, the MRI characteristics of active NRs and Wilms tumors may change with therapy. The rests and tumors often become dark on T2 or STIR examination, suggesting progressive sclerosis including hemosiderin deposition, hyalinization, or fibrosis. Lesions that remain bright on T2 and enhance with gadolinium have on occasion prompted resection and been confirmed as active Wilms tumor or hyperplastic NRs. It has been shown that there was a correlation between the MRI appearance of NRs and their eventual conversion to Wilms tumor. However, there has not been a prospective study with central review of images evaluating the utility of MRI in predicting conversion of NRs to Wilms tumor.

Treatment of Diffuse Hyperplastic Perilobar Nephrogenic Rests

Nephroblastomatosis or DHPLNR has not been formally studied by either the NWTSG or SIOP. As a consequence, patients are treated in various ways, some with multiple chemotherapeutic agents, some not at all. Treatment of DHPLNR is controversial due to the lack of data regarding the outcome of large numbers of children with this diagnosis. Often repeat biopsies and imaging studies are needed in these children to monitor disease progression. Initial observation of DHPLNR has been rarely reported. Most children with DHPLNR have been treated with chemotherapy, with radiation reserved for lesions that fail to regress. Surgery depends on the size and pathologic progression of the disease.

After initial treatment, partial nephrectomy is possible and the disease should be resected. If not, the children should be treated as if they have bilateral tumors. Data have shown that about 50% of children had DH-PLNR up to 5 years following diagnosis.

Lung Metastasis

Traditional outcomes for patients with lung metastasis have been defined by CXR imaging. Patients with lung metastasis in North America have been treated with adjuvant chemotherapy and 1200 cGy radiation to both lung fields. They are considered stage IV. However, chest CT scans are now the standard thoracic imaging modality. Lesions are detected on CT scans that are not seen on CXR. The clinical significance and surgical management of these smaller lesions has been evolving and has driven the revisions to the management of pulmonary lesions in children with WT. In 1997 a report from St. Jude's hospital concluded that the variability in interpretation of thoracic CT scans in WT limits the predictive utility of these studies. Based on this report, a variety of therapies were given to children with CT lesions. In some cases the children were treated based on the local stage of the tumor. Alternatively, others were classified as stage IV and received radiotherapy. Two recent studies have addressed these issues. The first review suggests that patients with pulmonary lesions detected by CT only and treated with only two chemotherapeutic agents have an inferior outcome compared to those treated with three drugs irrespective of whether they received pulmonary radiation. A second study (by the author) examined the pathology of these supposed benign lesions. Almost two thirds of the children had tumor on biopsy. Thus, CT-only lesions are not invariably tumor, demonstrating the need for histopathologic confirmation. Biopsy remains critical until radiographic techniques allow differentiation between benign and malignant lesions (Fig. 7).

New therapy for children with pulmonary lesions will be response based. Chemotherapy with two agents will be given first and the lesions will be reimaged at 6 weeks. If lesions are still present, more intensive and toxic therapy including radiotherapy will be given. There will be three times a surgeon may be asked to intervene in a child with a pulmonary lesion. The first is at diagnosis, likely a small single lesion. If the tumor is stage I (vs. stage IV), the child may be eligible for surgery alone (or less toxic chemotherapy) to obtain

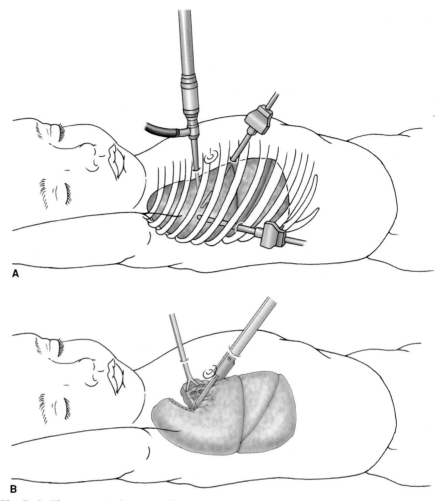

Fig. 7. A: Thoracoscopic biopsies of lung metastasis are now routine. After computed tomography localization, the ports should be placed in a triangular fashion to facilitate removal of the tumor. **B:** Wedge resection using Endo-stapling of a lung nodule.

a cure. The second will be after the first round of chemotherapy if lesions shrink but do not go away completely. It would be valuable to assess the histology of the lesion prior to giving radiotherapy. The third situation is if tumor remains after both chemotherapy and radiotherapy, requiring surgical resection for cure. Most WT metastases are peripheral and superficial.

Many of these lesions can now be fully excised by video-assisted thoracic surgery. The child under general anesthesia is placed in a lateral position. Small 3- or 5-mm ports are inserted in a triangular pattern around the lesion to facilitate removal. An endoscopic GIA-30 stapler 2.5 mm is used to excise the tumor with a wedge margin of normal lung. An air leak from the edge of the staple line can be oversewn with a continuous 000 chromic catgut lock stitch. The lesion can be brought out either through a trocar or an endoscopic bag.

For larger lesions (e.g., right middle lobe mass) or for those wishing to perform

an open procedure, a standard posterior lateral thoracotomy incision for exploration of the chest can be used. Under general anesthesia the child is placed in the lateral position. A posterior lateral incision is made using the tip of the scapula as a guide. Hemostasis is maintained using electrocautery. The latissimus dorsi muscle is divided with the electrocautery. The auscultatory space is entered, and the fifth interspace is identified. The serratus anterior muscle is divided along the line of the interspace. The chest is opened by incision of the intercostal muscles above the rib. The pleural space is entered, and a Finochietto retractor is inserted. The lesion should then be identified. The pleura over the major fissure is incised, and the pulmonary artery identified. The pulmonary arteries to the right middle lobe should be identified. The vessels should be carefully mobilized using a blunt right-angle dissector. The vessels should be ligated using 000 silk ties and stick sutured with a 000 silk. Next, the middle lobe branch of the superior pulmonary vein is identified and ligated in similar fashion. The bronchial arteries are identified and double-tied with 000 silk. This should result in the middle lobe being on a pedicle of the middle lobe bronchus. The bronchus is dissected free and proximal closure is performed using a GIA-30 stapling device. The remaining lung including the staple line should be placed under water. The lung is then lung expanded to look for an air leak. A chest tube is placed below the incision and to 10 to 15 cm of negative water pressure after the chest is closed. The operative filed is inspected for bleeding prior to closing. To approximate the ribs 0 polyglactin paracostal sutures are used. The muscles layers are closed using 00 polyglactin sutures. The subcutaneous tissue is approximated with interrupted 4-0 polyglactin sutures, and the skin, running suture of the same material.

RESULTS

Through the multidisciplinary management of Wilms tumor survival of children has improved over the last several decades. Currently more then 90% of children survive 5 years (compared to 30% in the 1930s) after their diagnosis, with 85% being cured. Nevertheless, there are populations of patients who do poorly, particularly those with locally recurrent Wilms tumor. Survival in this group is below 40%. The primary objective of clinical trials on Wilms tumor has evolved to a risk-based management. Therapy for those children with low-risk tumors is reduced to decrease unwelcome long-term side effects without reducing cure rates. Alternatively, new strategies, including treatment intensification, for patients with high-risk tumors are sought to further improve outcome.

SUGGESTED READING

Beckwith JB. Children at increased risk for Wilms tumor: monitoring issues. *J Pediatr* 1998;138:377.

Coppes MJ, Arnold M, Beckwith JB, et al. Factors affecting the risk of contralateral Wilms tumor development: a report from the National Wilms Tumor Study Group. *Cancer* 1999;85(7):1616.

D'Angio GJ. Pre- or post-operative treatment for Wilms tumor? Who, what, when, where, how, why—and which. *Med Pediatr Oncol* 2003;41:545.

Ehrlich PF. Wilms tumor: progress to date and future considerations. *Expert Rev Anticancer Ther* 2001;1:555.

Ehrlich PF, Ritchey ML, Hamilton TE, et al. Quality assessment for Wilms tumor: a report from the NWTS-5. *J Pediatr Surg* In press

Grosfeld JL. Risk-based management: current concepts of treating malignant solid tumors of childhood. *J Am Coll Surg* 1999;189:407.

Kalapurakal JA, Dome JS, Perlman EJ, et al. Management of Wilms' tumour: current practice and future goals. *Lancet Oncol* 2004;5:37.

Miser JS, Tournade MF. The management of relapsed Wilms tumor. *Hematol Oncol Clin North Am* 1995;9:1287.

Neville H, Ritchey ML, Shamberger RC, et al. The occurrence of Wilms tumor in horseshoe kidneys: a report from the National Wilms Tumor Study Group (NWTSG). *Pediatr Surg* 2002;37(8):1134.

Paulino AC, Wen BC, Brown CK, et al. Late effects in children treated with radiation therapy for Wilms tumor. *Inter J Rad Oncol* 2000;46:1239.

Porteus MH, Narkool P, Neuberg D, et al. Characteristics and outcome of children with Beckwith-Wiedemann syndrome and Wilms tumor: a report from the National Wilms Tumor Study Group. *J Clin Oncol* 2000;18:2026.

Ritchey ML, Pringle K, Breslow N, et al. Management and outcome of inoperable Wilms tumor: a report of the National Wilms Tumor Study Group. *Ann Surg* 1994;220:683.

Shamberger RC, Guthrie KA, Ritchey ML, et al. Surgery related factors and local recurrence of Wilms tumor in the National Wilms Tumor Study 4. *Ann Surg* 1999;229:292.

Shamberger RC, Ritchey ML, Haase GM, Intravascular extension of Wilms tumor. *Ann Surg* 2001;234(1):116.

Tournade MF, Com-Nougue C, Voute PA, et al. Results of the Sixth International Society of Pediatric Oncology Wilms' tumor trial and study: a risk-adapted therapeutic approach in Wilms' tumor. *J Clin Oncol* 1993;11:1014.

WEB SITES

American Academy of Pediatrics: www.aap.org

American Association of Pediatric Surgery: www.eapsa.org

American College of Surgeons: http://www.facs.org/

Children's Oncology Group: www.childrensoncologygroup.org

International Society of Pediatric Oncology: http://www.md.ucl.ac.be/siop/

Nongastrointestinal Transabdominal

EDITOR'S COMMENT

Wilms tumor is one of the most common tumors in childhood and, given the amount of work that has gone into Wilms tumor, one thinks of Wilms tumor and the number of cooperative studies that have taken place in its treatment and compares it to the national and, as a matter of fact, international, of breast cancer. The results are really quite striking. Except for bilateral tumors and tumors associated with nephrogenic rests, the survival is in the range of 90% and increasing. This is the type of treatment that is individualized for each patient with the result that one can expect the best outcome known at the particular time. Of course, as further studies take place, the constant updating of the various Wilms tumor oncology programs make certain that patients get the most up-to-date treatment and an appropriate combination of chemotherapy, radiation therapy, and surgery.

The role of the surgeon is very carefully defined in this chapter. While nephrectomy is perhaps the mainstay of surgical therapy, surgeons who are more adventurous have done partial nephrectomies and even segmental, as it were, nephrectomies of relatively small tumors. Whether or not the outcomes in more localized resections are as good as those with nephrectomy is not clear. What is clear, however, is that if there is tumor spill, the prognosis is considerably reduced. While in other places in this volume, for example, in carcinoma of the rectum, there have been great advances in restorative function up to and including excision of part of the rectal sphincter in an effort to avoid a permanent colostomy, the results in the restorative approach in Wilms tumor do not seem to be as good as they are, for example, in carcinoma of the rectum.

Part of the issue appears to be how big the tumor is. Since the tumor tends to occur in small children and the tumors are discovered either by pediatricians or parents, it is not surprising that as the tumor gets larger, the prognosis is worse. Indeed, in less fortunate populations as far as health care, morbidity, and the outcome of surgery in large tumors, even if they are pretreated, is concerned, size does matter. This is the point made by Hadley and Shaik (*Pediat Surg Int* 2006;22:409), who reported 67 patients whose tumor was greater than 1 kg. They make the point that as the tumor gets larger, more organs are involved and there's more of a necessity to undergo resection.

Their experience at the University of KwaZulu-Natal in South Africa is at variance with the experience expressed here, and that is the Wilms tumor does not invade adjacent tumors. I suppose one could say the tumor does not invade adjacent tumors when it is of reasonable size. When it is large, however, it may invade adjacent organs, requiring their sacrifice. In some of the photographs in the children operated on after one, two, or three cycles of dactinomycin and vincristine, the tumor varied between 10% and 16% of the infant's total mass. While there was no relationship between the patient's mass and mortality, it approached but did not satisfy significance. Notably, despite spills in 21% of the patients, which resulted in increased incidence of recurrence, 63% of the patients were alive and disease free 8 months to 12 years off treatment. Of the others, 21% are known to have died and a further 11% are lost to follow-up and presumed to have died. A very succinct summary of the current treatment is given by Arya et al. in a two-page paper, indicating the current form of therapy for various stages of tumor, that can be read quickly and easily and gives one an excellent

(continued)

summary based on the various study groups (*Br J Urol* 2006;97:899).

An unsolved problem is that of anaplastic histologic Wilms tumor, and this is summarized by Dome et al. (*J Clin Oncol* 2006;24[15]:2352); almost 2,600 patients were enrolled into the National Wilms' Tumor Study-5, of whom 11% had anaplastic histology. Stage I had favorable histology (92.4% survival) but decreased to 82% in stage II and only 33% in stage IV.

Finally, the problems of nephrogenic rests and heterogeneity and the pathogenesis of Wilms tumor were reviewed by Breslow et al. (*Pediatr Blood Cancer* Available at: . Accessed May 12, 2006) dealing with patients with either intralobar or perilobar nephrogenic rests. Multifocality decreased the mean age of the development of the tumor by 18 and 10 months and anaplastic histology increased it by 3, 10, and 16 months. Over 90% of the multifocal tumors occurred in the presence of demonstrated intralobar or perilobar rests.

They explained the various bimodalities on this basis. The nephrogenic rests, which are diffused premalignant lesions, remain an unsolved problem in Wilms tumors and require aggressive therapy, and clearly outcomes are not as good as they are in those with more favorable histology. Additional studies hopefully will result in a systematic approach enabling these patients to experience as good an outcome as favorable histology.

J.E.F.

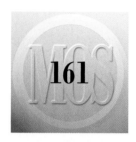

161 Genitourinary Tract Trauma

JACK W. MCANINCH AND VIRAJ A. MASTER

INTRODUCTION

The genitourinary system, encompassing the kidney, ureter, bladder, urethra, and external genitalia, is commonly injured in both blunt and penetrating trauma. Approximately 10% of all traumatic injuries seen in the emergency department involve the genitourinary system, but these injuries may be hard to identify. Early, thorough assessment allows for accurate staging, which then guides treatment and is essential in preventing serious complications. In this chapter, an evidence-based approach to diagnosis and management has been used. A detailed analysis of all genitourinary trauma articles published worldwide between 1966 and 2002 was conducted by an invited panel of surgeons (and chaired by J.W. McAninch), with subspecialty interests in traumatic and reconstructive urology, which was convened by the World Health Organization at the 2003 Stockholm Société Internationale d'Urologie meeting. Each paper from the primary literature was analyzed according to its numerical level of evidence classification, from randomized prospective clinical trials to case reports. Consensus papers were written on trauma to each genitourinary organ. As the editor of *BJU International* wrote (in a preface to the ureteral trauma consensus paper), "This is quite a unique document, of interest to all urologists, not only as a consensus of how this condition should be managed, but also as a model of how to review publications." Evidence-supported diagnostic algorithms for adult blunt injury and pediatric blunt injury are shown in Figures 1 and 2, respectively. Penetrating abdominal

trauma, especially gunshot wounds, will certainly be evaluated in the operating room. Treatment and further diagnostic algorithms for injuries to specific areas of the genitourinary tract are presented later in the chapter.

RENAL TRAUMA

The kidney is the genitourinary organ most commonly injured due to external trauma, found in approximately 5% of abdominal trauma cases. Advances in staging techniques resulting from increased use of computed tomography (CT) scanning and increased awareness based on outcomes research of the kidney's capacity for healing have permitted the vast majority of these injuries to be successfully managed nonoperatively by the surgical consultant. Nonetheless, certain severely injured kidneys are best managed by exploration and reconstruction, with nephrectomy reserved for life-threatening hemorrhage or kidneys that have been injured beyond repair. Ultimately, the objective of managing these patients is to prevent significant hemorrhage and retain enough functioning nephron mass to avoid end-stage kidney failure. A secondary goal is to avoid complications specifically attributable to the traumatized kidney.

Staging of Renal Injuries

Approximately 90% of renal injuries result from blunt trauma—usually falls from great heights, motor vehicle accidents, and violent assaults. Most of these injuries are minor and rarely require surgical exploration. At San Francisco General Hospital,

only 2% of all bluntly injured kidneys required exploration or repair. Pediatric kidneys as well as congenitally abnormal kidneys (cystic kidneys, hydronephrotic kidneys) are more susceptible to major injury secondary to blunt mechanisms. Although only 10% of renal injuries result from penetrating trauma, up to 55% of these injuries will require exploration or repair. This is usually due to a more severe renal injury, associated intra-abdominal injuries, incomplete preoperative radiographic staging, or a combination of these factors.

The American Association for the Surgery of Trauma (AAST) has created a renal organ injury scale that correlates with patient outcomes and allows appropriate and selective management to be undertaken (Table 1). The renal injury classification is one of the few classification schemes that has been prospectively validated and found to correlate directly with need for surgical intervention. Grade 1 injuries include subcapsular hematomas and renal contusions (Fig. 3). Grade 2 injuries involve small lacerations into the renal cortex. Grade 3 injuries extend through the corticomedullary junction. Grade 4 injuries consist of either injury into the collecting system or renal vascular injuries such as main renal artery or vein injury with contained hemorrhage, or segmental vessel injury. Grade 5 injuries include kidneys with pedicle avulsion off the great vessels, as well as completely shattered kidneys.

Clinical staging begins with history and physical examination, including the determination of whether the patient has been in shock as well as assessment for presence of hematuria. Based on these criteria, a

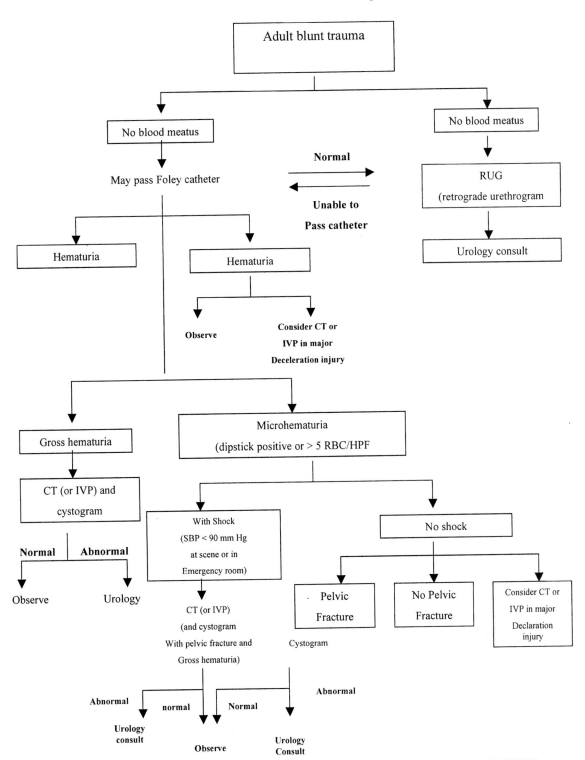

Fig. 1. Algorithm for staging blunt trauma in adults. CT, computed tomography; HPF, high-power field; IVP, intravenous pyelogram; RBC, red blood cell; SBP, systolic blood pressure. (Adapted from Santucci RA, Wessels H, Bartsch G, et al. Evaluation and management of renal injuries: consensus statement of the Renal Trauma Subcommittee. *BJU Int* 2004;93:937.)

subset of patients likely to have significant renal injury may be identified. This subset may then undergo radiographic staging in order to completely stage the injury and determine whether operative management is indicated (Figs. 4 and 5).

History should focus on the mechanism of trauma (blunt [Fig. 4] or penetrating [Fig. 5]), as well as presence of significant deceleration, which should raise suspicion for significant renal injury. In penetrating trauma, knowledge of type of bullet (high

vs. low velocity) or knife used in the assault may assist in prediction of degree of renal injury. On physical examination, the presence of shock (defined as systolic blood pressure <90 mm Hg) should be recorded. The lowest recorded systolic blood pressure

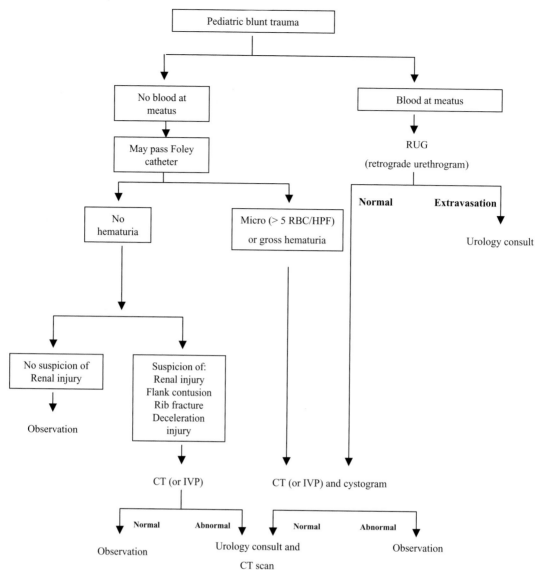

Fig. 2. Algorithm for staging blunt trauma in pediatric patients. CT, computed tomography; HPF, high-power field; IVP, intravenous pyelogram; RBC, red blood cell.

TABLE 1. AMERICAN ASSOCIATION FOR THE SURGERY OF TRAUMA ORGAN INJURY SEVERITY SCALE FOR RENAL TRAUMA

Grade	Injury	Description
I	Contusion	Microscopic or gross hematuria, urologic studies normal
	Hematoma	Subcapsular, nonexpanding without parenchymal laceration
II	Hematoma	Nonexpanding perirenal hematoma confined to renal retroperitoneum
	Laceration	<1 cm parenchymal depth of renal cortex without urinary extravasation
III	Laceration	>1 cm depth of renal cortex without collecting system rupture or urinary extravasation
IV	Laceration	Parenchymal laceration extending through the renal cortex, medulla, and collecting system (meaning extravasation)
	Vascular	Main renal artery or vein injury with contained hemorrhage
V	Laceration	Completely shattered kidney
	Vascular	Avulsion of renal hilum, which devascularizes kidney

Note that the injury scale is advanced one grade for bilateral injuries up to grade III. For more information, go to www.aast.org/injury/injury.html.

is critical in determining the need for radiographic imaging in adult blunt renal trauma. Clearly, a patient in shock who cannot be resuscitated may require urgent laparotomy, thus bypassing radiographic staging of suspected renal injury, and will require intraoperative staging. The abdomen, flank, and back should be carefully examined. Flank tenderness or ecchymosis as well as lower rib fractures may indicate underlying renal injury. In penetrating trauma, entry and exit wounds may be a helpful indicator that the kidney has been injured.

Hematuria is the most common sign of penetrating and blunt renal trauma. However, importantly, the presence of hematuria and degree of hematuria does not correlate consistently with degree of renal injury. This is particularly true in

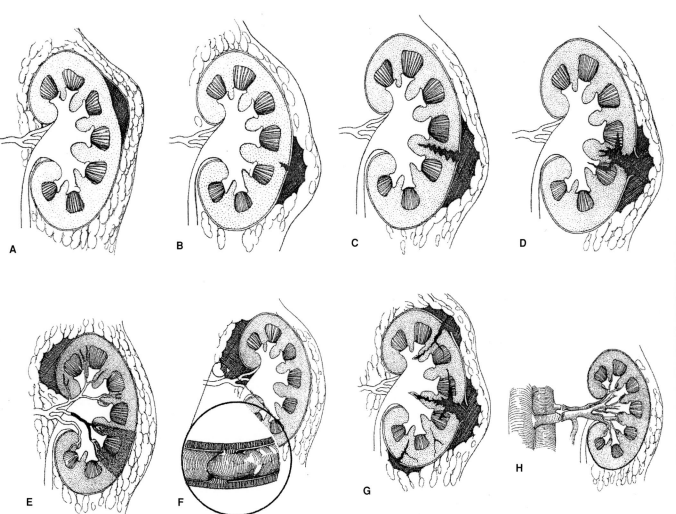

Fig. 3. Renal injury classification. Renal injuries are classified by the American Association for the Society of Trauma Organ Injury Scale. Grades 1 and 2 are considered minor renal injuries, only rarely requiring intervention, while grades 3, 4, and 5 are considered major renal injuries. **A:** Grade 1 is contusion or contained subcapsular hematoma without parenchymal laceration. **B:** Grade 2 is a nonexpanding, confined perirenal hematoma or cortical laceration less than 1 cm deep without urinary extravasation. **C:** Grade 3 is a parenchymal laceration extending greater than 1 cm into the cortex, but without urinary extravasation. **D:** Grade 4 can be parenchymal or vascular injury. Parenchymal grade 4 injuries are those with a laceration extending through the corticomedullary junction and into the collecting system. A segmental vessel may also be lacerated. **E:** Grade 4 vascular injury consists of a segmental renal artery thrombosis without a parenchymal laceration. Renal arteries are end-arteries and the area of parenchyma subtended by the injured segmental artery will be ischemic. **F:** Grade 5 injuries are multiple and consist of shattered kidneys, pedicle avulsion, or main renal artery thrombosis. These are life threatening by nature. Main renal artery thrombosis is generally due to intimal disruption with resultant thrombosis, which can be observed in the close-up of the figure. **G:** Grade 5 injury can also be a "shattered" kidney, consisting of multiple major lacerations. **H:** Avulsion of the main renal artery and/or main renal vein is also a grade 5 injury. (Adapted from Nash PA, Carroll PR. Staging of renal trauma. In: McAninch JW, ed. *Traumatic and reconstructive urology.* Philadelphia: W.B. Saunders, 1996.)

penetrating injuries, where a significant percentage of patients with significant renal injuries may have no hematuria. It is imperative that the first voided or catheterized specimen be analyzed, because hematuria may clear rapidly. Either dipstick or microscopic analysis may be performed.

Radiographic Staging

Using the clinical information outlined above, the indications for radiographic im-

aging may be tailored to detecting patients with a significant chance of having a major renal laceration (AAST Grades 3 to 5). Based on our experience at San Francisco General Hospital, we recommend imaging the following categories of patients, although it must be emphasized that clinical judgment continues to be paramount:

1. Penetrating trauma: Abdomen, flank, or back injury with ANY degree of hematuria, particularly when the course of

the missile appears to involve the kidney or ureter.

2. Blunt trauma with either gross (visible) hematuria or shock (defined as any recorded systolic blood pressure <90 mm Hg): Patients having sustained blunt trauma with microhematuria only can safely avoid renal imaging.

3. Blunt trauma in the setting of significant deceleration injury, for example, falls from heights or motor vehicle accidents: This mechanism of injury has

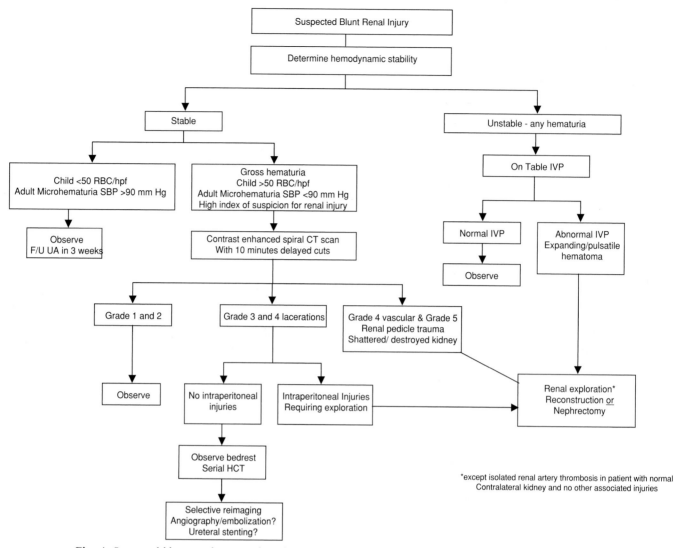

Fig. 4. Suspected blunt renal trauma algorithm. CT, computed tomography; HCT, hematocrit; HPF, high-power field; IVP, intravenous pyelogram; RBC, red blood cell; SBP, systolic blood pressure. (Adapted from Santucci RA, Wessels H, Bartsch G, et al. Evaluation and management of renal injuries: consensus statement of the Renal Trauma Subcommittee. *BJU Int* 2004;93:937.)

been associated with a higher incidence of ureteropelvic junction disruption as well as renovascular trauma.

4. Pediatric penetrating injury or blunt trauma with microhematuria greater than 20 red blood cells (RBCs) per high-power field (HPF): There is increasing evidence that the adult imaging criteria outlined above will identify the majority of significant renal lacerations in children, but this remains controversial. The surgeon should continue to maintain a low threshold for renal imaging in the pediatric population.

Contrast-enhanced CT scanning has replaced intravenous pyelography (IVP) as the imaging modality of choice in renal trauma patients. CT is noninvasive and offers rapid

and accurate detection of renal injuries, as well as associated injuries to other organs. CT defines depth and extent of lacerations, a functioning contralateral kidney, the presence of associated hematoma, and contrast extravasation, which suggests injury through the collecting system, as well as any devitalized renal parenchyma. Consideration must be given to each of these factors when deciding upon a treatment plan.

Helical (or spiral) CT scanning has been supplanting traditional CT scanning because of its speed in the trauma setting. The patient may pass through the scanner in a few minutes. This has limited use in fully staging renal injuries, because contrast may not have reached the renal calyces or renal pelvis before the images are obtained. Significant collecting system in-

juries may thus be missed. We routinely obtain a set of delayed images at 10 minutes in order to visualize the entirety of the collecting system down through the bladder. If this is not possible, a plain abdominal radiograph (kidney-ureter-bladder [KUB]) at this time may add complementary information to the CT scan. While CT may accurately demonstrate parenchymal lacerations, it has limited use in staging renovascular injuries. A renal vein laceration may be suspected by the finding of hematoma medial to the renal hilum. Adjunctive radiographic imaging techniques include renal ultrasound, nuclear scintigraphy, magnetic resonance imaging (MRI), and retrograde pyelography. None of these is recommended as a first-line study in the acute setting.

EDITOR'S COMMENT

This chapter, from a well-known trauma center, written by a senior author who is recognized as an expert in urologic injury, is intended to provide individuals who may not be in academic or level I trauma centers with an algorithm for treating patients with urologic and/or renal injuries. Although the authors state that as many as 10% of patients that are seen in the emergency room may have genitourinary injuries, other surveys suggest that the proportion of trauma patients with renal injuries is between 1.4% and 3.25% (Wessells H, et al. *J Trauma* 2003;54[3]:423). Although Wessells et al.'s paper dealt only with renal trauma, it is somewhat lower than has heretofore been proposed.

Not surprisingly, especially in the area of renal injury, the tendency has been to treat more injuries nonoperatively. One of the reasons for the adoption of the nonoperative approach to even vascular injuries is that, as the authors state, successful renal salvage after major renovascular injury occurs only in 25% to 35% of patients at best (Knudson MM, et al. *J Trauma* 2000;49:1116). The major factor in determining the ultimate outcome is the time to reperfusion; there is a small window with significant impairment of long-term renal function following 3 hours of total and 6 hours of partial warm ischemia. To make it worse, the absence of late hypertension, seemingly a sine qua non definition of a successful repair, occurs in 50% of renal vascular injuries managed nonoperatively but in 57% of patients that were revascularized, which, at the very least, is not statistically significant. A good example of this with excellent imaging is seen in an article by Lawrentschuk and Bolton (*Urology* 2005;65:386) in which the posterior branch of the renal artery is clearly seen as thrombosed in Figure 1, with confirmatory reformatting in Figure 2. Figure 3 shows a CT scan 3 months after injury with revascularization clearly seen as a revascularized posterior branch and atrophy of the posterior segment of the kidney. The patient, however, remained normotensive, which, given the tone of the various articles, would be counted as a success.

The emphasis on nonoperative care of these patients; the gradations of injury from the American College of Surgeons Trauma Committee and the American Association for the Surgery of Trauma presented in a renal injury classification that is pictured in the adjacent figure; and a good summary of graphic presentation of the levels and grades of renal injury are given by Harris et al. (*Radiographics* 2001;21:S201). That same paper proposes that as far as renal injury is concerned, the principal indications for the use of CT in the evaluation of blunt renal trauma include (a) the presence of gross hematuria; (b) microscopic hematuria associated with shock, which they define as a systolic blood pressure of less than 90 mm of mercury; and (c) microscopic hematuria associated with a positive result of diagnostic peritoneal lavage. Foley (*Eur J Radiol* 2003;45:S73) began with illustrating the contrast time of the renal circulation, which is very rapid, and pointing out that the kidney has a very high percentage of cardiac output, with 25% of the circulating contrast bolus passing through the renal circulation. Preferential

arterial flow to the renal cortex (90% of the renal blood flow) and rapid glomerular filtration complete the underlying bases of imaging. Foley pointed out that patients with macroscopic hematuria and pelvic fractures should be evaluated initially by a retrograde urethrogram, which is standard practice. If the urethra is intact, a bladder catheter should be placed and the catheter clamped so that there is sufficient distension of the bladder to 300 or 400 mL to detect urine extravasection. The CT scan should then be performed at a three-phase study: (a) an initial noncontrast study to detect intraparenchymal hematomas that may confuse normal renal parenchyma on the postcontrast examination; (b) a dynamic phase study to detect lacerations and vessel injuries (segmental or pedicle); and (c) delayed postcontrast study to detect contrast leakage into the perirenal or pararenal spaces signifying either ureteric disruption or pelvicaliceal disruption. Although MRI has been compared to CT scan in the evaluation of blunt renal trauma (Leppaniemi A, et al. *J Trauma* 1995;38[3]:420), this article written in 1995 suggests that MRI was not superior.

With respect to the kidney and exploration, it does appear in the cases that are explored that nephrectomy is a very frequent outcome. Wessels et al. (*J Trauma* 2003;54[3]:423) noted that in their study, the nephrectomy rate was 64% and was notably higher than the 11% to 47% reported in the literature. Nonoperative treatment of renal injury in nonacademic centers was carried out in 93%, versus 81% in academic centers. While 8% of the patients received renorrhaphy, 11% received nephrectomy. In contrast, in nonacademic centers, for those 7% explored, 5% underwent nephrectomy and 2% renorrhaphy. It is not clear whether the outcomes of this study reflect more severe patients in the tertiary centers or other factors.

The question of how to deal with a grade 5 injury or perhaps a grade 4 is still controversial. Early renal vascular control has been advocated to reduce the likelihood of renal loss, but given what the settings are in renal trauma, this approach has not been universally adopted as put forth in this chapter (McAninch JW, Carroll PC. *J Trauma* 1982;22:285; Gonzales RP, et al. *J Trauma* 1999;47:1039). Nonoperative renal trauma management has been espoused by many experienced centers (Altman AL, et al. *J Urol* 2000;164:27; Matthews LA, Spirnak JP. *Sem Urol* 1995;13:77; and from the authors' institution, Wessels H, et al. *J Urol* 1997;157:24).

Traveling down the urologic tract, Best et al. (*J Urol* 2005;173[4]:1202) summarized 57 patients treated at Los Angeles County with an injury severity score of 15 and a revised trauma score of 7.38. Penetrating injury in 55 cases, including gunshot wounds in 52 and stab wounds in two, and only two motor vehicle accidents were treated. An intraoperative diagnosis was made in 44 cases, or 77%, and 50, or 88%, required complex repairs or an adjunct procedure, including stents in 58%, ureteroureterostomy in 35%, ureteroneocystostomy with a psoas hitch 18%, and external diversion in 16%, and a variety of cystostomies and nephrostomies. Eighty-nine percent of the patients survived with no deaths related to ureteral injuries.

Traveling again down the urologic tract, Santucci commented on whether or not a suprapubic tube is necessary. The original article written by Parry et al. from Grady Memorial Hospital (*J Trauma* 2003;54:431) reviewed 51 patients, 28 treated by suprapubic tubes and transurethral catheters and 23 receiving only a transurethral catheter. There was no difference in outcome, and although the patients with transurethral catheters had the catheters in place for 11 days longer than those with suprapubic tubes that had a safety valve, there might be a case for suprapubic tubes in a difficult repair of the bladder or an unrepairable bladder (Santucci RA. *Int Braz J Urol* 2004;30[4]:344). Similar studies were reported by Ally et al. (*J Trauma* 2003;55:1152), Volpe et al. (*J Urol* 1999;161:1103), and Thomas (*Am Surg* 1998;64:77). A rare case of delayed bladder rupture in a 17-year-old was reported by Laufik et al. (*Am J Radiol* 2005;184:S99) with a nice series of CT scans.

Injuries to the urethra remain a problem, and as the authors nicely point out, strictures are the result of the injury to the postbulbar urethra. Two different approaches exist, the first again nonoperative, which the authors favor (Park S, McAninch JW. *J Urol* 2004;171:722) with just a suprapubic tube, and the second an endoscopic passage of a catheter. In the authors' series, up to 95% end up with a satisfactory result from the suprapubic tube approach only, and while Santucci wondered as to how realignment of the urethra could result in a worse outcome (*Int Braz J Urol* 2004;30[4]:345), it does appear that 9% of those treated with urinary diversion required urethroplasty and 17% with primary catheter realignment needed urethroplasty, although this was not statistically significant. However, the length of the stricture was much longer in patients managed with a urethral catheter. It does appear to be statistically significant, although in the article it is $P < .5$ rather than .05 (which it probably should be).

The incidence of missed injuries remains substantial (Zeron et al. *J Trauma* 2005;58[3]:533), in which 23% of the patients with pelvic fractures had concomitant urologic injuries missed. In several of the patients there was no blood in the meatus, and the prostate was said to be "normal in position." The authors stated, however, that there should be some recognition of the type of pelvic fracture that results in urethral injuries, and this should prompt more vigorous examination.

The authors have reminded us that in most patients with renal injuries, the endovascular approach has not been very satisfactory. An exception has been reported by Benson et al. (*Am Surg* 2005;71[1]:672).

Finally, adrenal injury has not been mentioned in this article, and Gabal-Shehab and Alagiri (*J Urol* 2005;173[4]:1330) analyzed almost 9,200 pediatric trauma cases and identified 20 adrenal injuries. Only three patients required transfusion, and no patient went to the intensive care unit or had operative intervention. Unfortunately, only two patients had follow-up CT, but in these patients hemorrhage was resolved. The message of this article was that these patients normally do not need intervention.

J.E.F.

Nongastrointestinal Transabdominal

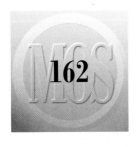

162

Supravesical Urinary Diversion

MATTHEW E. KARLOVSKY AND GOPAL H. BADLANI

A variety of temporary and permanent supravesical urinary diversion techniques are frequently used for benign, neuropathic, and malignant diseases of the lower urinary tract. Although there are numerous types of diversion—from a simple tube insertion to a complex continent diversion—their number continues to grow as none has achieved universal acceptance. No method yet fulfills all the principles of an ideal diversion: (a) preservation of renal function, (b) prevention or eradication of infection, (c) low perioperative and late complication rates, (d) minimal loss of gastrointestinal and sexual function, and (e) psychosocial acceptability. Nevertheless, judicious choice among the alternatives, according to the patient's specifics, gives good to excellent results. This chapter describes the types of urinary diversion that are currently most popular and discusses the indications for and pros and cons of each.

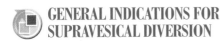

GENERAL INDICATIONS FOR SUPRAVESICAL DIVERSION

Obstruction and malignancy of the urinary tract are the most common indications for diversion. The most common malignant tumors leading to diversion are of the bladder, prostate, female reproductive tract, and colon. Urinary diversions are part of exenterative operations for malignant tumors in the pelvic region, such as during radical cystectomy. Nonmalignant causes of obstruction that lead to diversion include ureteral strictures, kidney or ureteral stones, retroperitoneal lesions with extrinsic compression, and fistulae. Less often, diversion is required because of severe pelvic trauma with extensive disruption of urinary and contiguous organs, scarring after radiation, or severe refractory interstitial cystitis. In the pediatric population, urinary diversion is necessary as a result of congenital anomalies (e.g., bladder exstrophy, cloacal malformations), spinal cord dysraphisms, or other congenital neurologic conditions.

Loss of urinary tract function for low-pressure storage or for efficient emptying is seen in patients with neuropathic bladder. Loss of volitional emptying can be managed successfully in many instances with clean intermittent catheterization (CIC). However, there remain patients who cannot be maintained with nonoperative therapy, including those with poor manual dexterity and those with progressive decompensation of the kidneys and ureters despite CIC due to poorly compliant or defunctionalized bladders. Inability to store urine for socially acceptable periods of time can be managed with a variety of behavioral and medical therapies. When these fail, urinary diversion may be one of the viable surgical interventions.

SELECTION OF THE PROCEDURE

All the diversionary procedures accomplish the same goal, namely the rerouting of urine. Some are more suitable than others for particular patients. The following sections address the main factors to be considered when selecting a diversionary procedure.

Ideally, the form of diversion is selected after one has chosen the curative treatment for the condition that made the diversion necessary. For malignancy, choice of diversion must respect oncologic principles and is tailored to findings either during preoperative workup or intraoperatively based on gross tumor extension, frozen section analysis, and tissue limitations. For example, if transitional cell carcinoma is found at the urethral margin on frozen section, a neobladder would be contraindicated. Radiated small bowel will redirect diversion reconstruction to either using large bowel or stomach, while a short mesentery that precludes low pelvic placement of a neobladder would redirect reconstruction to either a continent catheterizable pouch or a simple enterocutaneous conduit. If a neobladder is considered in either a male or female, the external striated urethral sphincter complex and its innervation must be preserved for future continence. Most importantly, all patients undergoing operative supravesical diversion must be prepared preoperatively for accepting the possibility that intraoperative findings may alter the surgical plan, resulting in an alternative diversion than planned.

PROGNOSIS

A more aggressive approach is justified in a patient who is expected to live for several years and should be offered a more complex urinary diversion in an attempt to reconstruct the urinary tract as much as possible. The patient with a poor prognosis should be offered the simplest procedure with quickest recovery, which avoids long postoperative courses and the increased incidence of reoperation. The need for postoperative chemotherapy and/or radiation in general does not preclude a more complex urinary diversion. After creation of a complex diversion, functional status is not diminished by the extent of the procedure, but rather is influenced by either the adverse effects of chemotherapy or the psychosocial adjustment to managing a continent pouch or neobladder.

PATIENT'S AGE

One must be concerned with the long-term preservation of renal function, the possible long-term effects of infection, the potential for delayed complications, the potential need for pouch or stomal revision, or the need for "undiversion," changing the type of diversion (i.e., from ileal conduit to a continent pouch or neobladder). Long-term survivors of treatment for malignancy at 5 years with refluxing (the standard) ileal conduits will see upper tract deterioration (hydroureteronephrosis and/or glomerular loss), symptomatic urinary tract infection (pyelonephritis), and urolithiasis in 40%, 50%, and 40%, respectively.

QUALITY OF RENAL FUNCTION

Incorporation of segments of intestine into the urinary tract produce metabolic derangements as a result of the interaction between intestinal mucosa and urine. These metabolic changes depend on which bowel segment is used (ileum, jejunum, colon, stomach), the length of the segment, duration of contact time between the segment's epithelium and urine, and the ability of the kidneys to compensate for the metabolic insult.

Due to the chronic exposure to urine, the absorptive properties of the (commonly) ileal and colonic segments are lost over time. Initially a reactive phase occurs, with mucous production. Absorption of mainly sodium and chloride and excretion of bicarbonate lead to hyperchloremic hypokalemic metabolic acidosis. This can be compensated for by normally functioning kidneys (serum creatinine <2.0 mg/dL); however, chronic bicarbonate loss promotes demineralization of bone with loss of buffers, demonstrated by elevate serum alkaline phosphatase. For patients with impaired renal function (serum creatinine >2.0 mg/dL), minimizing urine exposure to bowel is desirable.

Hyperchloremic acidosis may prompt diversion with gastric segments, as hydrochloride loss into the urine can mitigate the imbalance. Jejunal segments are rarely used due to their unique absorptive profile that leads to hypochloremic hyperkalemic acidosis.

BOWEL AS BLADDER SUBSTITUTE

Extensive resection of intestinal segments militates against further removal of bowel segment as this may lead to short-bowel syndrome and malabsorption. In such cases, complex diversion is contraindicated, and a short conduit or percutaneous renal diversion may be the only alternative. In addition, areas of irradiated bowel should be avoided because of its impaired vascularity and risk of poor healing.

Ultrastructural changes occur after prolonged bowel exposure to urine. Brush border and villi, the structures responsible for absorption, undergo significant atrophy. Paneth and goblet cells are rarely observed 4 years after diversion. Secretive function is lost as well. As mentioned above, different bowel segments vary in regard to solute absorption/secretion. Bowel length, surface area, contact time, pH, and solute concentration all impact metabolic consequences. Colonic absorption of chloride and secretion of bicarbonate is much greater than in the ileum, yet both these segments have equivalent sodium absorption. This has lead to the modern popularization of ileum as the preferred bowel segment.

Detubularization disrupts the intrinsic motility of the bowel as well as the contractile response to distention. As early as 1 year after detubularization, the interstitial Cajal cells in the myenteric plexus, which are responsible for normal peristalsis, are scarce and enteric nerve fibers are absent. The Cajal cells of the deep enteric plexus, responsible for distension-related contraction, remain intact for up to 3 years, but thereafter become rare.

Extensive loss of terminal ileum and/or the ileocecal valve can lead to oxalate wasting and predispose classically to struvite urinary stones. Cobalamin or vitamin B$_{12}$ may also be affected by loss of terminal ileum. Due to large body stores in the liver, deficiency may not become clinically apparent for 5 to 30 years, where megaloblastic anemia and neurologic disorders, such as lethargy, cerebellar ataxia, psychomotor retardation, and coma, can result. Once manifest, the neurologic insults are not reversible. A postoperative B$_{12}$ level below 200 pmol/L indicates a 50% risk of late cobalamin deficiency, at which point replacement should be instituted.

BOWEL PREPARATION PRIOR TO DIVERSION

Classic methods of preparing the bowel prior to diversion surgery have relied on mechanical cleansing with polyethylene glycol (PEG) and antibiotic prep using three doses each of erythromycin and neomycin base on the day before surgery with a strict liquid-only diet. Mechanical bowel prep is necessary to prevent retained particulate matter that may lead to recurrent infection and stone formation. However, abdominal pain, difficulty with completing the 4-L prep, and fatigue are cited as reasons for poor compliance with the usual 4-L PEG prep. Newer regimens include replacing PEG in favor of two doses of sodium phosphate, each 45 mL, starting at 3 p.m. and again at 9 p.m. the day before surgery, all while ingesting an 8-oz glass of water every hour until midnight. This regimen is better tolerated with less abdominal pain and fatigue, and has been judged to cleanse the bowel as well as, if not better than, PEG solution.

Sodium phosphate is, however, absolutely contraindicated in patients with renal insufficiency, symptomatic congestive heart failure, or liver failure with ascites. Other exclusionary criteria are elevated serum phosphate, decreased serum calcium, impaired gut motility, history of seizures, or myocardial infarction or stroke within the previous 6 months. PEG

is indicated in all patients with renal, heart, or liver insufficiency, and also in patients on bisphosphonates.

PSYCHOSOCIAL FACTORS

In the United States, there are enterostomal therapists, ostomy associations, and other sources of support for patients so that adjustment to a stoma is usually not a grave problem. However, for poorly educated patients and in geographic areas where support is unavailable, the stigma of a urinary stoma may be too great. In addition, in some parts of the world the medical supplies necessitated for a particular form of diversion may be too difficult to obtain or too costly.

The patient's understanding of different options of urinary diversion with their respective advantages and disadvantages requires significant educational effort. The patient's lifestyle, degree of physical and sexual activity, and cultural and religious concepts of body image play a crucial role in deciding which type of urinary diversion will provide the best quality of life.

IMPACT ON CANCER CONTROL AND LATE DE NOVO CANCER

Should complex urinary diversion be performed in those undergoing radical cystectomy and wide pelvic and iliac lymph node dissection from transitional cell carcinoma (TCC)? Survival is improved with meticulous lymph node dissection for those with node-positive bladder cancer at 5 years. Despite a local recurrence rate of 11%, only half of these patients experienced a disturbance of the orthotopic substitute during the last 6 months of life. It is well tolerated in patients who can anticipate normal neobladder function even with recurrence.

A urethral recurrence of TCC is 2% in contemporary series in patients with neobladders, which is improved over the historical figure of 10% urethral recurrences in patients with ileal conduits. No cancer-specific survival difference is noted between these two cohorts. However, when the urethra is involved, whether intraoperatively or at follow-up, a complete urethrectomy and alternate diversion is required.

Upper tract recurrences of TCC is an important consideration as it develops in approximately 5% of patients. About half of these occur at the ureteroenteric anastomosis. Evaluation of the distal ureters intraoperatively for carcinoma on frozen section will guide the surgeon to resect ureter until a negative margin is observed.

Extensive ureteral resection may be overcome with certain diversions that contain an afferent chimney (Studer neobladder) that can bridge a substantial ureteral deficit.

The development of a late "uroenteric" cancer at the anastomosis is a concern especially in patients diverted for benign conditions when young. When ileum is used for diversion, tumor development is rare, as opposed to colon cancer after ureterosigmoidostomy. The most common to develop are adenocarcinoma at the site of anastomosis, yet squamous cell and transitional cell carcinomas have been reported. The mechanism is believed to be due to the chronic bacteruria that produces N-nitrosamine from urinary nitrates, when urine is in contact with bowel flora. Chronic bacteruria is present in about 50% of all diversion patients. N-nitrosamine likely initiates the multistage process of neoplastic changes by causing irreversible DNA structural damage. Secondary neoplasms usually occur between 10 and 30 years after diversion; however, one report noted a latency of only 4 years. Prolonged storage of urine may be implicated in facilitating the chronic irritative changes. Questions have arisen whether frequent emptying, whether by voiding or CIC, may reduce the risk by decreasing contact time. Regardless of bowel diversion type, annual upper tract surveillance should be routine, with imaging and cytology. Yearly surveillance endoscopy of the bladder substitute is instituted after 10 years.

TYPES OF URINARY DIVERSION

The present techniques for urinary diversion can be classified as intubated, ureterocutaneous, ureterointestinal, ileal conduit, continent reservoir, and bladder substitution (Table 1).

Intubated Diversion

The distinction between temporary and permanent forms of urinary diversion is often arbitrary, but intubated procedures are in most instances considered an example of the former, primarily because they are used when the problem necessitating diversion is correctable or when the patient has a short life expectancy or is a poor surgical risk. Specifically, temporary intubated diversion may be of benefit in the following instances:

■ *Pyonephrosis.* Almost immediate objective improvement may be seen in septic patients after adequate drainage is achieved.

■ *Obstruction.* When surgical treatment is contraindicated. Recent myocardial infarction or other medical problems may prohibit a more definitive method of diversion. In these instances, intubated drainage provides relief of azotemia and facilitates control of infection.

■ *Unknown functional capacity* of an obstructed kidney. Intubated drainage can give the surgeon an excellent measure of the potential for recovery of function of an obstructed kidney by permitting differential creatinine clearance measurements on renal scans. The extent of renal function gain after establishment of appropriate drainage may make the difference between nephrectomy and reconstruction.

■ *Palliation* in azotemic patients with ureteral obstruction secondary to metastatic carcinoma for which potentially effective treatment is unavailable.

Internal Ureteral Stents

Ureteral stents, which extend from the renal pelvis to the bladder (Fig. 1), have been popular in patients with ureters compressed by a tumor, ureteral stones, and ureteral strictures. New designs have minimized the problems with stent collapse, encrustation, and migration.

The most popular stents are the hydrophilic-coated polyurethane double-J stents. They are available in various lengths and diameters, and they differ in their reactivity with the urothelium and in their relative stiffness. Stents are usually inserted retrograde through a cystoscope, but can also be inserted antegrade during a percutaneous nephrostomy or after a nephroscopic procedure, as well as during an open operation.

The principal advantages of ureteral stents are the minimal morbidity associated with their insertion and the fact that they can be inserted using local anesthesia. The principal disadvantages of ureteral stents are their continued tendency toward encrustation and obstruction with long-term use, which makes replacement necessary. Lower urinary tract symptoms due to irritation of the bladder as well as flank pain during voiding due to reflux may be bothersome features. Also, a single stent may provide inadequate drainage in extensive retroperitoneal disease.

Percutaneous Nephrostomy

Originally designed for assessment of renal function, the percutaneous nephrostomy has become one of the most accepted forms of temporary urinary diversion. Simply stated, the procedure involves passage of a catheter into the renal pelvis under fluoroscopic or ultrasonographic control, which can be done under local anesthesia. The resulting tract provides access for a multitude of procedures, such as nephroscopic examination and treatment of lesions, stone removal, incision of strictures, administration of drugs for cancer treatment, stone dissolution, and eradication of infections. Percutaneous nephrostomy is an alternative to cystoscopic retrograde placement of ureteral stents when the latter is impossible, as it often is when a large pelvic tumor obstructs the distal ureter.

Intravenous administration of antibiotics is advisable before the procedure, because manipulation of an obstructed kidney may readily produce septicemia. For fluoroscopy, the kidney is opacified with iodinated contrast medium administered intravenously at the time of the procedure or if renal function is poor, several hours beforehand. Alternatively, contrast medium can be instilled directly into the kidney through a 22-gauge ("skinny") needle directed under fluoroscopic control. The patient is then placed in a semioblique position so that the calyces are seen end-on on the fluoroscopic screen. An 18-gauge translumbar aortogram needle is inserted transparenchymally into the renal pelvis, usually through a middle or lower calyx to avoid entering the pleural cavity. The trocar is removed, and a 0.038-inch guidewire is inserted through the needle sheath until it curls in the collecting system. The sheath is removed, and a nephrostomy catheter is threaded over the guidewire into the renal pelvis after tract dilation (Fig. 2).

Many types of nephrostomy catheters are available as none is perfect. The standard 8 French pigtail catheter is too small caliber to provide adequate long-term drainage because it usually becomes obstructed with debris. Therefore, if long-term drainage is expected, a dilator should be inserted over the guidewire during the nephrostomy puncture to enlarge the tract and to accommodate a 14 French Malecot or balloon catheter. However, these have their own problems, such as obstruction of the collecting system by the balloon. Widely used these days is the Cope loop catheter (8 to 10 French), which is provided with a string that closes the loop after the catheter is optimally placed in the collecting system.

Percutaneous nephrostomy drainage is successful in 90% of the patients. Complications of nephrostomy puncture occur in

TABLE 1. METHODS OF URINARY DIVERSION

Method		Advantages	Disadvantages	Complications
Ureteral stent		Nonoperative insertion Excellent for temporary diversion No external collection device needed	Small intraluminal diameter predisposes to obstruction	Obstruction Infection
Percutaneous nephrostomy		Nonoperative insertion Adequate drainage Provides access to the kidney	Separate collecting device needed May be difficult to change Patient discomfort	Hemorrhage Infection Urine leak Pneumothorax
U-loop percutaneous nephrostomy		Nonoperative placement Easily changed Cannot be displaced Excellent drainage	Separate collecting device Patient discomfort	Hemorrhage Infection Urine leak Pneumothorax
Open nephrostomy		Allows exploration of perirenal space Excellent drainage	Separate collecting device needed Requires general anesthesia	Infection
Culaneous ureterostomy		May be temporary Requires no intestinal resection	Separate collecting device needed Requires general anesthesia Requires dilated ureter(s) for good results Prone to stomal stenosis	Stomal stenosis Infection Stones
Ureterosigmoidostomy		No collecting device needed Requires no intestinal resection	Requires adequate renal function and intact anal sphincter	Pyelonephritis and stones Hyperchloremic acidosis Adenocarcinoma of the colon
Ileal conduit		Best available long-term follow-up results Provides good drainage with minimal renal deterioration during first several years Does not require normal renal function	Allows ureteral reflux Long-term deterioration Collecting device needed	Stomal stenosis Infection Stones Ureteroileal stenosis
Ileal conduit		Intestine usually free of irradiated fields Suitable for direct anastomosis to the renal pelvis	Allows ureteral reflux Collecting device needed Requires normal renal function	Severe hypochloremic acidosis and azotemia

Nongastrointestinal Transabdominal

(continued)

TABLE 1. (*continued*)

Method		Advantages	Disadvantages	Complications
Sigmoid conduit		Can be used when pelvic exenteration is done Allows antireflux ureteral anastomosis Minimal stomal complications	Long-term follow-up data not available Cannot be used after pelvic irradiation	Infection Urelerosigmoid stenosis
Camey procedure		Voiding is per urethra No stoma	Frequent voiding during day and nocturanl incontinence Requires normal renal function Cannot be done in women	Incontinence Infection Hyperchloremic acidosis Stenosis of ureteral anastomosis
Studer neobladder		Voiding per urethra No stoma Low-pressure reservoir May be used in women Easily converted to ileal conduit	Requires adequate renal function High reoperation rate	Incontinence (nocturnal) Infection Stricture of the urethral anastomosis
Hautmann neobladder		Voiding per urethra No stoma Low-pressure reservoir Large-capacity reservoir May be used in women	Requires adequate renal function High reoperation rate	Incontinence (nocturnal) Infection Stricture of the urethral anastomosis
Mainz neobladder		Voiding is per urethra No stoma Can be used for continent diversion	Long-term follow-up data not available Requires normal renal function	Incontinence Infection Stenosis of ureteral anastomosis
Detubularized sigmoid reservoir ("doughnut")		Voiding per urethra No stoma	Long-term follow-up data not available Requires normal renal function	Incontinence Infection
Kock pouch		No collecting device needed Suitable for women Low-pressure reservoir	Long-term follow-up data not available Requires adequate renal function	Incontinence Infection Inability to catheterize stoma
Indiana pouch		No collecting device needed Low-pressure reservoir May be used in women Good continence mechanism	Requires adequate renal function High reoperation rate	Stomal stenosis Inability to catheterize stoma Infection

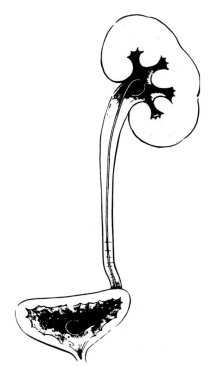

Fig. 1. Internal ureteral stent. The double-F stent drains the renal pelvis into the bladder.

complications; 6 died as a result of the operation, and another 74 died partly as a result of the operation. As an additional deterrent, only half the patients with regional or distant metastases obtained 2 months of useful life as a result of the operation. This is a rarely performed procedure today.

Surgeons are often faced with the philosophic dilemma of intervening in patients with terminal carcinomatous obstruction of the urinary tract, indeed, more often these days due to the low morbidity of percutaneous nephrostomy. However, the relevant question remains unchanged: Is it wise to intervene to prolong life or is it better to let the patient die of azotemia? Will the life that is gained by diversion be of acceptable quality? In answering this question, the following data may be helpful. The survival of patients who underwent palliative diversion with pigtail stents was studied in relation to the stage of the cancer. Patients with disease still apparently confined to the primary organ (8% of the series) had a 2-year survival rate of 88%, whereas in patients with local extension or regional nodal involvement (31% of the series), the rate was 18%, and in those with disseminated disease, it was only 2%. However, with percutaneous nephrostomy diversion, 65% to 85% of patients were able to leave the hospital, as opposed to 45% after open nephrostomy. The cell type of the cancer is not particularly useful in determining which patients with pelvic neoplasms will benefit, except in prostatic cancer, in which the endocrine sensitivity of many tumors means that patients can often expect many months of useful life if their urinary obstruction can be relieved. Another rule of thumb is to preserve renal function if chemotherapy, radiotherapy, or endocrine manipulation will confer a reasonable extension of life.

5% of patients, and the reported mortality is 0.2%, most deaths occurring in patients who are already severely ill. One must remain aware of the potential for infection, bleeding, urinary leak, or pneumothorax so that such complications can be promptly recognized and treated.

Before the development of percutaneous nephrostomy, urologists were often called on to do an open nephrostomy for palliative diversion in patients who were azotemic secondary to urinary obstruction by carcinoma. In such patients, open nephrostomy carried a high morbidity and mortality. In one series of 218 operations, 45% of patients had life-threatening

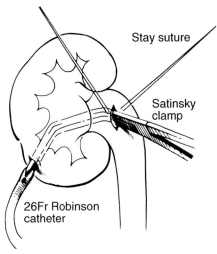

Fig. 3. Open nephrostomy. Satinsky clamp directed through a lower calyx, grasping catheter. (From Smith AD. Open and percutaneous nephrostomy. In: Whitehead ED, Leiter E, eds. *Current operative urology,* 2nd ed. New York: Harper & Row, 1983, with permission.)

Open Nephrostomy

The indications for open nephrostomy with its attendant hazards and complications have decreased dramatically since the introduction of percutaneous nephrostomy. Open procedures now are limited to those rare patients in whom percutaneous methods have failed or in whom some other operation is required (Fig. 3). Large drainage tubes—such as de Pezzer, Malecot, Robinson, Councill, or Foley catheters—are used. However, just as with nephrostomy tubes inserted percutaneously, these tubes may become blocked.

If long-term drainage is expected, an open U-loop nephrostomy is suggested as a way to avoid these problems. A Satinsky clamp is introduced (Fig. 4) and is used to pull the U-loop tube into the renal pelvis. The clamp, still holding the tube, is then redirected into an upper calyx and through the parenchyma. A U-loop nephrostomy can be placed also by percutaneous approach, accessing both the upper and lower pole simultaneously (see Fig. 4).

Cutaneous Urinary Diversion

Cutaneous ureterostomy clearly falls somewhere between temporary and permanent forms of diversion. It is most frequently used as a temporary measure in children who are in diapers and who have massive dilation of the upper urinary tract with sepsis or uremia commonly due to prune belly syndrome, posterior urethral valves, or massive ureteral reflux. Brought

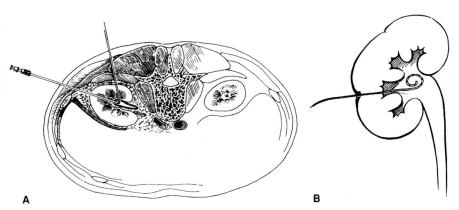

Fig. 2. Percutaneous nephrostomy. **A:** Cross section at the level of L2 shows skinny needle inserted in renal pelvis from a posterior approach and translumbar aortogram needle inserted by a transparenchymal approach. **B:** Percutaneous nephrostomy tube threaded into renal pelvis. (From Smith AD, Miller RP, Reinke DB, et al. Insertion of Gibbons ureteral stents using endourologic techniques. *Urology* 1979;14:330. © 1979 by Professional Medical Systems, Inc., with permission.)

Nongastrointestinal Transabdominal

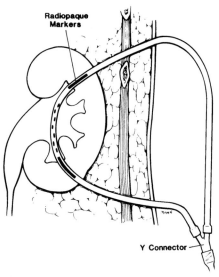

Fig. 4. A U-loop nephrostomy can be placed also by percutaneous approach, accessing both the upper and lower pole simultaneously.

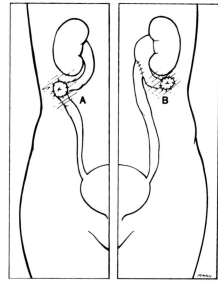

Fig. 5. Loop cutaneous ureterostomy. **A:** The most proximal loop of the redundant ureter is used. **B:** Y-ureterostomy. The proximal part of the ureter is brought out in an end ureterostomy, and the distal part is anastomosed to the renal pelvis.

out to the lower loin, it is ideal for infants because it decompresses the kidney, allowing optimal renal function and renal growth with time for unhurried roentgenographic and physiologic assessment of the urinary tract. Stomal care and symptomatic urinary tract infections are not a problem. Appliances are unnecessary if the child is still wearing diapers, and the peristomal skin rarely becomes inflamed. Most importantly, the urinary tract can almost always be reconstructed successfully.

In loop cutaneous ureterostomy, a cutaneous stoma made along the lateral wall of a dilated and elongated ureter while ureteral continuity is maintained, and the Y- or side-limb ureterostomy, in which the transected distal ureter is anastomosed to the renal pelvis after a proximal-end ureterostomy has been established, are the most popular ureterostomy techniques for children (Fig. 5). Cutaneous pyelostomy is an effective high diversion if the renal pelvis is large enough to be brought to the skin without tension. Moreover, the pyelostomy is easy to close, and the technique preserves the ureteral blood supply.

As a permanent form of diversion, particularly in adults, cutaneous ureterostomy has two disadvantages. The first is the need for two stomas if diversion is bilateral. Techniques developed to avoid this problem include the double-barreled infraumbilical stoma, over which a single collection device can be used, and joining of the medial borders of the ureteral ends combined with a Z-plasty technique in which skin is interposed to prevent

stenosis. Transureteroureterostomy and end-cutaneous ureterostomy also have been advocated (Fig. 6). The second problem is the propensity of the stoma to stricture. The poor ureteral blood supply frequently leads to distal ureteral slough, with recession of stricture of the stoma. This is

the primary cause of serious complications with this form of diversion and can be expected in approximately 60% of patients in long-term follow-up care. Once a stricture develops, intubation of the ureter is necessary, and this almost invariably leads to infection. Stricture is most likely if the ureter is 8 mm in diameter or less, if the stoma is flush with the skin rather than everted, and if the ureter or skin has been irradiated. To help prevent stricture, we and others advocate incorporation of a skin flap into the stoma: The distal 1 cm of ureter is spatulated and a U-shaped flap of skin is sutured to the area. The stricture problems associated with cutaneous ureterostomy have led many surgeons to abandon this operation. However, we believe that it still has a place, such as in poor-risk patients with greatly dilated ureters.

Ureterointestinal Diversions

The modern era of ureterointestinal diversion really began in 1911 with Coffey's description of a "tunneled" technique for implantation of the ureter into the intact colon. This technique, ureterosigmoidostomy, together with cutaneous ureterostomy, remained the most popular form of urinary diversion until 1950, when Bricker described the ureteroileal cutaneous operation and when the long-term

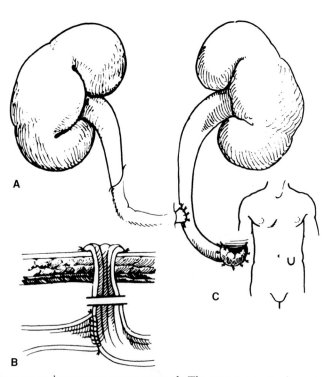

Fig. 6. Single stoma end-cutaneous ureterostomy. **A:** The narrower ureter is anastomosed side to end to the other. **B:** Note that the stoma is everted. **C:** U-shaped skin flap sewn into the spatulated ureter to prevent stomal stenosis.

TABLE 2. ONE-DAY INTESTINAL PREPARATION FOR URINARY DIVERSION
Clear liquid diet 24 h before surgery
Oral sodium phosphate (Fleet PhosphoSoda) 45 mL with four glasses of water at 3 p.m.
Repeat Fleet PhosphoSoda 45 mL six hours later with six glasses of water every hour in between
Neomycin, 1 g, and erythromycin, 1 g, orally at 1,2, and 11 p.m.
Intravenous fluids (usually 5% dextrose in 0.45 normal saline with potassium supplement)
Nothing by mouth 8 h before surgery

hazards of urinary diversion into the intact colon became increasingly apparent: Free reflux of fecal material to the kidneys or stenosis of the ureterocolic anastomosis, with high rates of pyelonephritis, stone formation, and loss of renal function; serious electrolyte imbalances; and late onset of neoplasm development. That same year, Leadbetter described a technique that built a submucosal tunnel with a direct mucosa-to-mucosa ureterocolonic anastomosis, and 2 years later, Goodwin described a transcolonic technique for preventing reflux by making a long submucosal tunnel. Leadbetter's and Goodwin's techniques are similarly effective in reducing the incidence of pyelonephritis, and one of these procedures should be used whenever ureterosigmoidostomy is performed.

For ureterosigmoidostomy, intestinal preparation is carried out as described in Table 2, except that neomycin retention enemas (200 mL of 1% neomycin sulfate) are given the night before and the morning of the operation. One or two large rectal tubes with side holes are inserted at either the beginning or the end of the operation to drain urine and stools during the first postoperative week.

After the sigmoid colon has been mobilized, the left ureter is brought anteriorly through the mesentery of the sigmoid. Both ureters are spatulated for a mucosa-to-mucosa anastomosis after a long submucosal tunnel has been made (Fig. 7). When the transcolonic (Goodwin) anastomosis is used, the anterior wall of the colon is incised vertically, and through this opening, both ureters are brought through separate submucosal tunnels in the posterior wall (Fig. 8). The anastomosis and ureters can be stented and the stents brought out through the anus.

With either the Leadbetter or the Goodwin anastomosis, acute pyelonephritis

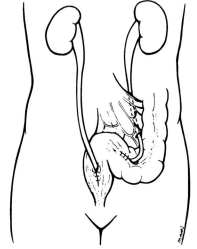

Fig. 7. Ureterosigmoidostomy. The left ureter is brought anteriorly through the mesentery of the sigmoid. Both ureters are spatulated for a Leadbetter anastomosis in the anterior taenia.

occurs in approximately 55% of patients. Obstruction of the ureterocolonic anastomosis occurs as a late complication in 32% to 62% of patients. The incidence of kidney stones is also high and increases with increasing length of the follow-up period.

Hyperchloremic hypokalemic metabolic acidosis, the most serious common complication of ureterosigmoidostomy, is reported in as many as 80% of patients. It is potentiated if the urine is in contact with the colonic mucosa for prolonged periods. In this situation, drainage of the colon by rectal tube quickly corrects the acidosis. To minimize electrolyte disturbances, frequent evacuation of the rectum

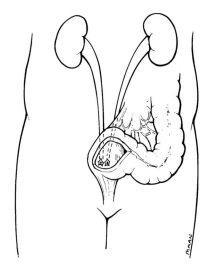

Fig. 8. Goodwin transcolonic ureterosigmoidostomy. The anterior wall of the colon is incised vertically, and both ureters are brought through separate submucosal tunnels in the posterior wall.

(during the night as well as during the day), a low-chloride diet, and supplemental sodium potassium chloride (e.g., Scholl solution) are recommended.

It is worth repeating again the importance of surveillance for de novo carcinoma at the uro-enteric anastomotic site. As many as 5% of patients may be affected. The mean lag period between the operation and the diagnosis of cancer is approximately 10 years in patients who were older than 40 years at the time of the operation and 21 years in patients younger than 40 years. Carcinogenesis requires the presence of urine, feces, urothelium, and colonic epithelium at the healing suture line. The most plausible mechanism is conversion of urinary nitrate to the carcinogen nitrosamine by fecal bacteria and conversion of nitrosamine to the even more active form, hydroxylated nitrosamine. Malignancy rarely appears if small intestine is used or in isolated loops of colon. To reduce the risk, ureteral stumps should not be left behind in the colonic wall when a ureterosigmoidostomy is revised or taken.

The various complications that can occur after ureterosigmoidostomy have led many urologists to abandon the operation. Nevertheless, the long-term results are good in properly selected patients, namely those with normal upper tracts, normal renal function, and adequate rectal sphincter tone. The greatest advantage of ureterosigmoidostomy is that no external appliance is required, a considerable plus in areas where medical supplies are difficult to obtain or patient acceptance of an external stoma is unlikely.

The Mainz group published a significant modification of the ureterosigmoidostomy. The essence of the Mainz pouch II is a U-shape folding of the sigmoid followed by detubularization. Suturing together the edges, a diverticulum-like cavity is created without the risk of compromising the blood supply. The ureters are implanted in this pouch. The pouch is fixed at the promontory, which reduces the risk of ureteral kinking and upper urinary tract dilation as it is sometimes observed after ureterosigmoidostomy. The detubularization brakes the peristaltic pressure wave in the bowel and protects the kidneys from reflux, inflammation, and stone formation.

Ureteroenteric-Cutaneous Diversion

Preparation of the Patient

A modified preoperative diet, extensive use of cathartics, and prolonged postoperative gastrointestinal inactivity accompany all permanent gastrointestinal diversion operations. Therefore, accurate preoperative assessment of nutritional and hydration status and correction of any deficiencies are imperative and may make the difference between a smooth and a stormy postoperative course. Preoperative assessment should include determination of total protein and albumin, as well as skin testing for the delayed hypersensitivity response. Anergic patients have a 70% septic complication rate from diversion operations and a 40% death rate if sepsis appears.

A healthy person can withstand at least a week of starvation if given adequate parenteral fluid and 100 g of glucose daily. However, many patients awaiting urinary diversion have for some time been unable to meet their caloric needs—which are elevated by chronic sepsis, cancer, or trauma—because of anorexia, weakness, or depression. These patients need to be converted to anabolic metabolism preoperatively with at least partial replenishment of their protein stores. This may require as much as 45 to 53 kcal/kg and 0.2 g of nitrogen per kilogram daily in a formula tailored to the patient's specific needs. We prefer to use hyperalimentation for this replenishment and continue it postoperatively until the patient is eating adequately.

Approximately 25% of patients awaiting an elective operation are dehydrated, as indicated by a low pulmonary wedge pressure measured by a Swan-Ganz catheter, even when there is no clinical evidence of hypovolemia. Therefore, in adults, we insert a central venous line 24 hours preoperatively and, after its correct position has been confirmed roentgenographically, hydrate the patient with Ringer lactate to a central venous pressure of 6 to 10 cm H_2O.

Preparation of the intestine begins 3 days before the operation (see Table 2) unless the patient has neurovesical dysfunction, in which case the preparation may need to be started 1 or 2 days earlier. We administer a second-generation cephalosporin preoperatively unless the patient has a history of endocarditis, a prosthetic device or graft, or an indwelling catheter, in which case we give an aminoglycoside and ampicillin.

The patient also must be prepared psychologically. Stomal care begins preoperatively, with teaching and counseling of the patient and family by the surgeon, nurses, and enterostomal therapy.

Ileal Conduit

Ileal conduit diversion, first described by Bricker in 1950, provided a welcome alternative for urologic surgeons weary of the complications of ureterosigmoidostomy and cutaneous ureterostomy. Heal conduit diversion has low incidences of infection; metabolic disorders, such as hyperchloremic acidosis; and long-term follow-up that has shown adequate preservation of renal function. The only contraindications are intrinsic small-intestinal disease or prior irradiation leading to radiation enteritis. The most common indication is loss of the bladder to cancer. Other indications include diversion

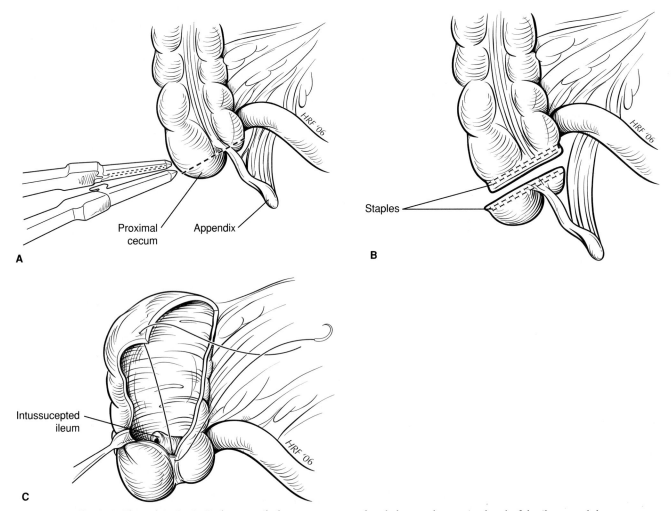

Fig. 9. Real conduit. **A–C:** Both ureteroileal anastomoses are placed close to the proximal end of the ileum, and the cutaneous stoma is performed at the distal end.

for refractory radiation cystitis and multiple failed repairs after vesicovaginal fistula.

The intestinal segment used for the conduit should be 15 to 20 cm long— long enough to reach from the sacral promontory to the abdominal wall skin. It derives its blood supply from a terminal branch of the superior mesenteric artery. The segment should end approximately 20 cm from the ileocecal valve to preserve the ileocecal artery and the various absorptive properties of the terminal ileum (Fig. 9).

The mesentery is divided at right angles to the intestine for approximately 10 cm distally and 5 cm proximally, thus making a broad vascular pedicle for the conduit. The longer distal length of mesentery is important so that the conduit can reach the skin. The isolated segment is placed posteriorly and the intestine reanastomosed anteriorly. The mobilized left ureter is brought to the right retroperitoneal space through a tunnel under the sigmoid mesentery, with care taken not to twist or angulate the ureter. Both ureters are then anastomosed to the proximal end of the conduit, end to side, with a single layer of interrupted 4-0 chromic catgut to all tissue layers. The proximal end of the conduit is anchored to the retroperitoneum, and the distal end is brought through the skin so that the conduit is placed in an isoperistaltic position. The conduit is anchored to rectus fascia with either two or four SAS sutures. The GIA autosuture instrument and intestinal staplers (TA-55) save considerable time in the division and reanastomosis of the intestine. However, we do not use staples in the proximal end of the conduit, because they may act as nidus for stone formation if they are in contact with urine. The ureters are stented (8 French single-J stent) and the stents brought out through the stoma. Stents are usually removed at follow-up between 2 and 3 weeks postoperatively.

Other important technical details of this operation include spatulation of the ureters to maximize the lumen at the anastomosis or, alternatively, the use of Wallace's technique of joining the ureters and then anastomosing them end to end with the proximal end of the conduit. The latter method is particularly well suited to the thick-walled dilated ureters produced by long-term obstruction. All mesenteric gaps should be closed to prevent later small-intestinal herniation and obstruction.

The technique of stoma construction is critical (Fig. 10). The stoma site should be selected before the operation and checked with the patient sitting, lying, and

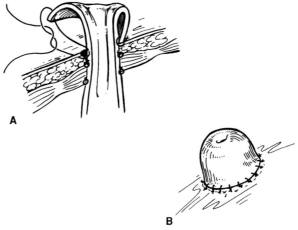

Fig. 10. Construction of the stoma. **A:** The conduit is sutured at the fascia level to prevent parastomal herniation. A separate layer of suture should incorporate the skin, the serosa, and the muscularis of the conduit at the level of the skin and at the end of the conduit. **B:** Bud nipple stoma after maturation.

standing. The site should be flat, unscarred, free of creases, and away from bony prominences and the umbilicus. Usually, the ideal site is just below a line between the umbilicus and the anterior iliac spine. The stoma should be placed higher in obese patients and in those with spinal abnormalities. A temporary bag can be worn preoperatively to assess the suitability of the site.

Two facts highlight the importance of proper construction of the stoma. First, from the patient's point of view, the appearance of the stoma is the most obvious sign of the surgeon's competence. Second, the incidence of stomal complications can be as low as 4% or as high as 50%, depending to a large degree on the care taken in construc-

tion. Bricker's original stoma was a simple orifice flush with the skin. Construction of a bud, as advocated by Brooke, was an advance in that it reduced stomal complications by providing a better appliance fit, by diminishing skin contact with urine, and by lessening stenosis. However, despite careful construction, a bud stoma may stenose. An alternative, especially for obese patients, is the Turnball loop stoma, which avoids most of the problems attending use of small intestine (Fig. 11). The chief problem with the Turnball stoma has been parastomal hernia. Nevertheless, comparison of standard buds with Turnball loops demonstrates the clear superiority of the latter.

Despite the durability and relative ease of construction, long term consequences

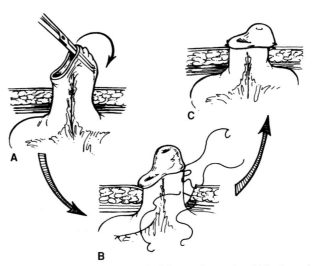

Fig. 11. Turnball loop stoma. **A:** The distal end of the conduit is closed. The loop should protrude 3 to 4 cm and is secured to the fascia. The loop is opened across the nonfunctional segment. **B:** The stoma is matured with interrupted sutures, including the skin, the seromuscular layer of the conduit, and the edge of the mucosa. **C:** Stoma after maturation.

of the "simple conduit" do result. A recent study reporting long-term outcomes with ileal loop conduits analyzed 131 patients considered long-term survivors, those surviving longer than 5 postoperative years. Sixty-six percent of patients develop conduit-related complications. The most common were related to kidney function/morphology (creatinine elevation or upper tract dilation) in 27%, stomal complications (parastomal hernia, stenosis or bleeding) in 24%, bowel complications (obstruction, diarrhea, or fistulae) in 24%, pyelonephritis in 14%, and urinary lithiasis in 9%. Those surviving longer than 15 years had a 50% rate of upper tract changes, and a 38% rate of urolithiasis. The true picture of conduit-related morbidity is borne out with long-term follow-up, which should include annual surveillance of the upper tracts and serum creatinine. The ileal conduit is a low-pressure reservoir; as long as urine flow is unobstructed at the level of the stoma and rectus fascia, complications such as hydronephrosis, azotemia, metabolic derangements, and stone formation can be minimized. Hydronephrosis is an expected development in at least half of conduit patients due to the free urinary reflux that occurs at the ureteral anastomoses. Reflux is minimized with good stomal outflow. Antireflux anastomosis does not change the glomerular filtration rate when compared to nonrefluxing conduits in two recent studies from Sweden. Conduit vascular insufficiency may lead to a poorly compliant "pipe-stem" loop that transmits detrimentally high retrograde pressures to the kidneys. Long loops increase urine contact time. Stomal stenosis can exacerbate both these scenarios with severe consequences on kidney function.

Ultimately, the imperfections with the straight conduit were the driving forces behind the development of alternative diversion strategies, such as continent cutaneous reservoirs and neobladders, as discussed below.

Jejunal Conduit

The jejunum is rarely used for urinary diversion, primarily because of the metabolic complications it entails. Jejunal conduits are contraindicated in patients with reduced renal function, those on low-salt diets, and those in whom a long loop would be required. They should be considered for patients with severe ileal radiation damage or those in whom there is need of compensation for short ureters. The surgical technique is similar to that for construction of an ileal conduit. Oral salt replacement is used when hyponatremic hypochloremic hyperkalemic metabolic acidosis develops.

Colonic Conduit Diversions

Colonic conduits have several advantages. Greater length is available for high loops. Because passage of urine through the conduit is mediated by mass peristaltic contraction of the colon rather than by peristalsis as in small-intestinal conduits, the conduit need not be placed in the isoperistaltic direction. Antireflux anastomoses are easier and more successfully accomplished. Furthermore, if the diversion is part of a total pelvic exenteration, the sigmoid colon can be used as the conduit and an end-colostomy can be made with the remaining distal colon, obviating intestinal reanastomosis.

Problems with deterioration of the upper urinary tract in children with ileal conduits have led to renewed attention to the value of the sigmoid colon as an isolated conduit with antireflux ureterosigmoid anastomoses. In some studies, this technique has reduced the incidence of pyelonephritis. However, long-term comparison data are not available, and some reports have shown no significant advantages over ileal conduits. Nonetheless, sigmoid conduit diversion is indicated for patients who require cutaneous diversion and who have normal upper tracts, for patients undergoing total pelvic exenteration for malignant disease, and for patients who require temporary diversion while serious but reversible bladder disease is being corrected. Overall, sigmoid colon is the most frequently used; however, transverse colon is a reasonable alternative in patients with prior pelvic radiation or compromised ureteral length.

Metabolic changes seen with colonic conduits are similar to ileum. Both bowel segments have equal absorption of sodium; however, chloride absorption and bicarbonate excretion are greater in colonic segments. This would make ileal loops the preferred conduit in the renally impaired.

Continent Urinary Diversions

The concept of a continent reservoir gained popularity among both patients and physicians because of the disadvantages of the ureterosigmoidostomy and the ileal conduit. Parallel to the development of orthotopic neobladders, the first attempt to create a continent reservoir was made in the 1950s by the Gilchrist group. They used the ileocecal segment to create an appliance-free cutaneous urinary diversion. Continence was based on the antiperistaltic function of the terminal ileum and the competence of the ileocecal valve. Various segments of bowel have been used (including small-bowel Kock pouch), and the continence and antireflux mechanism rely on different methods of imbrication, tapering, or intussusception. One of the initial advantages of these diversions over the neobladders was that they were the preferred continent diversion in women, prior to more recent evidence that they could equally be performed in women while maintaining continence and cancer control. This will be further addressed below.

A well-functioning bladder substitute, whether a catheterizable reservoir or a neobladder, needs a motivated patient and scrupulous surveillance postoperatively. In detubularized pouches, Laplace's law (pressure = tension / radius) states that the larger the radius, the lower the end-filling intrapouch pressure is. A spherical reservoir has maximum capacity for a given bowel segment, achieving a maximum volume–to–surface area ratio. This minimizes the reabsorptive surface and thus the metabolic complications. A low-pressure system mimicking the native bladder also helps protect against reflux and deterioration of the upper tracts while allowing socially acceptable intervals to pass between catheterization or voiding. In the initial postoperative period, pouches need to be drained more frequently every 2 to 3 hours; however, over time the emptying interval is increased to allow for capacity expansion, where a fully functional pouch can hold up to 500 mL.

Kock Pouch

In 1962, Kock first used a new type of pouch, taking advantage of the fixed direction of the peristaltic movements of the intestine. By splitting the intestine along its antimesenteric border and folding the split intestine twice, Kock forced the motor activity of the different parts to counteract one another. In 1967, Kock applied the technique to patients with ulcerative colitis who needed proctocolectomy. Partial continence was achieved by bringing the efferent limb of the intestine from the pouch obliquely through the abdominal wall, relying on the sphincter action of the rectus muscle. Continence, however, was not complete.

Application of this pouch as a urinary reservoir was not reported until 1975, at

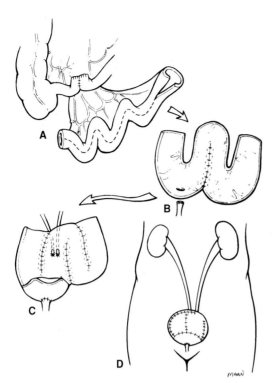

Fig. 18. Hautmann neobladder. The pouch is created from a 60- to 80-cm segment of ileum, sparing the terminal 15 cm. The bowel is detubularized along its antimesenteric border and fashioned into a "W" shape. A larger flap between the first and second limb is allowed to create a wider plate for anastomosis to the urethral stump. The ureters are reimplanted into the second and third limbs in a tunneled fashion. The pouch is then folded over to close on itself.

zation. Two neobladder-vaginal fistulae developed and were corrected transvaginally. More liberal preservation of the anterior vaginal wall and omental interposition were suggested to prevent fistula formation, especially for those who may receive adjuvant therapy for extensive disease.

Hautmann Neobladder

One of the most popular neobladders, the Hautmann neobladder, emerged from the need to further increase the volume of the pouch. By using 60 to 80 cm of detubularized ileum in the configuration of a "W" (Fig. 18), the average maximum capacity was 821 mL, with a mean resting pressure of 26.4 cm H_2O. Ureteral reimplantation is done directly into the pouch. Initial reports had intermittent catheterization rates of 4% of patients for postvoid residual volumes greater than 100 mL. A recent retrospective comparison of one surgeon's experience of both Studer and Hautmann neobladders from the University of Michigan was reported. Monte et al. found equivalent blood loss, pathologic stage, and rates of complications for both groups, but operative time was slightly longer with the Studer pouch, 5.9 hours versus 5.3 hours. In addition, total

continence, whether day or nighttime, was equivalent, but the Hautmann pouch had a large average capacity.

Mainz Pouch

The ileocecal segment has been used in several configurations to form a variety of neobladders and continent reservoirs. Because of its larger diameter than the ileum, the right colon requires less intestinal length removed from the gastrointestinal tract to obtain the same capacity as a small bowel pouch. The Mainz pouch is spherical and is constructed from a cut-open cecum, ascending colon, and two ileal loops (Fig. 19). The entire segment is detubularized, sacrificing the ileocecal valve. It is sewn together side to side in the shape of an incomplete W, and the ureters are implanted in the posterior tenia. An appendectomy is performed, and a buttonhole is performed at the most dependent part of the cecum, which is used for the urethrointestinal anastomosis. The rest of the procedure is similar to the ileal neobladder. This technique is also applicable for augmentation cystoplasty or construction of a continent reservoir with cutaneous stoma. Postoperative care is similar to the ileal neobladders, with

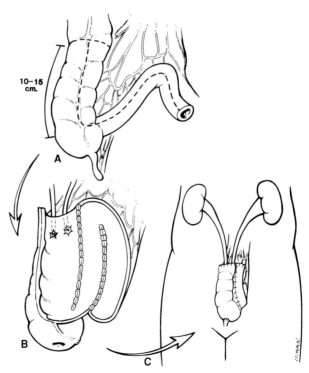

Fig. 19. Mainz neobladder. **A:** Ten to 15 cm of cecum and ascending colon with 20 to 30 cm of ileum is isolated. **B:** The entire segment is detubularized along its antimesenteric border, and a broad posterior plate is created by suturing the apposing edges to create a W. Tunneled ureterocolonic anastomoses are performed. **C:** A buttonhole incision is created at the base of the cecal portion for the urethrointestinal anastomosis. The neobladder is closed by folding the lateral limbs anteriorly and suturing in a continuous fashion.

Nongastrointestinal Transabdominal

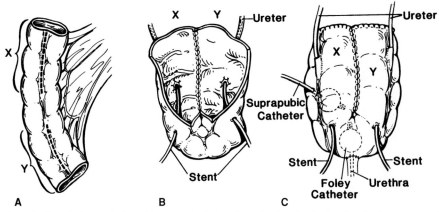

Fig. 20. Detubularized sigmoid reservoir ("doughnut"). **A:** The isolated colonic segment is folded in a "U" shape, the dependent portion facing the pelvis. The colon is incised along the medial taenia up to 4 cm from the anticipated urethral anastomosis. The posterior layer is sutured. An antireflux ureteral implant is performed. **B:** The posterior layer suture line is continued to the anterior layer. The cephalad end is also sutured. **C:** The completed reservoir is sutured to the urethra.

increased attention for frequent irrigation because of greater mucous production.

Detubularized Sigmoid Reservoir

The detubularized sigmoid reservoir ("doughnut") technique uses the same principle as the Mainz pouch but involves the sigmoid and descending colon. The advantages of this method are that the sigmoid easily reaches the urethra for a tension-free anastomosis, the alignment and tunneling of the ureters is easy, and the pouch is almost completely detubularized without the use of additional, less expendable segments of intestine (Fig. 20).

LAPAROSCOPY

Only recently have laparoscopy and robotic surgery been applied to radical cystectomy and urinary diversion. Even at high-volume centers the techniques are still evolving. Several types of diversions have been reported, including ureterosigmoidostomy, ileal conduit, and ileal neobladder. Some groups exteriorize the bowel, perform the diversion, and then return the pouch interiorly, while others report complete intracorporal construction of an ileal neobladder. Long-term oncologic control and continence rates will need to be compared to traditional contemporary open surgery to prove outcome equivalency.

Despite the absence of a perfect method for urinary diversion, the availability of many techniques ensures that at least one can be found that is suitable for each individual patient. A surgeon who is knowledgeable about the options and his or her skills will be able to achieve satisfactory results nearly all the time. Surgeon preference, operative time, ease of construction, and patient characteristics all influence the choice of urinary diversion and all must be considered for optimal outcomes.

SUGGESTED READING

Ali-El-Dein B, El-Tabey N, Abdel-Latif M, et al. Late uro-ileal cancer after incorporation of ileum into the urinary tract. *J Urol* 2002; 167:84.

Chang SS, Cole E, Cookson MS, et al. Preservation of the anterior vaginal wall during female radical cystectomy with orthotopic urinary diversion: technique and results. *J Urol* 2002;168:1442.

Ferguson KH, McNeil JJ, Morey AF. Mechanical and antibiotic bowel preparation for urinary diversion surgery. *J Urol* 2002;167:2352.

Gschwed JE. Bladder substitution. *Curr Urol Opin* 2003;13:477.

Hautmann RE. Urinary diversion: heal conduit to neobladder. Review. *J Urol* 2003;169:834.

Hemal AK, Abol-Enein H, Tewari A, et al. Robotic radical cystectomy and urinary diversion in the management of bladder cancer. *Urol Gun N Am* 2004;31:719.

Lee CT, Hafez KS, Sheffield JH, et al. Orthotopic bladder substitution in women: nontraditional applications. *J Urol* 2004;171:1585.

Lee KS, Monte JE, Dunn RL, et al. Hautmann and Studer orthotopic neobladders: a contemporary experience. *J Urol* 2003;169:2188.

Madersbacher S, Schmidt J, Eberle JM, et al. Long-term outcome of heal conduit diversion. *J Urol* 2003;169:985.

Matin SF, Gill IS. Laparoscopic radical cystectomy with urinary diversion: completely intracorporeal technique. *J Endourol* 2002;16(6):335.

Olofsson G, Kilander A, Lindgren A, et al. Vitamin B_{12} metabolism after urinary diversion with a Kock ileal reservoir. *Scan J Urol Nephrol* 2001;35:382.

Perimenis P, Burkhard FC, Kessler TM, et al. Heal orthotopic bladder substitute combined with an afferent tubular segment: long term upper urinary tract changes and voiding pattern. *Eur Urol* 2004;46:604.

Salomonowitz EK, Cragg AR, Lund G, et al. Nephrostomy tubes: insertion and replacement. In:

Shekarriz B, Shekarriz H, Upadhyay J, et al. Outcome of palliative urinary diversion in the treatment of advanced malignancies. *Cancer* 1999;85:998.

Skolarikos A, Deliveliotis C, Alargof E, et al. Modified ileal neobladder for continent urinary diversion: functional results after 9 years of experience. *J Urol* 2004;171:2298.

Stein JP, Daneshmand S, Dunn M, et al. Continent right colon reservoir using a cutaneous appendicostomy. *Urology* 2004;63:577.

Stein JP, Ginsberg DA, Skinner DG. Indications and technique of the orthotopic neobladder in women. *Urol Clin N Am* 2002;29:725.

Studer UE, Zingg EJ. Ileal orthotopic bladder substitutes: what we have learned from 12 years' experience with 200 patients. *Urol Clin North Am* 1997;24:4.

Webster C, Bukkapatnam R, Seigne J, et al. Continent colonic urinary reservoir (Florida pouch): surgical complications (greater than 11 years). *J Urol* 2003;169:1746.

EDITOR'S COMMENT

In this lovely chapter, the focus is rightly on the preservation of function in patients who require urinary diversion or substitution of some sort. The patients in whom these procedures are carried out have a catchall of urologic diseases, none of them good. They range from malignancy to interstitial cystitis to neurogenic bladder. The authors point out that the old-fashioned standard, which is an ileal conduit, leads to functional deterioration as well as stone formation and chronic infection. I am old enough to remember when the ileal loop first became popular, and it was regarded as a godsend. It was, at that time, but since that time we have learned, as the authors detail, that the preservation of function in patients who survive the malignancy and undergo, for

(continued)

example, exenteration carries with an impairment of renal function of about 50%. Thus, avoidance of a supravesical diversion is desirable.

In an effort to avoid urologic-damaging function in a group of patients with benign disease, Blaivas et al. (*J Urol* 2005;173:1631) reviewed 76 consecutive adults who underwent augmentation enterocystoplasty and continent diversion for benign disease. The study was carried out retrospectively, and outcomes assessed, for example, using a patient-satisfaction questionnaire, continence status, catheterization status, bladder capacity, bladder compliance, and detrusor instability. The largest group of patients included neurogenic bladder in 41 of the 76 patients. Following augmentation enterocystoplasty, mean bladder capacity increased from 166 to 550 mL and mean maximum detrusor pressure decreased from 53 to 14 cm of water. Serum creatinine level either improved or remained normal in all patients. Long-term complications were stomal stenosis or incontinence in 42% of patients with stomas, and there were recurrent bladder stones in 6%. Five of 71 patients (7%) had small bowel obstruction. One patient committed suicide, which I assume indicates that at least some aspect of his or her life was not thought to be of high quality.

Is age of any consequence as far as what type of diversion to do? Deliveliotis et al. (*Urology* 2005;66:299), reporting from Athens, analyzed 54 individuals older than 75 among 481 patients who underwent radical cystectomy between 1993 and 2002. Twenty-nine of these 54 patients underwent cutaneous ureterostomy (group 1) and ileal conduit urinary diversion was used in 25 patients (group 2). The latter group had a longer operating time, increased need for blood, longer stay in the intensive care unit, and a longer mean hospitalization time than patients with cutaneous ureterostomy. All these differences were statistically significant. Complications of all sorts, early and late, including medical and surgical, were more frequent in the group undergoing ileal conduit, which manifested complications of between 40% and 60% as compared with 14% and 24% in various categories in the group with cutaneous ureterostomies. One patient in the ileal conduit group died.

There have been a number of attempts to prevent ureteral stricture to avoid urinary diversion, including treatment of ureteral stenosis with a self-expanding nitinol stent covered with polytetrafluoroethylene. Thirty-seven stents were used in 20 patients during a 2-year period between 2001 and 2003; the stents were introduced retrograde under combined endoscopic and fluoroscopic guidance. Uretero patency was achieved in all 29 insertion procedures and maintained in most patients. Four

patients died of the neoplastic process within a year, and three and four stent migrations occurred in three patients, a 22% complication rate, but they responded to a new stent. These stents appeared to be resistant to calcification; there was nonobstructive mucous hyperplasia observed in 28% of the patients at the end of the stent without calcification.

One of the concerns about following performance of an orthotopic neobladder procedure, which is carried out during cystoproctostomy, is the rate of urethral recurrence, which is as high as 10% of patients in some reports, but more recent reports is considerably less. Nieder et al. (*Urology* 2004;64:950) analyzed their own results of a single-surgeon series of 226 patients with a mean age of 69 years who had undergone radical cystoproctostomy. Eight (3.5%) of the patients had undergone urethrectomy. Follow-up was 42 months; 108 patients had an orthotopic neobladder and 110 had supravesical diversion. Of the 218 patients between the two groups, eight (3.7%) developed urethral recurrence; seven had undergone supravesical diversion and one had an orthotopic neobladder. Seven of these patients underwent urethrectomy of the recurrence and were free of disease at the last follow-up. The other patient died of metastatic transitional cell carcinoma. The authors are reassured that recurrence or persistence of disease at the urethra after cystoprostotectectomy makes this a low-risk operation.

If one is carrying out a radical cystectomy and orthotopic neobladder construction in women, a problem may develop in those who are undergoing vaginal-sparing cystectomy. Rapp et al. (*Br J Urol Int* 2004;94:1092) reported on 4 of 37 patients in whom a seemingly minor injury in the anterior abdominal wall, which was closed, presented with postoperative fistulas. Three of the four patients underwent repair with either an obturator flap interposition or a two-layer repair. Two of the three procedures were ultimately converted to an ileal conduit or continent cutaneous diversion because of recurrence of the fistula. Thus, minor technical errors at the time of cystectomy can undermine an otherwise technically successful operation.

The group from Mainz and the Department of Urology at the Johannes Gutenberg University School of Medicine summarized their experience in 170 children and adolescents with a neurogenic bladder in a series of three articles (Stein et al. *Pediatr Nephrol* 2005;20:920, 926, 932). Twenty-four patients received an orthotopic reservoir, 14 of whom underwent orthotopic bladder and substitution with the ureteral reimplantation. The other 10 patients underwent bladder augmentation. Of these 24 patients, 8 of 10 had bladder augmentation and are continent, and all 13

patients with bladder substitution are continent during the day and 1 requires a pad at night.

The second group, reported in the second article, comprised 70 children and adolescents with a median age of 15 years who underwent an ileocecal pouch with an umbilical stoma (Mainz pouch I). Five died of unrelated causes. The upper urinary tracts remained stable or improved in 113 of the 118 renal units (kidneys) and complete continence was achieved in 97% of the patients with this continent cutaneous diversion. However, the revision rate was high, with incontinence of the outlet mechanism in 9%, stoma prolapse in 2%, stoma stenosis in 23%, pouch calculi in 15%, and ureteral stenosis in 16% of the renal units. Although the results are good, it comes at a cost of numerous reoperations.

A third group of 88 patients underwent colonic conduit, mostly in the period before urinary diversion. Of the 77 patients undergoing this operation, 11 died and the authors were unable to do follow-up; 3 of the deaths were related to continued renal deterioration. There were a number of revisions required, but these will not be detailed as this is an operative procedure that is not favored at the present time.

Finally, there are several articles about ureteral fistulae. For example, Alcaraz et al. (*Transplant Proc* 2005;37:2111) reported on 29 patients who developed ureteral fistulae that lasts more than 72 hours. Sixteen were managed endourologically and 13 required open surgery. The patients who underwent open surgery did well, and endourologic management was successful in 10 of 16 cases. Although a number were stented, the stenting with the double-J catheter proved to be of no advantage. In 13 of the 16 cases in which passage of contrast in the bladder was finally demonstrated after a number of corrections, the fistulae resolved in 10 cases, or 77%. Challacombe et al. (*Br J Urol Int* 2005;96:385) wrote about multimodal management of urolithiasis in renal transplantation. Twenty-one of the 2,085 patients who underwent rental transplantation at Guy's and St. Thomas' Hospital were reviewed when they developed urinary tract calculi. The incidence was 1% of the series. Ten of the 21 patients had an identifiable metabolic cause for the urolithiasis; two were caused by obstruction and two were stent-related. Thirteen of the 21 were treated by lithotripsy and 8 of these required multiple sessions. All patients were finally rendered stone-free. The results indicate that the contemporary methods, including lithotripsy, endourology, and finally open pyelolithotomy, will render even transplant patients, despite their somewhat precarious situation, stone-free.

J.E.F.

Nongastrointestinal Transabdominal

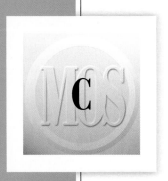

Gynocologic Surgery

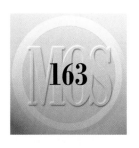

Cesarean Delivery

163

DAVID S. CHAPIN AND TAMARA C. TAKOUDES

BACKGROUND

Definition and History

The origin of the term *cesarean* is unclear, but the legend of Julius Caesar's "cesarean" birth is unlikely to be true. In those ancient times, cesarean delivery was universally fatal, and Caesar's mother was known to have lived for many years after his birth. The term may have derived from the Latin words *caedere* (to cut), and *caesons* (the term for children delivered by cesarean), or from the Roman law known as *Lex Cesare,* which mandated postmortem delivery so the mother and infant could be buried separately. The term "cesarean section" is redundant, derived from the Latin words *caedere* and *secare,* which both mean to "to cut."

The evolution of the current surgical technique is significant. Maternal mortality rates for cesarean birth prior to the 20th century approached 100%. Consequently, very few cesareans were performed. Cesarean delivery was combined with hysterectomy in the late 19th century in an effort to prevent maternal death. Well into the 20th century advances in surgical suture material, aseptic technique, anesthetic advances, the low-transverse incision, and antibiotics improved the safety of cesarean delivery. As a result, cesarean delivery rates increased in the United States from 4.5% of all deliveries in 1965 to 16.5% in 1980 to 24.5% in 1988 to 27.6% in 2003. Cesarean rates still vary widely based on geographic area and type of hospital (i.e., teaching vs. nonteaching). Currently, over 1 million cesarean deliveries are performed annually in the United States alone, making it is the most common surgical procedure performed today.

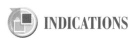

INDICATIONS

Cesarean delivery is indicated for fetal and/or maternal reasons, such as failure to progress in labor, fetal malpresentation, placenta previa, nonreassuring fetal monitoring, suspected macrosomia, active infections like herpes simplex virus or high-viral load HIV, vertical uterine incisions from previous deliveries, and certain fetal anomalies such as severe fetal hydrocephalus or fetal neck masses. The majority of cesareans are still primary with repeat cesarean as an indication for 37.5% of all cesarean births in 1997. A most controversial topic today is the "cesarean-on-demand"—elective, patient-choice cesarean birth. There are data suggesting less urinary incontinence and pelvic organ prolapse after elective cesarean, but the slightly increased morbidity and mortality associated with surgical delivery make the risk/benefit ratio for elective cesarean difficult to quantify. There is currently no standard recommendation regarding patient-choice cesarean. The American College of Obstetricians and Gynecologists states: "Although the evidence does not support the routine recommendation of elective cesarean delivery, we believe that it does support a physician's decision to accede to an informed patient's request for such a delivery" (ACOG Committee Opinion on Ethics 2003).

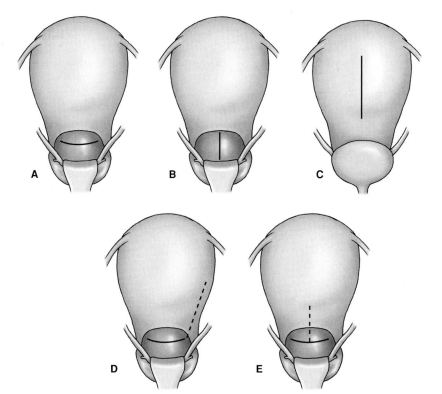

Fig. 3. Uterine incisions for cesarean delivery. **A:** Low-transverse incision. The bladder is retracted downward, and the incision is made in the lower uterine segment, curving gently upward. If the lower segment is poorly developed, the incision can also curve sharply upward at each end to avoid extending into the ascending branches of the uterine arteries. **B:** Low-vertical incision. The incision is made vertically in the lower uterine segment after reflecting the bladder, avoiding extension into the bladder below. If more room is needed, the incision can be extended upward into the upper uterine segment. **C:** Classic incision. The incision is entirely within the upper uterine segment and can be at the level shown or in the fundus. **D:** J incision. If more room is needed when an initial transverse incision has been made, either end of the incision can be extended upward into the upper uterine segment and parallel to the ascending branch of the uterine artery. **E:** T incision. More room can be obtained in a transverse incision by an upward midline extension into the upper uterine segment.

gestations. Care should be made to ensure a large enough uterine incision, especially in the preterm infant. With breech presentation, head entrapment may occur if the incision is too small.

Banking umbilical cord blood has become a common practice. The blood may be collected at the time of cesarean in order to harvest stem. There are many privately owned for-profit companies that will provide patients with kits for collection if notified in advance. The potential for banked cord blood use is not fully known and the likelihood of use in the routine obstetric patient is low (1:1,000 to 1:200,000). There is not yet an indication for routine banking of all cord blood, and the cost of such a program would be formidable.

The placenta should be spontaneously delivered with gentle massage of the uterine fundus and gentle cord traction. Manual removal increases the risk of postpartum endometritis and increases the likelihood of maternal/fetal hemorrhage, which can lead to red cell alloimmunization in future pregnancies, even in the Rh-positive patient, due to small blood group incompatibilities. If the placenta cannot be removed spontaneously or if hemorrhage ensues, manual removal may be achieved by the surgeon's hand creating a plane between the placenta and the uterine wall. After delivery of the placenta, using dry surgical gauze, the uterus should be wiped clean of all residual debris.

Uterine Closure and Control of Hemorrhage

After delivery of the placenta, hemorrhage should be controlled by rapid surgical closure of the uterine incision as well as intravenous oxytocin. Uterine incision closure can be accomplished by various means. To date, there is no absolute standard and variations in technique vary from hospital to hospital and regions of the world. Most surgeons prefer uterine exteriorization prior to surgical repair because this may be associated with decreased blood loss, but it may also be accompanied by increased patient discomfort. There is no increased risk of infection, and effective anesthesia usually prevents significant discomfort. Occasionally severe scarring, obesity, or patient discomfort prevents exteriorization. Pennington or Allis clamps can be used to grasp the edges of the incision for control of hemorrhage and identify the hysterotomy during surgical repair. Suture material should be an absorbable material such as Vicryl or Maxon (preferably size 0 or 1-0). If any extensions are identified, these should be closed first with a locking suture working toward the initial incision and then incorporated into the primary closure. The Kerr or Krönig uterine incision closure can be done by a single or double layer starting at one edge of the incision and proceeding to the other edge with locking sutures approximately 1 cm apart and 1 cm of tissue on each side. Most surgeons avoid incorporating the endometrium into the incision to theoretically prevent future development of adenomyosis, but little data exist to support this practice. The repair should ensure hemostasis, especially at the edges of the incision as this is the most likely area for bleeding postoperatively. A classical incision should be closed in multiple layers as the uterine wall is much thicker and multiple layers are required to reapproximate the tissue hemostatically.

The benefit or risk of single- versus double-layer closure of a low-transverse uterine incision is controversial. Many authors feel double layers may decrease the risk of future uterine dehiscence, but the data are confounded by lack of uniformity of suture material, technique, and definition of uterine dehiscence. Uterine dehiscence also is of such rare occurrence that it is difficult to study in a prospective fashion. Single-layer closure may cause less necrosis of tissue, decreased surgical time, and fewer sutures to control bleeding. If double-layer closure is done, it may be with a second imbricating suture incorporating 1 cm of tissue above and below the uterine incision in a vertical or horizontal (Lembert) fashion (Fig. 4). Most surgeons no longer reattach the bladder flap to the lower uterine segment because theoretically there is less risk of scarring of the bladder high on the uterus (decreasing the risk of bladder injury in future surgery), less risk of hematoma or abscess in the potential closed-off space, and less operative time. Ovaries and fallopian tubes should be inspected prior to return of the uterus to the abdominal space (if exteriorization

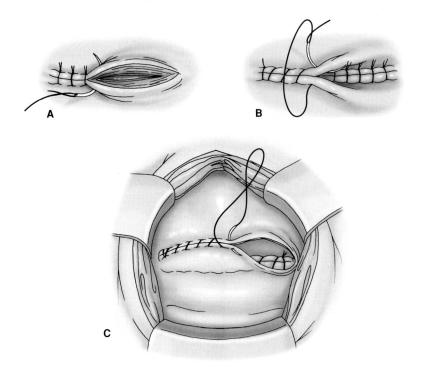

Fig. 4. Closure of a low-transverse incision. **A:** The first layer can be interrupted or continuous. **B:** A second inverted layer can be created by using a continuous Lembert or Cushing stitch, but is really needed only when apposition is unsatisfactory after application of the first layer. **C:** The bladder peritoneum is reattached to the uterine peritoneum with fine suture.

was done). There may be an exaggerated decidual reaction on the surface of the ovaries and fallopian tubes may appear very engorged. If ovarian pathology is suspected preoperatively or intraoperatively, consultation should be expedited so that removal can occur after cesarean delivery. Ovarian corpus luteum cysts need not be excised. Mature teratomas, large hydatid cysts of Morgagni, and suspected ovarian carcinoma should be removed. If a patient has preoperatively consented to permanent sterilization, this may be performed as well after delivery. A modified Pomeroy method is commonly used. A midisthmic portion of fallopian tube is grasped with a Babcock clamp, a 3-cm portion is doubly ligated with two free ties of 1-plain catgut, and this segment is removed with Metzenbaum scissors. The removed portions of fallopian tube must be sent to pathology to confirm that a complete cross section of tube was removed. Sterilization failures due to unintended ligation of the round ligament have been reported.

The uterus should then be replaced inside the abdomen with care not to disrupt any sutures. If inadequate space is found, the broad ligament vessels should be drained by holding up the uterus in the midline with care to alleviate pressure on the vascular sides and then gently rotating the uterus to allow for easy replacement. Clots of blood

and excess amniotic fluid should be removed from the peritoneal gutters with care prior to abdominal wall closure. A careful inspection of all areas, including the bladder, should be done to assess hemostasis. If blood is noted in the Foley catheter, retrograde filling via a three-way catheter can be done with methylene blue or sterile milk to assess for leakage of urine. If lacerations of the dome of the bladder are detected, repair should be performed with a double-layer closure of delayed absorbable suture. Urogynecologic or urologic consultation should be obtained if bladder laceration appears to involve the trigone or ureters.

If hemorrhage is not controlled primarily by uterine incision closure or uterine tone continues to be inadequate with increased blood loss during surgery, other measures must be taken. Increased concentrations of oxytocin may be given intravenously, but must not be in free water or as a rapid bolus because hypotension and water intoxication can occur. If uterine tone cannot be achieved by oxytocin, other uterotonics such as Hemabate (15-methyl prostaglandin F2α), Methergine (methylergonovine), or Cytotec (misoprostol) can be given. The first two are administered intramuscularly, and Cytotec is given as a rectal suppository. There are certain contraindications to giving Hemabate, such as asthma, and to giving Methergine, such as hyper-

tension or preeclampsia. Occasionally there is excessive bleeding in the placental bed, and this can be controlled locally with sewing the vessels prior to uterine incision closure. In cases where abnormal placentation or incomplete removal of the placenta is seen or suspected, as in placenta accreta, additional and rapid surgical steps must be taken. In the case where accreta was suspected preoperatively, additional surgical assistance can be requested from an oncologist or general surgeon. There are case reports of preoperative placement of uterine artery catheters so that interventional radiologists can inflate a small intravascular balloon or embolize vessels to control intraoperative hemorrhage. Uterine atony or placenta accreta is not usually anticipated, and these alternative procedures must be done quickly to control hemorrhage, often requiring emergency consultation.

The mainstay of surgical management for uncontrolled intrapartum hemorrhage remains hysterectomy, but in a gravida with a strong desire for future childbearing the surgeon must try to salvage the uterus. Blood and blood products must be readily available and the surgeon must be skilled in performing alternative procedures to preserve the uterus. Surgical alternatives to hysterectomy include bilateral vertical uterine artery ligation (O'Leary stitch), bilateral utero-ovarian vessel ligation, B-Lynch suture, or hypogastric artery ligation. The O'Leary stitch is accomplished with a single suture of 0 or 1-0 caliber placed in the uterus 2 cm medial to the uterine artery with the needle driven posterior to anterior at the level of the uterine incision (Fig. 5). If this is not successful, then bilateral utero-ovarian vessels may be ligated but with caution that if bleeding continues, each stepwise procedure increases blood loss and the potential for disseminated intravascular coagulation (DIC). Most surgeons would next attempt the B-Lynch suture, if atony is the cause of hemorrhage (Fig. 6). A large absorbable suture is placed bilaterally in the lower uterine segment and looped over the fundus in an attempt to physically compress the uterus. The last resort prior to hysterectomy in a stable but bleeding patient is a hypogastric artery ligation. The procedure is begun by pulling the uterus over the symphysis and opening the retroperitoneal space. The iliac bifurcation is identified and the internal iliac traced 2 to 3 cm downstream to avoid the posterior division of the artery. The anterior division of the artery is doubly ligated with a nonabsorbable suture; the vessel is not divided. Between 25% and 60% of patients require additional procedures. Serious

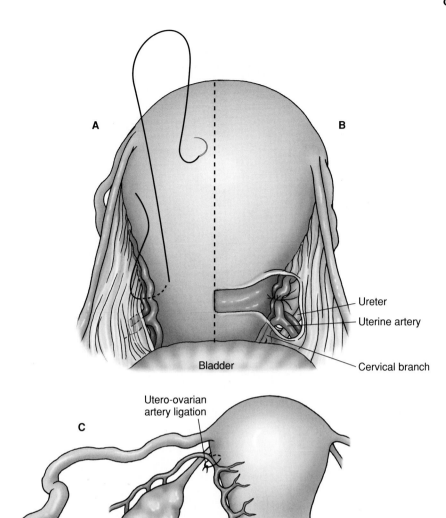

Fig. 5. Ligation of the uterine artery. **A,B:** This anterior view of the uterus demonstrates the placement of a suture around the ascending branch of the uterine artery and vein. Note that 2 to 3 cm of myometrium medial to the vessels has not been included in the ligature. The vessels are not divided. **C:** View of the sutured uterus.

rectus in the midline with one or two mattress sutures or close the peritoneum to allow more ease in future surgical cases. Data as to the benefit of these procedures are lacking.

All sites should be inspected for bleeding, including the underside of the rectus muscles, the fascia, and the subcutaneous space. The fascia is closed using an absorbable 0 Dexon or 0 Vicryl in a running fashion 1 cm apart and incorporating 1 cm of tissue width starting at the lateral corners and continuing toward the midline in a transverse incision. Hernias are more likely at the corners in Pfannenstiel or Maylard incisions, and therefore care should be taken to incorporate both layers of the fascia. Tissue necrosis occurs more easily here than on the uterus, so care must be taken not to make the sutures too close or too tight. A vertical incision may need to be closed with a delayed absorbable suture such as 0 Polyglycolic Dermal Suture (PDS).

If the subcutaneous tissue is more than 2 cm in depth, closure of the subcutaneous tissue with a 3-0 plain suture is appropriate. Data suggest a decreased risk of wound disruption and incidence of seroma. The skin may be closed with a subcuticular dermal suture of 4-0 Vicryl/Monocryl or staples. Staples are most commonly used because their use decreases operating time, but patient satisfaction may be increased with a subcuticular sutured closure. If increased risk of postoperative infection or bleeding is anticipated, a staple closure may be preferable, because it allows easier opening of only a portion of the incision. The patient's abdomen should be cleaned of the preoperative solution and a sterile bandage applied for 24 hours postoperatively. The uterus should be massaged prior to leaving the operating room to ensure that uterine tone is adequate and to prevent further clots from accumulating in the lower uterine segment as these may distend the uterus and prevent adequate uterine contractility.

Postoperative pain management should be given in the form of continued epidural anesthesia, long-acting morphine given through the epidural or spinal anesthetic, and/or intravenous medications, such as Toradol and/or narcotics.

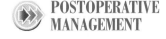

POSTOPERATIVE MANAGEMENT

Volume Status

Recovery from cesarean delivery is usually uncomplicated as most parturients are healthy preoperatively. Patients may require

---

morbidities include accidental ligation of the external iliac artery leading to necrosis of an extremity, laceration of the pelvic vessels, ureteral injury, and retroperitoneal hematomas (Fig. 7). Scant evidence exists that this procedure is efficacious, and most obstetricians are not familiar enough with the anatomy.

The postpartum or intrapartum hysterectomy is a procedure that must be done in cases of intractable bleeding, hemorrhage, or placenta accreta. The procedure itself is more complicated than the usual hysterectomy as the postpartum uterus is very large, the anatomy and location of routine landmarks (i.e., the ureter, uterine vessels, and the bladder) can be confusing,

and the patient may be unstable in many circumstances with ongoing blood loss and DIC. Surgical removal of the uterus must be done with appropriate blood product replacement, adequate anesthesia, and patient consent, if feasible. Supracervical hysterectomy is sufficient to stop the bleeding in most cases. Prior to surgical closure, all efforts must be made to correct coagulation defects and to avoid postoperative bleeding and need for re-exploration.

Abdominal Wall Closure

Multiple studies have failed to demonstrate any benefit of parietal peritoneal closure. Some surgeons reapproximate the

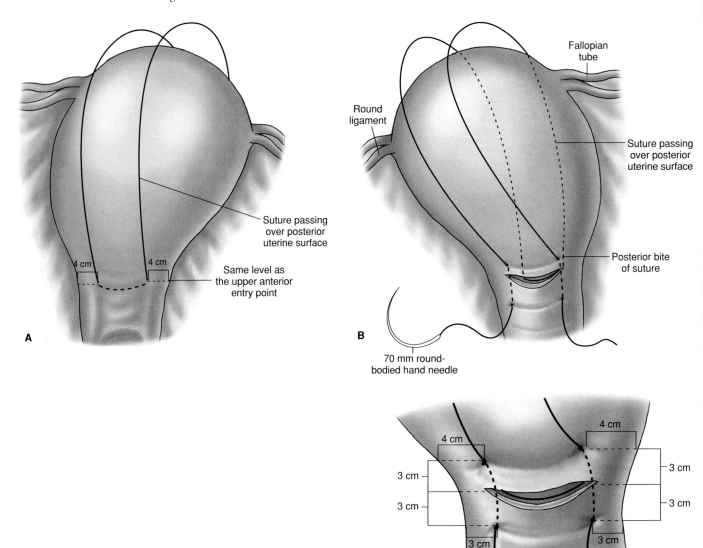

Fig. 6. A: The B-Lynch technique **B:** The B-Lynch suture technique for postpartum hemorrhage.

125 mL or greater per hour of intravenous fluids until oral intake is established. Indications for cesarean delivery must be taken into consideration when assessing fluid status and urine output. Routine hematocrits are not performed in most institutions unless blood loss was greater than anticipated or medical risk factors are present, such as preeclampsia, fever, low urine output, pulmonary edema, or renal or cardiac disease. The most common cause of fluid imbalance postpartum is an underestimation of blood loss from surgery. Postoperative bleeding and complications can occur in even the most routine cases, and careful evaluation of the postoperative patient should be done if signs of hypovolemia are present. Transfusion of blood is recommended in patients with symptomatic anemia and ongoing blood loss such as postpartum hemorrhage.

Intravenous fluids should be discontinued as soon as oral intake is established, usu-ally within 24 hours postoperatively. There are many studies supporting early feeding after most cesareans without awaiting flatus. If cesarean delivery involved bowel surgery or bowel injury, immediate oral intake is not offered. Ambulation is encouraged within 12 to 24 hours to decrease risk of postoperative thrombosis. Foley catheters are removed in approximately 12 to 18 hours in most patients without intraoperative bladder complications. Patients who are immobilized in an intensive care unit or who are unable to ambulate postoperatively require deep venous thrombosis prophylaxis in the form of pneumatic boot compression or subcutaneous heparin.

Pain

Many patients receive long-acting morphine in an epidural or spinal catheter. This allows for excellent pain relief for the first 24 hours in most cases. Additional nonnar-cotic medications such as Toradol can be given to these patients. Care must be given if any additional narcotics are used because the delayed absorption of long-acting morphine derivatives is variable and can lead to respiratory suppression. If spinal morphine is not used, patient-controlled analgesia (PCA) or intramuscular narcotics can be used until the patient tolerates oral intake. Pain medication is typically needed for 1 to 2 weeks postoperatively.

Infection

Infection is common after cesarean delivery, especially if the procedure was after rupture of membranes or labor. Ideally, prophylactic antibiotics are given in these cases, but this does not completely eliminate the occurrence of postpartum endometritis or pulmonary complications. The diagnosis of postpartum endometritis is clinical, based on fever above 100.4° F, fundal tenderness,

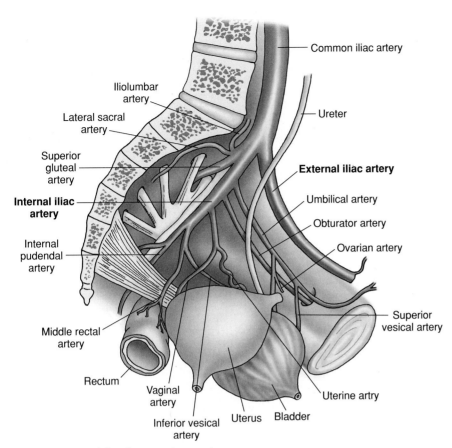

Common iliac artery

Iliolumbar artery

Lateral sacral artery

Ureter

Superior gluteal artery

External iliac artery

Internal iliac artery

Umbilical artery

Obturator artery

Internal pudendal artery

Ovarian artery

Superior vesical artery

Middle rectal artery

Rectum

Vaginal artery

Uterine artry

Inferior vesical artery

Uterus   Bladder

Fig. 7. The internal iliac (hypogastric artery).

foul-smelling discharge, and absence of alternative infections (i.e., wound infection, mastitis, or pneumonia). Treatment includes broad-spectrum intravenous antibiotics such as clindamycin and gentamicin or Zosyn until the patient is afebrile for 24 to 48 hours. If fever persists 24 to 48 hours after initiation of therapy, imaging studies, pelvic ultrasound, and computed tomography scans are recommended to evaluate for other fever sources such as hematomas, abscess collections, or thrombosis. If wound infection is apparent, wound exploration and culture may be necessary.

Postpartum Follow-up

It is important to discuss with the patient before discharge her emotions and her understanding of the indication for cesarean delivery. There are wide variations in patient reaction after cesarean birth including feelings of inadequacy, disappointment, and depression. In addition, if a trial of labor is contraindicated in the future due to a vertical uterine incision, it is prudent to educate the patient about this recommendation for future pregnancy. Patients are usually discharged 3 to 4 days

after delivery (third-party payers in the United States will usually pay up to 4 days for uncomplicated care). This time allows for patient recovery while learning how to care for a newborn and ensuring that breast-feeding is well established. Pain medication is usually a combination of narcotic analgesia (oxycodone or codeine) and ibuprofen unless there are allergies or contraindications. Most patients no longer need medications by 2 weeks after delivery. Routine activity is encouraged, although heavy lifting, tub baths, and vaginal penetration are avoided for at least 6 weeks. Driving is not recommended until the patient is off pain medications and minimal pain is present, usually about 2 weeks. Bleeding may normally persist for up to 6 weeks, with heavier bleeding noted with increased activity. Breast-feeding may alter this pattern with lighter bleeding but may also decrease vaginal lubrication, and the patient should be counseled that breast-feeding alone is not an adequate birth control option. Birth control should be reviewed and encouraged in all women not intending immediate conception after delivery since the timing of the first ovulation is unpredictable.

Fever or incisional drainage should prompt immediate contact with a medical provider. Follow-up appointments usually include a 2-week incisional check and 6-week postpartum examination. Additional follow-up may be necessary if any complications arise. Cesarean delivery requires careful postoperative follow-up even though the majority of patients have an uneventful recovery.

SUGGESTED READING

Bujold E, Bujold C, Hamilton EF, et al. The impact of a single-layer or double-layer closure on uterine rupture. *Am J Obstet Gynecol* 2002;186:1326.

Cetin A, Cetin M. Superficial wound disruption after cesarean delivery: effect of the depth and closure of subcutaneous tissue. *Int J Gynaecol Obstet* 1997;57:17.

Durnwald C, Mercer B. Uterine rupture, perioperative and perinatal morbidity after single-layer and double-layer closure at cesarean delivery. *Am J Obstet Gynecol* 2003; 189:925.

Ferrari AG, Frigerio LG, Candotti G, et al. Can Joel-Cohen incision and single layer reconstruction reduce cesarean section morbidity? *Int J Gynaecol Obstet* 2001;72:135.

Gilstrap LC, Cunninham EG, VanDorsten JP. *Operative obstetrics,* 2nd ed. New York: McGraw Hill, 2002:410.

Hamilton BE, Martin JA, Sutton PD. Births: preliminary data for 2003. *Natl Vital Stat Rep* 2004;53:1.

Hauth JC, Owen J, Davis RO. Transverse uterine incision closure: one versus two layers. *Am J Obstet Gynecol* 1992;167:1108.

Lasley DS, Eblen A, Yancey MK, et al. The effect of placental removal method on the incidence of postcesarean infections. *Am J Obstet Gynecol* 1997;176:1250.

Lynch C, Coker A, Lawal AH, et al. The B-Lynch surgical technique for the control of massive postpartum haemorrhage: an alternative to hysterectomy? Five cases reported. *Br J Obstet Gynaecol* 1997;104:372.

Magann EF, Chauhan SP, Bufkin L, et al. Intraoperative haemorrhage by blunt versus sharp expansion of the uterine incision at caesarean delivery: a randomised clinical trial. *BJOG* 2002;109:448.

O'Leary JA. Uterine artery ligation in the control of postcesarean hemorrhage. *J Reprod Med* 1995;40:189.

Petitti DB. Maternal mortality and morbidity in cesarean section. *Clin Obstet Gynecol* 1985;28:763.

Smaill F, Hofmeyr GJ. Antibiotic prophylaxis for cesarean section. *Cochrane Database Syst Rev* 2002;CD000933.

Wahab MA, Karantzis P, Eccersley PS, et al. A randomised, controlled study of uterine exteriorisation and repair at caesarean section. *Br J Obstet Gynaecol* 1999;106:913.

Wallin G, Fall O. Modified Joel-Cohen technique for caesarean delivery. *Br J Obstet Gynaecol* 1999;106:221.

Nongastrointestinal Transabdominal

EDITOR'S COMMENT

As indicated by Drs. Chapin and Takoudes, the cesarean section delivery represents one of the most common surgical procedures performed today; more than 1 million cesarean deliveries are performed annually in the United States alone. This chapter deals with fundamental surgical approaches following adequate prenatal care, operative considerations, and indications for cesarean delivery. Moreover, the authors depict graphically the variants of uterine incisions that should be considered for cesarean delivery (Fig. 3), and thereafter discuss the implications of each relative to its adequacy and practice throughout the world.

The induction of labor represents a commonly utilized medical practice. Zhang et al. (*Am J Obstet Gynecol* 1999;180[4]:970) indicated in a 1999 publication that its application has increased twofold in the past decade. Approximately one in every five births was induced in the United Kingdom, the United States, and Canada in 2000 (Thomas J, Paranjothy S. *National Sentinel Caesarean Section Audit Report: Royal College of Obstetricians and Gynecologists Clinical Effectiveness Support Unit.* London: RCOG Press, 2001; Curtin SC, Martin JA. Births: preliminary data for 1999. *Natl Vital Stat Rep* 2000;48[14]:1; Anonymous. Health Canada. *Health Services Cesarean Section Rate. Canadian Perinatal Report 2000.* Ottawa, Canada: Minister of Public Works and Government Services, 2000:19). Of recent, vaginal birth following cesarean delivery has been actively promulgated as a methodology to reduce the rising cesarean delivery rates evident in the United Kingdom and United States. As a consequence of this increase in the induction of labor as a common practice, vaginal birth following cesarean delivery rates increased and criteria were broadened for this technique such that women with prior cesarean were considered eligible for induction. Lydon-Rochelle et al. (*N Engl J Med* 2001;345[1]:3) and Wing et al. (*Obstet Gynecol* 1998;91[5 Pt 2]:828) provide reports of uterine rupture for women with prior cesarean undergoing trials of labor, and thereafter the concerns of patient safety were promulgated. Between 2000 and 2001, the Royal College of Obstetricians and Gynaecologists and the American College of Obstetricians and Gynecologists disagreed regarding the safety for induction of labor, particularly regarding the use of prostaglandins for women with prior cesarean section (Anonymous. *Induction of Labour.* London: Royal College of Obstetricians and Gynaecologists Clinical Effectiveness Support Unit, 2001:1; Anonymous. ACOG Committee Opinion. *Induction of Labor for Vaginal Birth after Cesarean Delivery.* Washington, DC: American College of Obstetricians and Gynecologists, 2002:679). The recent publication by

McDonagh et al. was designed to evaluate the risk and benefits for inducing labor in women with prior cesarean delivery (*BJOG* 2005;112:1007). These authors identified 14 fair-quality studies to compare spontaneous labor versus induction of labor to result in cesarean delivery. For women undergoing spontaneous labor, 20% had the cesarean procedure (range 11% to 35%) compared with 32% receiving oxytocin (range 18% to 44%). For studies utilizing prostaglandin (PGE)-2, spontaneous labor resulted in cesarean delivery in 24% (range 18% to 51%) compared with 48% with PGE-2 (range 28% to 51%). Importantly, there was a nonsignificant increase in uterine rupture among those induced compared with spontaneous labors. Further, there were no maternal deaths, and no significant enhancement of maternal complications. These authors concluded that women with prior cesarean delivery attempting a trial of labor requiring induction have a greater frequency of cesarean delivery and a slightly elevated risk of rupture compared with similar women with spontaneous labor.

The recent review by Horey et al. examined the effectiveness of information given to pregnant women to determine the adequacy of informed consent regarding cesarean birth (*Cochrane Database Syst Rev* 2005;4:1). Two randomized controlled trials with a total of 1,451 patients met inclusion criteria with aims to reduce cesarean births by encouraging women to first attempt vaginal delivery. About 70% or more women attempted vaginal delivery in both clinical trials, yet cesarean delivery exceeded 40%, at least 10% higher than optimal achievement. The authors determined that there was no significant difference between control and intervention groups for any of the outcomes measured: vaginal birth, elective/scheduled cesarean, and attempted vaginal delivery.

As indicated by Professors Chapin and Takoudes, the choice of the anesthetic agent utilized is determined by the anesthesiologist based on the clinical presentation and the maternal/fetal indications for delivery. Regional anesthesia is more commonly utilized for planned cesarean delivery and in the nonemergent presentation. The least common is local anesthesia alone, although additional options include spinal, epidural, combined spinal and epidural, or general anesthesia. For patients in whom general or spinal anesthesia is contraindicated, the authors prefer a slow-epidural anesthetic, such as in the case of maternal cardiac disorder or in the circumstance where there are indications to avoid rapid decrease in systemic vascular resistance.

The authors indicate in this review that various studies fail to demonstrate benefit of parietal peritoneal closure. Many surgeons reapproximate the rectus and midline fascia with mattress sutures for closure of the Pfannenstiel, Maylard, or midline ver-

tical closure. Data remain lacking as to the benefit of these procedures, but most surgeons prefer a closure with absorbable 0 Dexon or 0 Vicryl in a running fashion, incorporating approximately a 1-cm placement of the needles and purchase of approximately 1 cm of tissues from the cut surface edge. Herniation, as indicated by the authors, may be common at corners of the Pfannenstiel or Maylard incision; care must therefore be utilized to incorporate both layers of the fascia with closure. For vertical abdominal closures, sutures such as 0 PDS with delayed absorbable characteristics may be the more optimal choice of suture materials.

With presentation of progressive coagulopathy identified intraoperatively, an intrapartum hysterectomy should be performed. The postpartum hysterectomy is a procedure that must be done in cases of intractable bleeding, hemorrhage, or placenta accreta. As the postpartum uterus is quite large, this is a complicated procedure that presents with blood loss and difficulty with dissection of planes, due to the edema and distortion of anatomic landmarks, including the ureters, uterine vessels, and bladder. For ethical and litigious reasons, appropriate informed consent is needed before surgical removal of the uterus; before implementation of the procedure, provision of adequate blood replacement and planned anesthesia is essential. All efforts to correct the coagulation profile (international normalized ratio, prothrombin time, partial thromboplastin time) must be initiated prior to the surgical procedure to avoid postoperative hemorrhage and the necessity of re-exploration.

Gates and Anderson (*Cochrane Database Syst Rev* 2005;4:1) provided a comprehensive review: 1,993 women were included in a review of seven trials completed by meta-analysis. This extensive study confirmed no differences in the risk of wound infection, wound complications, febrile morbidity, or endometritis for women who had wound drains compared with those who did not. These authors concluded that there is evidence that cesarean sections may be about 5 minutes shorter, and that blood loss may be slightly less when drains were not used. These authors stated that there was no evidence in the seven small trials included to date to justify the routine use of wound drains at cesarean section. These studies did not address, and therefore no conclusions could be reached, whether wound drainage is of value when hemostasis is not adequate. Additional randomized prospective trials appear to be justified to examine the role of different types of wound drainage techniques at cesarean section.

K.I.B.

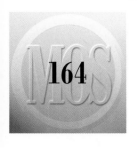

The Abdominal Hysterectomy

164

WILLIAM N. SPELLACY, MITCHEL S. HOFFMAN, AND
EVELYN G. SERRANO

INTRODUCTION

The hysterectomy operation is the second most common surgical procedure performed in the United States, with cesarean section being the most common. About 25% of hysterectomies are vaginal and the remainder abdominal operations. A small percentage of hysterectomies involve the use of laparoscopic techniques. It has been estimated that in the United States about 600,000 hysterectomies are performed annually at a cost of about $3 billion to $5 billion. Approximately one third of women 65 years of age have had a hysterectomy. The number of operations varies by year, geographic location, age, and race. The peak year for procedures was 1975, with more than 700,000 operations being done. The rate decreased in the 1980s as many new medical therapies became available to gynecologists. The highest rates are in the South and the lowest rates in the Northeast. This rate difference is 2.5-fold. The highest rate occurs in the perimenopausal age group of 40 to 50 years.

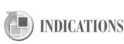

INDICATIONS

About 85% of hysterectomies are performed in the treatment of myoma, endometriosis, endometrial hyperplasia, cancer, or prolapse. Prolapse is usually corrected by vaginal hysterectomy, whereas most of the others are treated abdominally. Of the above indications, uterine myomas are the most frequent. Because myomas are more common in African-American women, they have a higher incidence of having an abdominal hysterectomy. Symptoms usually reported by women with these diseases are abnormal bleeding, chronic pelvic pain, abdominal mass, abnormal Papanicolaou (Pap) test, or pressure in the vagina. The frequency of hysterectomy is significantly higher in women who have been previously sterilized. This may represent the fact that they readily accept surgical therapy for their problems, including family planning. Except for cancer, surgery should not generally be the first approach to therapy.

Effective medical therapy exists for many of the benign diseases like myomas, endometriosis, and endometrial hyperplasia. Examples of these medical therapeutic agents are gonadotropin-releasing hormone agonists to establish early reversible medical castration for myomas and endometriosis, antiprogestins (RU486) for myomas, androgens (danazol) for endometriosis, and progestins for endometrial hyperplasia. Less extensive surgery is also available for these conditions like myomectomy, laparoscopic laser coagulation for endometriosis, dilation curettage for endometrial hyperplasia, endometrial ablation or progestin-type intrauterine devices for menorrhagia, and pelvic artery embolization for myomas. In general, the original complaint may be corrected by performing a hysterectomy, but on long-term follow-up, new problems can develop as a result of castration, such as weight gain, decreased libido, adhesions, and hot flashes.

PROCEDURE

Shaving the abdominal skin before surgery is usually unnecessary. A Foley catheter must be inserted into the bladder before surgery and attached to straight drainage. This reduces the size of the bladder and prevents incidental bladder damage when entering the lower abdomen and when taking the bladder off the lower uterine

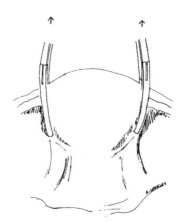

Fig. 1. Uterus is held and upward traction is exerted with Kocher clamps during the hysterectomy.

segment and cervix. Entry into the abdomen is usually by either a lower abdominal midline incision or by a transverse Pfannenstiel incision. It is important to incise the fascial layer down to the symphysis pubis if midline incision is used, as the lower portion of the incision is critical for adequate visualization of the cervix and vagina. The Pfannenstiel incision provides a more limited exposure and is contraindicated if there is a very large uterine mass or a bleeding tendency, or if inspection or surgery may be necessary in the upper abdomen. The advantage of the Pfannenstiel incision above the cosmetic absence of a visible scar is that it is less painful for the patient postoperatively and therefore allows earlier ambulation and recovery. There is no difference in dehiscence rates with a vertical or transverse incision.

Once the abdomen has been entered, inspection and palpation takes place. Assuming all the pathology is found to be limited to the uterus, then the bowel is packed out of the pelvis into the upper abdomen using moist packs to prevent serosal injury. Adhesions, if present, may need to be lysed either bluntly or sharply with scissors. A self-retaining retractor can then be fixed in place, giving good visualization of the pelvic structures. The uterus can be grasped and held with long clamps (e.g., Kocher) placed along the ovarian round ligaments at their uterine insertion (Fig. 1).

The initial uterine incisions on each slide should begin at the round ligaments. These are clamped, elevated, sutured, and then cut (Fig. 2). The external iliac vessels

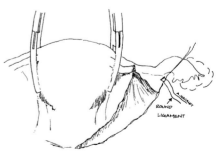

Fig. 2. The round ligaments are clamped, cut, and sutured bilaterally as the first step and initial incisions. This opens the retroperitoneal space.

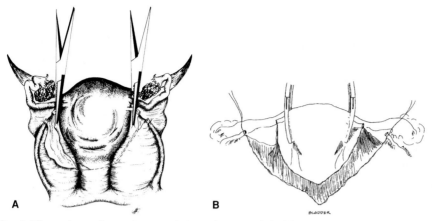

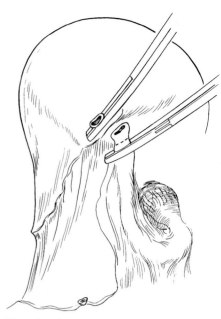

Fig. 3. The vesicouterine peritoneum is incised **(A),** and the bladder is pushed away from the cervix **(B).**

are in close proximity. Division of the round ligament lateral to the utero-ovarian vascular anastomosis avoids hemorrhage and facilitates isolation of the upper vascular pedicle. One small artery (Sampson artery) runs under this ligament and should be included in the suture. Back bleeding is prevented by the uterine-holding clamps. The pelvic peritoneum can then be opened laterally ahead and behind the round ligament. This peritoneal incision is carried from each side completely across the front of the uterus at the vesicle uterine fold (Fig. 3A,B). This allows the bladder to then be bluntly pushed in the midline inferiorly off the cervix. If there are any adherent areas, they must be sharply dissected in order to prevent bladder injury. This is commonly a problem in women who have previously had low segment transverse cesarean sections. If bladder damage is suspected at any time during the operation, the bladder should be filled with a sterile colored solution, which will quickly identify a cystotomy. One easily obtained solution that will not permanently stain the tissues is sterile nursery formula. Dyes like methylene blue can also be used, but if there is a cystotomy, the spilled dye will attach to the pelvic tissues and they will remain stained during the remainder of the operation.

The surgeon can then bluntly dissect the retroperitoneal space posterior to the round ligament. This will allow visualization of the iliac vessels on the lateral pelvic wall and the ureter on the medial peritoneal fold. A decision about retaining or removing the ovaries should be discussed with the patient prior to surgery. In general, if the ovaries are normal and the woman is 50 years of age or older, it is recommended that they be removed. Removal of ovaries in younger women will reduce their estrogen and androgen hormone levels and is not routinely done un-

less there is obvious gross ovarian pathology, a strong family history of ovarian cancer, or a disease process where ovarian hormones either aggravate the disease or may in fact harbor the disease, such as with endometriosis or chronic pelvic infection.

If the ovaries are to be removed, then the infundibulopelvic ligaments need to be identified bilaterally, doubly clamped with instruments like the Heaney clamps, cut, and ligated (Fig. 4). Because there are many large vessels in these ligaments, they are first ligated with a free tie, and then a suture ligature is placed distal to that first tie for permanent closure. This prevents the formation of a hematoma if the needle should penetrate a vessel. If the ovaries are to be preserved, the uteroovarian ligaments are clamped, cut, and ligated in a similar manner (Fig. 5). These ligaments

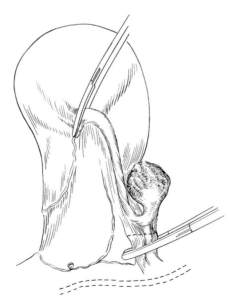

Fig. 4. The infundibulopelvic ligaments are identified, clamped, cut, and sutured if the ovaries are to be removed. Care is taken to avoid the ureter.

Fig. 5. The utero-ovarian ligaments are clamped, cut, and sutured when the ovaries are to be preserved.

should be clamped as close to the uterus as possible to reduce ovarian blood flow disruption and ovarian hypofunction.

The broad ligament support of the uterus is then excised from the top of the uterus in a series of clamps onto the cardinal and then vaginal mesentroid ligaments below the cervix (Fig. 6). The number of clampings needed will depend on the uterine size and cervical length. Because the ureter passes approximately 1.5 cm lateral to the uterus and under the uterine artery, it is important to keep the clamp applied close to the uterus. When clamping tissue in curved areas of the uterus the Heaney clamp is useful, whereas when clamping in straight areas as along the cervix a straight Ballantine clamp is helpful. Clamping occurs in sequence down the broad ligament to the upper vaginal cuff area. After each clamp the tissue is cut and then ligated with a transfixation ligature. Each suture is cut after it is tied. In general, absorbable (Vicryl, chromic) 0 or 1 suture is used.

The hysterectomy can be done with complete removal of the cervix, which is the usual procedure (Fig. 7), or the cervix can be left in place in a subtotal hysterectomy (Fig. 8A,B). If the latter procedure is selected, cervical disease should have been excluded with a normal preoperative pelvic examination and Pap test. Retaining the cervix may be elected in some patients based on the theory that the cervix is important for orgasm or pelvic wall support. If there is difficulty in dissecting off the

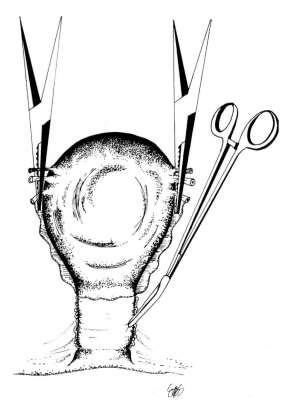

Fig. 6. The broad ligament is clamped close to the uterus at the cervical uterine lower segment where the uterine artery enters the uterus. These pedicles are clamped, cut, and sutured bilaterally. Staying close to the uterus avoids damage to the ureters.

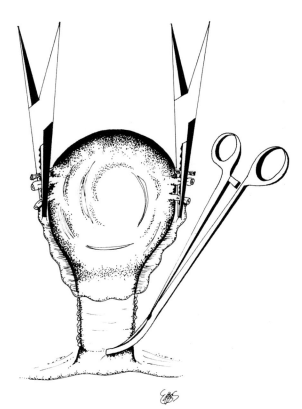

Fig. 7. In the total hysterectomy the vagina is clamped below the cervix, cut, and sutured.

bladder or if the patient develops significant intraoperative problems like cardiac arrhythmias, the surgeon may decide to shorten the operative time and leave the cervix. In some cases of advanced ovarian cancer the cervix is retained to prevent cancer growth into the vagina. When the cervix is left, the endocervical canal should be excised or cauterized to prevent later bleeding from retained endometrium.

When the cervix is to be removed with the uterus, the end of the cervix can be palpated and a bulge can usually be seen at this area of the vaginal apex. Heaney clamps can be placed across the vaginal cuff and when the tissue is cut, it will be clear that the vagina has been entered. Using a scissor like the Jorgenson type allows the vaginal apical cuff to be totally cut across. Inspection of the uterus will determine if the entire cervix is in the operative specimen. The vaginal cuff can then be grasped with clamps (e.g., Kocher) including both the vaginal mucosa and fascia. The cut edge will have small bleeders, but the main arterial systems are at 3 and 9 o'clock as ascending branches of the pudendal artery. The cuff can be closed with running stitches (Fig. 9A,B) or it can be left open. In the latter case the lateral angles can be sutured with a Ball-type stitch to obstruct those ascending arteries and secure the vagina to the cardinal ligaments. The cut edge can then be made hemostatic with a running locking suture (Fig. 10A,B). If the vaginal cuff is left open, the peritoneum should be used to cover the opening to prevent bowel herniation into the vagina. Less granulation tissue is present in the vagina postoperatively if Vicryl suture is used on the cuff. An advantage of leaving the cuff open is that pelvic drains can be placed if there has been infection or excessive bleeding, and pelvic collections of fluid postoperatively can be easily drained if they occur. Oncology follow-up may also be facilitated.

After removal of the specimen, the pelvis should be inspected and hemostasis obtained. If the vaginal cuff has been left open, a Betadine-soaked sponge is inserted into the upper vagina as soon as the uterus is removed to decrease the vaginal bacterial contamination of the pelvis. This sponge is removed from the lower vagina after the abdomen is closed. The pelvis can then be copiously irrigated with warm normal saline. If the ovaries are retained, the ovarian ligaments can be sutured to the round ligament stumps to prevent them from falling into the cul-de-sac and producing pain and dyspareunia (Fig. 11). There is no need to reperitonealize the entire pelvic surgical area except if the vaginal cuff is left open. Nonclosure of the

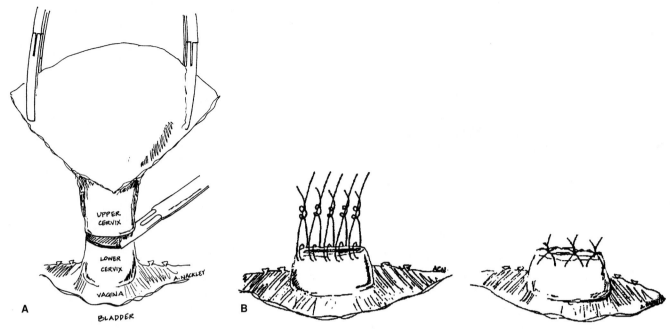

Fig. 8. A,B: In the subtotal hysterectomy the surgeon cuts across the cervix and leaves the cervical stump in place. The cervical stump cut surface is sutured to obtain hemostasis.

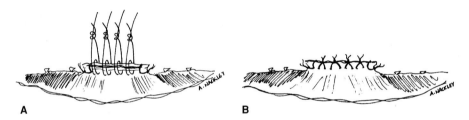

Fig. 9. A,B: The vaginal cuff can be closed after total hysterectomy with running sutures.

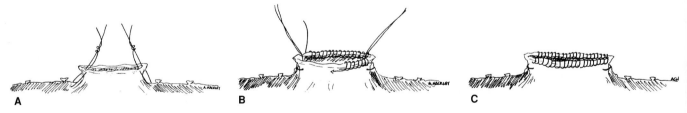

Fig. 10. A–C: The vaginal cuff can be left open after total hysterectomy. The angles are sutured to the cardinal ligaments and the cut edge is secured with a running suture.

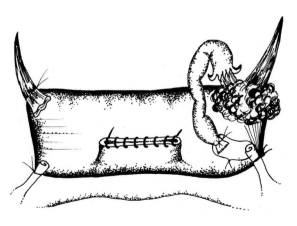

Fig. 11. The ovarian ligament is sutured to the round ligament if the ovaries are not removed, keeping them out of the cul-de-sac.

pelvic peritoneum results in shorter operative time and probably fewer postoperative infections and fluid collections.

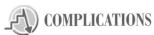

COMPLICATIONS

An abdominal hysterectomy has the usual surgical risks of bleeding and infection. For most procedures the anticipated blood loss should not be excessive, and usually is no more than 500 mL. The major sites for postoperative infection will be the vaginal cuff, the wound, the urinary tract as a result of the indwelling catheter, and the lungs (atelectasis or pneumonia) if general anesthesia is used. The use of short-term prophylactic antibiotics has been shown to significantly reduce the occurrence of cuff and wound infection and is recommended. Our routine is to give one dose of a cephalosporin parenterally 30 minutes before the skin incision is made. A second dose is administered if the surgery exceeds 4 hours or the blood loss exceeds 1,500 mL.

Intraoperative Complications

The majority of complications that occur with abdominal hysterectomy are common to laparotomies in general and especially to pelvic surgery in women. Structures that are occasionally injured during hysterectomy include the bladder, ureter, intestine, and lumbosacral nerves (Table 1). In addition, the pelvis is a highly vascular area with significant potential for hemorrhage. Postoperatively, occult injury to a viscus may become evident in the form of a vaginal fistula. Nerve injury is usually noted in the early postoperative period. Care should be taken with self-retaining retractors, especially in thin women where the lateral blades may impinge upon the femoral nerve as it exits from the caudal-lateral aspect of the psoas muscle. Postoperative infection specific to hysterectomy takes the form of a vaginal cuff cellulitis or abscess.

The pelvic ureter and the bladder have an intimate anatomic relationship with the uterus. Through knowledge of these relationships, injury is avoided by isolation of the gonadal vessels from the ureters before ligation, careful dissection of the bladder from the cervix and anterior vaginal fornix, and the keeping of clamps and sutures as close to the cervix to avoid the lateral soft tissue where the ureters course. When there is significant pathologic distortion or inflammation of the pelvic organs, the anatomic relationships are less reliable, predisposing to urologic injury. Other factors that predispose to urologic injury during hysterectomy are intraoperative hemorrhage and poor exposure. Adnexal pathology, especially with fixation in the posterior lateral pelvis and inflammation involving the lateral pelvic peritoneum (especially if also retroperitoneal), makes isolation of the gonadal vessels difficult. Opening the retroperitoneum above the pathologic process allows the surgeon to identify the ureter and trace it down. Injury of the ureter occasionally occurs at this level and can usually be managed by ureter-ouretorostomy. More commonly, the ureter is injured along its course through the paracervical tissues and is best managed with a ureteroneocystostomy. Less significant ureteral injuries may be managed by simple deligation, with or without stenting. If concern exists about ligating the ureter, verification of patentcy can be done by giving 5 mL of indigo carmine intravenously and observing the dye entering the bladder from the ureteral orifice by cystoscopy.

The urinary bladder is more likely to be injured during hysterectomy when inflammation or prior surgery (e.g., cesarean section) has distorted the plane between the bladder and cervix. In such circumstances, leaving a bit of a cervical tissue on the bladder is usually the best approach. An inadvertent cystostomy should not be closed until the hysterectomy is completed; this facilitates a more appropriate path of dissection and avoids later tension on the cystotomy closure. It is sometimes preferable to open the dome of the bladder so that sharp dissection can be done with a clear identification of the trigone and bladder wall. When a cystotomy occurs near the vaginal fornix, it is close to the trigone. If there is concern about the integrity of the bladder or unexplained significant hematuria during the operation, then approximately 100 mL of a dilute dye solution can be placed into the bladder to see if peritoneal leakage occurs.

The segment of intestine most commonly injured during the actual hysterectomy is the rectosigmoid colon. Several pathologic conditions (pelvic inflammatory disease, ovarian cancer, endometriosis) may obliterate the posterior cul-de-sac, resulting in dense adherence of the rectosigmoid colon to the posterior aspect of the uterus. As with the bladder, sharp dissection leaving a small amount of uterus on the colon works well.

The uterus, as would be expected from its function, is a highly vascular organ. Along its entire length, anastomosing branches of the gonadal and internal iliac vessels supply and drain the uterus. These numerous vessels run within the lateral uterine attachments, and it is not practical to isolate them. Rather, hemorrhage is avoided by careful attention to clamping, dividing, and ligating these ligaments. It is especially important to keep the clamps tight against the uterus and avoid large spaces between pedicles. This is made more difficult in the presence of significant pathologic distortion (e.g., large lower uterine segment leiomyomata, adnexa densely adherent to the posterior broad ligament as seen with pelvic inflammatory disease or endometriosis) and with poor exposure (e.g., markedly obese patient). When hemorrhage is encountered, rather than attempting prompt hemostasis, it is usually best to proceed with the hysterectomy in a careful but expeditious manner. Continued bleeding is usually from the more caudal blood supply and hemostasis occurs as this is ligated. When a large myomatous uterus interferes with distal exposure, it is best to ligate the gonadal and uterine vessels and then perform a supercervical hysterectomy. Occasionally, doing myomectomies improves exposure, and the hysterectomy then becomes an easier operation. With greatly improved exposure, removal of the cervix becomes practical. Clamping or ligating bleeding from the paracervical tissues endangers the ureter. One can carefully grasp the bleeding site with an Allis clamp, gently apply traction to the midline away from the ureter, and then carefully place a suture ligature.

Postoperative Complications

A significant though occult injury of the bladder becomes manifest as urinary leakage through the vaginal cuff. Depending on the mechanism of injury, this may be immediate or delayed, but will usually present within the first 10 days after surgery. The diagnosis is readily made by placing dilute methylene blue solution through a Foley catheter while observing for leakage through the vaginal cuff.

Unrecognized injury of the ureter may also present postoperatively with leakage of urine through the vaginal cuff. However, the patient may develop ureteral obstruction without leakage, and this is fre-

TABLE 1. INTRAOPERATIVE COMPLICATIONS OF HYSTERECTOMY	
Complication	**Incidence (Range)**
Bladder injury	0.3% (0.3%–1.1%)
Ureteral injury	0.2% (0.07%–0.4%)
Bowel injury	<0.5%
Postoperative hemorrhage	0.8%

quently asymptomatic. If concern arises after the surgery, a simple test is to measure the blood creatinine level. One ligated ureter will raise the creatine about 0.8 mg/dL for 2 days. The diagnosis is confirmed with intravenous pyelography.

Postoperatively, serous fluid or blood may accumulate at the operative site (above the vaginal cuff, between the bladder and rectosigmoid colon). This collection is contaminated by bacteria from the vagina and occasionally develops into an abscess. Important risk factors for postoperative vaginal cuff cellulitis or abscess include prolonged surgery and excessive blood loss. Prophylactic antibiotics have dramatically reduced the risk of this complication. Patients who develop an abscess present up to several weeks postoperatively with fever and lower pelvic discomfort. Drainage can usually be accomplished through the vaginal cuff.

Absent anticoagulation, significant postoperative bleeding will usually manifest within the first 24 hours. Along with the usual signs of hemorrhage, the patient will present with vaginal bleeding, high drain output, or increasing abdominal distention, but hemodynamic instability may be the first indication. The usual source is a branch of the internal iliac system, often from the vaginal cuff itself. Management options include careful observation with transfusion as deemed necessary, reoperation (sometimes a couple of transvaginal cuff sutures work), or percutaneous arterial embolization after arteriography.

As with any abdominal operation, postoperative small bowel obstruction may develop. The site of obstruction is usually the ileum adherent to the operative site (pelvis) or abdominal wound. At the completion of hysterectomy, placement of the sigmoid colon and cecum over the raw pelvis and the omentum between the intestines and abdominal wound may help prevent this complication.

During abdominal hysterectomy, a component of the lumbosacral plexus may be damaged. Femoral neuropathy is by far the most common. The usual mechanism is thought to be ischemia or neurapraxia as a result of prolonged compression by a self-retaining retractor. Patients at risk are those who are thin, have poorly developed rectus abduminus muscles, have diabetes, and have a low transverse abdominal incision. The patient reports weakness (usually unilateral) of the leg, often stating that her knee "gives out" upon ambulation. Neurologic examination confirms the diagnosis. Management includes neurologic consultation and physical therapy. It must be emphasized that careful restricted ambulation under the guidance of a physical therapist is important to prevent a fall. Prevention of this injury is based on proper retractor placement to avoid compression of the nerve as it traverses and exits the psoas muscle.

Other postoperative complications may occur, including deep vein thrombosis (DVT), pulmonary emboli, wound dehiscence, and bowel herniation through the vaginal apex. Women who are at high risk for any of these complications may need specific prophylactic measures. For example, women who have had a DVT during pregnancy or during estrogen treatment are at risk for having a congenital coagulation disorder. They need screening for protein C, protein S, activated protein C resistance (factor V Leiden), antithrombin III, prothrombin G 20210 A mutation, methylene tetrahydrofolate reductase mutation (MTHFR), and anticardiolipins. If any of the thrombophilic tests are positive, then prophylactic anticoagulation is recommended. Women with a postoperative serosanguineous wound discharge are at risk for wound disruption and dehiscence and appropriate wound review is necessary.

SUMMARY

The abdominal hysterectomy operation is a very common surgical procedure, used as a final treatment modality for many gynecologic diseases after more conservative therapies have failed. Preoperatively, decisions about removal of the cervix or ovaries must be made with all concerned. With properly performed techniques there are few complications expected.

SUGGESTED READING

Aslan P, Brooks A, Drummand M, et al. Incidence and management of gynaecological-related ureteric injuries. *Aust N Z J Obstet Gynecol* 1999;39:179.

Cardosi RJ, Cox CS, Hoffman MS. Postoperative neuropathies after major pelvic surgery. *Obstet Gynecol* 2002;100:240.

Carlson KJ, Miller BA, Fowler FJ Jr. The Maine Women's Health Study: I. Outcomes of hysterectomy. *Obstet Gynecol* 1994;83:556.

Carlson KJ, Nichols DH, Schiff I. Indications for hysterectomy. *N Eng J Med* 1993;328:856.

Colombo M, Maggioni A, Zanini A, et al. A randomized trial of open verus closed vaginal vault in the prevention of postoperative morbidity after abdominal hysterectomy. *Am J Obstet Gynecol* 1995;173:1807.

Gupta JK, Dinas K, Khan KS. To peritonealize or not to peritonealize? A randomized trial at abdominal hysterectomy. *Am J Obstet Gynecol* 1998;178:796.

Helstrom L, Lundberg PO, Sorbom D, et al. Sexuality after hysterectomy: a factor analysis of women's sexual likes before and after subtotal hysterectomy. *Obstet Gynecol* 1993;81:357.

Jones DED, Shackelford DP, Brame RG. Supracervical hysterectomy: back to the future? *Am J Obstet Gynecol* 1999;180:513.

Kovac SR. Guidelines to determine the route of hysterectomy. *Obstet Gynecol* 1995;85:18.

Learman LA, Summitt RL, Varner RE, et al. A randomized comparison of total or supracervical hysterectomy: surgical complications and clinic outcomes. *Obstet Gynecol* 2003;102:453.

Nahas EAP, Pontes A, Nahas-Neto J, et al. Effect of total abdominal hysterectomy on ovarian blood supply in women of reproductive age. *J Ultrasound Med* 2005;24:269.

Pearl ML, Rayborn WF. Choosing abdominal incision and closure techniques: a review. *J Reprod Med* 2004,49:662.

Somkuti SG, Vieta PA, Daugherty JF, et al. Transvaginal evisceration after hysterectomy in premenopausal women: a presentation of three cases. *Am J Obstet Gynecol* 1994;171:567.

Soper DE, Bump RC, Hurt WG. Wound infection after hysterectomy: effect of the depth of subcutaneous tissue. *Am J Obstet Gynecol* 1995;173:465.

Wilcox LS, Koonin LM, Pokras R, et al. Hysterectomy in the United States, 1988-1990. *Obstet Gynecol* 1994;83:549.

EDITOR'S COMMENT

Professors Spellacy, Hoffman, and Serrano of the University of South Florida discuss in detail the second most common surgical technique performed in the United States; the authors indicate that cesarean section is the most common procedure at present.

Hysterectomy most frequently uses an abdominal approach to remove *both* the uterus and the cervix (total hysterectomy) or the uterus alone (subtotal hysterectomy). The former operation is more common and approximately one quarter of all hysterectomies are

vaginal approaches. The authors indicate that approximately 85% of all hysterectomies performed are utilized in the treatment of endometriosis, uterine myomas, endometrial hyperplasia, cancer, or cervical and uterine prolapse. As the African-

(continued)

American population has a higher frequency of uterine myomas, this population has a higher frequency of abdominal hysterectomy. The authors correctly indicate that there are effective medical therapies that exist for various benign presentations; these include endometriosis, endometrial hyperplasia, and myomas. First-line therapies (e.g., RU486 for myomas, androgens for treatment of endometriosis, and progestins for hyperplasia) should be considered and utilized prior to surgical intervention.

Recently, Lethaby et al. assessed and compared outcomes with subtotal hysterectomy versus total abdominal hysterectomy in the therapy of benign gynecologic conditions (*Cochrane Library* 2006;3:1). As the total hysterectomy is the more common procedure, this study sought outcomes that systematically compared the total procedure to the subtotal approach. In review of the three randomized controlled trials for women undergoing either the total or subtotal hysterectomy for benign disease, 733 participants were included. These outcomes suggested no differences in rates of incontinence, constipation, or measure of sexual function. This meta-analysis did not confirm the perception that subtotal hysterectomy offers improved outcomes for sexual, urinary, or bowel function when compared to the total abdominal approach. It would appear that there is advantage in the recovery time, as well as decreased intraoperative blood loss, but women having the subtotal hysterectomy were more likely to experience cyclic bleeding for up to a year following surgery when compared to the total resection approach. As noted by these authors, one of the expected disadvantages of total hysterectomy has been an increase in postoperative vaginal vault prolapse. However, in this study by Lethaby et al., an increase in postoperative vaginal vault prolapse was not confirmed, although the authors cautioned that the trials may have been statistically underpowered to adequately assess this outcome. (Clinically, prolapse may appear years following total hysterectomy; these data suggest that long-term follow-up is essential to assess whether preservation of the cervix afforded superior protection for prolapse compared to the total hysterectomy approach.)

Professor Spellacy et al. depict in the figures abdominal entry by either a low abdominal midline or the transverse Pfannenstiel incision. The latter approach does provide the surgeon a more limited exposure, and as indicated by the authors, is contraindicated when more extensive intra-abdominal exploration is planned or necessary (e.g., large uterine mass, intra-abdominal bleeding, necessity of exploration of upper abdominal contents). Nonetheless, the Pfannenstiel incision is a time-honored, historic surgical approach that achieves cosmesis and affords rapid ambulation and recovery; in the majority of cases, this incision is less painful than the midline hypogastric exposure. The authors appropriately identify that there is no statistical difference in dehiscence rates between the two incisions.

The recent addition to the armamentarium of the gynecologist has been the laparoscopic hysterectomy, which has three subdivisions: (a) laparoscopic-assisted vaginal hysterectomy (LAVH), (b) total laparoscopic hysterectomy (TLH), and (c) laparoscopic hysterectomy (LH). The LAVH includes vaginal hysterectomy assisted by laparoscopic procedures that *do not* include uterine artery ligation. LH is the laparoscopic procedure in which uterine artery ligation is included, and the TLH includes no vaginal component of the procedure and the vaginal vault is sutured laparoscopically. Johnson et al. recently assessed the most common surgical procedures utilized for hysterectomy and provided analyses of the three common approaches to hysterectomy, including abdominal hysterectomy, vaginal hysterectomy, and laparoscopic approaches (*Cochrane Library* 2005;1:1). These authors utilized various Web-based search engines that have relevant citation lists to evaluate hysterectomies conducted by randomized trials that compare one surgical approach with another. These authors identified 27 trials inclusive of 3,643 participants with independent selection of trials and data extraction following Cochrane guidelines. In this detailed analysis that was statistically powered for anatomic differences, data suggested that the vaginal hysterectomy should be performed in preference to the abdominal hysterectomy approach when possible. Moreover, when the vaginal hysterectomy is not possible, or if determined by the gynecologist not to be the safest technical approach, the laparoscopic technique may avoid the necessity for abdominal hysterectomy. However, the length of the surgical procedure increased with the extent of the surgery performed laparoscopically and correlated with the laparoscopic time of the procedure, particularly when the uterine arteries were divided laparoscopically. Johnson et al. determined that there is a steep learning curve for the procedure, and the laparoscopic approach does require greater surgical expertise. These authors recommend, and we concur, that the selected surgical approach to hysterectomy must be an informed consent provided by the gynecologist that allows the woman to be informed of this decision by her surgeon relative to benefit and risk. These authors further determined that research is required that fully explores all relevant outcomes, particularly those of long-term results with randomized controlled trials that minimize bias reporting. Clearly, there will be evolution and increasing expertise that applies laparoscopic approaches, but these evolving techniques should only be undertaken in clinical centers with adequate expertise to ensure equivalent outcomes.

K.I.B.

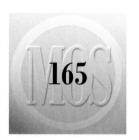

165

Radical Hysterectomy

YOUNG BAE KIM

INTRODUCTION

Radical hysterectomy and bilateral pelvic lymphadenectomy is the standard operation for early cervical cancer. Wertheim developed the modern technique for radical hysterectomy in the early 20th century, and in the 1940s Meigs added routine pelvic lymphadenectomy to the procedure, thereby increasing its curative potential. Initially described as a very morbid operation, radical hysterectomy can now be performed with an acceptably low rate of serious complications. Advances in modern surgical technique, as well as those in anesthesia, transfusion, and antibiotics, now allow the operation to be performed with a rate of serious morbidity approaching 1%. As a result, radical hysterectomy and bilateral pelvic lymphadenectomy is a viable alternative to radiation for the definitive treatment of some patients with FIGO stage Ia, Ib, and IIa cervical cancer.

A randomized study has shown that radical hysterectomy and radiation both result in 5-year survival rates of 85% in early cervical cancer. Therefore, the choice of treatment for a given patient rests with other considerations. Radical surgery has a number of potential advantages over radiation. It allows preservation of ovarian function. It also allows better preservation of sexual function relative to radiation. It is associated with fewer long-term complications than radiation, particularly with respect to chronic diarrhea, tenesmus, and urinary tract and bowel fistulas. Radical hysterectomy does have the disadvantage that it is not as widely applicable as radiation. Poor surgical candidates, such as those who are medically compromised or morbidly obese, may be better served with radiation. Radical hysterectomy is also associated with more acute complications compared to radiation, such as infection, thromboembolism, and ureteral injury.

Radical hysterectomy differs from simple (or total) hysterectomy in that the tissues surrounding the cervix are removed along with the uterus and cervix. This includes the cardinal ligaments, uterosacral ligaments, and upper vagina. While these tissues do not appear very impressive in the final specimen, the additional work necessary to remove them is considerable. During the operation, more time is spent in mobilizing the surrounding organs, namely the bladder, ureters, and rectum, than in removing the specimen. In addition, pelvic lymphadenectomy, while not strictly speaking a part of radical hysterectomy, is almost always performed in conjunction with radical hysterectomy when treating cervical cancer. The final result of radical hysterectomy and pelvic lymphadenectomy is a classic Halstedian operation, with radical resection of the primary tumor and resection of the draining lymph nodes.

Early cervical cancer is by the far the most common indication for radical hysterectomy and pelvic lymphadenectomy. However, a number of other indications exist for which this operation is suited. These include stage I vaginal cancers limited to the upper vagina and stage II endometrial cancers with gross cervical involvement. Somewhat more controversial is the use of radical hysterectomy for small, centrally recurrent cervical cancers occurring after previous treatment with radiation. Many surgeons feel that these patients have a better chance of long-term survival with pelvic exenteration.

There has been a long-term trend toward decreasing the radicality of radical hysterectomy in the hopes of decreasing morbidity while at the same time preserving curative potential. The most important example of this is the adoption of the Wertheim method over more radical operations. Going a step further, many surgeons now routinely perform an even less radical procedure, termed modified radical hysterectomy. A randomized clinical trial demonstrated that modified radical hysterectomy is associated with less morbidity and similar rates of cure in patients with stage Ib and IIa cervical cancer. One limitation of this study was the high rate of adjuvant radiation, which may have negated the effects of any differences in surgical technique between the treatment arms. Nevertheless, many surgeons advocate modified radical hysterectomy for patients with smaller tumors (<1 to 2 cm). The purpose of this chapter is to describe both radical hysterectomy and modified radical hysterectomy in detail, highlighting important points that allow these inherently difficult operations to be performed with success. Other recent developments include a resurgence of interest in vaginal approaches to radical hysterectomy, the incorporation of laparoscopy, and radical trachelectomy. These procedures are beyond the scope of this chapter, but they do offer the possibility of minimally invasive treatment and

sparing of fertility without compromising the chance for cure.

Although radical hysterectomy is intended to be definitive treatment for early cervical cancer, some patients are at significant risk for recurrence with surgery alone and benefit from adjuvant therapy. Patients with positive pelvic lymph nodes, parametrial involvement, and positive surgical margins should be offered pelvic radiation with concurrent platinum-based chemotherapy. Adjuvant therapy may also be considered for other high-risk patients such as those with large tumors, deep stromal invasion, or lymphovascular space invasion, although the data supporting treatment of these patients are not as strong. The management of patients with large (stage Ib2) cervical tumors is controversial, with some surgeons favoring a primary surgical approach with or without adjuvant chemoradiation and others favoring chemoradiation alone. This question is currently being addressed by a randomized clinical trial.

INITIAL STEPS

General anesthesia is induced. A single dose of antibiotic administered before incision is usually sufficient for prophylaxis, although a repeat dose may be given if the operation exceeds 4 hours. Pneumatic compression stockings, minidose heparin, or both may be used for thromboembolism prophylaxis.

The patient is placed in dorsal supine or low lithotomy position. Examination under anesthesia is performed to exclude the presence of disease beyond the cervix and upper vagina. Rectal examination is particularly important in order to exclude disease extension into the cardinal ligaments. Cystoscopy and proctosigmoidoscopy may also be performed at the discretion of the surgeon to exclude disease extension into the bladder or rectum. Any findings suspicious for disease extension beyond the cervix and upper vagina should prompt abandonment of the operation in favor of radiation.

A Foley catheter is placed (some surgeons favor a suprapubic catheter). A vertical midline or low transverse incision may be used. Two transverse incisions, the Maylard and Cherney, provide excellent pelvic exposure. A vertical incision is preferable when the surgeon plans to sample the para-aortic lymph nodes. Once inside the peritoneal cavity, the abdomen and pelvis are thoroughly explored manually and visually. Any evidence of metastatic disease should prompt abandonment of the procedure if confirmed histologically. Particular

attention is paid to the area around the cervix, including the posterior cervix and cul-de-sac. A formal para-aortic lymph node sampling, while favored by some surgeons, is associated with low yield and is therefore not standard. Peritoneal washings are sometimes performed, but the significance of positive washings in this setting remains unclear.

RADICAL HYSTERECTOMY

A Buchwalter or similar self-retaining retractor may be placed to expose the pelvis. Femoral neuropathy is a risk of using such retractors, but this risk can almost be eliminated by ensuring that there is room between the bottoms of the blades and the psoas muscles. The bowel is displaced cephalad using moist laparotomy packs. The uterus is grasped with a triple hook or Kelly clamps and placed on cephalad tension. The round ligaments are suture-ligated and divided. Absorbable suture, commonly 0 Vicryl, is used throughout the operation. The broad ligaments are opened in a cephalad and caudad direction lateral to the gonadal vessels, and the ureters are identified along the medial leaves of the broad ligament (Fig. 1). They are most readily identified as they enter the true pelvis and cross over the bifurcation of the common iliac arteries.

The pararectal and paravesical spaces are then developed. These are avascular potential spaces that allow the peritoneum over the pelvic sidewall to be mobilized safely, thus exposing the pelvic sidewall vessels and the course of the ureters. The pararectal space is bounded by the external and internal iliac vessels laterally, the ureter medially, and the cardinal ligament anteriorly. Using either a single finger or a dissecting instrument, the common iliac artery bifurcation is identified and the space just medial to this is opened, resulting in displacement of the ureter medially. Care is taken to ensure that the dissection remains medial to the internal iliac artery. The dissection follows the hollow of the sacrum caudad and curves slightly medially toward the rectum. The space may be opened to the level of the levator plate.

The paravesical space is bounded by the external iliac vessels laterally, the bladder and superior vesical artery medially, and the cardinal ligament posteriorly. Again using either a finger or a dissecting instrument, the space just medial to the most distal aspect of the external iliac vein is developed, displacing the bladder medially. The space is followed medially and caudad along the pubic symphysis toward the levator plate.

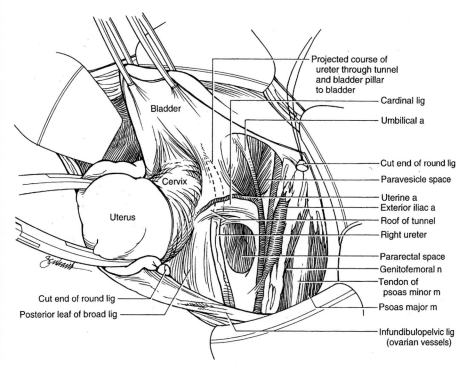

Fig. 1. The paravesical and pararectal spaces are developed. The cardinal ligaments are assessed for tumor extension. The uterine artery is ligated at its origin from the internal iliac artery.

chemoradiation afterwards. This approach may allow for improved sexual function compared with radiation alone, as the latter necessarily includes a very high dose of vaginal brachytherapy. We generally perform the pelvic lymphadenectomy after radical hysterectomy.

The cardinal ligament is dissected down to the uterine artery, which is then ligated at its origin from the internal iliac artery (Fig. 2). The uterine artery is reflected above the ureter. The ureteral dissection, the most critical part of the operation, then commences. The ureter is dissected off the peritoneum near the uterosacral ligament, taking care to preserve its surrounding adventitial blood supply. A small wavy vessel is often seen adjacent to the ureter and should be preserved. The ureter is then freed of its peritoneal attachments. This is facilitated by cephalad traction on the uterus and posterior traction on the ureter's adventitia. The ureter should not be handled directly. The "tunnel," through which the ureter courses lateral and anterior to the cervix, is then dissected, freeing the ureter (Fig. 2). It is crucial that the dissecting instrument remain in close proximity to the ureter in order to avoid significant bleeding that can ensue and obscure the field. The instrument is best placed just superolateral to the ureter. Once a pedicle is established, it may be ligated directly or after transection between clamps. The latter method is facilitated by specialized clamps developed by Casey.

The last part of the tunnel is composed of the bladder pillars, which are fibrovascular

Once the space is open, the superior vesical artery is readily apparent as it enters the lateral dome of the bladder. Care must be taken to avoid bleeding in the prevesical space just medial to the paravesical space.

Now the surgeon must make the final assessments for resectability prior to completing the planned operation. The vesicouterine fold of peritoneum is incised and the bladder is dissected down the anterior cervix and upper vagina in an avascular plane. This is best accomplished with sharp dissection or electrocautery to minimize bleeding and trauma to the bladder. Any tumor extension through the anterior cervix will be evident at this point. Such a finding indicates unresectability. The cardinal ligaments are then palpated with two fingers, one in the paravesical space and one in the pararectal space. This "web" of tissue comprises the condensation of fibrovascular tissue lateral to the cervix constituting the cardinal ligament (the term parametrium is often used synonymously). Any palpable disease in the cardinal ligaments also indicates unresectability. Finally, the pelvic lymph nodes are assessed, and any grossly suspicious nodes are sent for frozen section. Most surgeons abandon the radical hysterectomy if grossly positive lymph nodes are encountered. There is some evidence that debulking such nodes prior to closing improves the chances for cure.

Some surgeons now proceed with pelvic lymphadenectomy, the rationale

being that the finding of microscopically positive pelvic lymph nodes would result in abandonment of the operation. However, the yield is low if the nodes are grossly normal, and the technique of intraoperative frozen section is inaccurate and cumbersome. Furthermore, many surgeons would complete the radical hysterectomy with microscopically positive pelvic nodes and recommend adjuvant

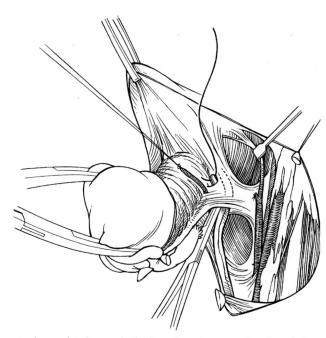

Fig. 2. The ureteral tunnel is dissected. The ligated uterine artery is reflected above the ureter.

Nongastrointestinal Transabdominal

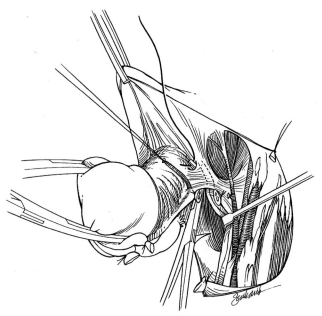

Fig. 3. The last part of the tunnel is dissected and the ureter is completely freed to its insertion into the bladder.

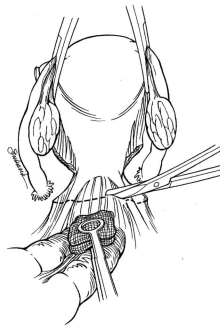

Fig. 4. The posterior peritoneum is incised and the rectum dissected off the posterior vaginal wall.

attachments of the bladder to the lateral aspects of the cervix. The pillars are exposed initially with the bladder dissection. Further anterior dissection of the pillars can facilitate the ureteral dissection, but care must be taken to avoid injuring the numerous small vessels within. The ureteral dissection is completed to the insertion into the bladder (Fig. 3). The surgeon must be careful to end the tunnel dissection once the bladder is reached, as the ureterovesical junction is not always obvious. The ureter, having been unroofed from its tunnel, is now dissected out of its cardinal ligament bed completely.

If the adnexa are to be removed, the gonadal vessels are now isolated above the ureters and ligated. If the adnexa are to be conserved, the utero-ovarian pedicles are isolated and ligated. The posterior dissection then commences (Fig. 4). The recto-vaginal fold of peritoneum is incised, taking care to avoid the ureters. The incision crosses both uterosacral ligaments and the upper cul-de-sac. The rectum is dissected down the posterior vagina in an avascular plane. This can often be accomplished with gentle blunt dissection, with care taken to avoid direct pressure on the rectum. Excessive force can result in unintentional entry into the posterior vaginal wall, which is quite thin. The uterosacral ligaments are cleared of the rectum. Some bleeding from the rectal pillars may ensue, but this is generally not problematic.

The specimen is now removed. It is helpful to palpate the cervix to ensure an adequate margin of vagina. The uterosacral ligaments are taken with clamps, cut, and suture-ligated at roughly their midpoints, taking care to avoid the rectum (Fig. 5). The cardinal ligaments are similarly divided near the pelvic sidewalls, taking care to retract the ureters laterally (Figs. 6 and 7). The vagina is clamped below the cervix and the specimen is removed. The vaginal margin may now be assessed. A 1- to 2-cm margin of vagina is generally adequate, but a larger margin should be obtained if there is disease extension to the upper vagina. The vaginal margin commonly appears smaller in the removed specimen than it does in vivo. The vaginal cuff is closed with transfixion sutures at the angles and figure-of-eight sutures in between (Fig. 8).

If the adnexa have been conserved, they are sometimes transposed out of the pelvis into the lower abdomen in case

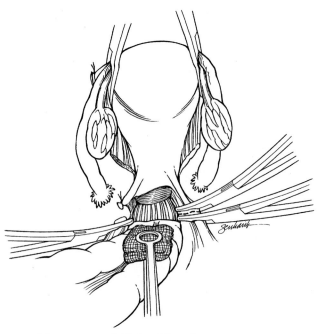

Fig. 5. The uterosacral ligaments are divided and ligated.

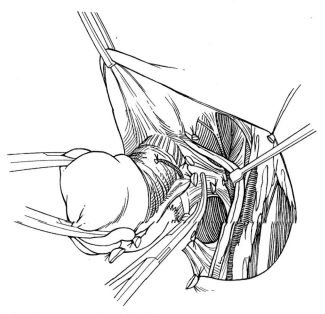

Fig. 6. The cardinal ligaments are divided and ligated.

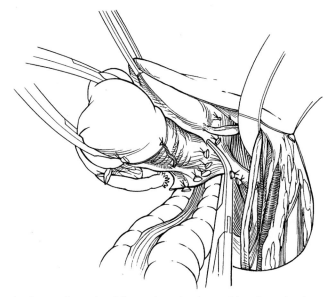

Fig. 7. The vagina is cross clamped and the specimen is transected just above the clamps and removed.

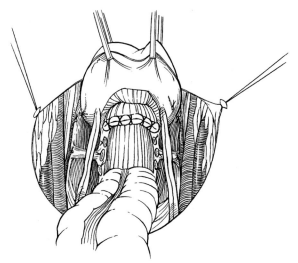

Fig. 8. The vaginal cuff is closed with suture.

radiation is necessary postoperatively. This procedure results in preservation of ovarian function in about 50% of patients needing pelvic radiation. The adnexa are mobilized on their vascular pedicles and tacked to the lower paracolic gutter peritoneum with nonabsorbable suture.

At this point, the bladder, rectum, and ureters are inspected for injury. All structures should appear intact and well vascularized. The ureters should be peristalsing freely and of normal caliber. If there is any question of an injury, further evaluation is performed. The bladder may be assessed by distension with methylene blue or sterile milk through the Foley catheter. The ureters may be assessed by intravenous injection of indigo carmine and visualization of urine emanating from the ureteral orifices, preferably via cystoscopy or alternatively via cystotomy at the dome of the bladder. Absence of dye extravasation into the pelvis should also be confirmed. Although rarely necessary, the rectum may be evaluated by insufflation via proctosigmoidoscopy after filling the pelvis with fluid. If an injury is identified, appropriate repairs are performed.

PELVIC LYMPHADENECTOMY

Pelvic lymphadenectomy is almost always performed in conjunction with radical hysterectomy for cervical cancer. Complete removal of the pelvic nodes rather than sampling is the goal. The operation is accomplished with sharp dissection or electrocautery, and hemoclips are often used for hemostasis and possibly to decrease the risk of lymphocysts.

The peritoneum is opened from the mid-common iliac artery to the deep circumflex iliac vein (Fig. 9). These landmarks constitute the cephalad and caudad limits of the dissection, respectively. A self-retaining retractor is used to expose the pelvic sidewall and retract the ureter medially. The dissection begins just medial to the genitofemoral nerve, which courses lateral and parallel to the external iliac artery. The lymph node–bearing tissues are mobilized medially off the external iliac artery and vein (Fig. 10). The obturator fossa is entered just below the external iliac vein. The surgeon should be aware of a possible accessory obturator vein off the external iliac vein, present in about 10% of patients (Fig. 11). This branch may be ligated to facilitate exposure of the obturator fossa. The dissection is carried under the external iliac vein toward the pelvic sidewall to the psoas muscle, separating the node bundle from the vein completely. The external iliac vein

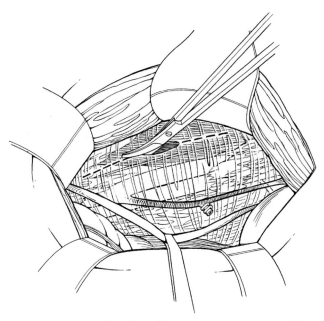

Fig. 9. The peritoneum over the pelvic sidewall is opened over the external iliac artery.

may be carefully retracted for exposure. The external iliac nodes may be taken separately or in continuity with the obturator nodes. The obturator nodes are then mobilized off the obturator nerve, which courses in the middle of the obturator fossa. It is important to avoid injury to this nerve, as it is vital for adduction of the lower extremity. Care should be taken to remove all lymph nodes above the nerve, including those in the genu between the external and internal iliac vessels and in the most distal aspect of the obturator fossa just proximal to obturator foramen. The lymph node bundle can often be grasped and pulled medially while sweeping it off the obturator nerve and internal iliac vessels with fine scissors. This allows the obturator nodes to be removed, often as a single specimen, without cutting any tissue, thereby

minimizing bleeding and the risk of obturator nerve injury. There may be a few obturator lymph nodes below the nerve, which some surgeons remove after ligating the obturator vessels (Fig. 12). The distal common iliac nodes are then removed just lateral to the common iliac artery. Particular care is taken on the right, where the right common iliac vein is lateral to the artery. Once the dissection is completed, the genitofemoral nerve, obturator nerve, superior vesical artery, and ureter should all be clearly visible and uninjured. It is not necessary to place drains or close the peritoneum. These steps have not been found to decrease lymphocyst formation.

Hemostasis is confirmed. The fascia is closed with a continuous permanent or delayed absorbable suture.

MODIFIED RADICAL HYSTERECTOMY

Modified radical hysterectomy differs from radical hysterectomy only in the amount of paracervical tissue that is taken. Although the indications for modified radical hysterectomy are somewhat controversial, many surgeons feel it is the procedure of choice for patients with small tumors (1 to 2 cm) confined to the cervix. Modified radical hysterectomy offers the potential advantages of shorter operating times, less blood loss, and decreased overall morbidity, including bladder dysfunction. As with radical hysterectomy, a complete pelvic lymphadenectomy is almost always performed in conjunction with modified radical hysterectomy.

There are only a few important technical differences compared to radical hysterectomy. The uterine artery is ligated over the ureteral tunnel rather than at its origin (Fig. 13). Once the tunnel is unroofed, the ureter is only partially mobilized from its tunnel bed, enough that the cardinal ligament medial to the tunnel may be taken with the specimen (Fig. 14). The uterosacral ligaments are ligated close to the cervix, and a smaller vaginal margin is taken.

 POSTOPERATIVE MANAGEMENT

Patients are advised to ambulate immediately to minimize pulmonary and thromboembolic complications. Diet may be advanced as tolerated. Evidence of bowel function is not a prerequisite to this. Oral pain medications are started as soon as the patient is tolerating oral intake. The urinary catheter is left in place during the

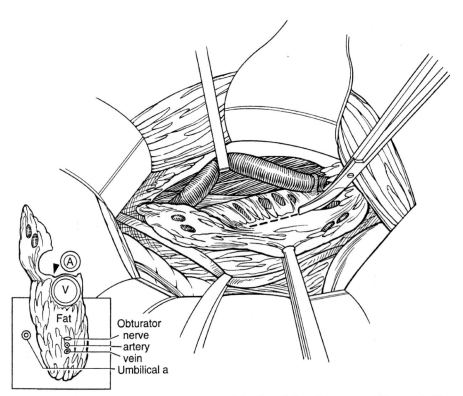

Fig. 10. The lymph node–bearing tissues are mobilized medially off the external iliac vessels. The obturator space is entered just below the external iliac vein.

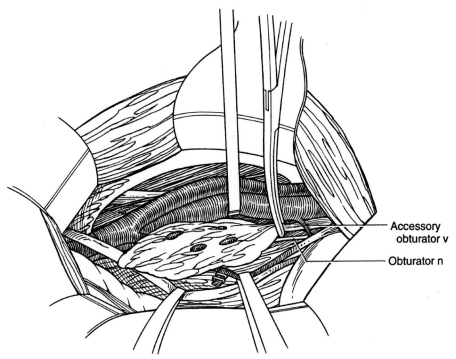

Fig. 11. The obturator nodes above the obturator nerve are removed.

most common sites of injury are the ureter, bladder, nerves, major vessels, and rectum. Sequelae of the most common injuries, to the ureter and bladder, include sepsis, fistula, loss of renal function, and re-operation. Injury can also delay or proscribe adjuvant therapy. Maintenance of a clear surgical field, gentle tissue handling, and careful dissection of surgical planes will minimize, though not eliminate, operative injury. The single most important determinant of outcome after operative injury is whether the injury is detected intraoperatively. Therefore, whenever an injury is suspected, careful evaluation as described above should be performed before closure of the abdomen.

POSTOPERATIVE COMPLICATIONS

Both short- and long-term complications are not uncommon following radical hysterectomy. The most common immediate complications are wound infection, thromboembolism, and ileus. Voiding dysfunction is expected and is therefore arguably not a complication. Likewise, febrile morbidity, although common, is of concern only insofar as it may be indicative of something more serious. In the immediate postoperative period, the surgeon should be particularly attuned to signs or symptoms suggestive of thromboembolism, and should have a low threshold for evaluating patients with imaging studies. Timely diagnosis of

immediate postoperative course due to anticipated voiding dysfunction. Using this approach, most patients may be discharged within 3 days following surgery.

Although some patients require catheter drainage for 3 weeks or more, most require only a week. This will depend to some extent on the radicality of the operation. We typically use a Foley catheter and have a home visiting nurse remove it a week after surgery. We have found that patients rarely need to return for catheter replacement due to voiding difficulties.

INTRAOPERATIVE COMPLICATIONS

The most common intraoperative complication is blood loss. The literature indicates that average blood loss is highly variable but is large, almost 1 L. Blood loss is probably dependent on patient selection and surgeon experience. The most problematic bleeding typically occurs during the ureteral dissection. Surgeons who exercise particular caution here are often rewarded with minimal blood loss and a clear surgical field. The ureter is surrounded by small, easily injured blood vessels as it courses through its tunnel into the bladder trigone. Once bleeding occurs, it can be difficult to control since the ureter is in close proximity. Often the only way to stop the bleeding is to hurriedly complete the

ureteral dissection, a circumstance that places the ureter at risk of injury. Transfusion is often necessary, but should be avoided if possible due to concerns, although unproven, that this can adversely affect prognosis.

Operative injury is another major concern, occurring in about 2% of cases. The

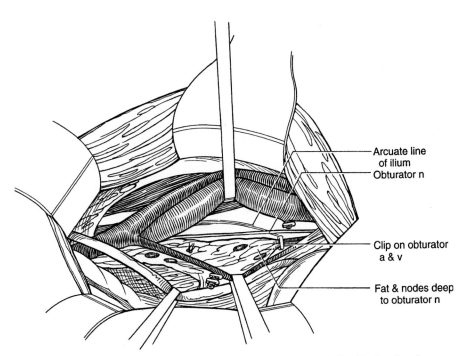

Fig. 12. The obturator nodes below the obturator nerve are removed after ligating the obturator artery and vein.

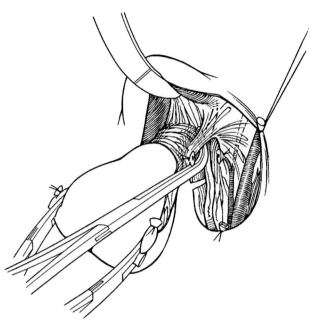

Fig. 13. The uterine artery is ligated at the level of the ureter.

this potentially fatal complication can be lifesaving.

Far less common but perhaps more dreaded, urinary tract fistula should be considered if a patient complains of watery vaginal discharge. Physical examination, testing with dye and tampons, and imaging studies such as contrast-enhanced computed tomography (CT) are diagnostic. A common first step is to instill the bladder with methylene blue after inserting a tampon in the vagina. Absence of dye on the tampon excludes a vesicovaginal fistula. Next, indigo carmine is injected intravenously. Further absence of dye on the tampon excludes a ureterovaginal fistula. It is important to recognize that a positive bladder dye test is diagnostic of vesico-

vaginal fistula but does not exclude a concomitant ureterovaginal fistula. Further evaluation, usually with cystoscopy and retrograde ureterography, is necessary. Prompt recognition of a fistula can decrease associated morbidity and in some cases even allow immediate reoperation and repair.

Ureteral obstruction after radical hysterectomy may be caused by direct operative injury or adhesions. Potential signs and symptoms include unexplained fever, flank pain, and prolonged ileus. Ureteral obstruction can occasionally be subclinical and come to light only upon discovery of a nonfunctioning kidney. Unilateral ureteral obstruction classically does not cause an elevation in creatinine, but a

Mayo Clinic study showed that most patients do in fact experience a modest, transient creatinine elevation in the first 2 postoperative days. Unilateral obstruction is not associated with a change in urine output, but of course bilateral obstruction can result in anuria. Ureteral obstruction can be diagnosed by renal ultrasound or CT. The primary concerns in management are preservation of renal function, control of any urine leak (e.g., urinoma), and ultimately repair. The obstructed ureter may be stented either retrograde or antegrade, or a percutaneous nephrostomy may be placed. Just as with fistula, prompt recognition of ureteral obstruction may allow immediate reoperation if clinically indicated.

Potential delayed complications include lymphocysts, lymphedema, sexual dysfunction, and bowel obstruction. Symptomatic lymphocysts are rare now that most surgeons do not close the pelvic sidewall peritoneum. Chronic lymphedema is surprisingly uncommon after pelvic lymphadenectomy in unirradiated patients but can be problematic in patients treated with radiation. Patients often experience some change in sexual function after radical hysterectomy, but severe dyspareunia as a result of a shortened vagina is not common with modern surgical techniques. As stated already, a vaginal margin of 1 to 2 cm is all that is necessary in most patients. Certainly patients receiving radiation rather than radical surgery are at higher risk of this complication. In addition, postoperative adjuvant radiation probably increases the risk of sexual dysfunction beyond that of surgery alone. If the ovaries are removed, this can result in dyspareunia from decreased vaginal lubrication, but this problem is readily corrected with estrogen, either topical or systemic. Estrogen use is not associated with cervical cancer risk and is not contraindicated in cervical cancer patients. Small bowel obstruction occurring after radical hysterectomy is usually caused by adhesions, although recurrence must always be considered. The risk of obstruction is increased in irradiated patients.

SUGGESTED READING

Casey M. A new vascular clamp for radical pelvic dissection. *Am J Surg* 1977;134:434.

Estape R, Angioli R, Wagman F, et al. Significance of intraperitoneal cytology in patients undergoing radical hysterectomy. *Gynecol Oncol* 1998;68:169.

Helmkamp B, Krebs H, Corbett S, et al. Radical hysterectomy: current management guidelines. *Am J Obstet Gynecol* 1997;177:372.

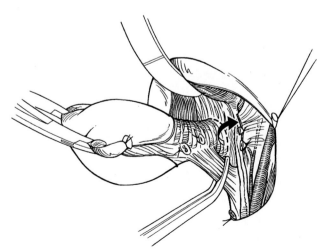

Fig. 14. The ureter is partially mobilized laterally, enough to take an adequate amount of cardinal ligament.

Landoni F, Maneo A, Colombo A, et al. Randomised study of radical surgery versus radiotherapy for stage Ib-IIa cervical cancer. *Lancet* 1997;350:535.

Landoni F, Maneo A, Cormio G, et al. Class II versus class III radical hysterectomy in stage IB-IIA cervical cancer: a prospective randomized study. *Gynecol Oncol* 2001; 80:3.

Lopes A, Hall J, Monaghan J. Drainage following radical hysterectomy and pelvic lymphadenectomy: dogma or need? *Obstet Gynecol* 1995;86:960.

Monk B, Tewari K, Gamboa-Vujicic G, et al. Does perioperative blood transfusion affect survival in patients with cervical cancer treated with radical hysterectomy? *Obstet Gynecol* 1995;85:343.

Morrow CP, Curtin JP. *Gynecologic cancer surgery.* Philadelphia: Churchill Livingstone, Harcourt Brace and Co, 1996.

Peters W, Liu P, Barrett R, et al. Concurrent chemotherapy and pelvic radiation therapy compared with pelvic radiation therapy alone as adjuvant therapy after radical surgery in high-risk early-stage cancer of the cervix. *J Clin Oncol* 2000;18:1606.

Rettenmaier M, Casanova D, Micha J, et al. Radical hysterectomy and tailored postoperative radiation therapy in the management of bulky stage 1B cervical cancer. *Cancer* 1989;63:2220.

Sedlis A, Bundy B, Rotman M, et al. A randomized trial of pelvic radiation therapy versus no further therapy in selected patients with stage IB carcinoma of the cervix after radical hysterectomy and pelvic lymphadenectomy: a Gynecologic Oncology Group study. *Gynecol Oncol* 1999;73:177.

Sevin B, Ramos R, Gerhardt R, et al. Comparative efficacy of short-term versus long-term cefoxitin prophylaxis against postoperative infection after radical hysterectomy: a prospective study. *Obstet Gynecol* 1991;77:729.

Trimbos J, Franchi M, Zanaboni F, et al. 'State of the art' of radical hysterectomy; current practice in European oncology centres. *Eur J Cancer* 2004;40:375.

EDITOR'S COMMENT

As indicated by Professor Kim of the Beth-Israel Deaconess Medical Center, Boston, the standard procedure for early cervical carcinoma is the radical hysterectomy, inclusive of bilateral pelvic lymphadenectomy. Currently, this operation is completed with minimal occurrence of serious operative morbidity and mortality. This improvement in operative outcome stems from advanced surgical approaches and applications of blood transfusions and antibiotics, with state-of-the-art anesthesia. As indicated by Dr. Kim, the radical procedure with bilateral nodal dissection is the sanguine alternative to radiation as a definitive therapy of eligible patients with FIGO stage IA, IB, and IIA cervical carcinoma.

As comprehensively reviewed by the author, the radical hysterectomy completed for malignant conditions of the cervix and the uterus requires mobilization of the bladder; this procedure is necessary to remove the upper vaginal canal, and to create adequate margins of resection. Thakar and Sultan (*Best Practice Res Clin Obstet Gynaecol* 2005;19[3]:403) recently reviewed the effects of hysterectomy on pelvic organ dysfunction, a condition that would be expected with this radical surgical approach. All said, women can now be reassured that the *simple* hysterectomy generally results in progressive improvement of pelvic organ function for as long as 2 years following the procedure. It would appear from very large studies that significant postoperative morbidity in terms of the pelvic organ dysfunctional syndrome is not as common after the *simple* procedure as after a *radical* procedure. This observation is evident as the ligaments and nerves that innervate the uterus and the cervix are interrupted, sparing some nervous innervation of surrounding structures. This is evident as in the radical hysterectomy, ligaments are divided laterally and have a greater frequency of pelvic organ dysfunction. This outcome is noted in the report by Thakar et al. (*J Obstet Gynaecol* 1998;3:267) in 1998, in which a survey of a large number of gynecologists in the United Kingdom suggested that total abdominal hysterectomy affected bladder, bowel, and sexual function more so than the subtotal (abdominal) hysterectomy. In the North American study by Zekam et al. (*Obstet Gynecol* 2003;102:301), most respondents confirmed that *neither procedure* offered any benefit with respect to the pelvic organ dysfunction; over one third felt that subtotal hysterectomy offered some protection against the development of prolapse. As damage to the autonomic nerves play a critical role in the cause of the pelvic organ dysfunction syndrome, as well as colorectal motility following radical approaches, Maas et al. (*Acta Obstet Gynecol Scand* 2005;84:868), from the Netherlands, advocate the nerve-sparing modification to allow sacrifice of only the medial branches of the hypogastric nerves. The anterior portion of the plexus of nerves of the uterosacral ligaments should be spared in this (anterior) portion of the plexus, as division of the same leads to macroscopic reduction in nerve innervation. This practice will hopefully diminish pelvic organ dysfunction syndromes.

As indicated above, the radical or modified radical hysterectomy is performed for early-stage disease (FIGO stages I and II). Further, the incidence of pelvic recurrence following the radical procedure and bilateral node dissection varies, and is dependent upon patient-specific risk factors. Survival rates for these patients range from 6% to 77% (Friedlander M, Grogan M; U.S. Preventative Services Task Force. *Oncologist* 2002;7:342), which represents a function of patient co-morbidity and patient-specific risk factors often evident in heterogeneous nonrandomized retrospective analyses. However, in the absence of poor prognostic factors (e.g., large tumor size, stromal invasion, lymphovascular infiltration, positive margins, positive parametrial invasion, positive nodes, etc.), a significant percentage of patients will still develop pelvic recurrence of their disease. In the recent retrospective study by Grigsby (*Radiation Med* 2005;23[5]:327), patients treated with radical hysterectomy and nodal dissection with a pelvic recurrence had a 5- and 10-year survival rate of 74% and 50%, respectively. Sites of failure for approximately one third of these patients occurred in the pelvis or in distant sites, and may require reoperation for obstructive large and/or small bowel recurrence. These authors recommend consideration of adjuvant chemotherapy for these patients with distant site failures.

It is unclear the role of sentinel lymph node mapping in the management of early cervical cancer. Like many organ sites that have previously been pioneered (e.g., breast, melanoma), the recent report by Roca et al. (*Eur J Nucl Med Mol Imaging* 2005;32:1210), of Barcelona, suggests that sentinel lymph node staging has a high negative predictive value, which may be incorporated into clinical routine (the laparoscopy or open surgery); this initial study is near the achievement of validation of its clinical value. Should such technology be confirmed in large prospective randomized studies, the application of the sentinel lymph node technique may diminish the number of bilateral pelvic lymphadenectomies planned *without* its application.

Roy et al. (*Best Practice Res Clin Obstet Gynaecol* 2005;19[3]:377), of Quebec, have admonished the gynecologic oncology community that before this minimally invasive approach becomes widely accepted, laparoscopically assisted vaginal radical hysterectomy must be comparable with standard abdominal (open) approaches. However, after more than 10 years of experience with the laparoscopically assisted technique, these authors stated that both vaginal and abdominal radical hysterectomies are comparable in terms of side effects and complications. Clearly, the choice of the procedure should be based on the experience of the surgeon and desires of the patient; the dexterity gained in the laparoscopic approach represents the key to performing fertility-sparing approaches. Consideration of the laparoscopic approach should be reserved principally for the young affected with early-stage cervical carcinoma who desires future pregnancies. Increasingly, gynecologic oncologists experienced in the technique will be able to safely offer the vaginal radical procedure, which almost certainly will be a technique that is offered internationally in the near future (Cibula D, et al. *Gynecol Oncol* 2005;97:707).

K.I.B.

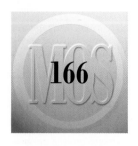

166

Surgical Management of Ovarian Carcinoma

ARLAN F. FULLER, JR.

THE PATHOGENESIS OF EPITHELIAL OVARIAN TUMORS

In the United States, ovarian carcinoma is the leading cause of genital tract cancer death among women, and its incidence rises steeply with increasing age after menopause. Two of the major reasons for the high case fatality rate in ovarian carcinoma are the early spread of the disease and its absence of symptoms, leading to late diagnosis in the majority of patients. Fully two thirds of patients have evidence of intra-abdominal spread to peritoneal surfaces or to the omentum at the time of diagnosis.

Much of this problem of silent transcoelomic dissemination of tumor arises from the pattern of histogenesis of epithelial ovarian cancer. Ninety-five percent of all ovarian carcinoma is epithelial in derivation, not arising from the germ cells (2.5%) or from the gonadal stroma (2.5%), but from the overlying serosal surface of the ovary. The pathogenesis is associated with ovulation, such that invagination of surface epithelium at the site of ovulation leads to the formation of an inclusion cyst thought to be the precursor of the carcinoma. As the female pelvis is open to the outside environment through patent fallopian tubes, particulate carcinogens may be incorporated into the cysts. This behavior accounts for the increased risk of ovarian carcinoma known to exist in women who dust their perineum with talc and for the decreased risk associated with prior tubal ligation or the use of oral contraceptives.

Formation of the epithelial inclusion cyst deep to the ovarian cortex is associated with appearance of immunohistochemical markers characteristic of malignancy. The development of invasive carcinoma parallels development of the müllerian duct into the epithelial tissues of the upper genital tract (Fig. 1). As the müllerian duct is formed in the embryo from invagination of the coelomic epithelium and develops into the fallopian tube, uterine corpus, and cervix, so too does the nascent cystic ovarian neoplasm progress to its respective serous, endometrioid/clear cell, and mucinous histotypes, recapitulating these müllerian structures.

It becomes intuitively clear that ovarian cancer is *not* really cancer of the ovary! It is cancer of the epithelial surface that is derived from and contiguous with the surrounding pelvic peritoneum. Fully 10% of the patients seen at the Massachusetts General Hospital with serous papillary carcinoma involving the pelvic viscera and omentum have disease that is histologically identical to epithelial carcinoma of the ovary and spreads in the same manner, but these patients either have no evidence of ovarian involvement or have a minor degree of involvement of the surface of the ovarian cortex. These lesions are termed *serous papillary tumors of peritoneal origin* and may actually represent a malignancy of polyclonal origin, etiologically distinct from the primary ovarian lesions that are monoclonal. It is not surprising, therefore, that prophylactic removal of both ovaries will greatly reduce, but not eliminate all risk of "ovarian" cancer in women at high genetic risk. Hence, in consenting patients at high risk for risk-reducing bilateral salpingo-oophorectomy, one must keep this observation in mind and

caution the patient that continued surveillance will be necessary.

PATTERNS OF METASTATIC DISEASE IN OVARIAN CARCINOMA

Dissemination of ovarian carcinoma from the early primary ovarian tumor predominantly occurs through transperitoneal spread. Exfoliated tumor cells typically implant first in the paracolic gutters and on the right hemidiaphragm. The negative pressure associated with respiratory movement of the diaphragm over the liver creates a flow of peritoneal fluid that is absorbed at this site. Because some epithelial ovarian carcinomas actually may begin on the surface of the ovarian cortex, transperitoneal spread may occur early in the natural history of the disease. In fact, if the tumor begins as a primary peritoneal neoplasm on the surface of the pelvic peritoneum, then peritoneal spread begins de novo. Implantation and growth of ovarian carcinoma on the diaphragm leads to the obstruction of lymphatic flow and contributes to the accumulation of ascites. That process is also facilitated by the influence of vascular endothelial growth factor production by the ovarian malignancy as part of the process of angiogenesis. Poorly differentiated tumors also commonly spread along ovarian lymphatics to regional nodes at the para-aortic level as well as to pelvic nodes. In patients with anaplastic ovarian tumors, regional spread to the para-aortic nodes at the origin of the gonadal arteries may be the only site of metastatic disease. The pattern of lymph node metastasis in patients with stage III (abdominal spread) ovarian cancer and any nodal metastasis is such that 25% of patients will have pelvic nodal involvement only, 25% will have para-aortic nodal involvement only, and 50% will have both pelvic and para-aortic nodal disease.

Early spread of ovarian carcinoma is classically identified in the right paracolic gutter and on the right hemidiaphragm. Several typical patterns of spread are identified with more advanced disease: some patients may present with disease solely in the omentum, some with "oligo" metastatic

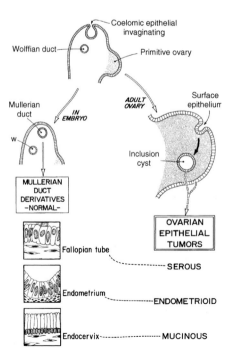

Fig. 1. Müllerian origin of the epithelial ovarian carcinomas.

prognosis, and prudent management demands adequate sampling of a substantial proportion of the lesions identified. Complete removal of all macroscopic lesions *should* be the goal, both to excise the tumor itself and also to ensure that a more aggressive metastatic lesion is not missed. Only a small proportion of women with borderline tumors will have invasive implants and present a risk of recurrence and death.

Monitoring of the typical patient with noninvasive implants—the patient with a stage III tumor of borderline malignancy—would involve regular pelvic examinations and quarterly CA-125 levels for the 1st year. After that time, progressively longer follow-up intervals would be appropriate. Routine CT scans in the absence of a rising CA-125 level, even for nonserous tumors, would not appear to be indicated.

Chemotherapy for these patients with advanced or recurrent disease is unlikely to produce any dramatic and sustained responses because of the low-grade nature of these tumors, their functional similarity to the corresponding normal tissue, and the low-growth fraction assayed in vitro. There is some evidence, in fact, that chemotherapy may actually induce more aggressive behavior, presumably causing further malignant progression with dedifferentiation as a consequence of the mutagenic effects of the chemotherapeutic agents. Hope in the future for biologic agents that will promote (re)differentiation in these minimally deviant tumors may represent the best opportunity for disease control.

SURGERY FOR ADVANCED OVARIAN CARCINOMA: OVERVIEW

At the time of diagnosis, ovarian carcinoma presents with the greatest tumor burden of any solid tumor; a kilogram or more of tumor may be distributed in the pelvis and upper abdomen, along with several liters of ascites. Although the epithelial ovarian tumors are considered quite responsive to primary chemotherapy, with response rates in the 80% to 90% range in untreated individuals, the dominant variable predictive of long-term survival is the amount of residual disease present at the conclusion of the initial surgical procedure. The validity of less than total excision in the presence of obvious metastatic disease appears to violate basic tenets of surgical oncology and has often been questioned. Nonetheless, it has been subjected to careful scrutiny during the

last 3 decades and consistently has been documented as the dominant prognostic factor in studies of patient survival, whether treatment involves chemotherapy or radiation therapy. Essentially every clinical study has documented that the extent of residual disease outweighs even surgical stage in its prognostic importance.

Griffiths, in a National Cancer Institute monograph, demonstrated that patients with bulky intra-abdominal spread of ovarian cancer who underwent extensive cytoreduction to minimal residual disease had the same median survival time as those patients who had the same amount of minimal residual disease, but did not require extensive surgical cytoreduction. We have similarly examined the outcome of patients requiring multiple resections at the time of primary surgery and have contrasted that with the outcome of patients requiring much more limited resection. As long as the amount of residual disease remained the same at the conclusion of surgery, there was no difference in survival, whether the patient had a simple hysterectomy, bilateral salpingo oophorectomy and gastrocolic omentectomy, or, in addition, splenectomy, transverse colon resection, rectosigmoid resection, small bowel resection, and resection of enlarged pelvic and para-aortic nodes. The theoretical explanation employed to support this observation is that surgical cytoreduction removes bulky tumor that is either constitutively drug-resistant, or one that is resistant because of poor drug penetration into a large tumor

mass. In addition to this effect, reduction from a 5-cm tumor mass to a 5-mm tumor mass represents a four log tumor cell reduction, from 10^{11} cells to 10^7 cells, decreasing the amount of chemotherapy needed for tumor control based on first-order kinetics of cell kill.

There is a threshold, however, above which surgical resection does not incrementally improve survival; that appears to be a largest residual tumor mass of 1.0 to 1.5 cm. Resection of disease to that level or below does improve survival time, and there is a further increment in survival with every additional decrement in residual disease, down to the microscopic level. Traditionally, resection to a largest residual mass of 1.5 cm or less has been termed *optimal* cytoreduction, in the sense that resection to this level or below improves survival. As the Latin root for "optimal" is "best," one should reserve that term for *complete* cytoreduction. The appropriate term for cytoreduction to the threshold level or below is *adequate*, as it is adequate for improvement in survival. In common use, however, the reasonable compromise is to call complete cytoreductive surgery complete; anything else is incomplete, either optimal or suboptimal. As noted in Figure 3, patients who underwent complete cytoreduction had a 5-year survival in excess of 75%, and patients who had macroscopic residual disease, but less than 1 cm in size, had an approximate 30% survival, and patients with residual disease greater than 1 cm but less than 2 cm had only a 15% 5-year survival. This retrospective study from the Mayo Clinic underscores the primacy

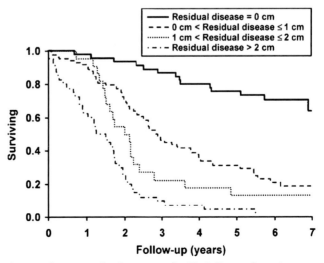

Fig. 3. Survival curves for patients by the extent of residual disease after primary surgical therapy. (From Aletti GD, Dowdy SC, Gostout BS, et al. Aggressive surgical effort and improved survival in advanced-stage ovarian cancer. *Obstet Gynecol* 2006;107:77, with permission.)

of complete cytoreductive surgery in the surgical management of this disease.

The success of cytoreductive surgery depends on the metastatic pattern of the tumor spread as well as the experience of the surgeon. Rarely is the pelvis the site of residual disease after incomplete cytoreduction. The challenge to the gynecologic oncologist is the resection of metastases to the upper abdomen. Common sites of surgical failure are the root of the small bowel mesentery, nodal disease above the celiac axis involving the lesser curve of stomach and the left lobe of liver, and perihepatic disease on the right as well as peripancreatic disease involving the C-loop of the duodenum. Although there may be an element of patient selection for surgical exploration, the proportion of patients who undergo "adequate" cytoreductive surgery should be in the 80% to 90% range; approximately half of these patients should have no more than 2 to 3 mm residual disease. We would anticipate that 30% to 40% of patients undergoing cytoreductive surgery will have all grossly visible disease resected; that is, complete cytoreduction. My personal experience is that 90% of patients will have resection to largest residual disease of 1.0 cm or less. More than one third of these patients will have no gross residual disease. We have documented this beneficial effect of surgical cytoreduction for patients with primary serous papillary peritoneal cancer, primary tubal cancer, and for patients with primary endometrial cancer in which there is a component of extensive peritoneal spread. Further documentation of the positive effect of the attitude of the gynecologic oncologist also comes from the Mayo Clinic, where, in another article, they have documented that Mayo Clinic surgeons performing radical surgery in more than 50% of patients had a median survival of their patients that was more than double that of their counterparts who performed radical surgery in less than 50% of the patients (Table 3).

There is recent evidence as well that subsequent cytoreduction may offer additional survival benefit for those patients who did not have adequate initial resection of gross disease. One arbitrarily defines "interval" cytoreduction as that carried out after a partial course of chemotherapy intended to reduce tumor volume to a resectable level. On the contrary, "secondary" cytoreduction refers to that procedure carried out for persistent or recurrent disease after completion of a full course of primary chemotherapy. The European study authored by van der Burgh demonstrated

in a prospective controlled trial that patients who were unsuccessfully treated with primary surgery could benefit from a planned surgical intervention after preliminary chemotherapy. Following suboptimal primary surgery and three cycles of chemotherapy with *cis*-platinum and cyclophosphamide, patients were randomized to interval cytoreductive surgery and three cycles of chemotherapy or chemotherapy alone. There was a statistically significant improvement in relapse-free survival of 6 months in the group with interval surgical resection. Moreover, the survival curve for patients found to have less than 1 cm disease at the time of exploration for interval debulking was essentially the same as for those patients who underwent secondary tumor resection to reach that optimal level (Fig. 4).

Prior exposure to chemotherapy, however, does alter the threshold at which surgical resection improves survival, as one might expect. In a later review of his personal experience, published posthumously,

Griffiths noted that the use of even three cycles of preoperative chemotherapy reduced the threshold of residual disease associated with a complete pathologic complete response at second-look laparotomy. After preoperative chemotherapy, only one of nine patients with minimal disease of 3 to 5 mm was determined to have a pathologic complete response. Without preoperative chemotherapy, eight of ten patients with the same amount of residual disease at the end of surgery did achieve a pathologic complete response. The proportion of pathologic complete responses in patients with residual disease of 0 to 2 mm was no different, suggesting that the threshold for improvement in survival after three cycles of chemotherapy dropped from 1 cm to 3 to 5 mm (Table 4).

Such a benefit of secondary resection also exists for patients with an isolated recurrence that can be completely resected after some interval following postoperative chemotherapy. Typically, these patients include individuals with CT evidence of

TABLE 3. CORRELATION BETWEEN TWO SUBGROUP OF SURGEONS AND RESIDUAL DISEASE (RD) IN PATIENTS WITH STAGE IIIC OVARIAN CANCER[a]

Surgeon (Surgery Performed)	RD = 0 Macro	RD <1 cm	RD = 1–2 cm	RD >2 cm	Median Survival (years)
Radical surgery in <50% of the patients	23.72	39.10	11.54	25.64	2.53
Radical surgery in >50% of the patients	23.68	63.16	10.53	2.63	5.9

[a]Number of patients = 194. $P = 0.008$; Pearson chi-square.
The last column represents the median survival in these two groups ($P = 0.04$; log rank test).
From Aletti GD, Gostout BS, Podratz KC, et al. Qvarian cancer surgical resectability: relative impact of disease, patient status, and surgeon. *Gynecol Obstet* 2006;100:33.

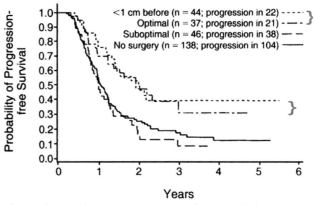

Fig. 4. Effect of interval cytoreduction on progression-free survival; the European Organization for Research and Treatment of Cancer study. (From van der Burg ME, van Lent M, Buyses M, et al. *N Engl J Med* 1995;332:629, with permission.)

TABLE 4. RESPONSE (AT SECOND LOOK) TO POSTOPERATIVE TREATMENT BY RESIDUAL SIZE AND PREOPERATIVE CHEMOTHERAPY (1975–1985)[a]

Response	Size mm			
	0–2	3–5	6–10	>10
Preoperative chemotherapy				
Complete	8	1		
Partial	5	5	2	1
Progression		3		3
Total	13	9	2	4
No preoperative chemotherapy				
Complete	8	8	3	
Partial	2	2	7	6
Progression			1	2
Total	10	10	11	8

From Griffiths CT, Parker LM, Lee S, et al. The effect of residual mass size on response to chemotherapy after surgical cytoreduction for advanced ovarian cancer: long-term results. *Int J Gynecol Cancer* 2002;12:323.

localized nodal recurrence, splenic recurrence, or solitary extraperitoneal lesions. The longer the free interval from prior chemotherapy, the greater the likelihood that complete surgical resection will be associated with prolonged survival, particularly if there has been limited prior exposure to cytotoxic chemotherapy.

Eisenkop et al. reported their experience with 106 patients who had disease recurrence more than 6 months after completion of chemotherapy. They examined both the probability of successful cytoreduction and the survival after diagnosis of recurrence. In multivariate analysis, the size of the largest residual tumor mass, preoperative chemotherapy with "salvage" chemotherapy, and preoperative performance status influenced the likelihood of success in surgical reduction to minimal residual disease. In univariate analysis, site of disease in the pelvis, a solitary site of recurrence, an asymptomatic state, and the absence of physical findings all influenced cytoreductive success, as might be expected, given that they all reflect the preoperative extent of disease. The overall survival was influenced by the disease-free interval. With a disease-free interval of 6 to 12 months as the baseline for comparison, the 13- to 36-month interval was associated with a risk ratio for recurrence of 0.16. With a disease-free ratio of more than 3 years, the risk ratio for recurrence dropped to 0.08. It is of note in this study that 83% of patients did not have ascites at the time of recurrence, suggesting a strong selection bias. In further support of this contention, the median survival from the time of recurrence in the group without preoperative

salvage chemotherapy was 47 months from the time of diagnosis of recurrence. It has been my personal experience that the success of secondary cytoreduction for tumor recurrence also highly depends on the extent of the original surgical procedure. When the primary surgical procedure is carried out by a community-based obstetrician–gynecologist or general surgeon, extensive retroperitoneal surgery has generally not been performed. Because of the predominant intraperitoneal spread of ovarian cancer, re-exploration via the extraperitoneal route is typically successful and unimpeded by extensive adhesions. In a similar manner, a Gynecologic Oncology Group study of interval cytoreduction

similar to the van der Burgh/European Organization for Research and Treatment of Cancer study did not demonstrate any advantage to surgical intervention, presumably because these patients were initially explored by a gynecologic oncologist, and subsequent surgery by an individual of similar training did not offer any strategic or therapeutic advantage.

Given the progressive development of drug resistance in this group of ovarian cancer patients treated with chemotherapy, it is not surprising that the outcome of secondary cytoreduction depends even more on the surgeon's ability to completely remove all residual disease, if possible. In patients with a limited number of sites of recurrent disease, the most vigorous attempt at complete cytoreduction is certainly warranted. In patients with multiple sites of "oligo" metastatic disease, again, an aggressive approach to resection of all disease is a prerequisite to success. In patients with extensive intra-abdominal disease, a preliminary trial of cytotoxic chemotherapy is generally appropriate; in part, so that one can have a sense of the in vivo drug response prior to an attempt at complete surgical resection. Obviously, any attempt at surgical resection in the presence of drug resistance has little benefit, except for the palliation of bowel obstruction. A German cooperative study looking at secondary cytoreduction confirmed that observation, noting that the only improvement in survival came among that group of patients whose recurrence was completely resected with no residual disease. All others, irrespective of the amount of residual macroscopic disease, had the same poor outcome (Fig. 5).

Nongastrointestinal Transabdominal

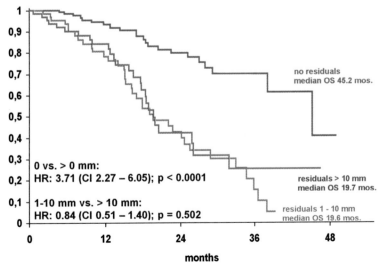

Fig. 5. Surgical end points. (From Pfisterer J, Harter P, Canzler U, et al. The role of surgery in recurrent ovarian cancer. *Int J Gynecol Cancer* 2005;15[suppl 3]:195, with permission.)

These extensive surgical procedures in patients with nutritional debility secondary to great tumor burden or intensive chemotherapy have generally been supported in the past with perioperative total parenteral nutrition (TPN). Our current approach to postoperative management has been facilitated by early postoperative feeding of elemental diet. Not all patients, however, are candidates for postoperative enteral feeding, even with elemental diet. We have chosen to use perioperative TPN for patients with extreme nutritional depletion as measured by serum albumin of less than 2.5 g/dL. The use of en bloc extraperitoneal resection of the ovarian mass(es), uterus, bladder peritoneum, and rectosigmoid colon with the involved cul-de-sac peritoneum has reduced the incidence of pelvic recurrence and late gastrointestinal obstruction, while permitting primary anastomosis in all patients.

 PREOPERATIVE PLANNING

When the patient is referred with the clinical picture of ascites, crampy abdominal pain, and distention with a palpable pelvic mass, the preoperative diagnosis of ovarian carcinoma is typically one of exclusion. What one seeks to exclude, therefore, are those lesions for which surgical exploration will not be beneficial. Attention to the patient's history of upper gastrointestinal symptoms may help to exclude those patients with occult gastric cancer. Should there be any question, an upper gastrointestinal series or, preferably, upper gastrointestinal endoscopy, will be a useful adjunct to the abdominal pelvic CT scan that is part of routine preoperative evaluation. CT scanning has particular value preoperatively in identifying occult liver metastases or extensive retroperitoneal invasion above the celiac axis by tumor that might otherwise contraindicate primary cytoreductive surgery. The CT scan may also exclude a clinically occult primary pancreatic neoplasm with intraabdominal metastases.

Preoperative physical examination is important in the identification of the extent of pelvic disease insofar as one can best identify infiltration of the pelvic sidewall or invasion of the very low rectovaginal septum that may present challenges to primary surgical resection. Although this extent of disease in the pelvis is not a contraindication to extensive cytoreductive surgery, it certainly requires surgical skills and experience in en

bloc resection of the intraperitoneal pelvic viscera, as will be described. In the event that one encounters a positive stool test for occult blood, colonoscopy may be useful in the exclusion of a primary colonic tumor; however, surgical intervention with colonic resection is still necessary. On rare occasions when there is a considerable anterior extent of the pelvic tumor and the question of extrinsic bladder involvement, cystoscopy can exclude those patients with unresectable disease invading the bladder base. In patients with severe irritative bladder symptoms, one may also exclude a primary bladder cancer, although this typically would not present with extensive intra-abdominal disease without a prominent history of hematuria. Except for overt obstruction of one or both ureters, there is little indication for preoperative ureteral catheterization. The typical lesion associated with ureteral obstruction will be a bulky intraperitoneal tumor with penetration through the peritoneum at the level of the uterine vessels. This is a common presentation of carcinoma arising in endometriosis involving the pelvic peritoneum. Occasionally, bulky nodal metastases may also cause extrinsic compression; direct invasion of the pelvic ureter is much less common. Preoperative ureteral decompression may reduce the risk of trauma to that dilated ureter. One should not have to rely on a ureteral catheter for the identification of the pelvic ureter: if the ureter is uninvolved by tumor, it is easily palpable; but if it is encased in tumor, a ureteral catheter provides little reassurance, as it is rarely palpable.

The preoperative preparation of the patient should include a forthright discussion of the diagnosis and management, with specific attention to the technique and importance of removing all gross residual tumor. Informed consent should specifically address the importance of complete surgical cytoreduction and the small but real risks associated with this surgical procedure, including those associated with gastrointestinal resection, omentectomy, and retroperitoneal node dissection. As one evaluates the medical status of the patient preoperatively, it is important to identify the occasional patient with liver disease and ascites associated with an elevated portal venous pressure. Patients with severe right heart failure may also present with ascites; surgical exploration for a pelvic mass may be relatively contraindicated. Both congestive heart failure and severe liver disease are associ-

ated with an elevated CA-125 level in the absence of ovarian cancer, and may lead to exploration for benign ovarian disease in a patient with substantial medical contraindications to laparotomy. Even in the presence of malignant ascites, these and other medical contraindications to primary extensive surgery, such as severe chronic obstructive pulmonary disease, emphasize the value of primary chemotherapy in the palliation of this disease. The so-called "neoadjuvant" chemotherapy will control the ascites and reduce tumor masses, providing substantial symptom relief, although not the same long-term control of disease achievable with combined surgery and chemotherapy.

The bowel preparation, consisting of mechanical and antibiotic "cleansing" of the lower intestinal tract, is an essential part of the preoperative treatment as, in my experience, two thirds of patients with advanced ovarian cancer presenting with bulky tumor masses ultimately require at least en bloc rectosigmoid resection in continuity with the ovarian tumor in order to achieve complete surgical cytoreduction. One must be cautious with the bowel preparation, of course, in the presence of partial small or large bowel obstruction; a prolonged clear liquid diet and gentle catharsis may be more appropriate.

As is true of all of our gynecologic cancer patients, the patient is positioned on the operating table in the modified lithotomy position in which both lower extremities are abducted with knees flexed, the so-called "ski" position (this term refers to the initial use of skis to support the legs in this abducted position). The benefits of this position include intraoperative access to the perineum as well as the opportunity for a third principal surgeon at the operating table. In addition to providing a position for transanal anastomosis, the surgeon at the perineal position is ideally situated to carry out a para-aortic node dissection with both assistants retracting laterally from above. The Foley catheter is not placed until the patient is completely prepared and draped. In this manner, one has access to the catheter in order to fill or empty the bladder as needed to facilitate the anterior pelvic dissection. Should cystoscopy be necessary intraoperatively, this too may be performed easily.

The choice of abdominal incision is relatively straightforward: a relatively short paramedian incision, near the midline, to permit initial abdominal exploration. Once the ascites, if present, has been drained and the resectability is determined, the incision can be extended to the pubis and to the xiphoid process, if necessary. As the kinetics of ascites formation is relatively slow, initial fluid replacement need only compensate for the increase in venous compliance as the abdominal fluid is removed. We generally employ a retractor that can be fixed to the operating room table, either the Bookwalter or Omni device, so that one may obtain maximal retraction in the upper quadrants or optimize retraction toward the pubis without the instrument always migrating toward the middle of the incision.

As far as operating instrumentation is concerned, my preference is for bipolar coagulation as a means of intraoperative hemostasis, particularly for node dissection, for retroperitoneal dissection of the bladder and ureters, as well as for hemostasis in general. The use of bipolar cautery permits rapid and efficient dissection without the need to stop and change instruments for hemostasis. Typically, one can perform both bilateral pelvic node dissections and bilateral para-aortic node dissections without the need for any adjunctive hemostasis. Unlike monopolar cautery, the effective current between the tips of the two electrodes avoids the risk of distant dissemination of current while maximum current density between the tips of the forceps. The use of gastrointestinal stapling devices has further facilitated the safety and effectiveness of gynecologic surgery for ovarian cancer. As the most frequent segment of bowel resected for ovarian cancer is the rectosigmoid, the use of end-to-end anastomosing (EEA) instrument permits rapid and safe reanastomosis of the pelvic colon. At the level of the transverse colon, or in the small bowel, we prefer the use of the 60-mm linear stapler used in a triangulating fashion. This creates an everted anastomosis with no reduction in the diameter of the intestinal lumen. In recent years, all of the patients with these anastomoses have been managed without postoperative nasogastric decompression. In my latest series of patients treated with early postoperative chemotherapy, of 125 patients, 80 women had a total of 105 bowel resections with no leaks, despite the use of chemotherapy targeted to begin on the 5th postoperative day.

Preoperative Evaluation Should Include a Discussion of Intraperitoneal Therapy

The Gynecologic Oncology Group has demonstrated a 16-month improvement in median overall survival time (66 vs. 50 months) in a randomized prospective trial of patients who have undergone optimal (<1.0 cm residual disease) surgical cytoreduction followed by intraperitoneal chemotherapy with cis-platinum and paclitaxel, compared with patients having similar chemotherapy via an intravenous route. This improvement in survival occurred despite both toxic and mechanical complications of intraperitoneal chemotherapy that prevented 58% of patients assigned to this therapy from completing the planned six cycles of treatment. The current clinical challenges are to optimize the delivery of this therapy and, in particular, to minimize catheter complications that prevent completion of treatment.

Preliminary evidence suggests that the use of the No. 9.6 French vascular catheter and reservoir is associated with a lower risk of complications than the use of the No. 14 French Tenckhoff catheter and intraperitoneal reservoir. Because of the risk of bacterial contamination of the catheter or reservoir in the presence of intestinal surgery, current recommendations are for placement of the catheter and reservoir at an interval after primary surgery that involves intestinal resection. This can typically be performed laparoscopically, and an extensive slide set documenting my technique for this procedure is available on the Gynecologic Oncology Group web site.

As the optimal time for placement of the catheter and reservoir is during the primary operative procedure that does not involve intestinal resection, it is important to discuss this option with the patient who has any significant risk of ovarian carcinoma. This permits informed consent as well as the opportunity to seek the ideal placement above the costal margin, where there is stable access to the reservoir and yet placement in a position that is comfortable for the patient.

The Initial Exploration and Assessment of Operability

Once the ascites has been drained, upper abdominal exploration begins. One evaluates the omental "cake," frees up small bowel adhesions from its underside, and mobilizes the attachments to the paracolic gutter. This procedure permits evaluation of both the small and large bowel centrally. One can then proceed centrifugally, evaluating the paracolic gutters and subdiaphragmatic spaces as well as the liver surface, stomach, and splenic capsule. Here it is not unusual to find omental tumor

extending to the splenic hilum, but this is usually resectable without splenectomy unless there is extensive capsular involvement. Once the upper abdomen has been evaluated, mobilization of a small bowel from the pelvic inlet helps to identify the local extent of pelvic disease. In most cases, the ovarian tumor will extensively involve one or both pelvic side walls (Fig. 6A,B); for this reason, the proper approach to the pelvis in a patient with advanced disease will be an extraperitoneal one.

Prior to any pelvic dissection, the gastrocolic omentectomy is first begun. If the transverse colon can be easily mobilized from the underside of the omental mass, that should be done first. In the event that the tumor invades the transverse colon, the most prudent approach is to leave that dissection for last and begin working from lateral to medial, freeing up the omentum from the paracolic gutters and from the splenic and hepatic flexures. One then divides the omentum from the greater curve of the stomach, entering the lesser sac just to the left of midline, and dividing the vessels while working toward the previously opened paracolic gutters. Then, with the omentum remaining attached only to the transverse colon, one can dissect from lateral to medial, mobilizing the omental mass from the mesocolon and from the bowel wall. If necessary, one can remove a segment of transverse colon at this point and perform a triangulated everting anastomosis with the linear stapler. With three stay sutures oriented at 120-degree intervals, beginning at the mesocolon, three firings of the TA 60 stapler (3.5 mm) across the everted full-thickness bowel walls will produce a secure anastomosis in a very short time. Given the extent of surgical cytoreduction required, the time saved in the use of surgical staplers is extremely valuable, as is the security of the anastomosis created with this technique.

Once the omentum has been resected, examination of the small bowel may lead to further resection with a similar closure technique using the TA 30 stapler. Any peritoneal disease, particularly disease involving the paracolic peritoneum, should be resected at this time, although resection of diaphragmatic peritoneum will be left until later. This choice of sequence—removing any central tumor first and then widely opening the paracolic peritoneum—will facilitate pelvic dissection by exposing the lateral pelvic sidewalls and protecting the ureter, at the same time removing any bulky intra-abdominal mass, so that the bowel may be packed up

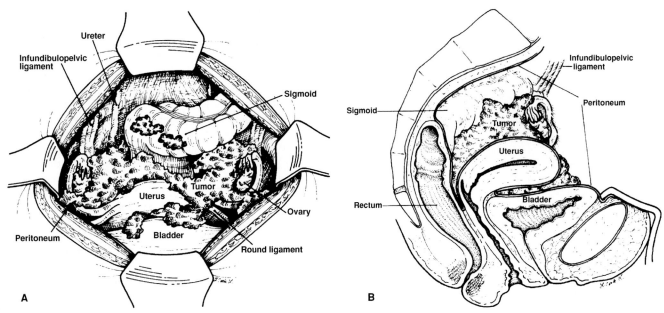

Fig. 6. A: Anterior view of the pelvis at the time of initial abdominal exploration. **B:** Sagittal view of the pelvic cavity. The tumor obliterates all intraperitoneal tissue planes to the level of the cul-de-sac.

into the midabdomen when the Book-walter retractor is inserted.

An extraperitoneal approach to the pelvis begins in the paracolic gutters. Opening the paracolic peritoneum along the lateral border of the ascending and descending colon permits high division of the ovarian blood supply and identification of the proximal ureter, optimizing orientation in the retroperitoneum prior to beginning pelvic dissection. With control of the ovarian blood supply, one can now mobilize the sigmoid colon and open the left paravesical and pararectal space. On the right side, one mobilizes the cecum and the terminal ileum medially from the paracolic gutter and superiorly from the right pelvic brim. Once the right pararectal and paravesical spaces have been opened to the pelvic floor, the only step remaining in the circumscription of the pelvic inlet is mobilization of the involved bladder peritoneum from the underlying bladder muscularis. As shown in Figure 6B, in surgical stage III disease, the bladder peritoneum is frequently involved by surface implants of ovarian carcinoma; however, even when confluent, it invariably remains confined to the peritoneal surface with an edematous plane superficial to the bladder muscularis that permits easy dissection, using the bipolar cautery for hemostasis. At this point, if it is clear that rectosigmoid resection is appropriate, division of the sigmoid colon is carried out as distally as possible with the GIA stapler. The sigmoid mesocolon is

divided along with the presacral peritoneum, as shown in Figure 7A and B. All of this dissection has been facilitated with hand-held retractors; at this point the Bookwalter retractor is inserted to optimize exposure at the periphery of the pelvis.

Once the fixed retractor is inserted, view of the pelvis is similar to that shown in Figure 7A: the tumor appears to be contained in a peritoneal bag. The ureters are now identified above the pelvic brim, at the bifurcation of the common iliac artery, and are mobilized laterally, away from the pelvic peritoneum all the way down to the uterine arteries using bipolar cautery for hemostasis. The presacral peritoneum can now be elevated up from the sacral hollow; one can typically mobilize the entire pelvic contents anteriorly at this point. Completion of the bladder peritoneal dissection is now performed. Once the paravesical spaces have been opened and the edge of the normal peritoneum identified anterior to the tumor mass, that edge is now grasped with Allis clamps and sharply dissected from the underlying bladder muscularis to the level of the cervix. Hemostasis with bipolar cautery should be completely sufficient for this dissection.

As the uterine vasculature has now been exposed anteriorly by reflection of the bladder peritoneum, the posterior peritoneal surface is now dissected away in continuity with the mobilization of the cul-de-sac peritoneum. The ureter has

already been mobilized laterally and posteriorly away from the uterine pedicle. The uterine vessels can now be divided just anterior and medial to the ureter and, in similar manner, the paracervical ligaments may be divided extraperitoneally, permitting the dissection posterior to the cervix to separate the anterior cul-de-sac peritoneum from the vaginal muscularis as shown in Figure 8B. With a cervix separated from the peritoneum, it is then divided from the upper vagina, once the latter is clamped. The vaginal apex is closed with the sutures left long to permit countertraction anteriorly as the cul-de-sac is mobilized from the remaining posterior vaginal wall.

With the cervix divided from the vagina, grasped with a triple hook, and retracted in a cephalic direction, the appearance of the pelvis is shown in Figure 8A and B. In Figure 8A, one can discern that the cul-de-sac tumor has been mobilized up from the anterior rectal wall and the middle rectal vessels have been divided prior to the anticipated division of the specimen from the distal rectum. The lateral view, Figure 8B, demonstrates the mobilization of the cervix and cul-de-sac peritoneum from the anterior aspect of rectum below the level of transection; it also shows the extent of posterior presacral dissection to the level of the coccyx. At this point, with no residual peritoneum in the pelvis and with the paravesical and pararectal spaces well developed, bilateral pelvic node dissection can be easily and

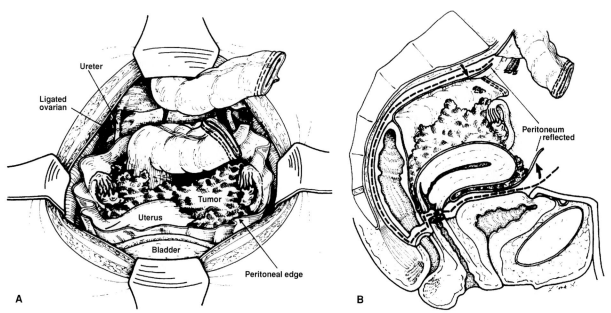

Fig. 7. A: The dissection is started at the pelvic sidewalls, freeing the ureters laterally and dissecting the peritoneum from the bladder muscularis. The infundibulopelvic ligaments are ligated above the pelvic brand after identification of the ureters. **B:** The *dashed line* indicates the plane of dissection. Beginning anteriorly, the peritoneum is dissected from the bladder. The hysterectomy is performed after lateral mobilization of the ureters and, prior to its transection from the vagina, the rectovaginal space is bluntly developed.

simply accomplished. Beginning with mobilization of the iliac vessels and associated nodal tissue from the psoas muscle laterally, the external iliac artery and vein are sequentially skeletonized from their midportion distally to the femoral canal and then the obturator space is widely dissected, identifying the obturator nerve and removing all nodal tissue anterior to it and the hypogastric vessels. Keeping the ureter medial, dissection is then carried up along the hypogastric vessels to the common iliac artery and vein. Once dissection has been completed at this level and hemostasis is secure, the common iliac vessels are dissected to the bifurcation of aorta.

Prior to carrying out reanastomosis of the sigmoid colon, or descending colon to

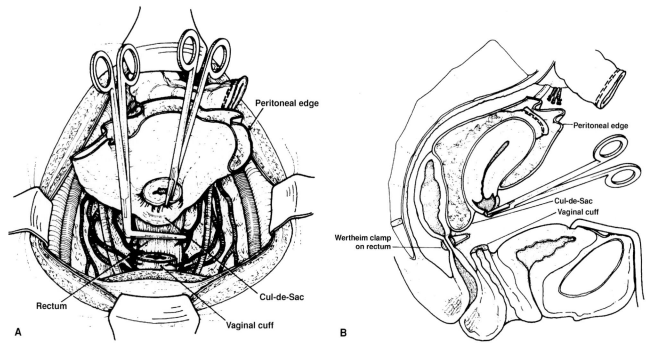

Fig. 8. A: The entire peritoneal envelope, including the anterior and posterior cul-de-sac with the cervix, is retracted anteriorly so as to expose and skeletonize the upper rectum. **B:** The lateral view demonstrates the anterior and posterior exposure of the upper rectum levels that facilitate transection of the upper rectum and removal of the specimen. Note that the Wertheim clamp is placed above the point of resection.

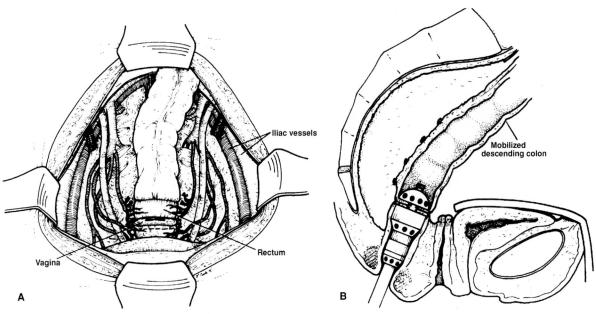

Fig. 9. A: Anterior view of the pelvis at the completion of the procedure. All pelvic peritoneum, associated tumor, lymph nodes, and the intrapelvic peritoneal organs have been removed. **B:** The distal end of the rectosigmoid is transected and stapled below the tumor; bowel continuity is restored using an EEA stapling device.

the upper rectum, para-aortic node dissection is now carried out in two parts. With the Bookwalter retractor moved to a slightly more cephalic position, first on the left side, the descending colon is mobilized medially with its mesentery, both to expose the left para-aortic nodes and to mobilize the colon for its pelvic anastomosis. Assuming that there will be no gross residual disease within the abdominal cavity, para-aortic node dissection is necessary to ensure complete removal of disease. The nodes should be excised up to the level of the origin of the left ovarian artery and the confluence of the left ovarian vein with the left renal vein, a common site for isolated nodal metastases from a primary left ovarian carcinoma. On the right side it is possible to elevate the cecum and descending colon as well as the root of the distal small bowel in a cephalic direction to expose the vena cava, right side of aorta, and left renal vein. Again, the nodes are dissected from a caudal to cephalic direction to the level of the origin of the right gonadal vessels.

In patients with extensive, bulky para-aortic nodal disease, it is not unusual to find nodal metastases in the aortocaval sulcus, posterior to the vena cava, and posterior to the aorta on the left. In patients in whom nodal metastases extend above the left renal vein, medial reflection of the descending colon from the splenic flexure down may not provide sufficient exposure. In this case one can mobilize the spleen and pancreas medially to expose

the nodes about the celiac axis and superior mesenteric artery on the left. Mobilization of the left kidney on its pedicle will similarly give access to the upper retroaortic area. On the right side one can first mobilize the hepatic flexure and second, perform a Kocher maneuver to improve access to the upper infrahepatic inferior vena cava. One can also explore the right side of aorta through the lesser sac. In the absence of significant vascular injury, all hemostasis can be achieved with use of bipolar coagulation.

Once node dissection has been completed, one may choose to use an ultrasonic surgical aspirator or similar device to remove any isolated peritoneal implants. Although this may be employed on the diaphragm, it is our preference to excise the diaphragmatic peritoneum if there is any substantial number of tumor implants. It is important to recognize that the involvement of diaphragmatic peritoneum may be as evident on the posterior surface in the retrohepatic area as it is anteriorly. Based on past experience with isolated recurrence in the retrohepatic peritoneum, we have assiduously sought to resect all of the peritoneal disease from this site. One begins this resection by dividing the ligamentum teres and incising the triangular ligament almost back to the suprahepatic inferior vena cava. With placement of the Bookwalter retractor obliquely above the right costal margin, retracting this structure upward and providing manual countertraction on the liver medially, one can

now place Allis clamps on the diaphragmatic peritoneal edge and dissect this structure down from the underlying diaphragmatic muscle all way to the central tendon. One can also dissect laterally and posteriorly to join the previous dissection in the right paracolic gutter and posterior hepatic peritoneum. Residual disease on the central tendon of the diaphragm or on the liver surface can be removed with the ultrasonic surgical aspirator.

Once dissection of all residual peritoneal tumor has been completed, the end of the descending or sigmoid colon can be resected back to healthy tissue and prepared for transanal anastomosis using the EEA stapler in routine fashion as described in Figure 9A and B. Great care is taken to ensure that the anastomosis is not on tension and is well vascularized. A single suction catheter is placed in the pelvis adjacent to the anastomosis. The integrity of the staple line is assessed by examination of the two rings of large bowel removed in the stapling device and by pumping air into the rectum with a bulb syringe after filling the pelvis with warm saline, looking for bubbles issuing from the anastomosis.

Although the extent of disease in some patients does not require en bloc resection of the rectosigmoid with the intraperitoneal viscera, approximately two thirds of our patients do present with the bulk of their intrapelvic disease on the rectosigmoid colon. Given the alternative course of piecemeal dissection of individual nodules

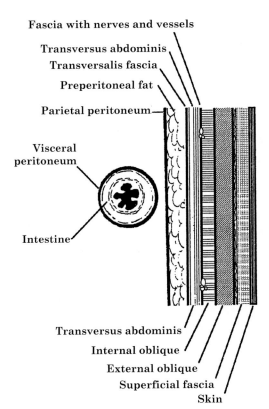

Fig. 2. Highly schematic section of the superficial and deep anterolateral and posterolateral abdominal walls. (From Colborn GL, Skandalakis JE. *Clinical gross anatomy.* New York: Parthenon Publishing Group, 1993, with permission.)

or left of the midline. The ring is formed by all layers of the abdominal wall (Fig. 7). If the opening is too small to permit reduction of the herniated intestinal loops, the defect occasionally needs to be enlarged by incising the lower edge of the ring. The capacity of the abdominal cavity, rather than the diameter of a constricting ring, is the limiting aspect for returning abdominal organs to the body cavity and repair of the defect.

SPIGELIAN HERNIA

Spigelian hernia occurs along the linea semilunaris of Spieghel (Fig. 8). There has been confusion in the literature about the linea semilunaris and the linea semicircularis (semilunar fold of Douglas). Hollinshead wrote, "Lateral ventral herniae are called spigelian hernias because they are said to occur along the Spieghel (Spigelius') line, which is generally regarded as synonymous with the semilunar line." We agree with Hollinshead, and believe that the confusion arose because most spigelian herniae occur at the site of intersection of the linea semilunaris and the linea semicircularis (Fig. 8B).

The linea semilunaris is usually understood to be the lateral border of the rectus sheath, although Spieghel intended it to be the line of transition between the muscular fibers and the aponeurosis of the transversus abdominis muscle. These two lines define a "semilunar zone" from 0.3 to 3.7 cm wide, in which a spigelian hernia may take place, anywhere from above the level of the umbilicus to the symphysis pubis (Fig. 8A).

If the hernia lies at the intersection of the linea semilunaris (of Spieghel) and the linea semicircularis (Douglas), the ring is formed by the aponeurosis of the internal oblique muscle and the aponeurosis of the transversus abdominis muscle (Fig. 8B, C). If the hernia is above the linea semicircularis, but below the umbilicus, the ring is almost the same. If the hernia is above the level of the umbilicus, the defect is formed by a tear in the transversus abdominis muscle and a defect of the aponeurosis of the internal oblique muscle. The neck of the hernia may be tough and rigid; the sac may be covered by preperitoneal fat.

If incarceration occurs, a transverse incision should be made just above the swelling. Keep in mind that the sac is under the aponeurosis of the external oblique muscle, which should be carefully incised. An oblique incision of the aponeurosis following the direction of the fibers is anatomically most sound. The procedures for umbilical herniorrhaphy should be followed.

GROIN HERNIA

There are four groin herniae: indirect, direct, external (anterior) supravesical, and femoral. All of them originate from the fossae of the anterolateral abdominal wall (Fig. 9). To understand these herniae and the formation of the rings, knowledge of the anatomy of the inguinal canal is essential (Fig. 10).

Boundaries of the Inguinal Canal

Anterior: The aponeurosis of the external oblique muscle and (more laterally) the

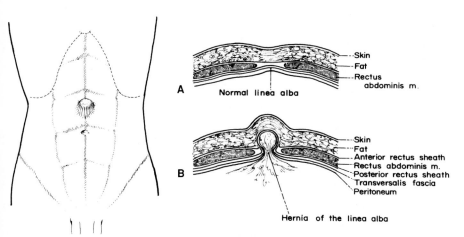

Fig. 3. Epigastric hernia. **A:** Transverse section of the normal body wall above the umbilicus. **B:** Herniation through the linea alba above the umbilicus. (From Skandalakis JE, Gray SW, Akin JT Jr. The surgical anatomy of hernial rings. *Surg Clin North Am* 1974;54:1227, with permission.)

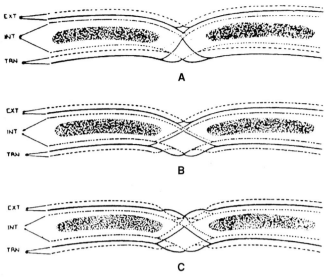

Fig. 4. Patterns of decussation at midline aponeurotic area (linea alba). **A:** Single anterior and single posterior lines of decussation (30%). **B:** Single anterior and triple posterior lines of decussation (10%). **C:** Triple anterior and triple posterior lines of decussation (60%). EXT, external oblique; INT, internal oblique; TRN, transversus abdominis. (From Askar O. Surgical anatomy of the aponeurotic expansions of the anterior abdominal wall. *Ann Royal Coll Surg Engl* 1977;59:313, with permission.)

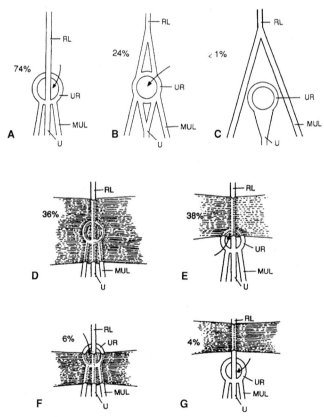

Fig. 5. Variations in umbilical ring (UR) and umbilical fascia seen from posterior (peritoneal) surface of body wall. **A–C:** Variations in disposition of umbilical ligaments. Arrows indicate path of hernia. **A:** Usual relations (74%) of UR, round ligament (RL), urachus (U), and medial umbilical ligaments (MUL). RL crosses UR to insert on its inferior margin. **B:** Less common configuration (24%). RL splits and attaches to superior margin of UR. **C:** Rare configuration (>1%). RL branches before reaching UR. Each branch continues with the medial umbilical ligament without attaching to UR. **D–G:** Variations in presence and form of insertion of umbilical fascia. **D:** Thickened transversalis fascia forms umbilical fascia covering UR (36%). **E:** Umbilical fascia covers only superior portion of UR (38%). **F:** Umbilical fascia covers only inferior portion of UR (6%). **G:** Although present, umbilical fascia does not underlie UR (4%). Fascia is entirely absent in 16% of cases (not shown). (From Orda R, Nathan H. Surgical anatomy of umbilical structures. *Int Surg* 1973;58:454, with permission.)

internal oblique muscle. Remember, there are no external oblique muscle fibers in the inguinal area, only aponeurotic fibers.

Posterior: In approximately 75% of subjects, the posterior wall (floor) of the canal is formed laterally by the aponeurosis of the transversus abdominis muscle and the transversalis fascia; in the remainder, the posterior wall is transversalis fascia only. Medially, the posterior wall is reinforced by the internal oblique aponeurosis.

Superior: The roof of the canal is formed by the arched fibers of the lower (roof) edge of the internal oblique muscle and by the transversus abdominis muscle and aponeurosis.

Inferior: The inferior wall of the canal is formed by the shelving lower border of the inguinal ligament (Poupart) and the lacunar ligament (Gimbernat).

Indirect Inguinal Hernia

An indirect hernia can be congenital or acquired. Herniation takes place through the deep ring. The sac follows the spermatic cord in males and the round ligament in females.

Boundaries of the Deep Ring

There is a normal defect in the transversalis fascia and transversus aponeurosis shaped like the uppercase Greek letter lambda (Λ). The anterior and posterior arms are a special thickening of the transversalis fascia, forming a sling (Fig. 11). However, the formation of the ring is not so simple. The inferior border is formed by another thickening of the transversalis fascia and transversus aponeurosis—the iliopubic tract—which is in some cases only weakly aponeurotic.

Remember: The anterior (superior) arm (crus) is formed by the transversus abdominis arch. The posterior (inferior) arm is formed by aponeurotic fibers from the iliopubic tract.

Boundaries of the Superficial Ring

The external (superficial) ring (Fig. 12) is a triangular cleft in the aponeurosis of the external oblique. The base is related to the pubic crest. Its margins are formed by two crura, superior (medial) and inferior (lateral). The superior crus is formed by the aponeurosis of the external oblique and the inferior crus by the inguinal ligament. To be more specific, the medial crus is attached to the lateral border of the rectus sheath and to the tendon of the rectus abdominis muscle in a form whose structure is subject to considerable variation. The lateral crus is attached to the pubic tubercle.

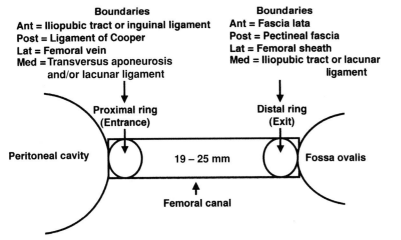

Boundaries
Ant = Iliopubic tract or inguinal ligament
Post = Ligament of Cooper
Lat = Femoral vein
Med = Transversus aponeurosis
and/or lacunar ligament

Boundaries
Ant = Fascia lata
Post = Pectineal fascia
Lat = Femoral sheath
Med = Iliopubic tract or lacunar
ligament

Proximal ring
(Entrance)

Distal ring
(Exit)

Peritoneal cavity

19 – 25 mm

Fossa ovalis

Femoral canal

Fig. 14. Highly diagrammatic presentation of the femoral canal.

The entrance to the femoral canal from the peritoneal cavity is guarded by the femoral ring (proximal ring), whose boundaries are:

Anterior: Iliopubic tract and inguinal ligament
Posterior: Ligament of Cooper (pectineal ligament)
Lateral: Femoral vein
Medial: Transversus aponeurosis or lacunar ligament, or both

The exit of the femoral canal to the fossa ovalis is guarded by the distal ring, whose boundaries are:

Anterior: Fascia lata and cribriform fascia
Posterior: Pectineal fascia
Lateral: Femoral sheath
Medial: Iliopubic tract or lacunar ligament

If there is incarceration, a small incision should be made to divide the inguinal ligament anteriorly or to divide the lacunar ligament medially. The incision of the inguinal ligament is preferred because the lacunar ligament is only 0.5 to 1.0 cm in length; division of the lacunar ligament may not enlarge the ring sufficiently.

We prefer the division of the inguinal ligament also because an aberrant obturator artery, found in more than 30% of cases and arising from the inferior epigastric artery, or, even more frequently, an aberrant vein, may pass across or medial to the femoral ring in the edge of the lacunar ligament rather than lateral to the ring. Injury to the aberrant obturator artery causes bleeding that is obvious in the recovery room. Injury to an aberrant obturator vein may not be immediately obvious.

If the approach is made from above the inguinal ligament, and thus through the floor of the inguinal canal, the aberrant obturator can be seen clearly, and the lacunar ligament can be cut safely.

POSTEROLATERAL ABDOMINAL WALL (LUMBAR AREA)

The posterolateral abdominal wall is bounded as follows:

Above, by the lower ribs
Below, by the iliac crest
Posteriorly, by the vertebral column (five lumbar vertebrae)
Laterally, by a vertical line starting from the anterior superior iliac spine and traveling upward

The posterolateral abdominal wall is formed by:

- Posterior muscles:
  Psoas
  Quadratus lumborum
  Iliacus
  Transversus abdominis
  External and internal obliques
- Fascia (thoracolumbar)
- Diaphragm (superior portion of posterolateral wall)

The area in the lumbar region related to the posterolateral abdominal wall herniae is formed by the superior and inferior lumbar triangles (Fig. 15).

Boundaries of the Lumbar Area

Anterior: Posterior border of the external oblique muscle
Posterior: Erector spinae muscles (sacrospinalis muscle)

Superior: Twelfth rib
Inferior: Iliac crest

Formation and Boundaries of the Lumbar Triangles

Hernial Ring of the Superior Triangle (of Grynfeltt) (Lesshaft Space)

Base: Twelfth rib and serratus posterior inferior muscle
Anterior (abdominal): Posterior border of the internal oblique muscle
Posterior (lumbar): Anterior border of sacrospinalis muscle
Floor: Aponeurosis of the transversus abdominis muscle arising from the fusion of the layers of the thoracolumbar fascia
Roof: External oblique and latissimus dorsi muscles

If incarceration occurs, the ring of the superior triangle can be enlarged by medial or lateral incision midway between the twelfth rib and the iliac crest.

Hernial Ring of the Inferior Triangle (of Petit)

Base: Iliac crest
Anterior (abdominal): Posterior border of external oblique muscle
Posterior (lumbar): Anterior border of latissimus dorsi muscle
Floor: Internal oblique with contributions from the transversus abdominis muscle and posterior lamina of the thoracolumbar fascia and the internal oblique muscle
Roof: Superficial fascia and skin

If incarceration occurs, the ring of the inferior triangle can be enlarged by medial or lateral incision of the thoracolumbar fascia.

INCISIONAL HERNIA

It is not possible to provide a generalized description of the ring in an incisional hernia because each case is different. The ring may be small or large, the result of any incision of the anterolateral or posterolateral abdominal wall (Fig. 15).

PELVIC WALLS

The pelvic walls are formed by four walls: anterior, posterior, right lateral, left lateral; and by a floor.

Anterior Wall

The anterior wall is formed by the pubic bones and the pubic symphysis.

Nongastrointestinal Transabdominal

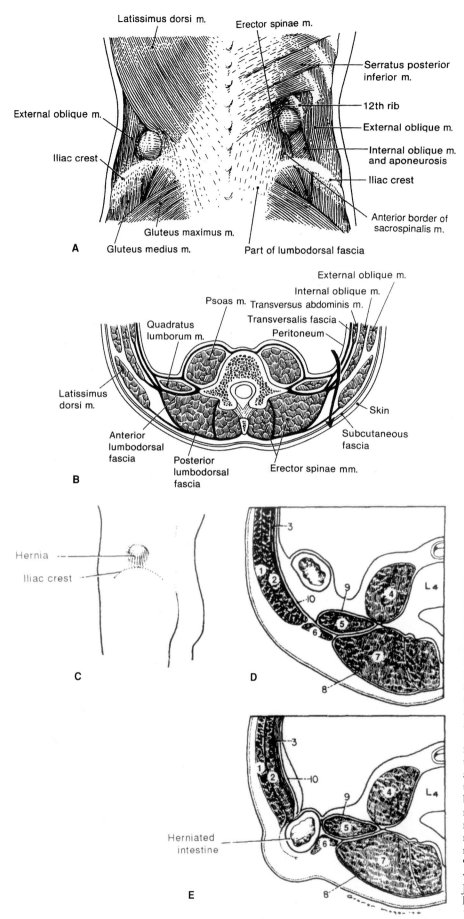

Fig. 15. A: Left: An inferior hernia through Petit triangle. The base of the triangle is formed by the iliac crest. Right: A superior hernia through the Grynfeltt triangle. The base of the inverted triangle is formed by the 12th rib. m, muscle. **B:** A diagrammatic cross section through the posterior body wall in the lumbar region. Arrow indicates the pathway of a superior lumbar hernia. m, muscle. (From Skandalakis LJ, Gadacz TR, Mansberger AR Jr, Mitchell WE Jr, Colborn GL, Skandalakis JE. *Modern hernia repair.* Pearl River, NY: Parthenon, 1996, with permission.) **C:** Hernia through the inferior lumbar triangle. **D:** Normal relations of the descending colon and the left posterolateral abdominal wall in cross section. **E:** Herniation of the descending colon through the inferior lumbar triangle. 1, external oblique muscle; 2, internal oblique muscle; 3, transversus abdominis muscle; 4, psoas muscle; 5, quadratus lumborum muscle; 6, latissimus dorsi muscle; 7, sacrospinalis muscle; 8, posterior layer of lumbodorsal fascia; 9, anterior layer of lumbodorsal fascia; 10, transversus abdominis aponeurosis. (From Skandalakis JE, Gray SW, Akin JT Jr. The surgical anatomy of hernial rings. *Surg Clin North Am* 1974;54: 1227, with permission.)

Posterior Wall

The posterior wall is formed by the sacrum and coccyx, sacroiliac joints, piriformis muscles, part of the pelvic diaphragm, and several ligaments.

Lateral Walls

The hip bones and the obturator foramen, with its membrane, form the lateral pelvic walls. The majority of the surface of the lateral pelvic walls is covered by the obturator internus muscles. The following anatomic entities are located medial to the obturator internus muscle: obturator nerve, obturator vessels, and branches of the internal iliac arteries and veins.

The obturator internus extends posteriorly from the lesser pelvis, through the lesser sciatic foramen, and then laterally toward the greater trochanter of the femur.

Pelvic Floor

The pelvic floor is simply the pelvic diaphragm (Figs. 16 and 17), which is formed by the levator ani muscles, the coccygeus muscles, and the superior and inferior fascial layer that covers the muscles. The levator ani is formed by three muscles: pubococcygeus, puborectalis, and iliococcygeus.

SCIATIC HERNIA RINGS

There are three potential rings associated with the at-large sciatic hernia (Fig. 18). The suprapiriformic and infrapiriformic rings are associated with the greater sciatic foramen, above or below the piriformis muscle. The subspinous ring is associated with the lesser sciatic foramen.

Boundaries of the Sciatic Hernia Rings

Suprapiriformic Ring

Anterior: Sacroiliac ligament
Inferior: Upper border of piriformis muscle
Lateral: Ilium
Medial: Sacrotuberous ligament and upper part of sacrum

If incarceration occurs, the piriformis muscle should be transected by a posterior and inferior incision (downward and outward). Remember that the greater sciatic foramen is the "Monemvassia" (only gate) of the gluteal area. The surgeon must exercise care to avoid damaging any of the structures that lie in or pass through the foramen:

- Piriformis muscle
- Superior gluteal nerve and vessels

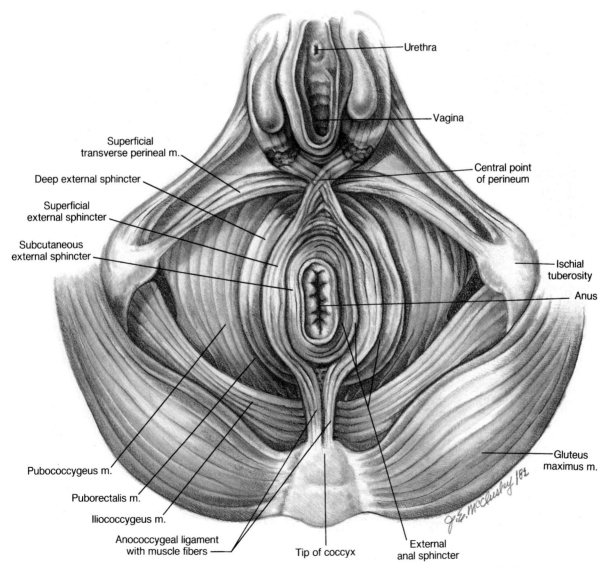

Fig. 16. Female pelvic diaphragm, seen from below. m, muscle. (From Gray SW, Skandalakis JE, McClusky DA. *Atlas of surgical anatomy for general surgeons.* Baltimore: Williams & Wilkins, 1985, with permission.)

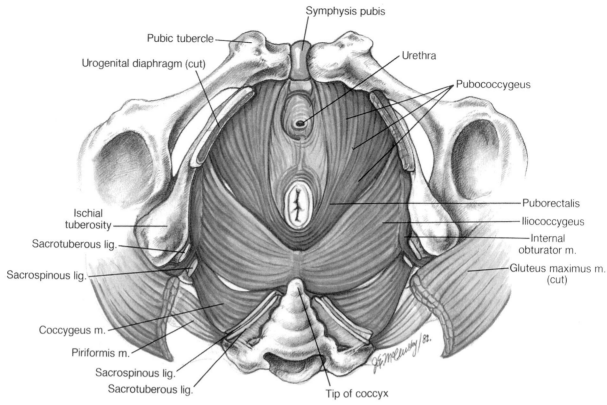

Fig. 17. Male pelvic diaphragm, seen from below. lig, ligament; m, muscle. (From Gray SW, Skandalakis JE, McClusky DA. *Atlas of surgical anatomy for general surgeons.* Baltimore: Williams & Wilkins, 1985, with permission.)

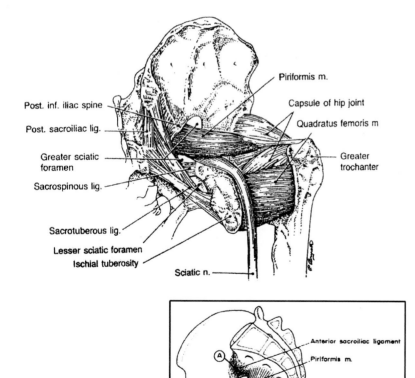

Fig. 18. Right lateral external view of pelvis. The greater sciatic foramen transmits the piriformis muscle and sciatic nerve. **Inset:** Sites of potential herniae through the sciatic foramina. A, suprapiriformic sciatic hernia; B, infrapiriformic sciatic hernia; C, subspinous sciatic hernia through the lesser sciatic foramen. (From Skandalakis LJ, Gadacz TR, Mansberger AR Jr, et al. *Modern hernia repair.* Pearl River, NY: Parthenon, 1996, with permission.)

- Inferior gluteal nerve and vessels
- Pudendal nerve and internal pudendal vessels
- Posterior femoral cutaneous nerve
- Nerve to the internal obturator muscle
- Nerve to the quadratus femoris muscle
- Sciatic nerve

Infrapiriformic Ring

Above: Lower border of piriformis muscle
Below: Sacrospinous ligament
Posterior: Sacrotuberous ligament
Anterior: Ilium

With incarceration, the piriformis muscle should be transected by upward and inward incision. Keep in mind the proximity of the vessels and nerves passing through the greater sciatic foramen (see previous section).

Subspinous Ring

Anterior: Ischial tuberosity
Superior: Sacrospinous ligament and ischial spine
Posterior: Sacrotuberous ligament

If incarceration occurs, incise the obturator internus and gemellus muscles, as necessary (Fig. 19).

OBTURATOR HERNIA RING

There is confusion in the literature about the definition and the anatomic entities involved in the formation of the obturator hernia (Figs. 20 and 21).

Boundaries of the Obturator Area

Superior: Superior ramus of the pubic bone
Lateral: Hip joint and shaft of femur
Medial: Pubic arch, perineum, and adductor musculature
Inferior: Origin of the adductor magnus from the ischiopubic ramus

Boundaries of the Obturator Foramen

The obturator foramen is formed anteriorly and inferiorly by the rami of the ischium and pubis. It is closed by the obturator membrane, except for a small area, the obturator canal.

Boundaries of the Obturator Canal

Superior and lateral: Obturator groove of the pubis

Inferior: Free edge of the obturator membrane and the internal and external obturator muscles

The obturator canal is the ring of the obturator hernia. It is a tunnel 2 to 3 cm in length, which begins at the pelvis and passes obliquely downward to end outside the pelvis in the obturator area of the thigh. The obturator artery, vein, and nerve pass through the canal. If incarceration occurs, an incision should be made at the lower margin of the ring.

PERINEUM

The perineum is defined as the area enclosed by and beneath the pelvic outlet. It is separated from the pelvic cavity by the pelvic diaphragm. The perineal boundaries are the following anatomic entities:

Anterior: Pubic symphysis and its arcuate ligament
Posterior: Coccyx
Anterolateral: Ischiopubic rami and ischial tuberosities
Posterolateral: Sacrotuberous ligaments

Nongastrointestinal Transabdominal

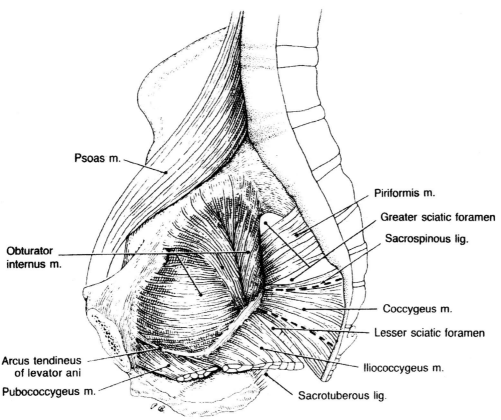

Fig. 19. Right pelvic wall with deep muscles and sciatic foramina. (From Skandalakis LJ, Gadacz TR, Mansberger AR Jr, et al. *Modern hernia repair.* Pearl River, NY: Parthenon, 1996, with permission.)

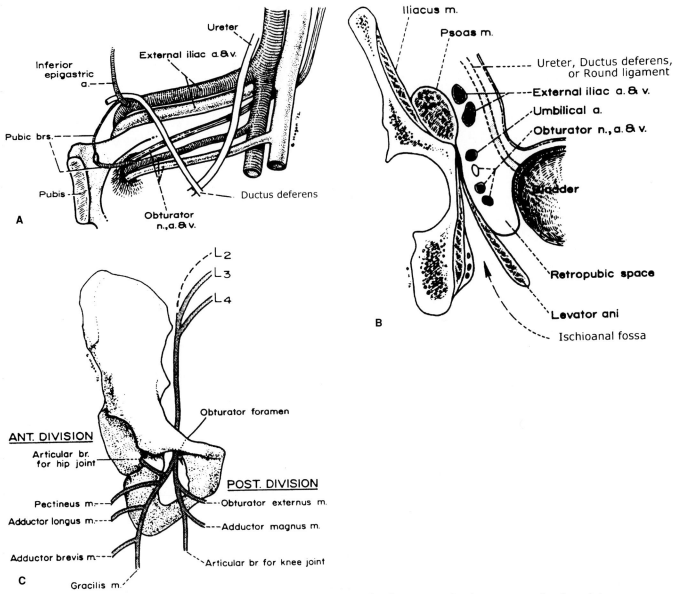

Fig. 20. A: View of the medial wall of the male pelvis showing the obturator canal and structures passing through it. **B:** Diagrammatic coronal section of the lateral wall of the male pelvis showing the relation of the obturator nerve, artery, and vein to other pelvic structures. (From Gray SW, Skandalakis JE, Soria RE, Rowe JS Jr. Strangulated obturator hernia. *Surgery* 1974;75:20, with permission.) **C:** The course and distribution of the right obturator nerve. (From Skandalakis PN, Skandalakis LJ, Gray SW, Skandalakis JE. Supravesical hernia. In: Nyhus LM, Condon RE. *Hernia*, 4th ed. Philadelphia: JB Lippincott, 1995;400, with permission.)

The maximum depth of the perineum is the inferior surface of the pelvic diaphragm; the superficial limit of the perineum is skin that is continuous with that covering the medial aspects of the thighs and the lower abdominal wall. The perineum is a diamond-shaped region. A transverse line between the right and left ischial tuberosities divides the diamond into an anterior urogenital triangle and a posterior anal triangle.

The perineum is one of the most complicated anatomic areas of the human body. We strongly advise the reader to study the section on the perineum in *Skandalakis' Surgical Anatomy: The Embryologic and Anatomic Basis of Modern Surgery.*

PERINEAL HERNIA RING

A primary perineal hernia may occur anterior or posterior to the superficial transverse perineal muscle (Fig. 22).

Anterior Perineal Hernia Ring

The ring is located anterior to the superficial transverse perineal muscle through the urogenital diaphragm into a triangle formed by the bulbospongiosus muscle medially, the ischiocavernous muscle laterally, and the transverse perineal muscle posteriorly. The sac passes between the ischiopubic bone and the vagina, producing a swelling in the posterior half of the labium majus.

If incarceration is present, the deep transverse perineal muscle, including both layers of the urogenital diaphragm, should be incised.

Posterior Perineal Hernia Ring

The ring is located posterior to the superficial transverse perineal muscle, through

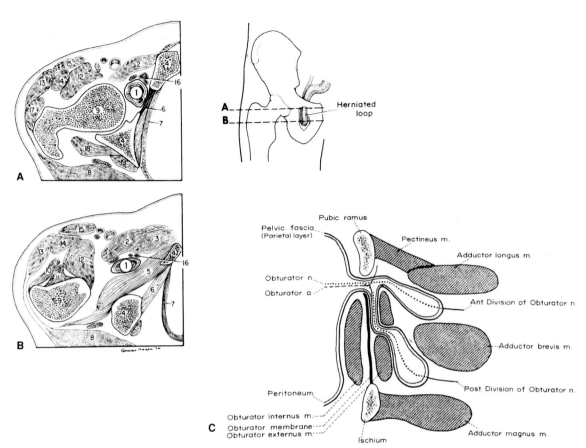

Fig. 21. Obturator hernia. Two levels, (**A** and **B**), are shown in cross-section inset. 1, herniated loop of intestine; 2, pectineus muscle; 3, adductor brevis muscle; 4, ischiopubic muscle; 5, obturator externus muscle; 6, obturator internus muscle; 7, levator ani muscle; 8, gluteus maximus muscle; 9, femur; 10, vastus lateralis muscle; 11, vastus intermedius muscle; 12, psoas muscle; 13, tensor fasciae latae muscle; 14, rectus femoris muscle; 15, sartorius muscle; 16, obturator vessels and nerve; 17, gluteus medius muscle; 18, gemellus inferior muscle; 19, gemellus superior muscle. (From Skandalakis JE, Gray SW, Akin JT Jr. The surgical anatomy of hernial rings. *Surg Clin North Am* 1974;54:1227, with permission.) **C:** Diagrammatic sagittal section through the upper thigh showing the ring and the potential pathways of the hernial sac. (From Gray SW, Skandalakis JE, Soria RE, Rowe JS Jr. Strangulated obturator hernia. *Surgery* 1974;75:20, with permission.)

the levator ani muscle, or between the levator ani and the coccygeus muscles. Koontz stated: "It usually emerges halfway between the rectum and the tuberosity of the ischium." If the levator ani muscle is not attached to the obturator fascia by the connective tissue band known as the arcus tendineus fascia pelvis, a gap (the hiatus of Schwalbe) is formed: "It is important because a process of pelvic peritoneum may be pushed through the hiatus into the suprasegmental space, and in this way occurs a hernia into the ischiorectal fossa" (McGregor and DuPlessis). This opening is referred to by gynecologic surgeons as a paravaginal defect.

Division of the levator ani muscle by a small incision is sufficient to release an incarcerated viscus. Care must be taken, however, to avoid the pudendal nerve, which lies in the perineum just deep to the levator ani.

DIAPHRAGM

The diaphragm is a musculotendinous organ that separates the abdominal cavity from the thoracic cavity. The muscular part is peripheral whereas the tendinous part, the so-called central tendon, is located centrally.
Remember:

- The foramen for the inferior vena cava is located in the central tendon.
- The esophageal hiatus is bordered by the right crus of the diaphragm in the area of the 10th thoracic vertebra. It transmits:
  Esophagus
  Both vagal trunks
  Branches of the left gastric vessels
  Some lymphatic vessels
- The aortic hiatus is formed by the right and left crura and the median arcuate ligament, which connects the two crura anterior to the aorta.
- There are several small openings in the diaphragm that never (if use of the word "never" is permitted) produce herniation.

HIATAL ESOPHAGEAL HERNIA (SLIDING HIATAL AND PARAESOPHAGEAL)

The muscular parts of the diaphragmatic crura and their fasciae are, for all practical purposes, responsible for the genesis of the esophageal hiatus because they form the anterior and lateral margins of the hiatus. In approximately 50% of patients, the hiatus is formed by the right and left limbs of the right crus; in the remainder, both right and left crura participate in the formation of the hiatus. Therefore, the ring must be considered to be muscular.

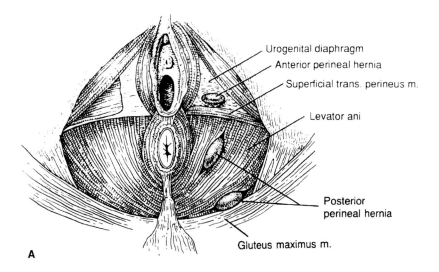

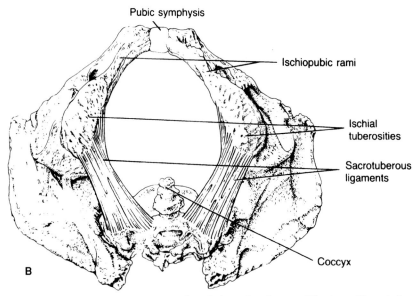

Fig. 22. A: The female perineum seen from below, showing possible sites of herniation. **B:** Boundaries of the perineum seen from above. This diamond-shaped area can be divided by a line connecting the ischial tuberosities into an anterior (urogenital) triangle and a posterior (anal) triangle. (From Skandalakis LJ, Gadacz TR, Mansberger AR Jr, et al. *Modern hernia repair.* Pearl River, NY: Parthenon, 1996, with permission.)

Two inconstant ligaments should be mentioned. Anteriorly, the transverse ligament of the central tendon is the point of union of the two limbs of the right crus. Posteriorly, the median arcuate ligament joins the crura just above the celiac axis. In approximately half the cadavers with hiatal hernia that we studied, we found the median arcuate ligament to be well developed. The origin of the crura from the vertebrae was tendinous, but in nine of ten cases, the tendinous part was posterior and medial (Fig. 23).

If incarceration is present, a left lateral incision must be made toward the central tendon to avoid injury to the phrenic nerve. The left phrenic nerve supplies the left half of the right crus and the left leaf and left crus of the diaphragm. A hernial sac is always present.

CONGENITAL DIAPHRAGMATIC RINGS

Bochdalek (Posterolateral) Ring

The Bochdalek defect (ring) is located at the lumbocostal trigone, just above and lateral to the left lateral arcuate ligament (lumbocostal arch). Therefore, it is located at the posterior portion of the diaphragm, and practically touches the 10th and 11th ribs. If the hernial ring is small, it is muscular. If the ring is larger, the central ten-don participates in the formation of the ring (Figs. 24 and 25).

The choice of approach to the diaphragm in any particular case is beyond the scope of this chapter. The surgeon should always be prepared to perform a thoracoabdominal incision if the preferred abdominal approach proves inadequate.

The diaphragm should be incised laterally from the margin of the ring toward the periphery. The surgeon should be familiar with the description by Merendino et al. of incisions that avoid severing branches of the phrenic nerve (Fig. 26). If a sac is present, it should be excised.

Morgagni (Retrosternal) Ring

The attachment of the diaphragm to the posterior surface of the xiphoid process by two narrow slips on either side of the midline and to the seventh costal cartilage lateral to the xiphoid process produces three gaps, one medial and two lateral. These are known as the sternocostal triangles, the foramina of Morgagni, or the spaces of Larrey. The boundaries of the hernial ring are as follows:

Anterior: Costal cartilage and xiphoid process
Lateral and posterior: Diaphragm
Medial: Diaphragm

According to Laberge et al., an upper abdominal approach is preferred. With incarceration, a lateral incision to enlarge the ring is performed. This approach avoids injury to the phrenic nerve.

Pericardial Ring

The pericardial ring is located at the fusion of the central tendon and the pericardium.

Eventration of the Diaphragm

The muscular layer of one diaphragmatic leaf is absent or greatly reduced with eventration of the diaphragm. There is no hernial ring associated with this condition.

PERITONEAL CAVITY AND THE ANATOMIC ENTITIES WITHIN

The reader should study the anatomy of the peritoneal cavity and the anatomic entities associated with it, such as:

Omentum
Mesentery
Several Foramina
Several Fossae

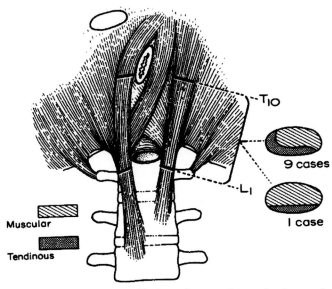

Fig. 23. The crura consist of both tendinous and muscular tissue; only the tendinous portion holds sutures. (From Gray SW, Rowe JS Jr, Skandalakis JE. Surgical anatomy of the gastroesophageal junction. *Am Surg* 1979;45:575, with permission.)

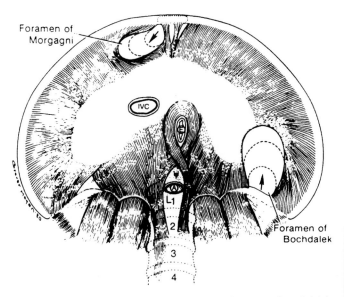

Fig. 24. The diaphragm from below, showing foramen of Bochdalek and foramen of Morgagni. Arrows indicate path of herniation. A, aorta; E, esophagus; IVC, inferior vena cava.

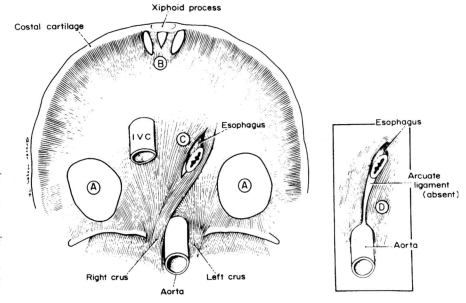

Fig. 25. Diaphragmatic herniae. A, foramina of Bochdalek (site of posterolateral hernia); B, foramina of Morgagni (site of anterior hernia); C, esophageal hiatus (site of hiatal hernia). IVC, inferior vena cava. (From Skandalakis JE, Gray SW, Akin JT Jr. The surgical anatomy of hernial rings. *Surg Clin North Am* 1974;54: 1227, with permission.) **Inset:** D, posterior enlargement of the esophageal hiatus to form the site of an aortohiatal hernia.

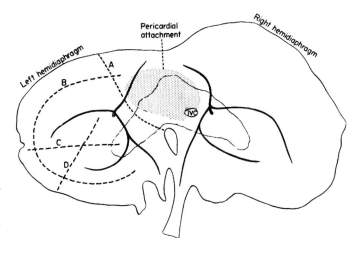

Fig. 26. Solid lines show the distribution of branches of the phrenic nerve (view from above). Broken lines show "safe" areas of the diaphragm where incisions may be made without any significant effect on diaphragmatic function. A, diaphragmatic component of a combined abdominothoracic incision extending down the esophageal hiatus; B, circumferential incision; C and D, incisions extending from lateral (midaxillary) and posterior costal areas into the central tendon. IVC, inferior vena cava. (From Merendino KA, Johnson RJ, Skinner HH, et al. The intradiaphragmatic distribution of the phrenic nerve with particular reference to the placement of diaphragmatic incisions and controlled segmental paralysis. *Surgery* 1956;39:189, with permission.)

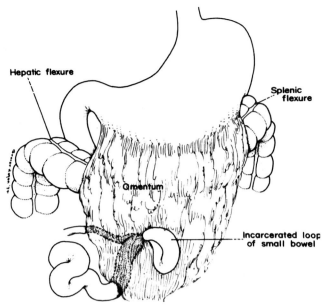

Fig. 27. Transomental hernia. (From Skandalakis JE, Gray SW, Akin JT Jr. The surgical anatomy of hernial rings. *Surg Clin North Am* 1974;54:1227, with permission.)

Transomental Hernia

The transomental hernia passes through the greater omentum. The surgical anatomy of the ring appears in Figure 27. The ring is formed entirely by omentum. A vessel usually lies in one edge of the ring. Incise the omentum between clamps.

Transmesenteric Hernia

A transmesenteric hernia may pass through the mesentery of the small bowel,

the transverse mesocolon, the pelvic (sigmoid) mesocolon, or the falciform ligament. The mesenteric ring may be located in the mesentery of the small intestine, the transverse mesocolon, or the sigmoid mesocolon (Fig. 28). At least one free edge of the ring is usually formed by a branch of the superior mesenteric or inferior mesenteric artery. Because there is no sac and the obstructed loop is invisible, decompress the dilated loop only and do not incise the neck. Vascular injury must be avoided.

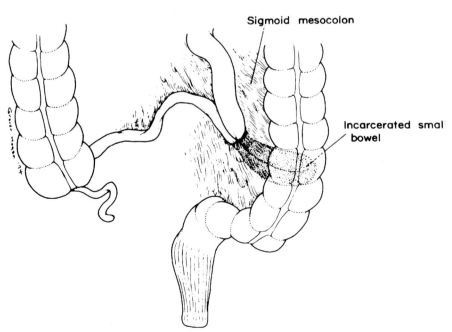

Fig. 28. Transmesenteric hernia. (From Skandalakis JE, Gray SW, Akin JT Jr. The surgical anatomy of hernial rings. *Surg Clin North Am* 1974;54:1227, with permission.)

FORAMINA AND FOSSAE

Hernia through the Epiploic Foramen of Winslow

The boundaries of the foramen of Winslow (Fig. 29) are:

Superior: Caudate process of liver and inferior layer of coronary ligament
Anterior: Hepatoduodenal ligament containing portal vein, hepatic artery, and common bile duct (cystic duct is also present in free edge of lesser omentum)
Posterior: Inferior vena cava
Inferior: First part of duodenum and transverse part of hepatic artery

For the incision, after clamping and decompressing the proximal intestinal loop, open the hepatogastric omentum. Do not incise the neck; the authors do not advise ligation of the hepatic artery. Remember that there is no excuse for dividing the neck of the sac.

Hernia through the Paraduodenal Fossae (Paraduodenal Hernia Rings)

Right Paraduodenal Hernia

The mouth of the sac lies behind the superior mesenteric artery and vein or the ileocolic artery at the base of the mesentery of the small intestine (mesentericoparietal fossa of Waldeyer) (Fig. 30). The mouth opens to the left. The sac is directed to the right and usually lies in the retroperitoneal space behind the right mesocolon or transverse mesocolon. The boundaries are:

Superior: Duodenum
Anterior: Superior mesenteric vessels or ileocolic vessels
Posterior: Lumbar vertebrae

When incarceration occurs, the incision must be in the lower part of the mouth of the sac to avoid vascular injury. If vascular damage appears inevitable, the surgeon should open the mesentery and decompress the proximal intestinal loop before attempting reduction.

Left Paraduodenal Hernia

The mouth of the sac usually lies behind the inferior mesenteric vein and the left colic artery at the left of the fourth part of the duodenum at the duodenojejunal flexure (Fig. 30A). The mouth opens to the right. The sac is directed to the left and usually lies in the retroperitoneal

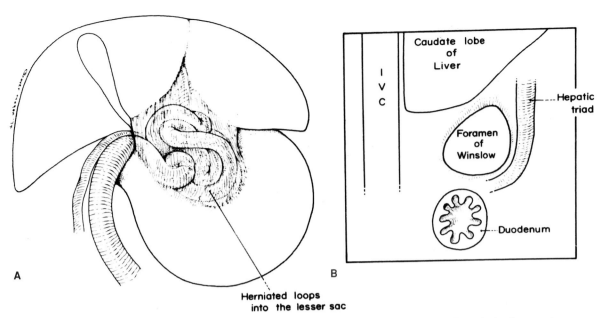

Fig. 29. Hernia through the epiploic foramen of Winslow. **A:** The intestines have passed through the foramen into the lesser peritoneal sac (omental bursa). **B:** Diagram of the structures surrounding the foramen of Winslow. IVC, inferior vena cava. (From Skandalakis JE, Gray SW, Akin JT Jr. The surgical anatomy of hernial rings. *Surg Clin North Am* 1974;54:1227, with permission.)

space behind the left mesocolon. The boundaries are:

Superior: Duodenojejunal flexure or the beginning of the jejunum, pancreas, and renal vessels
Anterior: Inferior mesenteric vein and left colic artery

Right: Aorta
Left: Left kidney

The incision should be made in the lower part of the mouth. McNair advised division of the inferior mesenteric vein. A downward incision of the mouth avoids this sacrifice.

Hernia through the Pericecal Fossae

The pericecal fossa is the most important boundary of the superior ileocecal fossae in the presence of the ileocolic (ileocecal) fold. This fold is formed by an anteriorly located semilunar elevation of the ileocolic mesentery that contains the anterior

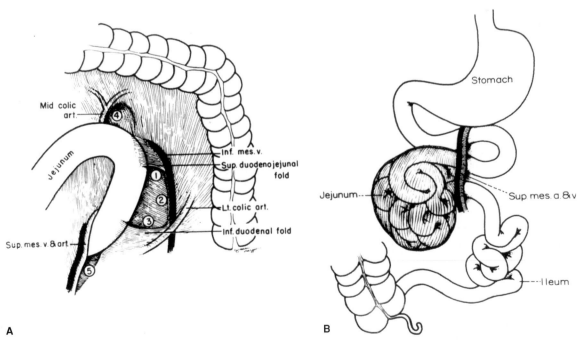

Fig. 30. Paraduodenal herniae. **A:** The five most constant sites of paraduodenal herniae: 1, 3, 4, 5, right paraduodenal herniae; 2, left paraduodenal hernia. The jejunum has been turned to the right. mes, mesenteric. (From Sims WG, Skandalakis JE, Gray SW. Right paraduodenal hernia into the fossa of Waldeyer. *J Med Assoc Ga* 1971;60:105, with permission.) **B:** A right paraduodenal hernia into the (mesentericoparietal) fossa of Waldeyer (site 5 in **A**). (From Skandalakis JE, Gray SW, Akin JT Jr. The surgical anatomy of hernial rings. *Surg Clin North Am* 1974;54:1227, with permission.)

branch of the ileocolic artery. The hernial sac travels under the right mesocolon or under the descending colon (Fig. 31). The surgeon must avoid the ileocolic and right colic arteries when incising the hernial ring. Aspiration of the proximal loop may be prudent.

The inferior ileocecal fossa has a prominent anterior ileoappendicular fold. This fold occasionally contains the ileoappendicular artery. The hernial sac is found under the cecum.

The paracolic fossa is located at the right gutter, resulting from nonfusion of the lateral and posterior walls of the ascending colon. The hernial sac travels under the proximal ascending colon.

Internal Supravesical Hernia

An internal supravesical hernia is a highly unusual phenomenon; the posterior supravesical hernia is especially rare. There are several sites of herniation in the supravesical fossa (Fig. 32). Through these sites, the hernial sac passes in front of, beside, or behind the bladder (Fig. 33).

We have performed dissections in fresh cadavers in an attempt to gain insight into hypothetical paths of herniation and the boundaries of possible hernial ring formation. Our own classification is based on theoretical pathways for the hernial sac, which we present as anatomic speculations, not clinically reported cases:

1. Anterior supravesical
   a. Retropubic (Fig. 33)
   b. Invaginating (Fig. 34)
2. Right or left lateral supravesical (Fig. 35)
3. Posterior supravesical (Fig. 33)

Note: For all practical purposes, there are three types of possible internal posterior supravesical herniae in the male patient (Fig. 36), and two possible types in the female patient (Fig. 37).

Anterior supravesical, retropubic, and invaginating hernial rings are similar. The boundaries can be described as follows:

Superior: The upward continuation of the vesicoumbilical fascia and its fusion with the transversalis fascia and the peritoneum

Inferior: Fold of vesical fascia and peritoneum

Lateral: Lateral umbilical ligament and peritoneum

Medial: Medial umbilical ligament and peritoneum

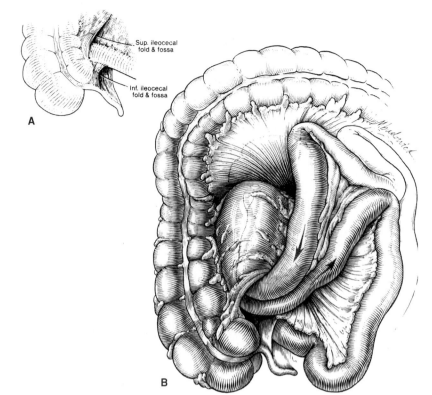

Fig. 31. Hernia into the superior ileocecal fossa. **A:** Superior and inferior ileocecal folds forming fossae. (From Skandalakis JE, Gray SW, Rowe JS. *Anatomical complications in general surgery.* New York: McGraw-Hill, 1983, with permission.) **B:** An intestinal loop trapped by the right mesocolon during fusion with the peritoneum of the body wall. (From Skandalakis LJ, Gadacz TR, Mansberger AR Jr, et al. *Modern hernia repair.* Pearl River, NY: Parthenon, 1996, with permission.)

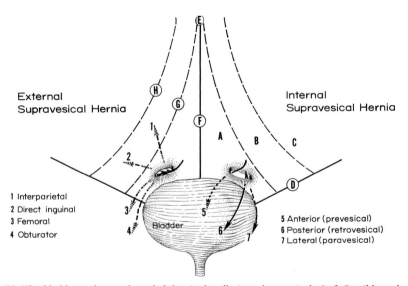

Fig. 32. The bladder and anterolateral abdominal wall viewed posteriorly. Left: Possible pathways of external supravesical herniae. Right: Possible pathways of internal supravesical herniae. A, supravesical fossa with mouth of supravesical hernia; B, medial fossa; C, lateral fossa; D, inguinal ligament; E, umbilicus; F, middle umbilical ligament (obliterated urachus); G, medial umbilical ligament (obliterated umbilical artery); H, lateral umbilical ligament (inferior [deep] epigastric artery). (From Skandalakis PN, Skandalakis LJ, Gray SW, Skandalakis JE. Supravesical hernia. In: Nyhus LM, Condon RE. *Hernia,* 4th ed. Philadelphia: JB Lippincott, 1995;400, with permission.)

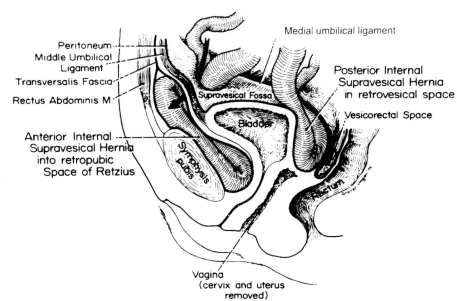

Fig. 33. Composition of anterior and posterior internal supravesical herniae. Most are of the anterior type. Arrow shows path of posterior hernia in a patient who previously had undergone a hysterectomy. (From Skandalakis JE, Gray SW, Burns WB, et al. Internal and external supravesical hernia. *Am Surg* 1976;42:142, with permission.)

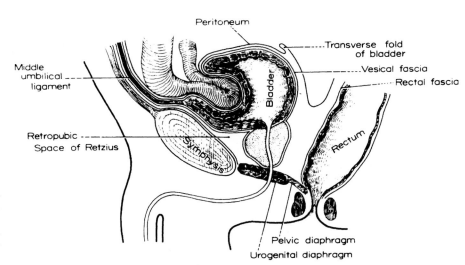

Fig. 34. Invaginating type of anterior internal supravesical hernia. (From Skandalakis PN, Skandalakis LJ, Gray SW, Skandalakis JE. Supravesical hernia. In: Nyhus LM, Condon RE. *Hernia*, 4th ed. Philadelphia: JB Lippincott, 1995;400, with permission.)

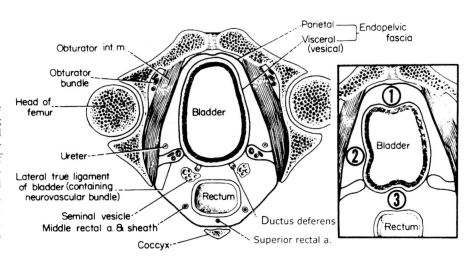

Fig. 35. Highly diagrammatic section of the body at the level of the acetabulum showing some of the landmarks of the spaces around the bladder. **Inset:** 1, location of sac in anterior internal (int.) supravesical hernia; 2, location of sac in lateral internal supravesical hernia; 3, location of sac in posterior internal supravesical hernia. (From Skandalakis PN, Skandalakis LJ, Gray SW, Skandalakis JE. Supravesical hernia. In: Nyhus LM, Condon RE. *Hernia*, 4th ed. Philadelphia: JB Lippincott, 1995;400, with permission.)

Nongastrointestinal Transabdominal

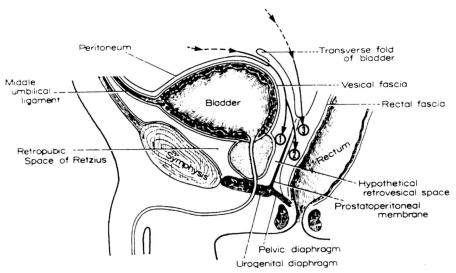

Fig. 36. Three possible pathways of posterior internal supravesical herniae in men (*arrows*). 1, path of true retrovesical hernia; 2, path of retrovesical hernia; 3, path of hernia through rectovesical pouch. (From Skandalakis PN, Skandalakis LJ, Gray SW, Skandalakis JE. Supravesical hernia. In: Nyhus LM, Condon RE. *Hernia,* 4th ed. Philadelphia: JB Lippincott, 1995;400, with permission.)

Boundaries of the retrovesical hernia ring are:

Superior and anterior: Vesical fascia and peritoneum of posterior bladder wall
Inferior and posterior: Transverse vesical fold

In all internal supravesical herniae, if enlargement of the ring is necessary, we recommend incising the posterior margins upward because of the anatomy of the area.

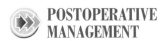 **POSTOPERATIVE MANAGEMENT**

Retroanastomotic Hernia

Markowitz, an authority on iatrogenic retroanastomotic herniae, stated: "Con-struction of each gastrojejunostomy, either as a procedure by itself or as a step in the performance of a partial gastrectomy, re-sults in the formation of an internal her-nial ring which may be the cause of severe difficulties in the immediate or distant postoperative period."

Hernia after Retrocolic Gastrojejunostomy

The surgical anatomy of the hernial ring after retrocolic gastrojejunostomy is seen in Figure 38A. The boundaries of the ring are:

Anterior: Gastrojejunostomy and efferent or afferent jejunal loop (depending on whether the afferent loop is attached to the lesser or the greater curvature of the stomach)
Posterior: Posterior parietal peritoneum
Superior: Transverse mesocolon and pos-terior wall of the gastric remnant
Inferior: Ligament of Treitz and duode-nojejunal peritoneal fold

In case of incarceration, no incision should be made. An enterostomy should be performed to facilitate reduction of the loop. Recurrence is prevented by closure of the ring.

Hernia after Antecolic Gastrojejunostomy

When the afferent loop is attached to the greater curvature of the stomach (Fig. 38B), the boundaries of the ring are:

Anterior: Gastrojejunostomy and afferent jejunal loop
Posterior: Greater omentum and meso-colon
Superior: Transverse colon and mesocolon
Inferior: Ligament of Treitz and duodeno-jejunal peritoneal fold
When the afferent loop is attached to the lesser curvature of the stomach, the boundaries of the ring are:
Anterior: Afferent jejunal loop with its mesentery
Posterior: Omentum, transverse colon, and mesoduodenojejunal peritoneal fold
Inferior: Jejunum with its mesentery

With incarceration, no incision of the ring is required. Enterostomy facilitates reduction.

Table 1 gives a summary of the surgical anatomy of hernial rings as presented in this chapter.

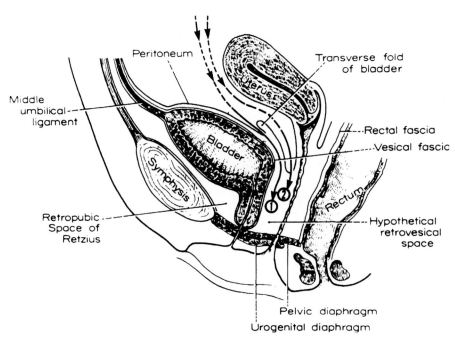

Fig. 37. Two possible pathways of posterior internal supravesical herniae in women (*arrows*). 1, path of true retrovesical hernia; 2, path of hernia through vesicovaginal pouch. (From Skandalakis PN, Skandalakis LJ, Gray SW, Skandalakis JE. Supravesical hernia. In: Nyhus LM, Condon RE. *Hernia,* 4th ed. Philadelphia: JB Lippincott, 1995;400, with permission.)

TABLE 1. SURGICAL ANATOMY OF HERNIAL RINGS

Hernia	Definition	Boundaries	If Incarcerated
Anterolateral Abdominal Wall			
Epigastric (ventral)	Defect of linea alba anywhere from xiphoid to umbilicus	Medial edge of right or left rectus sheath (anterior and posterior laminae as well as lateral edge of muscle between) may form lateral border	Superior or inferior incision of linea alba; rarely lateral incision of anterior lamina of rectus sheath
Umbilical	Incomplete closure of early natural umbilical defect; absence of umbilical fascia	Superior and inferior—linea alba Lateral—rectus abdominis muscle	Isolate sac; ligate through superior or inferior incision of linea alba
Omphalocele	Herniation of intraperitoneal viscera into open umbilical ring	Umbilical cord; hernial sac covered by double layer of membranes (amniotic outside, peritoneum inside, Wharton jelly in between)	Right or left horizontal incision
Gastroschisis	Defect of anterior abdominal wall to right or left of the midline	Layers of the abdominal wall	May need to incise the lower edge of the ring
Spigelian	Herniation along the linea semilunaris of Spieghel (line of transition between the muscular fibers and the aponeurosis of the transversus abdominis muscle) anywhere above level of umbilicus lateral to the symphysis pubis	*If at intersection of linea semilunaris (Spieghel) and linea semicircularis (Douglas), or above the linea semicircularis but below and lateral to the umbilicus:* aponeurosis of internal oblique muscle and the aponeurosis of the transversus abdominis muscle *If above the level of the umbilicus:* ring is formed by tear in the transversus abdominus muscle and a defect of the aponeurosis of the internal oblique muscle	Transverse incision above swelling; oblique incision of aponeurosis of the external oblique muscle following the direction of the fibers
Groin—indirect	Herniation through the deep (internal) inguinal ring following the spermatic cord in male patients and the round ligament in female patients; may herniate through superficial (external) ring	*Boundaries of deep ring:* anterior and posterior—thickening of transversalis fascia "sling" inferior—iliopubic tract *Boundaries of superficial ring:* triangular opening of aponeurosis of external oblique composed of superior (medial) and inferior (lateral) crura; base of triangle is pubic crest	If at deep ring: internal oblique retracted medially by upward incision; open sac and release incarceration
Groin—direct	Herniation through floor of inguinal canal—covered by transversalis fascia and aponeurosis of the transversus abdominis muscle	Located at medial fossa	Rarely, through external ring; treat as indirect hernia incarceration
Groin—external supravesical	Herniation between midline and lateral umbilical liga-ment	Partially or totally occupying the supravesical fossa	Treat as indirect hernia incarceration
Femoral	Herniation through femoral canal (consisting of proximal ring and distal ring)	*Proximal ring:* anterior—iliopubic tract, inguinal ligament, or rarely, both Posterior—ligament of Cooper (pectineal ligament) Lateral—femoral vein Medial—insertion of iliopubic tract *Distal ring:* anterior—fascia lata Posterior—pectineal fascia Lateral—femoral sheath Medial—iliopubic tract or lacunar ligament	Small incision to divide inguinal ligament anteriorly; alternatively, divide the lacunar ligament medially; in the latter case, be aware of an aberrant obturator artery (30%) passing medial to the femoral ring in the edge of the lacunar ligament

Nongastrointestinal Transabdominal

(continued)

TABLE 1. (continued)

Hernia	Definition	Boundaries	If Incarcerated
Posterolateral Abdominal Wall (Lumbar)			
	Herniation through superior and inferior lumbar triangles	*Superior triangle:* base—12th rib and serratus posterior inferior muscle Anterior—posterior border of the internal oblique muscle Posterior—anterior border of sacrospinalis muscle Floor—aponeurosis of transversus abdominis muscle Roof—external oblique and latissimus dorsi muscle	Enlarge ring of the superior triangle by medial or lateral incision midway between the 12th rib and the iliac crest
		Inferior triangle: base—iliac crest Anterior—posterior border of external oblique muscle Posterior—anterior border of latissimus dorsi muscle Floor—internal oblique with transversus abdominis muscle and posterior lamina of thoracolumbar fascia of internal oblique	Enlarge ring of the inferior triangle by medial or lateral incision of the thoracolumbar fascia
Incisions	Varies according to the incision	Various	Incision of the ring is determined by topography
Pelvic Walls and Perineum			
Sciatic—suprapiriformic	Herniation through greater sciatic foramen above piriformis muscle	Anterior—sacroiliac ligament Inferior—upper border of piriformis muscle Lateral—ilium Medial—sacrotuberous ligament and upper part of sacrum	Posterior and inferior (downward and outward) incision of piriformis muscle; be aware of other structures in greater sciatic foramen
Sciatic—infrapiriformic	Herniation through greater sciatic foramen below piriformis muscle	Above—lower border of piriformis muscle Below—sacrospinous ligament Posterior—sacrotuberous ligament Anterior—ilium	Anterior and superior (upward and inward) incision of piriformis; be aware of other structures in greater sciatic foramen
Sciatic—subspinous	Herniation through lesser sciatic foramen	Anterior—ischial tuberosity Superior—sacrospinous ligament and ischial spine Posterior—sacrotuberous ligament	Incise obturator internus muscle
Obturator	Herniation through the obturator canal	Superior and lateral—obturator groove of the pubis Inferior—free edge of obturator membrane and the internal and external obturator muscles	Incision at lower margin of ring; be aware of obturator artery, vein, and nerve as they pass through the canal; inspect for aberrant obturator vessel(s)
Perineal—anterior	Herniation anterior to the superficial transverse perineal muscle	Medial—bulbospongiosus muscle Lateral—ischiocavernous muscle Posterior—transverse perineal muscle	Incise deep transverse perineal muscle, including both layers of the urogenital diaphragm; sac passes between ischiopubic bone and the vagina; in male patients, very rare
Perineal—posterior	Herniation posterior to the superficial transverse perineal muscle	Ring formed through levator ani, or between the levator ani and coccygeus muscles	Small incision to divide the levator ani muscle

(continued)

TABLE 1. (continued)

Hernia	Definition	Boundaries	If Incarcerated
Diaphragm			
Hiatal esophageal (sliding or paraesophageal)	Herniation through diaphragmatic crura	In 50%, right and left limbs or the right crus; in remainder, both right and left crura are involved	Left lateral incision toward the central tendon (avoid injury to the phrenic nerve); hernial sac is always present
Diaphragmatic rings			
Congenital—Bochdalek (posterolateral)	Herniation through the lumbocostal trigone (above and lateral to left lateral lumbocostal arch)	Located at the posterior portion of the diaphragm close to 10th and 11th ribs; if large, the central tendon is involved	Incisc diaphragm laterally from margin of ring toward periphery (avoid branches of phrenic nerve)
Congenital—Morgagni (retrosternal)	Herniation through the sternocostal triangles (foramina of Morgagni)	Anterior—costal cartilage and xiphoid process Lateral and posterior—diaphragm Medial—diaphragm Ring located at fusion of central tendon and pericardium	Lateral incision to enlarge the ring (avoid phrenic nerve)
Pericardial ring	Herniation through the central tendon of the diaphragm and the pericardium	Various	Incision of the ring is determined by topography
Peritoneal Cavity and Anatomical Entities within			
Transomental	Herniation through greater omentum	Bordered entirely by omental tissues	Incise omentum between clamps since a vessel will usually lie in one edge of the ring
Transmesenteric	Herniation through mesentery of small bowel, transverse mesocolon, pelvic mesocolon, or the falciform ligament	Ring may be located in mesentery of small bowel, the transverse mesocolon, or the sigmoid mesocolon; at least one free edge of the ring is usually formed by a branch of the superior mesenteric or inferior mesenteric artery	Decompress dilated loop; do not incise the neck
Foramina or Fossae			
Epiploic foramen of Winslow	Herniation through the foramen	Superior—caudate process of liver and inferior layer of coronary ligament Anterior—hepatoduodenal ligament Posterior—inferior vena cava Inferior—first part of duodenum and transverse part of hepatic artery	After clamping and decompressing the proximal loop, open the hepatogastric omentum; do not incise the neck
Right paraduodenal	Herniation through right paraduodenal fossa	Superior—duodenum Anterior—superior mesenteric artery or ileocolic artery Posterior—lumbar vertebrae	Incise lower part of the mouth of the sac (sac lies behind the superior mesenteric artery or ileocolic artery at the base of the mesentery of the small intestine)
Left paraduodenal	Herniation through left paraduodenal fossa	Superior—duodenojejunal flexure or the beginning of the jejunum, pancreas, and renal vessels Anterior—inferior mesenteric vein and left colic artery Right—aorta Left—left kidney	Incise lower part of the mouth of the sac in downward fashion (sac lies behind the inferior mesenteric vein and the left colic artery to the left of the fourth part of the duodenum)

Nongastrointestinal Transabdominal

(continued)

TABLE 1. (continued)

Hernia	Definition	Boundaries	If Incarcerated
Superior ileocecal	Sac under right mesocolon or descending colon	Ileocolic (ileocecal) fold: formed by an anteriorly located semilunar elevation of the ileocolic mesentery by the anterior branch of the ileocecal artery	Avoid the right ileocolic and right colic arteries
Inferior ileocecal	Sac under cecum	Anterior ileoappendicular fold	Avoid the ileoappendicular artery present in the fold; avoid injury to ascending colon
Paracolic	Sac under proximal ascending colon	Paracolic fold located in the right gutter	
Internal Supravesical			
Anterior supravesical	Herniation of the supravesical fossa in front of the bladder	Superior—the upward continuation of the vesical fascia and its fusion with the transversalis fascia and the peritoneum Inferior—fold of vesical fascia and peritoneum Lateral—lateral umbilical ligament and peritoneum Medial—medial umbilical ligament and peritoneum	Incise the posterior margins upward
Retrovesical (posterior supravesical)	Herniation of the supravesical fossa behind the bladder	Superior and anterior—vesical fascia and peritoneum of posterior bladder wall Inferior and posterior—transverse vesical fold	Treat as anterior supravesical
Postsurgery —after retrocolic gastrojejunostomy	Two potential spaces are created; upper: above the mesocolon; lower: posterior to the gastric remnant	Anterior—gastrojejunostomy and efferent or afferent jejunal loop Posterior—posterior parietal peritoneum Superior—transverse mesocolon and posterior wall of the gastric remnant Inferior—ligament of Treitz and duodenojejunal peritoneal fold	No incision should be made; perform an enterostomy to facilitate reduction and closure of the ring
Postsurgery After antecolic gastrojejunostomy (when afferent loop is attached to the lesser curvature of the stomach)	Rare, but more common than herniation of loop to greater curvature	Anterior—afferent jejunal loop with its mesentery Posterior—omentum, transverse colon, and mesoduodenojejunal peritoneal fold Inferior—jejunum with its mesentery	
After antecolic gastrojejunostomy (when afferent loop is attached to the greater curvature of the stomach)	Information is scant because the herniation is so rare	Anterior—gastrojejunostomy and afferent jejunal loop Posterior—omentum and mesocolon Superior—transverse colon and mesocolon Inferior—ligament of Treitz and duodenojejunal peritoneal fold	No incision should be made; perform an enterostomy to facilitate reduction

n patients who had previous lower abdominal operations. It is now widely acknowledged that prior lower abdominal operations is a contraindication to TEP repair, and with maturation of the TEP experience, those injured patients likely would not be considered candidates for a TEP repair today.

CONCLUSION

The TEP hernia repair is our preferred laparoscopic technique. As with most laparoscopic procedures, it has a significant learning curve. It is associated with the short-term benefits of decreased rate of infection, hematoma, pain, paresthesia, and quicker return to normal activities when compared with the open mesh repair. The recurrence rates between the TEP repair and open mesh repair are equivalent, and we believe that, with more time, the TEP recurrence rate may even be shown to be superior to that of open repairs.

In the properly selected patient, the authors believe laparoscopic TEP repair is the best inguinal hernia repair we can provide.

SUGGESTED READING

Davis CJ, Arregui ME. Laparoscopic repair for groin hernias. *Surg Clin North Am* 2003; 83:1141.

EU Hernia Trialists Collaboration. Laparoscopic compared to open methods of groin hernia repair: systematic review of randomized controlled trials. *Br J Surg* 2000;87:860.

Ferzli GS, Freeza EE, Pecoraro AM Jr, et al. Prospective randomized study of stapled versus unstapled mesh in a laparoscopic preperitoneal inguinal hernia repair. *J Am Coll Surg* 1999;188:461.

Grunwaldt LJ, Schwaitzberg SD, Rattner DW, Jones DB. Is laparoscopic inguinal hernia repair an operation of the past? *J Am Coll Surg* 2005;200(4):616.

Hamilton EC, Scott DJ, Kapoor A, et al. Improving operative performance using a laparoscopic hernia simulator. *Am J Surg* 2001;182:725.

Liem MSL, Van Der Graff Y, Van Steensel, et al. Comparison of conventional anterior surgery and laparoscopic surgery for inguinal hernia repair. *N Engl J Med* 1997; 336:1541.

McCormack K, Scott NW, Ross S, et al. Laparoscopic techniques versus open techniques for inguinal hernia repair. Cochrane Database Syst Rev 2003;CD001785.

McKernon JB, Laws HL. Laparoscopic repair of inguinal hernias using a totally extraperitoneal prosthetic approach. *Surg Endosc* 1993;7:26.

Memon MA, et al. Meta-analysis of randomized clinical trials comparing open and laparoscopic inguinal hernia repair. *Br J Surg* 2003;90:1479.

Neumayer L, et al. Open mesh versus laparoscopic mesh repair of inguinal hernia. *N Engl J Med* 2004;350:1819.

Ramshaw, et al. A comparison of the approaches to laparoscopic herniorrhaphy. *Surg Endosc* 1996;10:29.

Smith AI, et al. Stapled and nonstapled laparoscopic transabdominal preperitoneal (TAPP) inguinal hernia repair. *Surg Endosc* 1999; 13:804.

Stoppa RE. The treatment of complicated groin and incisional hernias. *World J Surg* 1989;13:545.

Wright D, Paterson C, Scott N, et al. Five year follow-up of patients undergoing laparoscopic or open groin hernia repair: a randomized controlled trial. *Ann Surg* 2002; 235:333.

Nongastrointestinal Transabdominal

EDITOR'S COMMENT

No procedure is so hotly debated among general surgeons than the repair of the inguinal hernia. With nearly 700,000 groin hernia repairs performed annually in the United States, this is a bread-and-butter operation that has undergone radical changes during the last 2 decades. Classic tissue herniorrhaphies were replaced by "tension-free" techniques using mesh. Mesh repairs were further revolutionized with the introduction of laparoscopy in the early 1990s. Multiple prospective randomized trials have now shown that laparoscopic inguinal hernia repair is associated with shorter recovery times and less pain than open repairs. Although complication rates are similar, with managed care, direct hospital costs are an ever-increasing concern with the laparoscopic approach.

Large, scrotal, incarcerated, and strangulated hernias are best done with an open approach. Therefore, proper patient selection relies on the history and physical examination. Patients will usually complain of an intermittent bulge in the groin. For laparoscopic repairs, the fascial defect of the hernia should ideally be no larger than a silver dollar so that wide mesh overlap can be achieved. Scrotal hernias will result in bothersome scrotal seroma after laparoscopy even if the pseudosac is inverted, and should be avoided. Failure to reduce the hernia will prevent creation of the preperitoneal working space. If fever, tachycardia, exquisite tenderness, erythema, and obstructive symptoms are present, an irreducible hernia is likely strangulated and warrants immediate open operative intervention. Inability to tolerate general anesthesia is an absolute contraindication to laparoscopy.

On physical examination the diagnosis of hernia can sometimes be difficult. Herniography is a technique whereby a small amount of contrast material is injected into the peritoneal cavity and radiographs are taken during a Valsalva maneuver. Herniography has been advocated as a useful imaging study in patients with groin pain and no evidence of a hernia on physical examination. Computed tomography and ultrasound scanning may help exclude other causes of groin masses. When diagnosis has been ambiguous, I have been surprised on several occasions in which diagnostic laparoscopy clearly identified small hernias and rendered them asymptomatic after mesh repair. Laparoscopy allows routine inspection of the contralateral side and often detects hernias that would otherwise go unappreciated.

With traditional anterior open approaches, the goal of all repairs is to close the myofascial defect through which the hernia protrudes. The classic tissue repairs (Marcy, Bassini, Shouldice, and McVay) use permanent suture to reinforce the internal inguinal ring and the floor of the inguinal canal. The Lichtenstein and Plug/patch repairs employ prosthetic mesh. In a landmark study by Liem et al., the TEP was compared with the open repair that the surgeon was most comfortable performing. The laparoscopic repair was shown superior to the best open repairs.

Lichtenstein emphasizes that classic repairs suture together tendinous structures, which are not normally in apposition and thus create suture-line tension and may be the ultimate cause of early recurrence. The Lichtenstein repair reinforces the transversalis fascia forming the canal floor without attempting to use any attenuated native tissues. The largest study to date comparing laparoscopic and Lichtenstein hernia repair is a Veterans Affairs multi-institutional study. In this chapter, Dr Rattner briefly explains inconsistencies with this study compared with numerous other randomized prospective studies. The reference by Grunwaldt in the "Suggested Reading" section further discusses concerns with the Veterans Affairs study.

Two techniques have proven effective and have emerged as the most popular: the transabdominal preperitoneal (TAPP) and the totally extraperitoneal (TEP) methods. These repairs approach the myopectineal orifice posteriorly, similar in anatomical perspective to the open preperitoneal approaches of Stoppa. Understanding of the anatomy from this perspective is crucial in order to avoid a number of complications, mainly vascular and nerve injuries. Care must be taken to avoid injury to the external iliac vessels located in the "triangle of doom" bounded by the vas medially and the gonadal vessels laterally. Spiral tacks should not be applied posterior to the iliopubic tract to avoid nerve entrapment in the "triangle of pain" bounded by the gonadal vessels and iliopubic tract. Laparoscopy provides a clear view of the entire myopectineal orifice, and repairs of both inguinal and femoral hernias can be performed.

The TEP technique gains access to the groin via a completely extraperitoneal approach, and is my preferred repair for bilateral, recurrent, and unilateral inguinal hernias because patients recuperate with less pain and have a faster return to full activity. We use specialized operating rooms that permit two monitors at the foot of the bed. Having two monitors provides comfortable viewing for both surgeon and assistant. Before starting the operation, placing the patient in the Trendelenburg position may help reduce the hernia and facilitate later creation of a preperitoneal space with the dissecting balloon. Dr. Rattner favors blunt dissection with the laparoscope to create a preperitoneal space for TEP repairs, but a dissecting balloon is usually em-

(continued)

ployed. The balloon will pass easily if in the proper plane, and should never be forced. Before insufflating with air, I will keep one hand on the pubis to prevent dissection above the pubis by the balloon. Contrary to Dr Rattner, I will place the inferior 5-mm port three fingerbreadths above the pubis so two thirds of the mesh will ultimately rest on the anterior abdominal wall. Wide mesh overlap lessens the need for spiral tacks. Lastly, the peritoneum should never be allowed to slip under the mesh because this may favor recurrence.

In patients with previous open groin repairs and lower abdominal operations, a TAPP repair provides excellent visualization of the inguinal hernia. If during TEP procedure the peritoneum is violated, I may convert to a TAPP approach. Dr. Rattner points out that the TAPP procedure uses traditional intra-abdominal laparoscopic access and affords the benefits of easier visualization and rapid inspection of both groins. Dr. Rattner advocates full skeletonization of the cord to avoid missing small indirect hernias. The mesh should generously overlap all defects. TAP requires meticulous closure

of the peritoneum with staples, tacks, or, best, running suture.

Laparoscopic repairs are effective and safe. Numerous trials provide encouraging results, showing recurrence rates of 0% to 6%. The incidence of complications associated with laparoscopic repairs is comparable to or better than that of open repairs, especially after the learning curve has been overcome. Models and simulators have been developed to better train surgeons in inguinal anatomy and laparoscopic technique.

For laparoscopic repairs, the reasons for recurrence are surgeon inexperience, inadequate dissection, insufficient prosthesis size, insufficient prosthesis overlap of hernia defects, inadequate fixation, prosthesis folding or twisting, missed hernias or lipomas, and mesh dislodgement secondary to hematoma formation. Recurrence is directly related to surgeon experience, with failures occurring much more frequently early in the surgeon's learning curve. Incomplete dissection can result in missed indirect hernias and missed cord lipomas. Inadequate dissection can also limit the size of mesh that can be used or result in incomplete fixation

or folding. I strive to use a 12 × 15 cm piece of mesh to ensure a 3-cm overlap of all hernia defects. Except for the smallest hernias, I routinely tack the mesh into at least the Cooper ligament to prevent early migration of mesh. For larger defects, I will tack the mesh into the anterior abdominal wall.

Open repairs have long-standing and well-proven results, are associated with low morbidity and disability, can be more easily performed under local anesthesia, and do not require laparoscopic skills. Nevertheless, laparoscopic approaches are clearly indicated in bilateral and recurrent hernias because this approach provides access to both groins with no additional incisions. Furthermore, the laparoscopic repair avoids scarred anterior tissue planes and potential cord injury after failed open repairs. Many surgeons who perform TEP regularly offer this approach to their patients who have unilateral nonrecurrent hernias. Laparoscopic TEP is advantageous, but surgeons untrained in laparoscopy should either refer to a laparoscopic surgeon or perform the open operation that they do best.

D.B.J.

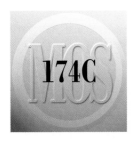

Groin Hernia Repair: Kugel Technique

ROBERT D. KUGEL

Arguably the most commonly performed general surgery procedure, hernia is clearly a significant problem and usually constitutes a major part of the typical general surgery practice. Although the argument continues regarding when it is necessary to operate on a groin hernia, it is obvious that this problem will continue to demand a prominent position in the general surgeon's practice.

Unfortunately, the attention given to this problem by the average general surgeon has not always been consistent with the frequency with which it is encountered and the seeming importance it plays as a percentage of general surgery practice. This may be due to the fact that it is not necessarily the most glamorous procedure or the sometimes frustrating nature of management of the hernia and the not infrequent and annoying complications that can occur. It might also be due to the relatively low reimbursement for hernia surgery. How few are the surgeons that count hernia surgery as the favorite part of their practice?

Fortunately, advances in hernia surgery in the last 15 years have greatly expanded the opportunities for success with hernia surgery. Previous centuries have seen the primary focus on reduction of a

high risk of recurrence. With the new "tension-free" repairs, when performed properly, the risk of recurrence can be reduced to very low levels. In addition, other factors affecting the disability associated with the groin hernia and the surgical repair of groin hernias are also being addressed.

Proper performance of whatever technique selected is a key element in success with hernia surgery. This requires attention to detail. The surgeon who approaches hernia surgery as a nuisance procedure will likely get results accordingly. The newer techniques require a thorough understanding of the technique involved and groin anatomy. Unfortunately, both of these seemingly obvious points are too often neglected.

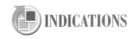 **INDICATIONS**

The Kugel repair is a tension-free, minimally invasive yet open, preperitoneal or posterior groin hernia repair. It is effective in and applicable to the treatment of indirect and direct inguinal hernias as well as femoral hernias. It is particularly useful for the treatment of recurrent groin hernias

after a previously failed anterior repair. With experience, it can be used selectively in patients having undergone prior radical prostatectomy or pelvic radiation, but should be avoided in patients with recurrence after failed laparoscopic groin hernia repair.

When speed of recovery is a factor, this technique allows for the fastest possible return to regular work and other activities without restrictions. It further minimizes the risk of nerve injury and associated burdensome chronic pain syndromes.

While not generally recommended for use in the younger pediatric population, the technique is useful in older teenagers. Although these hernias are almost always congenital and treatable with a simple high ligation of the hernia sac, this technique offers certain advantages worth considering in this patient population. The nearly full-grown teenager appears to tolerate this tension-free repair very well. It can generally be done with no significant increase in morbidity than that typically experienced with a simple high ligation procedure. Rather than simply treating the immediate problem, the patient has hopefully been protected from any future groin hernia on the surgical side.

PATIENT SELECTION

A key element in successful hernia surgery is proper patient selection. This relates to several areas of concern: Do all patients with a hernia require surgery? What is the proper procedure for an individual patient? And not least of all, does every patient with a groin complaint have a hernia?

Certainly, not every patient with a groin hernia requires surgical treatment. Elderly, debilitated, and inactive patients with asymptomatic hernias may best be left alone. With rare exceptions, symptomatic patients should all be treated. There is some debate about whether healthy and asymptomatic patients should be treated. The debate, as it evolves, will revolve around several factors. One of these is cost. Is it cost effective to surgically repair every hernia, and would this cost offset the sometimes increased cost of treating patients deferred who then develop a more complicated problem? Other factors will include age and health of the patient, type of work activity and risk of complications developing in an untreated hernia, location of the patient (do they live in a remote area or travel out of a preferred treatment area), increased difficulty of repair of a deferred and possibly larger hernia, and morbidity of the repair itself.

While the bias of this presentation is that this technique is useful for the majority of groin hernias, there are instances where it would not be an appropriate technique (see Indications) and even instances where it might not be the best technique. Although the repair is great for bilateral hernias and can be performed perhaps as easily as any other in obese patients, it might be easier to treat the morbidly obese patient with bilateral hernias using a laparoscopic approach. The point is, the surgeon should be prepared to treat each patient individually and have more than one procedure with which he or she is expert and even be willing to refer when appropriate. The surgeon should not try to force every patient into a single procedure or a single procedure on every patient, because there are always exceptions.

The final point involves a far too common occurrence, particularly but not exclusively among young surgeons. Not every patient with groin pain needs surgery. The groin area is particularly susceptible to injury. Muscle and ligamentous tears and strains can cause groin pain and even result in chronic pain, which will not improve with a hernia operation. Early, small, and occult hernias do exist and can be particularly difficult to diagnose, especially with femoral hernias. These can cause pain but in the absence of clear physical findings for a hernia, patience is prudent. Special caution is warranted in patients with a very short history of symptoms or a very long history of symptoms who do not demonstrate appropriate physical findings. Ultrasound is sometimes helpful but much too frequently overread. Caution is appropriate here if the surgeon is to avoid the not uncommon patient complaint after surgery that "the pain is worse now than before the surgery" or even that "the mesh must be causing the pain."

THE MESH PATCH

The Bard Kugel Patch (Davol, Cranston, RI) was developed to facilitate performance of the procedure. Although it started out as a simple, single layer of mesh it became progressively more complicated as it evolved in order to make performance of the procedure practical.

The patch is composed of two overlapping layers of a knitted, monofilament polypropylene mesh material that have been ultrasonically welded together (Fig. 1 and 2). Two concentric welds near the outer edge of the patch serve to contain a single polyester fiber spring or stiffener that helps the patch to unfold after placement and then maintain its intended configuration. This polyester "spring" is made a slightly greater diameter than the diameter of the space created between the top and bottom layer of mesh, which means that it is under tension when the patch is constructed.

One centimeter of mesh material extends beyond the outermost weld into which have been cut multiple radial slits. This outer fringe allows the patch to conform and fill more perfectly the irregular spaces and structures encountered in the preperitoneal space, particularly where the patch will fold back over the iliac vessels.

In the center of the patch is a single transverse slit, in the anterior layer only, which is utilized for insertion and positioning of the patch. Just beyond the anterior slit and inside of the inner of the two welds are multiple 3-mm holes through both layers of the patch. These serve to allow tissue-to-tissue contact through the patch for purposes of increasing friction and resistance to movement of the patch after placement. This is further augmented by several small V-shaped cuts associated with some of these holes in the anterior layer only. These cuts create a triangle of mesh, which tends to "pop up" when the patch is placed and then act as "sutureless" anchors for the patch.

There are two common sizes used for groin hernias. The small patch is 8 × 12 cm and the medium patch is 11 × 14 cm. The small patch is probably adequate most of the time, although the larger patch does provide a little greater margin for error and is preferred for use with very large hernias, especially direct hernias.

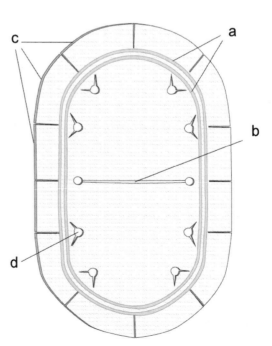

Fig. 1. Hernia mesh patch.

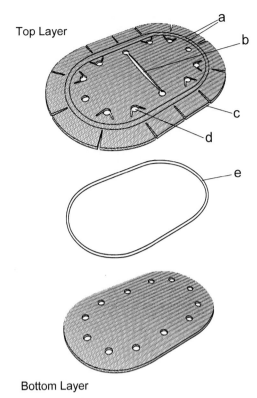

Fig. 2. Hernia mesh patch (exploded view).

OPERATIVE PROCEDURE

Anesthesia

Local Anesthesia

This procedure can usually be performed quite easily under local anesthesia and may be the preferred choice in certain high risk patients. It is useful to mix a rapid-acting agent (i.e., 1% xylocaine) with a long-acting agent (i.e., 0.5% bupivacaine) in a 50:50 ratio, neutralizing the acidity a little with the addition of a small amount of sodium bicarbonate. The addition of intravenous sedation may be necessary in some patients to keep the patient sufficiently comfortable. Furthermore, it is prudent to spray the local anesthetic mixture into the preperitoneal space as the dissection progresses. Very obese patients and those bilateral hernias or recurrent hernias may be more challenging if the surgery is performed under local anesthesia.

It is always advisable to inject a long-acting local anesthetic preemptively, prior to the incision, when performing the operation under general anesthesia and at the end of the procedure when using regional anesthesia.

General Anesthesia

This is the anesthetic of choice for patients who may, for one reason or another, be unable to cooperate fully. It is usually the back-up option of last resort. The primary disadvantage, other than any associated medical risk, is the limitation on the ability to test the repair at completion. This can be an important issue, and therefore may eliminate general anesthesia as the first choice for the majority of patients.

Regional Anesthesia

This is the preferred choice for most patients, with epidural anesthesia being somewhat preferred over spinal anesthesia. It is usually very effective and well tolerated. Both spinal and epidural anesthetics can be administered in a short-acting form, which should allow the patient to depart the surgical facility in quick fashion. The epidural anesthetic has the added advantage for redosing when a catheter is left in place during the procedure. This not only allows for a minimal initial dose, but also for the administration of additional doses, if needed, which is particularly useful with bilateral hernias. Furthermore, epidural anesthesia usually results in less muscle paralysis, enabling the patient to respond somewhat more forcefully when testing the repair following completion.

PATIENT PREPARATION

It is, of course, wise to have patients discontinue all aspirin-like products at least a week before surgery and anticoagulants 3 to 5 days prior to surgery when possible. The only lab and radiographs obtained would be those specific to the individual patient.

Use of prophylactic antibiotics is warranted in high-risk patients such as those with valvular heart disease or prosthetic joints. The slightly higher incision location and limited dissection associated with this procedure appears to have limited the infection risk, and no clear advantage for routine use of antibiotics has been demonstrated. The routine use, however, involves little added risk or cost and can therefore be used per the surgeon's personal preference, but regular use may be doing more to treat the surgeon than the patient.

A limited shave of the incision area is followed immediately by an antiseptic prep, which includes the lower abdomen and groin, including the scrotum.

The surgical procedure is easy to perform, with the patient in the supine position in most cases. Exposure may be improved, however, by placing the patient in a slight Trendelenburg position and rotating the patient away from the operative side.

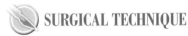 **SURGICAL TECHNIQUE**

Although there are certain aspects of the repair peculiar to the type of hernia encountered, the basic repair is the same regardless of the type of hernia and the mesh patch is placed in the same fashion and into the same position in every patient.

This repair is not usually difficult to perform, but for many surgeons the repair can be more difficult to learn than an anterior repair because of a lack of familiarity with the anatomy both in the posterior space and from this angle of approach. Understanding the anatomy is key to the successful performance of this procedure. For this reason, when learning this procedure the surgeon is well advised to consider a "hands-in" experience with another well-trained surgeon who has successfully completed at least 50 procedures and preferably more than 100. Ideal first patients are those of "average" size or on the thin side where the anatomy should be clearly visible. Avoid recurrent hernias or especially large scrotal hernias in the first 10 or 15 cases. When the first cases are scheduled in a manner to allow the surgeon time to more leisurely explore the field and investigate the anatomy, the experience will prove to be much more pleasurable and informative.

Not recommended for the first few cases are patients who have undergone

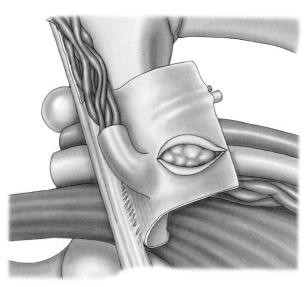

Fig. 13. Femoral hernia (skin and subcutaneous tissue removed, left groin).

If the gauze sponge was left under the malleable retractor to help restrain the peritoneum, it should be removed at this time. The malleable retractor is removed next and it is then inserted through the transverse slit in the mesh and used to complete insertion of the patch until it just drops into the preperitoneal space (Fig. 17).

After the malleable retractor is removed, the patch should tend to spring open. An index finger is then inserted over the top of the patch, pushing all edges of the patch into position. The finger is used to follow the entire outer edge of the patch to ensure that it has opened completely and that there are no kinks or sharp bends in the outer ring. Any sharp bends in the outer ring of the patch indicate a failure of the patch to fully deploy. In this situation, the patch has either not been inserted into the proper plane or more likely the dissection pocket is too small and needs to be enlarged. Small fibrous bands interfering with patch deployment may simply be bro-

ken up with careful digital manipulation, but if this fails to free up the patch sufficiently enough to allow it to completely open, it may be necessary to remove the patch in order to rework the pocket.

When properly placed, the patch should roughly parallel the inguinal ligament and extend medial over to the symphysis pubis and lateral and superior beyond the transversalis incision and split internal oblique muscle by a couple of centimeters. The posterior edge of the patch should lay back onto the iliac vessels about 2 to 3 cm posterior to the internal ring. The anterior slit in the patch should lie under the inferior epigastric vessels. (Fig. 18)

In this position, the patch will end up sandwiched between the peritoneum on one side and the transversalis fascia, the cord structures (or round ligament in the female), internal ring, femoral canal, and the Cooper ligament on the other side. The upper edge of the patch should lie under the upper edge of the incision in the transversalis fascia and thus protect against an incisional hernia through this space. When the medial edge of the patch extends over to the symphysis, the Hesselbach triangle should be completely covered along with the femoral canal and the internal ring. This results in a "total repair".

Closure

A long-acting local anesthetic is sprayed into the preperitoneal space prior to closure. The transversalis fascia is then next loosely closed with a single interrupted stitch with an absorbable suture, which "catches" the anterior layer of the patch near the medial–superior edge of the patch but just inside of the two tissue apposition holes in the patch. This is intended as a "restraining" stitch and not a fixating stitch. The goal is to restrain movement of the patch in an anterior direction but not deform the patch as can occur if the stitch is tied too tightly (especially in heavier patients with thicker preperitoneal fat). Multiple fixating stitches create two-point fixation, which is believed to interfere with hydrostatic tissue forces that develop when the two wet tissue surfaces are allowed to more perfectly conform to the patch. These tissue forces are believed to be important to proper patch stability.

The internal oblique muscle is not sutured to avoid potential nerve injury but simply allowed to reapproximate naturally. Great care should be taken, as well, when closing the external oblique fascia if nerve injury is to be avoided. A simple running stitch with an absorbable suture is sufficient here. Additional local anesthetic can

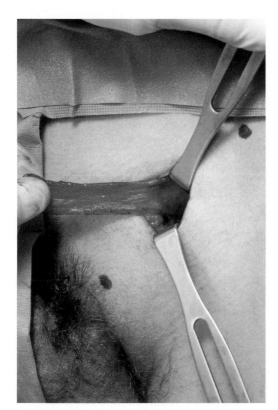

Fig. 14. Creating the preperitoneal pocket with an indirect hernia sac (left groin).

Nongastrointestinal Transabdominal

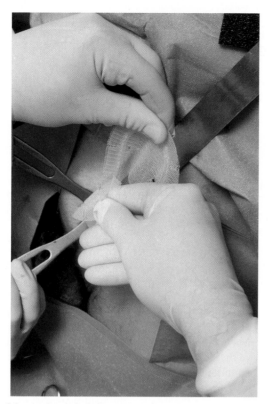

Fig. 15. Insertion of the mesh patch (left groin).

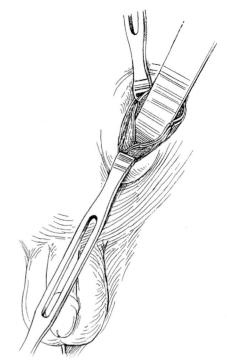

Fig. 17. Completing insertion of the patch using the malleable retractor (left groin).

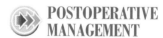

be infiltrated at this time and the remainder of the wound closed per the surgeon's preference.

An inguinal examination can be performed while encouraging the patient to cough to test the repair, and this is a worthwhile exercise to ensure proper patch placement and further to identify any possible missed "lipoma of the cord," which it may be wise to remove if found. Application of a pressure dressing will help to minimize hematoma formation and ecchymosis.

POSTOPERATIVE MANAGEMENT

With a short-acting regional or local anesthetic and limited sedation the patient can usually be discharged to home within a couple of hours. After general anesthesia, the patient may require a longer period of observation. The night of surgery the patient is encouraged to be ambulatory but to go slow and eat light.

The day following surgery, the patient is encouraged to ambulate somewhat more vigorously. While no specific restrictions are placed on the patient regarding activity, including lifting, the patient is cautioned that his or her greatest discomfort can be expected during the first 2 days and that it should taper off rapidly thereafter. Patients are asked to increase their activities a little

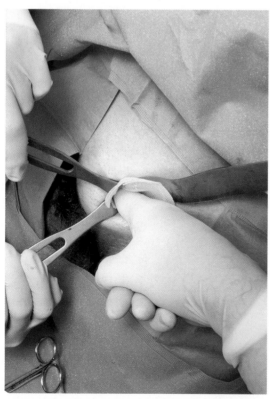

Fig. 16. Insertion of the mesh patch using a single index finger over a malleable retractor (left groin).

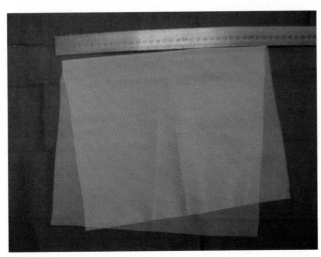

Fig. 3. A piece of the polyester Dacron mesh used for the prosthesis—supple, sticky, available in very large dimensions, and cheap.

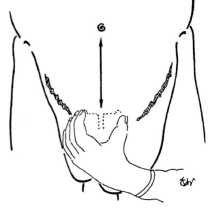

Fig. 5. The midline subumbilical incision in a patient with a bilateral recurrent groin hernia. The left hand of the surgeon easily finds the two pubic tubercles by palpation and, thereby, the inferior middle point of the incision.

suffering ventilatory insufficiency may need progressive pneumoperitoneum. The operation for the insertion of the giant prosthesis requires general, spinal, or epidural anesthesia. We advise surgeons against the use of local anesthesia, but point out that Wantz uses it in a unilateral half-cut GPRVS.

The following equipment should be present: mounted peanut swabs for the retroperitoneal separation; straight valve retractors for retraction of the abdominal wall; Ombredanne forceps or snares for handling the spermatic cord; a sterile ruler, straight scissors, and eight curved Kelly forceps for the measurement, cutting, and no-touch handling of the prosthesis; small suction drains; and slowly absorbing synthetic sutures.

Operation for a Typical Bilateral Hernia in a Male Patient

Midline Preperitoneal Approach

The patient lies in a slight Trendelenburg position. The surgeon and nurse stand on one side and the assistant on the other. After antiseptic preparation of the skin, an adhesive plastic shield is used to protect the incision from skin contamination. The abdominal wall is incised in the midline (Fig. 5). The umbilicoprevesical fascia is cut along its entire length with Mayo scissors.

The preperitoneal and prevesical cleavage is begun inferiorly and medially in the space of Retzius with a mounted swab. Dissection progresses laterally under the rectus abdominis muscle on the side

opposite the surgeon and posteriorly to the inferior epigastric vessels. Cleavage continues downward, anterior (ventral) to the bladder, to the prostatic fossa, and behind the iliopubic ramus in the space of Bogros. The pedicle of the hernia is isolated on the side opposite the surgeon, either distinct from the spermatic cord (in direct inguinal or femoral hernias) or connected to it (in indirect inguinal hernias) (Fig. 6). The iliopsoas muscle and external iliac vessels within their sheath are exposed. This dissection does not require delicate pressure, even in re-recurrent hernias, and is not problematic for the surgeon regardless of level of experience. The hernial sacs are treated differently according to the degree of adhesion to the neck of the myopectineal orifice. In instances of primary treatment of moderate-sized hernias, continuous moderate traction followed by resection or turning inside out can be sufficient. Conversely, a strong adherent sac of a multirecurrent hernia with a large neck sometimes needs to be freed by scalpel or scissors, with a finger introduced through an opening in the peritoneal infundibulum to assist the dissection.

After the sac has been treated, the preperitoneal cleavage is continued easily and quickly below the external iliac vessels and laterally along the psoas muscle. It is of no use to continue this work upward beyond the line of Douglas, where the peritoneum is adherent and prone to tearing. The cleavage of the spaces of Retzius and Bogros is done quickly and easily, with a single, flat retractor placed under the abdominal wall and the surgeon's left hand, displacing peritoneum.

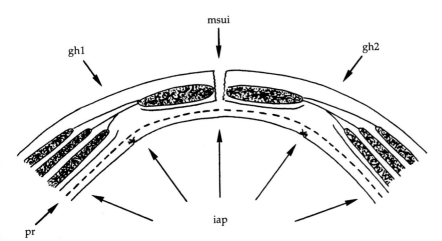

Fig. 4. Schematic horizontal cross section of the lower part of the abdominal wall showing how intra-abdominal pressure (iap) fixes the prosthesis (pr). msui, midline subumbilical incision; gh1 and gh2, groin hernias 1 and 2.

Nongastrointestinal Transabdominal

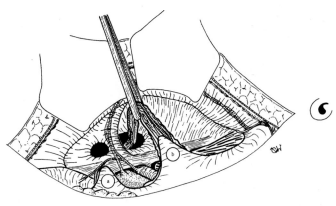

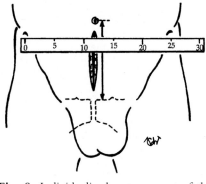

Fig. 8. Individualized measurement of the prosthesis.

Fig. 6. Intraoperative view of the retroparietal cleavage on the right side of a patient with a pantaloon hernia; a, direct, and b, indirect inguinal sacs after their reduction dorsally. The head of the patient is on the right.

The parietalization of the components of the spermatic cord greatly simplifies the placement of the giant prosthesis so that opening the mesh to allow passage of the spermatic cord is not required. For this purpose, the spermatic cord is retracted with a snare so that scissors easily separate the funicular elements from the peritoneal envelope. Beginning at the retroperitoneal convergence of these structures, freeing is performed with mounted swabs. At this stage, one can see an areolar sheath of triangular shape—which is the retroparietal segment of the funicular sheath—that is carefully preserved; the medial margin contains the ductus deferens and the lateral margin contains the spermatic vessels (Fig. 7). When the funicular elements are relaxed, they appear parietalized, and no pedicle can be seen crossing the preperitoneal and prevesical cleavage spaces.

Now the surgeon changes sides to achieve the retroperitoneal cleavage on the opposite side, which proceeds as described previously.

Placement of the Giant Prosthesis

The prosthesis should be measured directly on the patient to allow the implantation of the largest piece possible. The correct transverse dimension of the prosthesis is equal to the distance between the right and left anterosuperior iliac spines, minus 2 cm, and the correct vertical dimension is equal to the distance between the umbilicus and the pubis (Fig. 8). The mean dimensions are 26 cm transversely and 15 cm vertically. The prosthesis is then cut into a chevron shape according to the patient's measurements. A no-touch technique is mandatory. The chevron shape allows the prosthesis to run beyond the musculopectineal orifices and to correspond to the line of Douglas (Fig. 9). Before being inserted, the mesh is briefly soaked in povidone-iodine solution.

The giant prosthesis is then simply spread out in place by grasping its corners and the middle of each side with eight long Kelly forceps (Fig. 10). Figure 11 aims to help the surgeon to under-

stand the main principle of the operation and shows the relation of the wide bilateral prosthesis with the visceral sac and the spermatic cords. The prosthesis is first positioned on the side opposite the surgeon. While the assistant lifts and retracts the abdominal wall, the surgeon displaces the peritoneum with his or her left hand toward himself or herself and upward, thereby opening the cleavage plane. Placement is achieved by pushing the prosthesis into position with the Kelly forceps. The forceps on the middle lower margin of the mesh are placed first between the pubis and the urinary bladder, followed successively by the forceps on the inferior lateral corner, the middle point of the lateral margin, and finally the upper lateral corner (Fig. 12). The forceps are pushed as far as possible under the abdominal wall, thereby unfolding the mesh and placing it at the inferior, lateral, and posterior limits of the

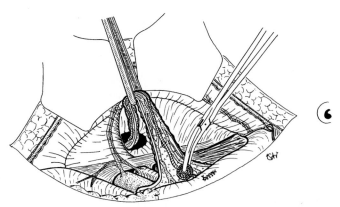

Fig. 7. Parietalization of the right cord elements. At the end of its separation from the peritoneum, the triangular funicular sheath contains and protects the spermatic vessels laterally (**right**) and the ductus deferens medially (**left**). The head of the patient is on the right.

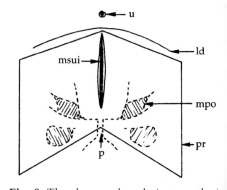

Fig. 9. The chevron-shaped giant prosthesis (pr), the angled superior margin of which fits the line of Douglas (ld) and inferior points overlap the two musculopectineal orifices (mpo) and anchor the prosthesis downward. The midline subumbilical wound (msui) is also protected. u, umbilicus; p, pubic symphysis.

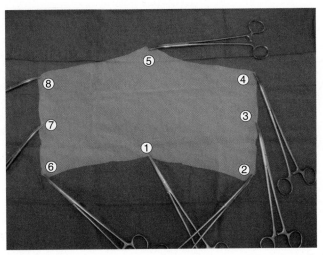

Fig. 10. Photograph of the chevron-shaped prosthesis grasped by eight long Kelly forceps for its no-touch handling and easy correct placement. The numbers 1 to 8 indicate the order of placement of the clamps, beginning on the right side of the patient.

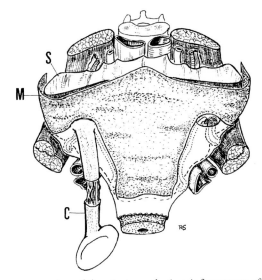

Fig. 11. Schematic representation of the giant prosthetic reinforcement of the visceral sac after parietalization of the spermatic cords contained in their preserved spermatic sheaths. C, spermatic cord; M, giant bilateral mesh prosthesis; S, visceral sac.

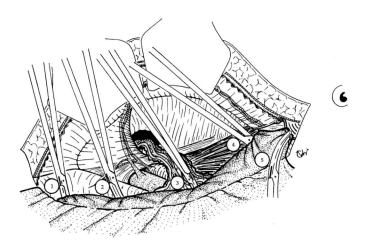

Fig. 12. Placing the right part of the bilateral prosthesis in the right side of the patient, as seen by the surgeon. The order of placement of the Kelly clamps is indicated by the numbers 1 through 5.

retroperitoneal dissection (Figs. 13 and 14). In this way, the prosthesis envelops the peritoneum on the side opposite the surgeon.

When the forceps have been pushed as far as possible, the assistant immobilizes them until the surgeon removes his or her left hand, thereby allowing the visceral sac to resume its normal position. The retractor of the abdominal wall is also removed at this time. The Kelly forceps are then loosened and withdrawn by carefully slipping them against the deep surface of the abdominal wall, in the same position as that used to place them initially. The surgeon again changes sides and repeats the same procedure on the other side.

This method of implantation leads to full unfolding of the Dacron mesh, which now widely envelops the peritoneum and extends well beyond the limits of both the myopectineal holes, and also protects the midline subumbilical incisional wound. One single stitch of slowly absorbing material fixes the middle of the upper edge of the mesh to the lower margin of Richet's umbilical fascia (Fig. 15).

Closure and Drainage

When necessary, suction drains are installed anterior to the prosthesis (Fig. 16). If the hernia is voluminous, it may be worthwhile to position one or two suction drains in the scrotum.

Closure of the midline incisional wound is then achieved using No. 3 to No. 5 slowly absorbing synthetic material. The subcutaneous fat is approximated with fine absorbable sutures while the skin is closed with fine monofilament nylon.

One should be reminded that, in the course of this technique, no direct repair procedure is done on the hernial orifice, per se. The surgeon's work consists of simply achieving wide cleavage of the retroperitoneal areolar spaces and cutting out an appropriately large piece of mesh to envelop the endoabdominal fascia in the area of the hernial orifices on both sides and the midline wounds, thereby preventing the recurrence of the hernia or median wound dehiscence.

Postoperative Care

The patient is urged to go about early unrestricted activity; this is easy because there is little postoperative discomfort. Slow-acting heparin is used for the first few days after the operation. Prophylactic antibiotic therapy is now routinely used by legal obligation in France (cephalosporin of

Nongastrointestinal Transabdominal

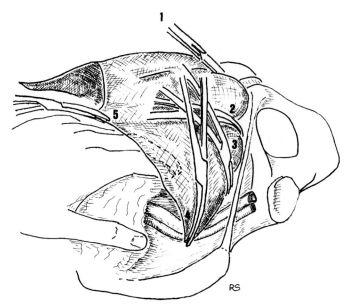

Fig. 13. Schematic representation of the placement of the right part of the bilateral prosthesis, as seen by an observer watching the operation from the right side of the patient, after virtual removal of the abdominal wall muscles. The order of placement of the Kelly clamps is indicated by the numbers 1 through 5. (Modified from Fig. 6–27 of Wantz GE. Atlas of hernia surgery. New York: Raven Press, with permission.)

first-generation flash). Suction drains and dressings are removed on the 2nd postoperative day. The patient is discharged from the hospital on the 2nd to the 5th postoperative day.

TECHNICAL VARIATIONS

The surgical procedure can be altered in several ways.

1. The Pfannenstiel incision proposed by Rignault is of cosmetic interest. It carries some risk of superficial nerve injury and hematomas.
2. When the hernial contents adhere to a scrotal sac, dissection and reduction are greatly simplified by freeing them through a separate inguinal incision (Fig. 17). The fundus of the sac can be left in the scrotum with an attendant

risk of seroma, which is prevented by suction drainage.
3. A Trendelenburg position is helpful in operating on obese patients.
4. The preperitoneal approach obviates most of the problems related to sliding hernias. The peritoneal sac is electively opened and the contents are reduced. Adequate resection of the sac is easy. The prosthetic repair protects well against the hazards resulting from a usually very large hernial orifice.
5. The simultaneous treatment of associated pelvic-abdominal intraperitoneal or extraperitoneal lesions—such as iliac incisional hernia, hydrocele, varicocele, or ovarian cysts—is possible if no contaminated procedures are envisioned.

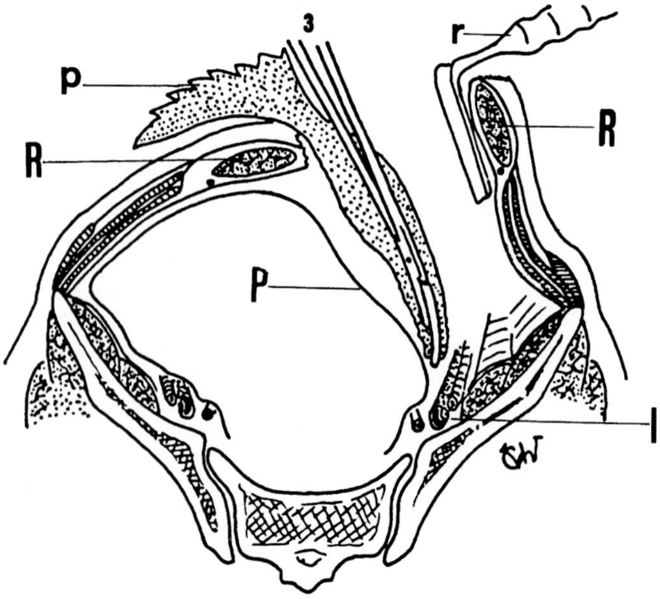

RESULTS

In 1984, I reviewed a series of 1,628 patients with 2,224 groin hernias operated on from 1970 to 1984 to compare the results of four techniques: the Bassini-Shouldice operation (BSO), the McVay-Cooper ligament repair (MVR), the inguinal patch (IP), and the GPRVS. The patients were 16 to 103 years of age. The mean age was 55.8 years for men and 61.5 years for women. The sex ratio was 5.3 men to 1 woman. The clinical and anatomic types of the hernias were as follows: 38.9% were indirect inguinal hernias, 29.8% were direct inguinal hernias, 7.6% were groin eventrations, 5.5% were femoral hernias, and 18.2% were diverse miscellaneous hernias. Of the hernias, 814 (36.6%) were bilateral (407 patients) and 349 (15.6%) were recurrent. Operation was performed on 153 patients (9.3%) for acute complications. The BSO technique was used to treat 109 hernias (5.0%), the MVR to treat 564 (25.3%), the IP to treat 215 (9.6%), the GPRVS to treat 1,223 (55%), and other techniques to treat 113 (5.1%).

POSTOPERATIVE COURSE

An uncomplicated postoperative course was noted in 97 (89%) patients who had BSO, 512 (90.7%) who had MVR, 191 (88.9%) who had IP, and 1,126 (92%) who had GPRVS. Hence, similarly favorable postoperative courses have been observed for every technique. The BSO was used for some complicated hernias, and GPRVS was used for the most unfavorable ones. Hematoma rates reported were 3.66% after BSO, 3.25% after IP, and 5.15% after

Fig. 14. Schematic horizontal cross section of the lower part of the abdomen showing the correct positioning of the third (right mediolateral) Kelly forceps, pushed posteriorly and vertically toward the iliac vessels. 3, right mediolateral Kelly forceps; I, iliac vessels; p, prosthesis; P, peritoneal sac; r, retractor; R, recti muscles.

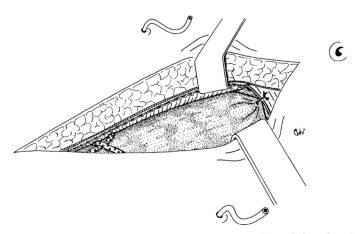

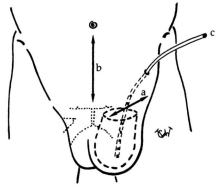

Fig. 15. The giant prosthesis has been placed on both sides. A single stitch fixes the middle of the superior margin of the prosthesis to the umbilical fascia of Richet.

Fig. 17. Direct upper scrotal incision (a) combined with the medial subumbilical route for freeing adherent contents of a scrotal sac (b). c, Scrotal suction drain.

GPRVS. This represents no significant difference between the techniques in the incidence of hematoma formation.

The sepsis rates were 4.58% after BSO, 2.3% after IP, and 2.15% after GPRVS. It should be noted that the BSO was used for complicated hernias.

Other complications observed were 28 (1.7%) chest infections: 10 after herniorrhaphies, 16 after GPRVS, and 2 after IP; 6 (0.27%) instances of phlebitis: 3 after MVR and 3 after GPRVS; and 3 (0.13%) pulmonary embolisms: 1 after an MVR and 2 after GPRVS.

During the 1st postoperative month, 26 deaths occurred, a mortality of 1.59%. Seventeen patients (2.5%) died after herniorrhaphies, 2 (0.93%) after IP, and 7 (0.57%) after GPRVS. All patients who died were elderly people with acutely complicated hernias.

In 1989, in another personal series of 529 GPRVS repairs, I reported 2.1% of hematomas, 1.3% of sepsis, and no death. These data can be considered the results of improved indications of GPRVS.

FOLLOW-UP STUDIES

Follow-up studies lasting 2 to 10 years were conducted on 1,664 hernias treated surgically, or 74.8% of all hernias. Of these 1,664 hernias, 113 (6.8%) had recurred: 16.5% after BSO, 11.1% after MVR, 11.5% after IP, and 1.4% after GPRVS. These recurrences after GPRVS happened at the beginning of our experience because the prostheses were too small or had slits in them. It should also be emphasized that the recurrence rate after 1 year increased to 27.8% of the total number after BSO and 31.4% after MVR, whereas no worsening of the results was seen after GPRVS.

Among the sequelae observed were six instances of testicular atrophy and 55 instances of pain, all of them after IP.

The late migration of the bladder after a preperitoneal prosthesis was placed during a prostatectomy obliges me to condemn the use of a giant prosthesis when septic maneuvers are performed simultaneously.

Finally, the personal 1984 series study emphasizes the favorable results of the preperitoneal prosthetic repair of groin hernias when compared with other techniques. Moreover, the results obtained by other surgeons are in agreement with our personal observations. In 1989, while checking the recurrence rates in another personal series involving 529 repairs with GPRVS, I noted a rate of 0.56% for primary repairs and 1.1% for recurring hernia repairs.

REMARKS

The risk of sepsis is not caused by the implantation of heterogeneous material and should no longer militate against the use of such material. A strict discipline is an efficient rule for avoiding septic complications. When faced with any kind of superficial infection, one must reopen the wound, even more so when a deeper sepsis occurs that is related to the prosthesis. It was never necessary to remove the prosthesis when the abscess could be correctly drained. Some patients, who were sent to us from other hospitals with late sepsis and fistulae, needed fistulography followed by a thorough surgical excision of the sinus tract.

GPRVS is a logical method. The Dacron mesh acts as an artificial endoabdominal fascia that prevents recurrences and at the same time protects all weak points of the lower part of the abdominal wall. The benign nature of the operation leads to a simple postoperative course, and the technique has many intraoperative advantages: simplicity of a quick incision, nonbloody dissection of the retrofascial spaces, good exposure of the hernia, facility of the parietalization of the elements of the spermatic cord, no dangerous maneuvers (no threats to the iliofemoral vessels), and no need to close the hernial orifice or fix the prosthesis. All these allow a short operation (20 to 40 minutes for a bilateral hernia).

Although I advise against locoregional anesthesia because of the increased septic risk incompatible with the use of a prosthesis, I recommend epidural anesthesia for patients who have respiratory problems. Again, I mention that Wantz uses local anesthesia for unilateral half-cut GPRVS in a day-surgery setting.

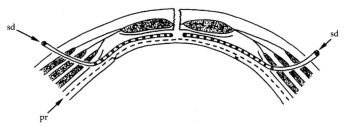

Fig. 16. Horizontal cross section of the lower part of the abdominal wall, showing the position of the suction drains (sd) in front of the giant prosthesis (pr) in a patient with a bilateral hernia.

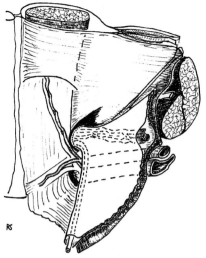

Fig. 18. The triangular retroparietal segment of the right spermatic sheath, containing the spermatic vessels (laterally) and the ductus deferens (medially).

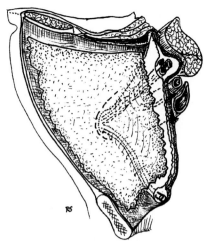

Fig. 20. Correct procedure for separation: the right part of the prosthesis has not been slit and is separated from the iliac vessels by the spermatic sheath.

Giant prosthetic repair is not a question of a major operation for a simple illness but of an operation correctly adapted both to the cure of certain hernias that have become more serious and to ensuring that they do not recur. The efficiency of GPRVS has been proved by our results and by the experiences of other surgeons. Groin hernias are a deficiency disease, and the general concept behind their repair is to conveniently reinforce the deficient tissue or replace what is missing. Why not use a mesh and a simple technique?

As for recurrences, there were six in my 1984 series. Early in my staff experi-ence, we used too small a piece of Dacron mesh; the hernias that recurred did so around the lower or lateral edge of the prosthesis. Reoperations by the inguinal approach permitted efficient fixation of the questionable edge of the prosthesis to the iliac fascia or the Cooper's ligament.

What about a further operation? All intraperitoneal procedures can be per-formed without any technical change, but an open operation on the bladder or prostate must take into consideration retroparietopubic sclerosis, which necessi-tates separating the bladder from the pu-bic bone with a xyster. The iliac vessels may be involved by the periprosthetic scar sclerosis if the foreign material is placed directly in contact with them; this may be an obstacle to the approach to these ves-sels in vascular surgical procedures, organ transplantation, or lymph node dissection. Fortunately, this consequence can be avoided by two simple but important technical details: (a) carefully preserving the triangular spermatic sheath around the ductus deferens and the spermatic ves-sels (Figs. 18–20) as a natural means of covering and protecting the iliac vessels; and (b) not slitting the mesh to let the cord pass through (see Fig. 19), but plac-ing it posteriorly to the cord contained in its own sheath, thus separating the vessels from the mesh by the thickness of the spermatic sheath.

For more than 25 years, in agreement with the work of Rives, I have also devel-oped the use of giant mesh prostheses for the repair of large incisional hernias (LIHs). The basic principles of the technique are roughly the same as those applied to groin hernias: large pieces of mesh deeply inter-posed between peritoneal sac and wall, widely reinforcing and overlapping the weak area. Intra-abdominal pressure is not the sole factor in the appearance and devel-opment of incisional hernias, however. The role of a kind of progressively bursting torque usually leads to a wide muscular di-astasis. Therefore, the surgeon must work not only to close the defect, but also to re-construct a reinsertion tendon for the sep-arated muscles (Fig. 21).

It is mandatory that before the opera-tion, the surgeon take care to evaluate and

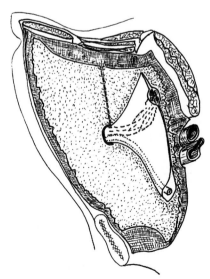

Fig. 19. A wrong slitting of the right part of the prosthesis, which is in contact with the right iliac vessels.

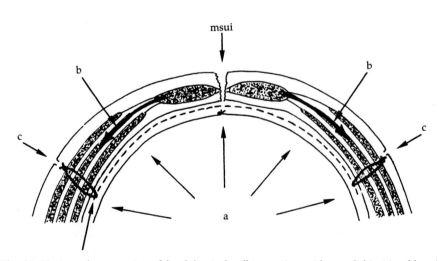

Fig. 21. Horizontal cross section of the abdominal wall in a patient with a medial incisional hernia treated by prosthetic repair. The intra-abdominal pressure contributes to the face-to-face reinsertion of the muscles on the interposed prosthesis. **a,** Arrows show the action of intra-abdominal pressure. **b,** Arrows show the disrupting torque related to the action of the lateral abdominal muscles. **c,** Bury-ing incisions for subcutaneous suturing of the prosthesis. msui, midline subumbilical incision.

manage the dangerous problems linked to large hernias that affect respiratory, circulatory, visceral, and spinal functions by adapting the preparation of the patient. When intraoperative or postoperative difficulties are foreseeable, I use pneumoperitoneum before the operation, with satisfactory results.

The results of prosthetic repair of LIHs are unsurpassable, as proved by a study of 409 LIHs in a series of 616 incisional hernias treated between 1971 and 1985. Of the 409 hernias, 208 were LIHs (collar diameter, >10 cm), 132 were medium-sized incisional hernias (collar diameter, 6 to 10 cm), and 69 were incisional hernias with multiple orifices. The incisional hernia was a primary occurrence in 296 cases, a recurrence in 52, and a re-recurrence (two to six times) in 61. Of the 409 patients, 389 underwent a prosthetic repair (289 primary, 48 recurring, and 52 re-recurring) and 20 underwent a nonprosthetic repair because of either general or septic risks. Of the 389 who underwent prosthetic repairs, 346 patients (89%) had uncomplicated courses, as did 17 (85%) of the 20 who had nonprosthetic repairs. The sepsis rate was 6.1% for prosthetic repairs and 5% for nonprosthetic repairs; none of the prostheses was removed, and all sepsis healed after treatment of the complication. The mortality rate related to general risks was 2% after prosthetic repairs and 5% after nonprosthetic ones. Findings after a mean follow-up of 5.5 years were available for 257 prosthetic repairs (67.5% of survivors) and 15 nonprosthetic repairs (79% of survivors). The success rate among control patients treated for LIH was 91% (234 patients) after prosthetic repair and 33.3% (5 patients) after non-

prosthetic repairs. In the whole series of 616 incisional hernias, the success rate was 85.5% for prosthetic repairs and 48% for nonprosthetic repairs. These results confirm those from other authors' series, and they are similar to those of Rives. They perhaps may encourage experienced surgeons to use retromuscular prostheses for repairing all types of incisional hernias, not just LIHs, and also all medial hernias with a risk of recurrence.

Without ruling out suture techniques used in simple hernias, I frequently use GPRVS in the treatment of recurrent and complex groin hernias. The Dacron mesh used in large pieces is comparable to a kind of nonabsorbable endoabdominal fascia that virtually prevents all recurrences. The comparative results of the four different techniques applied to groin hernias are, in my experience, evidence in favor of prosthetic repair. The precautions aimed at eliminating septic incidents are especially important, but simply relevant to correct surgical asepsis. I believe it is not possible to ignore the extraordinary possibilities offered by prostheses in the surgical treatment of groin and large incisional hernias. Moreover, as Nyhus has said, hernia repair should continue to be individualized, after a hoped-for, universally accepted classification; thus, I think that GPRVS will be used in the future to cure difficult cases of groin and ventral groin hernia.

ACKNOWLEDGMENTS

I would like to express my gratitude to Dr. Christian Warlaumont, a hernia surgeon and a friend, for having studied one of my series in his medical thesis and pro-

viding his artistic talents (Figs. 1, 2, 5–9, 12, 14–17, 21).

SUGGESTED READING

Fruchaud H. *Anatomie chirurgicale des hernies de l'aine.* Paris: Doin, 1956.

Houdard C, Stoppa R. *Le traitement chirurgical des hernies de l'aine.* Paris: Masson, 1984.

Nyhus LM, Condon RE, eds. *Hernia,* 4th ed. Philadelphia: Lippincott, 1995.

Rives J. Major incisional hernias. In: Chevrel JP, ed. *Surgery of the abdominal wall.* Paris: Springer-Verlag, 1987:116.

Rives J, Lardennois B, Hibon J. Traitement moderne des hernies de l'aine et de leurs récidives. *Tech Chir Appareil Dig* 1973;1(40110):1.

Schumpelick V, Kingsnorth AN. *Incisional hernia.* New York: Springer-Verlag, 1999.

Stoppa RE. The treatment of complicated groin and incisional hernias. *World J Surg* 1989;13:545.

Stoppa RE. Advances in the care of large incisional hernias. *Hospimedica* 1992;5:43.

Stoppa R, Henry X, Canarelli JP, et al. Les indications de méthodes sélectionnées dans le traitement des éventrations postopératoires. *Chirurgie* 1979;105:276.

Stoppa R, Petit J, Abourachid H, et al. Procédé original de plastic des hernies de l'aine: l'interposition sans fixation d'une prothèse en tulle de Dacron par voie médiane sous-péritonéale. *Chirurgie* 1973;99:547.

Stoppa R, Ralamiaramanana F, Henry X, et al. Evolution of large ventral incisional repair: the French contribution to a difficult problem. *Hernia* 1999;3:1.

Stoppa RE, Rives JL, Warlaumont CR, et al. The use of Dacron in the repair of hernias of the groin. *Surg Clin North Am* 1984;64:269.

Stoppa RE, Warlaumont CR. The preperitoneal approach and prosthetic repair of groin hernia. In: Nyhus LM, Condon RE, eds. *Hernia,* 3rd ed. Philadelphia: JB Lippincott, 1989:199.

Wantz GE. *Atlas of hernia surgery.* New York: Raven, 1991:101.

Nongastrointestinal Transabdominal

EDITOR'S COMMENT

This chapter is the embodiment of the response of the surgeon to the concept initially proposed by Fruchaud, that of the myopectineal orifice through which most hernias protrude through the abdominal wall. Rives and Stoppa proposed what is here—the ultimate answer to the weakened myopectineal orifice. They reasoned and argued that the pressure on hernias is from posterior to the peritoneum, and it makes little sense, therefore, to try and fix them from anterior, when actually the pressures that form the hernias are from dorsal, not ventral. Most of the traditional repairs—the Bassini, the Shouldice, the McVay-Anson Cooper's Ligament Repair—fix the hernia from ventral to

the forces that result in the protrusion of tissue through the myopectineal orifice.

In truth, many of the other chapters in these volumes also bespeak the need to provide a prosthesis dorsal to the hernia defect, whether or not one deals with plug repair by Gilbert, the prosthesis by Kugel, or a whole series of similar types of repairs (totally endoscopic preperitoneal [TEPP], transabdominal preperitoneal [TAPP]). This chapter takes the bull by the horns, as it were, and uses a giant prosthesis of sticky Dacron, perhaps less supple than polyester, which must be handled with care and which may shrink less, thus perhaps decreasing the postoperative pain from shrinkage, and interposes it between the

peritoneum and the defective myopectineal orifices. Because it is sticky, it requires the use of Kelly clamps to place it, and it is held in place just at one area, at the superior part of the middle of the mesh, with a single suture.

One of the things that Professor Stoppa points out is that in large scrotal hernias and in other hernias that have resulted in the loss of domain, a pneumoperitoneum is necessary. I agree entirely. If one has large amounts of viscera that have lost their right of domain and replaces them in the peritoneum, especially in people with impaired respiratory function, as seems to be common in most of the series, an abdominal compartment

(continued)

syndrome may result. I generally carry out a pneumoperitoneum by placing a port, very similarly as one would place a port for chemotherapy, within the abdomen, and refill the peritoneum with at least 1, and perhaps 2 L of air weekly and repeatedly, which generally enlarges the peritoneal capacity enough so that neither abdominal compartment syndrome nor respiratory insufficiency from a high diaphragm results.

One possible deficiency of this repair is its need for a somewhat longer length of hospital stay than traditional repairs. Although Wantz has done this on one side under a local anesthetic, one doubts that a prosthesis of this size can be placed under local, and one needs epidural, spinal, or general anesthetic. Length of stay according to this chapter is 2 to 5 days, and in other reports in the literature it is between 3 and 6 days. In the United States, this might be shortened to less than 2 days, but under no circumstance would it be day surgery.

In Professor Stoppa's results of his early review of 1984, the initial mortality recorded was 1.6%. Many of these patients were elderly, and so one could explain it on that basis. Another phenomenon, however, that one sees in elderly patients is that they have had a hernia for a long time, sometimes a very large hernia, which has not bothered them. However, when something does become bothersome, they request that the surgeon fix their hernia because they think that in doing so, it will correct whatever is really bothering them, which in fact may be anything from myocardial ischemia to carcinoma of the pancreas. Thus, significant mortality such as 1.6% is not surprising. Preoperative judgment, however, should weed out these patients so that a careful history should reveal that there are perhaps other symptoms. In his latest series, however, Professor Stoppa reports a much lower mortality.

With the exception of Wantz and the TEPP and TAPP, done laparoscopically, the open Stoppa Rives repair does not appear to have gained much traction in the United States, at least as far as I am aware. It does, however, appear to enjoy significant popularity worldwide. Maghsoudi and Pourzand (*Ann Saudi Med* 2005;25:228) reported on 234 patients, almost all of whom were men, with 420 inguinal hernias, of which 186 were bilateral. Patients' mean age was 60 years; almost half had one or more significant co-morbid conditions. Many of these patients had undergone surgery for one or two recurrences. Postoperative stay averaged 2.2 days and, similar to the author's, the operative time was 45 minutes. A less than 1% recurrence rate was reported. They deny postoperative neuralgia, chronic pain, testicular atrophy, or mesh infection, and there was no mortality. They are believers. Similar believers are from the University of Mumbai, India (Thapar V et al. *J Postgrad Med* 2000;46:80), who reported a much small series with 31 patients, mean age of 58, a slightly longer operative time at 65 minutes, and a slightly longer length of stay, 3.5 days, which may be social. No mesh infections or deaths were reported in four minor complications, with a 15-month follow-up.

From Holland, Beets et al. (*Br J Surg* 1996; 83:203) reported 75 patients with 150 bilateral hernias, of which by far the largest majority (126) were recurrent. Sixty patients (94%) of the surviving patients—indicating the advanced age of these patients—underwent a physical examination after 5.7 years. Two months after the operation, one patient had a recurrence, which appeared to be technical. The remainder did not recur at up to 6 years. Huang (*J Formos Med Assoc* 1999;98:122) proposed a somewhat different point of view in which unilateral first-timer recurrent hernias were treated by modified Shouldice technique. Multiple recurrences or bilateral hernia were treated with the Stoppa giant prosthesis. Interestingly, in the Shouldice group, a 4 × 10 cm preperitoneal mesh was used to reinforce the repair. I am not entirely certain what I would call this repair as it is a mesh repair underlying a Shouldice repair. The average hospital stay was 3 days for the unilateral repair and 6 days for the Stoppa procedure. The recurrence rates for the unilateral and Stoppa groups were 6% and 2%, respectively. Although there was one fatal myocardial infarction, the recurrence rates were low enough that the author proposes to use a modified Stoppa unilateral repair for the first-time recurrence and a giant prosthesis for subsequent recurrences.

Taken together, this repair seems to have a great deal of evidence for recommendation, but it is certainly a more extensive dissection than most of the plug and patch repairs, as well as the Lichtenstein tension-free repair, which appears to be the gold standard in the United States. Further experience with all of the plug-and-patch, TEPP, and TAPP, as well as giant prosthesis, should enable us to come to a conclusion following the basic Fruchaud myopectineal orifice hypothesis, and how best to deal with it.

J.E.F.

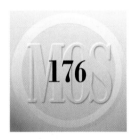

Lichtenstein Tension-Free Hernioplasty

176

PARVIZ K. AMID

Weakening of the abdominal wall tissue as one of the causes of inguinal hernias was suspected by Cooper as far back as 1800. The matter was emphasized again in 1922 by Harrison when he wondered why dozens and hundreds of men show hernias at 50–60 years after their active life is over. Need for prosthetic reinforcement of weakened abdominal wall tissue was recognized by Billroth, musing . . . "If only the proper material could be created to artificially produce tissue of density and toughness of fascia and tendon, the secret of the radical cure for hernia would be discovered." However, early generation of prosthesis resulted in disastrous complications from rejection and infection. It was not until the introduction of polypropylene mesh by Usher in 1959 that Billroth's dream was realized.

With the necessity of prosthesis for the repair of inguinal hernia in mind, and focusing on the principle of "no tension" (considered one of the great principles of surgery by Halstead), the Lichtenstein group popularized routine use of mesh in 1984 and coined the term "tension-free hernioplasty." During the rapid evolution of hernia surgery throughout the past decade, it was left to Nyhus to remove the previous generation's fear of infection and rejection of prosthesis, which he did when he stated in 1989, "My concerns relative to the potentially increased incidents of infection or rejection of polypropylene mesh have not been warranted to date."

Today, understanding the role of protease-antiprotease imbalance in the pathogenesis of groin hernias has led to a new grasp of the understanding of the pathology of groin hernias and the causes of their surgical failure. There is morphologic and biochemical evidence that adult male inguinal hernias are associated with altered collagen type I to type III ratio. These changes lead to weakening of the fibroconnective tissue of the groin and development of inguinal hernias. To use this already defective tissue, especially under tension, is a violation of the most basic principles of surgery. Furthermore, the tension resulting from approximation of the transverse tendon to structures, such as the inguinal ligament or iliopubic tract, may result in widening of the femoral ring and development of iatrogenic femoral hernias.

In the tension-free hernioplasty, instead of suturing anatomic structures that are not in apposition, the entire inguinal floor is reinforced by insertion of a sheet of mesh. The prosthesis that is placed between the transversalis fascia and the external oblique aponeurosis extends well beyond the Hesselbach triangle in order

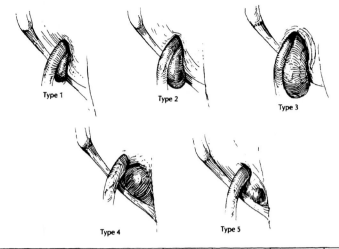

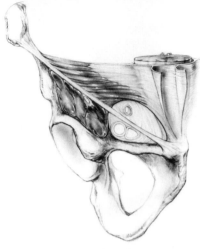

Type	1	2	3	4	5
Internal ring	<1FB	1FB	>1FB	Norm	Norm
Peritoneal sac	Y	Y	Y	N	N
Canal floor	I	I	DES	DES	DES (IFB)

Fig. 3. Gilbert classification for inguinal hernias. I, intact; FB, fingerbreadth; Norm, normal; N, no (peritoneal sac absent); Y, yes (peritoneal sac present); DES, destroyed.

Fig. 4. Myopectineal orifice. (From Wantz GE. *Atlas of hernia surgery.* New York: Raven Press, 1991, with permission.)

Nongastrointestinal Transabdominal

the peritoneum to reherniate. Cooper described the EOA as the "outer barrier" to the inguinal canal. Halsted's repair forfeited protection by that barrier, which in turn, gave up the "step-down" effect for the spermatic cord, considered to be another protective feature of the normal anatomy of the groin. Shouldice, of Toronto, reincarnated Bassini's original operation, mostly performing it using local anesthesia. The Shouldice operation became the "gold standard" and remained so until tension-free hernia repair with mesh was introduced.

Usher of Texas, in 1960, reported suturing a polyethylene mesh inlay patch deep to the transversalis fascia to do a "tension-eliminating" inguinal hernia repair. Lichtenstein of California, in 1970, used a polypropylene mesh as a rolled plug to perform "two-suture" plug repair of femoral hernias. Newman of New Jersey developed a tension-free technique for inguinal hernia using a polypropylene mesh onlay patch that he sutured over the posterior wall. Lichtenstein and Amid popularized Newman's technique to become a frequently used open-mesh tension-free procedure for groin hernias worldwide.

From 1958 until 1976, I used the modified Bassini technique with general or spinal anesthesia to repair all inguinal hernias. I estimate that it failed in 15% of primary hernias and 25% (or more) of recurrent hernias. After a visit to the Shouldice Hospital in Toronto in 1976, I began to use local anesthesia and to do the Shouldice repair using 3-0 Prolene suture instead of

metal wire. My failure rates of primary repairs dropped to less than 2% and of recurrent hernias to 8%. Encouraged by the work of Shockett in 1984, I began using polypropylene mesh routinely as an underlay supplement to the Shouldice operation for all primary and recurrent hernias. By placing a fortifying swatch of polypropylene mesh beneath the transversalis fascia, deep to the first suture line of a Shouldice repair, I reduced my own failure rate to less than 0.5% for primary hernias and to 3% for recurrent hernias. Even before the open tension-free anterior repair of inguinal hernias became popular, open posterior repairs attracted surgeons' interest through the works of Nyhus of Chicago and Condon of Milwaukee. They described musculoaponeurotic sutured repairs, sometimes with added mesh. Stoppa and Rives of France pioneered the concept that bilateral groin hernias can be repaired by widely wrapping the peritoneal bas with large mesh netting (giant reinforcement of the visceral sac), thereby blocking the viscera from entering any defect through either myopectineal orifice (MPO). The privilege of visiting and operating with Rene Stoppa in Amiens further convinced me that the ideal place to position mesh is in the properitoneal space, between the force of the hernia and the defect in the abdominal wall.

FUNCTIONAL CONSIDERATIONS

All groin hernias protrude through the MPO, a window in the lower abdominal

wall surrounded by musculoaponeurotic structures (Fig. 4). The MPO is bounded medially by the lateral edge of the rectus muscle and its fascia, superiorly by the transversus abdominus muscle, laterally by the iliopsoas muscle, and inferiorly by the pectineal ligament. It is divided into smaller inguinal and femoral windows by the inguinal ligament anteriorly and the iliopubic tract posteriorly. Groin hernias occur because of poor collagen content in the MPO. The hernia that presents clinically is in that part of the MPO that initially gives way to intra-abdominal pressure. When performing any repair, one should consider the plasticity of the canal's posterior wall and the deformation effect on vulnerable tissues that surround that defect. Appreciation of these factors is important to the long-term success of any repair in which a prosthetic device is used.

Preformed or handmade mesh plugs can be placed in the internal ring of indirect hernias or in the defect of direct hernias. The problem created by a plug in any primary hernia repair is that the remainder of the canal's unprotected posterior wall, medial and lateral to the plug, becomes subjected to an imbalance of plasticity. It is thereby rendered to have greater risk of herniation. The boundaries of the lateral triangle are the deep epigastric vessels, the middle third of the inguinal ligament, and a line from the junction of the upper and middle thirds of the inguinal ligament to where the deep epigastric vessels cross the lateral edge of the rectus muscle. It has been my observation that the majority of recurrences following pure tissue repairs presented in the medial triangle just above the pubic tubercle. Although half of tissue

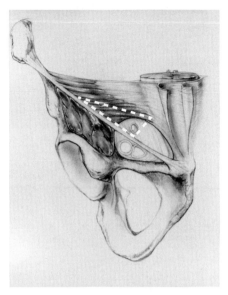

Fig. 5. Lateral triangle of the groin.

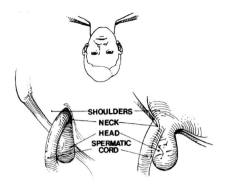

Fig. 6. Head, neck, and shoulders of the peritoneal sac.

repairs that failed occurred within 5 five years, other failures happened much later, some presenting decades after the original repair. Failures following prior mesh repairs presented more commonly in the lateral triangle and became clinically evident within 2 years following the initial repair (Fig. 5). The reason for failure following mesh repair is that the mesh used initially did not cover the entire MPO, leaving the unprotected area vulnerable. Anterior patches of sufficient size that are fixed far enough lateral to the internal ring and medial to the pubic tubercle will prevent recurrences through the entire superior pane of the MPO. Medial and lateral recurrences are seen if mesh is used that does not cover those areas. It is clear that an anterior patch acts as a lid, not as a stopper. Neither the plug nor the anterior patch techniques affords any measure of protection against femoral herniation.

CURRENT REPAIR OF INGUINAL HERNIAS

The basic principle of every type of indirect inguinal hernia repair is the reduction of the herniated peritoneum and its contents to within the abdominal cavity, and the prevention of herniation by restoring the competency of the internal ring. To be successful, the repair must permanently prevent passage of any intra-abdominal viscus to outside the musculoaponeurotic plane of the abdominal wall. The portion of peritoneal sac that resides within the deep inguinal ring of an indirect inguinal hernia must be completely reduced. In the management of a longer peritoneal

sac or one densely adherent to the spermatic cord, its proximal portion should be divided, leaving its distal portion undisturbed. The proximal portion is fully dissected from the cord and from the investing fibers of the transversalis fascia. It is then ligated and reduced. Regardless of how the distal portion of the sac is treated, meticulous dissection including the true neck of the sac is required to free it from the investing attachments of the transversalis fascia at the musculofascial threshold of the deep ring (Fig. 6). Further, the "shoulders" of the sac must be separated from the transversalis fascia to make a space for the prosthetic mesh. Completion of the repair requires absolute prevention of any portion of the intra-abdominal peritoneal sac from protruding through the deep inguinal ring.

Of the technical modifications I have made during the past 20 years, each has principally placed a swatch of polypropylene mesh into the properitoneal space (Fig. 7). The mesh, as in each posterior hernia repair, becomes fixed against the abdominal wall by intra-abdominal pressure. Since 1985 I have used this principle to successfully repair all primary and most recurrent

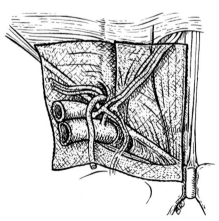

Fig. 7. Posterior view of mesh covering entire myopectineal orifice.

indirect inguinal hernias. My original techniques, and its two later generations, embrace this same important principle: when the patient's intra-abdominal force is harnessed and applied against the mesh patch that has been interposed between the peritoneum and the transversalis fascia, it will hold the patch in place to fortify the entire MPO. Each generation of my technique of indirect inguinal hernia repair incorporates the same three features: (a) the deep (internal) inguinal ring is an available and convenient passageway to be used to get to the properitoneal retromuscular space (Bogros space), (b) polypropylene mesh is an excellent permanent barrier to protect the deep inguinal ring, and (c) the body's intra-abdominal pressure is sufficient to permanently fix the mesh in its properitoneal position (Pascal's principle). Until April 1998, I used a tension-free polypropylene umbrella patch technique to repair all indirect inguinal hernias. I used the Shouldice repair with a reinforcing underlay mesh patch (not tension-free) to repair all direct hernias. In 1997, as a consultant to the Ethicon Company (Somerville, NJ), I designed the details of a bilayer connected mesh device to repair all types of direct and indirect inguinal hernias through an open anterior approach. This device is currently known as the Prolene polypropylene Hernia System. In its first generation it was available in three sizes.

Current Technique

 PREOPERATIVE PLANNING

When it is indicated, medical evaluation and clearance is requested. Aspirin and nonsteroidal anti-inflammatory drugs are stopped 10 days before surgery. If the patient takes Coumadin, it is stopped 5 days before surgery, and clotting evaluation is obtained on the day before the operation. All other medications are continued up until midnight before surgery. The patient is advised to shower the morning of surgery using a parachlorometaxylenol-impregnated sponge to bathe the abdominal and groin areas. On check-in to the preoperative suite, an intravenous route is established with Ringer's lactated solution. Hair in the operative site is clipped with an electric razor. I previously reserved routine perioperative antibiotic prophylaxis for patients 65 years and older. Recently, for no scientific reason, but strictly in response to the increase in professional liability exposure, I have adopted this policy for patients of all ages. One-half hour

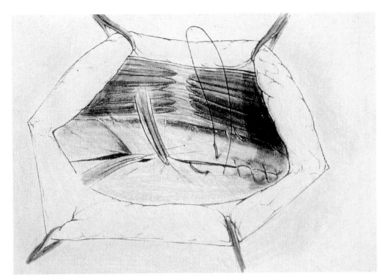

Fig. 7. Posterior sheath closure.

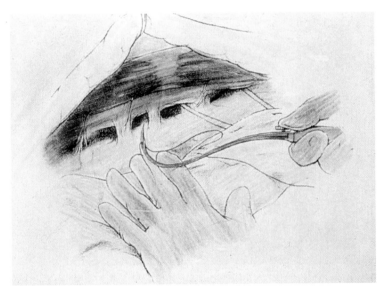

Fig. 8. Reverdin needle.

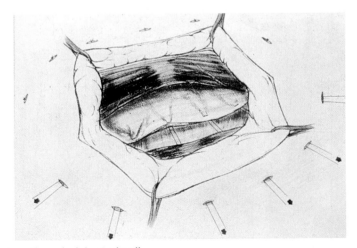

Fig. 9. Sutures through abdominal wall.

The rectus muscles and fascia are closed in the midline to cover the prosthesis. This is a critical step since this procedure has wound problems such as epidermolysis, necrosis, or infection up to 20% of the time and it is catastrophic if the prosthesis gets infected. Drains are placed in the subcutaneous space and any excess skin and fat are excised to give a good cosmetic result. We then close the dermis with interrupted 4-0 PDS sutures and the skin with staples that are removed 3 days later. We do not close the subcutaneous layer since this only leads to fat necrosis.

Intraperitoneal Rives-Type Repair

The previously described method of repair was developed in order to place a large piece of mesh behind the hernia defect but to keep it off of the viscera since the only two meshes available at the time were uncoated polyester and polypropylene. As mentioned earlier, there are now several meshes that can be safely placed in contact with the viscera, and this now allows an intraperitoneal placement of the mesh. This can be done as in the classic Rives repair with the interrupted sutures being brought up through the skin, but we developed a method where the suturing is continuous and done below the skin. The technique, developed in the early 1990s, utilized ePTFE mesh since it was the only mesh at that time that could be safely placed against the viscera. After the incision is made, the hernia sac is entered and adhesiolysis is done just as in the classic Rives repair. Once all of this is done, skin and subcutaneous flaps are developed on both sides back into good fascia and far enough laterally so that the rectus muscles and fascia can be approximated to cover the mesh after it has been implanted (Fig. 10). The proper size of mesh is determined by bringing the two mobilized rectus muscles to the midline with Kocher clamps. We then measure 6 to 8 cm laterally onto good fascia on either side to determine the width needed and similar overlap into good fascia superiorly and inferiorly. One or more disposable visceral retractors ("fish") are wrapped in a moist laparotomy sponge (it can be trimmed to fit and we remove the rigid plastic bar for easier removal) and placed in the abdominal cavity over the intestines. The mesh is then placed in the abdominal cavity and a #1 or #2 Prolene on a large needle that is 60 cm long is placed at the 6 o'clock position as a "U" stitch through the mesh and through the fascia back at the previously determined point and the suture is tied. A similar separate suture is placed at the 12 o'clock position and tied, thus anchoring the mesh in such a way that the following suture placement will not pull it too much to one side or the other (Fig. 11). The suture (either one) is then run in a continuous fashion as a series of "U" stitches going through the mesh and through the strong fascia (at the predetermined point) in a clockwise fashion (Fig. 12). When only 3 to 4 cm is left the visceral retractor and lap are removed and a malleable is used to ensure no bowel is caught in the suture line. The sutures are tied and there is now a large piece of mesh behind the defect with broad overlap into good fascia (Fig. 13). The rectus muscles and fascia are brought to the midline and sutured to cover the mesh to protect it from wound problems and to provide a functional and cosmetic result (Fig. 14). Closure is just the same as described in the classic Rives method. Figure 15 is a laparoscopic view of what this open repair looks like when completed.

We have done hundreds of repairs using both methods, and the advantage of the intraperitoneal approach over the classic Rives method is that it is quicker to do, there is less dissection, and it is more cosmetic in that there are no skin punctures where the sutures are pulled through. Seroma formation occurs with both techniques and suture pain is similar. Wound complications are the main morbidity and occur in 10% to 20% of cases. Gillion et al. compared placement of ePTFE in the classic Rives fashion with the intraperitoneal method and found equivalent results. The intraperitoneal approach should not be done if the patient has had previous aortic aneurysm repair since the blood supply to the skin and fat will have been interrupted and these flaps may not survive. Infection of the mesh can be limited by the methods described but still will occur more often than the laparoscopic approach.

Most all midline IHs can be repaired with the classic or modified Rives method. The surgeon must be careful to anchor the mesh to the Cooper ligament in the case of the true parapubic hernia wherein the lower border of the hernia is the pubic bone and no fascia exists. Similarly, in the subxiphoid hernia where there may be only rib or sternum, the mesh has to be anchored to a solid structure; otherwise, it is doomed to failure.

PARASTOMAL HERNIA

Parastomal hernia repair has a recurrence rate of 60% to 80% based on which study you read. Rubin did an extensive evaluation and found that suture repair gave a

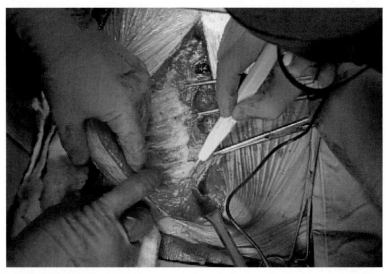

Fig. 10. Skin and subcutaneous flaps.

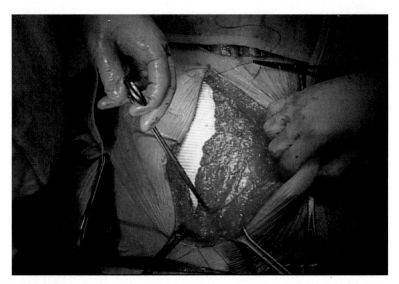

Fig. 11. Stay sutures.

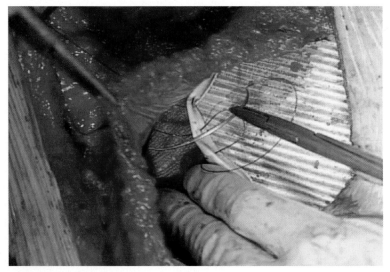

Fig. 12. Running sutures started.

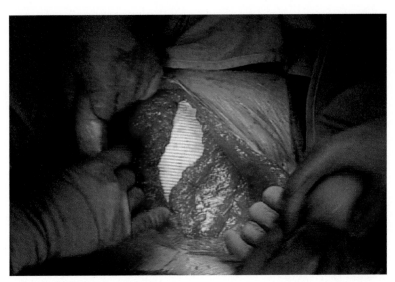

Fig. 13. Completed 360-degree suture.

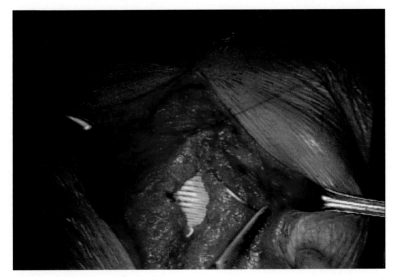

Fig. 14. Closure of rectus muscles.

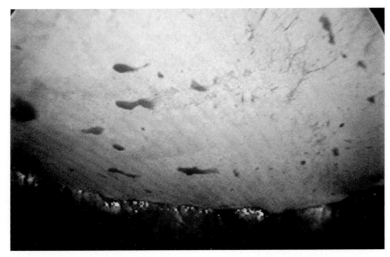

Fig. 15. Laparoscopic view of open repair.

76% recurrence, relocation of the stoma led to a 33% recurrence (and 52% got a new incisional hernia), and mesh repair had a 30% recurrence. The most important thing then is to first try to prevent the initial hernia from forming at the time of stoma formation. Sugarbaker has described a method to anchor the stoma to fascia 360 degrees, which helps prevent hernia formation. Another method recently (2004) described in a randomized, prospective trial evaluated taking a 10-cm piece of lightweight PPM and cutting a cross in the middle through which the bowel will be brought. The mesh was placed in a retrorectus fashion. There were 54 patients randomized and follow-up was up to 38 months. Fifty percent of the no-mesh stomas formed hernias, whereas only one hernia formed in the mesh group. There were no complications or infections of the mesh.

Once the hernia forms then proper initial repair is critical. As previously mentioned mesh is critical for successful repair but it needs to be placed in a certain fashion. The majority of surgeons learn to cut a keyhole in the mesh and wrap the tails around the bowel. This should NOT be done since the slit for the keyhole is a weak point that will then lead to a recurrence through the slit. A better method was described by Sugarbaker in the 1970s and consists of taking a piece of mesh and suturing it to the peritoneal surface, overlapping the defect in all directions. No slit is cut; the bowel is simply tunneled out one side of the mesh and lays between the peritoneum and the mesh. The mesh is sutured at the perimeter 360 degrees and on either side of the bowel (Fig. 16). Sugarbaker reported no recurrences and no complications from the mesh at 4 to 7 years of follow-up. The Sugarbaker repair has been our repair of choice and has led to a low recurrence rate, and we have had no mesh infections or erosions. A new mesh made by Bard specifically for parastomal hernias is now available, but it is too new to say anything about recurrence rates, etc.

DENERVATION FLANK BULGE

The denervation flank bulge (DNFB) occurs when a flank incision transects the intercostal nerves that are trophic to the abdominal muscles. The muscles become thin and fibrotic and lose their tone. This leads to a bulge that is often mistaken for a hernia. There can be a concomitant true fascial defect in addition to the denervation bulge, and a computed tomography

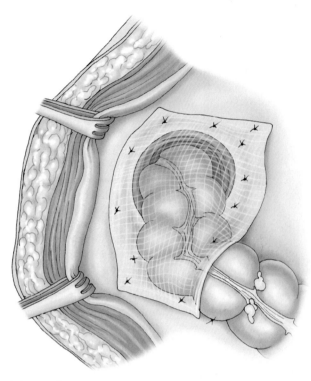

Fig. 16. Sugarbaker repair.

scan is usually required to differentiate these problems. It is critical to do so because the true hernia can be repaired using the intraperitoneal technique previously described but the denervation bulge cannot be definitively repaired. If one operates on the DNFB, the surgeon will see the thinning of the tissues without any true fascial defect. The thinned tissue can be removed and a prosthetic placed, but the patient should be warned that there is a good chance the bulge will slowly reappear since the muscles will not regain their tone. We have operated on many patients with the DNFB and the best results are seen in those who have a true hernia in addition to the bulge.

REFERENCES

Amid P. Polypropylene prosthesis. In: Bendavid R, ed. *Abdominal wall hernias.* Berlin, Heidelberg: Springer-Verlag, 2001:272.

Anthony T, Bergen P, Kim L, et al. Factors affecting recurrence following incisional herniorrhaphy. *World J Surg* 2000;24(1):95.

de Vries Reilingh TS, Van Goor H, et al. Components separation technique for the repair of large abdominal wall hernias. *J Am Coll Surg* 2003;196(1):32.

Flament JB, Palot JP, Burde A, et al. Treatment of major incisional hernias. In: Bendavid R, ed. *Abdominal wall hernias.* Berlin, Heidelberg: Springer-Verlag, 2001:508.

Franklin Jr ME, Gonzalez Jr JJ, Michaelson RP, et al. Preliminary experience with a new bioactive prosthetic material for repair of hernias in infected fields. *Hernia* 2002;6:171.

Gillion JF, Begin GF, Marecos C, et al. Expanded ePTFE patches used in the intraperitoneal or extraperitoneal position for repair of incisional hernias of the anterolateral abdominal wall. *Am J Surg* 1997;174:16.

Helton WS, Fisichella P, Berger R, et al. Short-term outcomes with small intestinal submucosa for ventral abdominal hernia. *Arch Surg* 2005;140:549.

Hesselink VJ, Luijendijk RW, deWitt JH, et al. An evaluation of risk factors in incisional hernia recurrence. *Surg Gynecol Obstet* 1993; 176(3):228-233.

Klinge U, Klosterhalfen B, Muller M, et al. Foreign body reaction to mesh used for the repair of abdominal wall hernias. *Eur J Surg* 1999;165:665.

Klinge U, Klosterhalfen B, Schumpelick V. Vipro®: a new generation of polypropylene mesh. In: Bendavid R, ed. *Abdominal wall hernias.* Berlin, Heidelberg: Springer-Verlag. 2001:286.

Law N. Expand polytetrafluoroethylene. In: Bendavid R, ed. *Abdominal wall hernias.* Berlin: Verlag-Verlag, 2001:279.

Leber GE, Garb JL, Alexander AI, et al. Long-term complication associated with prosthetic repair of incisional hernias. *Arch Surg* 1998;133:378.

Luijendijk RW, Hop Wim CJ, van den Tol MP, et al. A comparison of suture repair with mesh repair for incisional hernia. *N Engl J Med* 2000;343(6):392.

Ramirez OM, Girotto JA. Closure of chronic abdominal wall defects: the components separation technique. In: Bendavid R, ed. *Abdominal wall hernias.* Berlin, Heidelberg: Springer-Verlag, 2001:487.

Recent advances in incisional hernia treatment. *Hernia* 2000:4.

Soler M, Verhaeghe PJ, Stoppa R. Polyester (Dacron®) mesh. In: Bendavid R, ed. *Abdominal wall hernias.* Berlin, Heidelberg: Springer-Verlag, 2001:266.

Sugarbaker P. Peritoneal approach to prosthetic mesh repair of paraostomy hernias. *Ann Surg* 1985:344.

Van't Riet M, Steyerberg EW, et al. Meta-analysis of techniques for closure of midline abdominal incisions. *Br J Surg* 2002;89:1350.

Voeller GR. New developments in hernia repair. In: Szabo Z, ed. *Surgical technology international XI.* San Francisco CA: Universal Medical Press, 2003:111.

Welty G, Klinge U, Klosterhalfen B, et al. Functional impairment and complaints following incisional hernia repair with different polypropylene meshes. *Hernia* 2001;5:142.

EDITOR'S COMMENT

Ventral hernias are almost always the result of abdominal incisions. The basic problem with the repair of ventral hernias is an absolutely horrendous recurrence rate, which approaches approximately 50% of suture repair of incisional hernias (Cassar K, Munro A. *Br J Surg* 2002;89:534; and Paul et al. *Eur J Surg* 1998;164:361), despite the fact that the introduction of mesh opened up a new era (Read. *Hernia* 2004;8:8; Usher FC et al. *Am Surg* 1958;24:969). Several personal series have recurrence rates of less than 10% (Kingnworth A, LeBlanc K. *Lancet* 2003;362:1561; and Morris-Stiff GJ, Hughes LE. *J Am Coll Surg* 1998;186:352). Nonetheless, the continued reporting of horrendous results from good surgeons have led Schumpelick's group (Junge K, et al. *Eur J Surg* 2002;168:67) to conclude that there is a defect in collagen types I and III, which leads to the continual breakdown of wound repairs. Finally, following this logic, the chapter arrives at the conclusion that the previous practices of either overlay of various types of mesh or intraperitoneal types of mesh will be replaced by mesh between posterior rectus muscles, above the fascia and peritoneum, which would avoid the overlay mesh propensity to infection and the intraperitoneal mesh with a tendency for bowel to adhere and result in late fistulas and extrusion and terrible wound problems.

(continued)

It is surprising that the initial introduction to this chapter starts with the supposition that following the repair of incisional hernias, long-term pain (58%) accompanies the use of Marlex mesh, especially the heaviest type of Marlex. Medium type of Marlex, which is less constrictive to the abdominal wall, has chronic pain of 16%, but the lightweight Marlex, which is associated with a Vicryl onlay and is absorbable, has a chronic pain of 4%. The reason for the long-term pain with Marlex appears to be a strong scar plate from thickened Marlex, associated with wound contraction, stiffness, and lack of mobility of the abdominal wall. My question is, Why didn't we recognize the fact that 58% of the patients to get a Marlex repair have chronic long-term pain? Is this the same kind of situation as the emergence of mesh inguinodynia, in which in doing reviews of patients with open repairs, the number of patients with chronic long-term pain following their open repairs has been reported at 22% versus between 22% and 33% for mesh, which is difficult to believe based on one's own personal experiences? Is this because surgeons didn't ask the patients about chronic pain, or because they were dismissive when patients said that they had some chronic discomfort, which apparently did not interfere with their way of life? If one is to believe these data, however, it suggests that there is real interference with the way of life. Perhaps it is because in the United States surgeons generally do not focus on lifestyle or what happens with patients who have chronic pain, provided that there is no recurrence. This is reminiscent of the story with postduodenal ulcer surgery, in which the Visick rating focused not only on symptoms of postoperative ulcer disease, but also occasionally on symptoms of dumping, etc.; however, the worst Visick rating, which was Visick 4, was reserved for recurrence of ulcer, whereas in fact it may be that some of the other disabling side effects of the postulcer surgery, such as severe dumping, were far worse than recurrence.

The authors also claim that the use of Interceed (Ethicon) is beneficial when combined with heavy or medium Marlex, and will decrease the invasion or ingrowth of the viscera. While I have no personal experience with Interceed in patients, in Cincinnati, where my practice also consisted of reoperative surgery, there was one surgeon who fancied himself a "reoperative surgeon" and used Interceed constantly. I saw a large number of those patients, and the results were not happy. Therefore, I would doubt very much whether Interceed is effective at preventing the ingrowth of viscera.

I do agree, however, that the ePTFE, or Goretex, generally results in no ingrowth of viscera. Indeed, if one uses Goretex on open fascia because one cannot get closure at all, there's a thin layer of scar tissue that grows under the fascia, and there's generally no ingrowth at all. As a matter of fact, when one reoperates on patients with a Goretex, one just cuts through the Goretex and sews it up. In general, the bowel is not adherent, and one need not fear the erosion into bowel with fistulas. On the other hand, there may be a problem with ePTFE. Recently I have seen four seemingly clean cases in which as near as one could tell, there were the usual precautions to prevent infection, including Hibiclens washes, clipping rather than shaving, use of Ioban, and then the use of a single dose of antibiotics given at the appropriate time. Nonetheless, infections supervene for reasons that are not entirely clear.

The author comes down heavily on laparoscopic repair for umbilical hernias using Ventralex. I must say I do not share his enthusiasm. One of the problems with laparoscopic repair is one gets fluid collections both above and below whatever the mesh is, including persistent mesh above, even if one uses a closed suction drainage, which I believe does increase the incidence of infection if it is left in for a period of time. In addition, especially if one uses the through-and-through sutures, as described by the author, pain is a very substantial part of the postoperative period, and the sutures are extremely painful. An alternative to both laparoscopic repair and the use of ePTFE in a suture repair is wide mobilization of the subcutaneous flaps, primary suture repair, and reinforcing with a number of layers of Vicryl, which are appropriately attached. The Vicryl is presumably absorbed in between 120 and 180 days. It relieves the tension on the repair, and also provides a good scar while it is being reabsorbed. I do believe it is a viable alternative to both laparoscopic repair, which I am not enamored with, and the underlay of various kinds of mesh, especially Marlex mesh, with whatever it is combined with to prevent visceral ingrowth. Long term, I believe the Marlex remains, and the material that is intended to prevent visceral ingrowth either tends to be removed during placement or else has less staying power than Marlex and fistulas recur.

A major issue for the surgeon and patient is patients who have lost the right of domain with a large hernia. Attempt to repair without increasing the capacity of the peritoneum results in respiratory insufficiency and abdominal compartment syndrome. To carry out such a repair and forcibly returning the small bowel into the peritoneal cavity will lead to very high diaphragms, respiratory insufficiency, and, not infrequently, increased abdominal pressure. The latter has been dealt with in other parts of this section. The author seems unhappy with repeated pneumoperitoneum. I use pneumoperitoneum after implanting a port in the abdomen, sometimes with a somewhat larger tube attached to it, and use the port repeatedly, say, pumping in a liter or two once every 2 weeks, in an effort to increase the capacity of the peritoneum. This often works reasonably well, provided one is patient and does it repeatedly.

I agree entirely that component separation needs to be part of every general surgeon's armamentarium, but it then depends on what is meant by component separation. To me, there are at least four components to a component separation. The first is wide mobilization of the fat and the skin of the anterior abdominal wall. The second is true visualization of the lateral aspect of the rectus sheath, and the incision through the external oblique. The third is sliding the rectus over, as the authors propose, and making certain that they meet in the midline. One can use a postrectus mesh, usually in my hands expanded Goretex, and then sew the muscles together and then the fascia together. The fourth is placing Vicryl mesh, as I previously described, in several layers to relieve the tension at the suture line, as well as formed scar, in an onlay fashion.

I have previously referred to preparation of the skin, and this is extremely important. My own routine is the use of Hibiclens for 3 days, clipping rather than shaving, use of Ioban after Iodine tincture, and prophylactic antibiotics, whichever is appropriate, either a single dose of first-generation cephalosporin such as 2 g of Kefzol or 1 g of Ancef, making certain if the operation goes beyond 3 hours that a repeat dose is given. I do not use the prophylactic antibiotics more than the perioperative dose for fear of *Clostridium difficile*, which is a problem.

Paajanen and Laine (*Hernia* 2005;9:62) have reported on 10 patients who are massively obese and who have been repaired with polypropylene mesh, and stressed the attachment that the open technique that they borrowed on was used by Rives and Stoppa, that is, placement of the mesh in the preperitoneal fashion, and attaching it to the ribcage, the semilunar line, and, if the hernia extends caudad, to the Cooper ligament. The complications, especially considering the emergency nature of some primary operations, were not too great. There were three wound infections, and polypropylene meshes were used between the rectus muscle and the underlying fascia. Other meshes were used as a composite, as well as other innovations.

The problem of lack of abdominal domain was addressed by Hendrikus et al. (*World J Surg* 2005; 29:1080), in which abdominoplasty, tissue expansion, and methods of augmentation were discussed, including prostheses and the use of local muscle flaps to improve the closure. Finally, Le and Bender (*Am J Surg* 2005;189:373) reported on 150 patients in an effort to reduce the ventral incisional hernia recurrence rate, which they state is as high as 33%. A consecutive group of 150 patients was repaired using the proposterofascia technique of mesh, à la Rives and Stoppa, and they give credit to George Wantz, who actually did travel to observe Rives and Stoppa and modified their technique slightly. In this study, despite the size of the patients at 32 body mass index, there was only one postoperative mortality, but there was a 9% postoperative infection rate, with two patients (1%) requiring mesh removal. Long-term evaluation has revealed three recurrences and three admissions with bowel obstruction, with one patient requiring surgical relief. No fistulas have been noted as yet, but follow-up is short.

Finally, as will be discussed elsewhere in this section, the bioabsorbable tissue scaffolds of porcine submucosal small intestine extracellular matrix (Surgisis Gold [Cook Biotech]) is proposed as acceptable for ventral hernial repair by Helton et al. (*Arch Surg* 2005;140(6):549). The authors point out that Surgisis is considerably less expensive than some of the other bioplatforms and, therefore, since few hospitals are reimbursed for this type of biodegradable mesh, they tend to use the least expensive type. The working hypothesis states that this will be used as scaffolding, and it finally will result in the cellular ingrowth of this type of scaffolding in the patients in which it is used. While it sounds promising, others have reported far less satisfaction with Surgisis and some of the other biodegradable scaffolding. True, they're less likely to get infected, are more likely to be compatible, and do not invade the viscera, but there seems to be no perfect biologic scaffolding as of yet.

J.E.F.

Nongastrointestinal Transabdominal

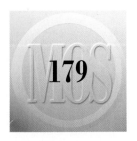

179

Laparoscopic Ventral Hernia Repair

BRUCE RAMSHAW

The laparoscopic approach for repair of ventral/incisional hernias was first reported in the early 1990s. Since that time, the technique has evolved into an accepted repair for the management of ventral/incisional hernias. The many reports of excellent clinical results have made laparoscopic ventral hernia repair one of the fastest growing minimally invasive techniques of the past several years.

The repair is based on the principles of the Rives-Stoppa open retrorectus tension-free mesh repair, in which the plane between the rectus muscle and the posterior fascia is dissected widely. Mesh is then placed posteriorly and fixed to healthy abdominal wall fascia using full–thickness permanent sutures. The laparoscopic approach differs, however, with mesh placement in the intra-abdominal cavity rather than in the retrorectus plane. Laparoscopic ventral hernia repair allows for clear visualization of the abdominal wall, wide mesh coverage beyond the defect, and secure fixation to healthy abdominal wall fascia, ensuring a successful repair.

This chapter will review the indications, contraindications, appropriate patient selection, technique, and postoperative care for laparoscopic ventral hernia repair. Particular attention will be paid to the management and avoidance of complications.

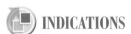

INDICATIONS

Although the appropriateness of mesh hernia repair in children is debatable, this chapter will focus on the technique for patients beyond puberty. Based on published studies, it is apparent that tension-free mesh repair for ventral hernias excels in terms of recurrence, even for the smallest primary hernia. Essentially any ventral hernia that can be repaired using an open tension-free mesh repair may potentially be repaired laparoscopically. Of critical importance during the surgeon's learning curve is patient selection for this procedure. In certain situations, such as the primary or first-time recurrent umbilical hernia in patients without previous abdominal operations, laparoscopic repair has the potential for minimal complications,

even early in a surgeon's experience. However, this same technique in a patient with many previous abdominal operations, especially in patients with previous intra-abdominal placement of heavyweight polypropylene mesh, can be a significant challenge for the most skilled laparoscopic surgeon. Bleeding, enterotomy, and other intra-abdominal organ injuries can be relatively common in patients with severe intra-abdominal adhesions. Of course, this is the case regardless of the approach, open or laparoscopic.

As mentioned, essentially all adult ventral hernias may be approached laparoscopically. However, depending on the surgeon's experience, relative contraindications may include active wound infection, loss of abdominal domain, and history of severe abdominal adhesions and/or previous intra-abdominal mesh placement. In patients with acute infection, alternatives to standard prosthetic mesh placement include laparoscopic placement of a biologic mesh or the use of a nonmesh repair, such as the components separation technique. Although rare with the current safety of general anesthesia, patients with significant cardiopulmonary disease or other medical problems may not be candidates for general anesthesia and, therefore, a laparoscopic repair. Hernias in these patients might be most appropriately managed nonoperatively, with abdominal binders and activity restrictions, to avoid unnecessary risks of surgery.

PREOPERATIVE PLANNING

In preparation for laparoscopic ventral hernia repair, patient education is imperative, especially in patients with complex and/or large hernias. It should be stressed that the laparoscopic ventral hernia repair combines the benefits of minimal recurrence and minimal wound complications. Yet, the postoperative pain may be significant and, except following repair of the smallest hernias, requires a hospital stay for pain management.

Other important patient education topics include potential for seroma formation, added incisions for suture fixation, and the potential for bowel injury as well

as the options for its management. This is especially important for patients with multiple previous abdominal surgeries, multiple previous ventral hernia repairs (especially with mesh), and patients with very large defects. The management of these patients can be aided by obtaining a preoperative computed tomographic scan to evaluate anatomy, and preoperative bowel preparation for decompression.

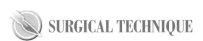

SURGICAL TECHNIQUE

POSITIONING AND PREPARATION

The patient is generally placed in the supine position with arms tucked at the side or on arm boards, depending on the size and location of the defect. Many hernias, especially larger ones, require the surgeon to move about during the procedure. In most situations, having the arms tucked out of the way allows more flexibility in handling instruments.

As opposed to most laparoscopic procedures, the surgeon, trocar, and monitor positions for a laparoscopic ventral hernia repair can be quite variable. For most long midline hernias, the initial access is lateral, and additional trocars are necessary on the contralateral side (Fig. 1). Monitors are placed on each side of the patient toward the head, or a single monitor is used at the foot, depending on the location and extent of the midline defect. For upper abdominal hernias, the monitors are located at the head of the bed, similar to placement for laparoscopic cholecystectomy. For lower abdominal hernias, the monitor is placed at the foot of the bed, similar to placement for a laparoscopic inguinal hernia repair. For a ventral hernia away from the midline, such as a spigelian hernia or an ostomy site hernia, the surgeon stands on the side of the patient opposite the side of the hernia, and the monitor is placed on the same side as the hernia (opposite the surgeon). The surgeon should make the operating room staff aware of this variability to avoid the potential for incorrect room setup.

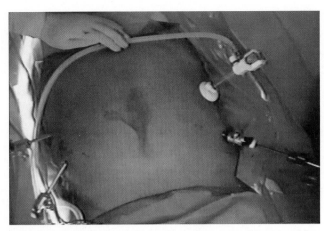

Fig. 1. Trocar placement in a patient with a long, midline, ventral/incisional hernia. The initial 10-mm access has been obtained just inferior to the left costal margin at the anterior axillary line. The 5-mm trocar is positioned inferiorly in the left flank at the anterior axillary line. Two 5-mm trocars are positioned in the right flank at the anterior axillary line after lysis of adhesions has allowed direct laparoscopic visualization for safe trocar placement.

Perioperative antibiotics are typically used, as well as an orogastric tube for gastric decompression and a Foley catheter for bladder decompression. Sequential compression devices are for deep venous thrombosis prophylaxis. Need for additional deep venous thrombosis prophylaxis is based on individual patient risk factors. The patient is shaved, prepared, and draped widely using an Ioban drape to avoid mesh to skin contact.

ACCESS AND PORT PLACEMENT

The initial access port is usually a 10-mm trocar. Use of a Verres needle or open technique for trocar placement should be based on the surgeon's experience. If a closed technique is chosen, an optical trocar is recommended. Because most of these patients have had previous abdominal surgery, accessing the abdomen away from previous incisions minimizes the risk of intra-abdominal injury. Three relatively safe areas for access include the subxiphoid midline, where the left lateral lobe of the liver usually protects other intra-abdominal organs, and each subcostal space at the anterior axillary line, where the presence of preperitoneal fat or intra-abdominal adhesions is rare.

Once safe access is obtained, the laparoscope is inserted and the abdominal cavity is explored. An angled scope is used to better view the anterior abdominal wall, where much of the procedure is performed. Typically, two to four 5-mm trocars are used for secondary ports. One or two are placed on the same side of the abdomen as the scope

for initial adhesiolysis, if necessary. Then, one or two 5-mm ports are placed, under laparoscopic visualization, on the contralateral side of the abdomen.

LYSIS OF ADHESIONS

The lysis of adhesions can be the most difficult and dangerous portion of this operation. Bleeding and injury to bowel or other organs may occur, especially in patients with multiple previous surgeries or previously placed intra-abdominal mesh. Typically, a plane is developed between the abdominal wall and the adherent abdominal contents to allow for safe, gentle, blunt and sharp dissection (Fig. 2A, B). Energy sources, including ultrasonic dissection devices, should be used only if bowel or other organs are clearly not adjacent or adherent to the abdominal wall. Delayed bowel injury can occur following the use of electrocautery, scissors, ultrasonic dissectors, or graspers. Thermal injury may be more difficult to identify during initial dissection. For centrally located hernias, no additional dissection is necessary prior to mesh placement. However, hernias located above, below, or lateral to the midabdominal wall may require additional dissection, such as division of the falciform ligament.

REDUCTION OF HERNIA CONTENTS

In most patients, reduction of hernia contents can be done safely with gentle traction using atraumatic graspers (Fig. 3A, B). External compression will assist with safe reduction. If bowel is incarcerated, or even possibly in a mass of incarcerated contents,

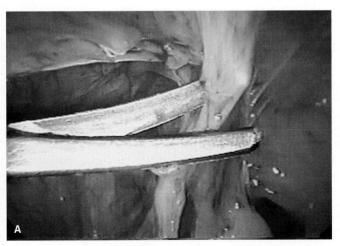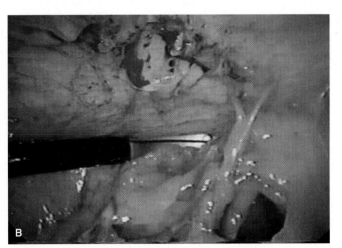

Fig. 2. Lysis of adhesions begins with sharp (**A**) and/or blunt (**B**) dissection in the plane between the abdominal wall and the adherent abdominal contents. Energy sources are avoided if bowel is potentially involved in the adherent tissue. Gentle traction with a grasper and/or external palpation with the nondominant hand can aid in this dissection.

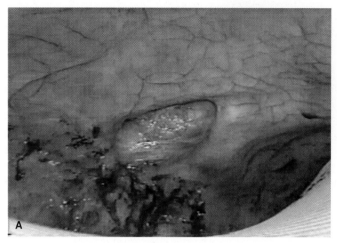
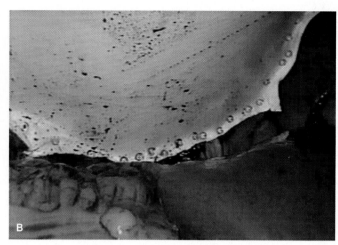

Fig. 3. Most surgeons attempt to achieve an overlap of mesh of at least 4 to 5 cm beyond the hernia defect in all directions. From a view above (**A**) and below (**B**) the mesh, an overlap of at least 5 cm is obtained in all directions for this small flank hernia.

care should be taken to avoid excessive tension with graspers to minimize the risk of bowel injury. For incarcerated omentum, the main risk during reduction is bleeding. The use of energy sources, clips, sutures, or endoloops may be required if bleeding occurs. In rare cases when incarcerated contents are not reducible, sharp division of the fascial edge of the defect will facilitate reduction. As in open surgery, the viability of reduced contents should be assessed. An open incision over the incarcerated hernia contents may be necessary to reduce or evaluate the incarcerated bowel and to perform a resection if the bowel is found to be nonviable. For umbilical and epigastric defects, reduction of preperitoneal fatty tissue may also be necessary.

HERNIA EVALUATION

Once the entire extent of the defect(s) is exposed and adequate dissection of the abdominal wall, allowing for wide mesh coverage, is achieved, the defect is measured. Especially in obese patients, it can be difficult to accurately measure the hernia defect because of the difference between the abdominal circumference at the skin and at the peritoneum. A piece of mesh measured and cut to size outside the abdomen would typically be larger than necessary when placed inside the abdomen and fixed to the peritoneum. Various tips will help to accurately measure the size of the defect at the peritoneal level. First, the abdomen can be deflated to minimize the difference in external to internal circumference of the abdominal wall. Spinal needles are also helpful when placed perpendicular to the abdominal

wall at the edges of the defect. Measurements between the spinal needles without the curvature of the abdomen will lead to more accurate measurements. The hernia defect can also be measured directly, using a suture or laparoscopic instrument, or by cutting a paper ruler lengthwise and placing it inside the abdominal cavity.

Typically, in the presence of multiple defects, the maximum distance between all defects is measured and one mesh is used to cover all defects. Occasionally, defects are separated by long distances of healthy abdominal wall, and in this scenario the use of two separate pieces of mesh may be more appropriate, based on the surgeon's judgment. For incisional hernia repair, it is recommended that the entire previous incision be covered with mesh unless there is no obvious hernia in a portion of the incision; adhesiolysis in this area would significantly increase the risks of the procedure.

MESH PREPARATION

The size of the mesh should allow for coverage beyond the edges of the defect by at least 4 to 5 cm in all directions (Fig. 4A, B). One reason for placing trocars laterally as far from the hernia defect as possible is to allow for this wide mesh coverage. Once the appropriate size of mesh is fashioned, markings are added for orientation and sutures to allow for accurate placement. Markings on the skin or Ioban drape should help localize the placement of the initial stay sutures. Typically, four sutures are initially placed in the mesh. Too many sutures will make it difficult to find the appropriate suture inside the abdominal cav-

ity, and too few sutures will not provide enough mesh fixation to simplify tack placement and additional suture fixation.

MESH PLACEMENT

After suturing the mesh, and marking the mesh and abdomen, the mesh is rolled up and brought through the 10-mm trocar or the wound itself, depending on the size of the mesh. A 5-mm grasper inserted through a trocar on the opposite side of the patient can be used to grasp the mesh through the 10-mm wound and pull it into the abdomen. A 5-mm laparoscope inserted through a third trocar may be used in order to visualize mesh placement.

MESH FIXATION

The mesh is then unrolled and proper orientation is verified. The sutures are brought out through small incisions in the skin using a suture–passing instrument to grasp each arm of the suture in a separate pass (Fig. 5A, B). The angle of the suture passer is slightly different with each pass, allowing the needle to exit the abdominal wall approximately 1 cm away from the first suture arm. In this manner, the suture is tied gently, approximating the anterior fascia and up to 1 cm of full–thickness abdominal wall to the mesh. The sutures are not tied down until all four have been placed and lifted to demonstrate the appropriate tautness of the mesh. If a suture is in an unacceptable position, it is dropped back into the abdominal cavity and brought out through another, more appropriate skin incision. Once the mesh is confirmed to be in a satisfactory position,

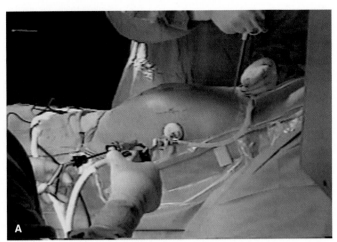
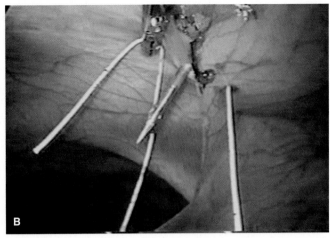

Fig. 4. A: With the mesh in the abdominal cavity, the suture passer is inserted through a small skin incision to grasp one arm of the suture. **B:** The suture passer will go through the same skin incision at a slightly different angle to exit the peritoneum, approximately 1 cm away from the first suture. Eventually, these sutures are tied gently to provide mesh fixation to abdominal wall peritoneum, muscle, and fascia.

the sutures are tied down to the anterior fascia. The sutures should be tied down gently to approximate, not strangulate, the tissue to minimize pain and the potential for a suture site hernia. Preinjection of local anesthetic at each suture site may also help minimize the pain.

The edge of the mesh is then fixed to the abdominal wall with tacks at approximately 1-cm intervals (Fig. 6A, B). Although the tacks may not provide long-term fixation, they stretch the mesh taut for additional suture fixation and help prevent internal herniation between the mesh and the abdominal wall. The tacker must typically be inserted into trocars opposite the mesh edge being tacked. Pressure is applied to the abdominal wall using the nondominant hand to approximate the edge of the mesh to the tacker at a 90-degree angle, ensuring appro-

priate tack placement. A tack that is not fired perpendicular to the abdominal wall may not be flush with the mesh. If a tack is only partially penetrates the mesh or falls into the abdominal cavity, it is removed, if possible, to avoid potential injury.

After the mesh is appropriately taut to the abdominal wall, additional full-thickness abdominal wall suture fixation may minimize the likelihood of recurrence (Fig. 7). Most experts recommend that sutures be placed from 3- to 5-cm intervals or up to 8- to 10-cm intervals, depending on the size and type of hernia defect. Small defects or "Swiss cheese" type of hernia defects, with most of the mesh approximating healthy abdominal wall, might require less additional suturing, with intervals of 8 to 10 cm. Large defects with less mesh approximated to the abdominal wall relative to the defect will

require more sutures at 3- to 5-cm intervals to minimize the risk of recurrence.

CLOSURE

After complete fixation of the mesh, the abdominal cavity should be explored for active bleeding or other injuries. The CO_2 is pushed out of the abdominal cavity and the fascia of the 10-mm incision is closed. Subcuticular sutures are used to close the skin of all trocar wounds, and sterile dressings are applied to all wounds, including the suture site wounds. However, prior to dressing the suture site wounds, a hemostat or other thin instrument should be used to elevate the skin of these incisions in at least two directions. This will help prevent the skin dimpling that can occur from the full–thickness abdominal wall sutures.

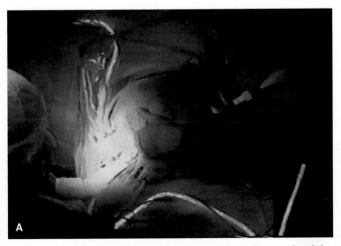
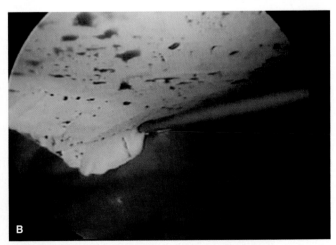

Fig. 5. A: The tacking device is brought into the abdomen through a trocar on the opposite side of the patient, using external compression to create a 90-degree angle between the tacker and the mesh. **B:** The tacker is placed at the periphery of the mesh, stretching the mesh taut while the abdominal cavity is inflated.

Nongastrointestinal Transabdominal

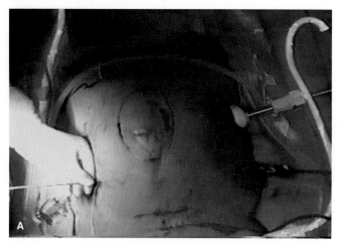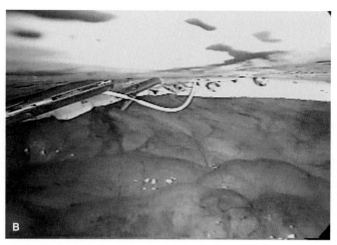

Fig. 6. After the mesh is taut from the initial suture fixation, and with tacks at 1-cm intervals around the circumference of the mesh, additional sutures are placed.

VARIATIONS OF HERNIA TYPES

Suprapubic Hernias

Suprapubic hernias require additional mesh coverage inferiorly into the pelvis, thus avoiding increased potential for recurrence when the mesh is fixed only to the pubis. The peritoneum is divided and dissected off the rectus muscles bilaterally down to the pubis. The peritoneum and bladder are then displaced posteriorly, exposing the Cooper ligament bilaterally. An extra 6 to 10 cm of mesh is placed into the pelvis and fixed permanently to the Cooper ligament bilaterally. Laterally, standard full-thickness abdominal wall suture fixation may be performed superior to the inguinal ligament bilaterally.

Lumbar/Flank Hernias

The patient is placed in the lateral position for lateral abdominal wall hernias. These hernias may occur primarily or, more commonly, they result from flank incisions after nephrectomy or iliac crest bone harvest. The peritoneum is incised and reflected medially to stay in the plane between the retroperitoneal organs and the paraspinal musculature.

After adequate dissection, mesh is fixed with full–thickness sutures to the paraspinous muscles between the costal margin and the iliac crest. Inferomedially, the mesh can be fixed with point fixation to the ipsilateral to the Cooper ligament and, with full-thickness abdominal wall sutures, superior to the inguinal ligament. Alternatively, the mesh can be fixed to the iliac crest with sutures through drilled holes, or with Mitek anchors. Superiorly, mesh is fixed up to the level of the diaphragm with full-thickness sutures subcostally and tacks to the abdominal wall posterior to the ribs up to the diaphragm. Standard fixation techniques are used for the medial and superior edges of the mesh.

Subxiphoid Hernia

Subxiphoid incisional hernias are frequently seen in patients with previous mediastinal tubes following coronary artery bypass graft or other cardiac surgery. In small subxiphoid hernias, the umbilicus may be used for the initial 10-mm trocar. As with most upper abdominal hernias, the falciform ligament should be divided to allow for mesh coverage flush with the anterior abdominal wall. Sutures are placed on either side of the xiphoid process with 6 to 10 cm of mesh left superior to the sutures, providing adequate overlap superior to the defect. Fixation of the mesh to the anterior abdominal wall superior to the xiphoid process can be accomplished with tacks and/or sutures placed intracorporeally, taking care to avoid mesh fixation into the diaphragm, especially in the vicinity of the heart. Additional sutures are placed immediately below the coastal margin bilaterally. Standard fixation techniques are used for the inferior and lateral edges of the mesh.

Parastomal Hernia

Parastomal hernias can be repaired laparoscopically, with minimal change in the previously described technique. Without cutting a slit in the mesh, the hernia is covered and the limb of bowel is brought out of the edge of the mesh (Fig. 7). Sutures are used to fix the mesh at either side of the bowel to prevent internal hernias. An alternate technique described by LeBlanc used two pieces of mesh with slits in opposite directions, designed to minimize the risk of recurrence through the mesh slit.

Fig. 7. Mesh fixation next to bowel coursing out from the edge of the mesh in a laparoscopic parastomal hernia repair.

Variations in Surgical Technique

NO SUTURES

Some surgeons have advocated laparoscopic mesh placement without suture fixation. Reasons to avoid the use of suture fixation include the potential for bleeding caused by the suture–passing instrument and the potential for postoperative pain caused by the suture. Carbajo et al. have described a "double crown" technique in which two circumferential rows of tacks are placed to provide fixation. Published results show low recurrence rates; however, suture fixation was used in selected patients. Other surgeons propose that sutures are unnecessary with certain types of heavyweight polypropylene mesh because of perceived ingrowth into the abdominal wall. Many cases of mesh migration and contraction with heavyweight polypropylene are seen clinically, and the fact that the mesh is being fixed to the peritoneum, not directly to the fascia, would argue for the use of suture fixation regardless of the type of mesh used.

CHOICE OF MESH

Laparoscopic mesh placement for ventral hernia repair requires a mesh with two unique characteristics. The side of the mesh toward the abdominal wall is usually placed directly on the peritoneum and, ideally, will incorporate through the peritoneum into the abdominal wall fascia with significant strength to minimize migration and, therefore, recurrence. On the visceral side, the mesh will ideally minimize adherence of the abdominal contents and, most importantly, prevent the ingrowth of any adherent organ to help eliminate long-term complications. These opposing characteristics make it difficult to create the ideal mesh.

Published reports of laparoscopic ventral hernia repair most frequently include the use of expanded polytetrafluoroethylene dual-sided mesh. The significant advantage of this type of mesh is the lack of ingrowth on the side placed toward the abdominal cavity. Although adhesions do occur on the smooth side, they are typically less aggressive and easier to lyse than those with other types of mesh.

A variety of "composite" types of mesh have been developed to promote ingrowth into the abdominal wall and prevent adhesions and/or ingrowth of the abdominal viscera. Products with heavyweight polypropylene on the abdominal wall side include those with expanded poly-

tetrafluoroethylene or absorbable antiadhesion film for the visceral side. There is also a composite polyester mesh with an absorbable collagen antiadhesion film for the visceral side. A potential advantage of the polyester composite is the ingrowth on the side toward the abdominal wall. Because polyester is hydrophilic, the ingrowth may occur without associated chronic inflammation, as seen with other heavyweight polypropylene mesh. A new mesh similarly allows ingrowth to the abdominal wall, but only with lightweight polypropylene, a material shown to have better ingrowth and less chronic inflammation than heavyweight polypropylene. The decreased density of the mesh and increased pore size is thought to account for this improvement. The visceral side is covered with absorbable cellulose to prevent adhesions and tissue ingrowth.

A group of biologic mesh materials have recently been introduced and may play a role in laparoscopic ventral hernia repair. Currently, its most common indication is during a repair in which the operative field is infected or contaminated because of previously placed mesh that has become infected, or after an enterotomy. There is little clinical data available to evaluate the biologic types of mesh at this time. It is thought that defects should be closed prior to biologic mesh placement. Maximum tissue approximation will help to promote tissue incorporation into the biologic scaffold.

INTRAOPERATIVE PITFALLS

Adhesions

The potential for increased difficulty and danger from severe dense adhesions has been mentioned. For the surgeon without significant laparoscopic experience, the best way to avoid complications associated with difficult adhesiolysis is to select patients unlikely to have complex adhesions.

Bleeding during adhesiolysis should be isolated and controlled with clips or endoloops, or possibly thermal energy when bowel or other organs are not near the site of bleeding. Bleeding that cannot be controlled laparoscopically requires that the procedure be converted to an open procedure.

As in open surgery, enterotomy during laparoscopic adhesiolysis is likely to occur at some point in a surgeon's experience. When encountering an enterotomy, the surgeon must use his or her best judgment, based on personal experience, and the patient's situation. Conversion to an open procedure is always an option and should not be considered a failure. Alternatively, a small incision

may be created to allow for repair of the enterotomy. Following abdominal wall closure, the procedure may proceed as a "laparoscopic-assisted" repair. For the experienced laparoscopic surgeon, a laparoscopic repair of the enterotomy, using laparoscopic suturing techniques, may be appropriate.

The decision whether or not to place mesh following an enterotomy also requires good judgment. The size of the enterotomy, degree of spillage, and the portion of the bowel injured all play a role in the decision. One option is to repair the injury and complete the adhesiolysis, but delay mesh placement. The patient is admitted to the hospital for observation and for administering of antibiotics, and returned to the operating room for laparoscopic mesh placement 2 to 6 days later. Placing a biologic mesh at the time of enterotomy repair is another option.

Suture Site Bleeding

The suture-passing instrument used to secure the mesh can cause bleeding in the abdominal wall. Direct pressure and/or tying the suture will usually stop this abdominal wall bleeding. If bleeding persists, additional sutures above and below the site of bleeding will most often control the bleeding.

 POSTOPERATIVE CARE

Patients are given clear liquids postoperatively and advanced to a regular diet as tolerated. Early ambulation is encouraged and return to normal activities is usually limited only by pain and discomfort. Patients with repair of relatively small ventral hernias often go home the day of surgery, and those with repair of larger ventral hernias require a hospital stay.

For large ventral hernia repairs, adequate pain control will almost always require intravenous narcotics. Pain management with an epidural catheter may also be considered in patients with large hernias. During the early postoperative period, pulmonary toilet with frequent use of incentive spirometry is encouraged, and SCD are maintained until the patient is ambulating. Patients who are ambulating well, tolerating a diet, and are able to control pain with oral analgesics alone are discharged from the hospital.

Complications

ILEUS

Patients requiring extensive adhesiolysis or those with very large defects are at risk for a postoperative ileus. Most patients with an ileus will require intravenous hydration and, possibly, suppositories or oral cathartics for return of bowel function. A nasogastric tube may be required for severe ileus.

SEROMA

The presence of a seroma is common, especially after repair of a large hernia defect. In general, seromas are not considered a complication. Most seromas resolve without therapy and rarely produce symptoms. It is important to explain to the patient that the "bulge" is not a recurrent hernia. Seromas are usually significantly improved within 6 to 8 weeks after surgery, although very large seromas can take several months to resolve. Rarely, a symptomatic or persistent seroma is aspirated. Sterile technique is essential to avoid secondary mesh infection.

SUTURE SITE PAIN

After the initial pain of the procedure resolves, it is not uncommon for patients to experience pain at one or more of the suture sites. Typically, this pain will resolve with time and conservative therapy. For severe or persistent suture site pain, an injection with the combination of short- and long-acting local anesthetic usually leads to resolution of the pain. Occasionally, repeat injections are required for permanent pain relief. Suture site pain can present or recur up to several months after the operation, usually resulting from increased activity. Suture site pain may be minimized with preinjection of all suture sites at the time of surgery and by tying knots gently to avoid tissue ischemia and nerve entrapment.

BLEEDING

Significant postoperative bleeding is rare because brisk bleeding is usually visualized during the procedure. In the largest study to date, less than 2% of patients required blood transfusions in the postoperative period. This could be a result of intra-abdominal bleeding from raw surfaces after extensive adhesiolysis or abdominal wall bleeding from injury to inferior epigastric vessels or muscular branches. This type of bleeding is almost always self-limiting and reoperation rarely results in identification of a specific source of active bleeding. The patient will often experience significant bruising in the pelvis and/or flanks as the hematoma resolves. As with all patients, suspected postoperative bleeding in a patient who is hemodynamically unstable

requires aggressive intervention for diagnosis and definitive treatment.

MISSED OR DELAYED BOWEL INJURY

A missed or delayed bowel injury should be suspected in a patient who has worsening abdominal pain and tenderness and begins to show signs of sepsis, such as elevated temperature and white blood cell count, tachycardia, and decreasing urine output and blood pressure, during the first few days after surgery. Other potential causes of the patient's worsening condition should be evaluated; however, an intra-abdominal source must be considered, especially in patients who required extensive adhesiolysis. Close monitoring and radiographic evaluation, including computed tomographic scan, may be appropriate in stable patients. The decision to reoperate should be made in a relatively short period of time, depending on the results of resuscitation, diagnostic testing, and close monitoring. However, a missed or delayed enterotomy and the resulting intra-abdominal sepsis can be fatal, even when diagnosed and treated in a timely fashion.

RECURRENCE

The recurrence rate for this procedure is excellent, compared with published results for a variety of open ventral hernia repairs. In the largest series of laparoscopic hernia repair, the recurrence rate was less than 5% and included cases performed during each surgeon's learning curve. The repair theoretically should have no recurrence if the basic principles of clear visualization, wide coverage, and secure fixation are practiced. The common causes of recurrence are technical: a missed hernia from lack of visualization of the entire abdominal wall, inadequate mesh coverage leading to mesh eventration out of the defect, and inadequate mesh fixation resulting in failure to cover the defect at one edge of the mesh, or migration of a portion or all of the mesh. Another mechanism of recurrence caused by failure of secure fixation can occur in giant ventral hernias. It is often necessary to sew multiple pieces of mesh together to achieve adequate coverage in patients with these defects. The suture used to sew two pieces of mesh together can break and result in a recurrence between two pieces of mesh. Use of interrupted permanent sutures in addition to running permanent sutures when multiple pieces

of mesh are required should minimize the potential for this mechanism of recurrence. Another rare cause of recurrence is a hernia at one of the permanent suture sites. Presumably, the likely causes in this situation are tension on the suture and/or ischemia of the tissue if the suture is tied too tightly. Tying knots gently and placing suture 1 to 2 cm from the edge of the mesh and allowing the mesh to cover the suture sites will help avoid this mechanism of recurrence.

CONCLUSION

The laparoscopic approach for ventral hernia repair has achieved widespread acceptance based on excellent clinical results, especially when compared with traditional open techniques. Combining a low recurrence rate with a low wound complication rate differentiates it from most open repairs. As with other advanced laparoscopic procedures, safe adoption of the technique requires appropriate training and patient selection. As experience is gained with this procedure, and with continued improvements in instrumentation, visualization technology, and mesh designed for the procedure, clinical results will likely continue to improve.

SUGGESTED READING

Carbajo MA, del Olma JC, Blanco JI, et al. Laparoscopic treatment of ventral abdominal wall hernias: preliminary results in 100 patients. *JSLS* 2000;4:141.

Constanza MJ, Heniford BT, Arca MJ, et al. Laparoscopic repair of recurrent ventral hernias. *Am Surg* 1998;64:1121.

DeMaria EJ, Moss JM, Sugerman HJ. Laparoscopic intraperitoneal polytetrafluoroethylene (PTFE) prosthetic patch repair of ventral hernia. Prospective comparison to open prefascial polypropylene mesh repair. *Surg Endosc* 2000;14:326.

Heniford BT, Park A, Ramshaw BJ, et al. Laparoscopic ventral and incisional hernia repair in 407 patients. *J Am Coll Surg* 2000;190:645.

Koehler RH, Voellwe G. Recurrences in laparoscopic incisional hernia repairs: a personal series and review of the literature. *JSLS* 1999;3:293.

LeBlanc KA. The critical technical aspects of laparoscopic repair of ventral and incisional hernias. *Am Surg* 2001;67:809.

LeBlanc KA, Booth WV, Whitaker JM, et al. Laparoscopic incisional and ventral herniorrhaphy in 1000 patients. *Am J Surg* 2000;180:193.

Ramshaw BJ, Esartia P, Schwab J, et al. Comparison of laparscopic and open ventral hernias. *Am Surg* 1999;65:827.

Toy FK, Bailey RW, Carey S, et al. Prospective, multicenter study of laparoscopic ventral hernioplasty. Preliminary results. *Surg Endosc* 1998;12:955.

Nongastrointestinal Transabdominal

EDITOR'S COMMENT

Laparoscopic ventral hernia repair is deceptively simple. Furthermore, the laparoscopic approach is gaining in popularity despite little-to-no level 1 evidence supporting this approach, compared with open mesh techniques. The basic steps are: gain access to the abdomen, adhesiolysis, and secure mesh. Yet, there are several concerns, and surgeons offering this operation should be cognizant of lessons learned.

Dr. Ramshaw is a recognized educator and has taught hundreds of surgeons this operation through regular courses across the United States. Unlike most laparoscopic procedures that boast decreased pain, this advantage has not been proven with laparoscopic ventral hernia repair. Dr. Ramshaw provides several tips that may be helpful in alleviating postoperative pain and avoiding recurrence.

One obstacle to learning more about laparoscopic compared with open approaches is that patients are unwilling to enroll in randomized prospective studies. Despite an institutional review board to study this question, as soon as I describe an open and a laparoscopic approach, the patient almost always chooses the " laparoscopic and convert if you must" option.

I do not offer the laparoscopic approach to all patients. I shy away from huge hernias. The laparoscopic approach requires a large sheet of mesh and wide mesh overlap. Folded mesh must be able to pass through a 10- to 12-port wound and ports must be placed lateral to the mesh on the abdominal wall. On the other extreme, very small 1-cm umbilical hernias may not need mesh and can be done as an open procedure through a small incision. Unless, the patient engages in very physical daily activity, I favor an open approach for small hernias.

I always will discuss the risk of enterotomy. Patients who have undergone previous abdominal operations are at a much higher risk of intestinal injury. The more previous operations to repair a hernia, the less inclined I am to advocate for laparoscopy when the patient is referred to me. Once patients are well informed, I am willing to take a look with the laparoscope if I can identify an area for safe insertion, usually the left upper quadrant. Two to three additional ports may be placed under laparoscopic visualization. If adhesions cannot be dissected with good visualization or if the hernia cannot be reduced without undo force, then conversion is clearly warranted. Enterotomy may be managed laparoscopically, but conversion should be considered. Injury may require delay in hernia repair, if there is contamination, or use of alternative mesh products such as bioabsorbables.

Although many surgeons use an Iodrape, this is probably unnecessary as long as the abdomen is prepared and draped. With the patient relaxed, I will palpate the hernial defect(s) and use a colored marker to outline defects. For small defects (<10 cm), a 3-cm mesh overlap will likely suffice; however, for larger hernial defects, a larger overlap of 5 cm is advisable to help avoid mesh migration and reherniation.

Surgeons vary as to mesh preference. Usually there is a smooth side to minimize adhesions and a side that promotes tissue ingrowth. I place corner stitches with long tails; between these, I space additional sutures approximately 5 to 8 cm apart, rather than pass additional sutures later. The spaghetti can usually be figured out. I fold the mesh like a letter, rather than roll it, as I find this easier to open. I will use a fascial closure device (Storz, Culver City, CA) as it is more durable than other devices I have used.

Once the mesh is affixed to the abdominal wall, a spiral tacker will prevent herniation. Dr. Ramshaw advocates 1-cm intervals, but I place my tacks a little further apart, but will have an inner and outer circle of tacks. Tacks must be flush with mesh or the tack can erode into bowel, especially if the patient experiences postoperative ileus. To achieve a flush tacking, I decrease the pneumoperitoneum pressure to 10 cm. I use my fingertips to depress the abdominal wall, and I fire the spiral tacker at 90 degrees. A misfire on the tack is usually caused by tacking at too much of an angle. Protruding tacks must be removed.

Some surgeons send patients home the same day, but I do not, unless in cases of few adhesions and a small hernia. Extensive adhesiolysis always risks bowel injury and a period of observation before discharge seems appropriate. Also, whether done open or laparoscopically, ventral hernia repair causes a lot of pain. I favor a patient-controlled analgesia overnight for most patients, and prior to discharge I want to enssure that patients are able to tolerate pain.

Dr. Ramshaw has several suggestions to decrease postoperative pain that are worthy of repeating. Local anesthesia is administered at all port sites but also injected at site of transabdominal sutures. He tries not to strangulate tissue with tacking sutures. I would also add that one should minimize the number of spiral tackers as these are also a source of discomfort. During the years, I have recommended an abdominal binder to potentially decrease postoperative seroma; many patients report that they feel more comfortable wearing an abdominal binder as well.

Laparoscopic method is an excellent operation to teach. Surgeons appreciate the concerns and consequences of adhesiolysis. The anatomy of the abdominal wall is understood. The principles of mesh overlap are the same. Therefore, laparoscopic ventral hernia repair is a good skill to learn for the general surgeon who is experienced in laparoscopic cholecystectomy. We have taught surgeons this procedure using inanimate models in the skills laboratory as it allows the student to practice sizing, preparing, and fixing the mesh. At our institution, we have used teleproctoring technology as well, and have found that this is a terrific way for surgeons early in their experience to tap into others' expertise.

Despite numerous prospective series and patient demand, the laparoscopic ventral hernia repair is not universally performed. Mesh companies really jack up the price of the product; therefore, in some facilities the laparoscopic approach becomes prohibitively expensive. Without randomized prospective studies, the cost benefit of this approach is difficult to justify to auditors. Meanwhile, studies such as the Veterans Affairs Laparoscopic Ventral Hernia Study are eagerly awaited.

D.B.J.

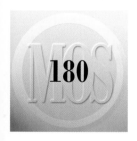

180 Biomaterials in Hernia Repair

JAMES R. DEBORD AND LISA A. WHITTY

From the beginning of modern anatomic hernia surgery, ushered in by Bassini in 1887, recurrences have plagued and frustrated surgeons of all ages, experiences, skills, and nationalities. Over the past century, it has become clear even to the most recalcitrant devotee of autologous tissue repairs that prosthetic biomaterials will sometimes be required to bridge or reinforce natural and unnatural defects in the integrity of the abdominal wall, inguinal canal, and chest wall.

The anatomic knowledge required of surgeons is nowhere more telling by its presence or absence than in the understanding of and surgical treatment of groin hernia. For almost 120 years this anatomic knowledge has been accumulated and surgical techniques devised to master the repair of groin hernia. In the best modern hands these techniques of primary repair have led to failures at rates for the most part considered unacceptable. The current widespread, worldwide use of prosthetics in groin hernia repair, while introducing a new unique set of problems and complications, has brought the failure rate for groin hernia repair to the low single digits.

Ventral incisional hernia repair is one of the most underrated, underappreciated, and undervalued operations in modern surgery. Since nearly all ventral abdominal hernias are incisional hernias, they represent surgical failure from the very beginning and occur in 10% to 20% of postlaparotomy patients. Primary repair of hernias greater than 4 cm in size may have failure rates (recurrence) nearing 50% due to multiple factors including technical issues of inappropriate or inadequate suture material, inadequate suturing technique (too small bites of fascia or inadequate suture length–to–wound length ratio), and poor surgical judgment with respect to the assessment of tension in the repair as well as biologic and demographic issues of obesity, malnutrition, chronic cough, smoking, old age, ascites, steroid therapy, chemotherapy, renal failure, diabetes, infection, and not fully understood abnormalities in collagen metabolism and tissue protease activity. Therefore, the augmentation of ventral incisional hernia repair by prosthetic biomaterials has become standard practice and has reduced the resultant recurrence rate to single digits in many reports.

The modern ascent of mesh utilization in hernia repair from scant and skeptical to common and acceptable has been a slow progression that has evolved over the past century. Through clinical research and trial and error, numerous biomaterials came into use over the years only to be abandoned for failure or excess complications. The modern surgical era has found useful and has depended upon three "surviving" biomaterials that have found widespread acceptance and use: Polypropylene mesh, polyester mesh, and expanded polytetrafluoroethylene (e-PTFE) patches. Numerous clinical publications in the surgical literature have documented the successful implantation of these biomaterials in inguinal and ventral hernia repair. With the markedly expanded use of prosthetics in hernia repair, we have seen an explosion in the past decade of commercial interest in this market. While this has yet to produce a totally new prosthetic material, it has led to the development of numerous variations and nuances of the three basic materials and some combinations of mesh types. These hybrid mesh products have attempted to marry the advantages of two different mesh materials into one product. Whether this is a victory of marketing over science remains to be seen.

One area where science has led to better mesh concepts has come from basic research on the bioactivity of mesh in tissue and the role of the inflammatory response in mesh incorporation, a better understanding of the biomechanics of the abdominal wall, and the influence of mesh on those mechanics. This has led to our current understanding that "less is more." In other words, less dense, lighter weight, larger pore size mesh, while still stronger than the abdominal wall, will result in less

inflammation, better incorporation, better abdominal wall compliance, possibly less scar contraction, greater abdominal wall flexibility, less pain, and therefore a better clinical outcome.

As we have utilized biomaterials to improve our outcomes with hernia repairs, difficult clinical problems remain, especially in the area of abdominal wall reconstruction in the presence of infection or contamination. This has promoted the recent development of biologic "mesh" products designed for use in these undesirable clinical situations. The most prominent of these biologic prosthetics currently are made from porcine intestinal submucosa or human cadaver dermis that is treated to result in an acellular collagen matrix that has inherent initial tensile strength but allows for host angiogenesis and cellular ingrowth that results in a biocompatible neofascia made of the patient's own tissue and collagen. Initial studies have shown these products to have clinical usefulness in complex reconstructions in infected or contaminated fields. With these biologic mesh products available there is less need for absorbable mesh such as polyglycolic acid (Dexon) or polyglactin (Vicryl). These absorbable meshes have variable clinical usage but may be helpful in desperate situations where their temporary nature is understood but acceptable under the circumstances.

While the ideal biomaterial for hernia repair has likely not yet been developed, a set of criteria for an ideal implantable prosthetic biomaterial has been established. The material

1. should not be physically modified by tissue fluids;
2. should be chemically inert;
3. should not excite an inflammatory or foreign body reaction;
4. should be noncarcinogenic;
5. should not produce a state of allergy of hypersensitivity;
6. should be capable of resisting mechanical strains;
7. should be capable of being fabricated in the form required; and
8. should be capable of being sterilized.

Since no single "ideal" operation exists for the cure of hernia, it is unlikely that a single "ideal" prosthesis to augment hernia repair will be developed that is universally adaptable.

The three biomaterials currently in widespread use throughout the world for hernia repair (polyester mesh, polypropylene mesh, and e-PTFE patch) are well tolerated by the body. All of these biomaterials, from a clinical perspective, meet, to a

great degree, the eight criteria previously outlined. None seems altered by tissue fluids, and while e-PTFE is clearly the most inert of these materials, none excites an inflammatory or foreign body reaction that interferes with its clinical applicability. None of these materials has been shown to be carcinogenic or to elicit an allergic reaction in tissues. While e-PTFE material strength and suture retention strength exceed those of polyester and polypropylene mesh, no clinical failures of any of these biomaterials have ever been reported due to mechanical prosthesis failure. Suture line failure has been reported many times, but this is always due to breakage of the suture material or pulling out of the suture–tissue interface, never the suture–prosthesis interface. All of these prostheses, then, appear to have adequate ability to resist the mechanical strains of clinical use. All three materials are readily available and may be fabricated in any form required by the defect to be repaired. All are clearly capable of being sterilized.

These three biomaterials have all been shown, both macroscopically and microscopically, to allow tissue ingrowth into the prosthesis. The more coarse macroporous meshes clearly differ from the smooth microporous e-PTFE patch in this regard. The polyester and polypropylene meshes incite a more proliferative, although disorganized, fibrous-collagenous response that many feel creates a more secure bond with the surrounding fascia. With time, scar tissue is well known to weaken and stretch and cannot be relied upon for the long-term integrity necessary for hernia repair. Therefore, the ultimate success of prosthetic herniorrhaphy with any of these three commonly used biomaterials must depend on the health of the surrounding fascia to which the prosthesis must be securely sutured, without undue tension, using adequate compatible suture material. The only prosthetic material that seems to elicit a strong, orderly, and organized collagen response, aligned in the direction of the stress applied, is carbon fiber–based material, which has had little clinical use reported.

The microporous e-PTFE patch does support tissue ingrowth into its internodal spaces, and this has been histologically well confirmed. When implanted as a replacement for the abdominal wall, without peritoneal coverage, the e-PTFE patch supports the rapid development of a mesothelial-like cellular monolayer that acts to "reperitonealize" the visceral surface of the patch. The resulting decrease in adhesion formation and bowel complications in this setting has been reported in numerous experimental and clinical papers.

Future biomaterials must meet three additional criteria to more nearly match the requirements for the ideal prosthetic material: They must be resistant to infection, provide a barrier to adhesions on the side of the material placed adjacent to the abdominal viscera, and respond in vivo more like autologous tissue, allowing tissue incorporation for good fixation and a strong lasting repair without encouraging the scarring and encapsulation problems seen with many of today's prostheses.

There is little doubt that infection remains the Achilles heel of implantation of any prosthetic material in human surgery and clearly is the leading cause of failure in hernia repair, no matter what biomaterial is used. Adherence of bacteria to the prosthetic material is the initial step in the pathogenesis of prosthesis colonization. Impregnation of broad-spectrum antimicrobial agents, such as silver and chlorhexidine, into implantable devices has been shown to reduce bacterial colonization. Systemic antibiotics often fail to prevent patch infections clinically because the drugs cannot penetrate the bacterial biofilm that forms on the surface of the prosthesis. This may lead to bacterial adherence to the prosthesis, resulting in infection and potentially fatal septic complications. Impregnation of silver and chlorhexidine into e-PTFE patches is now commercially available and may reduce bacterial colonization and subsequent infections, although this has not yet been proven by clinical trials.

Thus, it appears that an antimicrobial-impregnated prosthesis that allows well-organized fibrous ingrowth on one side and has antiadhesion properties on the other side would approach the brass ring of an ideal prosthetic biomaterial for abdominal wall reconstruction. Theoretically, the incorporation of cytokines or genes that promote or regulate the inflammatory response and collagen metabolism into prosthetics could further enhance the ideal biomaterial.

The tissue reaction to prosthetic biomaterials is "dose dependent" and most likely is influenced more by the physical properties of the mesh than the chemical properties of the underlying fiber material. Weight in g/m^2 of mesh and the surface area of exposed fiber are keys to biocompatibility of mesh in tissue. Surface area is a function of pore size and filamentous structure and is much reduced in monofilament versus multifilament mesh. Thus, biocompatibility of mesh increases with low weight, large pore size, and monofilament construction. No surgical mesh is totally inert and a chronic state of irritation exists in the tissue with all mesh.

For the working clinical surgeon, a theoretical and scientific analysis must boil down to the selection of an available prosthesis for a particular patient's hernia repair. Current clinical data supporting the successful use of polyester mesh, polypropylene mesh, and e-PTFE patches in hernia repair are readily available. In addition, the practical and subjective issues of "feel," "handling," "suturability," availability, and cost enter into the surgeon's final decision. A prudent surgeon considering all of the data might suggest the following:

1. For preperitoneal groin hernia repair and for anterior "tension-free" repairs, polyester, polypropylene, and e-PTFE prostheses are all satisfactory. Lightweight polypropylene mesh may be preferable.

TECHNICAL TIPS

a. Sutures to the Cooper ligament in preperitoneal repairs should be of permanent material.
b. Lightweight macroporous mesh may be sutured with absorbable sutures (0 to 2-0) in anterior tension-free repairs. Inferior-lateral sutures should incorporate the iliopubic tract as well as the shelving portion of the inguinal ligament.
c. In development, fibrin/biologic glues may allow for use of fewer sutures with anticipated less inguinodynia.
d. Tacking devices should be avoided in most cases or used sparingly with great care.
e. Mesh should overlap the pubic tubercle medially by 1 to 2 cm.
f. Mesh should be extended laterally under the external oblique aponeurosis several cm.
g. The mesh should have some mild laxity after being sutured to accommodate changes in the abdominal wall with increased postoperative intra-abdominal pressure. Do not suture the mesh "tight as a drum."
h. Plug devices should be securely sutured to reduce the risk of migration. A new bioabsorbable plug may prove beneficial in reducing plug complications.
i. The groin nerves should be identified and protected and entrapment by suture or mesh avoided.

2. For intraperitoneal placement of a prosthesis for inguinal or ventral hernia repair, by conventional or laparoscopic techniques, e-PTFE patches are preferred.

Some of the newer macroporous meshes bonded with antiadhesion films may prove satisfactory as well.

TECHNICAL TIPS

a. Intraperitoneal repair of inguinal hernia is not recommended.
b. Permanent transabdominal wall sutures are required for e-PTFE patches.
c. Tacking devices may be used for ventral hernia mesh fixation and to close gaps between fixation sutures.
d. A wide underlay (5 cm minimum) is advised.
e. The attenuated fascia should be preserved and closed over the mesh whenever possible in open repair.

3. For the Stoppa procedure of giant prosthetic reinforcement of the visceral sac, polyester mesh is preferred.

TECHNICAL TIPS

a. This is an excellent approach for recurrent, multiple recurrent, and bilateral hernias and in patients with inherent connective tissue disorders, since no sutures are required when large-size polyester mesh is used.
b. I have never done this operation. See Chapters 19 and 20 of Fitzgibbons and Greenburg's work in Suggested Readings for Technical Tips.

4. For ventral incisional hernia repair performed extraperitoneally, polyester, polypropylene, and e-PTFE prostheses are all satisfactory. Lightweight polypropylene mesh may be preferable.

TECHNICAL TIPS

a. This may be the best operation for ventral hernia repair when done properly.
b. The retromuscular, extraperitoneal placement of the mesh affords protection from visceral complications and leaves the mesh well away from potential contamination in the case of superficial wound infections.
c. Biologic mesh may be used to augment the posterior rectus sheath if it is inadequate to come together in the midline beneath the mesh. Absorbable mesh may also be used here if omental protection of the bowel is possible.
d. The retrorectus dissection is actually quite easy. Care needs to be taken to ensure good hemostasis.
e. Retrorectus dissection should extend to the lateral edge of the rectus abdominus muscle.

f. Lightweight macroporous mesh is best here and can be secured with absorbable sutures through the anterior rectus sheath or transabdominal via small skin incisions if subcutaneous dissection is avoided.

g. The linea alba is closed over the mesh to complete the repair.

5. For full-thickness chest wall or diaphragm defects, e-PTFE patches are preferred. The newer biologic meshes may be used in diaphragm repair.

TECHNICAL TIPS

a. Permanent sutures should be used.

6. For contaminated or grossly infected wounds or abdominal wall defects, polypropylene mesh may be preferred or absorbable mesh may provide adequate temporary closure. The newer biologic meshes have been successful also in the presence of infection.

TECHNICAL TIPS

a. These difficult problems continue to present opportunities for creative surgeons. A combination of open abdominal dressings, multiple lavages, vacuum-assisted wound care, and delayed closure techniques may provide the best solution currently to these complex contaminated abdominal wall defects.

There is no doubt that improvements and refinements in surgical biomaterials, based on further study of mesh construction parameters as well as the cellular reaction to prosthetic material in vivo, will lead us closer to the elusive "ideal" biomaterial for hernia repair. Regardless, surgeons will be wise to remember that prostheses, whatever their value, cannot replace a full knowledge of the underlying anatomy and pathology of hernia, or substitute for the exercise of time-honored principles of surgical technique and judgment.

SUGGESTED READING

Amid PK. Classification of biomaterials and their related complications in abdominal wall hernia surgery. *Hernia* 1997;l:15.

Bendavid R. The unified theory of hernia formation. *Hernia* 2004;8:171.

DeBord JR. The historical development of prosthetics in hernia surgery. *Surg Clin North Am* 1998;78(6):973.

Fitzgibbons RJ, Greenburg AG, eds. *Nyhus and Condon's hernia,* 5th ed. Philadelphia: Lippincott Williams & Wilkins, 2002.

Schumpelick V, Nyhus LM, eds. *Meshes: benefits and risks.* Heidelberg: Springer-Verlag, 2004.

EDITOR'S COMMENT

The reason for including this chapter is self-evident. Prosthetic materials have become a major part of hernia repair. Inguinal hernias have a finite recurrence when done by suture alone, and the recurrence rate is clearly less when some type of mesh or other material is used either with a suture repair or instead of a suture repair, as in the Lichtenstein tension-free repair, which seems to be the predominant repair at this point in time. Ventral hernia is, however, another issue. To put it simply, the recurrence rate of ventral hernia is extraordinarily high, probably higher than 50%. It is highly unlikely that weaknesses of collagen are responsible for this huge recurrence rate, but it is much more likely that this is a matter of the type of operation that is being undertaken, and what is being asked of weakened fascia. In addition, since a good part of my practice is gastrointestinal cutaneous fistulas, laparoscopic mesh repairs seem to have become a major source of gastrointestinal cutaneous fistulas, joining lysis of adhesions, inflammatory bowel disease, and cancer, as the fourth major source of gastrointestinal cutaneous fistulas. This, in my experience, appears much more likely with polyester and polypropylene (Marlex) meshes. Both are present in abundance in patients who undergo mesh repairs of hernias, either open or, more commonly, laparoscopically. As Dr. DeBord points out, ePTFE seems to have a layer of neoperitoneum that grows underneath, and adhesions are much less common. This is in keeping with my experience.

While Dr. DeBord seems to favor thin polypropylene, Demir et al. (*Surg Today* 2005;35:223) carried out experimental full-thickness 1.5 × 2.5-cm abdominal wall defects in 30 Sprague-Dawley rats, which were repaired with 2 × 3-cm polypropylene mesh (group 1), ePTFE—the double layer of polypropylene mesh (group 2), or polypropylene mesh with an oxidized cellulose adhesion barrier (Interceed, group 3). Two measurements of outcome were investigated: Mean adhesion scores and area involved by adhesions. The mean adhesions scores were 3.3, 1.3, and 0.7, respectively, and the area involved by adhesions was significantly greater in the standard polypropylene mesh group (group 1) and in group 2. However, the lowest incidence of both adhesions and area of adhesions favored group 3. The authors found, however, that PTFE not only impaired the tensile strength, but also induced fibrosis and inflammation. Thus, they favor the oxidized cellulose adhesion barrier attached to polypropylene.

Others have used different coatings. Champault and Barrat (*Hernia* 2005;9[2]:125) carried out either Lichtenstein repairs in 58 patients or laparoscopic procedures (total extraperitoneal hernioplasty/transabdominal extraperitoneal hernioplasty) utilizing an oat beta glucan coating of polypropylene mesh. They argued that glucan is an entirely natural plant product, and thus viral or prion contamination associated with the use of collagen of animal origin is not a problem. Patients were followed up for 2 years, by questionnaire. Ninety-five percent of the questionnaires were returned. Two years after operation, the recurrence rate was 1.9%, although it is not clear that all the patients were examined 2 years postoperatively. Ninety-four percent of patients had no pain; five percent had mild pain on movement; and one patient had moderate pain at rest. Thus, they argued that this is a satisfactory mesh with a theoretic advantage of being of plant origin.

Although the Lichtenstein tension-free repair appears to be the dominant type of repair, the PerFix plug has its adherents. Pikoulis et al. (*World J Surg* 2005;online first) reported 865 prosthetic repairs in 801 consecutive patients repaired with polypropylene PerFix plugs. The authors' excellent reported results, carried out by telephone interviews, included persisting inguinoscrotal paresthesia in 2% and neuralgia in 1%, which is very low. They also reported that the recurrence was 0.1%. However, Losanoff and Millis (*World J Surg* 2005;29[10]:1359) challenged these results, as they indicated that the Lichtenstein group abandoned the plug procedure 35 years ago, due to the frequency and severity of complications. They also pointed out that the known complications of plug hernia repair include the loss of 75% of the plug diameter; infection in between 5% and 9%; chronic postoperative pain; erosion of the femoral vessels, urinary bladder, or intestines; and plug migration into the scrotum. Pikoulis et al. responded to this criticism (*World J Surg* 2005;29[10]:1359), stating that their results were accurate. They also pointed out that they did not cover the pubic tubercle, which is a feature of the Lichtenstein repair. It is interesting, as one can see in my comments in other chapters in this section, that a major area of late recurrence is above and slightly lateral to the pubic tubercle. Thus, this important area is not covered by these individuals.

On the question of pain, they are less definite. They attempt to relate the incidence of pain to the material. As one who sees many of the chronic pain syndromes and rectifies them by triple neurectomy following mesh hernia repair, I have not noticed that the type of mesh makes any difference at all. All the meshes seem to entrap the nerves. Of course I have no denominator, so I do not know whether the incidence of one mesh entrapping the nerves is less than the others. In short, while I admire the persistence of Pikoulis et al., it does seem as if more careful follow-up would be in order.

The availability of biomaterials has been duly noted by the chapter authors. However, these are quite expensive, and it has not yet been established as to whether their results are superior. Indeed, several of the papers that will be quoted later in this commentary indicate that perhaps there are significant problems with some of them.

Does one require sutures in a Lichtenstein repair? Nowobilski et al. (*Eur Surg Res* 2004;36:367) randomized 46 males with unilateral inguinal hernias, which were repaired with a polypropylene tension-free procedure, anchored with 3/0 Dexon sutures in one group, and closing the skin with Dexon and Monosof, as compared to the other group in which the mesh was secured with butyl-2-cyanoacrylate adhesive, and the fascia and skin were also glued with the adhesive. Follow-up was only 4.7 months, and no recurrences were noted at that time. There was a statistically significant difference in pain score 24 hours after surgery, but not at

(continued)

proximally, or (c) various caustic treatments of the divided nerve ends. The later treatments have included laser treatment, electrofulguration, suture ligation, and various denaturing agents such as absolute alcohol and phenol.

There is little literature to support any of these treatments with sensory somatic nerves as described herein, and very few reports of postinguinal neurectomy neuroma occurrence. Nonetheless, a few minutes invested intraoperatively may be well worth the effort to prevent recurrence of the symptoms at a later date postoperatively.

The reported occurrence of typical pain following laparoscopic herniorrhaphy is explained by the same mechanism as the open repair, that is, entrapment or impingement upon these same nerves, particularly the genital branch of the genital femoral nerve. A large "unfurled" piece of mesh is usually tacked or anchored with metallic devices and these may involve not only the genital nerve branch, but also the more ventral inguinal nerves. Should this occur, repeat laparoscopy should reveal the involved nerve(s) and proximal neurectomy carried out. Neuroma prophylaxis might in this instance include suture ligation with or without nerve end fulguration. Application of a potentially harmful substance such as alcohol or phenol may not be justified in proximity to the femoral vessels and nerve.

Removal of implanted mesh and its hardware is a matter of personal preference, and if the entrapped nerves are easily visualized and can be dissected back proximally where they can be easily divided, then tedious dissection of mesh that is adequately controlling a hernia is probably unnecessary. However, if the mesh is large and encompasses one or more nerves, then effective treatment would require its removal.

Results of Treatment

The initial reports of inguinal neurectomy were in small series of patients in the early 1940s and were uniformly successful. Relatively few reports have appeared since then, suggesting either disinterest in reporting such patients or failure to recognize the problems that must predictably occur, given the large number of herniorrhaphies and suprainguinal incisions done each year. Risk factors for therapeutic failure are primarily seen in multiply recurrent hernias or in cases where not all of the nerves are located and divided. Collective reviews of the series that have been reported suggest an 80% to 90% success rate with few, if any, immediate or long-term problems.

SUGGESTED READING

Amid PK. A 1-stage surgical treatment for post-herniorrhaphy neuropathic pain: triple neurectomy and proximal end implantation without mobilization of the cord. *Arch Surg* 2002;137:100.

Callesen T, Bech K, Kehlet H. Prospective study of chronic pain after groin hernia repair. *Br J Surg* 1999;86:1528.

Heise CP, Starling JR. Mesh inguinodynia: a new clinical syndrome after inguinal herniorrhaphy? *J Am Coll Surg* 1998;187:514.

Madura JA, Madura JA II, Copper CM, et al. Inguinal neurectomy for inguinal nerve entrapment: an experience with 100 patients. *Am J Surg* 2005;189:283.

Picchio M, Palimento D, Attanasio U, et al. Randomized controlled trial of preservation or elective division of ilioinguinal nerve on open inguinal hernia repair with polypropylene mesh. *Arch Surg* 2004;139:755.

Starling JR, Harms BA, Schroeder ME, et al. Diagnosis and treatment of genitofemoral and ilioinguinal entrapment neuralgia. *Surgery* 1987;102:581.

Nongastrointestinal Transabdominal

EDITOR'S COMMENT

The fact that this chapter appears in this book indicates, at least in my experience, the unfortunate degree of nerve entrapment following the tension-free repairs and involving mesh. While not terribly common, it is sufficiently common that I see a fair number of these, and Dr. Madura has been able to collect a series of 100 patients in a relatively short period of time. From personal experience, I can tell you these patients are miserable, and their lives are ruined to a considerable extent. It is nagging, and in some patients, class A narcotic habituation has become an issue.

Most surgeons, including, unfortunately, the surgeon who has carried out the operation, do not deal with it, or rather refuse to deal with this, giving the patient no opportunity to get this under control other than going to pain clinics, in which habituation becomes more and more likely. The true incidence is not clear. It is probably somewhere between 5% and 15%, depending on the care with which the mesh is inserted. On the other hand, a nonmesh repair is no assurance of lack of posthernia or neuropathy pain. The ilioinguinal and iliohypogastric nerves are grasped with sutures during the repair and trapped with the posterior repair sutured to the pubic ramus, giving at least one cause of osteitis pubis, and inadvertently sutured during the external oblique closure. In the tension-free repair, the issue appears to be entrapment in the mesh as a major cause of inguinodynia. The two mechanisms are different. The genital branch of the femoral nerve is more likely to be entrapped at the exit of the inguinal canal, that is, at the external inguinal ring.

Diagnostic procedures are not numerous. While some have advocated nerve blocks, I have not used this in my diagnosis of these unfortunate patients. Twisting and turning, as indicated in Figure 3, putting these nerves on tension, is the usual way one makes the diagnosis, and one can try a series of nerve blocks with a small amount of steroid. The Xylocaine and Marcaine will give one an initial period of analgesia and tell you that you have hit the appropriate spot, but the steroid rarely makes any difference long term. Remember that the genital branch of the genitofemoral nerve runs along the cord and may be entrapped at the closure, and trying to inject the cord as it enters the scrotum may give the patient some relief there, but the entrapment is likely to be more proximal. There are other reasons for pain in the inguinal area, including the tears in the external oblique fascia, which David Mulder has reported on, being the team physician to the Montreal Canadians.

The appropriate therapy is outlined in the chapter, taking both the ilioinguinal and iliohypogastric nerves back to the point where they come out from the muscle and tying them with nonabsorbable sutures and using alcohol or phenol to prevent a distal neuroma. I do not know how often one finds neuromas when one re-explores entrapment by mesh. My own practice is to remove the mesh if it is not too difficult and does not damage the viability of the testicle or the vascularity of the cord. Since I, like Dr. Madura, find it difficult to really determine which nerve is involved, the femoral nerve is probably not a problem, although that is likely the most difficult of all the nerves to deal with. With the exception of the genitofemoral nerve difficulties, my impression is that the ability to relieve these patients' neuropathic pain is probably in the range of 80% to 90%.

Others have attempted to see whether routine ilioinguinal nerve excision in inguinal hernia repairs works (Dittrick GW, et al. *Am J Surg* 2004; 188:736). They reviewed 90 patients who underwent a Lichtenstein tension-free repair with onlay mesh. The patients were not matched nor were they equivalent. Sixty-six patients underwent excision and 24 patients nerve preservation. The incidence of neuralgia was significantly lower in the neurectomy group versus the nerve preservation group after 5 months (3% vs. 26%, $P < 0.001$). Paresthesia in the distribution of the ilioinguinal nerve was higher but not statistically significantly so in the neurectomy group (18% vs. 4%, $P = 0.1$). Lower incidence of neuralgia was maintained at 1 year (3% vs. 25%, $P = 0.003$) and the incidence of paresthesia again not higher. In both groups, the mean severity on a visual analog scale (0 to 10) was similar in the neurectomy and the nerve preservation patients at all end points (2 to 2.5 vs. 1 to 2.2). This trend was sustained for 3 years. While this is encouraging, it seems rather strange that one should undergo another procedure to carry out a tension-free repair. There is a substantial amount of postoperative neuralgia in the

(continued)

group that underwent the Lichtenstein tension-free repair. Is recurrence, if one does a continual suture and pays attention to the transversalis fascia, that much of a problem that one has to perform a neurectomy to do a tension-free repair? This strikes me as completely ridiculous.

Another effort to control postoperative pain following a total extraperitoneal (TEP) inguinal hernioplasty was carried out by Lau and Patil (*Arch Surg* 2003;138:1352), who studied 200 patients, again not randomized. Patients with less than a 4-cm defect were not stapled, and patients that had more than a 4-cm defect were, thus making the two groups not strictly comparable. However, there was no difference in outcome as far as neuralgia between the two groups. There are other pains that occur around the inguinal area.

Lateral femoral cutaneous neuralgia is something that one sees after any kind of abdominal operation and seems to vanish as mysteriously as it appears after 3 or 4 months. It is rare that this becomes a chronic problem. A very interesting anatomic study was recently reported by Dias Filho et al. (*Clin Anat* 2003;16:309), who traced the origin of the lateral femoral cutaneous nerve, with good illustrations, from the femoral nerve as it passed under the inguinal ligament. They point out that there are two layers of fascia and that the lateral femoral cutaneous nerve runs through an aponeurotic fascial tunnel beginning at the iliopubic tract and ending at the inguinal ligament, suggesting that the fascial structures proximal to the inguinal ligament may be implicated in the genesis of this neuralgia. They also demonstrated in their anatomic investigation of 26 embalmed cadavers that pseudoneuromas existed at the inguinal ligament. This adds some explanation to the origin of this mysterious malady. It is rare that surgical intervention is necessary.

J.E.F.

Vascular Surgery

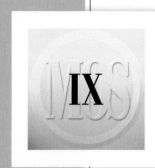

IX

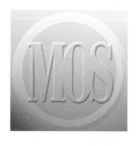

Introduction to the Endovascular Section

JOSEF E. FISCHER

Since the last edition, stenting, endovascular opening of thromboses, and the growth of minimally invasive surgery extended to vascular have revolutionized the field of vascular surgery. They have also created a new necessity for training, as the traditional open vascular training is relatively straightforward and similar to that of open general surgical training in the area of gastrointestinal and other open techniques. Endovascular surgery, which is the rapid growth area of the field, seems destined to continue to surpass open surgery as the field matures and changes.

Already there are indications that, for example, aortoiliac endovascular surgery, while having a slightly less long-term patency rate of, say, 97%, as compared to 99% in open aortoiliac surgery, is almost certain to improve with time as the technology advances. In the past 5 years, we have seen enormous strides in the nature of the stents, their seating capacity, the reduction of various types of endo leaks, and the ability to maintain long-term patency. This

will continue. The benefits to the patients, of which the most dramatic is the replacement of aortic aneurysmal resection, are striking. To me, who voluntarily stopped doing vascular surgery in 1976 because of a more profound interest in complicated gastrointestinal surgery and reoperative gastrointestinal surgery for fistulas, watching the continued performance of resection and grafting of aortic aneurysm meant 1 to 3 days in the intensive care unit (ICU), a 10-day hospital stay, a long incision from the xiphoid to pubis, and considerable morbidity. Contrast this with the overnight stay, a small groin incision, no stays in the ICU (but in an step-down unit), and, barring an occasional disastrous complication such as a retroperitoneal hole in the internal iliac artery due to a misplaced stent, really a benign postoperative course and low mortality.

Recognizing this, and recognizing that in our own excellent vascular division the number of open operations has remained stable, the endovascular procedures have in-

creased from three per month 2 years ago to about 100 per month, and are still climbing rapidly. Thus, in this edition, clearly in contrast to its predecessor, endovascular surgery plays a much more prominent part of the following sections. In neurosurgery, the growth of endovascular surgery is even more spectacular. A few individuals, such as Nick Hopkins, have revolutionized neurovascular surgery by producing a hybrid surgeon—one who is trained to do both endovascular neurosurgery intracranially and open intracranial neurosurgery for those very complicated lesions that do not lend themselves to endovascular neurosurgery. In a comparative study, it does appear as if the results are better for at least the majority of neurosurgical vascular lesions if done closed, that is, by endovascular neurosurgery. This has not yet reached the same level with endovascular peripheral surgery, but promises to head in that direction. As the technology improves, the results from endovascular surgery will almost certainly improve as well.

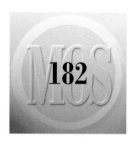

Carotid Endarterectomy with Shunt: Standard and Eversion Techniques

BRUCE L. GEWERTZ AND JAMES F. MCKINSEY

The techniques of carotid endarterectomy have been developed over some 50 years and are among the most standardized of all vascular surgical operations. This chapter will review the two most common endarterectomy procedures, herein termed "standard" (reflecting an axial arteriotomy extending the length of the atherosclerotic plaque) and "eversion" (referring to transection of the carotid bulb with traction extraction of the distal aspect of the plaque). We will also specifically consider the indications for the procedure with particular attention to the use and complications of

intraluminal shunting during the period of carotid occlusion.

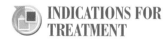

INDICATIONS FOR TREATMENT

A number of classic randomized prospective clinical trials have addressed the indications for and benefits of carotid endarterectomy in both symptomatic and asymptomatic patients. Consensus has been more clearly gained in symptomatic patients. Based on the classic North American Symptomatic Carotid

Endarterectomy Trial (NASCET) first published in 1991, it is now well accepted that symptomatic patients with bifurcation stenoses of greater than 70% diameter (calculated by comparing the diameter of the most narrowed area to that of the normal distal internal carotid artery) should be considered for treatment. It has been shown that such patients have at least a 30% incidence of stroke within 2 years. Most experienced surgeons extend these indications to symptomatic patients with greater than 50% stenoses, especially if the lesions are irregular, undermined, or extensive or if the patient has persistent symptoms despite suitable antiplatelet therapy.

The increased utility of nonsurgical approaches (i.e., carotid artery stenting with neuroprotection) has added an additional degree of complexity to the choice of therapy. In our practice, we favor operative treatment in those patients with relatively low operative risk, age less than 65 years, or anatomically unfavorable brachiocephalic anatomy, which might impair catheterization. Recent reports also suggest that patients greater than 80 years of age may have a higher incidence of complications from stenting and therefore may profit from operative rather than interventional therapy.

We prefer stenting with neuroprotection in those patients with high perioperative risk (usually due to cardiac compromise), age 65 to 80 years, anatomy that might make operation difficult (the infrequent very high carotid bifurcation), recurrent lesions, or an otherwise "hostile" neck (e.g., cervical radiation for malignancy). We also tend to employ stenting in those patients with unstable angina preparing for urgent cardiac surgery. In these circumstances stenting avoids both multiple operative procedures and/or simultaneous carotid and coronary revascularization.

The indications for treatment of asymptomatic lesions remain less firmly defined despite a large number of prospective studies. As a general rule, it is held that operative or interventional treatment of asymptomatic lesions should be reserved for good-to moderate-risk patients with stenoses of 70% or greater. The tendency to intervene is understandably greater in younger, healthier patients who could be expected to gain more benefit from any reduction in stroke risk. It is not yet clear whether the expanding options of nonoperative treatment will substantially change these decision patterns.

DIAGNOSTIC TESTS

Once a detailed neurologic and medical history is obtained, noninvasive carotid duplex scans are nearly always obtained. In properly validated laboratories, such tests can confirm the diagnosis and precisely quantitate both the degree of stenosis and the extent of the atheromatous lesions. Additional and valuable information is gained regarding the status of the contralateral carotid (involved in at least 50% of patients) and the direction of flow in the vertebral arteries. Some determination can also be made about the location of the bifurcation in relation to the cervical vertebrae and the presence of more proximal brachiocephalic disease.

Over the last 15 years, angiograms employing carotid catheterization have been used less frequently due to the well-documented fact that nearly one third of all strokes associated with evaluation and subsequent treatment of carotid lesions were associated with the diagnostic angiogram rather than the planned operation. Clinical experience has further suggested that when a thorough neurologic history documents unambiguous unilateral carotid territory symptoms and no confounding findings are noted on duplex examination, angiograms rarely reveal clinically important data. That said, the rapid development of computed tomography angiography (CTA) has rekindled enthusiasm for more extensive arterial imaging. With radiopaque contrast alone, and no risk of arterial embolization or occlusion, dramatic images of carotid lesions can be obtained while excluding intracranial aneurysms or stenoses or brachiocephalic involvement. These tests are most useful in those patients presenting with nonlateralizing symptoms, recurrent disease, bilateral carotid involvement, or vertebrobasilar insufficiency.

SURGICAL TECHNIQUE

Standard Endarterectomy

The common, internal, and external carotid arteries are exposed by an oblique anterior sternocleidomastoid incision. At all times, care is taken to avoid manipulation of the carotid bifurcation to minimize the risk of cerebral embolization. The facial vein is transected, allowing lateral retraction of the jugular vein. Deeper dissection of the adventitial plane of the common and internal carotid arteries is performed to the level of the hypoglossal nerve (Fig. 1A). If necessary, one or more muscular branches from the external carotid artery to the sternocleidomastoid muscle can be ligated, facilitating superior mobilization of the hypoglossal nerve (Fig. 1B). Even more important to distal exposure is the careful division of the smaller branches of the internal jugular vein that cross the internal carotid artery. This division should be performed before clamping and arteriotomy to allow complete and timely access to the distal internal carotid. If even more distal exposure to the skull base is required, transection of the posterior belly of the digastric muscle and subluxation of the mandible can be performed. The latter maneuver is needed in fewer than 5% of all cases.

The common carotid, internal carotid, external carotid, and superior thyroid arteries are all circumferentially dissected and isolated with vessel loops. If dissection of the proximal external carotid is likely to require undue manipulation of the carotid bifurcation, the vessel is simply exposed anteriorly to allow placement of an angled vascular clamp. Heparin is given systemically (100 units/kg of body weight), and vascular clamps are applied sequentially to the internal, common carotid, and external carotid arteries. Once the risk of distal embolization is eliminated, the carotid bulb is mobilized further. The vessel is rotated medially, and a lateral arteriotomy is begun in the common carotid artery and extended on to the internal carotid artery beyond the level of the atherosclerotic plaque or ulceration.

If an intraluminal shunt is required (see below), the clamp is removed from the distal internal carotid artery, and back-bleeding is controlled with tension on the vessel loop. The distal aspect of the balloon-tipped intraluminal shunt (already filled with heparinized saline) is inserted gently into the distal internal carotid artery beyond the level of the vessel loop. Retrograde flow through the shunt confirms appropriate positioning and allows washout of any debris or air (Fig. 1C). The balloon is gently and minimally inflated to decrease the risk of injury to the distal internal carotid artery; the device is maintained in place by "double looping" the vessel tape. If the diameter of the internal carotid artery is small, the balloon may not need to be inflated at all. A noncrushing clamp is placed on the distal limb of the shunt to control backbleeding. The common carotid artery is unclamped and controlled by digital pressure, and the vessel loop and the proximal aspect of the balloon-tipped carotid shunt are inserted into the common carotid artery. Blood is allowed to flush freely through the side of the shunt (i.e., the T limb). The proximal balloon is gently inflated and secured in place with the vessel loop. Once the proximal limb is adequately flushed and the entire shunt is inspected to ensure that there are no air bubbles or debris, the stopcock is rotated, and the clamp on the distal tubing is removed to restore perfusion to the internal carotid (Fig. 1D). Intermittent aspiration through the side arm of the shunt during the endarterectomy can be performed to confirm patency if the electroencephalogram (EEG) does not become normal within 5 minutes or if there

Vascular Surgery

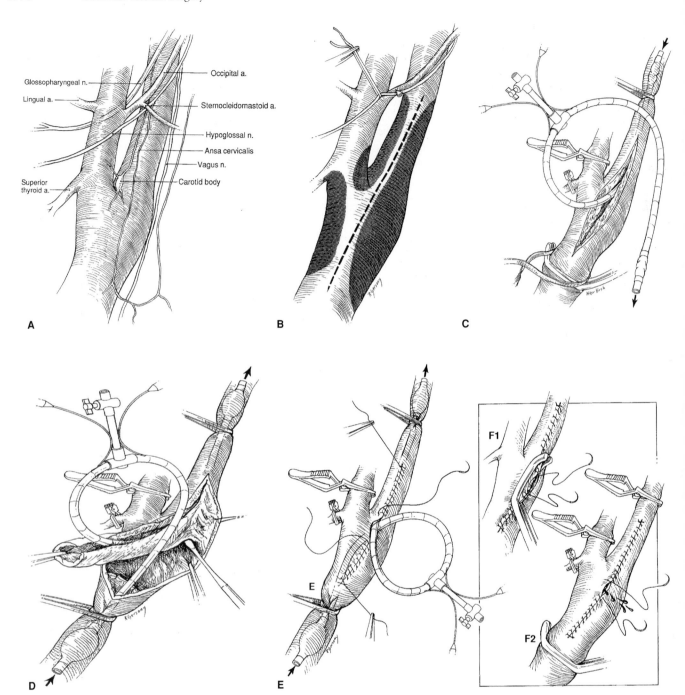

Fig. 1. A: The carotid bifurcation, with the carotid vessels shown in relation to major adjacent nerves. **B:** Division of the arterial branch to the sternocleidomastoid muscle facilitates superior mobilization of the hypoglossal nerve. The arteriotomy is made along the anterolateral side of the common carotid artery and extended distally along the internal carotid artery past the plaque. **C:** The distal aspect of the shunt is inserted into the internal carotid artery and secured in place with a vessel loop. Retrograde flushing of the shunt ensures proper position and removes any debris or air bubbles. **D:** Insertion of the proximal aspect of the shunt into the common carotid artery. Carotid endarterectomy is performed with the shunt in place. **E:** The primary closure after a successful endarterectomy with the shunt in place. Closely spaced single-filament 5-0 or 6-0 vascular suture is used. **F1:** A side-biting clamp is placed to allow immediate restoration of blood flow through the carotid endarterectomy site during closure. The clamp should be applied carefully to avoid direct injury to suture. **F2:** Completion of the primary closure of the endarterectomy site after removal of the shunt. Each vessel is transiently unclamped to clear the lumen. Flow is initially restored to the external carotid artery and then to the internal carotid.

is any unexpected change in frequency later in the procedure.

Throughout this entire sequence of maneuvers, it is important to remember that the speed with which the shunt is placed is of limited importance; ischemic injury is highly unlikely even if insertion times are 2 to 4 minutes. Furthermore, injury to the delicate distal internal carotid or embolization of air or debris will have much greater adverse effects. In short, the pace of the shunt insertion should be purposeful but not hurried.

The carotid endarterectomy is then performed, with elevation of the plaque at the deep medial endarterectomy plane and distal feathering of the plaque into the internal carotid artery. Tacking sutures are applied, if needed, at the distal end point. After completion of the endarterectomy and removal of all residual fronds of media, it must be determined whether the carotid artery is of adequate diameter for primary closure or whether a patch should be placed. In general, we place prosthetic vein patches in most female patients and smokers or in patients for whom the incised portion of the internal carotid artery is smaller than 3 mm in diameter. Irrespective of the nature of the closure, the repair is performed with the intraluminal shunt in place to ensure adequate cerebral perfusion; the shunt can also act as a temporary "stent" that effectively calibrates the lumen during closure (Fig. 1E). Once the arteriotomy is closed around the shunt so that the remaining sutures cannot be placed easily, the balloon of the distal shunt is deflated. A clamp is then placed on the shunt, the shunt is removed from the internal carotid artery, and a vascular clamp reapplied. Finally, the proximal balloon is deflated, and the shunt is removed entirely. All vascular clamps are transiently opened to flush the endarterectomy site, and the arteriotomy is irrigated with heparinized saline to cleanse the surface and remove all air bubbles. The small remaining portion of the arteriotomy is then rapidly closed (Fig. 1F2). Flow is initially directed to the internal carotid artery (after approximately five heartbeats) and then to the internal carotid artery. If a patient cannot tolerate even the brief period of carotid occlusion that is associated with this sequence, a side-biting clamp can be applied to the remaining length of the arteriotomy as soon as the shunt is removed (Fig. 1F1). This application allows restoration of blood flow while the closure is completed.

An occasional patient may present with an extensive plaque extending so far

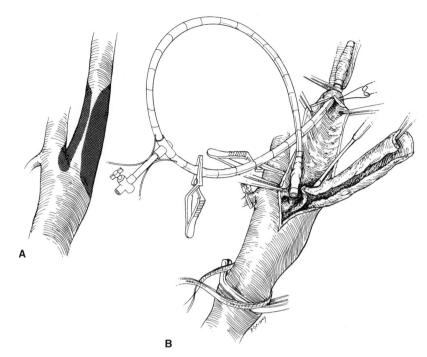

Fig. 2. A: Extensive stenosis of the distal internal carotid artery may prevent the safe and secure placement of the shunt. **B:** The distal endarterectomy is completed by placing tacking sutures, thus allowing the safe insertion of the distal end of the shunt. The proximal end of the shunt is inserted into the common carotid artery, and carotid endarterectomy is completed.

into the distal internal carotid artery that safe placement of the shunt is not possible until a distal endarterectomy is performed (Fig. 2A). In such circumstances, the distal end point should be completely visualized and tacking sutures placed if necessary. Although time is a factor, it is important to remember that the single most important element of the procedure is a technically perfect endarterectomy. Once the distal vessel is satisfactorily handled, the shunt can be inserted into the internal and common carotid arteries as described previously (Fig. 2B).

Eversion Technique

The procedure is identical to that described above until the arteriotomy is made. When using eversion technique, the surgeon transects the carotid bifurcation obliquely at the origin of the internal carotid artery (Fig. 3A,B). This requires complete mobilization of the carotid bulb in the periarterial plane after the clamps are applied. Care must be exercised to avoid injuring the vagus and glossopharyngeal nerves, which travel lateral and posterior to the bifurcation, respectively.

The atheroma is intussuscepted from the internal carotid artery by peeling back the deep media and adventitia of the distal vessel (Fig. 3C). With some experience, one

gains judgment regarding the necessary cephalad exposure of this vessel; with proper care, excellent distal exposure and endarterectomy end points can be obtained. Plaque removal usually requires a very short period of time. Once this is completed, a shunt can be placed if needed. The need for "tacking sutures" is assessed. Any atheroma in the external and common carotid is then removed in routine fashion.

If needed, the internal carotid stump is tailored and prepared for reanastomosis to the bifurcation. A single circular suture line is begun in the middle of the posterior wall and carried around the bulb (Fig. 3D–F). The primary benefit of this technique is the fact that no longitudinal suture line is placed in the small-diameter internal carotid artery. This avoids any needed for a patch and, at least in theory, might reduce postoperative recurrence due to intimal hyperplasia.

While the eversion technique has many surgical advocates, there is little if any evidence that either operative approach has advantages over the other. In our practice, we utilize the "standard" approach more commonly and reserve the eversion technique (a) for those instances where the internal carotid is elongated or kinked and reduction in length would be desired or (b) in those very few patients in whom prosthetic patch placement would

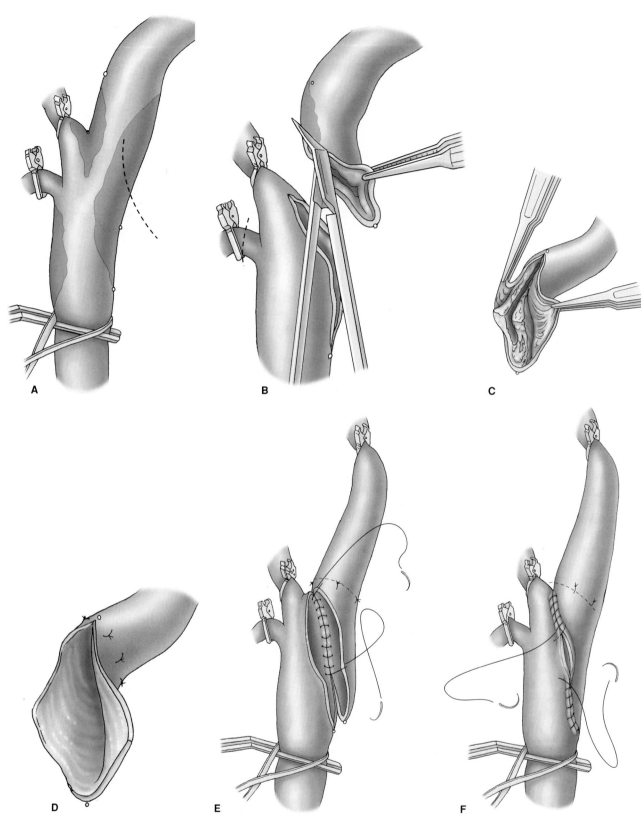

Fig. 3. A: After control and dissection of the carotid bifurcation, the origin of the proximal internal carotid artery is divided as it originates from the common carotid artery. The proximal incision is extended into the carotid bifurcation. This facilitates endarterectomy of the plaque. **B:** The internal carotid artery is opened up along its inner wall to the level necessary to straighten out any kink in the artery. **C:** An eversion endarterectomy of the distal internal carotid artery is carried out. The distal end point should be visualized. If needed, an intraluminal shunt can be placed, with care taken to straighten any coil or kink before advancing the shunt. **D:** Tacking sutures of interrupted 7-0 are used, if needed, to secure the distal end point, and the endarterectomized surface is carefully inspected. **E:** The spatulated internal carotid artery is then pulled down to straighten any kink. A primary anastomosis between the internal carotid artery and the common carotid artery is performed using continuous 6-0 monofilament suture. The back wall of the anastomosis is usually sewn from the inside of the artery. This provides the best visualization because rotation of the carotid may be cumbersome. **F:** Appropriate back flushing from the distal vessels is performed. The anastomosis is completed, and flow is restored to the external and then the internal carotid artery.

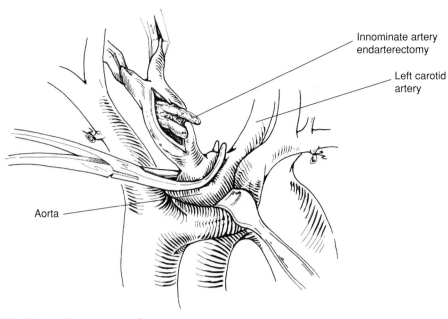

Fig. 3. Innominate artery endarterectomy.

innominate artery, (d) there is significant inflammation or adhesions due to radiation or arteritis, or (e) there is recurrence after prior endarterectomy.

INNOMINATE ENDARTERECTOMY

Intravenous heparin is administered at a dose of 1 mg/kg. The right common carotid artery is controlled before clamping the aorta to reduce the risk of cerebral embolism during manipulation of the arch (Fig. 3). The systemic pressure is maintained at or below a mean pressure of 65 to 70 mm Hg. An appropriate-shaped C-clamp, such as the Lambert-Kay or Lemole-Strong, is placed on the aorta at the base of the innominate artery. It should be noted that aortic pulsations may cause the C-clamp to migrate distally during the procedure leading to sudden, unexpected bleeding. The distal innominate artery or right subclavian and common carotid arteries are controlled. Shunting is not usually required during reconstruction of the innominate artery.

An endarterectomy of relatively isolated lesions avoids the risks associated with synthetic grafts. A longitudinal arteriotomy is made in the innominate artery to accommodate the endarterectomy. Traction sutures may be used to evert the arterial edges. The endarterectomy is carried out in the usual manner. Tacking sutures should be avoided unless absolutely necessary to avoid a distal intimal flap. The arteriotomy is closed with running 4-0 or 5-0 polypropylene suture. The

common carotid and subclavian arteries are back-bled and the innominate artery is forward flushed to removed debris and air. Trendelenburg position may facilitate the elimination of arterial air. Flow should be restored to the subclavian artery prior to restoring flow to the carotid to reduce the risk of cerebral atheroembolism. When

removing the C-clamp, it is necessary to maintain slight downward pressure toward the aorta to prevent the clamp from inadvertently injuring the suture line. It is usually appropriate to leave a suction drain in the mediastinum for 24 hours. The sternotomy is closed with wires in the usual manner. Postoperative chest radiographs should be obtained to detect occult pneumothorax.

INNOMINATE ARTERY BYPASS

The innominate artery is exposed for bypass in the same manner as undertaken for endarterectomy (Fig. 4). The aorta is usually selected for inflow unless the proximal innominate artery is completely free from disease. A soft location on the intrapericardial ascending aorta that is relatively free of disease is selected for the proximal anastomosis. Although some authors do not use heparin for the proximal anastomosis, we typically administer heparin 1 mg/kg prior to aortic clamping. A side-biting C-clamp is applied to the ascending aorta. A sufficient bite of aorta should be taken to accommodate separating the edges of the arteriotomy during suturing. An aortotomy is made with an 11 blade and the aortotomy is extended with a cardiac punch. An 8- or 10-mm low-porosity knitted polyester graft is usually selected

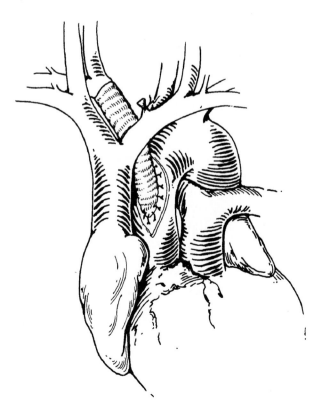

Fig. 4. Innominate artery bypass.

Vascular Surgery

for innominate reconstruction. The graft is soaked in antibiotic solution prior to implantation and care is taken to avoid contact with the skin. Polytetrafluoroethylene (PTFE) grafts are not typically used in this location due to needle hole bleeding that can be troublesome. The graft is beveled appropriately to avoid a right angle at the origin and sutured in place with a running 4-0 polypropylene suture. The graft is flushed by briefly releasing the aortic clamp to remove any air or debris from the aorta. The graft is clamped with an atraumatic clamp and then the aortic clamp is completely removed.

After obtaining distal control, the innominate artery is transected beyond the lesion. The origins of the subclavian and common carotid arteries are inspected to be certain that the plaque does not extend into these orifices. An end-to-end anastomosis is constructed between the end of the graft and the end of the innominate artery with 4-0 polypropylene suture. The graft is irrigated with heparinized saline to remove any particulate debris. Again, the distal vessels are back-bled and the graft forward flushed before restoring flow first to the subclavian artery and then to the carotid.

RIGHT SUBCLAVIAN OR COMMON CAROTID BYPASS

If the occlusive lesion extends into the proximal subclavian or common carotid arteries, the graft must be extended beyond the bifurcation of the innominate artery. If both the right subclavian and right common carotid artery must be revascularized separately, a bifurcated polyester graft is selected based on the diameter of the outflow vessels, typically 14 × 7 or 16 × 8.

Larger-diameter grafts are usually avoided due to the excessive arteriotomy that must be made in the aorta. The body of the bifurcated graft should arise from the most proximal section of the aortic arch and care should be taken to avoid kinking, particularly during closure of the sternotomy. Reul et al. have emphasized the importance of leaving a long body on bifurcated grafts and creating an oblique aortic anastomosis to reduce the risk of kinking. Some authors prefer to use branched custom-made grafts with diameters ranging from 7 to 10 mm rather than commercially available bifurcated grafts designed for aortofemoral grafting. There are no data that objectively differentiate these grafts, and thus graft selection remains the choice of the operating surgeon.

DIRECT RECONSTRUCTION OF INNOMINATE OR SUBCLAVIAN ANEURYSM

In the setting of aneurysm involving the innominate or right subclavian arteries, the same incision and exposure are employed as in occlusive disease, with the exception that more distal exposure is usually required (Fig. 5). Also, it should be noted that the vagus nerve and recurrent laryngeal nerve may be more difficult to expose at the flexion point between the normal artery and the aneurysm. It is usually unwise to perform complete circumferential dissection of the aneurysm, but this may leave intact significant branch vessels that must be ligated once the aneurysm is opened.

Aneurysm of the proximal subclavian artery often involves the origins of the internal mammary artery and the vertebral artery. If the contralateral vertebral artery is patent, ipsilateral vertebral artery ligation is well tolerated but reimplantation can be considered. It is uncommon to reimplant the mammary artery unless simultaneous or subsequent coronary bypass is anticipated.

DIRECT RECONSTRUCTION OF MULTIPLE AORTIC ARCH VESSELS

Direct reconstruction of multiple arch vessels is limited only by the surgeon's imagination and creativity (Fig. 6). In the setting of bilateral common carotid artery occlusion, an inverted bifurcated graft arising from the proximal aortic arch can be used to supply both carotid arteries (Figs. 7 and 8). Side branches to one or both subclavian arteries can be added to the parent graft as needed. If the distal anastomosis is planned at the level of the carotid bifurcation, some authors prefer to transect the common carotid artery and perform an eversion endarterectomy of the carotid bifurcation prior to completing the anastomosis. Others prefer to leave the carotid bifurcation in situ and perform a conventional carotid endarterectomy. The distal anastomosis of the aortic graft limbs incorporates the endarterectomy site in an end-to-side fashion.

It should be noted that approach to the left subclavian is severely limited through a median sternotomy. In most cases, it is easier to reconstruct the left common carotid artery directly and then perform a carotid-subclavian extra-anatomic bypass. Direct reconstruction of the origin of the left subclavian artery is best approached through a formal left thoracotomy.

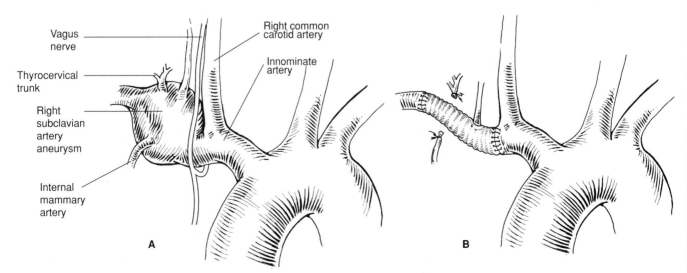

Fig. 5. Right subclavian aneurysm. **A:** Preoperative view. **B:** Postoperative view.

TABLE 1. INDICATIONS FOR ENDOVASCULAR REPAIR OF THE BRACHIOCEPHALIC TRUNKS IN 83 CONSECUTIVE PATIENTS

Anatomic Location	Indication (n)
Subclavian artery	
Internal mammary steal	27
"Claudication"	15
Vertebral-basilar ischemia with subclavian steal	10
Upper extremity embolization	4
Axillobifemoral bypass salvage	3
Pre-CABG (provide inflow for left internal mammary)	3
Provide access to aorta for another intervention	2
BP monitoring	1
Hemodialysis graft failure	1
Innominate artery	
Right arm "claudication"	5
Pre-CABG (provide inflow for right internal mammary)	1
Amaurosis fugax	1
Left common carotid	
Transient cerebral ischemia	6
Tandem internal carotid lesion	5
Asymptomatic	3

BP, blood pressure; CABG, coronary artery bypass graft.

TABLE 2. RELATIVE CONTRAINDICATIONS TO ENDOVASCULAR BRACHIOCEPHALIC RECONSTRUCTION

1. Extreme tortuosity
2. Lesions containing fresh thrombus
3. Lesions adjacent to an aneurysm
4. Subclavian arteries—lesions extending to the origin of the vertebral arteries
5. Innominate artery—lesions extending to the origin of the right common carotid or right subclavian arteries
6. Chronic occlusion of the left common carotid or innominate arteries
7. Heavily calcified lesions

the patient is brought to the endovascular lab and placed in the supine position. Both groins are prepared in a sterile fashion; for occlusions (but not stenoses) of the subclavian artery and for lesions involving the innominate artery, the left and right antecubital fossae, respectively, are also prepped. The authors' preferred technique follows that of Queral and Criado, published in the mid 1990s. Typically, an arch aortogram is performed prior to intervention in a 30% left anterior oblique projection to define the origins of the brachiocephalic trunks and to recognize any developmental anomalies that may exist. Great care must be taken to avoid embolization of air during the diagnostic study, which can be performed with 20 to 30 mL of iodinated contrast. Early in one's experience, the diagnostic arch study may be performed as a separate procedure prior to intervention to allow for careful, unhurried examination and preparation for the procedure.

For left subclavian lesions, retrograde percutaneous femoral access is obtained; following placement of a sheath, the patient is systemically anticoagulated to an activated clotting time (ACT) between 250 and 300 seconds prior to manipulation of wires and catheters in the aortic arch. Following arch aortography, a selective view of the left subclavian artery is performed with a simple "hockey stick" 5 French diagnostic catheter. Lesion length, character, and location of the vertebral and internal mammary arteries are carefully determined. With high-grade stenoses or occlusions, retrograde flow in these branch vessels may preclude adequate visualization until the lesion is crossed. A soft-tipped 0.035-inch guidewire is used to cross the lesion, and is advanced into the axillary artery. For chronic occlusions, a lubricious "glide" wire may be necessary to facilitate lesion crossing; in some instances, the lesion cannot be traversed in an antegrade fashion, and access from the brachial artery will be necessary to complete the procedure (Fig. 2). Once the lesion is crossed, a 7 French sheath *with its dilator* (70 or 90 cm in length, depending on patient body habitus) is advanced across the lesion; while these lesions can be predilated with a standard angioplasty balloon, this technique exposes the unstented (now patent) irregular artery to arterial flow, theoretically increasing the risk of distal embolization. It is the authors' preference, therefore, to cross the lesion with the sheath first, ensuring retrograde flow in the vertebral artery and theoretically reducing the risk of embolization. A balloon-expandable stent (typically 6 to 8 mm diameter) is then advanced across the lesion under the "protection" of the sheath, to prevent the stent

from becoming dislodged from the angioplasty balloon. As the sheath is withdrawn into the aortic arch and the stent exposed, contrast is injected through the sheath sideport to visualize the origins of the vertebral and internal mammary arteries and the subclavian–arch junction. The stent can be carefully repositioned as necessary to ensure that it does not cover the origins of these important branch vessels distally and that its proximal portion is 1 to 2 mm into the arch (for ostial lesions). Angioplasty and primary stenting are performed in a nearly all cases. A completion study can be performed through the sheath, which is then removed and hemostasis obtained with manual compression or with a closure device.

While left common carotid artery (CCA) lesions can be treated via an antegrade approach, the authors prefer to perform these interventions via a retrograde technique through a surgical cutdown. Under general or local anesthesia, a 2.5-cm incision is made in the base of the neck along the anterior border of the sternocleidomastoid muscle, and the common carotid artery exposed and isolated in a standard fashion. Following systemic anticoagulation, distal control of the common carotid is obtained with an atraumatic vascular clamp. The proximal CCA is controlled with a silastic loop, and a transverse arteriotomy performed. This technique (as opposed to direct puncture with an access needle) allows direct visualization of the guidewire as it passes into the vessel and avoids guidewire passage into a subintimal plane. A 7 French sheath is placed, and under direct fluoroscopic control, the guidewire is advanced into the aortic arch. Using a diagnostic catheter and a small amount of hand-injected contrast, the operator can confirm the presence of the system within the true lumen of the aortic arch. Over the guidewire, the sheath and its dilator are advanced into the arch. A balloon-expandable stent (typically 6 to 8 mm diameter) is then advanced across the lesion under protection of the sheath. As in the previously described subclavian intervention, the stent is positioned and then deployed so that its proximal portion is 1 to 2 mm into the aortic arch, to avoid "missing" the fibrocalcific lesion at the CCA origin, which typically includes the adjacent aorta. Occasionally, injection through the sheath will reveal contrast within a dissection plane in the arch adjacent to the target vessel; this iatrogenic dissection (created during predilation with the sheath) is repaired with stent deployment. The arteriotomy is then closed with interrupted polypropylene sutures after vigorous antegrade and retrograde vessel flushing (Fig. 3). While this particular

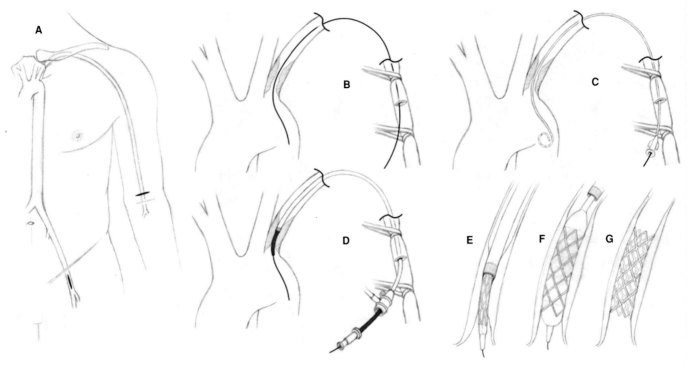

Fig. 2. Angioplasty and primary stenting of the left subclavian artery via left brachial approach.

technique does require a surgical incision, it essentially negates the risk of distal embolization. For tandem lesions involving the ostium of the left common carotid artery and the carotid bifurcation, we prefer to treat the CCA lesion first, place a temporary indwelling shunt if necessary, and then perform standard bifurcation endarterectomy.

The innominate artery can be approached from either the right brachial or femoral access sites. For "deep" arches where the innominate arises proximally on the arch, femoral access may be more difficult, and the right brachial is preferred. The same basic techniques of angioplasty and stenting are utilized regardless of approach, including predilation with a sheath and its dilator, delivery of a balloon-expandable stent to the lesion under protection of the sheath, and deployment after careful adjustment of stent position (Fig. 4). As the balloon is deflated

(following stent expansion and deployment), we typically perform temporary manual occlusion of the ipsilateral common carotid to avoid distal cerebral embolization. Because of the larger diameter (8 to 11 mm) of the innominate (compared to the common carotid and subclavian arteries), operators should be aware that many balloon-expandable stents will foreshorten when expanded to these larger sizes. Although others have reported on

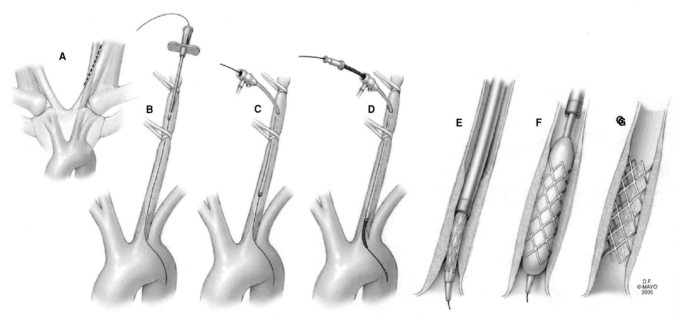

Fig. 3. Angioplasty and primary stenting of the left common carotid artery. Retrograde approach via common carotid cutdown.

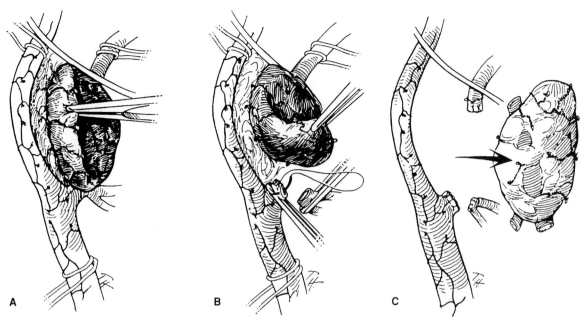

Fig. 9. When the tumor is very large or particularly adherent, division of the origin of the external carotid artery can be a useful maneuver. After detachment of the tumor from the internal carotid artery, the tumor is carefully separated from the bifurcation **(A).** Next, the origin of the external carotid is clamped and divided **(B).** This allows rotational mobilization of the lesion and ligation of nutrient tumor vessels, which are often encountered posteriorly in this location. Finally, division of the superior thyroid and distal external carotid artery (or its branches) allows for the safe removal of the carotid body lesion **(C).** Arrow indicates tumor.

discharged home on the first or second postoperative day. Before discharge, the skin staples are replaced with adhesive Steri-Strips and an appointment is made for the patient to return in 2 to 3 weeks for the first postoperative visit.

RADIATION THERAPY

For completeness, a comment regarding the use of radiation therapy, either as an adjunct or as a primary therapeutic option in the treatment of carotid body tumors, is appro-

priate. Traditionally, the statement has been made that cervical paragangliomas are not radiosensitive lesions. Very few clinicians have acquired sufficient experience to make sound conclusions regarding the efficacy of this treatment modality in this setting. Most

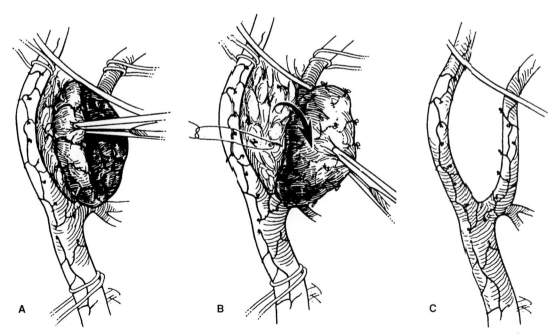

Fig. 10. Alternatively, with careful dissection, it is frequently possible to remove the carotid body tumor without sacrificing the external carotid artery or any of its main branches. Once again, the tumor is carefully separated from the bifurcation **(A).** Again, by rotating the lesion along the axis of the external carotid, nutrient vessels supplying the tumor posteriorly can usually be ligated easily **(B).** Finally, the carotid body tumor is meticulously dissected free, leaving the carotid bifurcation intact **(C).**

often, radiation is reserved for bulky, inoperable, or recurrent tumors, which may account for the disappointing reported results. There are, in fact, a number of sporadic reports indicating successful control of carotid body tumors by radiotherapy. Long-term follow-up for most of these anecdotal cases is currently not available. I admit little experience with this method of treating these tumors and, due to its safety and excellent documented long-term success, continue to recommend surgical resection for the majority of my patients. I acknowledge, however, that in poor surgical candidates with aggressive symptomatic lesions, radiotherapy may have a role in the management of carotid body tumors. This form of treatment requires further investigation.

COMPLICATIONS

An uncomplicated resection of a carotid body tumor is an extremely well-tolerated operation. The tissue trauma and operative blood loss are normally minimal, and patients are routinely discharged from the hospital on the second or third postoperative day. For this reason, perioperative complications are particularly discouraging and must be avoided at all costs. Operative intervention, particularly in the setting of a histologically benign neoplasm, continues to be justified only by keeping the operative morbidity and mortality of the procedure to a minimum.

Technical errors that occur during any operative procedure are preventable. As mentioned earlier, one major cause of technical complications occurring during the resection of carotid body tumors is inadequate hemostasis. Clamping of incompletely identified structures or the temporary occlusion of major cerebrovascular vessels can lead to cranial nerve or neurologic injuries.

As described previously in the Exposure and Extended Exposure Techniques sections, several peripheral nerves must be identified and protected during exposure of the carotid bifurcation. The frequency of injury to these structures is difficult to quantitate, but it is probably in the range of 1% to 15%. This difference is due at least in part to the variable expertise of the individual making the assessment. It must also be remembered that many cranial nerve deficits are related to tumor involvement and not caused intraoperatively. Once again, the importance of carefully examining these structures preoperatively cannot be overemphasized. Nonetheless, at least half of all postoperative cranial nerve injuries go unnoticed by the surgeon and the patient. The remainder of injuries are usually either very obvious or otherwise identified only after a detailed examination. Most of these injuries are not permanent. It should be acknowledged, however, that all cranial nerve injuries that occur during carotid surgery could be prevented if surgeons became familiar with the normal and possible abnormal anatomic neurovascular relationships and carefully protected these structures during the procedure.

RESULTS

Results after resections for carotid body tumors are excellent. However, this has not always been the case. Early series from the 1950s consistently reported a mortality of 5% to 15% of patients, cranial nerve injuries in 30% to 40% of patients, and significant cerebrovascular complications in as many as 10% to 20% of patients. Advances in preoperative diagnosis and localization, intraoperative anesthetic and surgical management, and postoperative care have all contributed to a significant decrease in these complication rates. Today, in experienced hands, a perioperative mortality of less than 0.5%, essentially no significant cerebrovascular sequelae, and a cranial nerve injury or other minor complication rate of no higher than 5% can be expected.

SUGGESTED READING

Bernard RP. Carotid body tumors. *Am J Surg* 1992;163:494.
Gardner T, Dalsing M, Weisberger E, et al. Carotid body tumors, inheritance, and high incidence of associated cervical paragangliomas. *Am J Surg* 1996;172:196.
Grufferman S, Gillamn MW, Pasternak RL, et al. Familial carotid body tumors. Case report and epidemiologic review. *Cancer* 1980;46:2116.
Hallett JW, Nora JD, Hollier LH, et al. Trends in neurovascular complications of surgical management for carotid body and cervical paragangliomas: a fifty-year experience with 153 tumors. *J Vasc Surg* 1988;7:284.
Kraus DH, Sterman BM, Hakaim AG, et al. Carotid body tumors. *Arch Otolaryngol Head Neck Surg* 1990;116:1384.
LaMuraglia GM, Fabian RL, Brewster DC, et al. The current surgical management of carotid body paragangliomas. *J Vasc Surg* 1992;15:1038.
McCabe DP, Vaccaro PS, James AG. Treatment of carotid body tumors. *J Cardiovasc Surg* 1990;31:356.
Nora JD, Hallett JW, O'Brien PC, et al. Surgical resection of carotid body tumors: long-term survival, recurrence, and metastasis. *Mayo Clin Proc* 1988;63:348.
Rabl H, Friehs, I, Gutschi S, et al. Diagnosis and treatment of carotid body tumors. *Thorac Cardiovasc Surg* 1993;41:340.
Sanghvi VD, Chandawarkar RY. Carotid body tumors. *J Surg Oncol* 1993;54:190.
Smith LL, Ajalat GM. Tumors of the carotid body: diagnosis, prognosis, and surgical management. In: WS Moore, ed. *Surgery for cerebrovascular disease.* New York: Churchill Livingstone, 1987:579.
Wax MK, Briant TDR. Carotid body tumors: a review. *J Otolaryngol* 1992;21:277.
Westerband A, Hunter GC, Cintora I, et al. Current trends in the detection and management of carotid body tumors. *J Vasc Surg* 1998;28:84.
Worsey MJ, Laborde AL, Bower T, et al. An evaluation of color duplex scanning in the primary diagnosis and management of carotid body tumors. *Ann Vasc Surg* 1992;6:90.

EDITOR'S COMMENT

In this nice review of the management of carotid body tumors, Dr. Moore draws on his extensive experience with this problem to carefully describe the evaluation and treatment of these unusual but highly vascular tumors. He clearly points out the indications for excision of these usually benign lesions and the value of preoperative imaging studies such as MRI and CTA in defining the vascular anatomy associated with carotid body tumors. He then extensively describes his approach to the surgical removal of these tumors and provides very useful illustrations to support this description. He also appropriately emphasizes the need to identify and protect the adjacent cranial nerves and to monitor cerebral perfusion particularly if temporary occlusion of the internal carotid artery is necessary.

The bar he sets in describing the results of surgical treatment of these tumors is high but appropriate, particularly the incidence of cranial nerve injury of less than or equal to 5%. Achieving these results requires good exposure, careful hemostasis, and a detailed knowledge of the surgical anatomy of the area between the carotid bifurcation and the base of the skull. Exposure of the area of the distal extracranial internal carotid artery close to the skull base can be facilitated by sublimating the mandible. However, in my experience, the amount of additional exposure gained by this maneuver is minimal and the other techniques described by Dr. Moore including extending the skin incision behind the ear, mobilizing or even dividing the sternocleidomastoid muscle, and dividing the posterior belly of the digestive muscle are of more value, although as pointed out by Dr. Moore, division of the digastric muscle puts the glossopharyngeal nerve at risk. Finally, it cannot be emphasized too strongly that hemostasis is critical to this procedure, and that although embolization of the extracranial carotid artery decreases the vascularity of carotid body tumor, it does not serve as a substitute for experience and good surgical technique in achieving the low complication rates that Dr. Moore describes.

J.M.S.

symptomatic TAAA, regardless of size. The primary concern is to prevent rupture, as patients who rupture have a markedly higher risk of mortality and complications, including renal failure and paralysis. The preoperative evaluation of patients with TAAA is important as most of these patients have co-morbid conditions that can affect their outcome. These patients often can have associated diseases that require intervention prior to TAAA surgery, such as carotid endarterectomy, coronary artery angioplasty or bypass, and pulmonary or renal optimization. After a thorough history and physical examination, standard studies are obtained, including electrocardiogram, chest radiograph, complete blood cell counts, coagulation tests, and a complete serum chemistry panel (electrolytes, blood urea nitrogen, creatinine, glucose, and liver profile).

Preoperative cardiac evaluation by an experienced cardiologist is essential because approximately 30% of the patients have associated coronary artery disease. Further cardiac evaluation usually comprises of a transthoracic echocardiogram, chemical stress test, and coronary angiography, depending on the patient's risk factors. We have found a correlation between a low left ventricular ejection fraction and worse patient outcome. In general for patients who require coronary artery stenting, 3 to 4 weeks of platelet inhibition (clopidogrel and aspirin) therapy is maintained to prevent acute in-stent thrombosis. Clopidogrel is stopped 5 to 7 days prior to TAAA repair. In patients who require coronary artery bypass prior to TAAA repair, we specifically avoid using the left internal mammary artery as a conduit, to obviate the possibility of cardiac ischemia in the event that aortic cross-clamping proximal to the left subclavian artery may be required during the TAAA repair (Fig. 5). Furthermore, the internal mammary artery can be an important collateral blood supply to the spinal cord. Patients who undergo coronary artery bypass usually require 4 to 6 weeks to recover before TAAA repair.

We have found that cerebrovascular diseases can have negative impact on patients undergoing TAAA surgery. Carotid duplex is used to screen for patients with occlusive plaque disease. Staged carotid endarterectomy is usually performed for severe carotid stenosis before TAAA repair. Preoperative consultation with a pulmonologist is helpful as well. Pulmonary

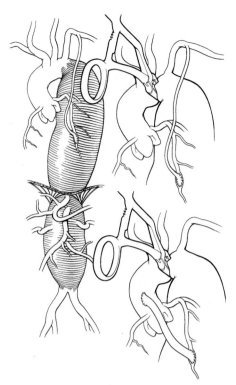

Fig. 5. We do *not* use the left internal mammary artery to bypass the left anterior descending artery in order to avoid cardiac ischemia should aortic cross-clamping be required proximal to the left subclavian artery at the time thoracoabdominal aortic aneurysm repair. In the presence of a saphenous vein graft to the left anterior descending artery, clamping proximal to the left subclavian artery can be done without the risk of coronary ischemia.

function tests and arterial blood gases provide good assessment of lung function and reserve. Preoperative pulmonary toilet consisting of breathing exercises and smoking cessation can have major impact on patient outcome. On occasions, bronchodilators and systemic steroids have been prescribed to improve pulmonary function preoperatively. Careful evaluation of the patient's renal function is mandatory because preoperative renal disease is well recognized to be a predictor of mortality, postoperative renal failure, and paralysis. In the past, we used serum creatinine as a measure for preoperative renal function. We found that approximately 9% of patients undergoing TAAA have pre-existing renal disease, which in turn is a risk factor for postoperative paraplegia and mortality.

However, we recently reviewed the incidence of pre-existing renal disease in our cumulative experience with 1,106 patients with TAAA. We found that the glomerular filtration rate (GFR) as estimated from the Cockroft-Gault formula,[1] which takes into account the patient's age, weight, and gender, is superior to serum creatinine both in detecting subclinical renal disease and predicting mortality. Based on GFR, approximately two thirds of our patients had stage 2 or 3 pre-existing renal disease according to the National Kidney Foundation's classification of chronic renal disease. More importantly, our study showed that 30-day mortality ranges from 5% in the best GFR quartile to 27% in the worst (Fig. 6). Contrasting serum creatinine alone to estimated GFR, mortality was 94/804 (11.7%) among patients with

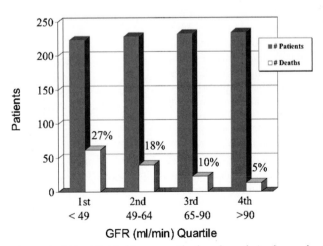

Fig. 6. Our patient population divided into quartiles based on their glomerular filtration rate along with the mortality for each quartile. Mortality correlated strongly with worsening renal disease ($P < 0.0001$).

[1](140 − age) × weight / 72 × serum creatinine × (.85 if female)

normal creatinine, compared with 13/234 (5.6%) among those with normal GFR. The use of potentially nephrotoxic agents, such as aminoglycosides, nonsteroidal anti-inflammatory medications, and iodinated contrast, is avoided when possible, particularly in patients with pre-existing renal disease. Notably, when iodinated contrast infusion is necessary in patients with chronic renal disease, we prescribe acetylcysteine and hydrate them well prior to the study.

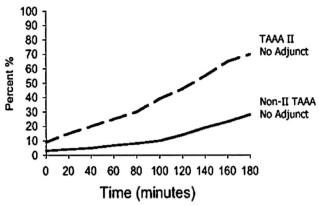

Fig. 7. Graph shows increased risk of neurologic deficit with prolonged clamp time during the clamp-and-sew era.

Operative Strategy and Techniques

The patient is brought to the operating room and placed initially in the supine position on the operating table. We cannulate the right radial artery for continuous arterial pressure monitoring. General anesthesia is induced. Endotracheal intubation is established using a double-lumen tube for selective right lung ventilation during surgery. The position of the endotracheal tube is confirmed endoscopically. We insert a sheath into the internal jugular or subclavian vein and float a Swan-Ganz catheter into the pulmonary artery for continuous monitoring of the central venous and pulmonary artery pressures. We place large-bore central and peripheral venous lines for fluid and blood replacement therapy. Temperature probes positioned in the patient's nasopharynx, rectum, and bladder record temperatures from these locations. We attach electrodes to the scalp for electroencephalogram and along the spinal cord and distal legs for somatosensory evoked potentials and motor-evoked potentials, to assess the central nervous system and spinal cord function, respectively. A detailed account of anesthetic management during TAAA repair is beyond the scope of this chapter. However, we emphasize the importance of maintaining adequate systemic arterial pressure with judicious blood transfusion, as organ perfusion greatly depends on the systemic circulation and correcting the obligatory acidosis related to visceral and lower extremity ischemia induced by aortic clamping.

SPINAL CORD PROTECTION

Paraplegia is the most dreaded complication arising from TAAA repair. When the descending thoracic aorta is cross-clamped, perfusion of the spinal cord is compromised not only because of interruption of pulsatile flow but also from a rise in cerebrospinal fluid (CSF) pressure. Methods of spinal cord protection aim to improve spinal cord perfusion during the ischemic clamp period and to restore and maintain pre-existing spinal cord flow after aortic graft replacement. Our strategy to provide spinal cord protection is a multimodality approach, using adjunct distal aortic perfusion, CSF drainage, and moderate hypothermia. In addition, we conduct the operation using sequential aortic clamping method and reattach all patent lower intercostal arteries. In the most recent review of our cumulative experience of patients undergoing TAAA and descending thoracic aortic aneurysm repair since 1992, the overall incidence of neurologic deficit is 3.3 % (36/1,106). Risk factors for postoperative neurologic deficit still include extent II TAAA, pre-existing renal disease, cerebrovascular disease, and older age. The use of the adjunct has increased the total aortic cross-clamp time by a mean of 12 minutes. More importantly, however, the use of adjunct was found to be protective, with the overall rate of neurologic deficit of 2.4% compared with 5.7% for patients in whom adjunct was not used (Fig. 7). Since we adopted this multimodality approach, the incidence of postoperative neurologic deficit has declined to 1.1% in the last quartile (years 2001 to 2004), for all extents of TAAA repair (Fig. 8). The decrease in neurologic deficit was most pronounced in extent II TAAA (from 21.1% during years 1991–1995 to 3.3% in the last 4 years).

CSF DRAINAGE

The increase in CSF pressure during the period of aortic clamp is thought to be related to a higher proximal arterial pressure and greater venous volume translocated from the lower body to the upper body. Although central venous pressure had been thought to correlate with CSF pressure, we

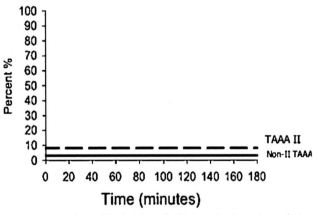

Fig. 8. Graph demonstrates that with the use of adjunct (distal aortic perfusion, cerebrospinal fluid drainage, moderate hypothermia), aortic cross-clamp time is no longer a significant risk factor for neurologic deficit. The incidence of neurologic deficit has declined to a rate of 1.1% for all TAAA extents. This reduction in neurologic deficit is most dramatic in patients with extent II TAAA (3.3%).

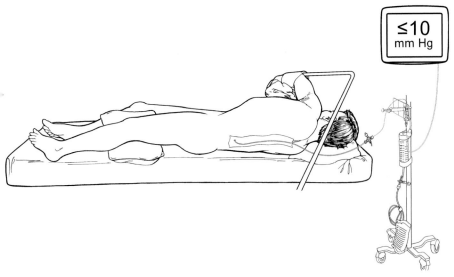

Fig. 9. Placement of the lumbar catheter in the third or fourth lumbar space to provide cerebrospinal fluid drainage and pressure monitoring.

have found no good predictors of CSF pressure, particularly during the aortic cross-clamp period. Hence, we measure CSF pressure directly using a lumbar drain placed in the subarachnoid space. To facilitate placement of the lumbar drain prior to the commencement of surgery, the patient is positioned on his or her right side, flexing the knees to open the space between the vertebrae. We insert a silastic catheter in the third or fourth lumbar space percutaneously, and advance it for approximately 5 cm (Fig. 9). We check the CSF pressure closely and drain CSF intermittently to maintain pressure below 10 mm Hg throughout the surgery and for 3 days postoperatively. Contraindications to placement of a lumbar catheter include active infection, coagulopathy, and rupture with hemodynamic instability.

THORACOABDOMINAL INCISION AND EXPOSURE

Once the lumbar catheter is in place, we readjust the patient's position on the operating table. The right lateral decubitus position is maintained on a bean bag, and the patient's shoulders are placed at right angle to the edge of the table, with the left hip flexed at approximately 60 degrees to allow access to both groins for exposure of the femoral arteries. The patient is cleansed and draped in the usual sterile fashion. We tailor the incision to fit the extent of the aneurysm (Fig. 10). A full thoracoabdominal incision begins between the spine and vertebral border of the left scapula, curves along the sixth rib across the costal cartilage in an oblique line to the umbilicus,

and then continues below the umbilicus to just above the symphysis pubis. Resection of the sixth rib facilitates exposure and is routinely performed for all TAAAs except extent IV. Usually, a full thoracoabdominal exploration is necessary for extents II, III, and IV. A modified thoracoabdominal incision begins in the same way as a full thoracoabdominal incision, but ends at the costal cartilage or above the umbilicus. A self-retaining retractor placed firmly on the edges of the incision maintains full thoracic and abdominal exposure during the procedure.

The left lung is selectively deflated. Mobilization of the descending thoracic aorta begins at the level of the hilum of the lung and continues cephalad to the

proximal descending thoracic aorta. We identify the ligamentum arteriosum and transect it, taking care to avoid injury to the adjacent left recurrent laryngeal nerve. We mobilize the middle descending thoracic aorta so that a distal clamp can be applied to allow distal aortic perfusion during the performance of the proximal anastomosis. The distal extent of the aneurysm is assessed and the distal extent of the exposure is determined accordingly. If the aneurysm does not involve the superior mesenteric artery, the diaphragm is simply retracted downward to expose the infradiaphragmatic aorta for clamping. When the aneurysm extends to the superior mesenteric artery and more distally, mobilization of the abdominal aorta requires partial division of the diaphragm and exposure of the retroperitoneum.

DIAPHRAGM PRESERVATION

We have found that diaphragm preservation during TAAA repair results in earlier weaning from mechanical ventilation and, consequently, a shorter length of hospital stay. Since 1994, rather than dividing the diaphragm, we cut only the muscular portion, leaving the central tendinous portion intact and preserving the phrenic nerve (Fig. 11A and B). This technique permits maintenance of pulmonary mechanics that more closely reflect normal function; hence, we are able to wean patients earlier from mechanical ventilation. After cutting only the muscular portion of the diaphragm, a retroperitoneal plane is developed, mobilizing the spleen, bowel loops, and left kidney to the right side of the abdominal aorta (medial visceral rotation).

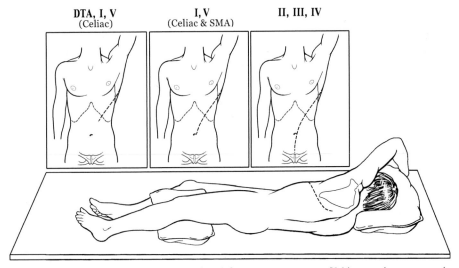

Fig. 10. Thoracoabdominal incisions tailored for aneurysm extent. SMA, superior mesenteric artery.

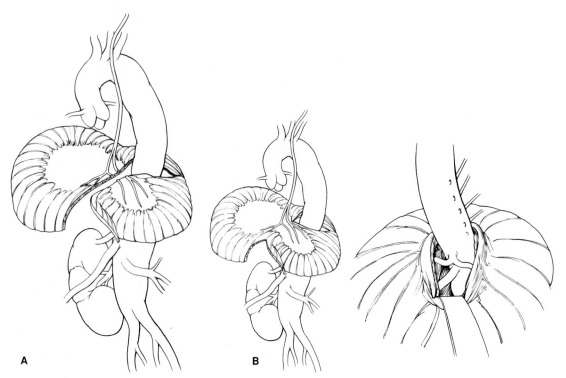

A   B

Fig. 11. A: Previously, we divided the diaphragm completely. **B:** We currently cut only the muscular portion of the diaphragm (**right**); the aortic hiatus can be retracted downward to expose the infradiaphragmatic aorta.

DISTAL AORTIC PERFUSION

Aortic cross-clamping not only endangers the spinal cord but also can lead to proximal systemic hypertension and left ventricular distension. Left ventricular distension can lead to increased wall stress and decreased subendocardial perfusion. To protect the spinal cord, reduce proximal hypertension, minimize cardiac ischemia, and "unload" the heart, we routinely use distal aortic perfusion. Afterload-reducing pharmacologic agents such as nitrates are frequently used to further protect the heart. However, we no longer use nitroprusside as an afterload reducing agent because we have observed precipitous systemic hypotension and paradoxical increase in CSF pressure associated with its use. Occasionally, severe cardiac dysfunction may require mechanical support using intraaortic balloon counterpulsation. To prepare for distal aortic perfusion, the patients receive a 1 mg/kg dose of heparin as an anticoagulant.

The pericardium is opened posterior to the left phrenic nerve to allow direct visualization of the pulmonary veins and left atrium (Fig. 12). The lower pulmonary vein is cannulated, and a cannula is inserted and connected to a BioMedicus pump with on-line heat exchanger (Fig. 13). The left common femoral artery is exposed and arterial inflow from the pump is established through the left common femoral artery. When the left femoral artery is not accessible (e.g., in

the presence of existing femoral prosthetic graft or severe arteriosclerotic occlusive disease), we cannulate the abdominal aorta or distal thoracic aorta instead. Distal aortic perfusion is initiated just before clamping of the aorta. The distal perfusion flow depends on the proximal pressure, and ranges from 500 mL to 2 L. We use passive moderate hypothermia (i.e., we let the patient's body temperature drift from 32°C to 34°C). We avoid dropping the body temperature below 32°C to prevent the occurrence of

ventricular arrhythmias. Our perfusion circuit includes a heat exchanger to permit active warming at the end of surgery to a nasopharyngeal temperature 36°C to 37°C.

SEQUENTIAL AORTIC CROSS-CLAMPING

We use sequential aortic cross-clamp to minimize ischemia to the spinal cord, viscera, and kidneys. We place the first padded

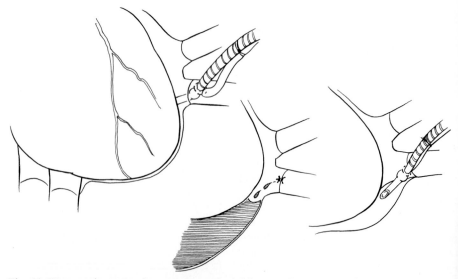

Fig. 12. We open the pericardium to expose the left lower pulmonary vein for cannulation. If the pericardium is not opened, the cannula may be inserted inside the pericardium but not into the pulmonary vein. In addition, decannulation can cause tamponade if the pericardium is not opened.

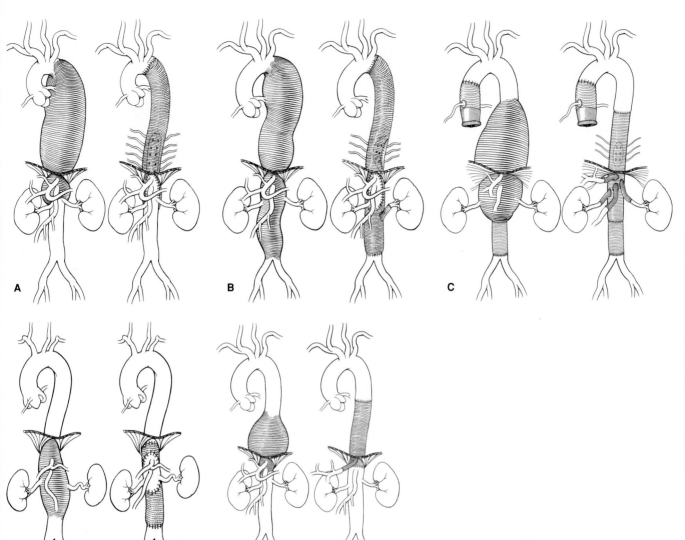

Fig. 15. Examples of TAAA repair according to extent. **A:** Extent I. The proximal anastomosis is just distal to the left subclavian artery. The patent lower intercostal arteries are reattached. The distal anastomosis is to the suprarenal aorta reattaching the celiac and superior mesenteric arteries. **B:** Extent II. The proximal anastomosis is just distal to the left subclavian artery. The patent lower intercostal arteries are reattached. The celiac, superior mesenteric, and right renal arteries are reimplanted together. The left renal artery is reimplanted via an interposition bypass graft; this is necessary because it is located far away from the remaining visceral arteries. On occasion, bypass is necessary to the right renal artery for the same reason. In the majority of the cases, however, the celiac, superior mesenteric, and right and left renal arteries can be reattached together as a patch/island. The distal anastomosis is to the infrarenal aorta, just above the bifurcation. **C:** Extent III. A patient with Marfan syndrome previously had a composite aortic valve-graft replacement of the ascending aorta, reimplantation of the right and left coronary arteries, and infrarenal abdominal aortic graft replacement (**left**). Graft replacement of the TAAA (**right**) included a proximal anastomosis at the level of the sixth intercostal space, reattachment of patent lower intercostal arteries, reimplantation of the celiac, superior mesenteric, right renal arteries, and left renal arteries via separate interposition bypass grafts, and the distal anastomosis is to the existing infrarenal aortic graft. In patients with Marfan syndrome, we use separate interposition grafts to reimplant the visceral and renal arteries individually to prevent the late development of patch aneurysm. **D:** Extent IV. The proximal anastomosis is to the abdominal aorta at the diaphragm. The celiac, superior mesenteric, and right and left renal arteries are reimplanted together as an island/patch. The distal anastomosis is to the infrarenal aorta, just above the bifurcation. **E:** Extent V. The proximal anastomosis is at the sixth intercostal space. The celiac artery is reimplanted via an interposition bypass graft. The distal anastomosis is to the abdominal aorta above the mesenteric artery. All lower intercostal arteries are occluded.

control, and close monitoring. Aortic surgery is avoided during the acute phase (that is the 14-day period after onset of pain) because of higher risks of mortality, bleeding, and paraplegia. However, for patients in whom surgical aortic graft replacement is indicated because of rupture or persistent pain, we use a number of modifications to our standard TAAA technique. First, we identify the true and false lumens. The true lumen is usually smaller and devoid of thrombus, whereas the false lumen usually contains a variable amount of thrombus. The partition between the two lumens is excised at each end of the aortic segment to be replaced (Fig. 17A). Before sewing the graft to the aorta, we run a 4-0 polypropylene suture to tack

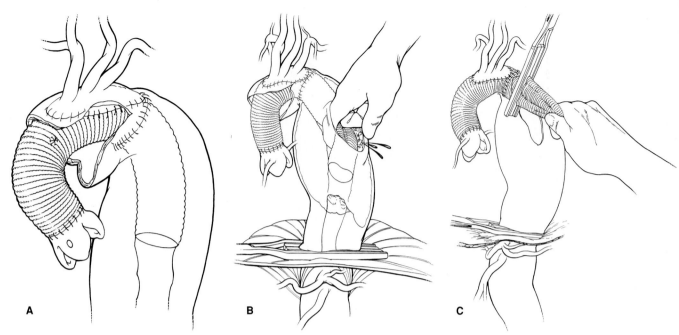

A   B   C

Fig. 16. Elephant trunk technique for extensive aortic aneurysm. **A:**Illustration of completed stage 1 elephant trunk. The ascending/arch aorta has been replaced using woven Dacron graft. The distal portion of the graft is left dangling in the descending thoracic aorta in preparation for the second stage. In stage 2, the proximal descending thoracic part of the aneurysm is opened, and the existing graft is quickly grasped (**B**) and clamped (**C**). The remainder of the surgery follows the standard technique for TAAA.

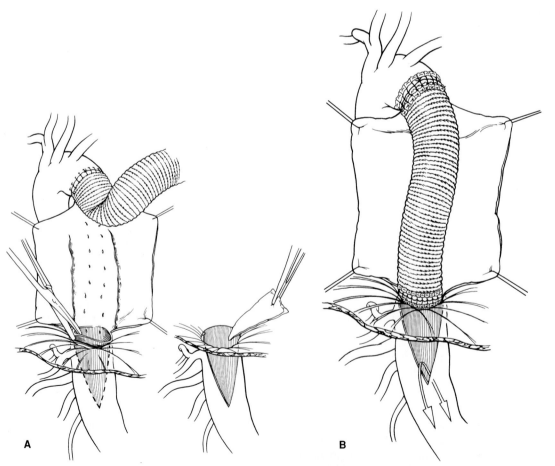

A   B

Fig. 17. It is imperative to identify the true and false lumens when there is dissection. **A:** The partition between the two lumens is excised. **B:** Interrupted pledgeted polypropylene sutures are placed liberally circumferentially on the posterior and anterior walls of the anastomoses for reinforcement.

down the dissected intima. The graft is then sutured to the aorta using running 4-0 polypropylene suture. In addition, we place interrupted pledgeted polypropylene sutures circumferentially on the posterior and anterior walls for further reinforcement (Fig. 17B). Although we always attempt to reattach the patent lower intercostal arteries during graft replacement of TAAA, we advocate ligation of patent intercostal and lumbar arteries in the acutely dissected aorta in order to avoid catastrophic bleeding associated with the friable tissues. However, patent lower intercostal arteries can be safely reattached in chronic dissection.

Our technique for repair of TAAA with chronic dissection is the same as the standard techniques already described for TAAA. Although chronic dissection had been a risk factor for paraplegia in the clamp-and-sew era, recent analysis shows that it no longer is a significant predictor for mortality or neurologic deficit with the use of adjunct.

All survivors of acute aortic dissection must be followed closely in the chronic phase. Serial imaging of the dissected aorta should be obtained prior to discharge from the acute care hospital, then at 1 month, 3 months, 6 months, 12 months following discharge, and yearly thereafter. Compliance with chronic antihypertensive therapy decreases the incidence of subsequent hospitalization and may reduce the progression of aortic dilatation. Patients who have persistent or recurrent pain should be considered for surgical aortic repair. Otherwise, surgical graft replacement of the TAAA is recommended when the maximal aortic diameter reaches 5 to 6 cm. In general, we replace all aneurysmal aortic segments with chronic dissection. Areas with chronic dissection that are nonaneurysmal can be observed with serial imaging.

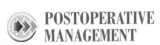

POSTOPERATIVE MANAGEMENT

In the intensive care unit, we continuously monitor the systemic arterial pressure, pulmonary artery pressures, cardiac index, mixed venous saturation, and pulse oximetry saturation. The patient's mean arterial pressure is maintained between 90 and 100 mm Hg to ensure good organ perfusion, particularly to the spinal cord. Chest tube drainage is monitored closely and blood loss is liberally replaced using packed red blood cells. We transfuse fresh-frozen plasma and platelets generously, especially if the patient is coagulopathic. On occasion, we have infused cryoprecipitates

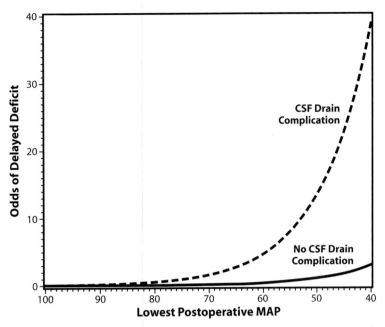

Fig. 18. Odds of delayed neurologic deficit by lowest postoperative mean arterial blood pressure (MAP), with or without cerebrospinal fluid (CSF) drain complication. Odds are referenced to one. For example, a patient with a mean arterial blood pressure of 40 mm Hg and a CSF drain complication would have 40:1 odds of delayed neurologic deficit.

and factor VII for severe disseminated intravascular coagulopathy. We use a heating blanket and blood warmer for transfusion therapy to maintain the patient's body temperature at 36°C to 37°C.

Delayed Neurologic Deficit

We try to wake the patient as quickly as possible to check his or her neurologic status. Postoperative neurologic deficit remains the most devastating complication following TAAA repair. Even after the patient recovers from anesthesia and is moving all extremities, we still have to be on the alert for delayed neurologic deficit. Delayed neurologic deficit refers to the onset of paraplegia or paraparesis after a period of observed normal neurologic function. As improved spinal cord protection during TAAA surgery has reduced the incidence of neurologic complications, onset of delayed neurologic deficit has emerged as an important clinical entity. We have observed delayed neurologic deficit as early as 2 hours and as late as 2 weeks (median, 2 days) following surgery. We have found no single risk factor responsible for delayed neurologic deficit. However, using multivariable analysis, we identified acute dissection, extent II TAAA, and renal insufficiency as significant preoperative predictors for delayed neurologic deficit. In a subsequent case-control study, postoperative mean arterial

pressure of less than 60 mm Hg and CSF drain complications were found to be predictors in the development of delayed neurologic deficit, independent of preoperative predictors (Fig. 18).

In the first 3 postoperative days, we monitor the CSF pressure closely. Approximately 10 to 15 mL of CSF is drained hourly to keep CSF pressure at 10 mm Hg or less. CSF drainage is discontinued on the 3rd postoperative day if the patient remains neurologically intact. To optimize postoperative spinal cord perfusion and oxygen delivery, we keep the mean arterial pressure above 90 mm Hg, hemoglobin above 10 mg/dL, and cardiac index greater than 2.0 L/min. If delayed neurologic deficit occurs, measures to increase spinal cord perfusion are instituted immediately. The patient is placed flat in the supine position, and patency and function of the drain is ascertained at once. If the drain has been removed, the CSF drainage catheter is reinserted immediately and CSF is drained freely until the CSF pressure drops below 10 mm Hg. The systemic arterial pressure is raised, banked blood is liberally infused, and oxygen saturation is optimized. CSF drainage is continued for at least 72 hours for all patients with delayed-onset neurologic deficit. Using this multifaceted approach, we have seen improvement in neurologic function in the majority of patients who developed delayed neurologic deficit.

Cardiopulmonary Care

Most of our patients are kept on mechanical ventilation the 1st postoperative night. We obtain a chest radiograph on arrival to the intensive care unit, routinely every morning if the patient is on mechanical ventilation, and as indicated. We start weaning the patient off mechanical ventilation on the 1st postoperative day. We consult with the pulmonologist for continued assistance with postoperative pulmonary care. Aggressive pulmonary toilet and incentive deep-breathing exercises are prescribed. Approximately 20% of patients require prolonged mechanical ventilatory assistance. Predictors of respiratory failure are advanced age, aortic cross-clamp time (greater than 60 minutes), number of packed red blood cells transfused, and tobacco use. When prolonged mechanical ventilation is deemed necessary, we favor early tracheostomy.

The consultant cardiologist also continues to monitor the patient's cardiac condition closely after surgery. We get an electrocardiogram immediately after surgery and as needed thereafter. Serum electrolytes levels, particularly potassium, magnesium, calcium, and phosphate, are checked regularly, and their derangements are treated aggressively to prevent cardiac arrhythmias. Approximately 10% of patients develop postoperative atrial arrhythmias. Treatment for atrial arrhythmias usually involves one or more of pharmacologic agents (amiodarone, beta-blockers, and calcium channel blockers). Occasionally, electrical cardioversion may be required in refractory cases or when there is associated hypotension.

Renal Failure

Urinary output is recorded hourly in the intensive care unit. Serum creatinine and blood urea nitrogen levels are checked at least daily. For patients who develop postoperative renal failure that require replacement therapy for fluid removal or clearance, we generally initiate early continuous venovenous hemodialysis if their systemic blood pressures are low or unstable. Alternatively, we start daily intermittent hemodialysis if the patients require renal replacement therapy but are otherwise normotensive. We have previously defined acute postoperative renal failure by an increase in serum creatinine of 1 mg/dL per day for 2 consecutive days or the need for hemodialysis. The overall incidence of acute postoperative renal failure is still approximately 18% after TAAA repair. Thirty-day mortality among our patients with acute renal failure is three

times higher than in patients without this complication. Approximately one third of our patients who develop acute renal failure remain on hemodialysis and, predictably, have a longer hospital stay.

Long-term survival for patients on hemodialysis is dismal. Our quest for a satisfactory method of renal protection has produced no definitive results. We have used several methods of renal protection, including different perfusion techniques and fenoldopam. Although there is some evidence that patients with cold visceral perfusion have superior survival and recovery rates, this strategy has not decreased the incidence of acute renal failure. Acute postoperative renal failure remains troublesome and the pursuit for the optimal method of renal protection continues to be one of our top priorities. This is especially important in view of our recent findings that subclinical pre-existing renal disease, based on preoperative GFR, is prevalent among patients with TAAA and a strong predictor for operative mortality.

Ancillary Care

In general, the patient resumes oral diet when regular bowel activity returns by postoperative day 2 or 3. For patients requiring prolonged mechanical ventilation, enteral feeding is given via a nasoduodenal feeding tube. At times, total parenteral nutrition is necessary for protracted ileus. The length of stay in the intensive care unit is approximately 3 or 4 days, depending primarily on the neurologic and pulmonary status of the patient. The patient is subsequently transferred to the telemetry floor. Physical therapy is initiated in the intensive care unit and continued throughout the patient's hospital stay. We give prophylaxis against deep vein thrombosis using low molecular weight heparin after removal of the CSF drain until the patient is fully ambulatory. Patients are discharged home once they resume normal daily activities, or are transferred to a rehabilitative facility if they still require further physical assistance.

The median length of stay for patients following TAAA is 15 days. After the patient is discharged, we recommend an annual follow-up with imaging to screen for the development of new aneurysm or graft-related pseudoaneurysm formation. The frequency of follow-up visits or imaging may vary, based on TAAA etiology. For example, patients with remaining unoperated aortic dissection, connective tissue disorders (Marfan or Ehler-Danlos syndrome), a family history of aortic aneurysm, or concurrent aneurysms may need closer surveillance.

SUMMARY

Successful surgical repair of thoracoabdominal aortic aneurysms remain a formidable task that requires not only an experienced surgeon but also a dedicated multidisciplinary team. Morbidity and mortality have declined, which we attribute to the adoption of the multimodality adjunct distal aortic perfusion and CSF drainage as well as the evolution of surgical techniques to include sequential aortic cross-clamp, intercostal artery reattachment, and moderate hypothermia. The application of our surgical approach and the use of adjunct have reduced the overall incidence of neurologic deficits following thoracoabdominal aortic aneurysm repair to 1.1%. The use of the adjunct appears to blunt the deleterious effects of prolonged aortic cross-clamp time, providing the surgical team a safety net to operate without rushing. Our current research goals are to improve renal protection and further decrease the incidence of neurologic deficits in extent II thoracoabdominal aortic aneurysms.

ACKNOWLEDGEMENT

We are grateful to Kirk Soodhalter for his assistance with the preparation of this manuscript.

SELECTED READING

Azizzadeh A, Huynh TTT, Miller CC, 3rd, et al. Postoperative risk factors for delayed neurologic deficit after thoracic and thoracoabdominal aortic aneurysm repair: a case-control study. *J Vasc Surg* 2003;37:750.

Borst HG, Walterbusch G, Schaps D. Extensive aortic replacement using "elephant trunk" prosthesis. *Thorac Cardiovasc Surg* 1983;31:37.

Cambria RP, Clouse WD, Davison JK, Dunn PF, Corey M, Dorer D. Thoracoabdominal aortic aneurysm repair: results with 337 operations performed over 15-year interval. *Ann Surg* 2002;236:471.

Clouse WD, Hallett JW Jr., Schaff HV, et al. Improved prognosis of thoracic aortic aneurysms: a population-based study. *JAMA* 1998;280:1926.

Engle J, Safi HJ, Miller CC 3rd, et al. The impact of diaphragm management on prolonged ventilator support after thoracoabdominal aortic repair. *J Vasc Surg* 1999;29:150.

Estrera AL, Miller CC 3rd, Huynh TTT, et al. Neurologic outcome after thoracic and thoracoabdominal aortic aneurysm repair. *Ann Thorac Surg* 2001;72:1225; discussion 1230.

Estrera AL, Miller CC 3rd, Huynh TTT, et al. Preoperative and operative predictors of delayed neurologic deficit following repair of thoracoabdominal aortic aneurysm. *J Thorac Cardiovasc Surg* 2003;126:1288.

Hasham SN, Willing MC, Guo DC, et al. Mapping a locus for familial thoracic aortic

POSTOPERATIVE CARE AND COMPLICATIONS

Despite modern advances in open AAA repair and intra- and postoperative care, morbidity ranges from 20% to 25% and mortality remains approximately 3% to 5%. Myocardial infarction is still the leading cause of single-organ associated early and late death. Postoperatively the patient should be aggressively rewarmed, hemodynamic stability should be maintained, and coagulation dysfunction should be corrected. The most common complications are pulmonary dysfunction (8% to 15%), myocardial infarction (2% to 8%), renal failure (5% to 15%) with dialysis (1% to 6%), colonic ischemia (1% to 2%), deep venous thrombosis (5% to 8%), bleeding (2% to 5%), distal embolization (1% to 4%), wound infection (1% to 5%), ureteral injury, and spinal cord ischemia (<1%). Postoperatively, a high index of suspicion of colonic ischemia should be maintained in patients with acidosis, abdominal distention, and/or guaiac-positive stools. Flexible sigmoidoscopy should be performed to document ischemia. If the patient's condition worsens, emergent colectomy and colostomy should be performed before sepsis and shock occurs. Paraplegia is exceedingly rare after infrarenal AAA repair but may occur in 1% to 2% after type IV TAAA repair due to interruption of flow to tributaries of the artery of Adamkiewicz, which supplies the spinal cord and is located 80% of the time between T7 and L1 vertebral bodies. Incidence of impaired sexual function manifested as either impotence or retrograde ejaculation after AAA repair is difficult to ascertain but has been reported to be from 10% to 25%. However, this is also reported to increase with time in this age group and is likely multifactorial. Other complications include graft infection (1%), aortoenteric fistulas (1.6%), pseudoaneurysms (3%), small bowel obstruction, and ventral hernias.

With endovascular grafting, the incidence of perioperative mortality is 0.4% to 2% with an overall 9% morbidity rate. One of the major factors affecting outcome is the durability of the repair, which has been hindered by the presence or development of persistent blood flow or pressurization within the aneurysm sac. These "endoleaks" (Table 5) have an incidence of 12% to 44% in different series and may lead to aneurysm rupture in 0.2% to 1% per year; therefore, lifetime surveillance must be performed in order to diagnose and treat this complication.

TABLE 5. CLASSIFICATION OF ENDOLEAKS

Classification	Failure Site	Treatment
Type I	Proximal or distal attachment zones Stent migration	Proximal or distal extension cuffs
Type II	Retrograde endoleaks Patent lumbar, IMA, intercostals, accessory renal, etc.	Percutaneous coil embolization Observe (may spontaneously close)
Type III	Midgraft component disconnection Fabric tear	Secondary endograft
Type IV	Graft wall porosity or suture holes	Secondary stenting (nonporous stent) Observe
Type V (Endotension)	High intrasac pressure without endoleaks shown	Secondary repair Open repair

IMA, inferior mesenteric artery.

The majority of all early endoleaks will disappear within the first postoperative month, especially type II endoleaks. Most physicians currently observe type II endoleaks in the absence of sac expansion. In the EVAR I trial the overall rate of reintervention was 15%, whereas in the EUROSTAR registry reintervention was performed in 10% per year and the rate of aneurysm rupture was 0.2% to 1% per year. However, EUROSTAR includes data from devices that are no longer in use. The Lifeline registry includes data from the IDE clinical trials of four FDA-approved devices (Ancure, AneuRx, Excluder, and Powerlink) and shows that freedom from AAA-related death was 98% at 6 years, freedom from rupture was 99% at 6 years, freedom from conversion to open repair was 95% at 6 years, and freedom from reintervention was 78% at 5 years. Persistence of an endoleak with aneurysm expansion or stent migration can usually be managed through a minimally invasive approach, but some may require conversion to an open repair. Other complications of EVAR include graft occlusion, arterial wall rupture, renal failure (due to contrast nephropathy or renal artery occlusion), distal embolization, and arterial dissection.

FOLLOW-UP

Close postoperative follow-up and lifelong surveillance is mandatory for patients who undergo EVAR. We routinely obtain CT angiograms at 1, 6, and 12 months followed by annually. CT is performed more frequently if an endoleak is present. After open AAA repair, a CT angiogram of the chest, abdomen, and pelvis is obtained postoperatively and every 5 years with more frequent testing to follow small thoracic or iliac aneurysms. Aneurysms of the proximal aorta, suture lines, or iliac arteries may be seen in up to 15% of patients at 8 to 9 years after open AAA repair.

SUGGESTED READING

Ailawadi G, Eliason JL, Upchurch GR Jr. Current concepts in the pathogenesis of abdominal aortic aneurysm. *J Vasc Surg* 2003;38 (3):584.

Brady AR, Fowkes FG, Greenhalgh RM, et al. Risk factors for postoperative death following elective surgical repair of abdominal aortic aneurysm: results from the UK Small Aneurysm Trial. On behalf of the UK Small Aneurysm Trial participants. *Br J Surg* 2000;87:742.

Brewster DC, Cronenwett JL, Hallett JW Jr., et al. Guidelines for the treatment of abdominal aortic aneurysms. Report of a subcommittee of the Joint Council of the American Association for Vascular Surgery and Society for Vascular Surgery. *J Vasc Surg* 2003;37: 1106.

Brown LC, Powell JT. Risk factors for aneurysm rupture in patients kept under ultrasound surveillance. UK Small Aneurysm Trial Participants. *Ann Surg* 1999;230(3):289; discussion 296.

Creech O Jr. Endo-aneurysmorrhaphy and treatment of aortic aneurysm. *Ann Surg* 1966;164(6):935.

Endovascular aneurysm repair versus open repair in patients with abdominal aortic aneurysm (EVAR trial 1): randomised controlled trial. *Lancet* 2005;365:2179.

Fillinger MF, Marra SP, Raghavan ML, et al. Prediction of rupture risk in abdominal

Vascular Surgery

aortic aneurysm during observation: wall stress versus diameter. *J Vasc Surg* 2003;37:724.

Hallin A, Bergqvist D, Holmberg L. Literature review of surgical management of abdominal aortic aneurysm. *Eur J Vasc Endovasc Surg* 2001;22:197.

Lederle FA, Johnson GR, Wilson SE, et al. Rupture rate of large abdominal aortic aneurysms in patients refusing or unfit for elective repair. *JAMA* 2002;287(22):2968.

Lederle FA, Johnson GR, Wilson SE, et al. The aneurysm detection and management study screening program: validation cohort and final results. Aneurysm Detection And Management Veterans Affairs Cooperative Study Investigators. *Arch Intern Med* 2000;160:1425

Lederle FA, Wilson SE, Johnson GR, et al. Immediate repair compared with surveillance of small abdominal aortic aneurysms. *N Engl J Med* 2002;346:1437.

Lifeline registry of endovascular aneurysm repair: long-term primary outcome measures. *J Vasc Surg* 2005;42:1.

Nesi F, Leo E, Biancari F, et al. Preoperative risk stratification in patients undergoing elective infrarenal aortic aneurysm surgery: evaluation of five risk scoring methods. *Eur J Vasc Endovasc Surg* 2004;28(1):52.

Schermerhorn ML, Finlayson SR, Fillinger MF, et al. Life expectancy after endovascular versus open abdominal aortic aneurysm repair: results of a decision analysis model on the basis of data from EUROSTAR. *J Vasc Surg* 2002;36:1112.

van Marrewijk CJ, Fransen G, Laheij RJ, et al.; EUROSTAR Collaborators. Is a type II endoleak after EVAR a harbinger of risk? Causes and outcome of open conversion and aneurysm rupture during follow-up. *Eur J Vasc Endovasc Surg* 2004;27(2):128.

EDITOR'S COMMENT

With all due respect to Dr. Debakey, one of the great surgeons of the 20th century, the first synthetic vascular graft was implanted by Dr. Arthur Voorhees and reported in a paper before the American Surgical Society in 1953. These initial grafts were constructed of vinyon-N and were simply tubes of material that were hand sutured into a cylinder. The understated work of Dr. Voorhees is an excellent example of applied surgical research. He first studied the use of silk material and then vinyon-N in animal models, where he documented the outcomes in a report in 1952 (Blakemore AH, Voorhees AB Jr. The use of tubes constructed from vinyon "N" cloth in bridging arterial defects—experimental and clinical. *Ann Surg* 1954; 40:324.). The subsequent published report of a series of successful implantations in the human was exciting news that marked a new era in vascular surgery. Over the ensuing years, several materials with various pore sizes, and textile structure were studied, among which Dr. Debakey's knitted Dacron velour fabric became quite popular. It was however, classic lab to bedside scientific investigation by Dr. Voorhees that resulted in the first synthetic graft repair of the human aorta.

The appropriate role of EVAR in the care of patients, is still unclear. I recall the comment a granddaughter of one of my patients made. After hearing the presentation of EVAR versus open repair, she turned to me and said, "In other words doc, one way he's cured, and one way he isn't." It is quite humbling when a patient can summarize profound clinical arguments with such a simple, pithy, statement that goes directly to the heart of the issue. Unfortunately, we have not had many reliable trials to determine the appropriate role of EVAR. Most disconcerting is the fact that EVAR does not seem to give better results in high risk patients than does open surgery. In a recent report summarizing information from several databases, the freedom from aneurysm related mortality was virtually identical at four years. What was not identical was the fact that the incidence of endoleaks at 4 years was 19% and the incidence of AAA sac enlargements was 11% at 4 years with EVAR. Time will tell, but this seems to be a high price to pay in the long run for avoidance of an abdominal incision. This field is now under such intense commercial pressure, that it is extremely difficult to obtain accurate data or to design high quality scientific trials. Such a trial would involve an entry point where randomization occurs very early and patients are then referred for EVAR or standard repair. Standard repair does not require the extensive evaluation required by EVAR, so all of that expense is unnecessary. Furthermore, in preparation for EVAR, arteriography is required and, it is often necessary to insert coils or other technology to occlude blood flow in one or both hypogastric arteries. I think it is extremely unlikely that we will ever see a trial where all of these data are included as part of the EVAR result. I suspect it will eventually require a system of computerized hospital records throughout the country before we can have the data necessary to make accurate decisions.

The authors provide some very helpful information about the details of open repair of suprarenal and infrarenal abdominal aortic aneurysms. These procedures can be carried out today in elderly, high risk patients with a high success rate, and the patient is cured. (Sicard GA, Zwolak RM, Sidawy AN, White RA, Siami FS. Endovascular abdominal aortic aneurysm repair: Long-term outcome measures in patients at high-risk for open surgery. *Journal of Vascular Surgery* 2006 Aug; 44(2):229–236.)

F.W.L.

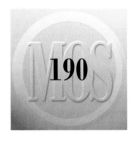

190

Ruptured Abdominal Aortic Aneurysm

FRANK POMPOSELLI AND BRANKO BOJOVIC

INTRODUCTION

No emergency in vascular surgery is more acute or lethal than rupture of an abdominal aortic aneurysm (AAA). Ruptured AAAs are the 15th leading cause of death overall and the 10th leading cause of death in men older than age 55 in the United States, claiming more than 15,000 lives annually. Although the true incidence of aortic rupture is difficult to determine, the mortality rate for patients arriving to the hospital alive ranges from 40% to 70%. When available autopsy data are taken into account, including patients who die before reaching the hospital, the true mortality rate is probably 90% or more. Although advances in anesthetic and surgical techniques have reduced the perioperative mortality to 2% to 4% for elective repair of intact AAAs, the surgical mortality rates continue to average 50% for ruptured AAA and have changed little in many years. Since aortic aneurysm is an insidious process rarely causing any symptoms prior to rupture, reduction in mortality for this condition depends primarily on timely recognition before the occurrence of rupture. Implementation of population-based screening for high-risk populations such as the recently approved SAAVE Act provides the best solution for reducing the occurrence of rupture.

Once rupture occurs, patient survival depends on prompt surgical intervention to control hemorrhage and aggressive and

Vascular Surgery

often complex postoperative critical care management. The development of endovascular aneurysm repair (EVAR) has radically changed the approach to elective repair of aortic aneurysm, reducing mortality, morbidity, and time to recovery for many patients treated by this approach. As experience with EVAR has grown, some centers have begun applying this technique to selected patients presenting with rupture. Although experience is limited, the rate of perioperative mortality has been lower than the expected rate of 50% to 70%, offering the promise of better outcomes for the first time in more than four decades. This chapter will review the diagnosis, treatment, postoperative care, and outcomes of contemporary treatment of ruptured abdominal aortic aneurysm.

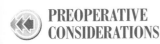

PREOPERATIVE CONSIDERATIONS

Diagnosis

The identification of a patient presenting with ruptured AAA is first and foremost a clinical diagnosis based on a careful history and physical examination. The classic triad for ruptured AAA presentation is severe abdominal or back pain, hypotension, and a pulsatile abdominal mass. Patients presenting with this constellation of symptoms and findings need no other evaluation and should proceed directly to surgery. In some patients the diagnosis may be far less obvious, presenting without hemodynamic instability and with less specific complaints including syncope, emesis, groin, and back or flank pain. Obesity may obscure palpation of the

aneurysm, making the diagnosis more difficult. In order to prevent a missed diagnosis and delay to treatment, it is important to have a high index of suspicion for the diagnosis in any patient over the age of 50 presenting with back, abdomen, or flank pain. When the physical examination is unclear, an abdominal ultrasound can be used as a quick adjunct to the history and physical examination, especially in the emergency department. Ultrasound is sensitive in identifying aneurysms and can be used to evaluate the aorta rapidly but is poor in determining the presence of aortic rupture. In stable patients where the diagnosis is suspected, a computed tomography (CT) scan (Fig. 1) is the most accurate method of detecting a ruptured AAA. Additionally, newer generation rapid multislice CT scanners can rapidly provide the needed anatomic information for the evaluation of some patients for endovascular options. Plain abdominal radiographs (KUB) continue to be performed on patients with abdominal pain and can be important in guiding the investigations in the emergency room. Aortic wall calcifications on the KUB confirm the presence of AAA in 75% of patients. Moreover, loss of a psoas shadow may be apparent in the presence of rupture.

Preparation

The preoperative patient management in cases of aortic rupture should be focused and expeditious. Two large-bore intravenous cannulas, suitable for high-volume blood transfusion, should be immediately established and blood drawn for routine laboratory data and typing and immediate

cross matching for 6 units of red blood cells. Rapid transport of the patient to the operating room must be immediately undertaken. Unnecessary time can be wasted in an ill-advised attempt at resuscitation of the patient prior to transport to the operating room. If a patient is stable with a "reasonable" blood pressure, large-volume infusions and/or the use of vasopressors to raise a slightly depressed blood pressure can only serve to accelerate the rate of bleeding, or worse, result in the loss of containment of the rupture by the retroperitoneal tissues, leading to rapid decompensation and cardiac arrest. It is important to remember that even in stable patients the situation can change quickly and that complacency can be deadly. The surgical team is responsible for maintaining a sense of urgency and the need to move as quickly as possible to surgery. The combined efforts of anesthesia, nursing, and technical personnel can quickly prepare the patient for operative intervention and definitive management. In the operating room a Foley catheter is inserted, and a broad-spectrum antibiotic is given. Rapid transfusion devices with the capacity to warm blood products and cell washing autotransfusion devices are useful and should be prepared if available. Hypothermia is a common problem in these patients and should be ameliorated by warming the room and covering the patient with a heated air-circulating blanket. The patient is prepped and draped widely from chest to midthigh. Unstable patients should be fully prepped and draped prior to induction of anesthesia, which often leads to rapid decompensation, necessitating immediate laparotomy so that aortic clamping or compression can be accomplished as quickly as possible. Moribund patients may require laparotomy prior to induction. After surgery has commenced, useful adjuncts such as nasogastric tubes and central venous, pulmonary artery, and radial arterial catheters can all be placed.

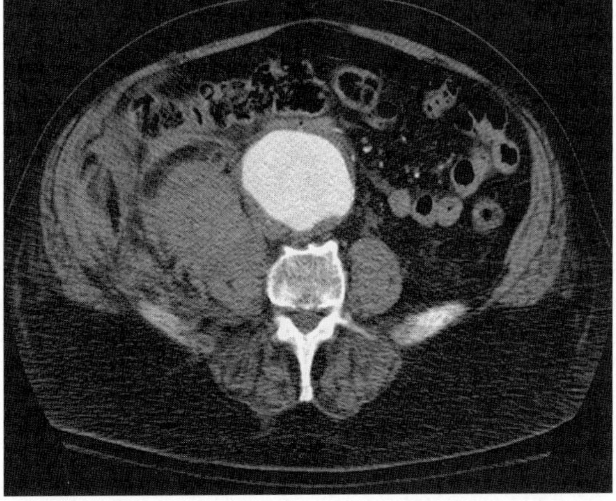

 ## SURGICAL TECHNIQUE

The immediate goal of the surgeon is to gain proximal control of the aorta. Although some surgeons use the retroperitoneal approach for ruptured aneurysm, most surgeons, including the authors, explore patients through a vertical midline incision extending from the xiphoid process to the symphysis pubis. If the patient's hemodynamic status deteriorates rapidly when the tamponade effect of the abdominal wall is lost with laparotomy, the surgeon

Fig. 1. Typical appearance of a ruptured infra-renal aortic aneurysm (AAA) on a contrast enhanced CT scan. Note the large hematoma to the right of the aorta, obscuring the right psoas muscle and displacing the bowel anteriorly.

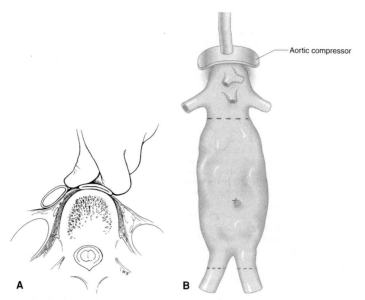

Fig. 2. A: Method of manually compressing the supra-celiac aorta against the spine for temporary proximal control. Alternatively a sponge stick, or **B**.) a commercially available aortic compressor can be used. (b. from Lindsay TF. Ruptured Abdominal Aortic Aneurysms. In: Rutherford RB, ed. *Vascular Surgery Vol 2*, 6th ed. Philadelphia: Elsevier Saunders, 2005:1480, with permission.)

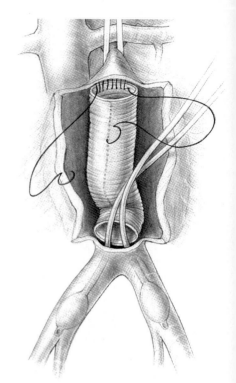

Fig. 3. Attempting to dissect out the iliac arteries in a large hematoma can be hazardous, risking injury to the iliac vein or ureter. An alternative is to gain control from within the sack by placing large diameter embolectomy catheters or a small foley catheter within the iliac artery orifice and carefully inflating the balloon. Over inflation can rupture the artery. (From Zarins CK, Gewertz BL. In: Zarins CK, Gewertz BL, ed. *Atlas of Vascular Surgery*. New York, NY; Churchill Livingstone Inc., 1989:69, with permission.)

can compress the aorta against the spine above the celiac artery (Fig. 2) while the anesthesia team "catches up" with resuscitation. The need for continuous communication between the surgical and anesthesia teams is critical to limit severe hypotension and shock from continued rapid blood loss without adequate replacement and/or excessive volume replacement once bleeding has been controlled.

Most ruptures occur posterior and lateral to the anterior surface of the aorta. In those cases the infrarenal neck of the aneurysm may be relatively free of the hematoma and can be approached in a manner similar to that for elective aneurysm repair. The transverse colon is retracted superiorly and the small bowel eviscerated or retracted to the right side of the abdomen. The retroperitoneum is incised over the aneurysm and the duodenum mobilized to the right by incising the ligament of Treitz. Dissection commences directly over the aortic pulsation by bluntly and sharply dissecting the overlying retroperitoneal tissues, exposing the wall of the aorta. All dissection should be directed superiorly, toward the neck of the aneurysm. Extending the dissection distally into the hematoma prior to gaining proximal control should be avoided as it can lead to loss of its containment, accelerating hemorrhage. If the region of the neck of the aneurysm is obscured by hematoma, much of the dissection and exposure can be done bluntly with surgeon's fingers avoiding sharp injury to adjacent structures. Dissection proceeds superiorly until the normal aortic wall is encountered. Usually this will be close to the point where the left renal vein crosses the anterior wall of the aorta, which should be identified to avoid inadvertent injury. The vein can be retracted superiorly slightly while the surgeon establishes a space on the lateral surfaces of the aorta with finger dissection in a longitudinal direction to permit placement of the aortic clamp. Almost always, the segment of aorta under the left renal vein is relatively normal in infrarenal aneurysms. Occasionally, the left renal vein may need to be divided to facilitate exposure of normal aorta. The vein should be divided close to the vena cava, preserving collateral flow through the left adrenal, lumbar, and gonadal branches. Attempting to encircle the aorta is dangerous and unnecessary, running the risk of injury to underlying lumbar arterial or venous branches or the posterior wall of the aorta itself. Once the aorta has been exposed for clamping, a dose of 3,000 to 5,000 units of heparin is given intravenously. If massive hemorrhage has occurred, heparin is not given due to the likelihood of severe coagulopathy. Once the aorta is clamped, the aorta is opened longitudinally and fully exposed. With the hematoma and aneurysm sack decompressed, the iliac arteries can be more easily exposed and clamped. Care must be taken to avoid injury to the adjacent vena cava and common iliac veins. As with the aortic neck, this is best accomplished by limiting dissection of the anterior and lateral surfaces of the arteries without trying to encircle them prior to clamping. We prefer the use of soft jaw clamps. If the iliac vessels are encased in hematoma, it is best to make no attempt to expose them at all, avoiding injury to both venous structures and the ureter. Control can be achieved with a large-diameter embolectomy balloon catheter placed into the lumen of the common iliac artery from within the aorta (Fig. 3). In some cases, backbleeding from the iliac arteries is so limited that no control is necessary.

Clinical circumstances, the extent of the retroperitoneal hematoma, and the size or shape of the aneurysm may necessitate modifications to the approach. In cases of severe hypotension or uncontrolled bleeding from intraperitoneal rupture, or whenever the surgeon feels that the extent of the hematoma or shape or size of the aneurysm makes conventional exposure too difficult or impossible, control of the supraceliac aorta can be obtained (Fig. 4). Exposure is undertaken by incising the gastrohepatic omentum to gain access to the lesser sac. The aortic pulse is palpated.

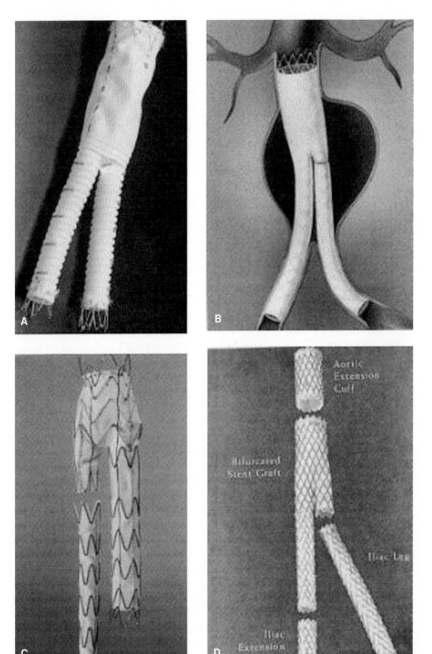

Fig. 9. Examples of commercially available stent grafts: Some are constructed as a single component including an aortic "body" with two iliac limbs. Most stent grafts in use today however are modular comprised of an aortic body with one attached iliac limb. The second limb must be attached or "docked" to the first component inside the patient. All grafts rely on radial force against the lumen of the aorta to maintain a water tight seal and keep it in place. Some designs incorporate a supra-renal bare metal stent and /or barbs to prevent distal migration. (From May J, White GH. Endovascular Treatment of Aortic Aneurysms. In: Rutherford RB, ed. *Vascular Surgery Vol 2*, 5th ed. Philadelphia: WB Saunders Company, 2000:1285, with permission.)

brachial or femoral artery and inflated in the distal descending thoracic or suprarenal aorta at the beginning of the procedure. Femoral cutdowns are then performed, sheaths inserted, and guidewires placed into the aorta. A calibrated flush angiography catheter is placed and an aortogram is performed to determine both the location of the renal arteries and iliac artery bifurcations as well as the length of device required. Two different strategies can be employed. One is to place a device from the aorta into one iliac artery (an aortouni–iliac device), occlude the contralateral common iliac artery, and perform a femorofemoral bypass (Fig. 11). This is generally simpler and quicker in most cases. The other is to place a conventional bifurcated device as used in elective repairs. This approach usually takes longer since some time is required to gain access to the docking limb of the aortic body with a guidewire in order to position and deploy the second iliac limb of the device. Many of the commercially available bifurcated devices have attachments available to convert a bifurcated device into aortouni–iliac systems.

Treating ruptured aneurysms with emergent EVAR requires significant expertise with elective endovascular aneurysm repair and an experienced endovascular team. Planning is the most important part of EVAR, and in the case of ruptured aneurysm, must be performed quickly. Nursing personnel must likewise be experienced and comfortable with the procedure and available 24 hours a day. The operating room must stock a full complement of the various sizes and lengths of the aortic device and its components as well as the various wires, catheters, and balloons most commonly used. The inventory required can cost several hundred thousand dollars and is probably only reasonable for hospitals with a substantial volume of elective procedures. These requirements coupled with the anatomic constraints make it likely that emergent EVAR for ruptured aneurysms will continue to be applied to a very selective group of patients in a similarly selective group of hospitals.

RESULTS

In spite of significant surgical advances and sophisticated anesthetic and critical care management, the outcome for patients suffering aortic rupture remains bleak. Mortality ranges from 25% to 75%, averaging approximately 50%. A bimodal pattern of mortality is seen in the postoperative period, with deaths secondary to

to custom fit the endograft to an individual patient's aortic and iliac anatomy. A segment of normal aorta distal to renal arteries must be present at least 1 cm in length for secure watertight attachment of the aortic component to the aorta. Inadequate seal zones will lead to leakage of blood between the device and the aortic wall (attachment site endoleak) and

continued exposure of the aneurysm sack to arterial blood pressure. Similarly, the iliac limbs must terminate in a segment of common iliac artery of suitable length and diameter or a distal attachment site endoleak will occur

Hypotensive patients can be stabilized with a large-diameter compliant angioplasty balloon catheter inserted through a

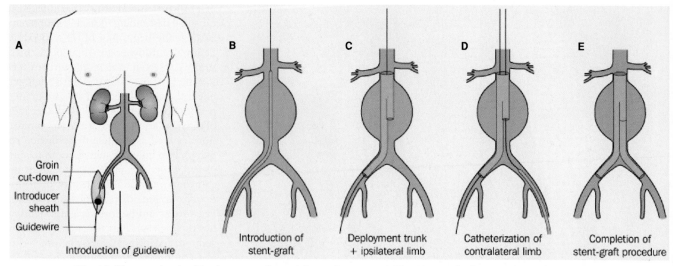

Fig. 10. The steps involved in placement of a modular aortic stent graft: The time involved in completing this procedure may not be feasible in an unstable patient with a ruptured AAA. (van Sambeek, et al. Abdominal Aneurysm-EVAR. In: Hallet JW Jr, Mills JL, Earnshaw JJ, Reekers JA, ed. *Comprehensive Vascular and Endovascular Surgery*. Mosby, 2004.)

hemorrhagic shock or myocardial infarction occurring within the first 48 to 72 hours and deaths from multiple organ system failure and sepsis occurring many days or weeks later. Patient, hospital, and surgeon factors have all been demonstrated to affect survival. Age greater than 80 years, systolic blood pressure less than 70 mm Hg, blood replacement greater than 3,500 mL, need for a suprarenal clamping, baseline renal insufficiency, and female gender have all been associated with higher rates of mortality. The lowest mortality rates are generally reported from tertiary centers who usually receive more stable patients accepted in transfer. Additionally, tertiary centers are more likely to have experienced vascular surgeons with greater exposure to both elective and ruptured aortic aneurysm surgery. In a recent study conducted in Ontario, Canada, other factors affecting mortality in both ruptured and elective AAA repair were compared over a 10-year period encompassing over 16,000 patients including 2,600 presenting with rupture. Mortality was 10-fold higher for patients with rupture (40.8% vs. 4.5%). For ruptured aneurysm significant predictors of lower survival included older age, female gender, lower socioeconomic status, repair of aneurysms on off hours, and surgeons with lower annual volumes of ruptured AAA and/or lack of vascular or cardiothoracic fellowship training. A similar study conducted in Maryland evaluating outcomes of ruptured AAA repair in 527 patients over a 5-year period found a nearly identical mortality rate of 43.2% and found that advanced age but not gender adversely affected mortality and that surgeons having performed at least 10 or more ruptured AAA repairs had lower mortality rates than surgeons with less experience.

Late survival following AAA repair is also adversely affected by the occurrence of rupture at initial presentation. Cho et al. from the Mayo Clinic evaluated the long-term survival and occurrence of late complications in 116 survivors of ruptured AAA repair. At 1, 5, and 10 years, survival rates were significantly lower for patients

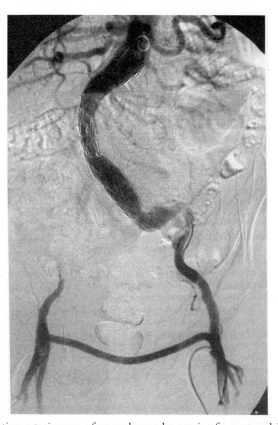

Fig. 11. Completion arteriogram of an endovascular repair of a ruptured infra-renal aortic aneurysm. In this case an aorto-uniiliac device was used. The contra-lateral common iliac artery is occluded with coils or similar device and a standard femoral-femoral bypass is performed to maintain blood flow to the right leg. This procedure is preferred in ruptured AAA repair due to the simplicity and speed with which the device can be placed compared to aorto-biiliac devices. (May J, White GH. Endovascular Treatment of Aortic Aneurysms. In: Rutherford RB, ed. *Vascular Surgery Vol 2*, 5th ed. Philadelphia: WB Saunders Company, 2000:1284.)

surviving rupture compared to a concurrent group of patients undergoing elective repair. Additionally, vascular and graft-related complications causing death occurred in 3% of the rupture group compared to 1% of the elective group.

While survival may be reduced in survivors of ruptured AAA, ultimate functional outcome appears to be reasonable once recovery is complete. In a comparatively small study of 81 survivors of rupture, Fisher et al. evaluated quality of life as measured by the SF-36 health status survey. Quality-of-life analyses showed that majority of survivors reported same or better quality of life compared to SF-36 norms for age-matched individuals.

The benefit of performing emergency endovascular repair for ruptured aneurysm remains unclear, although the results from single center studies and a global registry appear promising. To date, approximately 440 ruptured AAA have been repaired by EVAR with a procedural mortality of 18%. Extrapolating these results to the entire population of patients with ruptured AAA is difficult since selection criteria vary widely among centers, with some attempting to treat all suitable patients while others reserve it for stable patients or patients presenting when the personnel trained in EVAR are available.

The difficulties encountered in emergent EVAR for ruptured AAA are apparent from the recent results reported by Alsac et al. of a small but prospective series of 37 patients presenting with rupture where EVAR was attempted whenever possible. While 73% were found to be anatomically suitable for EVAR, only 46% ultimately had the procedure due to severe instability, poor anatomy, or lack of available appropriate endograft. Nonetheless, the EVAR-treated group had a 30-day mortality of 23.5% compared to 50% for the group treated with conventional open surgery.

CONCLUSION

Repair of ruptured aortic aneurysm remains a formidable challenge and continues to have a 10-fold or higher mortality than elective aneurysm repair. A high index of suspicion, immediate transport to the operating room, and early operative intervention remain the patient's only hope for survival. Technical excellence and avoiding complications are critical during surgery. The appropriate use of adjuncts like mesh closure of the abdomen, constant surveillance for colon ischemia, and aggressive critical management can improve the chances of survival in the postoperative period. The early results of endovascular repair appear promising and may ultimately change the treatment paradigm, but lack of availability of expert personnel and lack of equipment are significant obstacles to its widespread application.

SUGGESTED READING

Alsac JM, Desgranges P, Kobeiter H, et al. Emergency endovascular repair for ruptured abdominal aortic aneurysms: feasibility and comparison of early results with conventional open repair. *Eur J Vasc Endovasc Surg* 2005;30(6):632.

Alsac JM, Kobeiter H, Becquemin JP, et al. Endovascular repair for ruptured AAA: a literature review. *Acta Chir Belg* 2005;105(2):134.

Champagne BJ, Darling RC III, Daneshmand M, et al. Outcome of aggressive surveillance colonoscopy in ruptured abdominal aortic aneurysm. *J Vasc Surg* 2004;39(4):792.

Cho JS, Gloviczki P, Martelli E, et al. Long-term survival and late complications after repair of ruptured abdominal aortic aneurysms. *J Vasc Surg* 1998;27(5):813; discussion 9.

Dardik A, Burleyson GP, Bowman H, et al. Surgical repair of ruptured abdominal aortic aneurysms in the state of Maryland: factors influencing outcome among 527 recent cases. *J Vasc Surg* 1998;28(3):413; discussion 20.

Dueck AD, Kucey DS, Johnston KW, et al. Survival after ruptured abdominal aortic aneurysm: effect of patient, surgeon, and hospital factors. *J Vasc Surg* 2004;39(6):1253.

Johnston KW. Ruptured abdominal aortic aneurysm: six-year follow-up results of a multicenter prospective study. Canadian Society for Vascular Surgery Aneurysm Study Group. *J Vasc Surg* 1994;19(5):888.

Joseph AY, Fisher JB, Toedter LJ, et al. Ruptured abdominal aortic aneurysm and quality of life. *Vasc Endovasc Surg* 2002;36(1):65.

Mehta M, Darling RC III, Roddy SP, et al. Factors associated with abdominal compartment syndrome complicating endovascular repair of ruptured abdominal aortic aneurysms. *J Vasc Surg* 2005;42(6):1047.

Papavassiliou V, Anderton M, Loftus IM, et al. The physiological effects of elevated intra-abdominal pressure following aneurysm repair. *Eur J Vasc Endovasc Surg* 2003;26(3):293.

Rasmussen TE, Hallett JW Jr, Noel AA, et al. Early abdominal closure with mesh reduces multiple organ failure after ruptured abdominal aortic aneurysm repair: guidelines from a 10-year case-control study. *J Vasc Surg* 2002;35(2):246.

Vascular Surgery

EDITOR'S COMMENT

This is an excellent review of the management of patients with ruptured abdominal aortic aneurysms. The authors well describe the evaluation, surgical management, postoperative care, and outcomes of this true surgical emergency. Unfortunately, this is probably the most morbid problem encountered by vascular surgeons. In addition, as the authors point out, despite significant advances in the management of virtually every other disease of the vascular system, the mortality associated with this complex problem has remained essentially unchanged over the last 20 years (50% in hospital mortality, overall mortality 80% to 90%).

This seems to be due to the magnitude of the insult of aortic rupture and surgical repair in elderly patients with aneurysms and the significant comorbidities. Indeed, the systemic inflammatory response after repair of ruptured aortic aneurysms as measured by levels of circulating proinflammatory cytokines is the highest seen for any type of aortic surgery. In contrast, endovascular repair of both elective and ruptured aortic aneurysms is associated with a significantly lower inflammatory response and use of endovascular aneurysm repair may also be associated with a lower mortality, although most reports of this approach to date detail small, single center series where significant selection bias is highly likely. Regardless, the endovascular experience with this complex problem has taught us that "permissive hypotension" (systolic blood pressure under 100 mm) is acceptable and may even be beneficial as long as the patient is awake, that time to repair is not quite as critical as we once thought (almost 90% of patients survive up to 2 hours after hospital admission without treatment, *J Vasc Surg* 2004;39:788), and that the simplest, quickest repair possible, even if it has to be redone later in a more stable setting, will likely be associated with the best outcomes.

In the face of this high morbidity and mortality (and associated costs of therapy for overall benefit), multiple studies have also attempted to define factors that identify patients with ruptured aorta aneurysms who will not survive. Unfortunately, beyond cardiac arrest on presentation and possibly very advanced age, no specific factors have been shown to clearly identify those who will not survive repair, so we continue to be faced with treating a group of patients who will consume significant resources but few of whom will survive. Until we can understand and control the impact of profound physiologic and surgical stress, endovascular treatment of these problems seems to offer the only glimmer of hope for improved outcomes. However, we must continue to manage these critically ill patients until that hope potentially becomes reality, and following the principles and techniques described by Dr. Pomposelli will serve us and our patients with ruptured aneurysms well.

J.M.S.

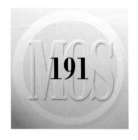

191

Aortic Endografting

GREGORIO A. SICARD AND JUAN C. PARODI

Endovascular repair has evolved as an important alternative and less invasive method for the treatment of patients with abdominal aortic aneurysms (AAAs). This minimally invasive technique has had a significant impact in the treatment of patients with AAA. Its widespread use has identified the advantages and disadvantages of this innovative technique. The device used for this technique, an endograft, is contained in a deployment catheter (sheath) and consists of a metal stent attached to a prosthetic graft material. This technique permits the sutureless aortic aneurysm exclusion by an endograft introduced through the femoral artery.

INDICATIONS

Endovascular aneurysm repair (EVAR) was initially reported by Dr. Parodi and collaborators in 1990 as an alternative for patients deemed unfit for open aneurysm repair as a result of significant co-morbidities. Although "unfitness for open surgery" is a common indication for EVAR, initial good results along with patient preference for a less invasive approach

have significantly expanded its use. The introduction of EVAR as a good alternative to open repair has not changed the indications for the treatment of AAA. Different than open repair, two strict anatomic requirements must be met prior to considering a patient to be a suitable candidate for EVAR: (i) a proximal aortic neck diameter below the lowest renal artery that ranges between 20 and 28 mm and 15 mm or more in length, and (ii) suitable iliac artery diameter to allow insertion of the device. These strict anatomic requirements demand precise preoperative imaging that permits accurate measurements of the diameter and length of the aorta from the level of the renal arteries to the common femoral arteries. This is best accomplished by thin-slice (1 to 3 mm) contrast abdominal and pelvic computed tomographic (CT) scan. Because of the frequently seen tortuosity of the infrarenal neck and iliac arteries, precise diameter measurement can best be accomplished when the thin-slice CT images are reconstructed in a three-dimensional field, which allows for center line measurement at the appropriate anatomic sites (Fig. 1A,B). Contrast CT scan can

identify the presence or absence of thrombus, calcification, or significant atheromatous disease in the aortic neck and/or iliac arteries that may interfere with an adequate endograft seal. Three-dimensional reconstruction of the thin-slice CT scan has practically eliminated the need for preoperative angiography. In patients with abnormal renal function, magnetic resonance angiography with gadolinium can be useful in providing all the anatomic information required.

There are currently four commercially available endografts in the United States: AneuR$_x$ (Medtronic Vascular, Santa Rosa, CA), Excluder (W.L. Gore, Flagstaff, AZ), Zenith (Cook, Inc., Bloomington, IN), and Powerlink (Endologix, Irvine, CA) (Table 1). All the current commercially available devices are self-expanding with a metal stent-based radial force and longitudinal strength. Each device has different construction in terms of the type of stent (nickel titanium alloy, cobalt chromium alloy, or stainless steel), the type and thickness of the graft material used (Dacron, expanded polytetrafluoroethylene), as well as, different attachment mechanisms at the proximal and/or distal landing zones. Even

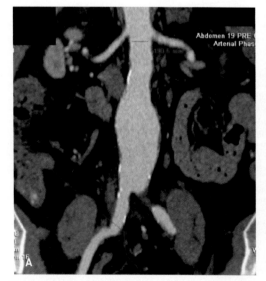
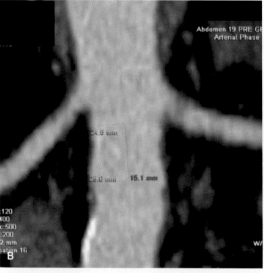

Fig. 1. A: Three-dimensional reconstruction of infrarenal abdominal aortic aneurysm with centerline measurement of distance from renal arteries to aortic and common iliac artery bifurcation. **B:** Magnified view with centerline base aortic neck diameter and length.

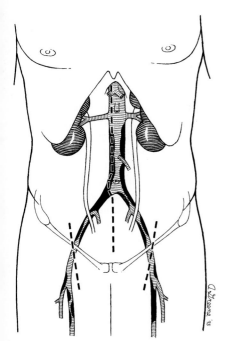

Fig. 1. Standard incisions for aortobifemoral bypass.

artery and then cephalad to the inguinal ligament. The lymph nodes and/or lymphatic tissue are best divided between clamps and then suture-ligated to minimize the possibility of a postoperative lymphatic leak with its associated risk of wound or graft infection. The caudal border of the inguinal ligament is partially divided directly over the femoral artery to ensure ample space for tunneling of the graft limb without compression. Dissection is then carried caudally to expose the common femoral artery bifurcation, and the proximal aspect of both the superficial and profunda femoral arteries are encircled with vessel loops (Fig. 2). Similarly, any sizable side branches of the femoral arteries are preserved and controlled with such loops. If significant occlusive disease is found in the proximal profunda femoris artery on the preoperative arteriogram or by intraoperative palpation, the vessel is exposed further caudally beyond the significant disease to allow concomitant profundaplasty at the time of distal anastomosis. This usually requires exposing an additional 2 to 3 cm of the vessel and necessitates division of one or more branches of the profunda femoral vein that typically cross the anterior surface of the proximal artery.

A midline abdominal incision is then created extending from the xiphoid to the pubis. After careful exploration of the intra-abdominal organs, the transverse colon and greater omentum are elevated and retracted cephalad, and the entire small bowel eviscerated and displaced to the right (Fig. 3). The descending and sigmoid portions of the colon are retracted laterally and caudally. After these maneuvers, the posterior parietal peritoneum overlying the infrarenal aorta is visualized, and this is incised along the longitudinal axis of the aorta starting between the duodenum on the patient's right and the inferior mesenteric vein to the left. Care is taken to avoid the plexuses of autonomic nerve fibers (Fig. 3B) that course primarily along the left anterolateral aspect of the infrarenal aorta and the proximal left common iliac artery. Careful dissection helps preserve these autonomic nerves and helps reduce the incidence of postoperative sexual dysfunction in male patients.

The retroperitoneal incision is extended cephalad and the ligament of Treitz is divided. This allows mobilization of the fourth portion of the duodenum off the aorta and facilitates visualization of the left renal vein as it crosses anterior to the aorta just below the renal artery origins. The left renal vein is an important landmark because the proximal graft anastomosis should be placed as close to it (and the renal arteries) as possible. This serves to minimize the potential for recurrent occlusive disease in the infrarenal aorta above the proximal anastomosis that could potentially compromise the late patency of the graft. The aortic dissection is extended distally just beyond the origin of the inferior mesenteric artery. This extent of aortic exposure is sufficient to allow construction of a proper proximal graft anastomosis and tunneling of each graft limb to the groin. Furthermore, it minimizes the dissection in the region of the aortic bifurcation itself, thereby reducing the possibility of autonomic nerve injury.

After completion of the aortic and femoral dissections, retroperitoneal tunnels are next made for passage of each graft limb from the aorta to the groins. Such tunnels are best made by gentle blunt dissection using both index fingers in a simultaneous fashion with one extending from the groin cephalad and the other from the aortic bifurcation caudal (Fig. 4A). Dissection should be kept on a plane directly anterior to the common and external iliac vessels to guarantee that the graft is subsequently placed posterior to the ureter. This is important because passage of the graft anterior to the ureter may lead to compression and obstruction of the ureter with hydronephrosis. When starting the tunnel in the groin, care must be taken not to tear the circumflex iliac venous branches that cross the distal external iliac artery just above the inguinal ligament. After appropriate tunnels have been created to both groins, a long blunt-tipped clamp is placed through the tunnel and a Penrose drain drawn through the tunnel (Fig. 4B). Elevation of both ends of the drain facilitates later passage of the graft limbs.

Proximal Aortic Anastomosis

A variety of prosthetic grafts are available for aortobifemoral bypass, including

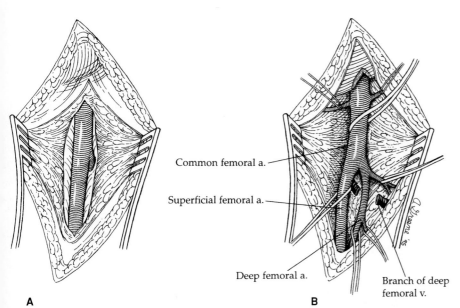

Common femoral a.

Superficial femoral a.

Deep femoral a.

Branch of deep femoral v.

A   **B**

Fig. 2. A: The common femoral artery is exposed from the inguinal ligament to the proximal portions of its superficial and profunda branches. **B:** More distal exposure of the profunda femoris usually requires division of one or more branches of the deep femoral vein that cross the artery anteriorly. The inguinal ligament has been partially divided to provide ample space for tunneling of the graft.

Vascular Surgery

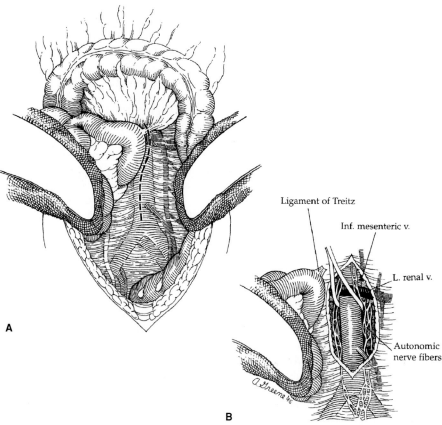

Fig. 3. A: Following evisceration of large and small bowel, the retroperitoneum overlying the aorta is opened from the aortic bifurcation to above the crossing left renal vein, and the ligament of Treitz is divided to allow mobilization of the duodenum off the aorta. **B:** The inferior mesenteric vein will often require division. Automatic nerve plexuses are preserved as best as possible, and dissection in the region of the aortic bifurcation is avoided.

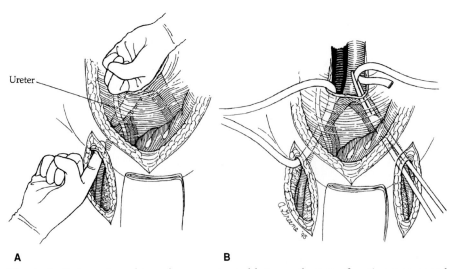

Fig. 4. A: Retroperitoneal tunnels are constructed between the area of aortic exposure and femoral artery dissection in each groin. Tunneling is best performed by simultaneous blunt finger dissection from above and below, immediately on the anterior surface of the iliac arteries. This ensures passages of the graft limb posterior to the ureter that usually crosses the iliac vessels at their bifurcation. **B:** After tunneling is completed, a long clamp is passed through each tunnel and a rubber Penrose drain is pulled through the tract. Anterior traction on the drain facilitates proper passage of the graft through the tunnel at a later stage of the procedure.

conventional Dacron (knitted and woven), coated Dacron (collagen, albumin, or gelatin), and polytetrafluoroethylene (PTFE). Available data do not suggest that any graft material or fabrication has superior patency, and selection is based mostly on the surgeon's personal preference.

Use of a properly sized graft is important to minimize the possibility of sluggish flow and deposition of excessive laminar thrombus that is likely to occur in an oversized graft. For aortoiliac occlusive disease, a 16 × 8 mm bifurcated graft (body diameter, 16 mm; limb diameter, 8 mm) is used most commonly, but a 14 × 7 mm prosthesis may be more suitable for patients with a relatively small-caliber aortoiliac segment (predominantly women). For most patients, an end-to-end aortic anastomosis (Fig. 5) is preferred for several reasons. First, because all blood flows through the graft, there is less chance of "competitive" flow through the native aortoiliac vessels that may potentially increase the incidence of graft limb thrombosis. Second, an end-to-end anastomosis is theoretically a hemodynamically superior configuration. It is associated with less perianastomotic turbulence and therefore a smaller likelihood of developing recurrent atheroma or an anastomotic aneurysm. In addition, the end-to-end anastomosis is less likely to cause distal atheromatous embolization and is easier to cover with retroperitoneal tissue after implantation than the end-to-side anastomosis, which tends to protrude anteriorly off the aorta. This consideration may reduce the potential for late graft-enteric fistula formation. However, end-to-side anastomosis may be advantageous in certain anatomic patterns of disease to be described subsequently.

After intravenous administration of 5,000 to 7,500 units of heparin, appropriate vascular clamps are applied to the aorta just caudal to the left renal vein and immediately caudal or cephalad to the inferior mesenteric artery (Fig. 5A). The aorta is then transected and a 3- to 4-cm long segment between the clamps is resected. Any patent lumbar artery branches arising from this segment are clamped and ligated. Care should be taken to maintain a resection plane immediately on the posterior wall of the aorta to prevent injury and troublesome bleeding from the adjacent lumbar veins.

The transected distal aortic end is next oversewn in two layers with a 3-0 vascular suture (Fig. 5B). If this segment is heavily calcified or diseased, a limited endarterectomy of the calcific plaque and use of Teflon-pledgeted sutures may be necessary

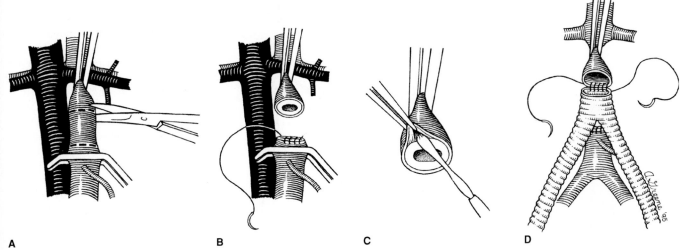

Fig. 5. A: Following administration of systemic heparin, the aorta is clamped proximally and distally, and a segment of aorta approximately 3 to 4 cm long is resected. **B:** The distal aorta is oversewn with an over-and-over running suture. **C:** Thromboendarterectomy of the proximal aortic cuff below the cephalad clamp may be necessary if a thickened or calcified intima and media compromise its lumen. **D:** Proximal anastomosis begun posteriorly with monofilament running vascular suture. The body or stem of the bifurcated graft is cut short, leaving a body that is only 3 to 4 cm in length so that it will occupy the area of the previously resected segment of native aorta.

to achieve a secure and hemostatic closure. The body of the bifurcated graft is tailored leaving approximately 3 to 4 cm from the bifurcation. This allows the short graft body to be situated in the bed of the resected aortic segment and facilitates closure of the retroperitoneum over the graft and separation of the anastomosis from the duodenum and other viscera. The short graft body also serves to advance the level of the graft bifurcation more cephalad and diminishes the takeoff angle of the graft limbs, thereby reducing the chance of kinking the graft at the origin of the limbs.

The divided proximal end of the aorta is inspected and thrombus or loose atheromatous debris removed. Standard graft anastomosis using a running 3-0 monofilament vascular suture is then performed (Fig. 5D). I usually start the anastomosis in the midline posteriorly using a double-armed suture. The anastomosis is performed in a running fashion extending both clockwise and counterclockwise approximately half the circumference of the aorta. A similar suture is then started on the midanterior aspect of the anastomosis and is similarly run in opposite directions. The anterior and posterior sutures are then tied to each other on the lateral aspects of the aorta to complete the anastomosis.

If the proximal, infrarenal aorta is significantly diseased and its lumen compromised, I often perform a thromboendarterectomy of the aortic stump up to the level of the proximal clamp (Fig. 5C). The remaining adventitial layer is often quite thin, but usually holds sutures well and allows a technically perfect anastomosis. In this circumstance, I always prefer to use an interrupted mattress suture technique with each suture bolstered by a Teflon pledget (Fig. 6).

After completion of the aortic anastomosis, the graft is clamped with an atraumatic vascular clamp (Fogarty soft-jawed clamp) and the proximal anastomosis tested

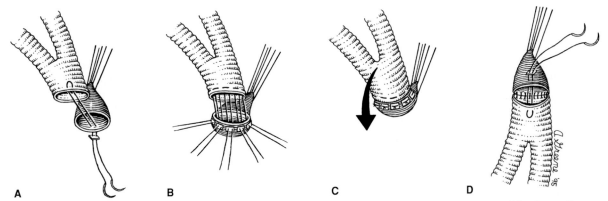

Fig. 6. Technique of interrupted mattress suture anastomosis, often useful for a fragile diseased aorta or following cuff endarterectomy, is illustrated. **A:** The graft is oriented with its limbs directed superiorly and the anastomosis begun by a double-armed mattress suture in the midline, each needle passed from the outside of the posterior graft wall, then from the inside of the posterior wall of the aorta, and finally through a pledget of Teflon felt. **B:** Placement of five such mattress sutures around the posterior one-half circumference of the graft and aorta, tied down over the felt pledgets, completes the back wall of the anastomosis. Care is taken to place each mattress suture immediately adjacent to its neighbor, with proper spacing achieved by altering the width of travel between the two limbs of each individual mattress suture. **C:** After the back wall is completed, the graft is flipped down into a proper anatomic position, and **(D)** the anastomosis is completed by insertion of a similar anterior row of mattress sutures.

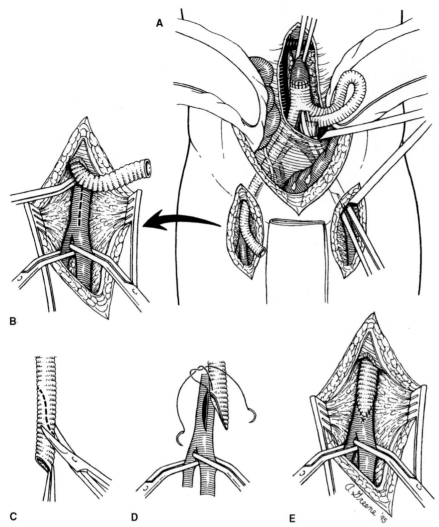

Fig. 7. A: Passage of graft limbs through the retroperitoneal tunnels. Elevation of the Penrose drain sling facilitates graft tunneling and ensures positioning behind the ureter. **B:** Location of common femoral arteriotomy in the absence of any significant profunda origin disease. **C-E:** Cutting graft to appropriate length and construction of femoral anastomosis.

by slow release of the proximal aortic clamp. If inspection reveals any leaks or defects, they are repaired with interrupted mattress sutures with pledgets. After a hemostatic and secure anastomosis has been verified, the proximal aortic clamp is reapplied and the graft thoroughly suctioned to remove any clot or debris.

Attention is then directed to the femoral region. The Penrose drains, previously placed in the graft tunnels, are elevated, and a long, blunt-tipped, slightly curved clamp such as a large DeBakey aortic clamp is passed from each groin incision to the region of the aortic dissection. The distal end of each femoral graft limb is then grasped with the clamp under direct vision, and each graft limb is pulled down through the tunnel (Fig. 7A). Care must be exercised to avoid twisting of the graft limbs. Fortunately, most of the bifurcated grafts have

stripes or marks that help to maintain the correct orientation. Again, it is important to ensure passage of each graft limb posterior to the ureter. This is usually best accomplished by properly constructing the initial graft tunnel immediately anterior to the iliac vessels and then elevating the Penrose drain "sling" that encompasses the ureter within the overlying retroperitoneal tissues during the actual pulling down of the graft limb. The ureter may be palpated at times as well. Gentle tension is applied to both graft limbs to eliminate any kinking or redundancy, but excessive tension must be avoided because this may contribute to late anastomotic aneurysm formation.

Femoral Anastomoses

Performance of a technically flawless femoral anastomosis is probably the most

important technical aspect of the aorto-bifemoral bypass and the most significant determinant of late graft patency. It is particularly critical to ensure unimpeded flow to the profunda femoris artery on each side. As previously emphasized, the majority of patients undergoing aortobifemoral bypass have diseased or occluded femoral arteries at the time of surgery. In other patients, progressive distal occlusive disease may result in later development of superficial femoral artery obstruction. Prolonged graft limb patency is therefore heavily dependent on profunda outflow. Hence, it is imperative to detect and correct any disease at the origin of the profunda at the time of the femoral anastomosis.

The femoral anastomosis is begun by occluding the proximal common femoral artery at the level of the inguinal ligament and the proximal superficial femoral and profunda branches using appropriate atraumatic vascular clamps. The anterior surface of the midcommon femoral artery is incised with a No. 11 scalpel blade and the femoral arteriotomy extended both proximally and distally with Potts scissors (Fig. 7B). The graft limb is gently stretched out with a slight tension and cut with a slightly curved bevel to a length appropriate to match the size of the arteriotomy. A standard vascular anastomosis is then performed with 5-0 monofilament vascular suture. I prefer to begin with a mattress suture placed at the "heel" of the graft. I usually tie this suture down and then continue the anastomosis in a running fashion down each side to its midpoint, but a "parachute technique" may be used if preferred. The direction of suture placement is always from outside to inside on the graft and inside to outside on the artery to minimize the chance that plaque or diseased layers of the vessel wall will be lifted or displaced and thus act as a potential obstructive flap. This is more apt to occur if the suture is passed from outside inside on the vessel wall. At the midpoint of each side of the anastomosis, the running sutures are tagged with a rubber-shod hemostat to maintain some tension on the suture line, and a new suture is begun at the "toe" of the graft and distal apex of the arteriotomy. This is tied down and run on both sides to meet the previously tagged sutures at the midpoint (Fig. 7D).

If the superficial femoral artery is occluded or any significant occlusive disease is detected at the orifice of the profunda femoris, a simple anastomosis to the common femoral artery alone is not recommended. In this situation, the femoral

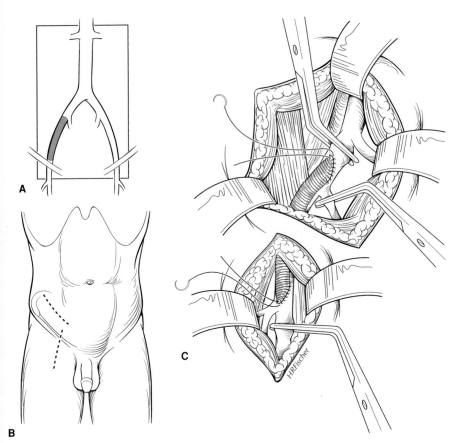

Fig. 13. A: Disease must be limited to the distal common iliac and/or external iliac artery, thereby allowing a proximal anastomosis to a relatively disease-free segment of proximal common iliac artery. **B:** Separate lower quadrant abdominal wall and vertical groin incisions are preferred. **C:** The in-line graft is placed retroperitoneally and tunneled posterior to the ureter for an end-to-side anastomosis to the femoral artery using the standard technique. (From Brewster DC. Direct open revascularization for aortoiliac occlusive disease. In: Zelenock GB, Huber TS, Messina LM, et al., eds. *Mastery of vascular and endovascular surgery*, with permission.)

the buttock musculature/surrounding skin, or cauda equina/lumbar plexopathy with neurologic deficit. The responsible mechanism is interruption of the pelvic blood flow. This has led to the generally accepted principle of maintaining flow in at least one internal iliac artery. The status of the pelvic circulation should be assessed during the operative planning as mentioned above, and consideration should be given to performing an end-to-side aortic anastomosis when indicated by the distribution of occlusive disease. Alternatively, one (or both) of the internal iliac arteries may be revascularized directly by using a limb of the bifurcated graft, then jumping off that limb down to the femoral artery in the groin with a second prosthetic graft.

Atheromatous debris may embolize at any time during the operative procedure, although the most vulnerable times occur when the vessels are manipulated such as during dissection or clamp application. The sequelae are dependent upon size of the debris and the distribution of the involved vessels. Macroscopic particles may

occlude the major, named vessels with the debris frequently lodging at the various arterial bifurcations. Fortunately, the majority of these are amenable to removal with a thromboembolectomy catheter. In contrast, the microscopic particles lodge in the corresponding sized vessels and are not usually amenable to removal or treatment. They can result in a wide spectrum of injury ranging from the classic "blue toe" to extensive tissue loss of the buttock and lower extremity. The potential for embolization may be minimized using the strategies outlined above in the technique section including rigorous flushing of the vessels before reperfusion with selective flushing into the pelvic and profunda femoris circulation before re-establishing flow to the superficial femoral artery.

Patients may develop ischemia of their lower extremities that may present either intraoperatively after completion of the bypass or during the early postoperative period. The specific concerns vary slightly with the temporal presentation but include atheroemboli, in situ thrombosis, and tech-

nical problems. The remedial treatment is contingent upon the precipitating cause, although it is imperative that all potential technical defects such as a twist/kink in the graft limb or a narrowed anastomosis be excluded. The femoral anastomosis is usually interrogated first and thromboembolectomy catheters are passed both proximally (graft limb/aorta) and distally (superficial/profunda femoral). A thromboembolectomy of the popliteal and tibial vessels through a below-knee popliteal artery exploration may be necessary if the femoral thromboembolectomy is unsuccessful and no obvious causes for the problem identified. Infrainguinal revascularization is occasionally necessary in patients with persistent lower extremity ischemia, although the morbidity/mortality rates of combined inflow/outflow procedures are significant.

Male sexual dysfunction can occur after aortoiliac revascularization due to either inadequate pelvic perfusion or interruption of the autonomic nerves that course over the distal aorta and common iliac arteries. The reported incidence ranges from 5% to 15%. Notably, the injury to the autonomic nerve results in the disruption of the internal sphincter mechanism and retrograde ejaculation. The status of the pelvic circulation should be factored into the operative plan and care should be exercised during the procedure to avoid injury to the responsible nerves. Furthermore, it is imperative that the potential for sexual dysfunction be discussed with patients preoperatively.

The incidence of wound complications after bypass to the femoral vessels is approximately 15%. Notably, the majority of these are wound breakdowns or wound healing problems rather than true wound infections per se. Local wound care measures including staple removal, limited debridement, and dressing changes are usually sufficient, although patients are also often started on antibiotics because of the proximity of the prosthetic graft. Multiple contributory factors have been identified, although few preventative strategies have been effective

POSTOPERATIVE MANAGEMENT

The immediate postoperative care after aortoiliac bypass is comparable to that after other major intra-abdominal vascular procedures. Patients are usually monitored in the intensive care unit on the night of their procedure then transferred to the general care floor. They are seen by the physical therapists when they reach the general care floor and are encouraged to start ambulating early. Their nasogastric tube is usually removed on the second or third postoperative day or when bowel function returns. Patients are usually discharged on their sixth or seventh postoperative day, but have to be sufficiently independent to care for themselves, eating adequately, and having normal bowel function. Patients are seen in the outpatient clinic biweekly until their wounds are healed and then at 6-month intervals indefinitely. Ankle brachial indices are obtained in the early postoperative period and at each 6-month follow-up visit.

The long-term outcome after direct aortoiliac revascularization is excellent. The reported patency rates after aortobifemoral bypass range from 80% to 90% at 5 years. The corresponding patency rates for aortoiliac endarterectomy are comparable, while those for unilateral iliofemoral bypass are nearly as good. Unfortunately, the long-term patient survival after aortoiliac bypass is only 75% and less than the corresponding age-matched controls. The majority of the late deaths are secondary to cardiovascular causes and further emphasize the importance of aggressive medical management of coronary artery disease and the associated risk factors for atherosclerosis. Approximately 5% of the patients develop anasto-

motic pseudoaneurysms, although the incidence is dependent upon the duration of follow-up and may exceed this value. These occur most commonly at the femoral anastomoses and can be related to technical errors, suture breakage, graft infection, and degeneration of the native artery, among other causes. The incidence of prosthetic graft infections after aortoiliac bypass is approximately 1% to 2%.

SUGGESTED READING

Brewster DC. Clinical and anatomic considerations for surgery in aortoiliac disease and results of surgical treatment. *Circulation* 1999;83(Suppl 1):42.

Brewster DC. Current controversies in the management of aortoiliac occlusive disease. *J Vasc Surg* 1997;25:365.

Brewster DC. Direct reconstruction for aortoiliac occlusive disease. In: Rutherford RB, ed. *Vascular surgery,* 6th ed. Philadelphia: Elsevier Saunders, 2005:1106.

Brewster DC. Technical features to simplify or improve aortofemoral or aortoiliac reconstructions. In: Veith FJ, ed. *Current critical problems in vascular surgery,* vol. 5. St. Louis: Quality Medical Publishing, 1993:278.

Brewster DC, Cooke JC. Longevity of aortofemoral bypass grafts. In: Yao JST, Pearce WFJ, eds. *Long-term results in vascular surgery.* Norwalk, CT: Appleton & Lange, 1993:149.

Brewster DC, Darling RC. Optimal methods of aortoiliac reconstruction. *Surgery* 1978;84: 739.

Brewster DC, Perler BA, Robison JG, et al. Aortofemoral graft for multilevel occlusive disease: predictors of success and need for distal bypass. *Arch Surg* 1982;117:1593.

Cambria RP, Brewster DC, Abbott WM, et al. Transperitoneal versus retroperitoneal approach for aortic reconstruction: a randomized prospective study. *J Vasc Surg* 1990;11: 314.

Corson JD, Brewster DC, Darling RC. The surgical management of infrarenal aortic occlusion. *Surg Gynecol Obstet* 1982;155:369

Crawford ES, Bomberger RA, Glaeser DH, et al. Aortoiliac occlusive disease: factors influencing survival and function following reconstructive operation over a twenty-five year period. *Surgery* 1981;90:1055.

DeVries, SO, Hunink MGH. Results of aortic bifurcation grafts for aortoiliac occlusive disease: a meta-analysis. *J Vasc Surg* 1997;26: 558.

Nevelsteen A, Wouters L, Suy R. Aortofemoral Dacron reconstruction for aortoiliac occlusive disease: 1 25 year survey. *Eur J Vasc Surg* 1991;5:179.

Rutherford RB. Options in the surgical management of aorto-iliac occlusive disease: a changing perspective. *Cardiovasc Surg* 1999; 7:5.

Szilagyi DE, Elliott JR Jr, Smith RF, et al. A thirty-year survey of the reconstructive surgical treatment of aortoiliac occlusive disease. *J Vasc Surg* 1986;3:421.

EDITOR'S COMMENT

Aortofemoral bypass for treatment of symptomatic aortic iliac disease is rapidly becoming one of the "dinosaurs" of vascular surgery, even in large referral centers such as Dr. Brewster's. However, despite most aortoiliac arterial occlusive disease being amiable to endovascular repair using angioplasty and stenting, there remains an occasional patient in whom endovascular therapy is either not possible because an iliac occlusion cannot be recanalized or contraindicated due to diffuse disease or a juxtare-

nal aortic occlusion. In such instances, aortobifemoral bypass, once one of the signature procedures of vascular surgery, is still required. In such instances, Dr. Brewster's careful and detailed chapter can serve as an excellent reference for this increasingly uncommon but remarkable durable procedure. His description and illustrations are excellent, and I would disagree with only minor details of his described technique, which would represent personal preference rather than any substantial differences.

Furthermore, the description of postoperative management and outcome of this excellent bypass procedure is also well done. Finally, the description of aortoiliac endarterectomy, though just as detailed and well presented, now is essentially obsolete in the endovascular age. Indeed, I do not believe our group has even considered this procedure, indicated primarily for isolated aortoiliac bifurcation disease, in the last 5 years.

J.M.S.

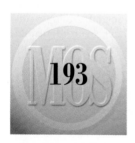

193 Axillobifemoral Bypass

GREGORY J. LANDRY, TIMOTHY K. LIEM,
GREGORY L. MONETA, AND LIOYD M. TAYLOR JR.

Freeman and Leeds performed the first extraanatomic bypass in 1952 using an endarterectomized superficial femoral artery tunneled subcutaneously to the contralateral femoral artery. The first axillofemoral bypasses for lower extremity ischemia were

independently reported by Blaisdell and Louw in 1963. Sauvage and Wood reported the first axillobifemoral bypass for bilateral lower extremity ischemia in 1966. Although axillobifemoral bypass has largely been regarded as a second-choice alterna-

tive to standard aortoiliac and aortofemoral reconstruction and has been replaced to a large degree by percutaneous endoluminal interventions in appropriate patients, it remains a reliable and durable option for lower extremity revascularization that should remain in the armamentarium of physicians performing vascular surgery.

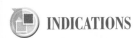

INDICATIONS

Axillobifemoral bypass has traditionally been reserved for the treatment of aortoiliac occlusive disease in patients with severe systemic illness increasing operative risk and in patients with local factors increasing the risk or difficulty of standard aortofemoral reconstruction. Examples of such local factors include prior aortoiliac procedures, prior radiation, extensive intra-abdominal adhesions, severe aortic calcification, abdominal malignancy, intra-abdominal infection, aortic or aortic graft infection, colostomy or ileostomy, and enterocutaneous fistula. While many aortoiliac revascularizations are now performed with percutaneous endoluminal therapy, axillobifemoral bypass remains a viable alternative in patients whose extent of disease is too great for percutaneous treatment.

PREOPERATIVE CONSIDERATIONS

Patients with aortoiliac occlusive disease of sufficient severity to warrant axillobifemoral bypass grafting typically have absent or weak femoral pulses. Noninvasive vascular examination of the lower extremities is helpful in documenting the severity of ischemia and level of distal disease. Lower extremity arteriography is routinely performed for elective cases but often is not essential in urgent or emergent cases. The adequacy of axillary inflow can be determined noninvasively in most cases. Segmental pressure measurements and Doppler analog waveforms are obtained at the level of the radial, ulnar, and brachial arteries in both arms. A pressure difference between arms greater than 15 mm Hg indicates significant occlusive disease. Upper extremity arteriography is performed when abnormalities are detected by noninvasive testing. Subclavian artery angioplasty with or without stenting is performed when indicated to improve axillary artery inflow. The right axillary artery is preferred for the axillary anastomosis, since the left subclavian artery has a higher reported incidence of developing atherosclerotic occlusive disease.

Prophylactic antibiotics, usually a first-generation cephalosporin, are administered immediately prior to surgery and continued for 24 hours. Aspirin therapy (325 mg/d) is started preoperatively and

continued indefinitely postoperatively. Patients with an identified hypercoagulable state or a history of multiple graft failures are treated with long-term warfarin anticoagulation.

TECHNICAL CONSIDERATIONS

Anesthesia

General anesthesia with endotracheal intubation is preferred. Monitored local anesthesia can be used in very high-risk unstable patients, although tunneling of the grafts requires supplemental sedation.

Patient Positioning

Patients are placed in the supine position with the donor arm abducted 90 degrees. This position maximizes the distance between the axillary and femoral arteries, thereby minimizing tension on the axillary anastomosis postoperatively. The supra- and infraclavicular regions, axilla, chest, abdomen, and femoral regions are widely prepped and draped. To minimize operative time, a multiple team approach is preferred if possible, with separate surgical teams operating simultaneously at each of the three operative sites.

Axillary Artery Dissection

The axillary artery is defined anatomically by the first rib proximally and the teres major muscle distally. It is convenient to define the parts of the artery by their relationship to the pectoralis minor muscle. The first, second, and third parts of the artery are medial to, posterior to, and lateral to the pectoralis minor muscle, respectively. There is one named branch, the supreme thoracic artery, arising from the first part of the axillary artery. Two branches (thoracoacromial and lateral thoracic arteries) emanate from the second part, and three (subscapular and medial and lateral humeral circumflex arteries) from the third part of the axillary artery. The axillary vein runs parallels to the course of the axillary artery and lies anterior and inferior to it. The brachial plexus nerves interdigitate with the axillary artery and its branches. The first part of the artery lies anterior to the brachial plexus. The divisions and cords of the brachial plexus lie anterior to the third part of the artery. The second part of the axillary artery is enveloped by the brachial plexus cords passing from posterior to anterior.

These anatomic relationships point out the advantages of using the first part of the

axillary artery for the proximal anastomosis. It is relatively fixed in position, is anterior to the brachial plexus, and has only a single collateral branch. An incision paralleling the course of the axillary artery is made approximately two fingerbreadths below the middle third of the clavicle. The fibers of the pectoralis major muscle are then bluntly separated, revealing the clavipectoral fascia, which is incised.

The pectoralis minor muscle is mobilized but not divided and serves as the lateral border of the dissection. The axillary vein is mobilized and retracted caudally to reveal the axillary artery, a step that requires ligation and division of the cephalic vein and other small venous branches along the cephalad portion of the vein. The thoracoacromial artery is left intact and used as the marker for the lateral corner of the anastomosis. Sufficient length of artery is dissected and mobilized medial to the thoracoacromial artery for the proximal anastomosis.

Femoral Artery Dissection

The femoral arteries are exposed through bilateral vertical groin incisions. The common femoral artery just prior to the common femoral bifurcation is the preferred site for the distal anastomosis; however, the choice of site for the distal anastomosis is based upon angiographic findings and patient circumstances. Accordingly, the distal graft anastomoses may be to the common femoral, deep femoral, or superficial femoral arteries. Occasionally, endarterectomy of the outflow vessels may be required. In special circumstances, distal anastomoses may be to more distal portions of the deep or superficial femoral arteries, and lateral approaches to these vessels may be used, especially in the presence of infection of previously placed femoral grafts. In obese patients, more distal anastomotic sites are sometimes preferred to minimize perianastomotic graft kinking when the patient is in a sitting position.

Axillofemoral Tunnel

A subcutaneous tunnel is begun at the ipsilateral femoral incision. The standard tunnel passes medial to the anterior superior iliac spine and then along the lateral aspect of the abdomen in the midaxillary line. The tunnel continues posterior to the pectoralis major and minor muscles into the axilla (Fig. 1). The use of the Oregon tunneler or similar tunneling device allows the tunnel to be made without the need

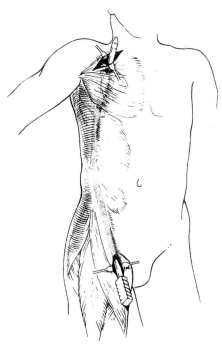

Fig. 1. Route of subcutaneous axillofemoral tunnel made with Oregon tunneler. The tunnel runs medial to the anterior superior iliac spine, along the midaxillary line, and posterior to the pectoralis minor muscle.

for counterincisions in all but unusually tall patients. An externally supported polytetrafluoroethylene (PTFE) graft (8 mm × 70 to 90 cm) is passed through the subcutaneous tunnel.

Femorofemoral Tunnel

A subcutaneous, suprapubic, inverted U tunnel is created between the two femoral incisions using a long, curved aortic clamp. The tunnel lies directly anterior to the external oblique and anterior rectus fascia. An externally supported PTFE graft (8 mm × 40 cm) is used.

Graft Anastomoses

The femoral-femoral bypass is performed first. After completion of the tunnels, intravenous heparin is administered at a dose of 100 U/kg. Bilateral end-to-side anastomoses are created to femoral arteriotomies with CV-5 or CV-6 PTFE suture. The arteriotomies are 2.5 times the diameter of the graft in length.

The axillary anastomosis is also performed in end-to-side fashion using CV-5 PTFE suture. A longitudinal arteriotomy on the anterior surface of the first part of the axillary artery, medial to both the pectoralis minor muscle and thoracoacromial artery, is made. The graft is

routed parallel and adjacent to the axillary artery posterior to the pectoralis minor muscle for approximately 8 to 10 cm before forming a gentle curve in the axilla to its inferior course (Fig. 2). This redundancy allows for arm extension, distributing any potential tension across the curve of the graft rather than at the proximal anastomosis. This is intended to prevent proximal anastomotic disruption. The distal end of the axillofemoral graft is then anastomosed in an end-to-side fashion to the cobra-head of the ipsilateral side of the femoral-femoral graft (Fig. 3). This configuration maximizes flow through the entire length of the axillofemoral graft. The final graft configuration is shown in Figure 4.

Hemostasis of needle-hole bleeding is obtained using topical spray thrombin and Gelfoam. Heparin is reversed with protamine sulfate at a dose of 1 mg/100 U heparin given.

Wound Closure

Following wound irrigation with bacitracin solution, all three incisions are closed in three layers. In the femoral incisions, running absorbable sutures are used to cover the grafts and the subcutaneous

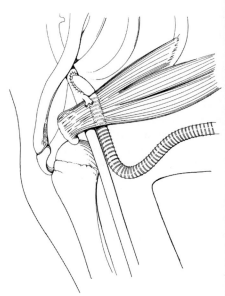

Fig. 2. Axillary anastomosis showing end-to-side graft anastomosis. The anastomosis is to the first part of the axillary artery. The graft is routed parallel and adjacent to the axillary artery posterior to the pectoralis minor muscle for 8 to 10 cm before forming a gentle curve to its inferior course.

tissue. The same sutures are used in the axillary incision to close the pectoral fascia and subcutaneous tissue. The skin is closed with a running absorbable subcuticular suture.

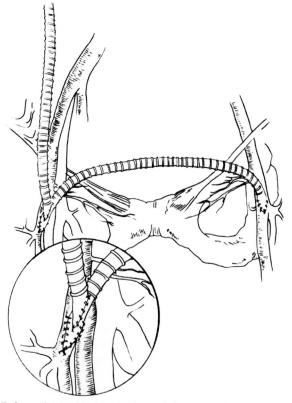

Fig. 3. Distal axillofemoral anastomoses. The femoral-femoral graft is anastomosed in an end-to-side fashion to the femoral arteriotomies. The distal end of the axillofemoral graft anastomosed in an end-to-side fashion to the femoral-femoral graft (inset).

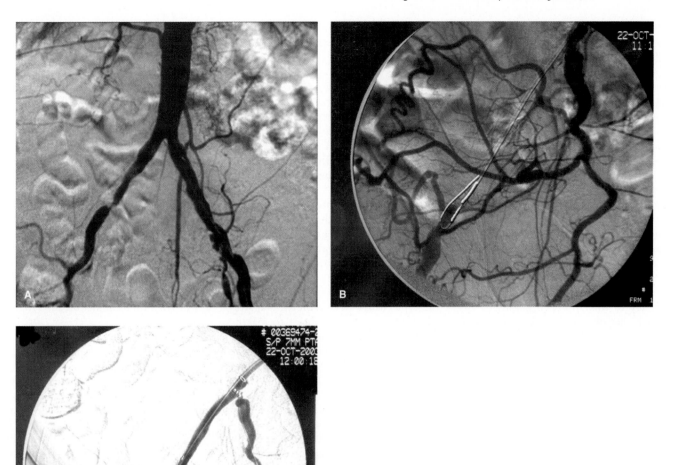

Fig. 4. A–C: Treatment of right chronic total external iliac occlusion using the Pioneer catheter to cross the occlusion followed by placement of two Fluency stent grafts from a contralateral approach.

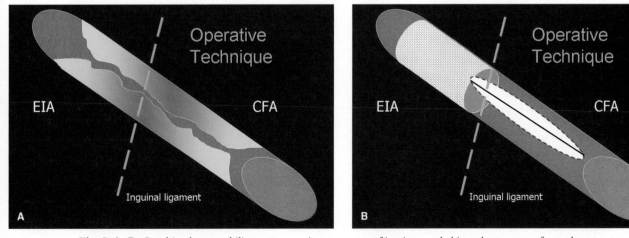

Fig. 5. A, B: Combined external iliac artery stenting or stent grafting is extended into the common femoral artery patch. Common femoral patch is extended just above the inguinal ligament.

other hand, patients with diffuse aortoiliac occlusive disease (TASC C and D lesions) will have markedly inferior patency with bare mental stenting when compared to aortobifemoral bypass. This is especially true in patients with diffuse aortoiliac occlusive disease that involves the external iliac arteries (Fig. 2). In these cases when open surgery is not a good option we have used stent grafting to treat such lesions. This has resulted in improved patency rates compared to bare mental stenting but remains less than aortofemoral bypass grafting. Of note is that patients who underwent stent grafting in conjunction with open femoral endarterectomy have improved patency compared to patients who underwent percutaneous placement of stent grafts. The midterm patency of this approach begins to approach that observed with aortofemoral bypass (Fig. 3). A likely explanation for this is that patients who undergo simultaneous femoral endarterectomy have improved outflow from the iliac system. This finding is what has prompted our more intense evaluation of femoral artery plaque burden prior to proceeding with iliac intervention.

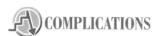 **COMPLICATIONS**

Complications can be categorized as dye related, sheath site related, and remote. Patients with preprocedure renal insufficiency are at greatest risk for postprocedure azotemia. In our practice patients with creatinine between 1.5 and 2.5mg/dL are treated preprocedure with N-acetyl-cysteine and intraprocedure bicarbonate infusion. In addition, we attempt to limit arteriography. Patients with creatinine greater than 2.5 mg/dL are treated with a combination of gadolinium, IVUS, and pre- and postprocedure pressure measurements.

The incidence of local wound complications related to sheath insertion is 1% to 3%. Accurate placement of the puncture site in the common femoral artery avoiding high or low puncture will limit this. It is our practice to attempt to close most femoral artery sheath insertions with a suture-type closure device. Iliofemoral arteriography is performed prior to making this determination. If the femoral artery is less than 7 mm or if significant calcification is present, then the sheath is removed after ACT has decreased to less than 200 and manual pressure applied.

Arterial rupture is an uncommon (<1%) but potentially serious complication. In most instances arterial rupture occurs in the setting of angioplasty or stenting of small heavily calcified external iliac arteries. When the procedure is performed under local anesthetic, patients will typically have significant flank or back pain, which will occur prior to arterial rupture, and further dilation should not be performed if placing bare metal stents. Patients under regional or general anesthetic will not have these symptoms. Arterial rupture can usually be treated with placement of stent grafts to seal the ruptured iliac artery (Fig. 6A,B). A balloon occlusion catheter may be needed to stabilize hypotensive patients. This may frequently need to be placed from the contralateral femoral artery in order to allow for upsizing the ipsilateral femoral sheath to a size sufficient to allow placement of a stent graft.

Distal embolization has been uncommon in the absence of aggressive predilation prior to iliac stent placement. We do not routinely assess the leg arteriographically before and after stent placement but rely on physical examination and Doppler evaluation.

SUMMARY

Iliac angioplasty and stent placement is the current first-line therapy for clinically significant isolated iliac stenosis. The results for more diffuse disease (TASC C and D) are inferior to aortobifemoral bypass but can be improved through the use of iliac stent grafts. Patients with heavy common femoral plaque burden should be treated with simultaneous femoral endarterectomy in combination with iliac stenting or stent grafting.

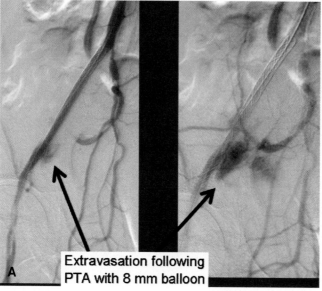
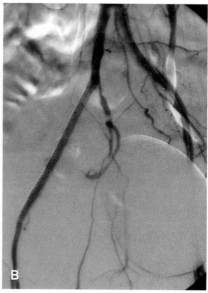

Fig. 6. Distal external iliac artery occlusion treated with stent graft resulting in rupture of the artery with blush on contrast. This was successfully treated with relining with second stent graft.

SUGGESTED READING

Nelson PR, Powell RJ, Walsh DB, et al. Early results of external iliac artery stenting combined with common femoral artery endarterectomy. *J Vasc Surg* 2002;35(6):1107.

Powell RJ, Fillinger MF, Bettmann M, et al. The durability of endovascular treatment of multisegment iliac occlusive disease. *J Vasc Surg* 2000;31:1178.

Powell RJ, Fillinger MF, Walsh DB, et al. Predicting outcome of angioplasty and selective

stenting of multisegment iliac artery occlusive disease. *J Vasc Surg* 2000;32:564.

Rzucidlo EM, Powell RJ, Zwolak RM, et al. Early results of stent-grafting to treat diffuse aorto-iliac occlusive disease. *J Vasc Surg* 2003;37:1175.

EDITOR'S COMMENT

As pointed out by Dr. Powell, endovascular treatment of symptomatic aortoiliac arterial occlusive disease is now the first line of therapy. Thus, the question now is not whether to treat iliac occlusive disease with endovascular techniques or open surgical bypass, but rather which patients with iliac disease to treat and which iliac lesions are appropriate for endovascular therapy. The answer to the first of these questions is relatively clear. Patients to be treated are those with hemodynamically significant iliac artery occlusive disease and appropriate symptoms. The low risk and good results associated with iliac angioplasty and stenting, as clearly outlined in this chapter, have lowered the threshold for evaluation and treatment of patients with symptomatic iliac occlusive disease using angioplasty and stenting to include essentially all patients with calf, thigh, and/or buttock claudication and lesions appropriate for endovascular treatment.

Definition of iliac lesions "appropriate" for endovascular therapy, the answer to the second question, is less clear, largely because continuing improvement in endovascular techniques and technology have resulted in improving outcomes for treatment of more challenging iliac lesions.

As noted by Dr. Powell, the TASC classification helps in defining the lesions appropriately for endovascular treatment, with treatment of TASC A and B lesions being associated with excellent results while treatment of C and D lesions is associated with poorer outcomes. Use of stent grafts and femoral endarterectomy as described by the author may result in improved outcomes after the treatment of TASC C and D lesions, but it is important to remember that the results presented to support that approach by Dr. Powell are based on retrospective review of a relatively small number of patients and thus are subject to significant selection bias. This approach may be

shown to improve results sufficiently to make iliac stent grafting for diffuse aortoiliac occlusive disease a first-line therapy, but that remains to be determined. Similarly, although Dr. Powell's preference for primary stenting of all iliac lesions is widely held by many interventionalists, data from a Dutch randomized trial of primary iliac stenting versus selective stenting for hemodynamically inadequate results after angioplasty alone showed no difference in immediate and long-term outcomes. Iliac angioplasty is now the first line of therapy for aortoiliac artery occlusive disease, and most patients can be treated with minimal risks and good results.

Overall, this is an excellent chapter describing endovascular therapy of iliac arterial occlusive disease that has revolutionized treatment of this problem. However, as noted above, there is still much to be learned.

J.M.S.

Vascular Surgery

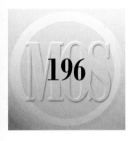

196

Embolectomy

THOMAS J. FOGARTY, BRADLEY B. HILL, AND CHRISTOPHER K. ZARINS

Although Harvey is credited with the recognition of the ischemic consequences of acute arterial occlusion, almost 3 centuries passed before the first successful arterial embolectomy was performed by Labey in 1911. The lack of initial enthusiasm for embolectomy can be traced to the high mortality and morbidity associated with the extensive dissection required to adequately remove the embolus and its distally propagated thrombus, as well as the frequent lack of clinical success. The surgical treatment of acute embolic arterial occlusion was greatly improved and simplified in 1963 by the introduction of the technique of balloon catheter embolectomy.

PATHOPHYSIOLOGY

The term *embolus* has its roots in the Greek word *embolos,* which means *projectile.* After the embolus dislodges from the luminal surface, it is carried through the

arterial tree until it impacts a site of luminal narrowing, usually at an arterial bifurcation. It is the location of the embolic occlusion and the events subsequent to its impaction that determine the eventual viability of the dependent structure.

When acute embolic occlusion occurs in a major artery, a soft coagulum of blood forms in the adjacent proximal and distal arterial segments secondary to stagnant flow. The occlusive process is thus extended as the clot propagates along the arterial tree, progressively embarrassing the important collateral pathways (Fig. 1). It has long been recognized that the extent of distal thrombotic propagation is the primary determinant of outcome after embolic arterial occlusion; failure to recognize and remove the distal thrombus results in incomplete restoration of circulation and possible loss of limb. In approximately one third of instances, distal circulatory stasis results in the development of discontinuous distal thrombosis. Backbleeding is an

unreliable indicator of distal patency. Its presence may be secondary to remaining unobstructed collateral vessels. Full-length passage of the embolectomy catheter is the only means of ensuring complete clot removal (Fig. 2).

Although most clinically significant emboli originate within the heart, the vessels of the lower limbs are the site of impaction in approximately 90% of the surgically treatable emboli (Fig. 3). The bifurcations of the aorta and femoral and popliteal arteries are the principal sites of impaction. Multiple emboli are more common than is generally accepted , and, in approximately 10% of instances, they involve more than one limb. Many smaller emboli undoubtedly lodge in well-vascularized "silent" arterial beds and are never recognized.

The tissues distal to the impacted embolus and associated thrombus are deprived of adequate oxygenation. Because of the sensitivity of peripheral nerve tissue

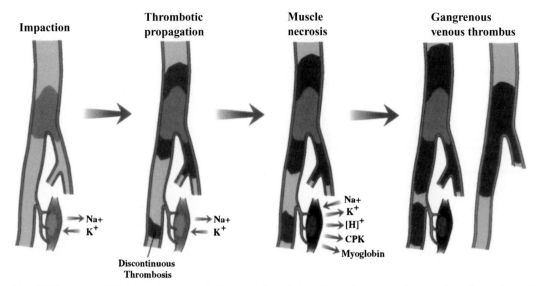

Fig. 1. The pathophysiology of acute embolic arterial occlusion. Ionic flux across the muscle cell membrane is shown. CPK, creatine phosphokinase.

to ischemia, pain and paresthesias are quickly noted in the affected limb. Continued cellular ischemia leads to anaerobic metabolism with local lactic acidosis and cell death, accompanied by nerve and muscle necrosis. Although local factors determine the rate of ischemic damage, diagnosis and therapy must be prompt because tissue necrosis may occur within 6 hours, and is a frequent occurrence after 12 hours of profound ischemia.

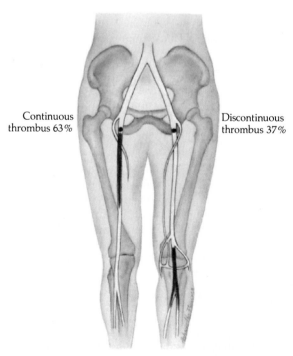

Continuous thrombus 63%

Discontinuous thrombus 37%

Fig. 2. Discontinuous distal clot propagation occurs in approximately one third of instances. Vigorous backbleeding could occur if the proximal clot alone were removed on the left side.

DIAGNOSIS

The sudden onset of symptoms of profound limb ischemia should immediately suggest the diagnosis of arterial embolus, particularly in a patient with atrial fibrillation, recent myocardial infarction, or abdominal aortic aneurysm. In more than 85% of instances, the clinical presentation and associated disease allow differentiation between embolic occlusion and acute arterial thrombosis. This differentiation is helpful in planning the surgical approach because additional vascular reconstructive techniques are often required with arterial thrombosis but are rarely needed with embolization. The characteristic clinical presentation of acute embolic occlusion is usually an abrupt onset without warning; it consists of the embolic syndrome of pain, pulselessness, pallor, paresthesias, and paralysis.

The initial examination should focus on the presence and amplitude of all arterial pulsations in the limb. The color and temperature of the limb, the presence or absence of sensation and proprioception, and the level of motor movement are recorded and related to the time of onset of pain. In addition, arterial blood flow should also be evaluated and recorded by Doppler technique. In most instances, the diagnosis can be confirmed and the site of impaction can be localized by history and physical examination alone. It is an almost universal finding that the site of embolic occlusion is the major arterial bifurcation immediately above the absent arterial pulsation.

Patients with suspected renal or visceral embolism should undergo preoperative arteriography. Arteriography may also be helpful in delineating the arterial morphology, if noninvasive studies suggest extensive atherosclerotic involvement. Time-consuming studies that may further compromise the ischemic limb, however, should be avoided.

Because virtually all patients with an arterial embolism have associated cardiac disease, a careful evaluation of cardiac status

CLINICAL PRESENTATION

Patients with aortic infection are septic. They present with fever and leukocytosis and complain of abdominal or back pain. Often a pulsatile abdominal mass will be detected. Patients are usually elderly individuals with pre-existing aortic disease, and males predominate over females. Often the recent history is positive for an antecedent episode of clinical sepsis related to enteritis, dental infection, bowel or gallbladder surgery, or drainage of localized abscess.

In patients without significant pain the presence of persistent, unexplained bacteremia and intermittent fever compels the physician to continue pursuing the diagnosis. Computed tomography (CT) scanning is the single most useful test to confirm a diagnosis of primary aortic infection. The presence of gas in the aortic wall or in the perianeurysmal tissues is pathognomonic for aortic infection. Other positive CT findings include fluid, edema, mass, or contrast enhancement within periaortic tissues consistent with local inflammation, retroperitoneal abscess, or spondylitis. If the diagnosis remains in doubt following CT scanning, then magnetic resonance imaging (MRI) may be performed. MRI is more sensitive in demonstrating edema and contrast enhancement within the perianeurysmal tissues. The vast majority of cases, however, are diagnosed utilizing a high index of suspicion based on the clinical presentation combined with definitive findings on CT scanning.

Typically, aneurysms caused by primary aortic infection appear saccular in configuration, as opposed to fusiform (Fig. 1). In one recent report of 46 patients with infected aortic aneurysms (20 suprarenal, 26 infrarenal), 80% of the aneurysms were described as saccular. Notably, aneurysm configuration did not appear to be predictive of perioperative mortality.

BACTERIOLOGY

Salmonella is frequently identified as the most common organism causing primary aortic infection. Curiously, the pathogenic mechanism for this consistent finding has never been clearly elucidated. While *Salmonella* can infect normal aortic tissue, the bacteria have a distinct predilection to seed diseased aorta, either atherosclerotic or aneurysmal. The risk of vascular infection complicating *Salmonella* bacteremia is estimated to be 10% to 25% in persons over 50 years of age. High-grade bacteremia manifest by multiple positive blood cultures is highly suggestive of focal intracardiac or intravascular infection.

While a review of published reports dealing with arterial infection identified *Salmonella* as the single most frequent organism causing primary aortic infection, *Staphylococcus* was a close second. In our practice, the organism most likely to cause primary aortic infection is *Staphylococcus aureus*. Other bacteria identified with some frequency as the cause for primary aortic infection include *Streptococcus* and *Escherichia coli*. Not surprisingly, the virulence

and resistance of the causative bacteria has an effect on overall patient outcome. For example, in our experience, clostridial aortic infection has been uniformly fatal. Of interest is a recent series of infected aortic aneurysms associating non-*Salmonella* infection with higher perioperative mortality.

SURGICAL TECHNIQUE

There are no prospective randomized studies investigating optimal surgical management of primary aortic infection. All surgeons agree with the principles of resection of infected aorta, wide debridement of periaortic tissue, drainage of established abscesses, and prolonged antibiotic therapy. Surgeons also generally agree that, with suprarenal aortic infection, in situ aortic graft placement is the most feasible and preferred option. However, with infrarenal aortic infection there is debate about the optimal method of lower extremity revascularization, specifically axillobifemoral bypass, through clean tissue planes versus in situ aortic graft placement. Lacking randomized studies, comparison between the two approaches is difficult and perhaps not a practical issue. Those cases with extensive local sepsis and abscess formation are usually treated with extra-anatomic bypass because of concern about secondary in situ prosthetic graft infection. Selected cases with minimal periaortic purulence can be managed with in situ graft placement. Unfortunately, in some cases the extent of periaortic purulence may be preoperatively underestimated. In addition, rare cases involving primary aortoenteric fistula requiring emergent surgery for control of hemorrhage are usually managed with in situ aortic graft placement.

With extra-anatomic bypass, it is preferred that the revascularization be performed through a clean surgical field prior to excision of the infected, infrarenal aorta. This approach obviously minimizes lower extremity ischemic time. Preoperative arteriography of the aorta and lower extremities is routinely performed when possible. The axillobifemoral bypass is performed using an externally reinforced, 8-mm polytetrafluoroethylene (PTFE) prosthesis (Fig. 2A). If there is a significant difference in arm systolic blood pressure, the axillary artery on the side of the highest pressure is used as the donor artery. If right and left arm systolic blood pressure is equal, then the right axillary artery is preferred due to the higher incidence of atherosclerotic involvement of the proximal left axillary artery. Through an infraclavicular incision,

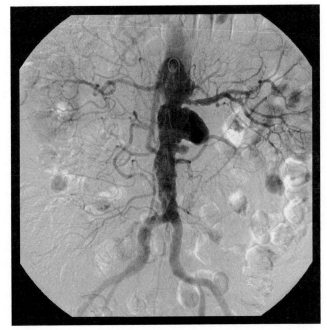

Fig. 1. Aortogram demonstrating a saccular, infected, infrarenal aortic aneurysm.

Vascular Surgery

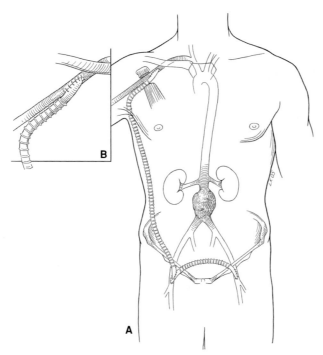

Fig. 2. A: Prosthetic right axillobifemoral bypass. **B:** Prosthetic graft routed adjacent and parallel to the axillary artery for a distance of 8 to 10 cm.

the proximal anastomosis is made end to side to the first portion of the axillary artery medial to the pectoralis minor muscle. The muscle is either reflected laterally or, if necessary, divided. The common femoral arteries are preferred for the distal anastomoses. The PTFE graft is tunneled subcutaneously from the femoral incision to the infraclavicular incision (Fig. 3). The graft is routed adjacent and parallel to the axillary

artery for a distance of 8 to 10 cm before passing in a gentle curve inferiorly to minimize axillary graft disruption (Fig. 2B). After the completion of the anastomoses, all the incisions are closed and excluded with adhesive dressings before approaching the infrarenal aortic infection through a midline incision.

Initial axillobifemoral bypass allows for an unhurried exposure of the aorta focusing on complete excision of the infected aorta, debridement of the proximal aortic wall and surrounding infected tissues, and secure closure of the infrarenal aorta utilizing generous bites with two separate rows of large monofilament sutures. A proximal row of continuous horizontal mattress sutures is preferred, followed by a distal row of continuous sutures placed in a simple running fashion over the end of the aortic stump (Fig. 4A). If feasible, circumferential dissection of the infrarenal aorta is performed prior to suture placement, enabling a secure aortic closure that is free of tension. Distally the aorta or common iliac arteries are oversewn in a similar fashion. Retroperitoneal abscesses are drained posteriorly through the left back or flank using soft rubber drains.

At times, more proximal extension of aortic infection may necessitate suprarenal clamping with placement of the aortic stump suture line just distal to the renal arteries. The left renal vein is mobilized and reflected cephalad or, if necessary, divided. In this instance, the proximal suture line is placed with the renal artery orifices under direct vision. A final, optional operative step involves coverage of the aortic stump and periaortic tissues with vascularized omentum delivered through the transverse mesocolon (Fig. 4B). Omental coverage may aid in promoting the resolution of localized infection and the healing of retroperitoneal tissues. Coverage of the distal aorta using a prevertebral fascial flap has been described but is not recommended due to concerns about additional dissection and potential for blood loss in the inflamed retroperitoneum. Avoiding unnecessary operative dissection minimizes the chance for major retroperitoneal venous injury.

With suprarenal aortic infection, in situ revascularization is favored as the most feasible option. In addition, some authors prefer in situ revascularization with infrarenal aortic infection as well. In situ revascularization is performed only after complete resection of the infected aorta and debridement of involved surrounding tissues. Selected patients with focal, saccular aneurysms may undergo aneurysm excision,

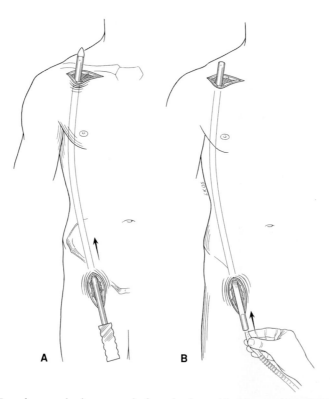

Fig. 3. A: Tunneler passed subcutaneously from the femoral incision to the infraclavicular incision. **B:** Prosthetic graft passed through the tunneler.

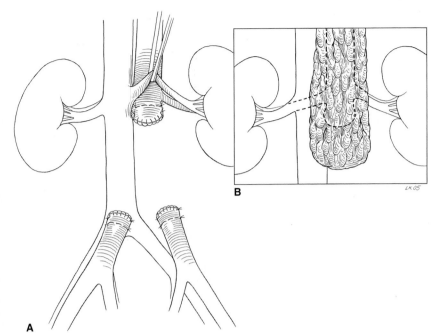

Fig. 4. A: Oversewn aortic stump with left renal vein reflected cephalad. **B:** Omental coverage of aortic stump.

aortic debridement, and patch (autogenous or prosthetic) closure of the aortotomy. A variety of bypass conduits have been used for in situ revascularization of primary aortic infection including conventional Dacron grafts, rifampin-soaked gelatin-impregnated polyester grafts, silver-coated polyester grafts, and cryopreserved arterial allografts. Although used more often in the management of prosthetic aortic graft infection, autogenous femoral vein has been utilized for aortoiliac reconstruction following resection of primary aortic infection. In addition, endograft repair in bleeding patients with primary aortoenteric fistula has been reported.

RESULTS

An exceptionally high mortality rate results when primary aortic infection is treated nonoperatively with antibiotics alone; however, long-term survivors have been reported. By contrast, with prompt operative treatment including resection of the infected aorta, revascularization, and long-term antibiotics, the perioperative mortality ranges from between 10% and 20%. Overall patient survival at 3 years following surgical treatment for all types of infrarenal aortic infection ranges from 60% to 70%. Axillofemoral prosthetic graft infection following treatment for primary aortic infection is less than 10%. With adequate debridement of the aortic wall prior to closure, the incidence of aortic stump infection and disruption is less than 2%. With in situ aortic grafting,

subsequent infection of the prosthetic aortic graft ranges from 10% to 30%.

SUMMARY

The rare patient with primary aortic infection presents a formidable challenge for any surgeon. Optimal management of these septic and critically ill patients includes a prompt diagnosis, appropriate antibiotics, and a technically demanding operative repair. In spite of an array of potential pitfalls and setbacks, the vast majority of primary aortic infection patients can be successfully managed with a reasonably good chance for long-term survival.

Abdominal Aortic Prosthetic Graft Infection

Prosthetic graft infections have been reported since abdominal aortic prosthetic grafting was first performed in the early 1950s. Aortofemoral grafts have a higher incidence of infection (2%) compared to aortoiliac grafts (less than .5%), since the groin area is frequently contaminated and prone to wound complications.

PATHOGENESIS

The vast majority of prosthetic graft infections occur as a result of bacterial contamination of the perigraft space around the time of original graft placement. During the early postoperative period, the fluid-filled

(blood, serum, lymph) perigraft environment is poorly perfused and relatively isolated from natural host defenses. These poorly vascularized, perigraft fluid collections serve as a receptive medium or "safe haven" for bacteria, enabling their survival and proliferation. Any early contamination of the perigraft space, even with relatively low numbers of bacteria, can lead to eventual prosthetic graft infection. Without early contamination, however, the prosthetic material becomes incorporated into surrounding, vascularized tissues, which functionally obliterates the perigraft space and after several months appears to render the graft more resistant to infection.

 ## CLINICAL PRESENTATION

Patients with aortic prosthetic graft infection may present early (weeks to months) or late (years) following original graft placement. In a recent series of patients with aortic graft infection the mean interval from graft implantation to presentation with infection was 56 months. Patient presentation is variable with an array of potential signs and symptoms including back and/or abdominal pain, anastomotic pseudoaneurysm, graft limb occlusion with ischemia, late wound infection, wound drainage from a sinus tract, fever, leukocytosis, or bacteremia. In addition, the rare patient with a prosthetic graft-enteric fistula typically presents with either sepsis or gastrointestinal bleeding.

CT scanning in patients with abdominal aortic prosthetic graft infection may demonstrate perigraft fluid and/or inflammation, which confirms the diagnosis and also helps determine the extent of graft infection. In addition, perigraft or intraluminal gas may be noted in patients with graft-enteric fistulae or patients with graft infection caused by gas-forming bacteria. During the early postoperative period, however, accurate CT scanning is problematic since perigraft fluid and, to a lesser extent, air are often present immediately following surgery. Postoperative, perigraft air should persist for only 7 to 10 days and retroperitoneal fluid collections normally are completely resolved after 6 or 7 weeks.

BACTERIOLOGY

Without exception, *Staphylococcus* is identified as the most common causative organism for aortic prosthetic graft infection. This fact is consistent with our understanding that the pathogenesis of prosthetic graft infection is related to bacterial contamination

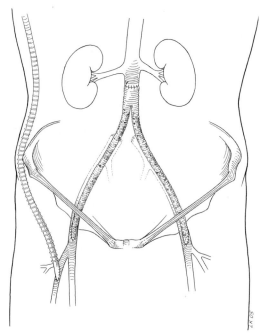

Fig. 5. Preliminary right axillofemoral prosthetic bypass routed lateral to the anterior superior iliac spine with distal anastomosis at the midprofunda femoral artery.

at the time of graft placement. *Staphylococcus epidermidis* is the slow-growing, slim-producing organism classically causing late, indolent graft infection. The more virulent *S. aureus* typically causes early graft infection and frequently is associated with overt signs of sepsis including fever and leukocytosis. Unfortunately, methicillin-resistant *S. aureus* is becoming more prevalent as a causative organism for prosthetic graft infection. Other bacteria not infrequently identified as causing prosthetic aortic graft infection include *E. coli, Pseudomonas,* and *Streptococcus* species. In contrast to primary aortic infection, *Salmonella* almost never is the causative organism for prosthetic graft infection.

SURGICAL TECHNIQUE

The surgical management of patients with an infected abdominal aortic tube or aortoiliac prosthetic graft is similar to that of patients with primary aortic infection. However, the surgeon managing a patient with an infected aortofemoral prosthetic graft is specifically challenged to perform lower extremity revascularization while contending with infection in the femoral region. Preliminary axillofemoral bypass in a patient with an infected aortofemoral prosthetic graft involves constructing the new femoral anastomosis to the profunda femoral artery (or superficial femoral artery) beyond the inguinal region through a

lateral incision distal to the original femoral anastomosis (Fig. 5). In these cases the PTFE axillofemoral graft is routed lateral to the anterior superior iliac spine circumventing the infected, original femoral incision. In cases of minimal groin sepsis, a prosthetic femorofemoral graft may be routed in a subcutaneous tunnel medial to

the original femoral incisions, avoiding the areas of infection. In selected cases with extensive femoral abscess/infection or extreme obesity, bilateral axillofemoral prosthetic grafts are utilized.

Recently, the autogenous femoral vein has become a popular conduit for use in infected fields. Indeed, the modern-day preferred method of revascularization for many patients with infected aortofemoral grafts is to construct the femoral-femoral component of the extra-anatomic bypass within the infected field using autogenous femoral vein (Fig. 6). This approach is utilized in patients with large femoral anastomotic aneurysm or abscess, or in any other aortic graft infection patient with significant groin sepsis. In these patients, avoiding the area of infection is problematic. Typically a preliminary, unilateral axillofemoral PTFE graft is routed, as previously described, outside the area of infection. The autogenous femorofemoral graft is constructed at the time the infected femoral anastomoses are exposed. Following detachment of the infected prosthetic limbs, the femoral arteriotomies are débrided and, if feasible, used as the anastomotic sites for the autogenous femorofemoral graft (Fig. 7). Frequently, however, in order to avoid localized inflammation or to prevent vein graft kinking, new sites for the femoral anastomoses are selected. The femoral vein is harvested from just distal to the profunda femoral

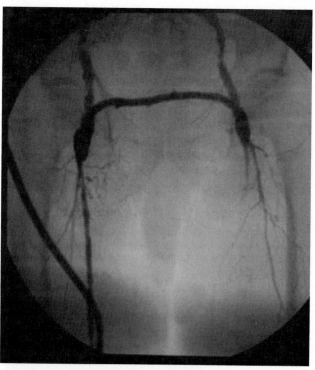

Fig. 6. Angiogram demonstrating right axillofemoral prosthetic bypass with the distal anastomosis to the superficial femoral artery and femoral-femoral bypass with autogenous femoral vein.

eries document excellent patency well above 90% at 10 years, though most have been judged on clinical grounds and not by strict repeated arteriography. Long-term follow-up should include blood pressure checks and serum creatinine, but given the above results, magnetic resonance arteriography or angiography is probably not indicated outside of a clinical suggestion of repair compromise.

Renal Artery Aneurysm Endovascular Interventions

In general, catheter-directed interventions for RAAs have had limited application, as the necks are wide and vessels small, with minimal margin for error. However, in select cases embolization of intraparenchymal aneurysms may be appropriate and a preferred alternative to partial nephrectomy. Similarly, endovascular stent graft placement is occasionally an acceptable therapy for proximal main RAAs, including dissections with a defined distal end point. A handful of case reports of endovascular techniques have been reported.

SUGGESTED READING

Centenera LV, Hirsch JA, Choi IS, et al. Wide-necked saccular renal artery aneurysm: endovascular embolization with the Guglielmi detachable coil and temporary balloon occlusion of the aneurysm neck. *J Vasc Interv Radiol* 1998;9:513.

Dzsinich C, Gloviczki P, McKusick MA, et al. Surgical management of renal artery aneurysm. *Cardiovasc Surg* 1993;3:243.

English WP, Pearce JD, Craven TE, et al. Surgical management of renal artery aneurysms. *J Vasc Surg* 2004;40:53.

Henke PK, Cardneau JD, Welling TH III, et al. Renal artery aneurysms: a 35-year clinical experience with 252 aneurysms in 168 patients. *Ann Surg* 2001;234:454.

Hupp T, Allenberg JR, Post K, et al. Renal artery aneurysms: surgical indications and results. *Eur J Vasc Surg* 1992;6:477.

Karkos CD, D'Souza SP, Thomson GJ, et al. Renal artery aneurysm: endovascular treatment by coil embolization with preservation of renal blood flow. *Eur J Vasc Endovasc Surg* 2001;19:214.

Love WK, Robinette MA, Vernon CP. Renal artery aneurysm rupture in pregnancy. *J Urol* 1981;126:809.

Mali WP, Geyskes GG, Thalman R. Dissecting renal artery aneurysm: treatment with an endovascular stent. *AJR Am J Roentgenol* 1989;153:623.

Martin RS 3rd, Meacham PW, Ditesheim JA, et al. Renal artery aneurysm: selective treatment for hypertension and prevention of rupture. *J Vasc Surg* 1989;9:26.

Pfeiffer T, Reiher L, Grabitz K, et al. Reconstruction for renal artery aneurysm: operative techniques and long-term results. *J Vasc Surg* 2003;37:293.

Rijbrock A, van Dijk HA, Roex AJ. Rupture of renal artery aneurysm during pregnancy. *Eur J Vasc Surg* 1994;8:375.

Stanley JC, Rhodes EL, Gewertz BL, et al. Renal artery aneurysms. Significance of macroaneurysms exclusive of dissections and fibrodysplastic mural dilations. *Arch Surg* 1975;110:1327.

Youkey JR, Collins GJ Jr., Orecchia PM, et al. Saccular renal artery aneurysm as a cause of hypertension. *Surgery* 1985;97:498.

Vascular Surgery

EDITOR'S COMMENT

This chapter exemplifies why the vascular surgical team at Michigan has gained such an outstanding international reputation in the management of renal artery disease. Their description of the incision and anatomic retroperitoneal approaches to the renal arteries and their description of autogenous repair should serve as an excellent guide for those surgeons engaged in these somewhat unusual procedures. As they note, there is some uncertainty about the indications for repair of renal artery aneurysms, other than in pregnant women or women of childbearing age, where the indication is very clear. An asymptomatic 2-cm main renal artery aneurysm in an elderly patient is probably of no significant concern. As they note, if a patient has an unusually large renal artery aneurysm and the opposite kidney is normal, nephrectomy is an effective and reliable treatment. As this is written, there is concern that these smaller, inconsequential aneurysms will become the object of a variety of endovascular treatment modalities, which may cause more harm than good. Finally, the authors make no mention of ex vivo repair and autotransplantation of the kidney for management of intraparenchymal aneurysms. With the excellent operative exposure they describe, along with bringing the kidney forward, few, if any, of these problems justify ex vivo management. As always, it gets back to that simple maxim of not doing harm.

F.W.L.

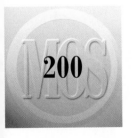

200

Renal Artery Intervention for Atherosclerotic Occlusive Disease

KIMBERLEY J. HANSEN AND K. TODD PIERCY

With the introduction of new antihypertensive agents specific to the renal angiotensin system and percutaneous renal artery angioplasty (PTAS) with endoluminal stenting, attitudes regarding open surgical intervention for atherosclerotic renovascular disease have changed. These new treatment alternatives have led many physicians to limit open surgical intervention to patients with (i) severe hypertension despite maximal medical therapy, (ii) anatomic failures or disease patterns not amenable to balloon angioplasty and stenting, or (iii) renovascular disease complicated by renal excretory insufficiency (i.e., ischemic nephropathy).

Our strategy for open operative management of atherosclerotic renovascular disease is outlined as follows:

1. Severe hypertension is considered a prerequisite for surgical intervention. Prophylactic repair of clinically silent, occlusive renal artery disease is not advised.

2. All clinically significant renal artery disease (i.e., associated with severe hypertension and/or excretory renal insufficiency) is repaired at a single operation. The exception to this approach is the individual who requires bilateral ex vivo renal reconstruction. In these cases, ex vivo operations are staged.

3. Direct aortorenal reconstruction is favored over indirect or splanchnorenal repair. Celiac axis disease accompanies renal artery disease in 40% of patients.

Up to 60% of patients require bilateral renal artery reconstruction and 30% require combined aortic repair.

4. Nephrectomy is performed infrequently. Nephrectomy is reserved for treatment of an unreconstructable renal artery lesion to a nonfunctioning kidney contributing to severe hypertension. Renal artery occlusions are reconstructed when a normal distal renal artery is present.

5. Simultaneous aortic repair is combined with renal artery reconstruction only when aortic disease is clinically severe. Aortic repair is not undertaken to provide an inflow source for renal reconstruction.

6. Regardless of the technique of reconstruction, each repair is assessed with intraoperative renal duplex sonography. Major defects requiring immediate revision are found in 10% to 12% of arterial repairs.

 PREOPERATIVE PLANNING

Patients who require multiple medications for hypertension may experience reduced medication requirements while hospitalized at bed rest. In this instance, hypertensive medications are reduced to minimum levels necessary for blood pressure control prior to operative repair. Both converting enzyme inhibitors and angiotensin receptor antagonists are discontinued. Preoperative and postoperative medical therapy for blood pressure control includes vasodilators (e.g., amlodipine) and selective β-adrenergic blocking agents (e.g., atenolol, metoprolol). Patients with severe hypertension (i.e., diastolic pressures exceeding 110 mm Hg) require postponement of operative treatment until pressure is brought under control. In the absence of excretory renal insufficiency, a combination of intravenous sodium nitroprusside and esmolol administered in an intensive care unit with continuous intra-arterial blood pressure monitoring may be required. Patients with significant heart disease, in combination with severe renal insufficiency, may require preoperative placement of invasive monitoring to optimize cardiac index and intravascular volume prior to operation.

Certain steps are common to almost every open renal artery procedure. Intravenous mannitol is administered during periods of aortic and perirenal dissection as well as before and after periods of renal ischemia. Small repeated intravenous doses are administered up to a total dose of 1 g/kg body weight. Prior to aortic or renal artery

cross clamp, 100 units of heparin per kilogram of body weight are administered intravenously and systemic anticoagulation is verified by activated clotting time. During periods aortic or renal cross clamp measurement of activated clotting time is repeated every 45 minutes and additional intravenous heparin administered as necessary. Protamine is not routinely administered at the conclusion of procedure unless required for hemostasis.

SURGICAL TECHNIQUE

Renal Artery Exposure

Open repair of atherosclerotic renal artery disease is most commonly made through a midline xiphoid to pubis abdominal incision. Extending the proximal incision 1 to 2 cm to one side of the xiphoid is required to obtain full exposure of the upper abdominal aorta and renal arteries (Fig. 1A). A fixed mechanical retraction system is advantageous, especially when combined aortorenal reconstruction is performed. Extended flank incisions coursing from the contralateral semilunar line, bisecting the ipsilateral costal margin and pelvic crest are useful for combined visceral renal artery reconstruction and ex vivo renal artery repair. When performed from an extended left flank incision, supraceliac exposure of the aorta is facilitated. In this instance, the ipsilateral flank is elevated on rolled sheets, the left arm is positioned posteriorly, and the surgical

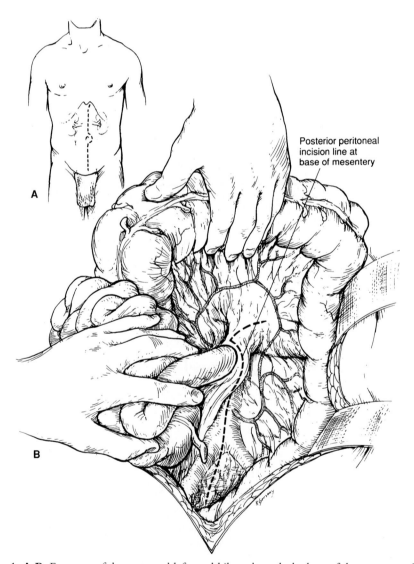

Fig. 1. A,B: Exposure of the aorta and left renal hilum through the base of the mesentery. Extension of the posterior peritoneal incision to the left, along the inferior border of the pancreas, provides entry to an avascular plane behind the pancreas. This allows excellent exposure of the entire left renal hilum as well as the proximal right renal artery. (From Benjamin ME, Dean RH. Techniques in renal artery reconstruction: part I. *Ann Vasc Surg* 1996;10:409, with permission.)

able is flexed. A left visceral mobilization provides access to the renal vasculature, the celiac axis, the superior mesenteric artery, and the supraceliac aorta. If required, the aortic crura can be divided allowing for extrapleural aortic dissection to the T$_{10}$ level of the descending thoracic aorta for proximal control and reconstruction.

When a midline abdominal incision is performed, the posterior peritoneum overlying the aorta is incised longitudinally (Fig. 1B). The ligament of Treitz is mobilized with care to identify visceral collaterals, which may course with the inferior mesenteric vein at this level (Fig. 1B). The duodenum is reflected to the patient's right to expose the renal vein, which is mobilized from the vena cava origin to renal hilum (Fig. 2A). By so doing, the inferior border of the pancreas is

also mobilized in an avascular plane, allowing exposure of the left renal hilum. Depending on the course of the left renal artery, the gonadal, adrenal, and lumbar renal branches of the left renal vein may be divided to retract the vein either superiorly or inferiorly (Fig. 2B). The proximal portion of the right renal artery can be exposed by this same approach. The entire retrocaval portion of the right renal artery can be exposed by ligating one or more pairs of lumbar veins (Fig. 2C).

When distal exposure of the renal artery is required or branch renal artery repair is planned, a transverse abdominal incision may be preferred. The right renal artery exposure is achieved by mobilization of the hepatic flexure of the colon combined with mobilization of the duodenum with an extensive Kocher maneuver (Fig. 3).

An avascular plane is entered anterior to the kidney, sweeping the duodenum medially (Fig. 4A). The vena cava is identified and the origin of the right renal vein is noted. The right renal artery usually courses posterior to the vein, which may be retracted either superiorly or inferiorly to provide the best exposure. Supernumerary renal arteries occur on both the right and left in 15% to 20% of patients. All arteries coursing anterior to the vena cava should be considered supernumerary or polar renal arteries to the right kidney and carefully preserved (Fig. 4B).

Aortic exposure proximal to the renal arteries is facilitated by partial division of the diaphragmatic crura. This maneuver allows exposure of the aorta proximal to origin of the superior mesenteric artery. Exposure and control of the aorta at this level is required during transaortic thromboendarterectomy.

OPEN RENAL ARTERY RECONSTRUCTION

No single method of open renal artery repair provides optimal reconstruction for all renal artery lesions. The method must be selected that best conforms to the patient and the disease process. However, of the three basic methods of renal artery repair (i.e., aortorenal bypass, transaortic thromboendarterectomy, and renal artery reimplantation), renal artery bypass is the most versatile. Saphenous vein is the preferred conduit for an isolated renal artery bypass in an adult. Hypogastric artery is selected for renal reconstruction in the child and adolescent. In the absence of satisfactory autogenous material and a renal artery of at least 4 mm in diameter, 6-mm thin-walled polytetrafluoroethylene provides patency equivalent to autogenous reconstruction.

Aortorenal Bypass

Regardless of the material chosen for aortorenal bypass, the proximal aortorenal anastomosis is performed first. A segment of infrarenal aorta proximal to the inferior mesenteric artery is controlled and an aortotomy created along the anterolateral aspect of the aorta. It is important to excise an ellipse of aorta with the length of the aortotomy at least three times the diameter of the renal artery conduit. Several applications of a 5.2-mm aortic punch can be used to create this ellipse. The proximal anastomosis is performed with continuous 6-0 polypropylene suture (Fig. 5).

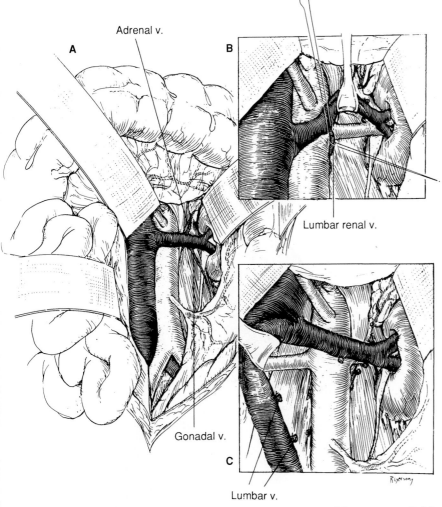

Fig. 2. A: Exposure of the proximal right renal artery through the base of the mesentery. **B:** Mobilization of the left renal vein by ligation and division of the adrenal, gonadal, and lumbar-renal veins allows exposure of the entire left renal artery to the hilum. **C:** Two pairs of lumbar vessels have been ligated and divided to allow retraction of the vena cava to the right, revealing adequate exposure of the proximal renal artery disease. (From Benjamin ME, Dean RH. Techniques in renal artery reconstruction: part I. *Ann Vasc Surg* 1996;10:409, with permission.)

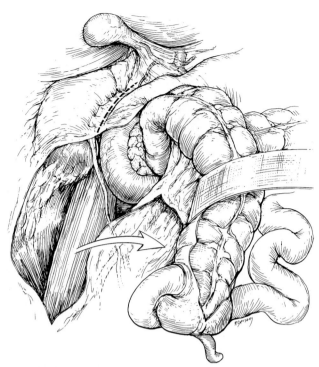

Fig. 3. With the right colon mobilized medially, a Kocher maneuver exposes the right renal hilum. (From Benjamin ME, Dean RH. Techniques in renal artery reconstruction: part I. *Ann Vasc Surg* 1996;10:409, with permission.)

In the past, distal graft to renal artery anastomoses were frequently created in an end-to-side fashion; however, distal end-to-end anastomosis is preferred. In this case, both conduit and renal artery are spatulated widely (two to three times the diameter of the renal artery) and the anastomosis accomplished with continuous 7-0 polypropylene suture. Prior to the completion of the anastomosis, the graft is flushed of air and debris and blood flow re-established to the kidney. In most instances, the warm renal ischemia time is 20 minutes or less.

Thromboendarterectomy

Transaortic thromboendarterectomy is particularly useful in patients with multiple renal arteries that demonstrate orificial atherosclerotic stenosis. Prior to undertaking thromboendarterectomy, the extent of atherosclerotic disease should be clearly defined. All visible and palpable renal artery atheroma should end within 1 to 1.5 cm of the aortic origin.

Thromboendarterectomy requires more extensive aortic exposure than aortorenal bypass (Fig. 6). The aorta proximal to the superior mesenteric artery should be exposed for control at this level (Fig. 6B). As discussed previously, this is facilitated by

partial division of the diaphragmatic crura. The superior mesenteric artery origin is exposed and controlled with an elastic loop. After preliminary control of each renal artery and after proximal and distal aortic control, the aorta is opened longitudinally to the base of the superior mesenteric artery (Fig. 6A). First a sleeve endarterectomy of the aorta is performed. The correct endarterectomy plane is best defined at the site of most advanced atherosclerotic disease. The aortic atheroma is divided sharply at the proximal and distal end points flush with the residual adventitia. Distal tacking sutures may be applied if necessary. Following sleeve endarterectomy of the aorta, an eversion type of endarterectomy of each renal artery is performed. The renal artery is everted into the aorta to allow the distal end point of the endarterectomy to be visualized (Fig. 6B). The aortic arteriotomy is then closed primarily with continuous 5-0 polypropylene suture.

As with thromboendarterectomy at all anatomic sites, this procedure is contraindicated by the presence of degenerative aneurysmal change of the aortic wall and aortic atheroma complicated by transmural calcification. This later condition is defined by gentle palpation of the aorta. Transmural calcification may feel like fine-grade sandpaper on palpation.

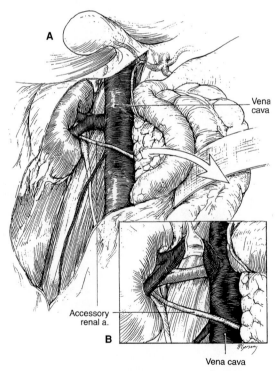

Fig. 4. A: Not uncommonly, an accessory right renal artery arises from the anterior aorta and crosses anterior to the vena cava. **B:** The right renal vein is typically mobilized superiorly for exposure of the distal right renal artery. (From Benjamin ME, Dean RH. Techniques in renal artery reconstruction: part I. *Ann Vasc Surg* 1996;10:409, with permission.)

Splenic artery aneurysms are most often asymptomatic. Vague epigastric or left upper quadrant discomfort is a nonspecific symptom attributed to these lesions. Roentgenographic demonstration of left upper quadrant, curvilinear, signet ring-like calcification may suggest the presence of a splenic artery aneurysm, but most are recognized as incidental findings during imaging studies, including computed tomography (CT), magnetic resonance angiography (MRA), and arteriography for unrelated diseases.

Rupture of bland splenic artery aneurysms occurs in less than 2% of patients. The mortality of rupture in nonpregnant patients is less than 25%. Rupture has been reported in more than 90% of aneurysms recognized during pregnancy, with a maternal mortality approaching 75% and fetal mortality exceeding 95%. However, many unruptured splenic artery aneurysms exist during pregnancy and go unrecognized clinically. Rupture often presents with hemorrhage into the lesser sac, with hemodynamic collapse as blood escapes through the foramen of Winslow. Lesser sac tamponade may postpone catastrophic intraperitoneal bleeding, which accounts for this so-called double rupture presentation.

Surgical treatment of splenic artery aneurysms is justified in pregnant patients and women of childbearing age, as well as in all patients with symptomatic aneurysms. Elective operations for asymptomatic splenic artery aneurysms 2 cm or greater in diameter are appropriate when operative mortality is less than 0.5%. If surgical therapy entails a prohibitively high risk, transcatheter embolization of the aneurysm represents an alternative form of management.

Splenic artery aneurysms are surgically approached through one of several anterior abdominal wall incisions. Extended right subcostal, transverse epigastric, and vertical midline incisions are all suitable, with the specific exposure selected depending on the patient's disease process and the planned procedure. Proximal aneurysms are best exposed through the lesser sac. Aneurysms in the midsplenic artery may be exposed with a retroperitoneal approach following pancreatic mobilization and elevation. Aneurysms located in the distal artery or splenic hilus are exposed with splenic mobilization (Fig. 1). Laparoscopic management of splenic artery aneurysms, especially in the distal splenic artery, may provide a less hazardous alternative to conventional operation.

Proximal and Midsplenic Artery Aneurysmectomy or Exclusion

Proximal splenic artery aneurysms are often treated by aneurysmectomy or exclusion with splenic artery ligation without arterial reconstruction (Fig. 2). This portion of the vessel is easily exposed by dividing the gastrohepatic ligament along the lesser curve of the stomach. Entering and exiting vessels are ligated, and the aneurysm is excised. If it is not embedded within pancreatic tissue, the aneurysm is not removed, but must be opened to ensure that all branches are ligated.

Certain splenic artery aneurysms, especially false aneurysms associated with inflammatory disease, may not be easily excised. False aneurysms occurring as a consequence of pancreatic pseudocyst erosions into the splenic artery, when responsible for active hemorrhage, are treated best by arterial ligation with monofilament suture from within the aneurysm. Internal or external drainage of a pseudocyst may be necessary after arterial ligation. Distal pancreatectomy, including the diseased artery, is often preferred when treating false aneurysms in patients who can tolerate the procedure.

Vascular Surgery

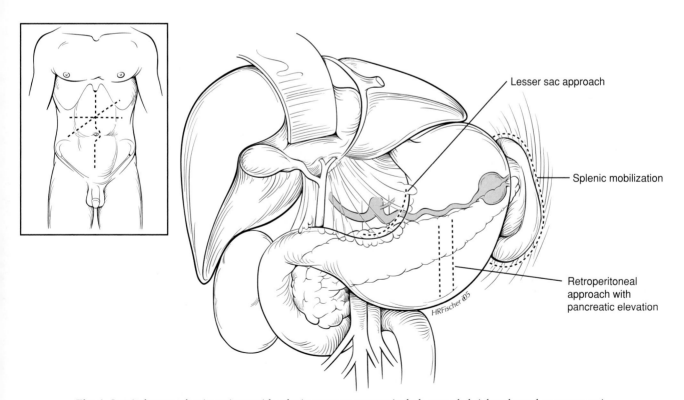

Fig. 1. Surgical approaches in patients with splenic artery aneurysms include extended right subcostal, transverse epigastric, and vertical midline incisions. Specific intra-abdominal exposure depends on the location of the splenic artery aneurysm. (From Stanley JC, Upchurch GR, Henke PK. Treatment of splanchnic and renal artery aneurysms. In: Zelenock GB, Huber TS, Messina LM, et al., eds. *Mastery of vascular and endovascular surgery.* Philadelphia: Lippincott Williams & Wilkins, 2006, with permission.)

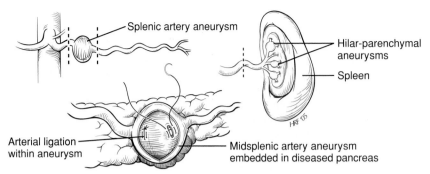

Fig. 2. Variations in surgical treatment of splenic artery aneurysms reflect the location and type of aneurysmal disease. (From Stanley JC, Upchurch GR, Henke PK. Treatment of splanchnic and renal artery aneurysms. In: Zelenock GB, Huber TS, Messina LM, et al., eds. *Mastery of vascular and endovascular surgery.* Philadelphia: Lippincott Williams & Wilkins, 2006, with permission.)

Hilar and Parenchymal Splenic Artery Aneurysmectomy or Exclusion

Historically, surgical therapy for most aneurysms within the hilus or substance of the spleen has been splenectomy. Standard surgical technique has usually been followed in these instances. However, splenic preservation to maintain host resistance with simple suture obliteration of distal aneurysms is preferable to splenectomy, even though segmental splenic infarction may subsequently occur.

Splenic Artery Aneurysm Endovascular Intervention

Percutaneous transcatheter embolization of splenic artery aneurysms, especially in high-risk patients with portal hypertension, is a preferred alternative to open operation. Careful follow-up of endovascularly coiled patients is mandatory. Splenic infarction and late rupture may occur. Nonsustained obliteration of the aneurysm as well as coil migration and erosion into the adjacent viscera are concerns that must be addressed in follow-up studies.

HEPATIC ARTERY ANEURYSMS

Aneurysms of the hepatic artery represent nearly 20% of splanchnic artery aneurysms and are often life threatening. Medial degeneration, trauma, and infection account for 24%, 22%, and 10% of hepatic aneurysms, respectively. Arteriosclerosis occurs in 32% of these aneurysms but is considered secondary, not causative. Interestingly, 17% of hepatic artery aneurysms encountered recently have occurred in patients undergoing orthotopic liver transplantation. In the latter group, women are affected twice as often as men. Excluding trauma, most hepatic artery aneurysms are

encountered in patients greater than 50 years of age.

Hepatic artery aneurysms are extrahepatic in 80% of cases, with 20% being intrahepatic. Generally, lesions that exceed 2 cm in diameter are saccular and smaller aneurysms are fusiform. In a review of 163 aneurysms in which the specific site of arterial involvement was documented, 63% arose from the common hepatic artery, 28% in the right hepatic artery, 5% in the left hepatic artery, and 4% in both left and right hepatic arteries. Excluding microaneurysms associated with systemic arteritis, hepatic artery aneurysms are usually solitary.

Symptomatic intact aneurysms often produce right upper quadrant or epigastric pain, similar to chronic cholecystitis. Severe pain may accompany acute aneurysmal expansion and be misdiagnosed as acute pancreatitis. Rupture occurs in less than 20% of cases. The 35% mortality from hepatic artery aneurysm rupture has not changed during recent years. Rupture occurs with equal frequency into the peritoneal cavity and hepatobiliary tree. Rupture into the latter results in hematobilia, manifest by biliary colic, periodic hematemesis, and jaundice. Erosion of hepatic artery aneurysms into the stomach, duodenum, and pancreatic duct occurs uncommonly. Extrahepatic rupture, usually of inflammatory aneurysms, frequently results in exsanguinating intraperitoneal hemorrhage.

Preoperative diagnosis of hepatic artery aneurysms may be difficult. Aneurysm calcifications are occasionally evident on abdominal plain film. Displacement or compression of adjacent gastrointestinal structures seen during barium contrast studies or endoscopic retrograde cholangiopancreatography (ERCP) may suggest the presence of these aneurysms. More often, CT, MRA, and arteriography have resulted in the incidental recognition of these aneurysms. All hepatic

artery aneurysms should be treated surgically unless inordinate operative risks are present.

Hepatic artery aneurysms are approached through an upper abdominal transverse, an extended right subcostal, or a vertical midline incision. The common and proper hepatic arteries are easily accessible through the lesser space. Initial palpation of these aneurysms within the hepatoduodenal ligament allows the surgeon to assess the relationship of the aneurysm to the common bile duct and portal vein, something that may prove difficult once dissection has begun. Proximal proper hepatic artery lesions should be dissected cautiously, with particular attention directed to the gastroduodenal artery and its pancreaticoduodenal branch, which often overlie and cross anterior to the common bile duct. Distal proper hepatic artery aneurysms near the hilus of the liver must also be dissected with great care to avoid bile duct injuries.

HEPATIC ARTERY ANEURYSM LIGATION

Common hepatic artery aneurysms can occasionally be treated successfully by aneurysm exclusion without reconstruction of the involved vessel. The extensive foregut collateral circulation through the gastroduodenal and right gastric arteries as well as the portal vein usually ensures adequate blood flow to the liver. If blood flow in the liver appears compromised after temporary hepatic artery occlusion, reconstruction of the aneurysmal vessel must be performed.

Hepatic Artery Aneurysmectomy and Primary Closure

Aneurysmorrhaphy is appropriate in certain instances of saccular aneurysms, especially in those associated with penetrating trauma (Fig. 3). Following dissection of the hepatic artery proximal and distal to the aneurysm, microvascular clamps are used to occlude the hepatic vessels. After aneurysmectomy, a primary closure is performed using fine monofilament cardiovascular suture in a continuous manner. Placement of the initial stitch at the distal apex of the arterial defect is critical in decreasing the chance for narrowing of the vessel as the repair commences.

Hepatic Artery Aneurysmectomy and Interposition Graft Repair

Fusiform and large saccular aneurysms of the proper hepatic artery are best treated by aneurysmectomy and formal reconstruction of the vessel. Interposition grafting is preferred (Fig. 4), with reversed autogenous saphenous vein being favored over prosthetic conduits. Vein grafts are carefully procured, gently handled, and flushed with heparinized blood before implantation. Careful dissection and isolation of the aneurysm is performed, with ligation and transection of the gastroduodenal and pancreaticoduodenal vessels if they are involved with the aneurysm. Digital control of entering and exiting vessels and early entrance into the aneurysm, with additional control using balloon catheters or rigid dilators from within, may be appropriate for large lesions and in those instances in which dissection of the artery from the surrounding biliary and venous structures might be hazardous. The anastomoses, with spatulation of the vein and artery, are carried out in a standard manner.

Hepatic Artery Aneurysmectomy and Aortohepatic Bypass

Aortohepatic bypass (Fig. 5) is preferable to other reconstructions if the common

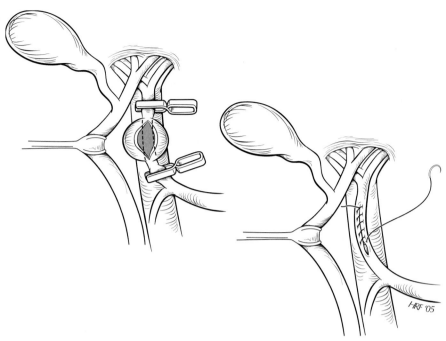

Fig. 3. Hepatic artery aneurysmectomy and primary closure. Certain saccular aneurysms with narrow necks may be treated by simple excision and closure of the arterial defect using a continuous monofilament suture. (From Stanley JC, Upchurch GR, Henke PK. Treatment of splanchnic and renal artery aneurysms. In: Zelenock GB, Huber TS, Messina LM, et al., eds. *Mastery of vascular and endovascular surgery.* Philadelphia: Lippincott Williams & Wilkins, 2006, with permission.)

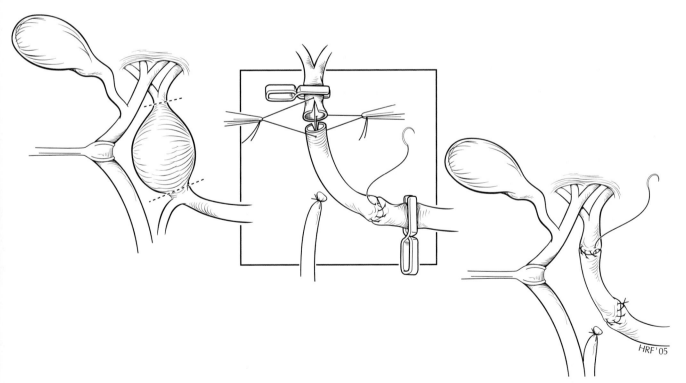

Fig. 4. Treatment of fusiform or large saccular hepatic artery aneurysms often requires an interposition graft. Autogenous saphenous vein is favored over prosthetic materials. The hepatic artery is spatulated anteriorly and the vein graft is spatulated posteriorly to allow for creation of an ovoid anastomosis. A fine continuous monofilament suture is preferred. Two initial sutures through the apex of the spatulation and opposite vessel are used for traction during completion of these anastomoses. (From Stanley JC, Upchurch GR, Henke PK. Treatment of splanchnic and renal artery aneurysms. In: Zelenock GB, Huber TS, Messina LM, et al., eds. *Mastery of vascular and endovascular surgery.* Philadelphia: Lippincott Williams & Wilkins, 2006, with permission.)

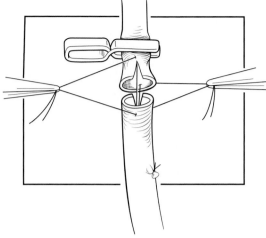

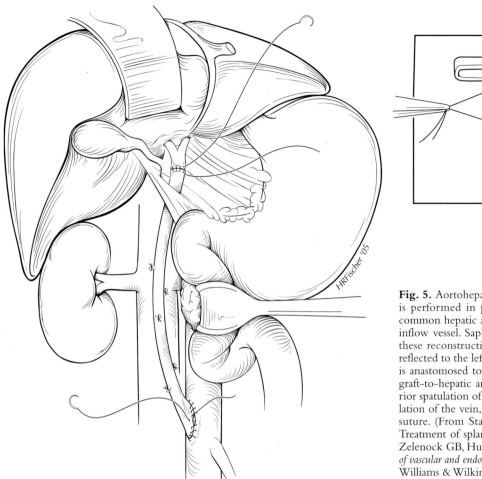

Fig. 5. Aortohepatic bypass for hepatic artery aneurysm is performed in patients with intrinsic disease of the common hepatic artery that precludes its ready use as an inflow vessel. Saphenous vein is the favored conduit in these reconstructions. The duodenum and pancreas are reflected to the left, exposing the aorta. The reversed vein is anastomosed to an anterolateral aortotomy. The distal graft-to-hepatic artery anastomosis is created after anterior spatulation of the hepatic artery and posterior spatulation of the vein, using a continuous fine monofilament suture. (From Stanley JC, Upchurch GR, Henke PK. Treatment of splanchnic and renal artery aneurysms. In: Zelenock GB, Huber TS, Messina LM, et al., eds. *Mastery of vascular and endovascular surgery.* Philadelphia: Lippincott Williams & Wilkins, 2006, with permission.)

hepatic artery is not a suitable inflow vessel for an interposition graft. This clearly would be the case when coexistent celiac artery stenosis was present. Following dissection of the aneurysm, an extended Kocher maneuver is performed to expose the aorta and inferior vena cava. A segment of saphenous vein, adequate in length for an aortohepatic bypass, is carefully procured. An anterolateral aortotomy is made approximately twice the diameter of the vein. The reversed vein graft is anastomosed to the aorta using a continuous monofilament suture. The distal hepatic artery beyond the aneurysm is occluded with a microvascular clamp, the proximal vessel is ligated, and the aneurysm is excised. The hepatic artery is spatulated anteriorly and the vein graft is spatulated posteriorly. Two initial fine monofilament cardiovascular sutures are placed in the apex of each spatulation and the free border of the adjacent vessel to serve as stay stitches. The anastomosis is completed with a continuous suture, after which the clamps are released and antegrade flow through the bypass is restored to the liver.

Hepatic Artery Aneurysm Endovascular Intervention

Endovascular transcatheter obliteration of hepatic artery aneurysms with balloons, coils, or thrombogenic particulate matter is a reasonable and often preferred alternative to open surgical intervention. It is recognized that in some cases, transcatheter embolization may only be transiently successful and repeated embolization or surgical therapy may be required to definitively treat these aneurysms. Therefore, these patients must be followed carefully.

SUPERIOR MESENTERIC ARTERY ANEURYSMS

Aneurysms of the proximal superior mesenteric artery (SMA) are the third most common splanchnic artery aneurysm, and account for 5.5% of these lesions. Men are affected nearly twice as often as women. Mycotic aneurysms secondary to bacterial endocarditis are relatively common, with nonhemolytic streptococci and a variety of pathogens associated with substance abuse serving as a source of the infectious agents.

SMA aneurysms also have been related to medial degeneration, periarterial inflammation, and trauma. Arteriosclerosis, when present, has been considered a secondary event rather than an etiologic process. SMA aneurysms, similar to most splanchnic artery aneurysms, are usually recognized during radiologic studies for other diseases. The majority of SMA aneurysms are symptomatic, with varying degrees of abdominal discomfort described. In many patients, the pain has been ascribed to intestinal angina.

SMA aneurysm rupture is rare. Gastrointestinal hemorrhage associated with these aneurysms usually reflects their acute occlusion and bleeding from areas of intestinal ischemia and mucosal sloughing. The unique location of SMA aneurysms near the origins of the inferior pancreaticoduodenal and middle colic arteries effectively isolates the distal small bowel circulation, should aneurysmal dissection or occlusion occur. It is in this setting that the usual collateral networks from the adjacent celiac and inferior mesenteric arterial circulations are lost.

EDITOR'S COMMENT

Professor Kenneth Cherry at the University of Virginia provides a succinct, comprehensive treatise that depicts the historical evolution of the management of chronic mesenteric ischemia, as well as its contemporary management. As discussed in the chapter, it was Dunphy at the Brigham Hospital, in 1937, who provided the seminal work that delineated the anatomic lesion and its subsequent physiologic injury that results from chronic mesenteric ischemia with progression to intestinal infarction and death. With the first description of SMA endarterectomy by Shaw and Maynard in 1958, the treatment of this anatomic lesion evolved into a more direct approach. Thereafter, prosthetic infrarenal bypass grafting to the SMA, in 1962, with subsequent retrograde venous bypass was described. With what was a brief flirtation with reimplantation and the saphenous vein bypass, subsequent use of the prosthetic graft for mesenteric reconstruction differentiated the advantage of this technique. Professor Cherry indicates that until the 1990s, the mortality was in the 7% to 10% range. However, it was Wylie and Stoney who advanced the application of the transaortic endarterectomy of the paravesicular aorta and mesenteric arteries, and also championed supraceliac aortic graft reconstructions to the celiac and superior mesenteric arteries. Moreover, Wylie and Stoney advocated the thoracoretroperitoneal approach, which has evolved currently to the abdominal incision with medial visceral rotation. Professor Cherry reiterates that the "accumulated experience" from different centers suggests that preferential high disease-free inflow coupled with attention to the celiac artery and the SMA represent the foundation for successful intervention. The author emphasizes the expectant poor outcomes when the vascular surgeon bases reconstruction on the severely diseased infrarenal aorta with attempt to avoid cross clamping at higher levels.

With evolution to minimally invasive aortic aneurysmal endovascular repair, the author suggests that the immediate controversy today is the consideration of *conventional open surgery* versus consideration of *endovascular repair* of the mesenteric lesion. In most series, mortality from endovascular repairs remains lower than with the "open" repair; similarly for all series, recurrence rates for the necessity of reinterventional surgery is higher. Thus, in many circumstances, the option to the surgeon for open versus endovascular repair is based upon patient age and co-morbidities, which enhance operative risk and subsequent mortality for the open procedure. We would agree that the young, healthy individual should be highly considered in the first operation for an open conventional approach. This is because the durability of conventional aortic reconstruction is superior with the open technique; as emphasized by the author, no long-term data for mesenteric angioplasty and stenting are available. Some surgical groups favor the "tailored approach" for revascularization to optimize patency and ensure long-term symptom-free survival. The report by Leke et al. from the University of Southern California, Los Angeles, advocated a variety of surgical techniques to provide durable relief of

chronic mesenteric ischemia. Their revascularization approach was tailored to arterial anatomy and includes bypass of the SMA alone, bypass to the celiac artery and SMA, SMA reimplantation onto the aorta, SMA/inferior mesenteric reimplantation, and transaortic endarterectomy of the celiac and superior mesenteric arteries. Leke et al. also included bypass grafts that originated from the supraceliac aorta; remaining bypass grafts originated from the left limb of the aortofemoral graft (Technical consideration in the management of chronic mesenteric ischemia. Presented at the Annual Meeting, Southern California Chapter of the American College of Surgeons, January 18–20, 2002, Santa Barbara, California).

Silva et al. recently reported on the outcomes of a consecutive series of patients with chronic mesenteric ischemia treated with percutaneous stent revascularization. (*J Am Coll Cardiol* 2006;47[5]:944). For 59 consecutive patients with mesenteric ischemia, stent placement was conducted in 79 stenotic mesenteric arteries (>70%). A consistent clinical follow-up indicated that 90% had anatomic evaluation with angiography or ultrasound after 6 months of the procedure. Procedural success by Silva et al. was 96% and symptom relief was significant (88%). All patients with recurrent symptoms had angiographic in-stent restenosis and were percutaneously successfully revascularized. These authors indicated a low procedural morbidity and mortality, and suggested that the endovascular approach is the preferred technique. This represents the largest series of endovascular approaches for chronic mesenteric ischemia. However, as indicated by Professor Cherry in this chapter, long-term benefits and symptom-free recurrence measured over a prolonged period is essential to determine its durability and success relative to the conventional open technique. Jimenez et al. of the University of Florida, Gainesville, sought to review the outcome of patients with chronic mesenteric ischemia that were treated with antegrade synthetic aortomesenteric bypass (*J Vasc Surg* 2002;35:1078). These authors graded outcome measures with functional capacity, and both graft patency and survival rates were determined with life-table analyses. For 47 patients undergoing aortomesenteric bypass, the in-hospital mortality rate was high (11%) and mean length of stay was 32 ± 30 days. However, at a mean follow-up of 31 months, all patients had relief of abdominal pain and 86% gained weight. The primary, primary assisted, and secondary 5-year patency of grafts using life-table analyses were 69%, 94%, and 100%, respectively. The 5-year survival rate was 74%. Thus, this procedure appears to be both effective and durable, which is evident with long-term survival and freedom from the symptoms of recurrent mesenteric ischemia. These authors emphasize that objective determination of graft patency is possible in the clinical setting with mesenteric duplex ultrasound scanning, which can be utilized to facilitate the identification of graft stenoses *prior* to evidence of graft failure and the clinical development of ischemic symptoms. Again, I would emphasize, as do the authors, that there is procedural-associated morbidity and mortality that is significant. Efforts that are focused to improve these outcomes and reduce adverse perioperative events have been the focus of many clinical groups in this complex subset of patients.

Similar advocacy for the transaortic endarterectomy technique for primary mesenteric revascularization has been presented by Lau et al. of the Brigham and Women's Hospital, Boston, MA (*Vasc Endovasc Surg* 2002;36[5]:335). In an effort to study safety and outcomes of primary mesenteric revascularization for mesenteric ischemia, these authors performed transaortic endarterectomy as a "trap door" endarterectomy. The principal clinical presentation for the procedure was abdominal pain and weight loss. Short ischemic times allowed an initial success rate for revascularization of 93%, with one early graft failure that was salvaged with urgent embolectomy without bowel resection. This group reports no hospital mortality with an overall morbidity that was significant at 50%. Of this cohort 93% achieved sustained relief of symptoms and overall survival rates were 85% and 77% at 1 and 3 years, respectively. This group advocates the transaortic technique as a safe, effective measure for elective primary revascularization for mesenteric ischemia. An added advantage of this approach is the opportunity for simultaneous revascularization for multiple visceral arteries, which may allow patient relief of symptoms when successful.

Similarly, Cho et al. of Henry Ford Hospital, Detroit, MI, addressed the controversial issues that determine late results following mesenteric artery reconstruction in the treatment of mesenteric ischemia (*J Vasc Surg* 2002;35:453). A 37-year experience from Henry Ford Hospital provided insight into the 48 patients studied who had undergone mesenteric artery reconstruction for symptoms of nonembolic origin. The most commonly performed procedure for acute mesenteric ischemia was the *single-vessel revascularization;* use of the single vessel was more common in the acute than in the chronic mesenteric ischemic presentation (91% vs. 48%; P = 0.001). Cho et al. reported a high perioperative mortality of 52% in the acute mesenteric group versus no mortality in the chronic mesenteric ischemic group (P <0.001). As for other clinics evaluating this patient group, major complication rates occurred in 60% of these patients, but freedom from recurrent rates in the survivors was 79% at 5 years and 59% at 10 years. Long-term survival following revascularization of the acute and chronic group was overall 77% at 5 years and 29% at 10 years. Importantly, these authors confirmed that there were no differences between the acute versus chronic ischemic groups relative to survival once successful revascularization had been completed. These authors concluded that although mesenteric artery reconstruction for the chronic variant of ischemia produces a low mortality rate (0% in their series), the acute mesenteric variant represents a lethal, frequently unheralded problem. Again, success of the revascularization for both presentations can be durable once successfully completed. Patency of the SMA is essential for prevention of symptomatic recurrences; thus, elective revascularization should be strongly considered in such patients with chronic mesenteric ischemia, as this will warrant long-term surveillance otherwise.

K.I.B.

Vascular Surgery

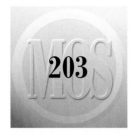

203

Superior Mesenteric Artery Embolectomy

C. KEITH OZAKI

Few clinical scenarios challenge the intellectual, technical, and clinical skills of the surgeon more than management of the patient with acute mesenteric ischemia. Several pathologic mechanisms can result in acute mesenteric ischemic syndromes, including embolism to the superior mesenteric artery (SMA), arterial dissections, mesenteric thrombosis (e.g., acute thrombosis of a chronic SMA atherosclerotic lesion), low-flow nonocclusive mesenteric ischemia, and mesenteric venous thrombosis. The following discussion focuses on SMA thromboembolism, which accounts for the majority of acute mesenteric ischemia cases, with the heart standing as the most common embolic source. Cardiac pathologies that predispose to thrombus formation include atrial fibrillation (especially in patients with anatomic abnormalities such as atrial dilation who are not anticoagulated or are underanticoagulated), recent myocardial infarction with mural thrombus formation, and ventricular aneurysm. Acute mesenteric ischemia remains a highly lethal clinical event, with mortality averaging 69% from several series. While uncommon, the incidence of this problem may increase with the aging population. A recent population-based series cites an incidence rate as high as 5.3 cases per 100,000 inhabitants per year.

The SMA arises from the anterior aorta typically 1 to 2 cm below the celiac artery, and 1 to 2 cm cephalad to the take off of the renal arteries. It usually originates at the level of the first lumbar vertebral body and passes inferiorly and to the right, posterior to the pancreas, and anterior to the fourth portion of the duodenum. This blood vessel, which in the adult is about the size of the fifth finger in diameter, supplies the distal duodenum, the small intestine, and the ascending and transverse colon. Early branches off of the SMA are the pancreaticoduodenal artery (which can serve as a major collateral network between the SMA and celiac axis in occlusive lesions that develop slowly) and the middle colic artery. Since the blood vessel changes caliber with the takeoff of these early branches, most clinically apparent emboli lodge near the origin of the

middle colic, leading to ischemia from the proximal jejunum to the splenic flexure. In 10% to 20% of the population, the right hepatic artery has a replaced origin from the SMA. The SMA terminates as the ileocolic artery. While acute occlusion of the celiac or the interior mesenteric arteries is usually well tolerated, acute SMA occlusion produces widespread infarction throughout the small bowel and colon.

With abrupt cessation of arterial inflow via the SMA, intestinal ischemia rapidly initiates within the well-vascularized bowel mucosa, where epithelial and endothelial cell damage lowers mucosal barrier function, leading to bacterial invasion, susceptibility to degrading enzymes, microcirculatory stasis, edema, and intravascular thrombosis. Bacterial and cellular toxins, inflammatory mediators such as cytokines, and particles from cellular death are released into the portal venous circulation and beyond, and drive systemic effects such as increased capillary permeability with edema formation and shock. Even after restoration of organ perfusion, the endothelial cell dysfunction often persists. The resultant ischemia-reperfusion syndrome drives distant multiple organ insufficiency or failure.

The key factor limiting progress in lowering the morbidity and mortality in acute mesenteric ischemia remains prompt diagnosis; thus, symptoms and signs deserve emphasis. A key to diagnosis is a high index of clinical suspicion in elderly patients, especially those with risk factors such as cardiac dysrhythmias, recent myocardial infarction, valvular heart disease, congestive heart failure, atherosclerosis, and malignancy. Patients typically note abrupt onset of constant epigastric or midabdominal pain, followed soon after by defecation (sometimes diarrhea and/or blood per rectum) and vomiting. The surgeon should also inquire about evidence of chronic symptoms such as postprandial cramping pain, change in bowel habits, and weight loss, since the distinction between acute versus acute-on-chronic disease may impact technical approaches to bowel revascularization. Finally, in the case of SMA embolization, approximately 25%

of patients give a history of prior embolic events (brain, leg, etc.).

Physical findings in acute mesenteric thromboembolism can be subtle and nonspecific. The abdomen may be distended with diminished intestinal peristaltic sounds. Classically, abdominal tenderness is less than expected from the patient's complaints of severe pain. Bloody fluid may be retrieved from a nasogastric tube and on rectal examination. Later in the clinical course, as the bowel progresses to infarction, the patient will appear toxic, with shock and peritonitis.

Laboratory tests also yield little sensitivity and specificity. Notable findings may include a leukocytosis with a predominance of immature white blood cells and a metabolic acidosis. D-dimer has been noted to have a high sensitivity for SMA occlusion, but the specificity is probably low.

Plain roentgenograms may be normal but occasionally demonstrate thickened intestinal walls, and in late stages gas in the intestinal wall or portal vein. While emerging as a useful modality in chronic occlusive disease, mesenteric duplex is often of limited benefit in the acute setting due to dilated, air-filled loops of bowel. In cases of diagnostic uncertainty, computed tomography (CT) scan with intravenous contrast screens for other pathologies. Relevant acute findings on CT scan include whether the contrast-filled SMA can be identified out to its peripheral branches and bowel abnormalities such as segmental bowel wall thickening. The diagnosis of mesenteric venous obstruction (which is managed primarily with anticoagulation and nutritional support unless it has progressed to significant bowel complications) is made via CT scan—a "halo" or "target" sign may be identified in the superior mesenteric vein.

Visceral biplanar arteriography can well define mesenteric anatomic occlusive lesions. However, angiography is not mandatory, and may result in modest delays that adversely affect outcome. In addition to anterior posterior views, a lateral view starting at the first lumbar artery can demonstrate the characteristic appearance of an embolus with a meniscus sign. Nonocclusive mesenteric ischemia (resulting from a depressed cardiac output and oxygen delivery) findings on angiogram include narrowing at the origin of branches of the SMA, spasm of arcade vessels, and impaired filling of intramural vessels. This syndrome is managed nonoperatively by intra-arterial instillation of dilating compounds.

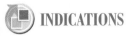 INDICATIONS

In cases where there has been a clear intra-abdominal catastrophe (which is often the case with acute mesenteric ischemic), extensive laboratory and radiographic testing unnecessarily delays bowel revascularization, leading to increased bowel loss and eventual patient mortality. Emergency laparotomy must proceed expeditiously as the patient is resuscitated and prepared for exploration. With less dramatic clinical presentations, symptomatic acute mesenteric embolus diagnosed by way of the algorithms outlined above warrants emergency exploration and bowel revascularization.

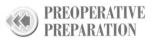 PREOPERATIVE PREPARATION

The surgeon's focus on clinical diagnosis, immediate laparotomy, and urgent bowel reperfusion via surgical interventions builds from the report of Klass over 50 years ago. Patients suffering acute SMA obstruction require multiple simultaneous interventions in preparation for the operating room. Yet none of these should stand as a rate-limiting step toward skin incision, since these patients can deteriorate rapidly and every minute of delay jeopardizes outcome. Upon diagnosis of acute mesenteric ischemia, the patient is systemically heparinized to minimize clot propagation. Activated clotting times throughout the operative period can ensure adequate systemic anticoagulation. Crystalloid infusion improves oxygen delivery, and electrolyte abnormalities can be addressed as the resuscitation proceeds. All available personnel should work to place hemodynamic monitors such as arterial lines, secure venous access, a Foley catheter, and a nasogastric tube. Simultaneously, the status of lower extremity pulses is documented since this patient subset often holds risk factors for lower extremity occlusive disease and may have embolized to the leg arteries, and aortic clamping may shower emboli distally.

In a warmed operating room, the patient is prepped from the nipples to the toes bilaterally since vein may be required for patch or conduit (femoral vein functions well for bypass conduit in the setting of

peritoneal contamination from gastrointestinal contents). The theater should be equipped with an activated clotting time machine to follow ongoing heparin anticoagulation. Once the airway is secured, intraoperative transesophageal echocardiogram can assess volume status and ventricular function and delineate cardiac anatomic abnormalities that may predispose to clot formation and embolization.

 SURGICAL TECHNIQUE

Typically the incision is made from the xiphoid bone to the pubis in the midline. Gangrenous or perforated bowel is immediately resected to reduce soilage. It must be emphasized that intestinal resection alone is not acceptable therapy when ischemic or infracted bowel is found at laparotomy, and a systematic interrogation into the potential cause of the bowel loss must be conducted. The pattern of ischemia is important to establishing diagno-

sis. Vascular compromise of the entire jejunum, ileum, and portions of colon stands as the hallmark of SMA occlusion at the origin. With an embolus to the SMA, there is often sparing of the first portion of jejunum due to some perfusion from the celiac branches via the pancreaticoduodenal artery. Patchy, segmental small bowel ischemia/infarction is consistent with showers of emboli or the vasospasm associated with nonocclusive mesenteric ischemia.

If gut vascular compromise is suspected, steps are initiated to assess the cause of impaired blood supply. Tilt of the operating room table to the right helps keep small bowel out of the surgical field, and self-retaining retractor systems such as the Bookwalter facilitate exposure. To evaluate the SMA, the omentum and transverse colon are lifted cephalad. All small bowel is then retracted to the right, and the sigmoid colon packed to the left (Fig. 1). The ligament of Treitz and the superior attachments of the duodenum are then sharply divided,

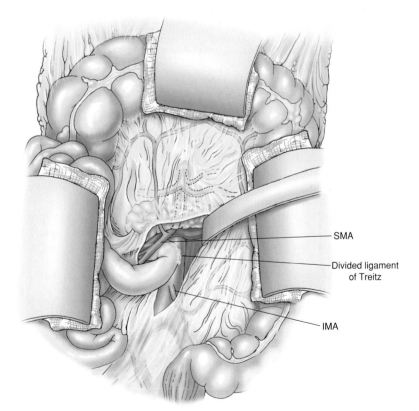

SMA

Divided ligament of Treitz

IMA

Fig. 1. Exposure of the SMA for embolectomy. The omentum and transverse colon are lifted cephalad. All small bowel is retracted to the right, and the sigmoid colon packed to the left. The ligament of Treitz and the superior attachments of the duodenum are sharply divided, with the goal of mobilizing the last portion of the duodenum to the right. Then, with four fingers behind the small bowel mesentery and with the thumb anteriorly, the SMA should be palpable near the base of the transverse colon mesentery.

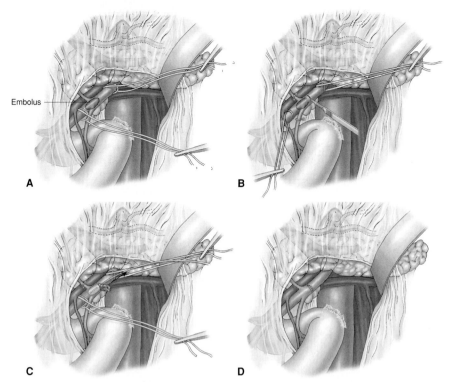

Fig. 2. Technique of SMA embolectomy using Fogarty balloon catheter. If normal blood supply via the SMA cannot be confirmed by palpation and Doppler examination, then the artery is surgically exposed, including ligation of overlying small blood vessels and lymphatics (Figure 203-2A). If large in caliber and an embolus is suspected, transverse arteriotomy offers the potential for simple closure (Figure 203-2B). Conversely, if bypass for occlusive disease may be necessary, the arteriotomy is best made longitudinally in the event that this site is needed as the distal anastomosis site for a bypass graft. Mechanical thrombectomy is completed using Fogarty balloon catheters (Figure 203-2C). The transverse arteriotomy is closed via simple interrupted closure using double-armed monofilament sutures so that the intima is re-tacked up from within (Figure 203-2D).

with the goal of mobilizing the last portion of the duodenum to the right (Kocher maneuver). Then, with four fingers behind the small bowel mesentery and with the thumb anteriorly, the SMA should be palpable at the base of the transverse colon mesentery. If a pulse is palpable, then continuous-wave handheld Doppler is used to ensure that there is diastolic flow and not just a water hammer pulse proximal to an occlusion.

If normal blood supply via the SMA cannot be confirmed via these algorithms, then the artery should be surgically exposed. Continuing the maneuvers above at the level of the transverse mesocolon base, the soft tissues overlying the artery are carefully dissected, including ligation of overlying small blood vessels and lymphatics (Fig. 2). The SMA has a larger caliber proximal to the middle colic origin, making for technically easier arteriotomy. An approximately 3- to 4-cm length of artery is exposed and elastic vessel loops placed for proximal and distal control. If large in caliber and an embolus is suspected, transverse arteriotomy offers the potential for simple closure. Con-

versely, if bypass for occlusive disease may be necessary (based on palpation of substantial atherosclerosis in the proximal SMA), the arteriotomy is best made longitudinally in the event that this site is needed as the distal anastomosis location for a bypass graft.

Mechanical thrombectomy is completed using appropriately sized Fogarty balloon catheters passed proximally and distally. To minimize trauma, the devices are passed into the large portion of the SMA and pulled back gently until one pass retrieves no further clot material. Extreme care must be taken to avoid blood vessel disruption in the peripheral SMA branches, which are soft and small. Tactile feedback regarding the radial balloon force on the blood vessel wall can only be inferred by resistance as the balloon is moved along the intima. Thus, the balloon should never be inflated while the catheter is stationary, but rather as the Fogarty is withdrawn.

A transverse arteriotomy is closed via simple interrupted closure using double-armed monofilament sutures so that the in-

tima is retacked up from within. Longitudinal arteriotomy usually requires a vein patch closure to prevent stenosis with the closure. If adequate inflow is not attained, then bypass grafting is appropriate. In the emergency setting externally supported prosthetic conduits are reasonable, assuming there is no enterotomy or enterectomy. The iliacs, infrarenal aorta, or supraceliac aorta (which tends to be spared from extensive atherosclerosis) may serve as inflow sites for such a bypass. If frank bowel infarction has occurred, then autogenous conduit lessens the chance of infectious complications. Femoral vein serves as a durable bypass material, and lies best with less opportunity for kinking if taken from the supraceliac aorta. While revascularization of both the celiac and SMA stands as a standard in operations for chronic mesenteric ischemia, it is reasonable to limit the procedure to the SMA alone in the acute setting to minimize operative duration and trauma.

After revascularization, at least 30 minutes should pass prior to determination of bowel viability. Clearly dead bowel is resected. Return of peristalsis indicates viable bowel. However, this clinical judgment can be quite difficult, and adjuncts in addition to close bowel inspection include listening for Doppler signals at the antimesenteric border and bowel fluorescence under Wood (ultraviolet) lamp examination after intravenous fluorescein infusion. Occasionally, injection of vasodilators and glucagon may be of benefit.

Despite these maneuvers, delineation of salvageable versus unsalvageable bowel often still remains obscure. In this setting, bowel ends can be stapled off or brought up as ostomies, and the abdomen closed in a single layer. A second-look operation is planned and carried out in 24 to 48 hours. During this time frame the patient's oxygen delivery and metabolic status is optimized. A second-look strategy commits the operative team to another procedure in 24 to 48 hours (even if the patient's clinical status improves dramatically). Conversely, if the patient's status deteriorates during this early operative period, further interrogation (such as angiogram to ensure optimal intestinal revascularization) and re-exploration (for signs of progression to transmural bowel infarction with subsequent complications) may be warranted sooner. Since these patients are often quite ill and the bowel viability may be in question, construction of a primary anastomosis may lead to subsequent dehiscence and enteric contents spillage in a critically ill patient. Therefore, the safest strategy is creation of stomas, which can be observed postoperatively for

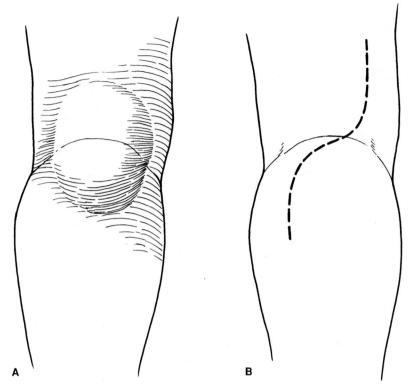

A **B**

Fig. 5. A: Popliteal saccular aneurysm. **B:** Incision to repair popliteal saccular aneurysm.

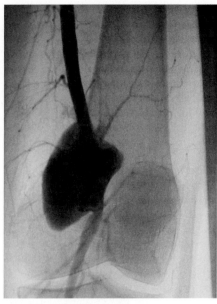

Fig. 7. Popliteal artery aneurysm.

by retracting the two heads of the gastrocnemius apart with or without division of the raphe.

After heparinization, the popliteal artery is clamped proximal and distally. The aneurysmal sac is opened longitudinally, and the geniculate branches are oversewn from within. Arterial reconstruction is performed with a portion of reversed lesser saphenous vein (Fig. 6). The greater saphenous vein may need to be harvested if the lesser saphenous vein is inadequate. Proximal and distal anastomoses are performed with the vein beveled, in an end-to-end fashion using 6-0 polypropylene suture. An adequate hemodynamic result is confirmed with intraoperative duplex scanning or arteriography (Figs. 7 and 8).

Popliteal artery aneurysms may also present with acute arterial occlusion. In most cases, percutaneous thrombolysis of the outflow vessels (not the aneurysm) is performed, followed by a femorodistal

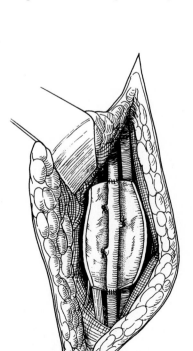

A **B**

Fig. 6. A: Exposure of popliteal saccular aneurysm. **B:** Repair of popliteal saccular aneurysm and graft.

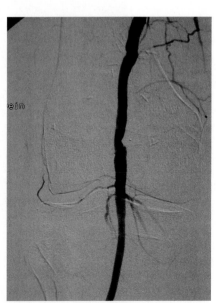

Fig. 8. Completion angiogram after an in situ replacement of the popliteal artery aneurysm with a reversed saphenous vein.

Vascular Surgery

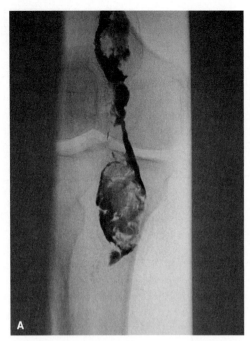
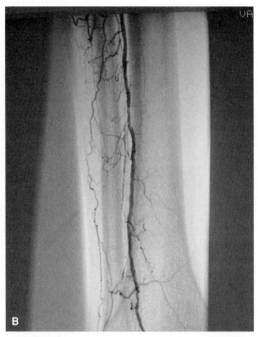

Fig. 9. A: Angiogram of a patient presenting with an acute limb ischemia with no obvious target (outflow vessel) and a popliteal artery aneurysm filled with thrombus. **B:** Following 12-hour infusion of urokinase, the patient has a visible anterior tibial vessel that can be used as a bypass target vessel.

bypass (see below). Patients with severe ischemia are best managed operatively with distal popliteal/tibial thromboembolectomy with balloon-tip catheters or, as is our preference, using catheter-directed or intraoperative thrombolysis. Occasionally, the distal arterial branch can be cleared by an infusion of urokinase (250,000 to 500,000 IU) into the occluded distal arterial tree. More often, isolated limb perfusion with a pump-oxygenator and large doses of urokinase is necessary.

ENDOVASCULAR MANAGEMENT

Endovascular techniques can be useful in the patient presenting with an acute thrombosis or distal embolization. In many of these patients presenting with an acute event, no obvious outflow vessels are seen.

In the absence of contraindications for the use of pharmacologic thrombolysis, the use of these agents may help define a target vessel for bypass (Fig. 9A,B). The goal of thrombolysis is not to remove thrombus from the popliteal aneurysm, but to dissolve distal thrombus in the outflow vessels to establish a target vessel for the bypass. Once a target vessel has been identified, a standard open surgical bypass with

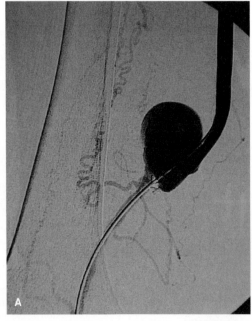
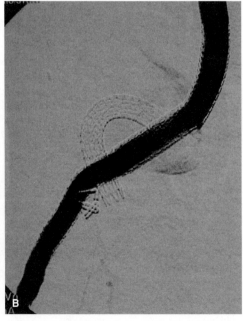

Fig. 10. A: Popliteal artery aneurysm. **B:** Popliteal artery aneurysm treated with a covered stent (Viabahn).

aneurysm exclusion is performed as described above.

The recent availability of numerous expanded polytetrafluoroethylene-covered stents has resulted in an interest in the use of covered stents for treating popliteal artery aneurysms (Fig. 10A,B). No prospective studies are available comparing the use of covered stents to open surgical options. Overall, stents perform poorly in the popliteal artery, due to external compression during flexion of the knee. Until more data are available, this technique should be limited to use in patients who are at poor risk for open surgical procedures and will be able to tolerate long-term warfarin anticoagulation.

SUGGESTED READING

Anton GE, Hertzer NR, Beven EG, et al. Surgical management of popliteal aneurysms: trends in presentation, treatment, and results from 1952–1984. *J Vasc Surg* 1986;3:125.

Borowicz MR, Robison JG, Elliott BM, et al. Occlusive disease associated with popliteal aneurysms: impact on long term graft patency. *J Cardiovasc Surg* 1998;39(2):137.

Braithmaite BD, Quinones-Baldrich WJ. Lower limb intraarterial thrombolysis as an adjunct to the management of arterial and graft occlusions. *World J Surg* 1996;20(6):649.

Carpenter JP, Barker CF, Roberts B, et al. Popliteal artery aneurysms: current management and outcome. *J Vasc Surg* 1994;19:65.

Dawson I, Sie RB, van Bockel JH. Atherosclerotic popliteal aneurysm. *Br J Surg* 1997; 84(3):293.

Duffy ST, Colgen MP, Sultan S, et al. Popliteal aneurysms: a 10-year experience. *Eur J Vasc Endovasc Surg* 1998;16(3):218.

Garramone RR Jr., Gallagher JJ Jr., Drezner AD. Intra-arterial thrombolytic therapy in the initial management of thrombosed popliteal artery aneurysms. *Ann Vasc Surg* 1994;8:363.

Illig KA, Eagleton MJ, Shortell CK, et al. Ruptured popliteal artery aneurysm. *J Vasc Surg* 1998;27(4):783.

Ouriel K. Posterior approach to poplitealcrural bypass: a useful approach. *Semin Vasc Surg* 1997;10(1):23.

Ouriel K. The posterior approach to poplitealcrural bypass. *J Vasc Surg* 1994;19(1):74.

Ouriel K, Rutherford RB. Popliteal aneurysm repair using a posterior approach. In: Ouriel K, Rutherford RB, eds. *Atlas of vascular surgery: operative procedures.* Philadelphia: WB Saunders, 1998:138.

Ouriel K, Shortell CK. Popliteal and femoral aneurysms. In: Rutherford RB, ed. *Vascular surgery,* 4th ed. Philadelphia: WB Saunders, 1995:1103.

Sapienza P, Mingoli A, Feldhaus RJ, et al. Femoral artery aneurysms: long-term follow-up and results of surgical treatment. *Cardiovasc Surg* 1996;4(2):181.

Sarcina A, Bellosta R, Luzzani L, et al. Surgical treatment of popliteal aneurysm. A 20-year experience. *J Cardiovasc Surg* 1997;38(4):347.

Shortell CK, DeWeese JA, Ouriel K, et al. Popliteal artery aneurysm: a 25-year surgical experience. *J Vasc Surg* 1991;14:771.

Thompson JF, Beard J, Scott DJA, et al. Intraoperative thrombolysis in the management of thrombosed popliteal aneurysms. *Br J Surg* 1993;80:858.

Van Sambeek MRHM, Gussenhoven EJ, van der Lugt A, et al. Endovascular stent-grafts for aneurysms of the femoral and popliteal arteries. *Ann Vasc Surg* 1999;13:247.

Varga ZA, Locke-Edmunds JC, Baird RN. A multicenter study of popliteal aneurysms. *J Vasc Surg* 1994;20:171.

EDITOR'S COMMENT

The authors have nicely summarized the demographics and indications for surgery for popliteal aneurysms. Surgeons should be familiar with a variety of technical and anatomic approaches to the popliteal aneurysm, depending on the specific circumstances. I agree with the authors that the posterior approach has many advantages when simple direct repair of the aneurysm is indicated by arteriography. My preference is to use an arterial tourniquet on the thigh to greatly simplify the dissection. The only additional caveat I would add is to watch for the sural nerve, especially when separating the two heads of the gastrocnemius muscle.

Surgeons should also feel completely comfortable managing popliteal aneurysms through the standard medial approach to the proximal and distal popliteal arteries, using a vein bypass graft around the aneurysmal segment, taking care to ligate the popliteal artery proximally and distal to the site of the aneurysm, which eventually leads to thrombosis

of the aneurysm. I suspect, but cannot prove, that taking the posterior approach, which eliminates the mass compression effects of the aneurysm, is advantageous in those circumstances in which the patient has evidence of venous compression by the popliteal aneurysm. The medial approach is especially advantageous when there are issues with thrombosis involved and there is a need to perform thrombectomy or intraoperative thrombolysis.

When a patient presents with critical ischemia, the most important element in operative planning is to obtain a precise runoff arteriogram. This is best accomplished with the arteriographic catheter positioned just proximal to the aneurysm, using digital subtraction angiography (DSA) techniques. The goal is to look for any runoff arterial segment that is suitable for a vein graft anastomosis. If a suitable target artery or even a segment of patent target artery is identified, in my view, the surgeon should proceed immediately with a vein bypass graft. At the time of performing the distal anastomosis,

thrombectomy or thrombolysis may be used, but the value of thrombolysis remains uncertain. Most surgeons have had an occasional dramatic success with thrombolysis in the management of popliteal aneurysms, as the authors describe. However, in my experience, thrombolysis has delayed surgery and, in the end, caused more problems than it solved. For the most part, I have regretted not proceeding directly with arterial reconstruction with or without thrombectomy, as dictated by the circumstances.

The use of stents and stent grafts to repair a popliteal aneurysm remains to be assessed. The alternative for such patients would be a simple direct repair with a short bypass graft. If a patient is deemed to be too high a risk for such a relatively simple procedure, it begs the question of whether anything should be done at all. Nonetheless, this is an area that will continue to be probed by surgeons and endovascular specialists.

J.M.S.

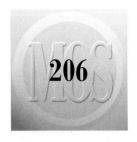

206

Reversed Vein Bypass Graft to Popliteal, Tibial, and Peroneal Arteries

ROBYN A. MACSATA, BYRON FALER, AND ANTON N. SIDAWY

As the average population age keeps increasing, atherosclerosis, in particular lower extremity occlusive disease, is on the rise. Patients presenting with rest pain, nonhealing ulcers, or gangrene are candidates for infrainguinal distal bypass for limb salvage. There are multiple ways to perform an infrainguinal vein bypass, including reversed, in situ, and translocated configurations. In this chapter, we will focus on reverse vein bypass advantages and disadvantages, techniques, and outcomes.

We find the reverse vein bypass technique to be most advantageous in patients requiring short bypasses. There are multiple benefits to this technique, most importantly, maintaining venous endothelial integrity. Because the vein is reversed, there is no need for valvulotomies, with the potential for endothelial damage and long-term consequences of intimal hyperplasia leading to graft thrombosis at these sites. Another benefit, seen in short bypasses, the best portion of the available vein may be used and relocated to the bypass site. For example, in a popliteal-to-tibial bypass, the larger thigh greater saphenous vein may be removed and placed in the distal leg for bypass. This also avoids long skin incisions in the distal aspect of the leg where the skin is often tenuous or even broken down and at risk for poor wound healing and infection secondary to ischemia.

There are two main disadvantages of the reverse vein bypass. First and most importantly, there is a size discrepancy between the inflow and outflow arteries and the ends of the vein used as conduit. This can create a problem at the proximal anastomosis, between the large arterial inflow vessel and the distal smaller aspect of the vein. In small-caliber veins, a postanastomotic stenosis may develop in the vein conduit, which leads to intimal hyperplasia. A second problem with reverse vein bypass is difficulty in treatment of an acute perioperative thrombosis. Secondary to the valves still being in place, passing of thrombectomy catheters is extremely difficult, and usually results in valvular endothelial injury, leaving the graft at risk for recurrent thrombosis.

PREOPERATIVE PLANNING

Many patients with lower extremity ischemia present with foot infections including abscesses and wet gangrene. These patients need to have thorough irrigation and debridement of their abscesses and infected tissue followed by a course of intravenous antibiotics before proceeding with revascularization. Only when these foot infections have completely cleared and the foot is believed to be salvageable does treatment for arterial ischemia proceed.

Adequate visualization of inflow and outflow vessels through high-quality preoperative arteriogram is essential in distal bypasses. To improve quality, arteriograms are obtained in an appropriate radiology suite using digital subtraction imaging. Selective catheterization to at least the external iliac artery is imperative to adequately visualize outflow vessels. Intra-arterial injections of papaverine or nitroglycerin help to vasodilate and better visualize outflow vessels. Lower extremity arteriograms are only complete once adequate visualization of the inflow and outflow vessels is achieved.

Preoperative venous mapping performed in the noninvasive vascular laboratory is not routinely performed; however, this can be particularly useful in a subgroup of patients. Vein is often in limited supply in patients who have had multiple venous harvests for cardiac or other peripheral bypass procedures, and vein mapping can identify the longest lengths of vein left available. Also, in patients requiring a long distal bypass, such as a common femoral artery to dorsalis pedis bypass, an adequate length vein may be identified preoperatively and help avoid the need for multiple harvests and venovenostomies. When preoperative vein mapping is done, all harvest sites are marked in the vascular laboratory, which decreases the need for multiple skin incisions and helps avoid large skin flaps at harvest sites, improving wound healing.

Arterial Inflow

Shorter bypasses require less vein conduit, which allows the surgeon to choose the best segment of the vein available, as well as decreasing the need for venovenostomies. Therefore, the inflow of venous bypasses is taken as distally as possible in the lower extremity. The common femoral artery is used when necessary; however, the profunda femoris, the superficial femoral artery, and the popliteal artery are all adequate sources of inflow and are used when available. Also, in secondary procedures, the common femoral artery may be previously dissected and used for bypass, making repeat dissection difficult. By using distal sources of inflow this challenging and often tedious dissection may be avoided.

Arterial Outflow

The most important determining factor for adequate distal outflow is the preoperative arteriogram. As mentioned previously, this makes high-quality arteriograms with adequate visualization of outflow vessels imperative. To decrease the length of our vein conduit, we choose the most proximal popliteal or tibial artery with the best runoff to the foot as our distal target vessel.

Venous Conduit

When deciding on portions of vein to harvest, the best available vein of appropriate length is used at all times. Multiple pieces of vein require venovenostomies to be performed and decreases long-term graft patency rates overall. This situation can be avoided by using shorter bypasses.

Our choices for venous conduit in order include ipsilateral greater saphenous vein, contralateral greater saphenous vein, arm vein, and lesser saphenous vein. Use of the contralateral greater saphenous vein is rarely associated with limb loss on the contralateral side; therefore, we do not hesitate to use this vein.

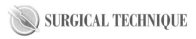 SURGICAL TECHNIQUE

Arterial Dissection

The common femoral as well as proximal superficial and profunda femoral arteries

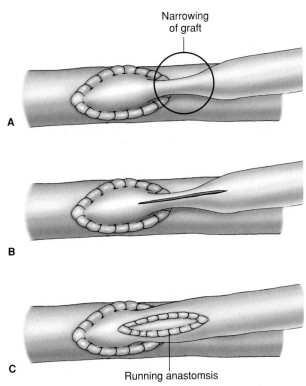

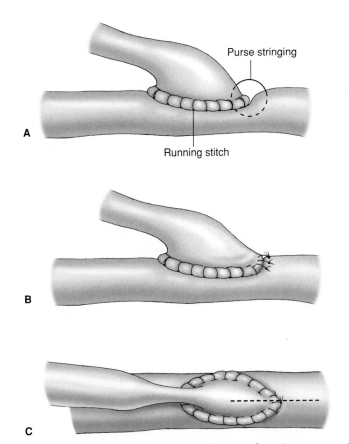

Fig. 7. Technique of patching proximal anastomosis. **A:** Conventional anastomosis is prone to narrowing in proximal portion of graft. **B:** Venotomy through area of narrowing. **C:** Narrowing alleviated with proximal venous patch.

Fig. 8. Technique of distal anastomosis. **A:** Standard technique of running anastomosis leaves toe of anastomosis prone to purse stringing. **B:** Interrupted sutures placed at toe of anastomosis prevents purse stringing. **C:** Interrupted sutures allow for opening of hood of anastomosis without unraveling of suture line.

conduit, and distal runoff are performed routinely. This is done by percutaneous cannulation of the proximal hood of the graft with a 20-gauge butterfly needle. The arteriogram is completed with intraoperative fluoroscopy using digital subtraction imaging and hand injection of contrast mixed half and half with saline. If distal visualization is not adequate, the butterfly needle is moved further distally in the graft, just above the distal anastomosis, and imaging is completed.

Skin Closure and Wound Management

Wounds are closed in as many layers as possible with interrupted or continuous 3–0 Vicryl sutures for subcutaneous tissue, taking care not to injure or compress the graft. In the femoral incision, we do not close the deep fascia secondary to possible graft compression. Distally, the deep compartments are also left open because of inevitable postbypass lower extremity edema and concern of compartment syndrome. The proximal skin is closed with staples and any distal tenuous skin is closed with interrupted vertical mattress sutures of 3–0 nylon. Dry dressings are placed and are removed 2 days postoperatively and left open to air, except for groin incisions, which are always covered with a dry dressing until healed. These groin wounds, especially in patients with a large pannus, are prone to breakdown and infection. All staples and sutures are removed 2 weeks later.

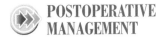

POSTOPERATIVE MANAGEMENT

Rarely are any foot procedures done at the time of distal bypass. All infected foot wounds are thoroughly irrigated and debrided and left open prior to revascularization. These open wounds are closed secondarily approximately 1 week after revascularization. Any amputations of dry gangrene are also completed approximately 1 to 2 weeks after revascularization, when lines of demarcation are clear.

Early ambulation with the assistance of physical therapy staff is encouraged as soon as the 1st postoperative day. Weight-bearing status is determined by any foot procedures required in the perioperative period.

We do not prescribe anticoagulation therapy to patients when autogenous vein is used, except low-dose aspirin. If patients have previously been taking Plavix or Coumadin, this is resumed on postoperative

Vascular Surgery

day 1 as long as no significant wound bleeding is noted.

Grafts are monitored closely during the perioperative period by evaluating distal pulses, graft pulse, or ankle brachial indices. If a graft is believed to be thrombosed clinically or if confirmed by duplex evaluation, the patient is immediately brought back to the operating room for re-evaluation. As discussed previously, one of the main drawbacks of the reverse bypass is difficulty with thrombectomy secondary to competent valves left behind. This makes passing of a thrombectomy catheter complicated, with the potential of endothelial injury at patent valve sites. In our practice, we have used the following technique for thrombectomy of reversed vein. A thrombectomy catheter is passed from the proximal to distal anastomosis in the direction of the blood flow, opening the competent valves. Next, distally, a second thrombectomy catheter is tied to the first, and the two catheters are fed distally to proximally, through the previously opened valves. The first thrombectomy catheter is untied and removed. The second thrombectomy catheter is then inflated and passed proximally to distally, performing the thrombectomy in the direction of the valves and therefore not injuring the competent valves.

Once the patient is discharged, routine long-term follow-up is scheduled for graft surveillance at 6 weeks postoperatively and then biannually. Any stenosis in the graft or at the anastomotic sites is further evaluated with arteriogram and treated to prevent graft thrombosis, either with endovascular angioplasty or open patch angioplasty.

Patency Rates

Several studies have evaluated the patency rates of reverse vein and in situ vein bypasses. In a review of the current literature, 2-year patency rates for reverse vein bypasses range from 69% to 82%, and 2-year patency rates for in situ vein bypasses are similar at 69% to 80%. Also, there is no difference in limb salvage rates between these two groups of patients. In both groups, the most significant determining factor in patency rates and limb salvage is the distal target vessel; those patients with infrapopliteal bypasses have significantly lower patency and limb salvage rates than both above-the-knee and below-the-knee popliteal bypasses. Also noted in the literature, the most common cause of graft failure in reverse vein bypasses is vein stenosis just adjacent to the proximal anastomosis. As we have discussed, this is secondary to the small diameter of the vein just distal to the proximal anastomosis, and this area should be thoroughly evaluated and treated, if necessary, at the time of reverse vein bypass placement. This size discrepancy is probably the best argument favoring in situ or transpositional vein configurations over reversed vein.

CONCLUSION

Using the preoperative planning, surgical techniques, and postoperative care described in this chapter, we find reverse vein distal bypasses to be a satisfactory technique for limb salvage in patients presenting with rest pain or gangrene. In our practice, we find this technique to be ideally suited for patients requiring short bypasses below the knee, allowing for the best segments of vein to be used while minimizing incisions in the distal aspect of the leg.

SUGGESTED READING

Ballotta E, Renon L, De Rossi A, Barbon B, Terranova O, Da Giau G. Prospective randomized study on reversed saphenous vein infrapopliteal bypass to treat limb-threatening ischemia: common femoral artery versus superficial femoral or popliteal and tibial arteries as inflow. *J Vasc Surg* 2004;40:732.

Bandyk DF. Infrainguinal vein bypass graft surveillance: how to do it, when to intervene, and is it cost-effective? *J Am Coll Surg* 2002;194(1 suppl):S40.

Berkowitz HD, Greenstein S, Barker CF, Perloff LJ. Late failure of reversed vein bypass grafts. *Ann Surg* 1989;210:782.

Bush HL Jr, Nabseth DC, Curl GR, O'Hara ET, Johnson WC, Vollman RW. In situ saphenous vein bypass grafts for limb salvage. A current fad or a viable alternative to reversed vein bypass grafts? *Am J Surg* 1985;149:477.

Cruz CP, Eidt JF, Brown AT, Moursi M. Correlation between preoperative and postoperative duplex vein measurements of the greater saphenous vein used for infrainguinal arterial reconstruction. *Vasc Endovascular Surg* 2004;38:57.

Dalman RL, Harris EJ, Zarins CK. Is completion arteriography mandatory after reversed-vein bypass grafting? *J Vasc Surg* 1996;23:637.

Faries PL, Teodorescu VJ, Morrissey NJ, Hollier LH, Marin ML. The role of surgical revascularization in the management of diabetic foot wounds. *Am J Surg* 2004;187:34S.

Harris PL, Veith FJ, Shanik GD, Nott D, Wengerter KR, Moore DJ. Prospective randomized comparison of in situ and reversed infrapopliteal vein grafts. *Br J Surg* 1993;80:173.

Lawson JA, Tangelder MJ, Algra A, Eikelboom BC. The myth of the in situ graft: superiority in infrainguinal bypass surgery? *Eur J Vasc Endovasc Surg* 1999;18:149.

Moody AP, Edwards PR, Harris PL In situ versus reversed femoropopliteal vein grafts: long-term follow-up of a prospective, randomized trial. *Br J Surg* 1992;79:750.

Sasajima T, Kubo Y, Kokubo M, Izumi Y, Inaba M. Comparison of reversed and in situ saphenous vein grafts for infragenicular bypass: experience of two surgeons. *Cardiovasc Surg* 1993;1:38.

Taylor LM Jr, Edwards JM, Phinney ES, Porter JM. Reversed vein bypass to infrapopliteal arteries. Modern results are superior to or equivalent to in-situ bypass for patency and for vein utilization. *Ann Surg* 1987;205:90.

Taylor LM Jr, Edwards JM, Porter JM. Present status of reversed vein bypass grafting: five-year results of a modern series. *J Vasc Surg* 1990;11:193.

Taylor LM Jr, Phinney ES, Porter JM. Present status of reversed vein bypass for lower extremity revascularization. *J Vasc Surg* 1986;3:288.

Watelet J, Cheysson E, Poels D, Menard JF, Papion H, Saour N, Testart J. In situ versus reversed saphenous vein for femoropopliteal bypass: a prospective randomized study of 100 cases. *Ann Vasc Surg* 1987;1:441.

EDITOR'S COMMENT

Despite a proliferation of endovascular procedures for infrainguinal occlusive disease, vein femoral-popliteal and distal tibial bypass will remain common and important operations for saving limbs in the increasing population of elderly patients with peripheral arterial disease. Many of these individuals, especially those in their 80s and 90s, do not have the classic atherosclerotic risk factors of smoking, dyslipidemia, hypertension, diabetes mellitus, and family history (genetic predisposition). They appear to have only age-related deterioration of their peripheral vasculature.

The operation described by Dr. Sidawy and his colleagues is the classic approach and is sound and effective. The differences that I point out are more differences of style rather than of substance. The first difference is that I prefer the nonreversed, translocated vein bypass. This avoids

(continued)

the discrepancy in size between the inflow and outflow arteries and the ends of the vein graft. As pointed out, the size discrepancy at the proximal anastomosis can lead to a stenotic area in the vein graft just distal to the "hood" of the vein graft that may need remedial patching as described by the authors. In addition, I think that fear of acute thrombosis from instrumenting the vein graft to disrupt venous valves and associated endothelial damage is more theoretical than real, and is probably outweighed by the superior hemodynamics of a conduit with valves rendered incompetent. (Walsh DB, et al. *J Surg Res* 1987;42:39; Chin AK, et al. *J Vasc Surg* 1988;8:316). However, I must admit that this is also a largely theoretical advantage and is not proven. Bottom line: both techniques are valid and it is impossible to argue that one approach is superior to another.

In this day and age, I don't think that it is necessary to obtain digital subtraction arteriography on all patients. High-resolution computed tomographic angiography (CTA) from multidetector row systems (Ouwendijk R, et al. *Radiology* 2005;236:1094), magnetic resonance angiography (Swan JS, et al. *Radiology* 2002;225:43), and even duplex ultrasonagraphy (Staffa, R, et al. *J Vasc Surg* 2006, in press) have been used by many to find distal "targets." All of these imaging modalities are less invasive than digital subtraction arteriography, and some are less expensive. Our approach has evolved to using CTA cou-

pled with prebypass angiography in the operating room when CTA doesn't adequately image distal arteries. CTA is rapidly improving and may replace conventional arteriography for most imaging needs.

As for tunneling, I prefer an anatomic approach rather than routing the vein bypass through the subcutaneum. The anatomic passage may require more dissection, but the deeply placed vein graft is less likely to get infected if there are wound complications. Wound infections are quite common in this population, and the subcutaneous vein bypass may disrupt if it becomes infected by contiguous wound sepsis that may be only a few millimeters away. This is rare, but it is a life-threatening problem when it occurs. The anatomic placement also makes the vein graft less vulnerable to kinking.

Wound complications may be avoided by harvesting the vein through carefully placed interrupted or "skip" incisions over the course of the vein. This technique is particularly useful in obese patients. The long "slash" to harvest vein is, in my opinion, to be avoided. Another approach that has some merit is the endoscopic harvest technique. This also reduces the incidence of wound complications from vein harvest but may be associated with increased trauma to the vein graft, has a bit of a learning curve, and may be cost-ineffective.

The final issue worthy of discussion is the role of antithrombotic therapy in the postoperative period and on long-term follow-up. A large, random-

ized trial from the Netherlands (the Dutch BOA Study) showed superiority of warfarin anticoagulation with a rather high INR (3.0–4.0) over aspirin therapy in maintaining patency (Dutch Bypass Oral Anticoagulants or Aspirin (BOA) Study Group, *Lancet* 2000;355:346; Tangelder MJD, et al. *J Vasc Surg* 2001;33:522). However, the benefit was marginal and a there was a significant and disturbing increase in the incidence of major hemorrhage in patients on warfarin therapy. In addition, a Veterans Affairs Cooperative randomized study showed an excessive incidence of bleeding complications in patients receiving warfarin (INR 2.0–3.0) plus aspirin versus aspirin alone, and no significant improvement in patency or any other outcomes (Johnson WC, Williford WO. *J Vasc Surg* 202;35:413). Thus, I prefer aspirin treatment for the majority of patients undergoing infrainguinal bypass unless the quality of the runoff or the bypass conduit is poor. In the latter group of patients I will use warfarin plus aspirin, particularly for reoperative bypasses. This strategy is based on a small, randomized trial that showed superior patency and limb salvage in patients with severely "disadvantaged" infrainguinal bypasses treated with this regimen (Sarac TP, et al. *J Vasc Surg* 1998;28:446). Patients treated with warfarin plus aspirin must be thoroughly reliable and monitored closely.

G.P.C.

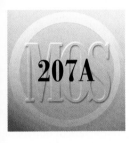

Use of Arm Vein Conduit for Lower Extremity Revascularization

ALLEN D. HAMDAN, AMY R. EVENSON, AND LORELEI GRUNWALDT

INTRODUCTION

The ipsilateral greater saphenous vein (GSV) is the conduit of choice for lower extremity bypass procedures. Given the utility of this conduit in coronary artery bypass grafting (CABG) and the high prevalence of co-morbid coronary artery disease in patients receiving CABG, the ipsilateral GSV may not be available for lower extremity revascularization. While some authors advocate the use of the contralateral GSV, the presence of synchronous and metachronous lesions of the contralateral lower extremity make use of the contralateral GSV unappealing in patients who have a high likelihood of requiring contralateral revascularization. For these reasons, it is important to be familiar with alternative conduits for use in patients with lower extremity ischemia when the ipsilateral GSV is unavailable or too short. Options for vascular conduit in these situations include the lesser saphenous vein (LSV), prosthetic conduit

(polytetrafluoroethylene, knitted polyester), composite or sequential grafts, or upper extremity veins.

The LSV may be a good choice for a short graft or as part of a composite graft using more than one vein segment; however, the LSV is generally smaller in diameter and not of sufficient length for a long bypass. Compared to any autologous conduit, prosthetic grafts have lower patency, higher infection rates, and worse results when they do occlude. Generally, aside from bypass to the above-knee segment of the popliteal artery, prosthetic grafts are used as a last resort. Sequential and composite grafts are used infrequently and are outside the scope of this chapter. It is our practice that after ipsilateral GSV, the arm vein is the next best choice for lower extremity revascularization. The similar size, ability to achieve adequate length, and ease of harvest allow for a great deal of flexibility when using this conduit. Although many of the same techniques and principles employed when using prosthetic grafts

or greater saphenous vein as conduits apply to the use of upper extremity veins, there are a number of issues and technical points that are specific to the use of arm veins.

 ANATOMY OF ARM VEINS

It is crucial to have a working understanding of the anatomy of the vessels and nerves of the upper extremity when the choice is made to use the arm vein as a bypass conduit. There is nothing more frustrating than searching for a vein when none is readily apparent and the incision has already been made (Figs. 1 and 2).

Cephalic Vein

The cephalic vein starts at the wrist on the dorsal surface of the forearm, crosses onto the anterior surface of the arm in the midforearm, and runs up the lateral aspect of the arm to the elbow. It is joined by multiple perforators and connects at the level of

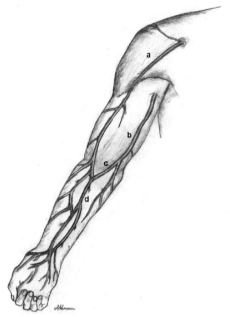

Fig. 1. Veins of the arm. *a:* Cephalic vein. *b:* Basilic vein. *c:* Median cubital vein. *d:* Median antebrachial vein.

the antecubital fossa via the median cubital vein to the basilic vein. The cephalic vein then continues up the lateral aspect of the anterior upper arm to the shoulder and into the deltopectoral groove. At the level

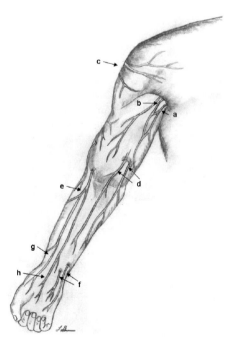

Fig. 2. Nerves of the arm. *a:* Intercostobrachial nerve. *b:* Medial brachial cutaneous nerve. *c:* Superior lateral brachial cutaneous nerve. *d:* Branches of medial antebrachial cutaneous nerve. *e:* Lateral antebrachial cutaneous nerve. *f:* Dorsal and palmar branches of ulnar nerve. *g:* Superficial branch of radial nerve. *h:* Palmar branch of median nerve.

of the clavicle, the cephalic vein pierces the fascia to join the axillary vein.

Basilic Vein

The basilic vein starts somewhat posteriorly on the medial forearm receiving multiple perforators before connecting to the cephalic vein via the median cubital vein. The basilic vein then extends up the medial aspect of the upper arm into the axilla and is joined by multiple branches draining the shoulder girdle to form the axillary vein. Due to its posterior location on the forearm, harvest of this portion can be challenging and always requires two surgeons. The upper arm basilica is much more easily removed by a single surgeon.

Venous Relations to the Nerves of the Upper Extremity

The cephalic and basilic veins course in the cutaneous plane of the arm superficial to the fascia overlying the muscular compartments. During dissection of these vessels, a number of superficial nerves are encountered. The distal cephalic vein is in close proximity to the superficial branch of the radial nerve at the level of the wrist. In the midforearm, the cephalic vein runs among the branches of the lateral antebrachial cutaneous nerve, a branch of the musculocutaneous nerve. In the upper arm, the cephalic vein crosses branches of the inferior and superior lateral brachial cutaneous nerves while at the level of the shoulder, it is deep to branches of the supraclavicular nerves. The basilic vein runs in proximity to the anterior and posterior branches of the medial antebrachial cutaneous nerves throughout its course in the forearm and upper arm. At the level of the axilla, the vein runs deep to the intercostobrachial and medial brachial cutaneous nerves. Careful dissection is required to avoid damaging the many nerves found in the course of these vessels and the resultant paresthesias, numbness, or neuroma formation that may accompany injury to these nerves.

◀◀ PREOPERATIVE PLANNING

In deciding which configuration of arm vein will be used for a specific bypass procedure, a number of factors must be considered. The characteristics of the various upper arm veins provide some guidance. If harvested onto the shoulder girdle, the cephalic vein is longer than the basilic vein. However, the cephalic vein is often

the place chosen for intravenous catheters and phlebotomy access, which can result in significant sclerosis or webbing. The segment of the vein in the forearm is most likely to be of substandard quality and tends to be smaller than the basilic vein, especially below the antecubital crease.

To select the proper arm vein construct it is paramount that the inflow and outflow targets are chosen ahead of time based on preoperative angiography. This requires a clear decision on both a best-case scenario for bypass (i.e., planned procedure if there was unlimited vein) as well as at least one or two alternative plans should there not be adequate conduit for the first-choice procedure. This will provide a realistic idea of the length of venous conduit required and whether it is likely to involve a continuous segment or require splicing.

The patient should undergo bilateral upper extremity vein mapping using duplex ultrasound to determine patency as well as vein diameter. In some cases, ultrasound will reveal wall thickening or sclerosis, but these findings are not always apparent. In general, diameters of 3 mm or greater are required for adequate upper extremity conduit. It is also important to pay attention to major size changes (i.e., a vein that is 3 mm in the antecubital fossa but only 1.5 mm in the upper arm) before deciding on which vein to harvest for bypass.

After adequate vein mapping and a clear understanding of the length of bypass required, a simple bedside maneuver can be performed to confirm a realistic approach to lower extremity bypass using umbilical tape. First, the expected length of the venous conduit on the surface of the patient's leg is measured. Then, the umbilical tape is placed on the arm and which choice of venous segments is most suitable is determined. This maneuver helps to avoid the situation where what appears to be adequate length of vein preoperatively is found to be inadequate during the harvest, requiring multiple venovenostomies to proceed. Finally, attention must be paid to the diameters of the vein conduit at sites of potential anastomoses. For example, the shoulder portion of the basilic vein is often greater than 5 mm in diameter and would be a poor choice to be sewn to a small dorsalis pedis artery, while it would be a great choice for the proximal anastomoses to the common femoral artery.

In constructing a lower extremity bypass, there are several choices of arm vein segments to choose from:

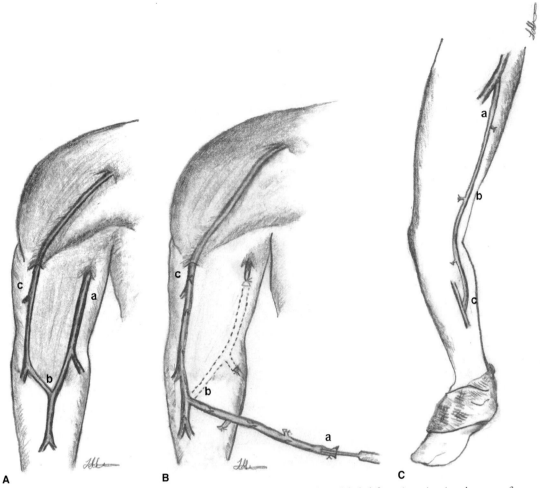

Fig. 3. Basilic–cephalic vein loop. **A:** Three points (*a, b,* and *c*) have been labeled for orientation in subsequent figures. *Point b* is the location at which the cephalic vein is divided in the forearm. The divided stump will later be used for insertion of the valvulotome. **B:** Harvesting of arm veins with mobilization of the basilic vein to become the inflow segment. The end of the vein is cannulated to facilitate subsequent valvulotomy. Before cannulation the end of the basilic vein may be everted so that the first valve can be excised with a scissors. **C:** The vein bypass graft in position. The proximal basilic segment is in the "nonreversed" orientation while the distal cephalic segment is in the "reversed" orientation. (Permission pending from LoGerfo FW, Paniszyn CW, Menzoian J. A new arm vein graft for distal bypass. *J Vasc Surg* 1987;5:889.)

1. Entire cephalic vein from wrist to shoulder
2. Entire basilic vein from posterior forearm to axilla
3. Cephalic–basilic upper arm vein loop connected via the median cubital vein (Fig. 3)
4. Cephalic vein in forearm to the median cubital vein in the antecubital fossa and then to the basilic vein to the axilla

In addition, there are multiple options involving splicing pieces of cephalic vein to basilic vein or segments of GSV or LSV. Ultimately, the goal is to obtain the best segment of vein for bypass and limit the number of venovenostomies required to attain a vein conduit of sufficient length for use in the lower extremity.

Once the harvest site is chosen, the arm vein must be protected. If the patient is in-house, instruct the team to place a sign over the bed that no intravenous catheters may be placed or blood draws performed on that arm. For elective patients, choose the arm that will be used and tell the patient to protect himself or herself from any blood draws or intravenous placements until the scheduled operation. Communication with the anesthesia team must be performed to avoid placement of intravenous or arterial lines on the side to be harvested.

Finally, it is worth mentioning the special circumstance of performing a bypass in a patient on hemodialysis with a functioning fistula. In the setting where another surgeon is involved in the long-term management of a patient's vascular access options, a discussion should occur between the teams before the use of arm vein conduit. Use of arm vein without consultation with the transplant team may limit the patient's options for future hemodialysis access. Alternate choices should be made in this setting.

INTRAOPERATIVE MANAGEMENT

Dissection commences with the arm vein harvest to avoid exposing arterial segments that cannot be reached with the available conduit. The patient is positioned with two arm boards with the arm extended and completely shaved and prepped to include the shoulder and axilla. Electrocardiogram leads are removed from the shoulder girdle. The radial arterial line as well as any other intravenous lines should be on the opposite side. If there has been a mistake with the arterial line being placed on the index side, use of additional tubing extending over the fingers and off the hand will prevent the tubing from pulling the arm from its straight positioning. The line may be prepped into the field or the prep stopped just proximal to the line site. Should an intravenous line be placed on the side to be harvested, it can be pulled out and the vein used if there are no other choices. However, with optimum planning and communication to the residents and nursing and anesthesia staff, this problem should not be encountered.

Depending on the segment to be taken, it is often easiest to find the cephalic vein at the wrist, and then follow it up the forearm. Dissection should proceed in the plane directly on top of the vein with the use of Metzenbaum scissors to spread underneath the skin and Mayo scissors to cut the skin. When performed with an assistant, this dissection can proceed very quickly. It is crucial to stay directly on top of the anterior surface of the vein and not leave extensive areolar tissue intact. Arm veins will be less formidable from a textural sense than a saphenous vein, so it is important to be able to visualize the intima and the adventitia without extraneous tissue. It is also important when dissecting the length of vein to spread in an anteroposterior fashion as opposed to medial-lateral. There are very few anterior branches, and this approach avoids the inevitable branch avulsion that may occur when the proper technique is not employed.

Based on preoperative vein mapping and on what length of vein is needed, it is often important to preserve the medial cubital vein. In the situation where the distal cephalic vein connected via the median cubital vein to the proximal basilic vein is to be used, creation of a continuous incision from the wrist to the upper arm results in unacceptable wound morbidity. Instead, creation of a skin bridge between the basilic vein incision above the elbow crease and the forearm cephalic incision allows for a fairly easy dissection under the skin bridge to free up the cephalic and median cubital veins and for them to be pulled into the upper arm incision. In addition, it is incredibly helpful to disconnect either the distal cephalic or basilic vein at the wrist, ligate it, and then place a Marks needle with heparinized saline and papaverine into the vein. With gentle distension, it is very easy to find the side branches for ligation and to have a poor man's assessment of the size and suitability of the venous conduit.

Another maneuver to consider is to perform in situ angioscopy. Angioscopy, in general, is mandatory for arm veins unless very short segments are to be used. The

high incidence of webbing in the areas of previous intravenous lines, and especially when the median cubital vein is part of the construct, mandates evaluation of the lumen of the vessel prior to its use. The routine use of angioscopy can be a sensitive method of detecting intraluminal problems that may not be obvious from external examination of the vein. In one series, intraluminal disease was noted in 62.8% of arm veins harvested for use in bypass. Identification of significant webs, stenosis, or sclerosis allows endoscopic or surgical interventions on troublesome segments and may allow for the conduit to be "upgraded," improving early graft patency. Prior to disconnection of a long length venous conduit, a sterile angioscopy set is brought onto the field, the vein is cannulated at the most distal location, and a bulldog clamp is placed on the vein at shoulder level. This is a quick look and is not meant to lyse valves, just to make sure there is not a segment that looks suitable from the outside but has dense webbing or significant sclerosis inside. Thus, before removing an entire cephalic vein and then realizing that a 5-cm segment in the forearm is unusable, the decision can be made to switch to the upper arm cephalic–basilic loop or alternate site. This is an attempt to avoid splicing together multiple pieces with venovenostomies. After harvest of the entire vein, a second angioscopy is performed on a sterile back table to lyse the valve segments. The vein is then placed in a heparin–papaverine solution on ice until the proximal and distal anastomoses are performed.

A special comment should be made about the technique of tying side branches in venous conduits, which is especially important in arm veins. Arm vein branches can be very fragile and tend to avulse causing fairly large defects when not handled properly. In addition, these branches can be short and stubby. Smaller ties are often better since they allow for direct apposition of the vein wall. Ideally, a 3–0 or 4–0 silk tie should be applied to the vein side and a clip or additional tie on the other end of the branch. The tie should not be directly flush but approximately 1 mm away from the vein wall to avoid narrowing. Narrowing can also occur with sloppy harvest when a great deal of connective tissue is left intact and pulled in with the tie. There should also be a large stump or cuff of vein branch distal to the tie so that when the vein is arterialized and distended, the tie will not pop off. Double ties are cumbersome and it is better to place a single, properly placed tie. Another common error occurs with the few large posterior branches encountered in the upper arm segment of the basilic vein; if the assistant tries to provide too much exposure and inadvertently bends the vein at an angle when the posterior branch is tied, it will significantly impinge on the wall and cause narrowing of the vein.

On occasion, a vein branch tie will be found to be impinging upon the lumen of the conduit (dumb-belling) (Fig. 4). This situation may become evident when the graft is distended either with heparin–papaverine solution via a Marks

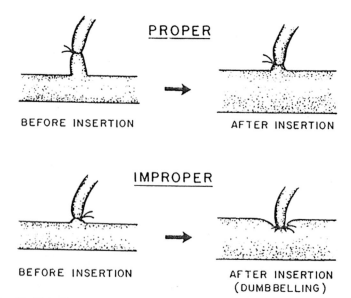

Fig. 4. Dumbbelling. Placement of side branch ties too close to the vein may result in dumbbelling of the vein. A technique to remedy this problem is described in the text. (Permission pending from Campbell DR, Hoar CS, Gibbons GW. The use of arm veins in femoral-popliteal bypass grafts. *Ann Surg* 1979;190:740.)

needle or after releasing the clamp on the proximal anastomosis. One way to salvage the situation is to use a fine curved snap and dissect away the excess areolar tissue inevitably caught in the tie and then cut this tissue with a tenotomy scissor. A word of caution, however, is to avoid this maneuver with the vein under full arterial pressure since arm veins are thin-walled and can be readily torn under these circumstances.

Several other points are worth mentioning about the harvest. As described above, there are several cutaneous nerves that are encountered during the dissection of the upper extremity veins. The best way to avoid these nerves is to stay directly on the vein and not to create any flaps. The nerve branches are much more apparent over the basilic vein, especially in the upper arm. In addition, meticulous hemostasis is important because a minimal hematoma will cause significant patient discomfort. A hematoma in the upper arm over the basilic vein can cause a median nerve compression syndrome. Closure of the vein harvest site is generally achieved with a subcutaneous layer of running 3–0 Vicryl. The skin is closed with either staples or a subcuticular closure. The arm is then placed in an ACE bandage from hand to shoulder prior to emergence from anesthesia.

In certain patients, the length of arm vein needed to perform the bypass would necessitate more than one venovenostomy regardless of choice of segment. If the patient has an adequately sized lesser saphenous vein (i.e. in the 3.0 mm range), it may be wise to start in the prone position, harvest the lesser saphenous vein, and close the leg prior to harvesting the arm vein. The two segments can then be spliced together with one venovenostomy.

Generally, as expected, the most proximal portions of the cephalic and basilic veins have the largest diameter. In fact, the proximal basilic vein may be quite large (up to 0.5 to 0.7 cm). Thus, when constructing the venous conduit, the proximal basilic vein may be suitable for in-flow anastomosis, but is often a poor choice for a distal anastomosis to the dorsalis pedis or distal tibial vessel because of size mismatch. This principle is most important in the cephalic–basilic loop (Fig. 3). The proximal basilic vein is harvested in continuity with the median cubital vein and proximal cephalic vein. A skin bridge is left intact over the cubital fossa whenever possible. Maintaining a short segment of the cephalic vein distal to its junction with the median cubital vein will allow for introduction of a valvulotome to lyse the valves of the basilic vein. Use of the larger proximal basilic vein

in the proximal anastomosis in the leg allows the smaller proximal cephalic vein to be used to bypass to the distal below-knee popliteal or tibial or peroneal vessels.

Whether the arm vein graft is tunneled or placed in the subcutaneous plane in the leg depends on the specific operation performed. However, since the arm vein is potentially more likely to develop a stenosis that may require either a jump graft or a vein patch angioplasty to salvage the graft, placement in a subcutaneous location is often advisable. For example, in performing a common femoral to anterior tibial artery bypass, use of a lateral approach to the anterior tibial artery with placement of the vein graft in a lateral subcutaneous tunnel allows easier access for future revisions to the graft.

The technique of venovenostomy deserves special comment. As many lower extremity bypass procedures that require arm vein conduit are reoperative cases that require a significant length of vein, it is not uncommon to need to perform venovenostomies to obtain an appropriate conduit. One technique to facilitate this challenging anastomosis is to use a clear French pediatric feeding tube placed through the vein across the area that is to be anastomosed. Both segments are spatulated and a suture tied at either end of the spatulation anteriorly and posteriorly. The sutures are then run toward each other and tied in the middle. The two-suture technique over a feeding tube minimizes any potential for twisting and ensures a reasonable lumen size. It is important, however, not to make too large a spatulation, especially when sewing a large basilic vein to a small cephalic vein. A large spatulation will result in a nearly 45-degree angle as the two pieces come together and can be a potential site for kinking or twisting resulting in poor flow characteristics.

POSTOPERATIVE MANAGEMENT

In addition to routine postbypass care, the patient's arm is elevated overnight with the ACE wrap left in place. The next

morning, the ACE wrap and dressing are completely removed. The wound is examined and then rewrapped for 1 or 2 more days. Any significant hematoma should be re-explored because it may be painful for the patient and can lead to severe wound problems as well as potential nerve damage. It is also important to counsel patients preoperatively about the potential for some numbness and paresthesias that can occur. However, it is very uncommon for any significant swelling to occur after the initial perioperative period. Skin staples are removed 10 to 14 days postoperatively depending on the patient's co-morbidities.

Postoperative graft surveillance is essential, but the appropriate intervals are debated. Our practice is to follow arm vein grafts more closely and often start surveillance at 6 weeks. This earlier time point has not been clinically proven, but it does make sense given the increased risk of graft failure using an arm vein conduit as compared to GSV. Correction of anastomotic or midgraft stenosis identified on standard follow-up prior to graft thrombosis allows improved secondary patency and limb salvage. Armstrong et al. reported that routine postoperative surveillance resulted in intervention (percutaneous transluminal balloon angioplasty or open surgical repair) on 48% of grafts resulting in a 3-year assisted primary patency rate of 91%.

OUTCOMES OF ARM VEIN CONDUIT IN LOWER EXTREMITY BYPASS GRAFTING

Numerous reports suggest the utility of arm veins in reconstruction of the vasculature of the lower extremity (Table 1). The largest series of arm vein conduits used in lower extremity bypass reported the results of 524 revascularization procedures. In this series, 85% of patients had diabetes mellitus and follow-up ranged from 1 month to 7.4 years with a mean of 24.9 months. Primary patency in this series was 80.2% at 1 year and 54.5% at 5 years, with limb salvage rates of 89.8% and 71.5% at 1 and 5 years, respectively. This series reported similar patency rates between composite and simple vein conduits.

TABLE 1.

Study	No. Patients	1-Year Patency	Limb Salvage
Campbell 1979	18	82%	N/A
Balshi 1989	33	73%	86%
Marcaccio 1983	104	71%	N/A
Holzenbein 1995	54	74.7%	90.7%

TABLE 2.

Graft Type	1-Year Primary Patency	3-Year Primary Patency	5-Year Primary Patency	1-Year Secondary Patency	3-Year Secondary Patency	5-Year Secondary Patency	1-Year Limb Salvage	3-Year Limb Salvage	5-Year Limb Salvage
Arm Vein	76.9 ± 4.8	70.0 ± 8.0	53.8 ± 8.7	77.5 ± 4.6	70.7 ± 7.5	57.7 ± 8.0	89.3 ± 3.7	80.5 ± 7.0	76.3 ± 9.9
Composite	59.5 ± 9.6	43.7 ± 12.4	0	59.8 ± 9.5	44.9 ± 13.1	0	73.9 ± 8.9	49.6 ± 14.3	0

From Faries PL, LoGerfo FW, Arora S, et al. Arm vein conduit is superior to composite prosthetic-autogenous grafts in lower extremity revascularization. *J Vasc Surg* 2000;31:1119. Figures are expressed in percent ± standard deviation.

The use of arm vein conduit compares favorably to the use of prosthetic grafts in lower extremity revascularization. Prospective follow-up of 506 arm vein and 234 prosthetic lower extremity bypass grafts demonstrated the superiority of arm vein conduit. Patency and limb-salvage rates varied by graft configuration with more proximal grafts achieving better 1- and 3-year values. For femoro-below-knee-popliteal grafts, 1- and 3-year primary patency was 92.9% and 72.8% for arm vein conduits compared to 83.4% and 55.5% for prosthetic grafts, respectively. For femorotibial bypasses, arm vein grafts provided 81.6% and 68.3% patency at 1- and 3-year follow-up, respectively, while prosthetic grafts afforded 58.0% and 41.4% patency over the same time periods. The 1- and 3-year limb-salvage rates were improved in the arm vein group in femorotibial bypasses at 91.1% and 81.4% as compared to 58.0% and 41.1% in the prosthetic group, respectively. The limb-salvage rates for femoro-below-knee-popliteal grafts trended toward better outcome with arm vein, but this difference was not significant. When compared to prosthetic-autogenous grafts, simple or multisegment arm vein conduit provides superior graft patency and limb-salvage rates (Table 2).

CONCLUSIONS

Ipsilateral greater saphenous vein is the conduit of choice for lower extremity revascularization. In the absence of an available GSV, the arm vein provides the best alternative due to the flexibility offered by this conduit. An understanding of the anatomy of the veins of the arm, mastery of specific techniques to harvest and prepare these vessels, and an intensive program of postoperative surveillance and intervention for failing grafts enables patency and limb-salvage rates comparable to bypasses using GSV.

SUGGESTED READING

Principal References

Faries PL, Arora S, Pomposelli FB, et al. The use of arm vein in lower-extremity revascularization: results of 520 procedures performed in eight years. *J Vasc Surg* 2000;31:50.

Faries PL, LoGerfo FW, Arora S, et al. A comparative study of alternative conduits for lower extremity revascularization: all-autogenous conduit versus prosthetic grafts. *J Vasc Surg* 2000;32:1080.

Faries PL, LoGerfo FW, Arora S, et al. Arm vein conduit is superior to composite prosthetic-autogenous grafts in lower extremity revascularization. *J Vasc Surg* 2000;31:1119.

Holzenbein TJ, Pomposelli FB, Miller A, et al. The upper arm basilic-cephalic loop for distal bypass grafting: technical considerations and follow-up. *J Vasc Surg* 1995;21:586.

LoGerfo FW, Paniszyn C, Menzoian J. A new arm vein graft for distal bypass. *J Vasc Surg* 1987;5:889.

Additional References

Armstrong PA, Bandyk DF, Wilson JS, et al. Optimizing infrainguinal arm vein bypass patency with duplex ultrasound surveillance and endovascular therapy. *J Vasc Surg* 2004; 40:724.

Balshi JD, Cantelmo NL, Menzoian JO, et al. The use of arm veins for infrainguinal bypass in end-stage peripheral vascular disease. *Arch Surg* 1989;124:1078.

Campbell DR, Hoar CS, Gibbons GW. The use of arm veins in femoral-popliteal bypass grafts. *Ann Surg* 1979;190:740.

Chew DK, Owens CD, Belkin M, et al. Bypass in the absence of ipsilateral greater saphenous vein: safety and superiority of the contralateral greater saphenous vein. *J Vasc Surg* 2002;35:1085.

Faries PL, Arora S, Pomposelli FB, et al. The use of arm vein in lower-extremity revascularization: results of 520 procedures performed in eight years. *J Vasc Surg* 2000;31:50.

Faries PL, LoGerfo FW, Arora S, et al. A comparative study of alternative conduits for lower extremity revascularization: all-autogenous conduit versus prosthetic grafts. *J Vasc Surg* 2000;32:1080.

Faries PL, LoGerfo FW, Arora S, et al. Arm vein conduit is superior to composite prosthetic-autogenous grafts in lower extremity revascularization. *J Vasc Surg* 2000;31:1119.

Holzenbein TJ, Pomposelli FB, Miller A, et al. The upper arm basilic-cephalic loop for distal bypass grafting: technical considerations and follow-up. *J Vasc Surg* 1995;21:586.

Holzenbein TJ, Pomposelli FB, Miller A, et al. Results of a policy with arm veins used as the first alternative to an unavailable ipsilateral greater saphenous vein for infrainguinal bypass. *J Vasc Surg* 1996;23:130.

LoGerfo FW, Paniszyn C, Menzoian J. A new arm vein graft for distal bypass. *J Vasc Surg* 1987;5:889.

Marcaccio EJ, Miller A, Tannenbaum GA, et al. Angioscopically directed interventions improved arm vein bypass grafts. *J Vasc Surg* 1983;17:994.

EDITOR'S COMMENT

Hamdan and Everson present an excellent description of a somewhat tedious operation. Their aggregate experience at Beth Israel Deaconess Medical Center with arm vein infrainguinal revascularization is probably unmatched in the United States. Vascular surgeons inexperienced in performing this operation would do well to carefully read this chapter. Despite the technical demands of harvest and preparation of arm vein conduits, the results of lower extremity bypass with these grafts are gratifying. Most of these patients have undergone previous procedures that have failed, and they have critical limb ischemia with rest pain and open, non-healing foot lesions. They are at the "end of the line" and are facing major amputation.

One feature that is implied but not explicitly pointed out by the authors is that these procedures are lengthy, often taking 4–6 hours. One must be patient, methodical and unrushed. There are a myriad of sequential, technical details that require careful and continuous attention. All of these are described well by the authors. One must also be prepared to alter the operative plan, be prepared to harvest other veins and to splice segments when necessary. For exceptionally long operations, I find that allowing breaks for members of the surgical team (myself included) to be important in maintaining focus. Hunger, hypoglycemia, a full bladder and a short temper are to be avoided!

Careful preoperative planning with complete, four-extremity vein mapping with duplex ultra-

(continued)

Vascular Surgery

sound is extremely important. When the upper extremity with the most suitable veins is identified, the patient is carefully instructed to not allow blood draws and intravenous lines in that arm. This is the best way to protect the veins from trauma. In obese patients, we have found intraoperative ultrasound useful in identifying where to place incisions for harvest and this prevents flaps and malpositioned incisions that can lead to significant wound problems.

We do not use angioscopy as described by the authors and I suspect that this modality is infrequently used by others. Excessive intraluminal instrumentation with both the valvulotome and the angioscope may be problematic unless this is frequently and routinely performed as is done in the authors' practice.

I prefer to ablate all valves with the Mills-Leather valvulotome if the vein has sufficient integrity to withstand this manipulation and instrumentation. Arm veins are thin-walled and ablating

the valves can lead to significant and irreversible damage by the valvulotome "digging" into the valve sinus and tearing through the vein wall. If the vein appears excessively fragile, I forgo attempts at valve ablation and simply place the vein in a reversed configuration. I do not think that the problem of size discrepancy at the proximal and distal anastomoses is a major impediment to reversing the arm vein graft and I use this configuration for most of these operations. This contrasts to my preference for not reversing saphenous vein grafts. In addition to having much greater structural integrity and being better able to withstand the valvulotome, saphenous veins usually have a larger size discrepancy at the ends.

There is a single point of disagreement that I have with the authors. We do not hesitate to harvest the contralateral greater saphenous vein when the ipsilateral vein is absent or inadequate. As pointed out by the authors, results of arm vein infrainguinal bypass are distinctly inferior to those performed with saphenous vein. To use arm vein when contralateral saphe-

nous vein is available on the hypothetical premise that a contralateral infrainguinal bypass or coronary revascularization may be necessary is, in my opinion, untenable. There are studies that have addressed this issue and have found the need for a subsequent contralateral infrainguinal bypass or aortocoronary bypass to be less than 24%. (Chew DK, Owens CD, Belkin M, Donaldson MC, Whittemore AD, Mannick JA, Conte MS. Bypass in the absence of ipsilateral greater saphenous vein: safety and superiority of the contralateral greater saphenous vein. J Vasc Surg 2002; 35:1085-1092; Poletti LF, Matsuura JH, Dattilo JB, Posner MP, Lee HM, Scouvart M, et al. Should vein be saved for future operations? A 15-year review of infrainguinal bypasses and the subsequent need for autogenous vein. Ann Vasc Surg 1998; 12:143-147) I suspect that the percentage is even less today with the increasing success of interventional, catheter-based techniques for coronary and lower extremity revascularization.

G.P.C.

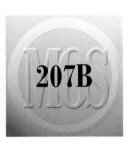

In Situ Vein Bypass

R. CLEMENT DARLING III, BENJAMIN B. CHANG, PAUL B. KREIENBERG, PHILIP S. K. PATY, SEAN P. RODDY, KATHLEEN J. OZSVATH, MANISH MEHTA, AND DHIRAJ M. SHAH

There is no question that the in situ use of the saphenous vein is on occasion tedious, time consuming, and demanding, but the surgeon's patience and persistence are rewarded with immediate bypass function in more than 95% of patients with the most diffuse and advanced stages of atherosclerotic occlusive disease.

PATIENT SELECTION

In selecting patients to be recipients of this investment of time and effort, one should be certain that the indications for it are clear (Table 1). Limb-threatening ischemia should be confirmed by noninvasive studies compatible with this degree of ischemia, and the diagnosis should exclude other causes of pain due to concomitant disease such as arthritis, diabetic

neuropathy, and neurocompressive syndromes. The most consistently accurate indicator of true ischemic rest pain is the characteristic history of pain (a) occurring in the forefoot, (b) awakening the patient from a sound sleep, and (c) relieved by dependency, walking, or both. A "nonhealing" ulcer should be present long enough with optimal care to be considered truly nonhealing. In the same sense, a gangrenous toe of and by itself may not be a manifestation of a critical degree of ischemia unless it is representative of the perfusion state of the foot. Preoperative arterial imaging should document the presence of multilevel disease, usually superficial femoral artery occlusion plus proximal or distal tibial involvement. Isolated superficial femoral artery occlusion alone rarely results in such a severe degree of ischemia. Similarly, operations for intermittent claudication are performed only with the full understanding by the patient that it is for functional improvement only and may prejudice long-term limb preservation, because distal reconstructions using vein have a rate of attrition of 5% to 7% per year. Once this vein is used electively, it is not available should limb-threatening ischemia develop in the future (although alternative autogenous conduits usually are).

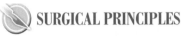 **SURGICAL PRINCIPLES**

Technically, the crucial issue in using the greater saphenous vein for arterial bypass is to remove the valvular obstruction to arterial flow. While this may be accomplished by excising and reversing the vein, leaving the saphenous vein in situ appears to be the most reliable method of achieving endothelial preservation, provided the valves can be rendered incompetent without injury to this friable endothelial cell monolayer. In addition, leaving the vein in situ requires interruption of venous side branches, some of which may become arteriovenous fistulae when the vein is arterialized, and the minimal mobilization of its ends for the construction of the proximal and distal anastomoses. The objective is to accomplish this maneuver with a minimum of operative manipulation of the vein and especially of the endothelial surface, with particular avoidance of circumferential shear. The simplest, most expedient, and least traumatic method of rendering the bicuspid venous valve incompetent is to cut the leaflets in their major axes while they are held in the functionally closed position by fluid or arterial pressure from above. This is the essence of the valve incision technique (Fig. 1).

TABLE 1. INDICATIONS FOR OPERATION

Indication	Patients
Claudication	526
Microemboli	48
Limb salvage	3,784
Aneurysm	129

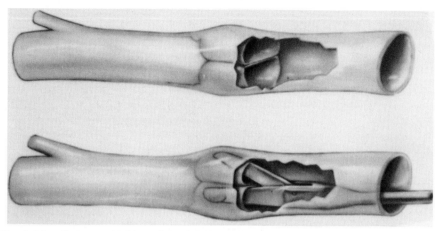

Fig. 1. Use of scissors with blunted tips for valve incision.

There is a widely held misconception that all techniques of in situ bypass produce comparable results. Since the resurrection of in situ bypass by the introduction of "valve incision" as the least traumatic method of rendering bicuspid venous valves incompetent, many surgeons have introduced their own variations of technique. However, common to virtually all is the use of the Mills valvulotome or an obturator-style cutter-disruptor (or both). The Mills valvulotome is the safest instrument for valve incision, largely owing to the limited area of contact between this instrument and endothelium. This is borne out by the excellent results—that is, less than a 5% failure rate at 30 days—whether it is used with the vein exposed or under angioscopic guidance. In Europe, closed in situ bypass has been largely carried out by means of retrograde sequential valve disruption with the Hall-Gruss and Cartier-Chevalier instruments, although the newer LeMaitre device has been used more recently with success. These instruments have two serious disadvantages: A mechanism that produces valvular incompetence by blunt tearing or avulsion of the valve leaflets, and, more significantly, these instruments are usually introduced and withdrawn through the distal divided end of the vein, which is invariably the portion of the vein smallest in diameter and most likely to be further narrowed by spasm when manipulated. These factors conspire to increase the likelihood of circumferential endothelial injury. Although the use of such instruments in this way is seductive in its simplicity, analysis of femoropopliteal bypasses using veins less than 4 mm in outside diameter or longer, low-flow bypasses carried to the crural arteries for limb salvage revealed a 15% to 20% 30-day failure rate. However, this has not been our experience.

The primary concerns of most surgeons embarking on the use of this procedure are identification and division of venous valves, as well as the location and interruption of side branches, which become arteriovenous fistulae when the vein is arterialized. This has led to two different approaches to the procedure.

The first approach is to expose the vein over its entire length so that all technical maneuvers are in direct view, which is basic to operative surgery. This technique provides familiarity and confidence in performing this new procedure. An alternative to this approach, at which we have arrived by evolution through this "open" method, is to use the intraluminal valve cutter on the thigh portion of the vein, because it is the largest and least tapered segment. This allows safe use of this "blind" technique if the vein is large enough for such a cutter to be free-floating, thereby minimizing the potential for endothelial abrasion. As in all operations, there are tradeoffs. The open approach carries a greater risk of injury to the vein directly and a greater chance of causing spasm and desiccation, in addition to an increase in problems with wound healing. The closed or blind approach is safe in 90% of operations if the cutter is used on only the large (>3.5 mm) segment of the vein and one has precise knowledge of the venous anatomy by ultrasonic mapping or venography. It is tempting to extend this blind approach to the smaller-diameter below-knee portion of the vein. This, however, exceeds the limit of its safety, because the risk of circumferential abrasion is greatly increased, not only because of decreasing vein size, but also because of the propensity of these smaller veins to go into spasm when manipulated. The retrograde valvulotome, because of its minimum potential for endothelial con-

tact, remains the safest instrument for valve incision in small veins.

The use of an angioscope has been advocated by some authors as a means of cutting the valve leaflets under direct vision. Although perhaps comforting, it may be unnecessary, because consistently safe and effective valve incision can be produced by a valvulotome or cutter. Furthermore, it is expensive and potentially injurious. The fear of a "missed" valve depends more on anatomy and experience than on currently available instrumentation.

The effect of arteriovenous fistulae on in situ saphenous vein bypass hemodynamics and patency has been of great concern to some, even to the point of regarding these as a frequent cause of in situ bypass occlusion. From the outset more than 30 years ago, it has been our practice to ligate only fistulae that conduct enough dye on completion angiography to visualize the deep venous system (Fig. 2). Most of the residual subcutaneous iatrogenic arteriovenous malformations produced undergo spontaneous thrombosis. We have studied more than 735 such bypasses, using duplex ultrasonic scanning to assess overall hemodynamic function. The results indicate a steady reduction in fistula flow, with no overall effect on distal perfusion. There is a small group of patients in whom high fistula flow is poorly tolerated, usually

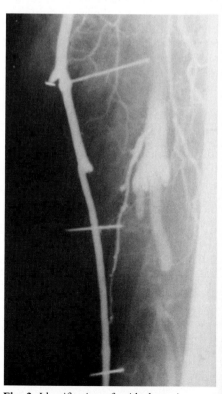

Fig. 2. Identification of residual arteriovenous fistulae by intraoperative angiography using a needle grid.

those with limited inflow capacity due to proximal stenosis or a small vein (<3 mm in outside diameter). In most patients, however, the flow capacity of the in situ conduit far exceeds the volume demanded by a fistula and adequate distal perfusion.

The allegation that fistulae are a potential cause of occlusive bypass failure is not true. The probable cause of failure in this setting is endothelial injury in the distal vein, the portion of the in situ conduit proximal to the fistula remaining patent because of flow to the fistula. For these reasons, we regard fistulae as at most an annoyance to the patient and the surgeon, but not as a crucial determinant of thrombosis of the bypass.

 PREOPERATIVE PLANNING

In the early experience, preoperative assessment of the greater saphenous vein was limited to physical examination of its below-knee pathway. Saphenous phlebography was adopted after the report by Veith et al. of its safety and use. It proved not only invaluable in the preparation of the vein in situ, but also mandatory if a valve cutter is to be used safely.

In more than 300 preoperative phlebograms of a remote vein on the dorsum of the foot after heparin pretreatment, venography has proved safe while providing the relevant information for the efficient planning of this procedure. However, this is now mostly of historic interest only.

Currently, transcutaneous mapping of the saphenous vein by B-mode duplex ultrasonography has been found to be a noninvasive and equally effective method of determining venous anatomy, provided that an experienced technician is available. This procedure provides a detailed three-dimensional map of the course of the saphenous vein, which can be traced onto the overlying skin. This map aids in the placement of skin incisions and the location of venous access points for instrumentation. Furthermore, it avoids the risks associated with phlebography and can be routinely performed in approximately 30 minutes. Our experience with more than 25,000 limbs studied in this way demonstrates that, in more than 95% of patients, B-mode imaging is the optimum technique of venous assessment. In the less than 5% of instances in which unexpected complex systems are encountered, an on-the-table intraoperative duplex study may be necessary.

In spite of these considerations, many surgeons remain resistant to these preoperative assessments, preferring to determine anatomic variations at operation. However, such attempts to define them by surgical dissection may often be frustrating and ineffective, leading to inappropriate excessive dissection, to failure and abandonment of the procedure, to an increased incidence of serious wound complications, and to an increased potential for spasm and other forms of injury to the vein.

Preparation for the operative procedure ideally should include the following:

1. Preoperative imaging angiograms (contrast, magnetic resonance, or duplex), including the ankle and foot with multiple views of the calf, not only to determine the true extent of disease in the vessels, but also to accurately differentiate the anterior tibial artery from the peroneal artery
2. Suitable duplex-generated vein map with vein quality, size, wall characteristics, wall thickness, or abnormalities noted
3. Marking the path of the saphenous vein on the skin
4. Assembly of the operating table so that the patient's foot is extended sufficiently to allow all surgical manipulations from the knee down to be performed with the surgeon in a comfortable sitting position and the arms resting on the table for proper use of microsurgical instruments

In addition, the following equipment is helpful for the optimum performance of tibial artery bypasses:

1. Operating loupes of at least 2.5 power and, ideally, 3.5 power with an extended field, each with comfortable and easily accommodated fields 7 to 8 cm in diameter and a comparable depth of field
2. A coaxial headlight, which provides ideal illumination required for optimal visual acuity
3. A Doppler ultrasonic flow detector with sterile 8- or 10-MHz probe, preferably with a 3-mm tip and/or intraoperative duplex
4. Microsurgical instruments, that is, forceps, needle holders, and scissors of the Castroviello type
5. A sterile orthopedic tourniquet cuff for use in place of occlusive vascular clamps or intraluminal balloons for control of calcified tibial vessels
6. Calibrated handleless clips for truly atraumatic control of the saphenous vein and tibial arteries (e.g., Yasargil neurosurgical microclips)
7. Items specific to the in situ procedure, in addition to the valvulotomes and

the cutter instruments: A sterile standard intravenous set; Dextran 40 or 70 in a compliant plastic bag; a pneumatic transfusion cuff; papaverine hydrochloride, 30 mg/mL and 1,000 U heparin; this solution is placed under 300 mm Hg and used on the operative field to dilate the vein through side branches to remove spasm

 SURGICAL TECHNIQUE

Although the common femoral artery has been considered the proper site for proximal anastomosis of all distal bypasses, there is evidence that use of the superficial femoral artery in patients undergoing limb salvage is equally satisfactory. Furthermore, technical circumstances, such as a previous surgical scar or exposure of the common femoral artery or its encasement with circumferential calcification, make the deep femoral (profunda femoris) or the superficial femoral artery a valid alternative inflow source. In spite of its less accessible anatomic location, the deep femoral artery is usually less affected with thick or calcified plaque than the common and superficial femoral arteries, and therefore frequently provides the most satisfactory site for proximal anastomosis.

It is best approached from the medial aspect (with the surgeon on the opposite side of the table) by incision of the subcutaneous tissue immediately over to the saphenous vein down to the underlying investing myofascia (Fig. 3). Dissection laterally in this fusion plane to the superficial femoral artery is bloodless. The fascia is incised over the superficial femoral artery and, if it is occluded, a segment of 3 to 5 cm can be excised, thus facilitating exposure of the deep femoral artery. The lateral circumflex femoral vein is divided, and the proximal deep femoral artery lies immediately deep to it (Fig. 4).

The most satisfactory site of proximal anastomosis is determined as well as the length of the proximal saphenous vein required to reach. If the common femoral artery is to be used as the inflow source, a complete dissection of the saphenous bulb and secure ligation of its branches are carried out. If additional length is required to facilitate anastomosis to the common femoral artery, a portion of the anterior aspect of the common femoral vein is removed in continuity with the saphenous bulb. An alternative is to preserve an appropriate length of the frequently present anterior branch at the saphenous bulb and incise it for use as a patch. The valve leaflets

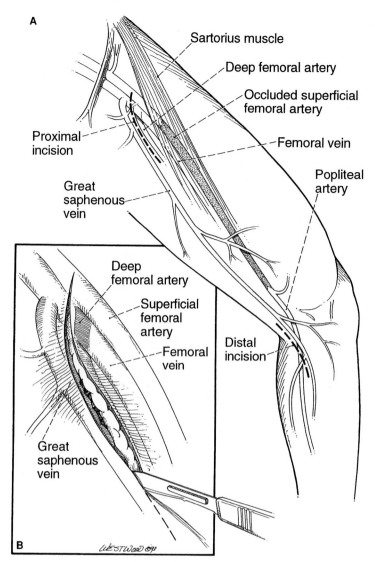

Fig. 3. A,B: Incisions for typical in situ bypass.

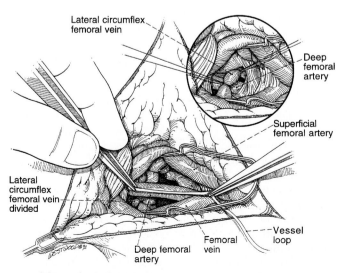

Fig. 4. Exposure of the profunda femoris artery.

at the saphenofemoral junction are excised, removing only the transparent portion, leaving the usually prominent insertion ridge intact. The second valve invariably present 3 to 5 cm distal to this location can be incised easily with a retrograde valvulotome through a side branch distal to the valve before the vein is divided or, alternatively, cut with scissors or an antegrade valvulotome through the open end of the vein, as is the valve immediately distal to the medial accessory branch. These valves are identified by gently distending the vein through its open end with dextran or heparinized blood and are cut with scissors while the valve is held in the functionally closed position by fluid trapped between the open end of the saphenous vein and the valve, with the thumb and index finger around the shank of the scissors.

The plane of closure of the valve cusps is invariably parallel to the skin. This dictates the orientation of all instruments in relation to the valve cusps.

If the cutter is to be used, a 3- to 5-cm incision is made 5 mm posterior to the position of the main saphenous vein below the knee, marked preoperatively on the skin, identifying a predetermined branch seen on the venogram and using it to gain access to the lumen of the saphenous vein. A 3 Fogarty catheter is introduced into the saphenous vein through this side branch and passed proximally (with the leg straightened) to exit through the open end of the vein. The catheter is then divided at an acute angle at the 20- or 30-cm mark, whichever is closest to the open end of the vein. The Leather valve cutter (2 or 3 mm) is threaded onto the catheter, and a 6 or 8 French catheter is then secured to the cutter with a loop of a fine suture (Fig. 5).

The leading cylinder of the cutter is drawn into the vein, providing a partial obturator obstruction to venous flow while permitting visualization of the cutting blade and minimal resistance in torque, thus allowing precise orientation of the cutting edges at 90 degrees to the plane of closure of the valves, that is, to the plane of the overlying skin surface. The catheter-cutter assembly is then drawn slowly distally while the dextran solution or blood is introduced through the catheter at 200 to 300 mm Hg pressure with a pressure seal provided by a 1-mm Silastic (polymeric silicone) vessel loop around the most proximal end of the saphenous vein secured by a small hemostat. This pressurized fluid column snaps each successive valve to the closed position so that the cusps are efficiently engaged by the blades of the cutter. A slight but definite

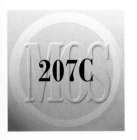

Secondary Infrainguinal Arterial Reconstruction

MICHAEL BELKIN AND DAVID K. W. CHEW

Infrainguinal arterial reconstruction using autogenous vein is an effective operation for limb salvage in patients with critical limb ischemia. However, despite reported cumulative graft patency rates of 76% at 10 years after infrainguinal bypass surgery, approximately 20% to 50% of patients will ultimately suffer graft failure. The majority of these patients present with a recrudescence of their original symptoms and, in most cases, will suffer limb-threatening ischemia. Approximately 10% of our patients undergo major amputation as their next intervention after failure of their infrainguinal bypass grafts. In most patients, however, an attempt at limb salvage through restoration of graft patency or repeat bypass surgery is appropriate.

The challenges of secondary infrainguinal bypass surgery after a previously failed reconstruction are well known to vascular surgeons. Extensive scarring in the operative field and a lack of ipsilateral greater saphenous vein, necessitating the use of alternative vein conduits present technical challenges to the surgeon. Furthermore, included in this cohort of patients with failed previous reconstructions are those patients with the most severe atherosclerosis, marked intimal hyperplastic response, poor-quality venous conduits, and hypercoagulable states. Therefore, it is not surprising that the published results of secondary bypass surgery in large series of patients are often inferior to those achieved with primary reconstructions. Given the complexities of secondary bypass surgery, a premium must be placed on effective graft surveillance and, when necessary, revision of the vein grafts to maintain bypass graft patency. In this chapter, we will review our graft surveillance protocol and strategies for revision of failing vein grafts. In addition, the selection of patients, operative considerations, and the technical strategies that may contribute to successful secondary arterial reconstructions will be discussed.

ETIOLOGY OF GRAFT FAILURE

A detailed understanding of the mechanisms of graft failure is important for the management of patients with occluded vein grafts. The etiology of vein graft occlusion generally varies with the interval from operation to the time of graft failure. Early graft occlusions, which occur within the first 30 days after bypass surgery, are usually attributable to errors of operative technique. These include technical errors (e.g., inadequate arterial flushing, clamp injuries, retained valves, vein graft injuries, anastomotic errors) as well as judgmental errors (e.g., employing inadequate inflow or outflow vessels, the use of inadequate venous conduit). Rarely, early graft thrombosis may be caused by graft surface thrombogenicity or unsuspected hypercoagulable states. Vein graft failure from 31 days to 18 months after surgery most frequently results from the formation of intimal hyperplastic lesions within the graft or at the site of an anastomosis. Finally, vein graft failure beyond 18 months after surgery is usually caused by the progression of atherosclerotic disease within the inflow or outflow vessels, ultimately leading to graft thrombosis.

GRAFT SURVEILLANCE AND REVISION

Routine periodic examination of the vein graft using duplex ultrasonography may detect subclinical lesions that predispose to graft thrombosis, permitting prophylactic revision of the graft to prolong its patency. Patient evaluation and duplex examination of the graft are performed at 1, 3, 6, 9, and 12 months postoperation and yearly thereafter. A recurrence of symptoms, change in character of the graft or distal pulses, or a decrease in the ankle-brachial index of more than 0.1, or pulse volume recording waveforms are indications of possible graft stenosis. Duplex ultrasound criteria of impending graft failure include decreased overall graft velocity (peak systolic velocity <25 cm/s in a normal-caliber graft) or focal increase in velocity (peak systolic velocity >300 cm/s, or an increase in peak systolic velocity in one segment of the bypass greater than three times that of an adjacent segment). A contrast angiogram or magnetic resonance angiogram should be performed to confirm the diagnosis and define the anatomy of the vein graft. Focal lesions (<3 cm) are best addressed using vein patch angioplasty. Occasionally, very short (<15 mm) lesions with flanking segments of normal-caliber vein undergo percutaneous balloon angioplasty. Long segmental lesions (>3 cm) generally require interposition vein grafting or jump-grafting around the anastomoses using autogenous vein. Transposition of the vein graft to a different vessel target may also be used if such an option exists. A recent review of our experience with revision of vein bypass grafts showed an overall 5-year primary patency from the time of graft revision of 49% ± 5%, secondary patency of 80% ± 4%, and limb salvage rate of 83% ± 4%. These durable results were similar among the different techniques of graft revision used. Tibial/pedal bypass grafts and grafts that were revised within 6 months of the index operation were associated with poorer long-term patency following graft revision.

MANAGEMENT OF EARLY GRAFT FAILURE

As noted previously, early postoperative vein graft failure is usually caused by a technical or judgmental error, and results in a recurrence of ischemic symptoms (often more severe than the preoperative state). If the patient is stable and an acceptable risk for reintervention, an attempt at restoration of graft patency is warranted. The etiology of graft failure can often be suspected based on the intraoperative findings at the time of the original operation as well as a review of the completion arteriogram. For example, the use of a marginal venous conduit or a history of vein wall trauma occurring during valve lysis at the original operation may indicate the cause of graft occlusion.

When vein graft failure is diagnosed within the first several days after operation, immediate return to the operating room is indicated to minimize adherence of the thrombus to the graft wall, propagation of thrombus into the outflow vessels, and ischemic injury to the vein graft itself. The patient is systemically anticoagulated with heparin, the proximal and distal graft hoods are opened, and the thrombus is gently extracted using a combination of heparinized saline irrigation through the graft and balloon catheter thrombectomy when necessary. Limited local installation of thrombolytic agents within the graft conduit or outflow vessels may be a useful adjunct. All potential defects are corrected with patch angioplasties, interposition grafts, or replacement of larger segments of graft with newly harvested vein. Intraoperative duplex scanning is useful to evaluate the graft for any residual defects. Short-term anticoagulation (2 to 4 weeks) is used in all patients and long-term anticoagulation with warfarin is employed selectively. This is particularly important for the small number of patients in whom no technical defects are identified. These patients have an increased incidence of unsuspected hypercoagulable states, among which antiphospholipid syndrome and heparin-induced platelet activation correlate most highly with early graft occlusion.

MANAGEMENT OF INTERMEDIATE AND LATE GRAFT FAILURE

A variety of important factors must be considered when confronted with a patient with a failed infrainguinal reconstruction beyond the perioperative period. If the patient does not have significant rest pain or ischemic ulceration, conservative nonoperative management may be preferred. At the other end of the spectrum are patients whose medical co-morbidities and general debility prohibit a major secondary infrainguinal reconstruction. In most patients, however, the goals of relieving pain and preserving function of a critically ischemic limb through a secondary bypass operation are appropriate. The surgeon must decide whether to attempt to restore patency to the failed graft or proceed to a new secondary bypass graft.

Restoration of patency of the bypass graft followed by revision of the graft is often desirable. This is achieved by removal of the thrombus, evaluation of the graft with angiography and/or duplex ultrasonography, and, finally, repair of the defects responsible for graft failure. The best results with this approach are achieved when the intervention occurs early (within 30 days) after graft thrombosis in bypass grafts that have been patent for more than 1 year.

Unfortunately, balloon-catheter thrombectomy of thrombosed vein grafts has seldom been rewarded with satisfactory long-term graft patency rates, with only 19% to 28% patency rates at the 5-year interval after reintervention for the failed graft. The failure of vein graft thrombectomy has led to considerable enthusiasm for the use of thrombolytic therapy in the initial management of patients with thrombosed vein grafts. Thrombolytic therapy offers several potential advantages. Completion arteriography after successful thrombolysis supplies the surgeon with a "road map" of the vein graft and may reveal the defect(s) responsible for occlusion. Additional advantages include the avoidance of balloon catheter-induced endothelial injury and the potential for more complete removal of thrombus from both the graft and outflow vessels. Following dissolution of the clot, revision of the graft is performed using one of the techniques listed here, depending on the anatomy of the culprit lesion.

In vein grafts that have been thrombosed for more than 30 days, thrombolytic therapy is less successful in restoring normal graft patency. In these cases, especially if the patient experiences a recurrence of critical limb ischemia, a new secondary bypass procedure should be considered.

SURGICAL EXPOSURE OF INFLOW AND OUTFLOW VESSELS

Exposure of previously operated blood vessels poses one of the greatest challenges of reoperative bypass surgery. Dense adherence of the vessels to surrounding scar makes the dissection tedious and time-consuming. As a general rule, minimal dissection should be performed to expose only a sufficient portion of the vessel to control flow and create an anastomosis. Great care must be taken to avoid breaching the outer layers of the arterial wall (subadventitial plane), which may compromise the integrity of the vessel wall and require an extensive local repair (such as with a patch angioplasty) before the vessel can be used as inflow or outflow for the new bypass. Scarring is usually most severe at areas of previous anastomotic sites. Prior prosthetic grafts are usually incorporated by a dense fibrotic capsule. It is best to enter this capsule directly with sharp dissection, which then allows easy separation of the graft from the remaining capsule with gentle blunt dissection. Following the graft toward the anastomosis, it is critical to avoid cutting the previous suture line during the dissection as the integrity of the anastomosis will be violated

and a pseudoaneurysm may result. Re-exposure of native blood vessels is best done by starting in an unviolated plane slightly more proximally or distally, and then following these vessels inward using careful sharp dissection through scar tissue. Staying as close to the vessel wall as possible (without entering the adventitia) will avoid potential injury to surrounding structures (such as nerves and veins).

The use of a sterile surgical tourniquet to achieve a bloodless field has greatly simplified the control of previously dissected vessels. This technique is employed for the re-exposure of the below-the-knee popliteal artery or more distal vessels. With this technique, only the anterior surface of the vessel sufficient for completing the anastomosis needs to be exposed. Circumferential control and dissection of extra length of vessels for placement of clamps or vessel loops are unnecessary. The patient is anticoagulated, the leg is elevated and exsanguinated with an Esmark bandage, and a sterile thigh tourniquet is applied at 250 to 300 mm Hg over a cotton thigh wrap. The outflow vessel is then incised and the distal anastomosis constructed in a minimally exposed surgical field that is unfettered with clamps or vessel loops.

Given the inherent challenges of re-exposure of blood vessels, it is best to avoid redissection of arteries whenever possible by selecting alternative inflow and outflow sites. Alternative inflow sites may include the superficial femoral artery (SFA) below the femoral bifurcation or the popliteal artery. Even in the setting of prior femoral to distal artery bypasses, the SFA may be relatively well preserved down to Hunter's canal. This vessel is easily exposed through a medial, midthigh incision, which is then carried down through the superficial fascia. The sartorius muscle is retracted posteriorly. The SFA pulse may then be felt through the adductor fascia, which is then incised (Fig. 1). The profunda femoris artery beyond the lateral circumflex artery may also be suitable as an inflow vessel and can be exposed by incising lateral to the sartorius muscle and carrying the dissection down between the superficial femoral vessels and the adductor longus muscle.

In selected situations, the proximal common femoral or distal external iliac artery may be used as the inflow artery. Although these sites have the disadvantage of lengthening the venous conduit necessary for bypass, they are easily exposed and are particularly suitable when the distal anastomosis may be constructed at the popliteal level. These more

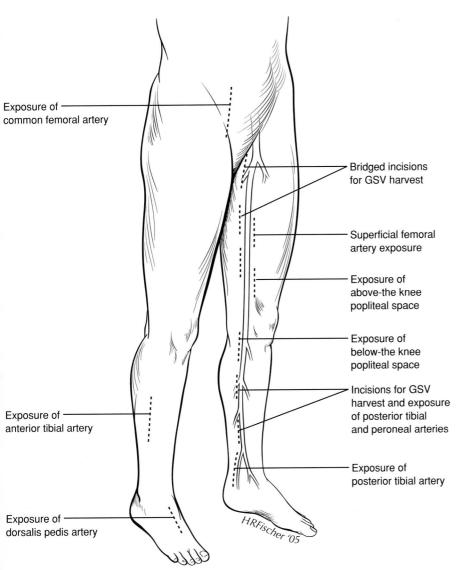

Exposure of common femoral artery

Bridged incisions for GSV harvest

Superficial femoral artery exposure

Exposure of above-the knee popliteal space

Exposure of below-the knee popliteal space

Incisions for GSV harvest and exposure of posterior tibial and peroneal arteries

Exposure of posterior tibial artery

Exposure of anterior tibial artery

Exposure of dorsalis pedis artery

HRFischer '05

Fig. 1. Exposure of the distal superficial femoral artery above the adductor canal is readily obtained through a medial-based longitudinal thigh incision. The incision is deepened by retracting the sartorius and adductor longus muscles posteriorly and the vastus medialis muscles anteriorly. The adductor fascia is incised and the artery is easily exposed above the adductor canal. (From Chew DKW, Belkin M. Open surgical revascularization for femoropopliteal and infrapopliteal arterial occlusive disease. In: Zelenock GB, Huber TS, Messina LM, et al., eds. *Mastery of vascular and endovascular surgery*. Philadelphia: Lippincott Williams & Wilkins, 2006.)

the results are inferior to those using autogenous vein in all reported reoperative series. Furthermore, the great majority of patients who require reoperative bypass surgery have distal vascular anatomy, which necessitates a below-the-knee popliteal or, more commonly, tibial-level bypass, which is clearly unfavorable for prosthetic grafts. Thus, vascular surgeons should strive to complete all reoperative bypass grafts with autogenous vein.

However, many patients undergoing reoperative bypass surgery lack ipsilateral greater saphenous vein (GSV) for the reconstruction. The situation may be even more complicated for those who have had GSV harvested for prior coronary artery bypass surgery. As a general principle, the reoperative bypass operation should be completed with the shortest bypass possible, using the best available autogenous vein conduit. A number of strategies are important in achieving these objectives.

Distal Origin Grafts

The use of grafts originating distal to the femoral bifurcation is an important strategy in achieving the shortest bypass possible, thereby minimizing the length of vein required. These grafts, which employ the SFA, popliteal, or even tibial arteries as inflow vessels, were once considered a compromise but are now recognized as an important technique in both primary and reoperative distal bypass surgery. This approach is particularly applicable in diabetic patients because of the relative preservation of the SFA and even popliteal artery despite extensive occlusions of the tibial arteries. Originating the bypass graft off the distal popliteal artery can allow a bypass to a tibial or pedal vessel with a single segment of remnant saphenous vein or ectopic vein. In selected cases, when autogenous vein conduit is in short supply, percutaneous endovascular techniques may be used to optimize the inflow into the SFA and popliteal vessels to allow for a distal origin graft, which would have not been possible otherwise.

Overall, the results of distal origin grafts are comparable with those of longer grafts originating in the common femoral artery. In a recent review from our group, the 5-year cumulative primary graft patency was 62% ± 4%, primary-assisted patency was 67% ± 4%, secondary patency was 73% ± 4%, and limb salvage was 81% ± 4%. These results were significantly better in patients with diabetes mellitus compared with patients without diabetes mellitus.

proximal inflow vessels should only be employed when there is unimpeded inflow into the profunda femoris artery. Because long-term limb salvage often hinges on patency of the profunda femoris artery, this vessel should be re-exposed and reconstructed (with a profundaplasty) whenever necessary as part of the secondary bypass procedure.

Avoidance of redissection is particularly important in exposure of distal outflow vessels. Re-exposure of tibial vessels is easily complicated by trauma to the arteries and accompanying venae comitantes. The tibial veins are often densely adherent to the artery and resultant bleeding

can make the exposure extremely difficult. In the majority of cases it is possible to expose new, more distal (or even more proximal) sites on the vessel. Similarly, alternative routes of exposure (such as lateral exposure of the peroneal artery with segmental fibular resection) may simplify exposure of distal vessel targets.

OPERATIVE STRATEGIES

Autogenous tissue should be used whenever possible and in most reoperative bypass procedures. Although some reasonable results have been reported in reoperative surgery using prosthetic grafts,

Autogenous Composite Vein Grafts

When there is insufficient length of a single segment of vein to complete a bypass procedure, splicing several vein segments together to form a composite vein graft may allow the bypass to be completed using purely autogenous tissue. Remnant GSV, arm veins (cephalic or basilic veins), or lesser saphenous vein may be spliced in various combinations to create a conduit that is long enough. Duplex ultrasound is useful in mapping out the availability and quality of arm and leg veins in order to guide the prioritization strategy in which these alternative vein conduits are used. Although it is preferable to splice only two segments, in some cases it may be necessary to join three or more segments to achieve sufficient length.

The general principles of composite vein grafting are to create a conduit with a larger diameter proximally and smaller diameter distally. Various combinations of reversed and nonreversed veins are used to create this continuous taper. In our practice,

vein grafts are used in a reversed orientation only if the caliber of the graft is uniform throughout. Nonreversed vein segments have their valves lysed prior to construction of the venovenostomy. This is best accomplished using the modified Mills valvulotome while distention of the vein (and valve closure) is maintained with an irrigating syringe (Fig. 2). Ideally, vein segments should have a minimum diameter of 3.5 mm; they should distend easily with irrigation and lack evidence of significant wall thickening and sclerosis/thrombosis. Vein segments that do not meet these criteria are excised. The venovenostomy is accomplished by cutting each vein at a 45-degree angle and then spatulating further to create a size match between the ends of the two vein segments. The anastomosis is started by anchoring the heel and toe of the anastomosis with two 7-0 polypropylene sutures (Fig. 3). Each side of the suture line is then completed while maintaining distraction on the vein segments to prevent purse-string constriction of the anastomosis. Once an adequate

conduit is prepared, the bypass operation can be completed in standard fashion. Careful intraoperative assessment of the completed bypass graft using arteriography or duplex ultrasonography is important to ensure a satisfactory technical result.

In our experience with 300 reoperative bypasses after failed previous reconstructions, approximately 16% required some form of composite vein bypass. In a larger series of 165 composite vein grafts, 75% of the bypasses were completed using two segments of veins whereas 25% required three or more segments. The overall 5-year cumulative graft patency rates were 44% ± 5% for primary patency, 63% ± 5% for primary-assisted patency, and 65% ± 5% for secondary patency. The overall limb salvage in patients with limb-threatening ischemia was 81% ± 5% at 5 years. Interestingly, grafts constructed of three or more segments performed equally well compared with those comprising two segments. However, composite vein grafts are characterized by the frequent occurrence of myointimal hyperplasia, equally distributed between the proximal, distal anastomoses and venovenostomies. Twenty-seven percent of grafts required revision for stenotic lesions identified by duplex ultrasound graft surveillance, stressing the need for careful long-term follow-up.

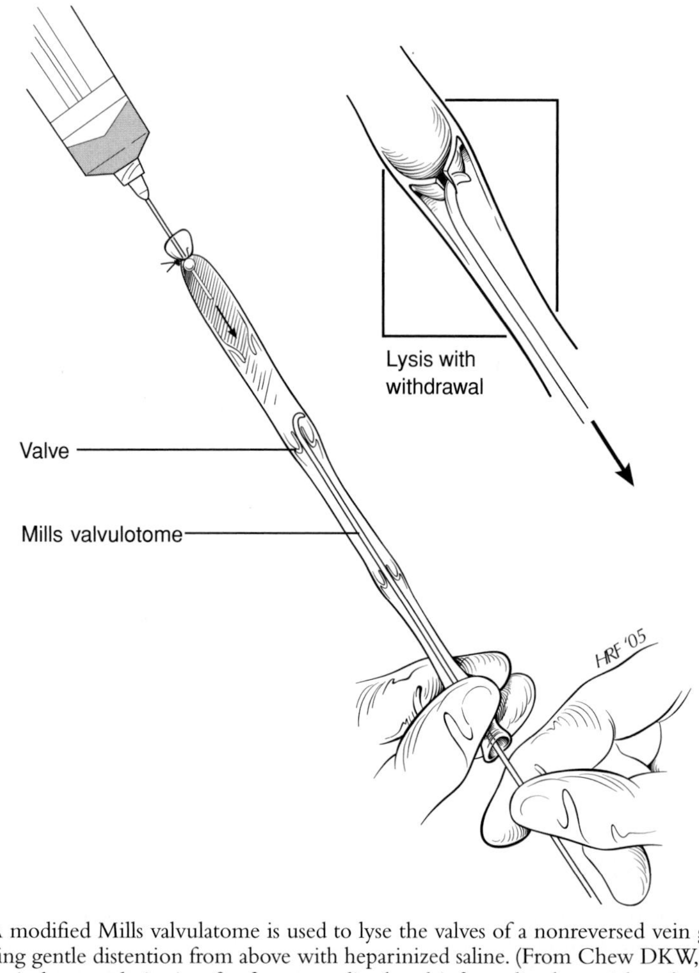

Bypass Conduits

Greater Saphenous Vein

In a minority of patients who have failed prior prosthetic grafts, the ipsilateral GSV may be employed as an in situ or other configuration graft. In most cases, however, the contralateral GSV is the best available conduit and may be translocated for use in a reversed or nonreversed (with lysed valves) configuration. The nonreversed configuration is generally preferred as it optimizes vein use as well as size match between the artery and vein at the proximal and distal anastomosis. The only contraindication for use of the contralateral GSV is the presence of significant contralateral limb ischemia with the impending need for contralateral revascularization. The trauma of contralateral GSV harvest may be minimized by the use of endoscopic vein harvest techniques, which has proven beneficial in coronary artery bypass surgery. In our series of reoperative bypass grafts, GSV (whether ipsilateral or contralateral) performed better than any other conduit with 5-year primary patency rates of 60% ± 7% and secondary patency rates of 69% ± 6%.

Despite the universal recognition that GSV is the optimal conduit for infrain-

Fig. 2. A modified Mills valvulatome is used to lyse the valves of a nonreversed vein graft while maintaining gentle distention from above with heparinized saline. (From Chew DKW, Belkin M. Open surgical revascularization for femoropopliteal and infrapopliteal arterial occlusive disease. In: Zelenock GB, Huber TS, Messina LM, et al., eds. *Mastery of vascular and endovascular surgery*. Philadelphia: Lippincott Williams & Wilkins, 2006.)

Valve

Mills valvulotome

Lysis with withdrawal

vein graft is initially sewn onto the arteriotomy, and the graft is then sewn onto a central venotomy. The Miller cuff consists of a venous "cylinder" sewn in an intervening segment between the artery and graft. The distal arteriovenous fistula aims to improve flow through the prosthetic graft.

 ## SURGICAL TECHNIQUE

When using prosthetics, there are a few rules that should be followed. As hemostasis is more difficult than when dealing with autologous tissues, it is important to maintain right angles with the needle and the graft. It is similarly necessary to "follow the curve of the needle," and not torque the tip. There are sutures specifically made to minimize needle-hole bleeding. Gore has developed a suture material made of PTFE, where the suture is the same size as the needle. Most surgeons, however, have found that the increased cost of such suture is not outweighed by a significant advantage.

One of the advantages of prosthetic grafts is the ability to grasp a full-thickness piece of the grafts, as there is no living endothelium to injure. As opposed to venous conduits, which may be stretched to accommodate a mismeasured arteriotomy, ePTFE cannot be stretched. As a result, it is generally safer to always err on the side of measuring a larger graft opening. Lastly, it is always important not to twist these grafts. Although it is more difficult to twist prosthetic grafts than autologous tissues, it is still possible. This is especially true in situations where multiple counterincisions are necessary. To prevent this, many prosthetic grafts have a printed vertical line. As with autologous tissues, "double-armed" sutures are preferred. If for no other reason, this helps in the event of damage to one needle tip. When tunneling grafts, the authors prefer to keep the grafts in a deep plane. This is especially important when dealing with extremity bypasses. By keeping these grafts in a deeper plane, they will be more resistant to infection in the event of wound complications. Such a tunnel location includes remaining deep to the sartorius muscle or between the heads of the gastrocnemius. When working with ePTFE, it is preferable to leave as many rings as possible without interfering with the anastomosis.

When sewing to the aortoiliac segment, the authors prefer to use Dacron. Dacron offers certain advantages secondary to its ease of handling, as well as flexibility. The diameter of the graft may be estimated based on previous experience, or may be sized with the aid of plastic "sizers." The relative benefits of end-to-end versus end-to-side configurations are covered elsewhere. As a general rule, we use 3-0 Prolene for aortic anastomoses and 4-0 Prolene for distal anastomoses.

When it comes to infrainguinal bypasses, we prefer ePTFE. This preference is secondary to its kink resistance (with the aid of the rings) and the theoretic advantage of complete thrombus removal. It must be re-emphasized, however, that there is no level 1 evidence to support this preference. For the femoral and popliteal anastomoses, the 6-0 Prolene is used. For tibial vessels, 7-0 Prolene is used.

Most research has focused on a way to reduce neointimal hyperplasia. As recirculation and therefore wall shear stress are primarily found opposite the heel and distal to the toe, this is felt to be largely responsible for neointimal hyperplasia. Enlarging the patch area aids in reducing the wall shear stress in the area. As a general rule, we aim for an anastomosis measuring 15 mm in length. Although the optimal anastomotic angle has not been conclusively demonstrated, most authors recommend an angle ranging from 40 to 45 degrees. Several methods of theoretically improving the patency rate of tibial vessel reconstructions have been mentioned previously. In both animal and human experiments, there has been no significant advantage between these various alternatives, and patency rates remain low despite their usage.

At Maimonides, we perform a combination of the techniques with a venous interposition and an arteriovenous fistula. This consists of performing an end-to-side anastomosis between the tibial artery and one of its corresponding veins. This anastomosis should measure approximately 15 mm in length. After this is completed, a 15-mm venotomy is made, onto which the graft is anastomosed. It is important not to extend the venotomy too close to the artery, as this could inadvertently extend distally across the entire vein. This technique combines two advantages conferred from the previously listed options. It helps to reduce the compliance mismatch with an intervening venous segment and helps to increase flow and therefore decrease wall shear stress with the presence of a fistula. It is important to look for both accompanying tibial veins during this procedure, as one is often atretic or phlebitic. It should be mentioned that this technique does require a more extensive and meticulous exposure of the arteries. Given the prohibitively poor patency rates, revascularization to pedal vessels with prosthetic conduits is not performed.

SUGGESTED READING

Principal References

Faries PL, Logerfo FW, Arora S, et al. A comparative study of alternative conduits for lower extremity revascularization: all-autogenous conduit versus prosthetic grafts. *J Vasc Surg* 2000;32(6):1080.

Hingorani AP, Ascher E, Marks NA, et al. A 10-year experience with complementary distal arteriovenous fistula and deep vein interposition for infrapopliteal prosthetic bypasses. *Vasc Endovasc Surg* 2005;39(5):401.

Johnson WC, Lee KK. Comparative evaluation of externally supported Dacron and polytetrafluoroethylene prosthetic bypasses for femorofemoral and axillofemoral arterial reconstructions. Veterans Affairs Cooperative Study #141. *J Vasc Surg* 1999;30(6):1077.

Additional References

Ducasse E, Fleurisse L, Vernier G, et al. Interposition vein cuff and intimal hyperplasia: an experimental study. *Eur J Vasc Endovasc Surg* 2004;27:617.

Kallakuri S, Ascher E, Hingorani A, et al. Hemodynamics of infrapopliteal PTFE bypasses and adjunctive arteriovenous fistulas. *Cardiovasc Surg* 2003;11(2):125.

Kannan R, Salacinski H, Butler P, et al. Current status of prosthetic bypass grafts: a review. *J Biomed Mater Res Part B Appl Biomater* 2005;74B:570.

Klinkert P, Post P, Breslau P, et al. Saphenous vein versus PTFE for above-knee femoropopliteal bypass. A review of the literature. *Eur J Vasc Endovasc Surg* 2004;27:357.

Laurila K, Lepantalo M, Teittinen K, et al. Does an adjunctive AV-fistula improve the patency of a femorocrural ptfe bypass with distal vein cuff in critical leg ischemia? A prospective randomised multicentre trial. *Eur J Vasc Endovasc Surg* 2004;27:180.

Miller J, Foreman R, Ferguson L, et al. Interposition vein cuff for anastomosis of prosthesis to small artery. *Aust N Z K Surg* 1984; 54:283.

Moawad J, Gagne P. Adjuncts to improve patency of infrainguinal prosthetic bypass grafts. *Vasc Endovasc Surg* 2003;37(6):381.

Rashid S, Salacinski H, Button M, et al. Cellular engineering of conduits for coronary and lower limb bypass surgery: role of cell attachment peptides and pre-conditioning in optimising smooth muscle cells (SMC) adherence to compliant poly(carbonate-urea) urethane (MyoLink) scaffolds. *Eur J Vasc Endovasc Surg* 2004;27:608.

Trubel W, Schima H, Czerny M, et al. Experimental comparison of four methods of end-to-side anastomosis with expanded polytetrafluoroethylene. *Br J Surg* 2004; 91:159.

Tyrrell M, Wolfe J. New prosthetic venous collar anastomotic technique: combining the best of other procedures. *Br J Surg* 1991;78: 1016.

Walsh M, Kavanagh E, O'Brien T, et al. On the existence of an optimum end-to-side junctional geometry in peripheral bypass surgery—a computer generated study. *Eur J Vasc Endovasc Surg* 2003;26:649.

Vascular Surgery

The authors have very nicely summarized the history of prosthetic arterial grafts, an area where, unfortunately, there has been little progress with regard to improvement in the base material since the introduction of Dacron 40 years ago. They correctly note that, in spite of strong individual personal preferences, there is no scientific evidence that favors Dacron, or the competitive material, ePTFE, in any location. For technical reasons, nearly all surgeons favor Dacron in the aortoiliofemoral system and ePTFE for infrainguinal grafts. Surgeons are under tremendous commercial pressure to accept evidence that one material or the other is better as far as thromboresistance is concerned, but this is not justified. Regardless of the nature of the surface, whether the surface potential is negative or positive, within a few seconds, the multivalent proteins of blood adhere to the surface and reduce that surface potential. This process goes on until the strength of the shear forces of the moving blood exceeds the strength of the electrochemical forces binding the proteins to the surface, the so-called zeta-potential or the surface potential at the plane of slip, which probably varies very little as a function of the base material. Shortly after that electrochemical attachment occurs, the coagulation proteins and platelets come into action to form a fibrin/platelet/red cell pseudointima. It probably proceeds until the shear forces exceed the strength of the procoagulant forces. Theoretically there is a zone, very near the ultimate surface, where the chemistry of the blood is slightly affected by the surface, known as the chemical boundary layer (i.e., the moving fluid that is chemically altered by the surface). As flow through the graft slows down, this chemical boundary layer becomes thicker, and the procoagulant surface or pseudointima also becomes thicker and eventually leads to full thrombosis of the graft.

This sequence of events is ultimately unrelated to the nature of the underlying surface. Furthermore, it is difficult to conceive of a surface that could be created that would be so biochemically active as to influence this process, such as by heparin binding to the surface. Such surfaces are effective only for a short time as the release of heparin is great enough as to overcome the procoagulant activities in the developing biochemical boundary layers. Nonetheless, the objective of developing biologically active surfaces is worthy of further study. In short, 40 years later, we have no surface that, because of its nature, alters the long-term prognosis of prosthetic arterial grafts, including biologic constructs such as umbilical cord vein grafts, etc. These fundamental principles of the interaction of blood with artificial surfaces should be in the knowledge base of all vascular surgeons and will prove helpful in dealing with various claims about patency rates, etc.

The authors mention the place of prosthetic grafts versus autogenous vein for femoral-popliteal reconstruction above the knee. I personally favor autogenous vein, when available, for this construct. In my years of experience, it has been extremely rare to come back and require a further reconstruction where loss of that segment of vein has proven to be any compromise. On the other hand, I have had to deal with infected prosthetic arterial grafts in that position and add that to the reasons I do not favor prosthetic arterial grafts for this procedure. The authors did not mention axillofemoral grafts, where a stronger argument can be made with regard to the ease of thrombectomy of ePTFE grafts. For that reason, probably most vascular surgeons favor ePTFE in this location. On the other hand, the lack of any "give" in the ePTFE graft requires some diligence with regard to the angle and construct of the proximal anastomosis since we and others have reported disruption of that suture line in the postoperative period due to positionally related tension.

The only point of disagreement I have with the authors is with regard to prosthetic grafts to tibial vessels with creation of an arteriovenous fistula. Having seen these patients after the prosthetic graft has failed and the fistulas remain patent, I have concerns about the downside risk of causing worse ischemia. In the absence of any evidence that this procedure is better than a prosthetic graft with some sort of autogenous cuff at the distal anastomosis, I do not recommend the procedure. Elsewhere in the book, I have indicated my preference for construct for an autogenous venous cuff when using a prosthetic graft to a tibial vessel, a procedure that should be resorted to only when sufficient autogenous vein, including arm vein graft, is not available.

The authors advocate a low-angle anastomosis between the prosthetic graft and host artery but acknowledge the absence of evidence to support this. I agree, and work from our laboratory with animal models does not support the idea that the flow field disturbance at the anastomosis is of significant importance in graft failure. The development of neointimal hyperplasia at the downstream anastomosis is more likely related to the presence of a foreign body, pulsatile suture line stress, and interaction of blood with the thrombogenic pseudointima in transit adding to cytokine stimulation of endothelium at the outflow anastomosis. This problem remains the Achilles heel of prosthetic arterial grafts.

F.W.L.

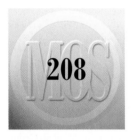

208

Dorsalis Pedis, Tarsal, and Plantar Artery Bypass

FRANK B. POMPOSELLI, JR., AND BERNADETTE AULIVOLA

INTRODUCTION

Arterial reconstruction to the arteries of the vessels in the distal ankle and foot has become commonplace in those patients with occlusive disease of the infrapopliteal vessels precluding a bypass to a more proximal vessel. Often, bypass to the dorsalis pedis (DP), tarsal, and plantar arteries is the only alternative to limb amputation, especially in patients with diabetes mellitus presenting with ischemic foot lesions. The usefulness of these bypass options in the diabetic population can be attributed to the characteristic pattern of tibial vessel occlusive disease seen in these patients. We have previously reported our results with DP bypass in 384, and subsequently in over 1,000, cases. In addition, we have documented the safety of DP bypass in patients with foot infection in the setting of ischemia. DP bypass has been demonstrated to be useful also in the healing of ischemic ulcers of the heel. Over the past decade, DP bypass comprised nearly 30% of all lower extremity arterial reconstructions on our service, which has a high number of patients with diabetes mellitus due to our affiliation with the Joslin Diabetes Center. This chapter will outline our evaluation and approach to foot-level arterial bypass.

PATIENT SELECTION

Foot bypass is reserved for patients with limb-threatening symptoms including rest pain, nonhealing ulcers, gangrene, or poor healing of toe amputations or other foot surgery due to arterial insufficiency. These procedures are not appropriate for intermittent claudication. In fact, claudication is rarely improved by pedal bypass since the arteries of the calf are occluded and rarely adequately perfused through the pedal circulation. Comprehensive, high-quality intra-arterial digital subtraction angiography (DSA) is a key component of the planning process for DP or other foot vessel bypass (Fig. 1). Appropriate evaluation of the lower extremity circulation includes imaging of the entire arterial tree from the renal arteries to the base of the toes in all patients with limb ischemia. Proper imaging of the foot vessels requires magnified anteroposterior and lateral views in order to fully ap-

Vascular Surgery

preciate the quality of the DP, tarsal, and plantar arteries to assess their potential use as outflow target vessels. Magnetic resonance angiography (MRA) is used infrequently, and is generally reserved for those patients who are unable to undergo DSA due to severe contrast allergies or renal insufficiency. However, some data suggest that occult foot vessels on DSA may be unmasked with MRA, resulting in successful bypass to these vessels. "Blind" operative exploration may be performed in the case of nonvisible foot arteries on DSA in cases where patency is suspected on the basis of an audible Doppler signal, although this is rarely required due to the precise imaging capabilities of modern DSA.

The decision to perform a DP bypass is made on the basis of several important anatomic and clinical factors. The goal of restoring a palpable foot pulse when possible in patients with diabetes and tissue loss is based upon our observation that this end point most reliably leads to healing and foot salvage in the setting of the compromised biology of the ischemic diabetic foot. If a more proximal outflow target artery cannot achieve that goal, preferential bypass to the DP artery should be considered. In situations of rest pain without tissue loss, the DP artery should be chosen as the outflow target vessel when it is the best-quality vessel for bypass or the only available outflow vessel

as determined on DSA evaluation. In circumstances where a more proximal outflow vessel would restore a palpable foot pulse and tissue loss is the indication, DP bypass is not necessarily the procedure of choice. In cases of tissue loss or gangrene, however, DP bypass is often chosen in preference to a patent peroneal artery, given the technical ease of this bypass configuration. However, when the peroneal artery is evaluated to be a superior target vessel to the DP artery on DSA, or when the length of available vein conduit is inadequate for bypass to the DP artery, peroneal bypass is performed. In cases of severe dorsal foot infection, or when the indication for arterial reconstruction is

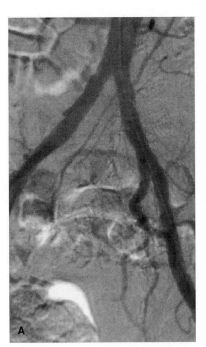
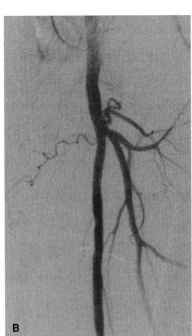
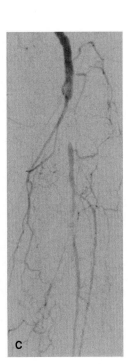
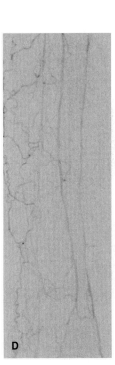

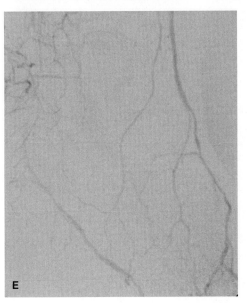

Fig. 1. Intra-arterial digital subtraction arteriogram demonstrating the characteristic pattern of occlusive disease in diabetes. The aorta, iliac arteries **(A),** superficial femoral arteries, and popliteal arteries **(B)** are uninvolved. The tibial/peroneal arteries **(C,D)** are diffusely diseased and the dorsalis pedis artery **(E)** is patent. (Reprinted with permission from Aulivola B, Pomposelli Jr. Dorsalis pedis artery bypass. In: Davies AH, ed. Fast facts—vascular surgery highlights 2002-03. Oxford: Health Press Limited, 2003:36.)

claudication alone, DP bypass is not preferentially performed. Bypass to the tarsal or plantar arteries is generally preserved for cases in which the DP artery is not a viable option for bypass outflow.

The majority of limbs requiring DP bypass have undergone previous ipsilateral limb revascularization. In our own unpublished collection of 124 tarsal or plantar bypasses over a 14-year period, approximately 18% had undergone previous bypass procedures and 5% had undergone previous DP bypass on the ipsilateral extremity. The most frequent indication for bypass in these patients was tissue loss, present in 95%, with ischemic rest pain in an additional 3% and failing graft in 2%. All had no other reasonable bypass outflow target, including the DP artery.

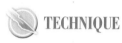

TECHNIQUE

Dorsalis Pedis Bypass

The overall strategy of DP bypass is designed to simplify the procedure and minimize the use of prosthetic graft material. The key principles include the use of distal inflow sites and short, translocated, saphenous vein grafts whenever possible. Short vein grafts with distal inflow have been demonstrated to result in acceptable limb salvage even in the face of poor arterial runoff and high outflow resistance. Bypass procedures originating from the femoral level with an intact saphenous vein are well suited for use of the in situ technique with angioscopy for valve lysis under direct visualization. Vein tributaries are ligated with silk suture. The use of an angioscope with a pump irrigation system facilitates valve lysis and allows for thorough evaluation of the vein conduit for webs or stenoses. The angioscope is inserted into the proximal end of the vein graft and a long flexible valvulotome is inserted from the distal end for valve lysis and vein graft inspection prior to performing the anastomoses (Fig. 2). Use of the pump irrigation system has been shown to decrease the amount of crystalloid infused while aiding in the clarity of the angioscopic examination. When the saphenous vein is unavailable, unusable, or of inadequate length, an arm vein is the preferred source of alternative conduit. When an arm vein is not available, the lesser saphenous vein may be used if the caliber and quality are thought to be adequate. Composite grafts composed of multiple vein segments may also be used, but are only required on occasion. The quality of arm and composite vein conduits should be evaluated with angioscopy. The importance of using the most distal appropriate inflow vessel is especially salient in cases of limited vein conduit. In these cases, every effort should be made to originate the graft from a distal inflow site, even in the presence of a diseased superficial femoral artery (SFA), as long as the extent of disease at this level is not thought to be hemodynamically significant. When significant SFA disease precludes this approach, a simultaneous femoral to popliteal bypass with a prosthetic graft and popliteal to DP bypass with vein may be indicated, if anatomically feasible.

The DP artery at a level just distal to the ends of the malleoli is usually located approximately 1 cm lateral to the extensor hallucis longus tendon (Fig. 3). Exposure of this artery is accomplished with a longitudinal incision directly over the Doppler signal of the artery on the dorsal foot. Occasionally, the artery may be located more laterally, underscoring the importance of careful examination of the preoperative DSA and use of Doppler to precisely locate the artery prior to making the incision. The dissection is carried through the extensor retinaculum, under which the DP artery lies. The DP artery gives rise to the lateral tarsal artery proximally and bifurcates more distally, at the level of the proximal first metatarsal. At this level, the DP branches into the deep plantar and first dorsal metatarsal artery. In most cases, the DP artery is amenable to bypass grafting between these two branch points. An internal luminal diameter of greater than 1 mm is optimal. The heavily calcified dorsalis pedis artery may be controlled with an intraluminal coronary occluder rather than vascular clamps or vessel loops. The distal anastomosis is completed with a 6-0 or 7-0 monofilament polypropylene suture on a small cardiovascular cutting needle. Management of extensive circumferential calcification has been described with a fracture technique, but we find that this is generally not necessary with the use of small cutting needles.

When an in situ vein graft is used, the graft is tunneled at a gentle angle between the saphenous vein harvest incision and the parallel dorsal foot incision used to expose the DP artery, never directly under the resulting skin bridge (Fig. 4). Foot wounds can be closed primarily without the use of advancement or rotational flaps, but must be meticulous, avoiding undue tension. Closure of these incisions is best

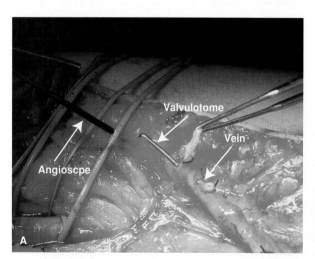

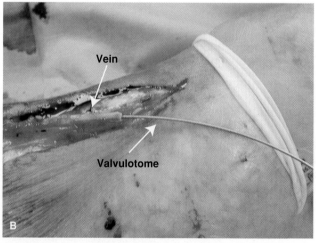

Fig. 2. Insertion of the angioscope into the proximal saphenous vein **(A)** and insertion of the valvulotome into the distal vein **(B)** for valve lysis under direct visualization. (Reprinted with permission from Aulivola B, Pomposelli Jr. Dorsalis pedis artery bypass. In: Davies AH, ed. Fast facts—vascular surgery highlights 2002–03. Oxford: Health Press Limited, 2003:36.)

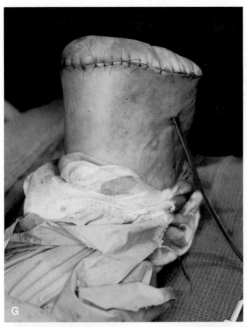

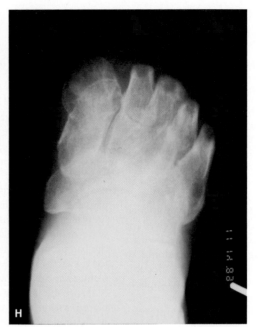

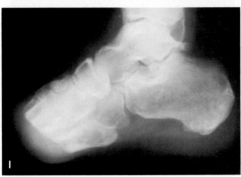

Fig. 8. Continued **G:** The plantar and dorsal skin flaps have been repaired with nylon simple interrupted sutures. A tube-low-suction drain is seen exiting the skin on the dorsolateral side of the foot. **H,I:** Anteroposterior and lateral radiographs, postoperative transmetatarsal amputation.

Fig 9. Long-term appearance of a well-healed transmetatarsal amputation. **A,B:** Satisfactory shape and contour of the right transmetatarsal amputation stump. The plantar skin is healthy with no evidence of elevated plantar pressure. The healed incision rests on the dorsum of the foot.

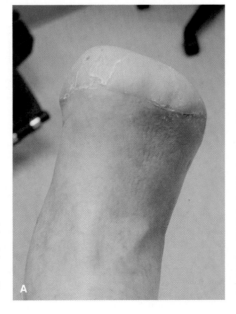

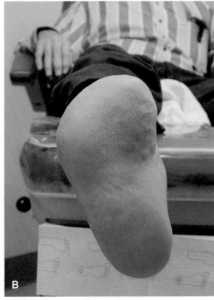

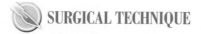

POSTOPERATIVE MANAGEMENT

Dressings consist of nonadherent fine mesh gauze (petrolatum, 3% Xeroform (Kendall) or Adaptic (Johnson & Johnson Hospital Products)) placed on the suture line, wide gauze sponges (4 × 8 s, with a long dorsal and plantar tail, secured around the stump), and combine pads for protection of the heel and lateral border of the foot. Dressings are held in place by 4-in. gauze bandages. A well-padded plaster posterior splint is applied to immobilize the foot and ankle. It is very important to protect the heel with a combine dressing and/or cast padding, so as to avoid the development of a decubitus ulcer. This is a preventable complication. The patient remains non–weight bearing with the affected extremity elevated to reduce postoperative edema and bleeding. Drains are generally left in place for 48 to 72 hours. Normal sterile saline moist-to-dry dressings are applied when there is persistent drainage from the wound or when portions of the wound remain open. Sutures and/or staples are removed after 21 days, and if the wound is healed, the patient is then placed in a short-leg fiberglass cast, a removable walking brace, or Multi-Podus Foot Orthosis (Restorative Care of America Incorporated, St. Petersburg, Fl) partial weight bearing for an additional 3 weeks. The patient gradually returns to full weight bearing in therapeutic-depth inlay footwear. Shoe modifications include a stump filler and stiffened outer sole. Consultation with a certified pedorthist will help with selection of the most appropriate footwear.

Transmetatarsal Amputation with Excision of Plantar Ulcer

Chronic nonhealing neuropathic plantar ulceration is often associated with the complications of soft tissue infection and osteomyelitis. Cases that are refractory to off-loading of the foot and conservative wound care may benefit from a modified transmetatarsal amputation with excision of the ulcer from the plantar flap. This technique can also be used in the absence of a plantar ulcer to remodel an excessively broad plantar flap, thereby avoiding redundant skin and unsightly dog ears.

SURGICAL TECHNIQUE

Ulceration Beneath the Central Metatarsal Heads

Following a standard TMA procedure, the plantar flap is revised as illustrated in Figures 10 and 11. The ulcer is completely enclosed in a triangle with its apex located proximally. Several Allis tissue forceps are applied to the distal flap and the wedge of skin is excised. It should be emphasized that the Allis clamps should only be placed on skin that is to be excised. A wide malleable retractor placed beneath the flap provides a firm supporting surface for the excision. The two segments of the plantar flap are then approximated with 3-0 absorbable simple interrupted sutures placed within the wound, and either 4-0 or 3-0 nylon simple interrupted sutures (+/− staples) in the skin. The dorsal and plantar flaps are closed over a TLS drain. Dressings, posterior splint, and cast are applied as for a basic TMA.

Ulceration Beneath the First Metatarsal Head

Following a standard TMA procedure, the plantar flap is revised as illustrated in Figures 12 to 14. The ulcer is completely enclosed in a triangle with its apex located proximally. The base of the wedge is located at the distal medial border of the

plantar flap. Excision of this wedge allows for easy repair of the plantar and dorsal skin flaps, with very little additional remodeling required.

COMPLICATIONS

Postoperative complications include infection, hematoma formation, seroma, skin necrosis, and wound dehiscence. Commonly, a triangular area of discoloration develops on the dorsal flap within 1 to 2 weeks after surgery and resolves spontaneously.

Open Transmetatarsal Amputation

Extensive forefoot infection or gangrene that extends onto the plantar skin may preclude a standard forefoot or midfoot amputation. In these cases, an open or "guillotine amputation" performed at the midmetatarsal level may be required. Guillotine amputations have a major disadvantage in that they require extensive revision. A better alternative is to fashion flaps in the usual manner but to leave the wound open, with the intent to perform a delayed primary closure. The main disadvantage of open procedures is the prolonged length of time for healing and the need for frequent dressing changes and débridement. Ideally, the wound will

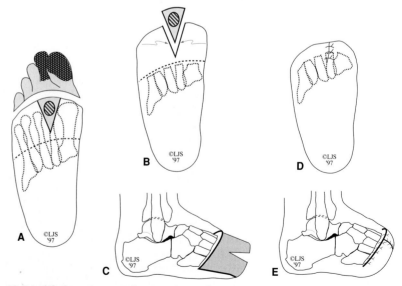

Fig. 10. Modified transmetatarsal amputation with excision of a plantar ulcer beneath the second metatarsal head. **A:** A triangular wedge is drawn on the skin, encompassing the plantar ulcer. **B:** The forefoot has been amputated and the triangular wedge of skin excised from the plantar flap. **C:** Appearance of the plantar flap prior to repair. **D:** The plantar flap has been repaired with simple interrupted sutures. **E:** Completed repair with approximation of the dorsal and plantar skin flaps. (From Sanders LJ. Transmetatarsal and mid-foot amputations. *Clin Padiatr Med Surg.* 1997;14(4):741, with permission from Elsevier Science).

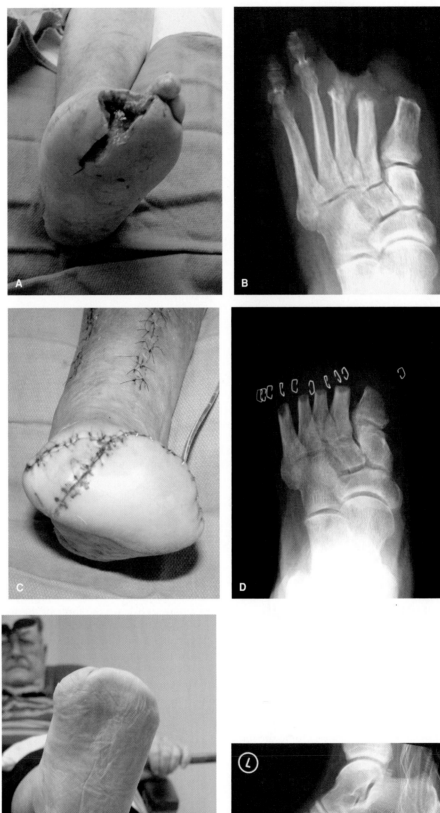

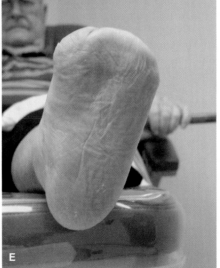

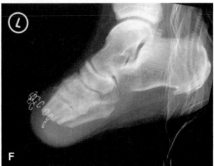

Fig. 11. A 71-year-old male with type 2 diabetes mellitus, peripheral arterial disease, peripheral neuropathy, and chronic renal insufficiency. Same patient as in Figure 2A,B, status post incision and, drainage of left foot with partial amputation of rays 1 to 3, and revascularization (popliteal artery to anterior tibial artery bypass). **A:** Preoperative transmetatarsal amputation of left foot; appearance of the foot 1 week following revascularization. **B:** Anteroposterior (AP) radiograph of left foot, status post incision and drainage with amputation of toes 1 to 3 and portions of the first, second, and third metatarsals. **C:** Completed transmetatarsal amputation with excision of the plantar wound and repair of the plantar flap. **D:** AP radiograph following transmetatarsal amputation. **E:** Appearance of the left foot, 1 year postoperative. **F:** Postoperative lateral radiograph, left foot.

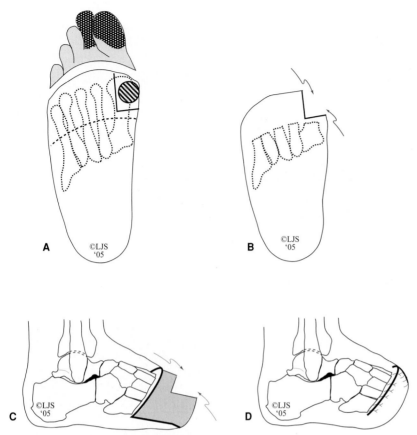

Fig. 12. Modified transmetatarsal amputation with excision of plantar ulcer beneath the first metatarsophalangeal joint. **A:** Plantar ulcer beneath the first metatarsal head, enclosed in a right triangle. **B,C:** Appearance of the plantar flap following transmetatarsal amputation with excision of a triangular wedge of skin. **D:** Completed transmetatarsal amputation with repair of the skin flaps.

form a healthy granulation tissue base that can support a split-thickness skin graft or heal by secondary intention.

Amputations Through the Midfoot

Lisfranc and Chopart amputations are frequently complicated by the development of equinus deformity. Equinovarus deformity is associated with the Lisfranc disarticulation. Amputation at the tarsometatarsal joints appears to be the most proximal level that allows for satisfactory function of the foot. Care must be taken to preserve the base of the fifth metatarsal with its tendinous attachments. The Achilles tendon should be lengthened, as necessary.

The Chopart midtarsal joint amputation has the advantage of producing less limb shortening than a Syme procedure because the talus and calcaneus are re-

tained. However, complications are commonly reported with the Chopart amputation. Severe equinus deformity develops due to loss of the tibialis anterior, long extensor, and peroneal tendons, with resultant failure to balance the force of the triceps surae. The resulting foot is short with a very small weight-bearing surface, and is at increased risk for further breakdown. Some authors advise reattachment of the tibialis anterior to the talus to prevent equinus deformity of the hindfoot. However, long-term results demonstrate inevitable development of equinus deformity, even with tenotomy of the tendo-Achilles.

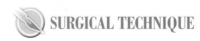 SURGICAL TECHNIQUE

Modified Lisfranc Amputation

Modifications of the Lisfranc amputation include preservation of the fifth metatarsal

base, and the second metatarsal base, in its intercuneiform mortise.

This procedure is performed in a manner similar to the transmetatarsal amputation, with the development of a longer plantar flap and short dorsal flap. The dorsal skin incision is made just distal to the first metatarsal-cuneiform joint and carried across the dorsum of the foot, ending just distal to the fifth metatarsal base. Occasionally it may be necessary to develop a longer dorsal flap to compensate for devitalized plantar skin. The medial and lateral incisions are carried distally along the metatarsal shafts to the necks of the metatarsals and then curved plantarly across the ball of the foot. The plantar flap is developed to the intended level of disarticulation.

The first metatarsal base is disarticulated from the medial cuneiform. Using a power saw and working from medial to lateral, the second metatarsal is transected at the level of the first and third cuneiforms, leaving its base intact in the intercuneiform mortise. The third and fourth metatarsals are then disarticulated, followed by transection of the fifth metatarsal, just distal to its base. Although the fifth metatarsal base will leave a prominence of bone, this generally does not cause a problem. Wound closure is performed in the same manner as described above for a TMA. Dressings and postoperative care are also the same. High-top shoes with a stump filler and mild rocker sole are well suited for this level of midfoot amputation.

OUTCOMES OF TRANSMETATARSAL AND MIDFOOT AMPUTATIONS

Of the levels of local amputation of the foot discussed in this chapter, the transmetatarsal amputation is the most successful with respect to functional outcomes, patient satisfaction, and long-term results. Transmetatarsal amputation preserves foot function, is cosmetically acceptable, does not require a prosthesis, and enables fitting with commercially available footwear. Amputations performed at the tarsometatarsal and midtarsal joint levels frequently result in deformity and difficulty fitting shoes. Limb salvage can be achieved, with functional outcomes, by the motivated patient and knowledgeable surgeon with the use of these procedures.

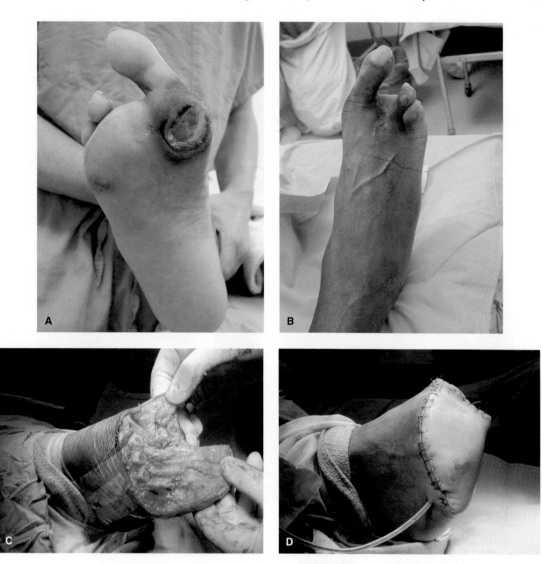

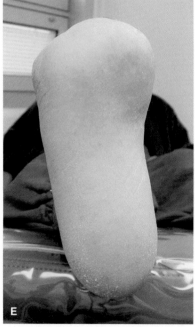

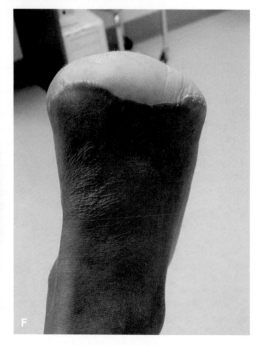

Fig. 13. Modified transmetatarsal amputation with excision of plantar ulcer beneath the first metatarsophalangeal joint. **A:** Full-thickness ulcer beneath the first metatarsal head, right foot. **B:** Dorsal view right foot, amputation of the second and third toes. **C:** Plantar flap prior to repair. **D:** Repair of plantar flap with closure of the transmetatarsal amputation. A small dog ear is present at the apex of the repair. This will flatten out and does not require excision. A drain exits from the lateral aspect of the foot. **E,F:** Appearance of the right foot at 18 months post–transmetatarsal amputation. Note the shape and contour of the stump and healthy appearance of the plantar flap.

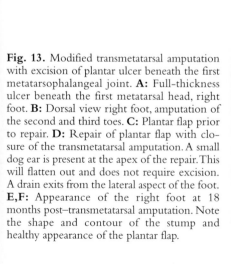

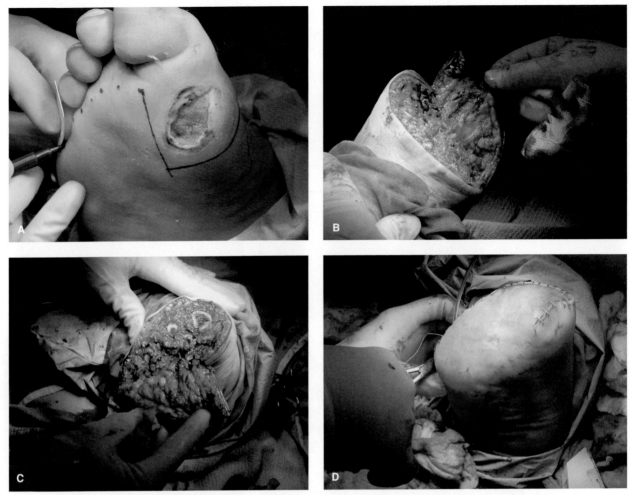

Fig. 14. Modified transmetatarsal amputation with excision of plantar ulcer, right foot, in a 49-year-old male with type 2 diabetes, dense peripheral neuropathy, and chronic (greater than 2 years' duration) nonhealing plantar ulcer, right foot. Biopsy revealed a verrucous squamous cell carcinoma. **A:** Full-thickness ulcer beneath the first metatarsal head right foot. **B,C:** Appearance of the plantar flap following excision of the ulcer. **D:** Completed transmetatarsal amputation with repair of the dorsal and plantar flaps.

SUGGESTED READING

Principal References

McKittrick LS, McKittrick JB, Risley TS. Transmetatarsal amputation for infection or gangrene in patients with diabetes mellitus. *Ann Surg* 1949;130(4):826.

Sanders LJ. Transmetatarsal and midfoot amputations. *Clin Podiatr Med Surg* 1997;14(4):741.

Sanders LJ, Dunlap G. Transmetatarsal amputation: a successful approach to limb salvage. *J Am Podiatr Med Assoc* 1992;82(3):129.

Smith DG. Amputation. Preoperative assessment and lower extremity surgical techniques. *Foot Ankle Clin* 2001;6(2):271.

Sanders LJ. Surgical approach to the diabetic foot. In: Edmonds ME, Foster AV, Sanders LJ, eds. *A practical manual of diabetic foot care,* 1st ed. Oxford: Blackwell Publishing Limited, 2003.

Additional References

Boulton AJM, Kirsner RS, Vileikyte L. Neuropathic diabetic foot ulcers. *N Engl J Med* 2004;351:48.

Centers for Disease Control and Prevention. CDC National Diabetes Surveillance System, Hospitalizations for Nontraumatic Lower Extremity Amputations. Available at: www.cdc.gov/diabetes/statistics/lea/index.htm. Accessed May 18, 2005.

Dalla Paola L, Faglia E, Caminiti M, et al. Ulcer recurrence following first ray amputation in diabetic patients: a cohort prospective study. *Diabetes Care* 2003;26(6):1874.

Durham JR, McCoy DM, Sawchuk AP, et al. Open transmetatarsal amputation in the treatment of severe foot infections. *Am J Surg* 1989;158(2):127.

Glass H, Rowe VL, Hood DB, et al. Influence of transmetatarsal amputation in patients requiring lower extremity distal revascularization. *Am Surg* 2004;70(10):845.

Hosch J, Quiroga C, Bosma J. Outcomes of transmetatarsal amputations in patients with diabetes mellitus. *J Foot Ankle Surg* 1997;36 (6):430.

Lavery LA, Lavery DC, Quebedeax-Farnham TL. Increased foot pressure after great toe amputation in diabetes. *Diabetes Care* 1995; 18(11):1460.

Lipsky BA, Berentdt AR, Deery HG, et al. Diagnosis and treatment of diabetic foot infections. *Clin Infect Dis* 2004;39(7):885.

Murdoch DP, Armstrong DG, Dacus JB, et al. The natural history of great toe amputations. *J Foot Ankle Surg* 1997;36(3):204.

Mwiipatayi BP, Naidoo NG, Jeffrey PC, et al. Transmetatarsal amputation: three-year experience at Groote Schuur Hospital. *World J Surg* 2005;29(2):245.

Pinzur M, Kaminsky M, Sage R, et al. Amputations at the middle level of the foot. *J Bone Joint Surg* 1986;68A:1061.

Pinzur MS, Sage R, Schwaegler P. Ray resection in the dysvascular foot. A retrospective review. *Clin Orthop* 1984;(191):232.

Reiber GR. Epidemiology of foot ulcers and amputations in the diabetic foot. In: Levin ME, Pfeifer MA, Bowker J, eds. *The diabetic foot,* 6th ed. St. Louis: C.V. Mosby Company, 2001.

Sanders LJ. Amputations in the diabetic foot. *Clin Podiatr Med Surg.* 1987;4(2):481.

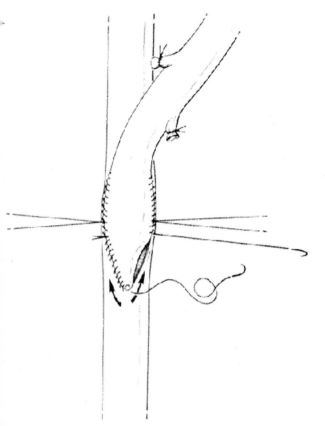

Fig. 4. The completed anastomosis.

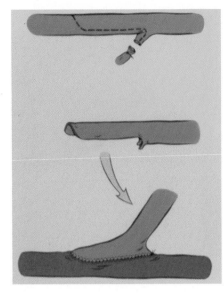

Fig. 6. Distal anastomosis of vein graft.

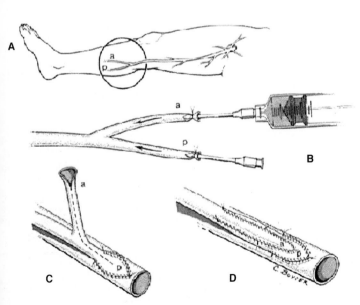

Fig. 5. Pedicle patch angioplasty.

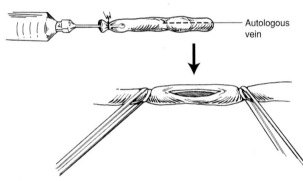

Fig. 7. A short piece of autologous vein is cannulated at its peripheral end and gently distended. The vein is then incised to match the arteriotomy in the tibial artery.

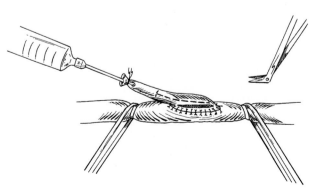

Fig. 8. The vein is then incised as indicated, but it is not completely transected.

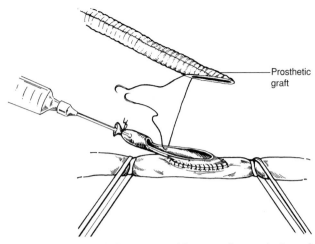

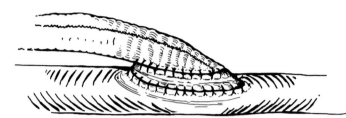

Fig. 9. An anastomosis is constructed between the prosthetic graft and the vein

Fig. 10. At the completion of the anastomosis, the vein segment is transected.

EDITOR'S COMMENT

Infrageniculate vein bypass remains one of the signature procedures of vascular surgery. All of us who do a substantial number of such bypasses have over the years developed tricks for making these often tedious and complex procedures easier. In this chapter, Dr. LoGerfo, a master surgeon for this type of procedure, shares some of his tips and tricks with us. These are useful procedures that he describes and are very well illustrated. My comments will be directed toward each of the tips or tricks and generally represent only my variations on the theme established by Dr. LoGerfo.

Stabilization of the vein for the distal anastomosis of a tibial bypass can be problematic. The proximal anastomosis is usually done first to allow pressurization of the vein for passage through the tunnel. Additionally, when multiple segments of vein are used to construct the graft, particularly multiple pieces of arm vein, assessing the hemostasis of the graft prior to placing it in the tunnel is essential. Dr. LoGerfo's technique for stabilizing the vein during the distal anastomosis is certainly helpful if a sufficient length of extra vein is available to leave the cannula in the vein. This approach also assumes that the vein has been placed in reversed fashion, which, as I will note later, we usually do not do. In contrast, if the amount of vein available is severely limited so that you need every millimeter, placing a stitch in the end of the vein while the heel portion of the anastomosis is done serves a similar purpose to the cannula that Dr. LoGerfo describes. This can be placed as a stay suture with a small clamp attached to it. Additionally, while Dr. LoGerfo describes the use of a parachute technique for the heel of the anastomosis, my preference has been to use a single horizontal mattress suture at the heel for these small anastomoses. This actually accomplishes the same mobility of the heel of the anastomosis as parachuting does without the risk of tearing the vein when the parachute suture is pulled down. Finally, if adequate

vein is available, it is most useful to fashion the toe of the anastomosis as the sutures are placed rather than cutting the ears off beforehand, again, as described by Dr. LoGerfo.

Dr. LoGerfo's pedicle patch angioplasty technique for enlarging a vein graft anastomosis is a helpful technique. However, this is a technique that we rarely use for several reasons. First, as previously noted, our approach has been to generally place vein grafts in a nonreversed configuration, thereby avoiding the problem of the "little end of the vein to the big artery." Additionally, in the patient who has limited venous conduit (as it seems all of our patients do), it is usually difficult to find a vein in which an appropriate branch is present at the appropriate place. Regardless, if such a vein branch is seen, this is a useful technique. A trick to make this type of patch anastomosis easier is to put two traction sutures at the corners of the "heel" of this anastomosis, thereby pulling this narrowest part of the patch open. These stitches can then be used in an alternating fashion to complete the anastomosis in a three fourths to one fourth fashion. Alternatively, a standard patch can be placed to enlarge a proximal anastomosis as Dr. LoGerfo notes or through a distal anastomosis if not only the patch but also the artery needs to be repaired. When a standard patch is placed and it passes through the anastomosis, it is important to remember that the anastomotic suture line that has been divided must be secured. In this situation, I generally use a "two-stitch technique," placing two double-armed stitches at each end of the patch and subsequently completing the anastomosis by using alternating portions of each of these sutures to complete each wall of the anastomosis.

Similarly, the use of a branch to accommodate a "high angle" of an in situ femoral popliteal bypass can be very helpful. However, tunneling the graft anatomically between the heads of the gastrocnemius muscle avoids the problem of the high angle altogether and also avoids the uncommon but significant problem of crimping of the graft by the medial

head of the gastrocnemius muscle. This problem is occasionally seen with in situ femoral popliteal bypass grafts when the vein is caught by the head of the muscle and the tibia as scarring ensues. When this occurs, forceful flexion or extension of the foot will occlude the graft and can cause recurrent claudication. Additionally, in its most severe form, injury to the vein will develop and either graft thrombosis or distal atheroemboli leading to limb loss can occur.

Finally, as Dr. LoGerfo notes, multiple techniques have been described for construction of a distal vein cuff in conjunction with a prosthetic femoral to below-knee popliteal or infrapopliteal bypass. However, to date, no one technique has been shown to be superior. As he notes, many of these techniques are complex; therefore, any simple technique including the technique that Dr. LoGerfo describes is useful when such a cuff needs to be done. The technique described by Dr. LoGerfo is useful when you have a short piece of adequately sized vein for construction of that cuff. In contrast, when the available vein is small, a true collar needs to be constructed by longitudinally incising the vein and suturing one wall of the incised vein around the arteriotomy in a continuous fashion, usually starting and ending on the front portion of the arteriotomy where the adjacent ends of the vein are then closed vertically to complete the collar. The prosthetic graft can then be attached to the collar in the usual fashion. Interestingly, despite all that has been written about the value of vein cuffs for improving prosthetic infrainguinal bypass graft patency, in the single randomized trial comparing prosthetic femoral popliteal bypass done with and without vein cuffs, only when the distal anastomosis was done to the below-knee popliteal artery was there any improvement in early or late patency associated with the use of the vein cuff (Stonebridge P. *J Vasc Surg* 1997;26:543).

J.M.S.

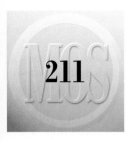

Major Lower
Extremity Amputation

MARK R. NEHLER AND PEGGE HALANDRES

INTRODUCTION

Despite advances in lower extremity revascularization with widespread use of alternate vein conduit and bypass to tibial/pedal targets, national registries including the Department of Veterans Affairs National Surgical Quality Improvement Program (NSQIP) and the 1980–2000 National Hospital Discharge Survey (NHDS) show no reduction in major lower extremity amputations in the United States. The aging of the U.S. population and the persistent trend for delayed and inconsistent referral to vascular surgery are major reasons for this. Therefore, major lower extremity amputation will continue to be a common operative procedure for the general and vascular surgeon.

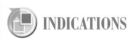 ## INDICATIONS

The three most common indications for major lower extremity amputation are acute limb ischemia, chronic critical limb ischemia, and major infection due to malperforans ulcers in diabetics with normal arterial circulation. The latter two have significant clinical overlap, with many diabetic patients with poor or marginal circulation and eventual limb loss suffering neuropathy and malperforans ulcers as an initiating event. Failure to recognize this leads to a significant amount of unnecessary limb loss due to delay in referral for potential revascularization (often following failed forefoot directed amputations), leading to limbs not considered salvageable due to extensive pedal necrosis.

Acute Limb Ischemia

Most occlusions in acute limb ischemia involve the popliteal or more proximal arteries. Therefore, amputation in acute ischemia is frequently at or above the knee level. In addition, significant muscle beds are usually threatened and most vascular surgeons attempt to salvage acutely threatened limbs if the outcome is in doubt, so many amputations in acute limb ischemia occur in patients suffering significant reperfusion injury with rhabdomyolysis

and renal damage. In addition, incisions from previous revascularization attempts may complicate planning the subsequent amputation and lead to delayed healing. Acute limb ischemia patients are often receiving anticoagulants for therapy of the underlying thrombotic or embolic event, further increasing the risk of hematoma and wound complications. Finally, many cases of amputation due to acute limb ischemia involve iatrogenic vascular injury or delay in diagnosis/referral, increasing the psychological complexity of the care and having medical legal implications.

Chronic Critical Limb Ischemia

The vast majority of major lower extremity amputations are due to critical limb ischemia (CLI). Unlike other areas of vascular surgery such as aneurysm disease and carotid disease, accurate guidelines on potential salvage of limbs based on revascularization potential and extent of necrosis are lacking. This leads to significant differences in practice patterns based on geography, access to vascular surgery and vascular imaging, and surgeon experience in the use of alternate vein conduit and bypass to tibial/pedal targets. More recently, many patients with CLI are undergoing partial or complete therapy with interventional techniques. Finally, unlike cardiac disease, there is no established route of access for suspected CLI to vascular surgery in modern health care systems, leading frequently to significant delay in referral and ultimate diagnosis. Therefore, eventual amputees with CLI fall in to two categories: (a) patients who are not offered revascularization either due to the extent of pedal necrosis on vascular presentation, failure to recognize CLI and futile forefoot amputations, and/or co-morbidities (medical and/or functional) that would preclude revascularization; and (b) patients who fail revascularization (either occlusion or ongoing pedal necrosis despite improved circulation). Most centers with aggressive limb salvage practice perform far fewer primary amputations than revascularizations, so that many patients with CLI who require amputation have had prior

revascularizations that have failed. Although several studies have demonstrated no effect of a failed infrainguinal revascularization on amputation level, below-knee amputations (BKA) after failed infrainguinal bypasses have greater wound complications and prolonged healing times.

Malperforans Ulcer/Normal Circulation

Younger diabetics with normal circulation who develop overwhelming foot infections are another major amputee group. Typical patterns include first or fifth metatarsal osteomyelitis from a chronic malperforans ulcer in that location. Patients with Charcot foot can have chronic ulceration at the midplantar area due to osteophytes and pressure points at the chronic midfoot fracture. Many of these diabetic amputees have had prior digit or ray amputations that may have healed, only to have another malperforans ulcer occur in the adjacent digit. The cause of eventual limb loss in this population is multifactorial. Poor compliance (often demonstrated in significantly elevated glycosylated hemoglobin values), obesity (increasing the pressure on the neuropathic foot when ambulatory), and inadequate footwear are major contributors. A less recognized but equally important cause is patient education. Many poorly educated diabetic patients assume that seeking health care for foot lesions will lead to a major amputation, and therefore delay care until a major amputation is inevitable, which continues to perpetuate this widespread fear.

 ## PREOPERATIVE PLANNING

General

Few vascular surgery procedures have the psychological and functional impact of a major lower extremity amputation. Amputation-free survival is considered the primary end point for any clinical trial for patients with critical limb ischemia. However, in clinical practice, a number of variables can markedly change this end point that has no relationship to efficacy of therapy. Understandably, patients often adamantly refuse amputation. Critical limb ischemia (the most common indication for amputation worldwide) rarely results in overwhelming infection and imminent patient death if left untreated. Therefore, patient pain tolerance is often the deciding variable. Many patients turn to unproven therapies in desperation. All of these issues increase amputation-free survival. Therefore, for many patients, the first step in preoperative preparation is acceptance of the procedure—which frequently takes days to weeks and sometimes multiple visits to answer questions and work through the various stages of grief and loss—for the patient and family members. Often consultation with rehabilitation medicine, physical therapy, prosthetics, and even other amputees is very helpful in preparing the patient and family for the realities of life as an amputee.

Standard evaluation with a thorough history and physical examination should be performed in all patients. Active congestive heart failure, unstable angina, or concurrent myocardial infarction must be addressed. In the absence of active cardiac symptoms, evidence of congestive heart failure on history or physical examination, or acute changes on electrocardiogram, thorough cardiac evaluation is not routinely performed. It is important to recognize that most patients presenting for amputation have had limited activity and may not manifest covert cardiac disease due to the lack of physiologic stress, so even minor symptoms should be very concerning.

Perioperative treatment with beta-blockade has been shown to be beneficial in perioperative management of patients undergoing revascularization for aortic and lower extremity disease. However, due to the shared risk factors, the positive impact of beta-blockers can likely be extrapolated to the amputation population. Management of associated hypertension, diabetes, and renal failure should be optimized. An aggressive approach to normalize glucose levels is essential to ensure proper wound healing. The timing of hemodialysis in relation to operation is important in managing fluids and electrolytes in the perioperative period. Perioperative nutrition is critical, as many patients are depressed, manifested by severe emaciation. Depressed patients not eating or participating in their postoperative rehabilitation programs are at risk for a host of complications including further nutritional depletion, incisional wound complications,

decubitus ulcers, contractures, and deep venous thrombosis (DVT).

Finally, due to relative inactivity and frequent hypercoagulable states in the amputation population, venous thromboembolism is a major source of postoperative morbidity/mortality. Recent data would indicate the incidence is 15%. In addition to the risk of fatal pulmonary embolism, postoperative DVT may cause severe stump swelling and impaired primary healing of the amputation. Routine DVT prophylaxis and/or careful perioperative screening for DVT with duplex scanning in amputation patients appears prudent.

Determination of Amputation Level

The goals of major lower extremity amputation are several: to eliminate the nonviable tissue, to provide a stump that has the best chance to heal, and to provide a stump with the best chance of long-term function—ambulation with a prosthesis. However, which of these factors is most important often depends on the age, baseline function, and co-morbidities of the patient. On balance, it is important to avoid additional operative procedures in this compromised group of patients. In all reported series, healing of an above-knee amputation (AKA) is more rapid and involves less incisional complications than healing a BKA. However, any chance at rehabilitation and prosthetic use in older vascular patients requires the knee joint. Finally, physicians and patients wish to preserve as much limb length as possible.

Worldwide, the ratio of AKAs to BKAs performed is one. Many AKAs are performed in patients with limited rehabilitation potential and significant co-morbidities, as the primary healing is better and there is a risk of knee contracture in BKAs done in patients who are unable to participate in postoperative physical therapy. Despite this, most patients are considered for BKA due to a variety of reasons, and the surgeon needs to determine if a BKA will heal primarily. A number of studies in the literature describe various circulatory measures to determine amputation level healing. As a general point, many of these techniques are not practical in clinical practice. A palpable pulse at a level immediately proximal to a proposed amputation has been associated with a 100% rate of healing. Most surgeons agree that a BKA without a femoral pulse is unlikely to do well. However, a palpable femoral pulse does not guarantee success. The clinical judgment of the operating surgeon (skin temperature, hair growth,

tissue bleeding, viable muscle, and wounds without tension) has been demonstrated to be reasonably accurate (75% to 85%) in several large clinical series (combined, around 1,000 patients). Finally, despite the plethora of research regarding the technical aspects of salvaging the knee joint, the sobering fact is that many vascular patients will take minimal advantage of this in rehabilitation.

Thermography, skin perfusion via radioisotope injection, and segmental pulse volume recordings (PVRs)/limb pressures have been used to try to improve on the success of clinical judgment in predicting BKA healing. Each has limitations ranging from clinically impractical (thermography and skin perfusion) to not accurate due to calcified vessels (PVRs and pressures) in many amputees. Arguably the most reproducible noninvasive test used to determine BKA healing is transcutaneous measurement of the partial pressure of oxygen ($TcPO_2$). Measurements are obtained in the supine position by placing an oximetry probe on the skin in question and heating the area to 44°C. The generation of heat results in local skin hyperemia, a decrease in flow resistance, and subsequent arterialization of capillary blood. The probe then records skin oxygen tension reflecting the true arterial oxygen pressure in the area in millimeters of mercury. Absolute measurements, measurements compared to a control location such as the chest, and measurements compared to transcutaneous carbon dioxide values have been reported. Various studies have shown that $TcPO_2$ measurements of greater than or equal to 30 mm Hg have an accuracy of 87% to 100% in predicting BKA healing. In addition, this technique can be used in patients with arterial calcification. However, supplemental oxygen can falsely elevate $TcPO_2$, and edema can falsely reduce $TcPO_2$.

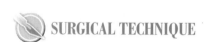 **SURGICAL TECHNIQUE**

Basic Principles

The authors follow several general principles in amputation surgery. When at all possible, tourniquets are used to minimize blood loss despite liberal use of the knife for dissection. All major vessels are suture ligated. We do not use bone wax for control of any bone marrow bleeding, for concern of leaving a foreign body and potential infection. We transect both the tibia and the fibula with a saw, to avoid any spiral fracture of the fibula. Major

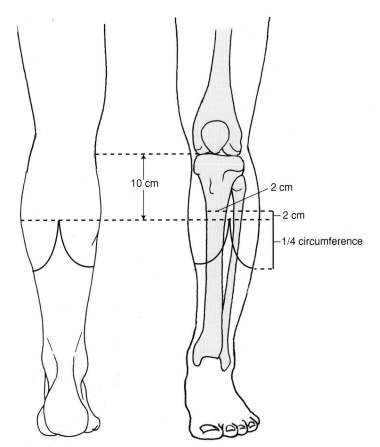

Fig. 7. Initial measurements for skin flap incisions in skew flap below-knee amputation.

forefoot procedures. Many patients are in the last months of their lives, and could be described as dying from the periphery inward. An episode of aspiration pneumonitis, subendocardial infarct, or exacerbation of congestive failure can easily prove to be fatal. Compounding the problem, amputations are rarely considered by anesthesia and/or surgeons as a case of the same

magnitude as a major vascular reconstruction or cardiac case.

In addition to the typical cardiovascular morbidities, patients undergoing major amputation are immobile both in the preoperative and perioperative periods. Not surprisingly, the incidence of deep venous thrombosis is high in this population, mandating some level of prophylaxis. As many

of these patients have underlying hypercoagulable states or undergo amputation for acute arterial thrombosis, anticoagulation is frequent, which often leads to bleeding complications. Finally, many diabetic patients require amputation for severe forefoot sepsis. These patients can suffer septic complications from delay in definitive removal of the septic focus and/or bacteremia at the time of the procedure.

Healing rates of BKA vary, but failure in 10% to 20% is widely reported. These patients often have one or more operations attempting to salvage the knee joint, followed by an eventual AKA. Amputation healing times are often measured in months rather than weeks. Part of the difficulty in wound healing is related to falls and stump trauma. However, even without postoperative trauma, CLI patients heal incisions below the knee poorly. Casting the BKA stump appears useful to reduce trauma and edema, but the single small trial using these devices did not demonstrate efficacy compared to standard protective bandages.

From the patient perspective, one of the most important morbidities of amputation is postoperative pain. Chronic postoperative amputation pain can be divided into two groups, residual limb (stump pain) and phantom limb pain. The prevalence is in the range of 50% to 80% of amputees. Both central and peripheral pain mechanisms appear to be involved, including ectopic activity originating from afferent fibers in a neuroma and cortical reorganization/spinal cord sensitization. For most patients, the pain is episodic in nature and not particularly troublesome. In approximately one in four of patients, however, the symptoms are very disabling. In addition, some data suggest that the duration and intensity of preamputation limb pain plays a role in early post amputation residual limb and phantom limb pain.

FUNCTIONAL OUTCOMES

A substantial amount of research has focused on preoperative evaluations to determine if a BKA will heal, with preservation of the knee joint and improved function and potential mobility. This is extremely relevant in the younger amputee population. However, the sobering fact is that many elderly patients will not be able to complete an arduous rehabilitation program to ambulate to any extent with a prosthesis. Much of this is related to the co-morbidities in the population as previously stated with regard to perioperative mortality. However, in the United States,

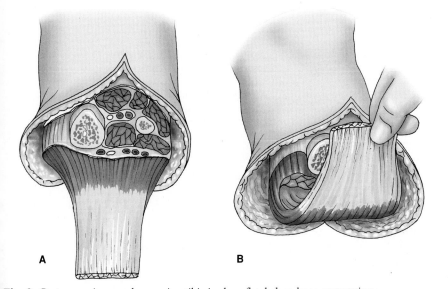

Fig. 8. Gastrocnemius muscle covering tibia in skew flap below-knee amputation.

Vascular Surgery

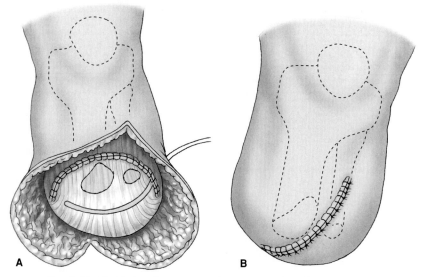

Fig. 9. Finished below-knee amputation stump in skew flap amputation.

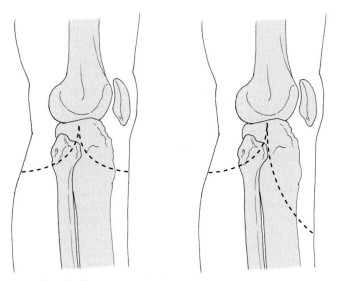

Fig. 10. Skin incisions for through-the-knee amputation.

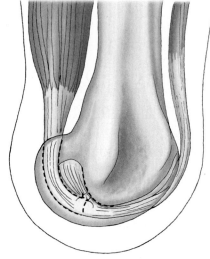

Fig. 11. Tendon reapproximation in through-the-knee amputation.

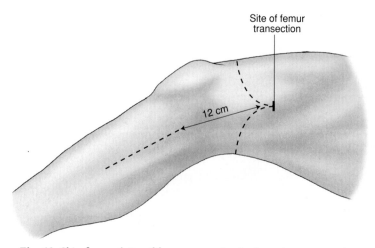

Fig. 12. Skin flaps and site of femur transection in above-knee amputation.

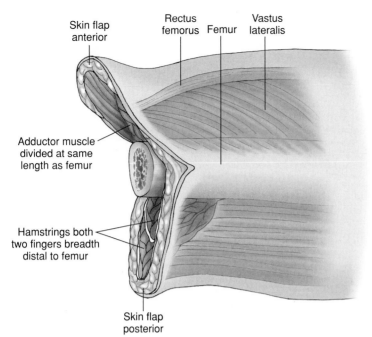

Fig. 13. Muscle division in relationship to femur division in above-knee amputation.

at 3 years, respectively, again emphasizing the palliative nature of these procedures in most patients. In addition to mortality, significant ongoing morbidity occurs in both the remaining stump (BKA) and contralateral limb following major lower extremity amputation. At 2 years, 15% of patients with an initially successful BKA will convert to an AKA, and another 15% will suffer a major contralateral amputation.

SUMMARY

Major lower extremity amputation is a common procedure. Despite the improvements in limb salvage, available data would indicate that the incidence is not decreasing. Based on results, it is one of the more complex operations performed. Careful selection of level based on circulation and functional issues, attention to detail in the operating room, and careful perioperative care are required to obtain good results in this often frail population.

SUGGESTED READING

Bacharach JM, Rooke TW, Osmundson PJ, et al. Predictive value of transcutaneous oxygen pressure and amputation success by use of supine and elevation measurements. *J Vasc Surg* 1992;15:558.

Dillingham TR, Pezzin LE, MacKenzie EJ. Limb amputation and limb deficiency: epidemiology and recent trends in the United States. *South Med J* 2002;95:875.

Feinglass J, Pearce WH, Martin GJ, et al. Postoperative and late survival outcomes after major amputation: findings from the Department of Veterans Affairs National Surgical Quality Improvement Program. *Surgery* 2001;130:21.

Nehler MR, Coll JR, Hiatt WR, et al. Functional outcome in a contemporary series of major lower extremity amputations. *J Vasc Surg* 2003;38:7.

Wagner WH, Keagy BA, Kotb MM, et al. Noninvasive determination of healing of major lower extremity amputation: the continued role of clinical judgment. *J Vasc Surg* 1988;8:703.

Yeager RA, Moneta GL, Edwards JM, et al. Deep vein thrombosis associated with lower extremity amputation. *J Vasc Surg* 1995;22:612.

the passage of the Americans with Disability Act in 1990 has improved wheelchair access by mandating it for public buildings. Frequently, elderly amputees choose to focus effort toward modifying the home to allow at least some mobility in a wheelchair. A recent review at our institution demonstrated that less than half of amputees were ambulatory postoperatively, but relatively few required transition to a care facility. A patient with a healed amputation (AKA or BKA) who can independently transfer and take a few limited steps but remains in the community is the end result for the majority of elderly amputees. The prevalence of vascular amputees that ambulate postoperatively declines over time due to a variety of issues. Finally, the occasional patient will fall and suffer a major fracture during prosthetic use.

Conversely, if patients are to have any realistic hope of extensive prosthetic ambulation postoperatively, the knee joint must be spared. Many of the AKAs performed are done so based on lack of rehabilitation potential rather than inability to eventually heal a BKA. One obvious question is the potential benefit of the knee joint in the nonambulatory patient. Although statements regarding improved transfer potential and balance are frequently made, the available data to support this are lacking. Thigh muscle atrophy has been noted to correlate with the length of the AKA stump. Balance is clearly an issue with prosthetic use, and has been widely studied. However, similar data regarding balance and wheelchair use are lacking. Finally, small series of the bilateral amputee (both above and below knee) have been reported. Ambulation is unusual, but pressure ulcers as seen in neurologically impaired patients do not appear to be a long-term issue.

NATURAL HISTORY

Patient survival in the NSQIP amputation series for BKA and AKA was 57% and 39%

Vascular Surgery

EDITOR'S COMMENT

Few procedures in surgery evoke more fear in a patient than a major amputation of the lower extremity. Moreover, these amputations are often performed under the most adverse of circumstances, either as a complication of acute arterial insufficiency, leading to myonecrosis, to control life-threatening sepsis or as the final stage of a long treatment course for chronic limb ischemia, usually with one or more failed attempts at limb revascularization. Pain, disfigurement, and loss of mobility and independence are some of the many reasons why patients have such a strong emotional response to major amputation. For these reasons, addressing the issue of amputation with a patient requires the surgeon to approach this topic with the utmost of compassion and empathy.

Oftentimes, amputation is looked upon as a clinical defeat, especially when following a failed attempt at limb revascularization. Nevertheless, for many patients who have suffered through weeks or months of rest pain, nonhealing wounds, ulcers,

(continued)

and/or gangrene in addition to one or more unsuccessful attempts at limb revascularization, the loss of pain and suffering from a successful amputation often results in a significant improvement in the overall quality of their lives, especially when they begin to walk again with a prosthesis. These issues need to be emphasized to the patient during the discussion of a proposed amputation and underscore its important role in the treatment of severe ischemia.

Drs. Nehler and Halandres have summarized the significant morbidity and mortality associated with major amputations, especially in patients with critical limb ischemia, and correctly emphasize the importance of meticulous technique, attention to detail, and excellent postoperative care to minimize these events. The practice of relegating major limb amputation to the most inexperienced member of the health care team is only mentioned to condemn it in the strongest of terms.

It has been said that any surgeon who performs a major limb amputation owes the patient the debt of rehabilitation. Although the functional outcome for major limb amputation will vary greatly based on the patient's baseline level of functioning, age, and associated co-morbidities, it is a good approach in most patients to assume that the patient has the desire and capability to walk with a prosthesis. As a result, planning to save the knee should be the fundamental goal in any patient in whom there is any potential for rehabilitation. In our experience, most patients who have been ambulatory prior to a successful below-knee amputation have a high likelihood of achieving some level of ambulatory function postoperatively. The same cannot be stated for patients who undergo an above-knee amputation, however, where the likelihood of walking with a prosthesis is considerably lower, especially for those over the age of 80. Based on these considerations, determining the likelihood of an amputation healing below the knee is critical to maximize the chances for successful rehabilitation while minimizing the need for multiple procedures. The authors correctly point out that none of the noninvasive modalities used to determine whether an amputation will successfully heal is entirely accurate. Transcutaneous oxygen measurements are perhaps the most popular across the country. However, in our experience, even TcPO$_2$ measurements are associated with a significant "gray area" where the likelihood of amputation cannot be successfully predicted. In addition, we have seen patients with low TcPO$_2$

measurements go on to heal with indices predictive of inadequate perfusion. As a result, we continue to rely on our clinical impression when determining the level of amputation. When the likelihood of healing is marginal, we will still usually attempt a below-knee amputation in any patient thought suitable for rehabilitation. While this results in two procedures if the below-knee amputation fails to heal, it maximizes the chance for saving the knee and has not increased perioperative mortality in our experience. In most patients with no rehabilitation potential, performing an amputation above the knee is usually preferred except under unusual circumstances.

Our approach to major limb amputation varies somewhat from that described by the authors. We never use tourniquets on patients with arterial occlusive disease. Although the Burgess long posterior flap procedure is the most popular method for performing below-knee amputations, on our own unit, we continue to use the fish mouth–shaped incision with equal anterior and posterior flaps. In our experience this technique is technically easier to perform than the long posterior flap procedure, and places the transverse incision directly over the end of the stump, as opposed to the anterior surface of the tibia, which can lead to flap breakdown and exposure of bone, particularly in thin patients with minimum amounts of soft tissue. Moreover, it usually results in a cylindrical-shaped stump without the bulbous end of redundant soft tissue that so frequently occurs with the Burgess technique. Stump swelling is less prominent and often resolves quickly and without the need for a compression device. When fashioning anterior and posterior flaps, the wound closes with more tension than the Burgess technique, but this can be obviated by cutting the tibia back enough to be certain that the wound closes easily. We routinely close our wounds with stainless steel skin staples and avoid the use of plaster casting in favor of a well-padded Velcro knee immobilizer.

Our approach to rehabilitation has changed dramatically. When all rehabilitation for amputation patients was done within the hospital, a below-knee amputation patient with a nicely healing wound would usually be fitted for a temporary prosthesis on postoperative day 5 and would be ambulating in parallel bars, under the supervision of our physical therapists, by the 10th postoperative day. Cost containment concerns in more recent times have required all amputation rehabilitation, including the fitting for the prosthesis, to be outsourced to inpatient skilled nursing facilities or rehabilitation hospitals. As a con-

sequence, rehabilitation has become more varied and out of our immediate control. Physiatrists at the local nursing facility or rehabilitation hospital determine when the patients can be fitted and begin walking with their prosthesis. Many favor a more protracted and conservative approach, with patients with having their fitting delayed for several weeks and not ambulating for as long as 2 to 3 months.

Above-knee amputations are, unfortunately, still frequently required, particularly in patients with critical limb ischemia with no likelihood for rehabilitation or inadequate circulation for healing below the knee. The authors state that worldwide, the ratio of below-knee to above-knee amputations is 1. However, in state-of-the-art vascular units, this ratio should be substantially greater than 1. On our unit, there is approximately a 3:1 ratio of below-knee to above-knee amputations. For those patients requiring above-knee amputations, the authors state that they favor the use of knee disarticulation, with preservation of the entire femur. We feel that for the typical ischemic patient requiring an above-knee amputation, this approach provides few advantages and greater chance of complications, compared to the more commonly performed transfemoral approach, which we have used routinely.

The authors' sobering statistics illustrate that mortality for major limb amputation remains significantly high, in spite of the many improvements and advances in the care of patients with peripheral vascular disease. On our own unit, the mortality for lower extremity arterial reconstruction is less than 2%. In a recent series of nearly 1,000 major lower extremity amputations over the last decade, our composite mortality for major amputations was 6%, including 16.5% for those performed above the knee and 5.7% for those below the knee. In longer follow-up, patients undergoing above-knee amputations and requiring amputations for sepsis or end-stage renal disease had significantly worse survival.

I agree completely with the authors that major lower extremity amputation has been, and will continue to be, a common and important treatment modality in patients with severe peripheral vascular disease. The technical simplicity of major amputations stands in contrast to the clinical complexity of the patients requiring them. Surgeons performing major amputations should accord them the same attention to detail as complex lower extremity arterial reconstructions.

F.P.

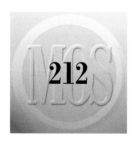

Contemporary Venous Thrombectomy

ANTHONY J. COMEROTA, STEVEN S. GALE, AND SANTIAGO CHAHWAN

INTRODUCTION

Although this is a techniques-related chapter, several background comments are warranted because of the controversy surrounding venous thrombectomy in the United States.

Patients with extensive deep venous thrombosis (DVT) suffer the most severe

consequences of the postthrombotic syndrome. Studies of the pathophysiology of the postthrombotic syndrome consistently have shown that patients with the combination of venous obstruction and valvular incompetence have the most severe postthrombotic consequences. Moreover, patients with iliofemoral venous obstruction, with or without distal venous

involvement, suffer the most severe consequences of their disease. Therefore, if unobstructed venous drainage from the leg into the vena cava can be restored, these patients enjoy a significantly better quality of life as a result of fewer postthrombotic sequelae. This has been shown with catheter-directed thrombolysis as well as venous thrombectomy. Therefore, it is

TABLE 1. TECHNIQUE OF CONTEMPORARY VENOUS THROMBECTOMY

1. **Identify cause of extensive venous thromboembolic process**
   a. Complete thrombophilia evaluation
   b. Rapid computed tomography scan of chest, abdomen, and pelvis
2. **Define full extent of thrombus**
   a. Venous duplex examination
   b. Contralateral iliocavagram
3. **Prevent pulmonary embolism (numerous techniques)**
   a. Anticoagulation
   b. Vena caval filter
   c. Balloon occlusion of vena cava during thrombectomy
   d. Positive end-expiratory pressure during thrombectomy
4. **Perform complete thrombectomy**
   a. Iliofemoral (vena cava) thrombectomy
   b. Infrainguinal venous thrombectomy (if required)
5. **Provide unobstructed venous inflow to and outflow from thrombectomized iliofemoral venous system**
   a. Infrainguinal venous thrombectomy (if required)
   b. Correct iliac vein stenosis (if present)
6. **Prevent recurrent thrombosis**
   a. Arterial venous fistula
   b. Continuous therapeutic anticoagulation
   c. Catheter-directed postoperative anticoagulation (if infrainguinal venous thrombectomy is required)
   d. Extended oral anticoagulation

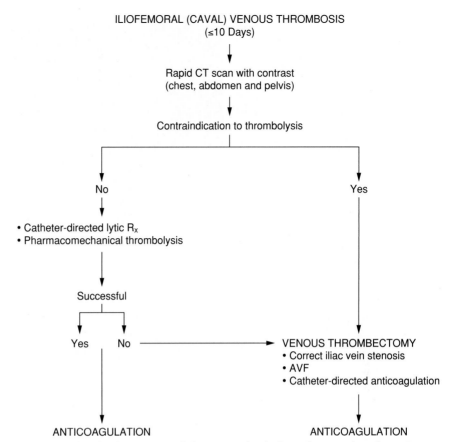

Fig. 1. Algorithm for the recommended treatment for iliofemoral venous thrombosis. CT, computed tomography; AVF, arteriovenous fistula.

important to adopt a strategy of thrombus removal as the critical first step in the care of these patients (Fig. 1).

Venous thrombectomy was largely abandoned in the United States because of two reports in the literature. Interestingly, the procedures were performed over 40 years ago at a time when "vascular" technique did not exist, vascular imaging was in its infancy, and anticoagulation was inconsistent. Unfortunately, current guidelines on the management of venous thromboembolism continued to focus on these outdated retrospective reports and overlooked more recent reports using contemporary vascular techniques. More importantly, guideline authors overlooked a multicenter *randomized* trial evaluating contemporary venous thrombectomy versus standard anticoagulation. Results of the Scandinavian randomized trial demonstrated significant benefit to those

undergoing operation, with fewer postthrombotic sequelae, increased iliac vein patency, lower venous pressures, and improved valvular function.

The technique of contemporary venous thrombectomy is designed to maximize the chance of a favorable patient outcome (Table 1) and is significantly different compared to the technique used in the early reports (Table 2).

TECHNIQUE OF VENOUS THROMBECTOMY

The principles of successful venous thrombectomy are briefly summarized in

TABLE 2. VENOUS THROMBECTOMY: COMPARISON OF OLD AND CONTEMPORARY TECHNIQUES

Technique	Old	Contemporary
Pretreatment phlebography/computed tomography scan	Occasionally	Always
Venous thrombectomy catheter	No	Yes
Operative fluoroscopy/phlebography	No	Yes
Correct iliac vein stenosis	No	Yes
Arteriovenous fistula	No	Yes
Infrainguinal thrombectomy	No	Yes
Full postoperative anticoagulation	Occasionally	Yes
Catheter-directed anticoagulation	No	Yes
Intermittent pneumatic compression postoperatively	No	Yes

Adapted from Comerota AJ, Gale SS. Surgical venous thrombectomy for iliofemoral deep vein thrombosis. In: Greenhalgh RM, ed. *Towards vascular and endovascular consensus.* London: BIBA Publishing, 2005.

Vascular Surgery

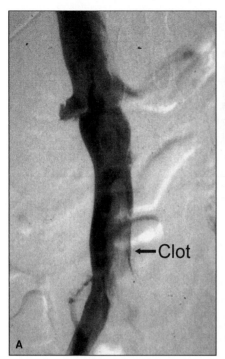
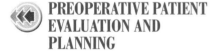
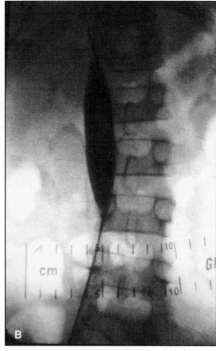
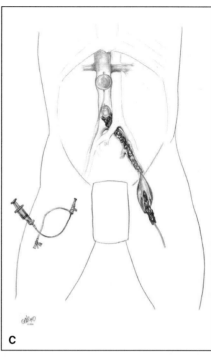

Fig. 2. A: Preoperative iliocavagram shows nonocclusive thrombus extending from the left iliofemoral venous system into the vena cava. **B:** A suprarenal balloon catheter was placed from the contralateral femoral vein and inserted under fluoroscopy. The balloon is inflated at the time of thrombectomy. **C:** Schematic of iliocaval thrombectomy performed with the double balloon catheter technique, protecting the patient from pulmonary embolism. (Reprinted from Comerota AJ, Gale SS, Technique of contemporary iliofemoral and infrainguinal venous thrombectomy. *J Vasc Surg* 2006;43:185–191, with permission from the Society for Vascular Surgery.)

Table 1. The important conceptual elements of the procedure are numbered sequentially, with methods to achieve these goals listed beneath each numbered item.

PREOPERATIVE PATIENT EVALUATION AND PLANNING

Patients with extensive iliofemoral venous thrombosis, which may involve the infrainguinal venous system and perhaps the vena cava, have a much more aggressive thrombotic process than the majority of patients treated for acute DVT. Oftentimes there is a reason for this degree of extensive thrombosis, which may include an underlying thrombophilia or tumor.

The full extent of thrombus (proximally and distally) should be defined preoperatively. The infrainguinal veins are well examined by venous duplex. We prefer a contralateral iliocavagram to evaluate the vena cava and iliac veins. Magnetic resonance venography or spiral computerized tomography (CT) with contrast may obviate the cavagram in some patients.

A rapid CT scan with intravenous contrast of the chest, abdomen, and pelvis is routinely performed. Asymptomatic pulmonary emboli (PE) are found in approximately 50% of the cases. Extending the

imaging from the chest to the abdomen and pelvis is an effective way to rapidly screen for other pathology. In addition to identifying the proximal extent of thrombus and PE, we have found patients with renal cell carcinoma, adrenal tumors, metastatic cancer to the liver, retroperitoneal lymphoma, iliac vein aneurysm, and congenital absence of the vena cava. Each of these findings had important implications for immediate and long-term patient care.

A full thrombophilia evaluation is requested upon initial examination, especially in patients with no other findings but venous thromboembolism (VTE) on CT scan. Blood is sent for fibrinogen, antithrombin III, protein C, protein S, factor V Leiden, prothrombin gene mutation, antiphospholipid/anticardiolipin antibody, factor VIII levels, and homocysteine. If the patient is already anticoagulated, antiphospholipid/anticardiolipin antibodies, factor V Leiden, prothrombin gene mutation, and homocysteine can be reliably performed. The results of the hypercoagulable evaluation are important for appropriate recommendations regarding the duration of anticoagulation.

Therapeutic anticoagulation with unfractionated heparin (UFH) is initiated after the blood samples are drawn for the thrombophilia evaluation and continued

throughout the procedure and postoperatively. Although low-molecular-weight heparin (LMWH) is as effective as UFH, intravenous UFH offers better temporal control of the degree of anticoagulation.

Vena caval filtration is generally not required; however, an exception may be the patient with nonocclusive thrombus in the vena cava or those with symptomatic PE. Also, patients can be protected from intraoperative PE by balloon occlusion of the proximal vena cava during the operative procedure (Fig. 2). The vena caval balloon can be positioned from the contralateral femoral vein using fluoroscopic guidance during preoperative iliocavagraphy. Once the balloon is properly positioned, it remains deflated until the time of thrombus extraction. During thrombectomy, the caval balloon is inflated and the thrombectomy performed with fluoroscopic guidance. Therefore, the operating room is always prepared for fluoroscopy with any necessary modifications in operating room table positioning. An autotransfusion device is also available during the procedure.

SURGICAL TECHNIQUE

Following the induction of general anesthesia, the entire involved leg, lower abdomen, and opposite leg to the knee are

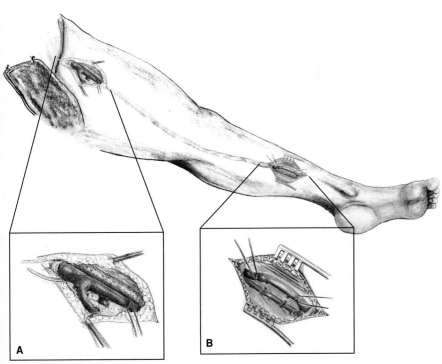

Fig. 3. A: Exposure of the common femoral, femoral, and profunda femoris veins. **B:** Exposure of the posterior tibial vein

other no. 4 balloon catheter is placed into the proximal end of the silastic sheath. A single operator applies pressure to the two balloons, which firmly secures the catheters inside of the sheath, providing protective passage distally through the clotted venous system and valves (Fig. 4B). The catheters exit the posterior tibial venotomy (Fig. 4C). A standard balloon catheter thrombectomy can then be performed in the direction of the venous valves (Fig. 4D,E). Repeated balloon thrombectomy (with a larger catheter if necessary) can be performed until no further thrombus is extracted. At this point, the infrainguinal venous system is vigorously flushed with a heparin–saline solution to hydraulically force residual thrombus from the deep venous system (Fig. 5). This is accomplished by placing a no. 14 to 16 red rubber catheter into the proximal posterior tibial vein and flushing with a bulb syringe. A vascular clamp is then applied below the femoral venotomy and the infrainguinal venous system is then filled with a large volume of dilute plasminogen

prepped into the field. In some patients both legs are prepped into the operative field. A longitudinal inguinal incision is made, exposing the common femoral vein to the inguinal ligament and saphenofemoral junction, which is dissected distally to expose the origin of the profunda femoris vein and femoral vein (Fig. 3A). A longitudinal venotomy is performed, frequently at the saphenofemoral junction. The exact location of the venotomy will depend upon the extent and location of the thrombosis. Since the femoral vein is distended, a longitudinal venotomy is preferred and can be closed primarily without compromising vein lumen.

If the infrainguinal venous system is thrombosed, the infrainguinal venous thrombectomy is performed first. Initially the leg is elevated and wrapped tightly with a rubber bandage. The foot is squeezed and dorsiflexed, and the leg is milked in an effort to remove clot from below. If these maneuvers are successful, the femoral vein below the venotomy is clamped. If unsuccessful, the distal posterior tibial vein is exposed to perform the infrainguinal venous thrombectomy (Fig. 3B). A no. 3 or 4 balloon catheter is passed proximally from below to exit the common femoral venotomy (Fig. 4A). The silastic sheath of a large intravenous catheter (12 to 14 gauge) is cut from its hub and slid halfway onto the balloon catheter that was passed from below. An-

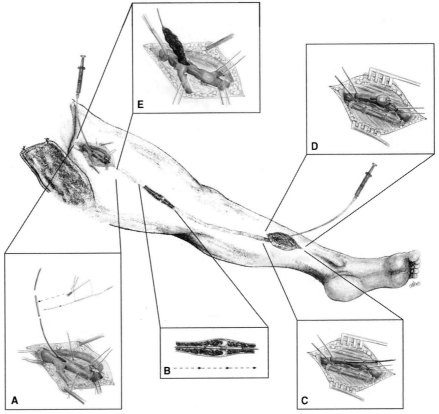

Fig. 4. Technique of infrainguinal balloon catheter venous thrombectomy begins with passage of a no. 3 or 4 balloon catheter from the posterior tibial vein proximally **(A)**, exiting the femoral venotomy. A silastic IV sheath is placed halfway onto the catheter and another no. 4 balloon catheter inserted into the other end of the sheath. **B:** The balloons are inflated to fix the catheter tips inside of the sheath with pressure applied by a single individual guiding them distally through the clotted veins and venous valves. **C:** Catheters and sheath exit the posterior tibial venotomy. **D:** The thrombectomy catheter balloon is gently inflated as the catheter is pulled proximally **(E)** to exit the femoral venotomy, extracting thrombus. (Reprinted from Comerota AJ, Gale SS, Technique of contemporary iliofemoral and infrainguinal venous thrombectomy. *J Vasc Surg* 2006;43:185–191, with permission from the Society for Vascular Surgery.)

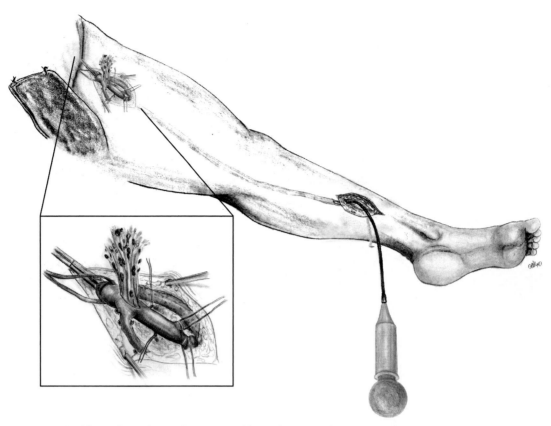

Fig. 5. A red rubber catheter (largest diameter possible) is placed into the posterior tibial vein and vigorously injected with a heparin-saline solution using a bulb syringe to flush residual thrombus. After flushing, the femoral vein is clamped and the leg veins injected with 150 to 200 mL of a dilute urokinase or rt-PA solution. (Reprinted from Comerota AJ, Gale SS, Technique of contemporary iliofemoral and infrainguinal venous thrombectomy. *J Vasc Surg* 2006;43:185–191, with permission from the Society for Vascular Surgery.)

activator solution. Commonly, 4 to 5 mg of rt-PA is diluted in 200 mL of saline and injected into the infrainguinal venous system. If the infrainguinal thrombectomy is not successful due to chronic thrombus in the femoral vein, or if there is evident recanalization and chronic disease of the femoral vein, it is ligated and divided just below its junction with the profunda. Patency of the profunda femoris vein must be ensured prior to ligation of the femoral vein. This maneuver prevents the certain venous reflux through the diseased femoral vein. Venous drainage through an unobstructed profunda system, which may have competent valves, offers a better chance at reducing postthrombotic sequelae.

The iliofemoral (and caval) thrombectomy is performed by using a no. 8 or 10 *venous* thrombectomy catheter. The catheter is passed partway into the iliac vein several times to remove the majority of the iliac vein thrombus before advancing into the vena cava. The proximal thrombectomy is performed under fluoroscopy using contrast to expand the balloon. This is especially important if a vena caval filter is present, if there is clot in the vena cava, or if the surgeon experiences resistance to catheter passage. The anesthesiologist applies positive

end-expiratory pressure during the iliocaval thrombectomy.

Following completion of the iliofemoral and vena caval thrombectomy, the iliofemoral system and vena cava are examined with intraoperative phlebography to ensure unobstructed venous drainage into the vena cava. Any underlying iliac vein stenosis is corrected with balloon angioplasty and, if necessary, a stent to maintain the desired luminal diameter (Fig. 6). If a stent is placed into the common iliac vein, it should be no smaller than 12 mm in diameter, with most being larger.

The venotomy is closed with a running fine monofilament suture. The proximal saphenous vein is exposed and frequently requires thrombectomy in anticipation of performing the arteriovenous fistula (AVF). The AVF is constructed by anastomosing the end of the transected proximal saphenous vein (or a large proximal side branch of the saphenous vein) to the side of the proximal superficial femoral artery. The anastomosis should be no greater than 3.5 to 4.0 mm in diameter. A piece of polytetrafluoroethylene (PTFE) graft (5 mm) or silastic is placed around the saphenous AVF and a large permanent monofilament suture is looped around the PTFE graft and

clipped, leaving approximately 2 to 3 cm in the subcutaneous tissue (Fig. 7A). This is performed to guide future dissection in the event that operative closure of the AVF becomes necessary. Although others have used the AVF as temporary and report closure by percutaneous occlusion, we view the AVF as permanent. Most patients tolerate the AVF well and the flow through this small channel often diminishes with time due to neointimal fibroplasia. Since approximately 15% of patients with early closure of AVFs have developed recurrent thrombosis, and since our patients have tolerated the AVF without difficulty, we believe that elective closure is not indicated.

Common femoral vein pressures are measured before and after the AVF is opened (Fig. 8). Pressures should not change. If the femoral vein pressure increases when the AVF is opened, the proximal iliac vein should be re-evaluated for residual stenosis or obstruction and the proximal lesion corrected. If the pressure remains elevated in the absence of proximal disease, the AVF should be constricted to decrease flow and normalize pressure.

If there appears to be notable serous fluid in the wound, a careful search for

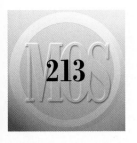

213 Vena Cava Filter Placement

MARC SCHERMERHORN AND KAKRA HUGHES

Venous thromboembolic disease occurs in an estimated 400,000 to 600,000 United States residents each year resulting in 50,000 to 200,000 deaths. Although treatment with anticoagulation remains the mainstay of therapy, clinical situations arise when anticoagulation is contraindicated or inadequate. In these instances, vena cava filters are used to prevent pulmonary embolism (PE).

INDICATIONS FOR FILTER PLACEMENT

The primary reason for placement of a vena cava filter is for the prevention of a potentially fatal PE. Table 1 shows the absolute and relative indications for vena cava filter placement. Patients with absolute indications have thromboembolic disease with a contraindication to anticoagulation or a complication or failure of anticoagulation. Those with relative indications are typically those without overt thromboembolic disease but with high risk for deep vein thrombosis (DVT) and a contraindication to anticoagulation. In this group of patients, it is particularly important that the potential risks and benefits be assessed on an individual basis.

TABLE 1. INDICATIONS FOR VENA CAVA FILTER PLACEMENT

Absolute indications
Thromboembolic disease with
  Contraindication to anticoagulation
  Recurrent thromboembolic disease
    despite anticoagulation therapy
  Significant complication of
    anticoagulation therapy

Relative indications
  Large, free-floating iliocaval thrombus
  Pre- or postpulmonary
    thromboembolectomy
  Thromboembolic disease with limited
    cardiopulmonary reserve
  Poor compliance with medications
  Thrombolysis of iliocaval thrombus
  High-risk trauma patients
    Head or spine injury
    Spine, pelvis, or long bone fracture
  Bariatric surgery

TYPES OF AVAILABLE VENA CAVA FILTERS

The first widely used inferior cava filter, introduced in 1972, was the original stainless steel Greenfield filter (also known as the Kimray-Greenfield filter). The device consisted of a cone of six stainless steel wires terminating in tethering hooks that anchored the device in the inferior vena cava (IVC). This design allowed two-thirds filling of the filter cone with only a 50% reduction of the filter's cross-sectional area, thereby allowing the fibrinolytic system to lyse the clot. It was initially inserted by venotomy, with the first percutaneous placement reported in 1984. Since then, the Greenfield filter has been improved and several generations of other vena cava filters have been developed. The characteristics of an ideal filter are listed in Table 2. However, the ideal filter does not exist, and each has advantages and disadvantages. Table 3 depicts some of the features of available filters in use today including profile, maximum caval diameter, magnetic resonance compatibility, and retrieval window.

PREPROCEDURE EVALUATION

After determining that a patient is an appropriate candidate for a vena cava filter, preoperative preparation includes physical examination to determine potential access sites

TABLE 2. CHARACTERISTICS OF AN IDEAL VENA CAVA FILTER

Nonthrombogenic, biocompatible
High filtering efficiency with no flow
  impedance
Secure fixation within vena cava
Ease of insertion
  Low profile
  Simple deployment
  Able to reposition
Magnetic resonance imaging compatibility
Low incidence of complications
  (migration, occlusion, perforation,
  insertion-site thrombosis)
Retrievable, with no time limit
Low cost

and venous duplex of bilateral lower extremity veins to assess for DVT. The right common femoral vein is our preferred access site; however, in the presence of a right-sided iliofemoral DVT, an alternate side would be chosen, typically the left common femoral vein or the right internal jugular vein. Routine laboratory analyses are obtained with particular attention to the patient's coagulation status and creatinine level.

INFERIOR VENA CAVA FILTER PLACEMENT TECHNIQUE

The common femoral vein is localized fluoroscopically using the femoral head as a landmark. The right groin is then anesthetized and the skin overlying the femoral vein is incised with a scalpel. Percutaneous retrograde cannulation of the right common femoral vein is then performed and a wire (Bentson wire or J-wire) is advanced into the IVC under continuous fluoroscopic visualization. A short No. 6 French sheath is advanced into the right common femoral vein using Seldinger's technique. An iliac venogram is performed to rule out iliac venous thrombosis, venous anomalies, and to define the location of the caval bifurcation (Fig. 1). A marker pigtail catheter is then positioned at the caval bifurcation, the image intensifier is repositioned to encompass from the caval bifurcation to the renal veins, and a cavogram is obtained (Fig. 2). This image allows measurement of caval diameter, assessment for caval thrombus, anomalous caval anatomy, the level of the caval bifurcation, and the likely level of the renal veins.

Next, using a C2 Cobra catheter, each renal vein is selectively cannulated to more clearly establish its location (Fig. 3). The length between the iliac bifurcation and the renal veins is noted. Most available filters are 60 mm in length or shorter, except the bird's nest filter, which is 80 mm long. IVC thrombus necessitates jugular access. Caval diameter less than 28 mm is acceptable for any of the filters in use today. The Gunther-Tulip and TrapEase/OptEase filters can be used in IVC diameters up to 30 mm. The bird's nest filter may be used in IVC diameters up to 40 mm. For an IVC diameter more than 40 mm (or >30 mm

Vascular Surgery

TABLE 3. CHARACTERISTICS OF AVAILABLE VENA CAVA FILTERS

Filter	Introducer Size (FR)	Maximal Caval Diameter (mm)	Magnetic Resonance Compatibility	Other
Greenfield	14	28	Safe	Greatest clinical experience
Bird's nest	12	40	Not recommended	IVCs[a] >30 mm
Simon nitinol	7	28	Safe	
Vena Tech	7	28	Safe	
TrapEase/ OptEase	6	30	Safe	OptEase is retrievable within 23 days
Gunther-Tulip	8.5 Femoral 7 Jugular	30	Safe	Nonspecific retrievable window
Nitinol Recovery	7	28	Safe	Nonspecific retrievable window

[a]IVC, inferior vena cava.

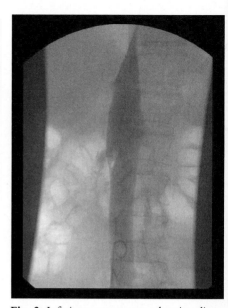

Fig. 2. Inferior venocavogram showing diameter and length of inferior vena cava and likely level of renal veins.

to avoid a bird's nest filter), one may consider placement of bilateral common iliac vein filters.

If the anatomy is appropriate, the IVC filter packaging is then opened and the short No. 6 French sheath is exchanged for the long delivery sheath that comes with each filter. This sheath is advanced until the marker at the sheath tip is just below the lowest renal vein. The dilator (and guidewire for all but the over-the-wire filters) is then removed. The filter is inserted into the long sheath and advanced until it is positioned within the end of the sheath. The position is verified fluoroscopically. Next, the filter is unsheathed by grasping and immobilizing the delivery system with one hand and pulling back on the sheath with the other hand. Simply unsheathing will deploy most filters, but some have an additional release mechanism after unsheathing to avoid "watermelon seeding." A completion spot film is then obtained to document final positioning (Fig. 4).

Suprarenal and Superior Vena Cava Placement

The infrarenal IVC is the preferred position for a vena cava filter placement, but situations arise when suprarenal placement may be considered, such as when a thrombus extends to the level of the renal veins. Suprarenal placement may also be considered in pregnant women to prevent the potential situation of the gravid uterus compressing an infrarenal IVC filter.

If a superior vena cava filter is to be placed for the prevention of PE from upper extremity DVT, placement proceeds following the steps described for the IVC filter. The ideal location is immediately proximal to the inominate vein. It is important to remember that, in this case, a femoral kit must be used for the jugular approach and a jugular kit for the femoral approach.

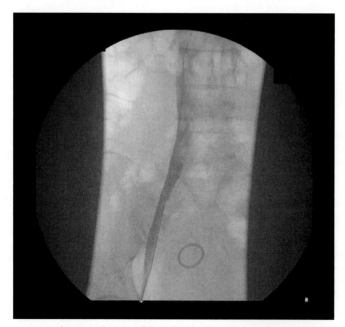

Fig. 1. Iliac venogram showing absence of thrombus in iliac veins and location of caval bifurcation.

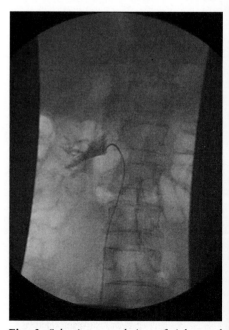

Fig. 3. Selective cannulation of right renal vein with C2 Cobra catheter to confirm its location.

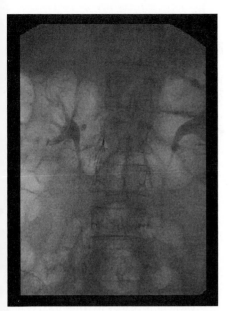

Fig. 4. Completion spot film documenting adequate placement of filter.

Inferior Vena Cava Filter Placement without Fluoroscopy

For patients who will not tolerate transfer to an appropriate endosuite, IVC filter placement may be performed using either intravascular ultrasound (IVUS) or duplex ultrasound. Duplex ultrasound-guided IVC filter placement requires an experienced technician to localize the renal veins and visualize the long sheath and IVC filter prior to deployment. Duplex ultrasound often does not allow visualization of the iliac veins and the entire cava to rule out thrombus or anatomic anomalies. Even in experienced hands it can be difficult to visualize the cava and renal veins adequately. However, IVUS allows excellent visualization of the iliac veins and the cava.

Experience is again requisite for appropriate identification of the renal veins. IVUS-guided filter placement may be performed with bilateral femoral vein punctures to allow visualization of the filter in the correct position below the renal veins just prior to deployment. Alternatively, a single puncture technique may be employed in which the IVUS probe is inserted into the long sheath, which is then positioned appropriately below the renal veins. The IVUS probe is then removed and the filter is inserted to the end of the sheath using a mark on the introducer system for the appropriate insertion distance within the sheath, and the filter is then deployed. Further details are available in the "Suggested Reading" list.

THE PREPIC TRIAL

The PREPIC (Prevention du Risque d'Embolie Pulmonaire par Interruption Cave) study, the only long-term randomized study of caval filter placement in the prevention of PE, had its 2-year results published in 1998. In this multi-institutional trial, 400 patients with venographically confirmed acute proximal DVT were randomized to treatment with anticoagulation (low molecular weight heparin for 8 to 12 days and a vitamin K antagonist for at least 3 months) alone versus anticoagulation and a permanent caval filter. At 12 days, there were two PEs in the filter group (1.1%) versus nine PEs in the nonfilter group (4/8%) (*P* = 0.03). At 2 years, there were 6 PEs in the filter group (3.4 %) and 12 PEs in the nonfilter group (6.3%) (*P* = 0.16). The incidence of recurrent DVT was 37 (20.8%) in the filter group and 21 (11.6%) in the nonfilter group (*P* = 0.02). These 2-year results suggested that caval filters provided significant additional short-term protection

from PE compared with anticoagulation, and that this benefit seemed to wane over time and was associated with an increased risk of recurrent DVT.

The 8-year results of the PREPIC trial, published in 2005, showed that there were 9 PEs in the filter group (6.2%) versus 24 PEs in the nonfilter group (15.1%) (*P* = 0.08). The filter group had 57 patients with DVT (35.7%) versus 41 (27.5%) in the nonfilter group (*P* = 0.042). The incidence of postthrombotic syndrome was similar: it was observed in 109 (70.3%) filter patients and 107 (69.7%) nonfilter patients at 8 years. Mortality was also similar: 103 filter patients had died, compared with 98 nonfilter patients. These results showed that at 8 years, vena cava filters reduced the risk of PE while increasing the incidence of DVT, and without effect on the incidence of the postthrombotic syndrome or on survival.

RETRIEVABLE/OPTIONAL FILTERS

The rationale for a temporary or retrievable filter arises from a desire to eliminate the increased risk of DVT associated with filters, as was shown in the PREPIC trial. Additionally, in many young trauma or orthopaedic patients the risk for thromboembolic disease exists for a limited time, and some have expressed concern about leaving a permanent device in such patients with a long life expectancy. Retrievable (or optional) filters are placed much like permanent filters, but are designed so that they may be retrieved in a separate percutaneous procedure. If desired, retrievable/optional filters also may be left in place permanently. Currently available retrievable filters are shown in Figure 5. The

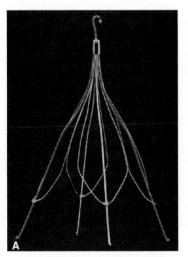
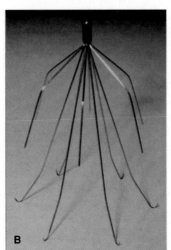
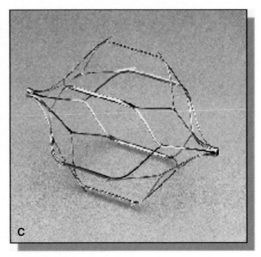

Fig. 5. Currently available retrievable filters. *Left to right:* Tulip, Recovery, and OptEase.

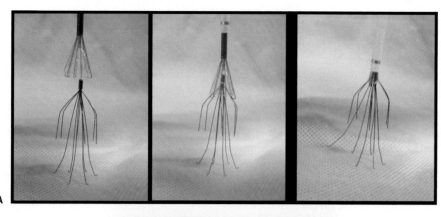

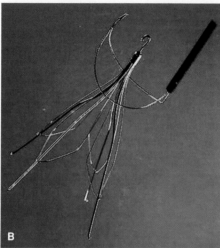

Fig. 6. Retrieval process for Recovery and for Gunther-Tulip filters.

SUGGESTED READING

Asch MR. Initial experience in humans with a new retrievable inferior vena cava filter. *Radiology* 2002;225:835.

Ascher E, Hingorani A, Tsemekhin, et al. Lessons learned from a 6-year clinical experience with superior vena cava Greenfield filters. *J Vasc Surg* 2000;32:881.

Connors MS 3rd, Becker S, Guzman RJ, et al. Duplex scan-directed placement of inferior vena cava filters: a five-year institutional experience. *J Vasc Surg* 2002;35:286.

Decousus H, Leizorovicz A, Parent F, et al. A clinical trial of vena caval filters in the prevention of pulmonary embolism in patients with proximal deep-vein thrombosis. *N Engl J Med* 1998;338:409.

Ebaugh JL, Chiou AC, Morasch MD, et al Bedside vena cava filter placement guided with intravascular ultrasound. *J Vasc Surg* 2001;34:21.

Greenfield LJ, McCurdy JR, Brown PP, et al. A new intracaval filter permitting continued flow and resolution of emboli. *Surgery* 1973; 73;599.

Greenfield LJ, Proctor MC. Supra-renal filter placement. *J Vasc Surg* 1998;28:432.

Kinney TB. Update on inferior vena cava filters. *J Vasc Interv Radiol* 2003;14:425.

Knudson MM, Ikossi DG, Khaw L, et al. Thromboembolism after trauma. *Ann Surg* 2004;240:490.

Millward SF. Temporary and retrievable inferior vena cava filters: current status. *J Vasc Interv Radiol* 1998;9:381.

Mobin-Uddin K, Smith PE, Martines LO, et al. A vena caval filter for the prevention of pulmonary embolus. *Surg Forum* 1967;18:209.

The PREPIC Study Group. Eight-year follow-up of patients with permanent vena cava filters in the prevention of pulmonary embolism: the PREPIC (Prevention du Risque d'Embolie Pulmonaire par Interruption Cave) Randomized Study. *Circulation* 2005;112:416.

Rosenthal D, Wellons ED, Levitt AB, et al. Role of prophylactic temporary inferior vena cava filters placed at the ICU bedside under intravascular ultrasound guidance in patients with multiple trauma. *J Vasc Surg* 2004; 409:58.

Sapala JA, Wood MH, Schuhknecht MP, et al. Fatal pulmonary embolism after bariatric operations for morbid obesity: a 24-year retrospective analysis. *Obes Surg* 2003;13:819.

Stein PD, Alnas M, Skaf E, et. al. Outcome and complications of retrievable inferior vena cava filters. *Am J Cardiol* 2004;94:1090.

Streiff, MB. Vena caval filters: a review for intensive care specialists. *J Intensive Care Med* 2003;18:59.

Whitehill TA. Current vena cava devices and results. *Semin Vasc Surg* 2000;13:204.

nitinol Recovery filter requires a special retrieval device, whereas the Gunther-Tulip and TrapEase filters are retrieved simply by employing a gooseneck snare and encapsulating the filter with a long sheath (Fig. 6). Several small studies have demonstrated the safety of retrievable filters, but there is currently no widely accepted consensus for the exact role of these filters in clinical practice.

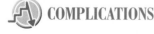 COMPLICATIONS

There are relatively few serious complications reported with vena cava filter placement. Fatal complications are rare, with a combined fatal complication rate of all filters reported at 0.12%. Recurrent PE is reported in the range of 2% to 4% (0.7% fatal PE). Most complications from insertion are related to bleeding (i.e., formation of a hematoma at the access site or superficial wound infection). Infection of the device is rare. Access-site thrombosis (i.e., formation of a DVT at the site of access) was first noted with the original Greenfield filter, which was delivered via a No. 29 French system. With lower profile delivery systems, however, a reduction in this has not yet been demonstrated. Some believe that this may be partially related to overzealous compression at the access site. In rare instances, complications such as filter migration and caval penetration may become clinically significant (e.g., perforation into the vascular or gastrointestinal systems).

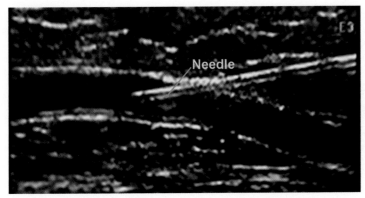

Fig. 9. Ultrasound image of needle access to vein.

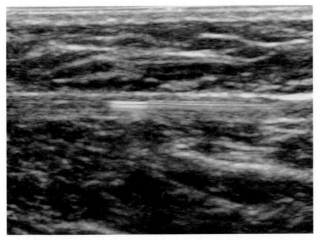

Fig. 10. Catheter tip in vein.

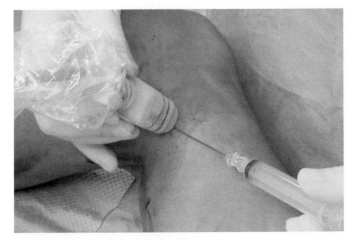

Fig. 11. Percutaneous access with ultrasound guidance.

and somewhat disfiguring, especially when extensive removal is required (Fig. 12). This can be a time-consuming technique depending on the extent of the varicose veins. With small clusters, this can be done with local anesthesia. In the case of more extensive lesions, general or spinal anesthesia may be required. Reimbursement from third-party payers is low; many clinicians regard this as a cosmetic operation and bill the patient directly.

Sclerotherapy

Sclerotherapy involves injection of a sclerosing agent such as hypertonic saline, polidocanol, or sodium tetradecol into the vein to irritate the inner wall of the vessel and cause its lumen to obliterate (Fig. 13). Results are better if compression is used for a period of time after the procedure (Fig. 14). A small needle is used for the injection and various lighting devices have been used to better identify the vein under treatment, especially the reticular vein. This is an effective technique in the case of minimal residual varicosities, but may require multiple treatments if the lesions are extensive.

Rotoblader Therapy

Powered phlebectomy (TriVex ablation) involves the insertion of two instruments through small incisions around patches of varicose veins. One is a light source (Fig. 15) that is coupled with a power injector to identify the veins (Fig. 16) and infuse a tumescent solution, which reduces the hematoma formation and protects the overlying skin as the vein is emulsified. The second device is a rotating ablator in conjunction with a suction apparatus, which emulsifies the vein and removes it. Less time is involved as compared with stab phlebectomy and the number of incisions required is greatly reduced. This is a very effective way to remove large and extensive varicosities, but in most instances will require either a spinal or general anesthetic. The procedure was evaluated on 114 patients (117 limbs) from four centers in Europe and four in the United States. In the study, 84% of the limbs seen were CEAP class 2; there were only 16% in classes 3 and 4. Accompanying greater saphenous vein ablation was performed in 67% of the limbs in the United States in 80% of those in Europe. The study showed the transilluminated, powered phlebectomy used in varicose vein removal was swift, efficacious, and produced good results.

Vascular Surgery

nearly always improved. However, in approximately half the cases, the varicosities remain. This is especially true in the case of larger varicosities. Most patients whose varicosities remain are not satisfied with the cosmetic result. In these patients, the varicose veins must be individually removed or ablated using one of the following techniques.

Stab Phlebectomy

Stab phlebectomy has been used for many years as a means of removing varicosities of the lower extremity. It involves multiple small incisions along the course of the varicose vein with avulsion using a variety of hooks and other specially designed instruments. The procedure is time-consuming

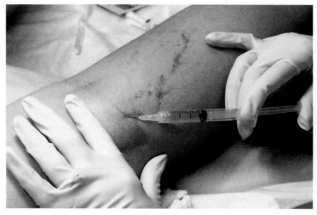

Fig. 12. Sclerotherapy injection.

Name	Location
TABLE 3. NAME AND LOCATION OF PERFORATOR VEINS	

Name	Location
Hunterian	Upper to mid thigh
Dodd	Lower thigh
Boyd	Upper calf or knee region
Cockett III	Mid calf
Cockett II	Lower calf
Cockett I	Ankle region

INCOMPETENT PERFORATING VEINS

Perforating veins direct blood flow from the superficial venous system to the deep system. They contain valves that prevent retrograde reflux from the deep system. Incompetence in the superficial valves results in reflux into the superficial venous network. There is an association between perforator vein incompetence and venous ulceration, although there is controversy as to whether interruption of these perforator veins as an isolated procedure is sufficient to reduce the recurrence of venous ulcers. In the majority of cases, perforators are interrupted in conjunction with greater saphenous vein ablation and it is difficult to isolate the contribution of each. Interruption of perforator veins alone has minimal effect on objective measurements of venous hemodynamic, and recent data suggest that ablation of the greater saphenous vein in conjunction with removal of multiple varicosities may be sufficient to ameliorate the deleterious effects of perforator vein incompetence.

CLASSIFICATION OF PERFORATOR VEINS

Perforating veins occur in the thigh and calf and have been given names by various investigators depending on their anatomic location (Table 3). Most surgically significant incompetent perforator are in the medial calf, and Stuart et al. provide a useful classification of incompetent medial calf perforating veins (Table 4).

It is generally accepted that in the thigh, ablation of the saphenous vein is sufficient to eliminate problems related to the thigh perforating veins. Also it is extremely unusual to get venous ulcerations in the thigh region. Calf vein perforator incompetence is the subject of greater controversy because most venous ulcers occur in the "gaiter" area or ankle region. Cockett's perforators are the major perforator veins in the calf. Surgical efforts to ligate them were described by Linton using a direct surgical approach. More recently the SEPS procedure (subfascial endoscopic perforator surgery) offers a means of visualizing and ligating the vein through an incision remote from areas of potential ulceration.

PERFORATOR SURGERY

In addition to excellent anatomic information concerning perforator veins in the lower extremity, Padberg provides a well-illustrated description of the SEPS procedure. TenBrook performed a comprehensive literature review of the surgical treatment of lower extremity venous disease

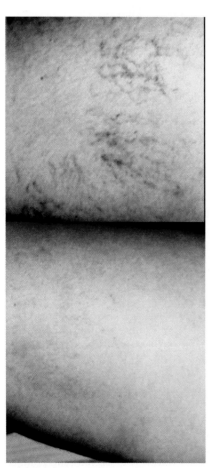

Fig. 13. Before and after sclerotherapy.

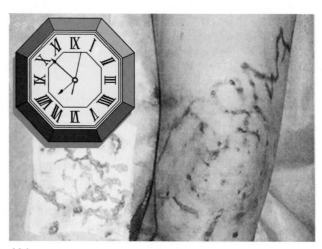

Fig. 14. Stab phlebectomy.

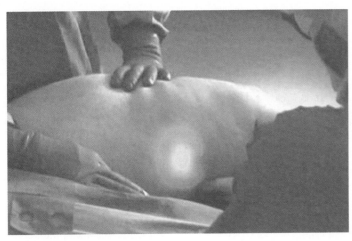

Fig. 15. TriVex light source.

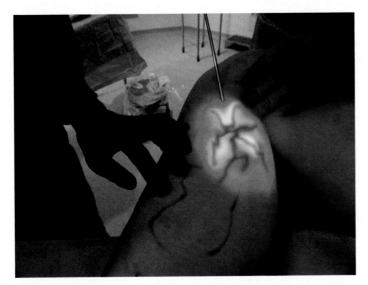

Fig. 16. Backlighted vein.

incorporating SEPS, and concluded that "surgical management of venous ulcer including SEPS with or without saphenous ablation, leads to an 88% chance of ulcer healing and a 13% chance of ulcer recurrence over the short term." What cannot be determined from this review is the isolated contribution of SEPS to this healing rate.

Rhodes analyzed the results of endoscopic perforator vein division in 26 patients and noted that 77% of them had both deep and perforator vein incompetence. His data confirmed that calf muscle pump function improved and venous incompetence decreased after SEPS associated with correction of superficial incompetence. His data also show that although significant clinical benefit was documented in those limbs treated with SEPS alone, objective hemodynamic improvement could not be documented. He concluded that adding SEPS to ablation of superficial reflux in patients with advanced chronic venous insufficiency was indicated.

Iafrati et al. stress an aggressive approach to superficial and perforating vein reflux in patients with CEAP class 5 and 6 disease. The authors performed the SEPS procedure on 51 limbs in 45 patients. Sixteen patients underwent SEPS alone and 35 had additional surgery on the greater saphenous vein, the lesser saphenous vein, or tributary varices. Among patients in whom the ulcers healed or were seen with healed ulcers, the 5-year ulcer recurrence rate was 13%. The authors were unable to differentiate the effect of SEPS versus superficial venous ablation on outcome.

VENOUS ULCERATION

Venous ulcerations of the lower extremity are a frequent occurrence and result in significant morbidity for a large number of patients. In addition, many of these individuals are unable to work because of this problem. Healing of venous ulcerations is a significant time and financial undertaking. Favorable results occur when strict attention is paid to wound care, compression, and judicious use of surgical procedures. The University of Oregon reported a 93% healing rate with venous ulcerations, and large cohort studies suggest that the general community does not fare as well. In one report, only 34% of patients were ulcer-free in a 5-year follow-up. In most cases, the recurrence of ulcerations is the result of poor patient compliance. After the lesion is healed, patients often pay less attention to the continued use of compression therapy by means of surgical-strength support hose.

TABLE 4. CLASSIFICATION OF PERFORATING VEINS	
Type	**Description**
I	Perforating veins fed by a refluxing saphenous vein in the presence of a normal deep venous system. In 80% of these cases, saphenous surgery will correct the outward perforator flow.
II	Perforating veins associated with isolated deep venous reflux. In this circumstance, direct surgical interruption may be necessary.
III	Perforating veins associated with mixed superficial and deep venous reflux. Saphenous surgery alone may be inadequate in this situation and SEPS[a] may be required to correct outward flow.
IV	Perforating veins associated with collateral circulation, which bypasses an occluded deep venous system. In this instance, perforator interruption with or without saphenous ablation may be detrimental to the patient.
V	Perforating veins in the absence of other venous reflux or obstruction.

[a]SEPS, subfascial endoscopic perforator surgery.

Vascular Surgery

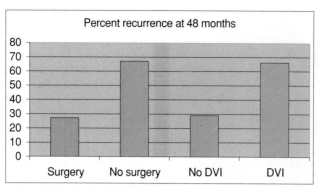

Fig. 17. Healing rates following correction of pathologies in various superficial venous systems.

Unusual causes of venous ulcerations should be searched for when more obvious causes are not forthcoming. For example, magnetic resonance or computed tomographic examination may demonstrate congenital absence of the inferior vena cava or obstruction of the left iliac vein secondary to arterial compression. This latter condition is known as May-Thurner syndrome, and its lack of recognition can result in significant long-term chronic venous insufficiency symptoms. This is especially tragic when it occurs in young female patients and is not treated appropriately with lytic therapy followed by the use of venous angioplasty with stent.

McDaniel et al. analyzed 99 limbs with CEAP class 6 chronic venous insufficiencies that had been evaluated with standing reflux duplex ultrasound scanning and air plethysmography. Corrective venous surgery was carried out in 37 limbs. The overall recurrence rate for venous ulcers was 37% at 3 years and 48% at 5 years. Patients who underwent venous surgery had a lower recurrence rate, as did patients without associated deep venous insufficiency (Fig. 17).

Surgical correction in these patients consisted of saphenous ligation accompanied by stripping from groin to knee for greater saphenous incompetence and ligation for lesser saphenous incompetence. Nine patients with perforator incompetence underwent open ligation early in the series and six had SEPS division in the last 3 years of the study. Six of the patients had autologous vein transplant.

Although the study includes patients with a wide variety of surgical procedures, the authors stress the fact that corrective venous surgery, when possible, reduces the rate of ulcer recurrence. Other factors associated with an increased risk of recurrence were the recurrence of pain, the presence of deep venous disease, increased venous volume, and increased venous-filling index.

Isolated Superficial Vein Incompetence

Although many practitioners believe that venous ulceration is invariably associated with incompetence of the deep venous system, a significant number of individuals with venous ulcers have superficial vein incompetence without associated deep venous insufficiency. Shami et al., using objective noninvasive laboratory data, showed that slightly more than half of their patients with venous ulcers had abnormalities of the superficial venous system and normal deep veins.

Bjellerup and Akesson divided patients with venous ulcers into two groups: 86 patients had healed ulcers and 91 patients had therapy-resistant ulcers. Venous insufficiency was the most common cause of ulceration in both subgroups, although the pattern of venous incompetence was different. Patients with isolated superficial disease constituted 68% in the first group and only 26% in the ulcer-resistant group. Thus, approximately 40% of venous ulcers are secondary to isolated superficial incompetence, and those patients had a better prognosis than those with an associated deep venous insufficiency.

MIXED SUPERFICIAL AND DEEP VENOUS INSUFFICIENCY

There are various theories as to the cause of superficial and deep venous insufficiency. Some investigators have suggested that superficial venous incompetence might cause overflow into the deep system through perforator vessels, the so-called "overload theory," resulting in deep venous incompetence. Puggioni et al. reported that saphenous vein ablation resulted in resolution of deep reflux in approximately one third of the 38 limbs they studied.

Ting et al. analyzed the hemodynamic changes after superficial vein surgery in patients with mixed superficial and deep ve-

nous insufficiency. They studied 78 patients with 102 operated limbs. In this study, superficial vein ablation consisted of flush saphenous ligation at the saphenofemoral junction without stripping, and stab phlebectomy for avulsion of varicosities. The venous-filling index, ejection fraction, and residual volume fraction improved significantly after superficial vein surgery. In addition, the proportion of limbs with deep venous insufficiency as determined by duplex scan decreased from 70% to 44%.

Sales and colleagues reviewed 45 patients who had symptomatic venous insufficiency and were found to have greater saphenous vein reflux. Reflux in the femoral vein was associated with reflux in the superficial venous system in 17 patients. All patients underwent removal of the greater saphenous vein and stab avulsion of varicosities. In 94% of the 17 patients, the coexistence femoral venous insufficiency completely resolved. The authors concluded that saphenectomy might be an effective means of correcting femoral venous reflux.

Finally, Padberg evaluated 11 limbs in ten patients with the CEAP class 5 or 6 venous insufficiency (ulceration or healed ulcer). All of the limbs had combined deep and superficial vein reflux. Clinical symptom scores decreased from 10 to 1.4 after superficial venous operations and there was a significant improvement in hemodynamic data. They concluded that surgical correction of the superficial problem significantly improved clinical symptoms and venous hemodynamics. They also thought that superficial and perforator vein ablation is an appropriate initial step in the management of combined deep and superficial venous incompetence.

It is clear from the investigation cited in the previous paragraph, that when feasible, the correction of superficial venous incompetence is warranted, even in the case of associated deep venous insufficiency. One caveat that must be stressed, however, is the fact that superficial venous ablation is not indicated in the case of obstruction of the deep venous system. The potential exists in this situation to markedly worsen the patient's symptoms.

PERFORATOR INCOMPETENCE

Perforator incompetence was discussed in the previous section of this chapter. It is frequently associated with symptomatic venous diseases of the lower extremity. Its significance, however, remains unclear. Stuart et al. evaluated the relationship between abnormal medial calf perforating vein structure and function and the clinical severity of chronic venous insufficiency. They used duplex ultrasound to determine the number, the diameter, and flow characteristics of medial calf perforating veins as well as the presence of deep and superficial reflux. They concluded that a deteriorating CEAP grade of chronic venous insufficiency is associated with an increase in the number and diameter of medial calf perforating veins. This is particularly true in those that permitted bidirectional flow. In those patients with isolated superficial venous reflux, ablation of the reflux allowed most perforating veins to regain competence, whereas perforating veins in patients with mixed superficial and deep reflux were generally not rendered competent by means of superficial venous surgery alone. Stuart et al. further stress that under the circumstances of mixed disease, SEPS is necessary to correct outward flow in medial calf perforating veins.

Other observers also believe that, in the case of superficial vein incompetence associated with perforator insufficiency, ablation of the saphenous vein results in resolution of perforator incompetence. Al-Mulhim et al. studied 57 limbs in 33 patients with isolated superficial venous reflux. Greater saphenous vein reflux alone was observed and 39, isolated short saphenous reflux in 4, and combined reflux in 14. Incompetent perforator veins were observed in 89.5% of the limbs, and 74.5% of these regained their competence postoperatively. The healing rates for all ulcerated legs were 80.7%. Results for individual venous situations is shown in Figure 18.

The authors performed flush litigation of the saphenofemoral junction with stripping of the long saphenous vein to just below the knee. The short saphenous vein was ligated but not stripped. No leg underwent any perforator surgery. The authors concluded that, in the absence of deep venous reflux, superficial venous surgery eliminated reflux in 74.5% of incompetent perforating veins.

Some surgeons recommend a SEPS procedure in association with ablative therapy of the superficial venous system in those patients with perforator incompetence. Others believe that in the absence of deep venous insufficiency removal of the superficial system alone is sufficient to deal with perforator incompetence. Mendes et al. evaluated patients with superficial and perforator vein incompetence and a normal deep venous system and noted significant improvement in both air plethysmography parameters and symptom scores after superficial ablative surgery alone. In their patient population, one-third with CEAP class 3 through 6 had disease confined to the superficial and perforator systems. In these patients, they performed saphenous vein stripping in conjunction with TriVex ablation of varicosities. They postulate that removal of varicosities using the rotoblader therapy actually performs extra fascial perforator ligation, and concluded that symptomatic chronic venous insufficiency caused by superficial and perforator vein incompetence, without deep venous insufficiency, can be treated with superficial ablative procedures alone.

More recent information would suggest that a normal deep venous system in conjunction with valvular disease in the superficial system is present alone or in conjunction with perforator insufficiency in as many as 50% of patients with venous ulcers. Most patients with superficial venous insufficiency and venous ulceration will benefit from ablative therapy of the involved saphenous vein, although those with a normal deep system do have better results with regard to recurrence of ulceration.

VENOUS BYPASS PROCEDURES

In individuals with obstructive lesions of the deep venous system, venous bypass operations have enjoyed some success. In the case of obstruction of the superficial femoral vein, the May-Husni or saphenopopliteal bypass procedure is an option, and with iliac vein occlusion, the Palma cross-femoral procedure may be performed. Patency can be a problem because veins have both low blood flow and low velocity rates. Some surgeons believe that an associated arterovenous fistula improves long-term patency.

ENDOPHLEBECTOMY

There is general agreement that ablative therapy of the superficial venous system is indicated in the presence of deep venous insufficiency in those patients with venous ulceration. However, ablative surgery in individuals with obstructed venous segments in the deep venous system may be harmful. Puggiono et al. describe a surgical disobliteration or endophlebectomy of chronically obstructed venous segments during various kinds of deep venous reconstructions. They performed the procedure on 23 deep venous segments to create a single lumen in individuals undergoing venous valve transplantation. The authors obtained a cumulative patency of 83% at 10 years in trabeculated veins.

VALVULAR RECONSTRUCTION

Reconstruction of the deep venous system has been used on occasion to restore competence to the vein and reduce venous reflux. Tissue valves have been used as well as transplants from the upper extremity. The results are mixed and beyond the scope of this chapter.

SUGGESTED READING

Al-Mulhim AS, El-Hoseiny H, Al-Mulhim FM, et al., Surgical correction of main stem reflux in the superficial venous system: does it improve the blood flow of incompetent perforating veins? *World J Surg* 2003;27:793.

Bjellerup M, Akesson H. The role of vascular surgery in chronic leg ulcers: report from a specialized ulcer clinic. *Acta Derm Venereol* 2002;82:266.

Cheshire N, Elias SM, Keagy B, et al. Powered phlebectomy (TriVex) in treatment of varicose veins. *Ann Vasc Surg* 2002;16:488.

Iafrati MD, Pare GJ, O'Donnell TF, et al. Is the nihilistic approach to surgical reduction of superficial and perforator vein incompetence for venous ulcer justified? *J Vasc Surg* 2002;36:1167.

McDaniel HB, Marston WA, Farber MA, et al. Recurrence of chronic venous ulcers on the basis of clinical, etiologic, anatomic, and pathophysiologic criteria and air plethysmography. *J Vasc Surg* 2002;35:723.

Mendes RR, Marston WA, Farber MA, et al. Treatment of superficial and perforator

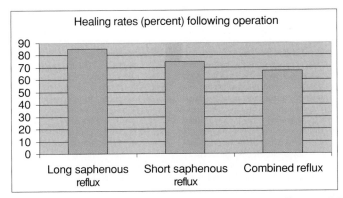

Fig. 18. Ulcer recurrence associated with surgery and deep venous insufficiency (DVI).

venous incompetence without deep venous insufficiency: is routine perforator ligation necessary? *J Vasc Surg* 2003;38:891.

Owens LV, Farber MA, Young ML, et al. The value of air plethysmography in predicting clinical outcome after surgical treatment of chronic venous insufficiency. *J Vasc Surg* 2000;32:961.

Padberg FT Jr. Surgical intervention in venous ulceration. Cardiovasc Surg, 1999. 7(1): p. 83–90.

Padberg, FT, Jr. Endoscopic subfascial perforating vein ligation: its complementary role in the surgical management of chronic ve-

nous insufficiency. *Ann Vasc Surg* 1999; 13:343.

Puggioni A, Lurie F, Kistner RL, et al. How often is deep venous reflux eliminated after saphenous vein ablation? *J Vasc Surg* 2003; 38:517.

Puggioni A, Kistner RL, Eklof B, et al. Surgical disobliteration of postthrombotic deep veins—endophlebectomy—is feasible. *J Vasc Surg* 2004;39:1048.

Stuart WP, Adam DJ, Allan PL, et al. The relationship between the number, competence, and diameter of medial calf perforating veins and the clinical status in healthy subjects and

patients with lower-limb venous disease. *J Vasc Surg* 2000;32:138.

Tenbrook JA Jr, Iafrati ML, O'Donnell TF Jr., et al. Systematic review of outcomes after surgical management of venous disease incorporating subfascial endoscopic perforator surgery. *J Vasc Surg* 2004;39:583.

Ting AC, Cheng SW, Wu LL, et al. Changes in venous hemodynamics after superficial vein surgery for mixed superficial and deep venous insufficiency. *World J Surg* 2001;25:122.

Welch HJ. Surgical options for the treatment of venous ulcers. *Vasc Endovascular Surg* 2004; 38:195.

EDITOR'S COMMENT

The chapter by Drs. Keagy and Mendes gives an excellent overview of superficial venous insufficiency, including a discussion of a number of the more controversial topics. A couple of additions to the chapter may be of some benefit. Because minimally invasive treatment of greater saphenous vein reflux has been performed for the last few years, there are a number of additional issues raised by that manner of therapy. The first involves duplex scanning performed as a diagnostic preoperative evaluation. During the duplex scan, the specific segments of greater saphenous vein reflux can be identified. It can be easily differentiated whether the reflux starts directly at the saphenofemoral junction and extends down to the calf, or if it starts in the middle or lower thigh. This will have obvious implications. In addition, because percutaneous techniques involve catheter placement, information about the tortuosity of the greater saphenous vein, location of the epigastric vein, distance of the greater saphenous vein to the skin surface and the size in centimeters of the greater saphenous vein are of import. More of the specifics regarding these values will be detailed later. In addition, duplex scanning can easily identify perforator veins, especially in the gaiter area, which is often problematic.

I believe it would be important to have some additional comments regarding the technique of greater saphenous vein stripping. It has been clearly shown that stripping is more advantageous from the standpoint of recurrence as opposed to simple ligation. A formal stripping involves ligation and transection of the four to five tributaries at the saphenofemoral junction. The greater saphenous vein at the saphenofemoral junction is then ligated flush. If the saphenous vein itself is varicosed at this location, a more definitive reconstruction at this location is required. The patient does not need to be heparinized. A Satinsky clamp is placed at the base of the patulous saphenous vein at the top of the femoral vein. Then, using a knife, the vein is disconnected, leaving a small cuff distal to the clamp. Then the cuff is then oversewn with Prolene in a running fashion. This avoids a patulous and static vein cuff sitting directly on the femoral vein. It does not cause any narrowing of the vein and allows the operation to proceed.

After treatment as previously described or flush ligation of the greater saphenous vein, the vein distal to the tie is incised either with a Metzenbaum scissors or a knife so that the anterior surface of the vein is fully open. I then favor stripping in a retrograde fashion from this location to the knee or low calf. The reason for this technique is that the distal incision can often be buried in the knee crease, it is easy with a couple of simple maneuvers, and it

avoids stripping of the distal saphenous vein from the ankle to the calf. There is some controversy concerning this matter, but the saphenous nerve anatomically is more closely approximated to the vein at the very distal location, and although it is very easy to strip antegrade from the ankle to the groin, the nerve can be injured during this maneuver. Neuropraxia can be very annoying to patients and can be permanent. In addition, it is fairly uncommon to have varicose vein clusters associated with the very distal portion of the saphenous vein.

On passing the stripper retrograde, there may be some competent or partly competent valves. These can be maneuvered by gentle force and by manipulating the leg, often bending it at the knee. In addition, counter pressure with your assistant or your other hand can allow you to navigate through the valves and down to the location of the knee. Then through a separate but very small incision the vein at the knee can be isolated with the stripper in place. It is then disconnected distally; you can either ligate at this location, or if you want to strip an additional portion of the saphenous vein, just pull it up through the wound taking care to skeletonize it so that the nerve is not attached. Then, after disconnecting the vein at the saphenofemoral junction, a small or medial stripper head is secured to the disposable stripper. It is tied to the vein and the vein is then stripped from the groin out through the knee. The patient should be in extreme Trendelenburg position, because in this position, manual pressure is held and a sterile ace bandage can be applied if you are planning on doing additional avulsions at this point. At the end of the procedure, using a laparotomy pad you can role whatever hematoma is apparent in the thigh and flush it out through the groin, cutting down on the bruising postoperatively. Passage of an epinephrine-soaked sponge through the tract is also a technique that has been advocated, but this is generally not necessary if you use manual pressure and extreme Trendelenburg position.

Two minor comments should be made about sclerotherapy as well as powered phlebectomy. When performing sclerotherapy for larger veins, greater than 1.0 mm, the patients need to be followed soon after. This vein will not ablate wall-to-wall, but will fill with clot; for a better cosmetic result, the patient should be brought back in 7 to 10 days and, through a simple stab with a No. 11 blade, the clot can be extruded. This is time-consuming and is one reason that I generally advocate the use of sclerotherapy only in the treatment of spider veins. As far as powered phlebectomy, although the results have been adequate in a number of series, there have been a number of patients who have developed permanent hemosiderin deposition of the skin, leaving pigmentation that is cosmetically unfavorable. The other is-

sue is "puckering," as both subcutaneous tissue and the veins are removed. The patient often has a dimple or indentation in the thigh that is very cosmetically unappealing. These potential complications need to be considered and described to the patients preoperatively.

Some additional comments on perforator disease and ulcers are warranted. There is a new treatment that is under trial for treatment of perforator veins. It is typically done after the superficial incompetence is treated, but the ulcer does not heal. The technique involves using a perforator catheter, which is similar to the radiofrequency ablation catheter used for VNUS closure. This is somewhat technically challenging, but can be effective. We are awaiting results of the trial before its use can be expanded.

Another important point about nonhealing ulcers is that even the experienced surgeon can be sometimes lulled into a sense of security based on the location of the ulcer (i.e., in the typical venous location). One needs to ensure that there is adequate arterial circulation based on palpable dorsalis pedis and posterior tibial pulses. There are patients with combined arterial and venous insufficiency and, even after treatment of the predominant venous problem, they will not heal. They will often then need treatment of their arterial circulation, which may be either catheter-based or surgical therapy.

Comment must be made about minimally invasive treatment of the greater saphenous vein.

During the last several years, percutaneous treatment of the incompetent greater saphenous vein has been expanded. Potential benefits of this therapy are (a) no incisions, (b) local anesthesia only, (c) no neuropraxia, and (d) potentially less recurrence. Because both of the treatments (radiofrequency ablation or VNUS closure and endovenous laser therapy) use catheters to occlude the vein, I will only discuss use of radiofrequency ablation in depth. The use of laser is a very similar technique with comparable results. The only potential problem with laser treatment is that it tends to be more painful for patients during the treatment and there is more chance for perforation and hematoma.

Preoperative vein mapping is done on all patients. The segments of venous reflux as well as the size of the vein and the depth from the skin surface are documented. In general, the injury current is about 4.0 mm, but to be safe it is ideal to have the vein more than 1.0 cm away from the skin surface during treatment. This, however, does not mean the resting baseline vein needs to be that deep because you would be using tumescent anesthesia to both encapsulate the vein in cold solution and create a heat sync, as well as pushing the vein away from the

(continued)

Vascular Surgery

skin surface. In addition, veins greater than 1.2 cm are generally not good candidates for radiofrequency ablation because of the likely higher deep vein thrombosis rate. Once you have documented that the patient is appropriate for treatment, the procedure can be scheduled in the office.

After consent, we generally give the patient 5 to 10 mg of oral Valium. The patient is then mapped with ultrasound guidance and a line is drawn over the greater saphenous vein. The access site at the knee or just into the calf is identified and EMLA cream is placed on the skin. The patient is prepared with S.T. 37 and draped in the usual fashion. After micropuncture technique, as the vein can be very small in this location, and the greater saphenous vein usually goes into extreme spasm, I find that using this technique the access failures have gone to 0. You can anesthetize the _____ with 1% lidocaine, although it is not necessary. The micropuncture wire is placed in the vein and confirmed on longitudinal ultrasound projection, and then directly over the micropuncture wire a No. 6 or 8 French sheath is delivered. This depends on the size of the vein. Then the radiofrequency ablation catheter is delivered to the saphenofemoral junction and pulled back below the epigastric vein, generally at a distance of 1.5 to 1.7 cm from the saphenofemoral junction.

With the catheter in place and the prongs open, tumescent anesthesia containing epinephrine, lidocaine, and bicarbonate is instilled using a Klein pump. It is very important that the tumescent is placed under the fascia as this gives you both maximum depth of the vein as well as creating a heat sync around the saphenous vein. If you just place it directly in the subqu above the fascia it will push the vein down, but the patient will still feel pain during the treatment. Using the Klein pump, you are able to treat the whole saphenous vein with three to four punctures, maximum. When the vein is more than 1 cm from the skin surface, the catheter is heated to 85°C to 90°C. The catheter is then pulled back approximately per minute. It is important that this is a continuous pull and not a stop, pull, stop motion.

After completion of the pullback, a repeat ultrasound is performed to make sure there is no deep vein thrombosis, and also to show occlusion of the greater saphenous vein. Pressure is held for approximately 10 minutes and an ace bandage is applied. We generally perform repeat ultrasound in 3 to 4 days. Note: it is important to state at consultations that approximately 30% to 40% of patients will need additional stab evulsions done at a separate time as some of the branch varicosities will shrink, but not completely resolve.

A.D.H.

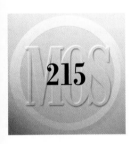

215

Venous Bypass

PETER GLOVICZKI AND ALESSANDRA PUGGIONI

Reconstruction of the occluded iliofemoral vein or the inferior vena cava (IVC) may be required in patients with chronic venous insufficiency (CVI). Iliofemoral venous occlusion is responsible for CVI in at least 10% of the patients afflicted by this disease. Endovascular treatment for iliocaval obstruction has progressed rapidly, and today venous stenting is the primary choice for treatment of benign iliac vein or iliocaval venous occlusions in patients who failed conservative compression therapy. Venous stenting is used for patients with malignancy only in those cases when excision of the tumor is not possible and the goal of therapy is palliation. In the last two decades results of open surgical reconstructions have also improved, and symptomatic patients who are not candidates or who failed endovascular reconstructions can be treated with venous bypasses to relieve venous outflow obstruction. Venous reconstruction is also performed in those patients who undergo excision of malignant tumors invading large veins like the IVC or the iliac veins. Patient selection for surgical treatment of the postthrombotic syndrome (PTS) can be challenging, since proximal occlusion is frequently combined with infrainguinal venous valvular incompetence. Thorough preoperative evaluation to identify significant venous outflow obstruction in these patients is essential.

ETIOLOGY

Chronic deep venous obstruction is usually the result of a previous acute deep venous thrombosis (DVT), although it can also be caused by retroperitoneal fibrosis; iatrogenic, blunt, or penetrating trauma; congenital venous anomalies; or benign or malignant tumors (Fig. 1). Compression of the left common iliac vein by the overriding right common iliac artery (May-Thurner syndrome) is a frequently overlooked cause of left iliofemoral venous thrombosis. May and Thurner observed secondary changes, such as an intraluminal web or "spur," in the proximal left common iliac vein in 20% of 430 autopsies. The most frequent primary malignant tumor is venous leiomyosarcoma; secondary tumors invading the vena cava include adenocarcinoma or liposarcoma. Renal carcinoma may extend into the IVC, and the tumor thrombus in some patients may reach all the way into the right atrium. Congenital suprarenal caval occlusion can occur due to webs or caval coarctation that may also present with associated hepatic vein occlusion (Budd-Chiari syndrome).

PATHOPHYSIOLOGY

During the acute phase of DVT, the thrombus in the vein activates the inflammatory cascade, which in turn promotes partial lysis of the thrombus and leads to recanalization. However, these processes are also responsible for damage to the vein wall and to the venous valves, leading to chronic obstruction and valvular incompetence. If collateral venous circulation in iliofemoral venous occlusion is inadequate, ambulatory venous hypertension develops due to a functional venous outflow obstruction. In PTS deep reflux and obstruction of multiple venous segments often coexists.

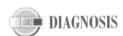 **DIAGNOSIS**

Patients with chronic iliac vein or iliocaval obstruction present with signs and symptoms of CVI. These include pain that frequently develops after exercise (venous claudication), swelling, varicosity, pigmentation, and skin changes (eczema, induration, ulcers) of the affected limb. Preoperative evaluation of CVI must focus on two major issues: Confirming the cause of chronic iliofemoral venous occlusion and establishing the presence and significance of poor venous outflow due to venous obstruction. The physician must exclude any abdominal or pelvic malignancy and consider May-Thurner syndrome as the cause of benign left iliac vein thrombosis.

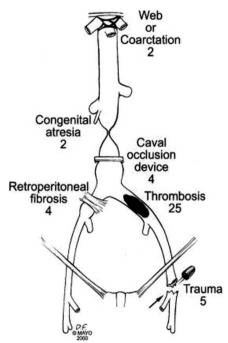

Fig. 1. Cause of venous occlusion in 42 patients who underwent open surgical reconstruction for nonmalignant venous occlusive disease. (Reprinted with permission from the Mayo Foundation.)

Venous duplex scanning should be performed in all patients with symptoms of CVI to help to define the location, cause, and severity of the underlying problem. Duplex scanning will diagnose both valvular incompetence and venous obstruction. Typical appearance of a post-thrombotic vein at duplex scanning is that of a thickened, hardly compressible vessel with damaged, incompetent valves and variable degrees of venous flow due to partial recanalization. Obesity and bowel gas may prevent good visualization of the common hepatic veins and the IVC with ultrasound.

Air or strain gauge plethysmography is designed to evaluate the global leg hemodynamics by measuring reflux, obstruction, and calf pump function. Decreased vein wall compliance in patients with PTS may interfere with proper evaluation of calf muscle pump function. Unfortunately, the site and the level of reflux cannot be localized with plethysmography. Plethysmography, however, is suitable to confirm functional venous outflow obstruction.

Magnetic resonance (MR) imaging and computed tomography (CT) scanning will identify any obstructing mass or tumor, and adding gadolinium for MR or intravenous contrast for CT will give the anatomy of the venous system. Contrast venography is still performed in most patients who undergo open surgical deep venous reconstructions or endovascular intervention. Ascending venography is both an anatomic and a functional study that provides the best "road map" of the deep veins of the limb, defines the sites of obstruction, and images the collateral venous circulation and the patterns of preferential flow. Descending venography under fluoroscopy permits evaluation of sites of reflux in the saphenous and deep system. Contrast venography is combined with direct venous pressure measurement to document a pressure difference between the femoral vein and the vena cava: A resting pressure differential of 5 mm Hg or greater is considered evidence for significant obstruction. A lower pressure at rest but an increase to 10 mm Hg after exercise is also a sign of functional obstruction: Exercise consists of 10 dorsiflexions of the ankles or 20 isometric contractions of the calf muscle. Intravascular ultrasound is used frequently today to assess the degree of iliac vein stenosis before stenting.

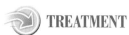 **TREATMENT**

Conservative Management

Symptoms of deep venous obstruction should be first treated with leg elevation, graduated compression stockings (30 to 40 mm Hg), and local wound care of venous ulcerations, if there are any. Compression garments result in variable degrees of success and mandate strict patients' compliance, which in a hot climate can be both distressing and difficult. The benefits of graduated compression stockings reside in their theoretic effects on venous hemodynamics, skin circulation, and calf muscle pump function. Randomized prospective studies demonstrated a 50% net risk reduction of developing PTS in patients wearing elastic compression stockings after DVT. Patients with persistent disabling symptoms, such as venous claudication, severe swelling, and nonhealing or recurrent ulcers not responding to conservative treatment, should be considered for endovascular or open surgical reconstruction.

Endovascular Treatment

Iliac or iliocaval stenting has become the primary treatment for chronic nonmalignant venous occlusions. Early and midterm results of endovascular technique, such as angioplasty and stenting, using most frequently self-expandable stents, have been good. Seventy-seven percent of the patients stented for iliofemoral occlusion were free of significant in-stent restenosis at 3 years in one study. Risk factors for restenosis were PTS, positive thrombophilia test results, and long stent extending below the inguinal ligament.

Open Surgical Treatment

Patients who are not candidates or who failed endovascular reconstructions can be treated with venous bypasses to relieve symptomatic venous outflow obstruction. Venous reconstruction is also performed in those patients who undergo excision of malignant tumors invading the vena cava or iliac veins.

Crossover Saphenous Vein Transposition (Palma Procedure)

Patients with symptomatic unilateral iliac vein obstruction are candidates for saphenous vein transposition (Palma procedure) (Fig. 2). With this technique, the contralateral saphenous vein is used for a crossover bypass to decompress venous congestion in the affected limb. The common femoral vein on the affected side is exposed first through a 6- to 8-cm long longitudinal groin incision. The collateral veins should be preserved if possible. The great saphenous vein of the contralateral leg is dissected through a 3- to 5-cm incision made in the groin crease, starting just medial to the femoral artery pulse. Tributaries of the saphenous vein are ligated and divided and the saphenous vein is mobilized in a length of about 10 to 12 cm. A short second upper-thigh incision is made to dissect a 20- to 25-cm long portion of the saphenous vein. Distally the vein is ligated, and proximal to the ligature it is divided and pulled up to the groin incision. Alternatively, endoscopic harvesting of the saphenous vein can also be performed, but the vein proximally should not be divided. It is essential to free up the saphenofemoral junction completely and dissect at least the anterior wall of the common femoral vein around the saphenous vein so there is no kink or buckle when the saphenous vein is pulled into the suprapubic tunnel. In some patients with a low saphenofemoral junction a kink is unavoidable: Excision of the saphenous vein with a 2-mm cuff from the common femoral vein and reanastomosis to the femoral vein with running 6/0 polypropylene suture, after turning the junction upwards 180 degrees, is the way to solve this problem. Before tunneling, a small Satinsky clamp is placed on the common femoral vein to allow distention of the saphenous

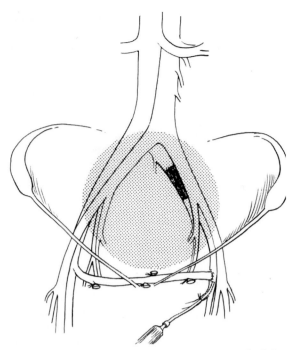

Fig. 2. Suprapubic saphenous vein transposition (Palma procedure) for left common iliac vein thrombosis. Bilateral groin incisions are performed to expose the left common femoral vein and the right saphenofemoral junction. The right saphenous vein is harvested open through short incisions in the thigh or using an endoscopic technique. The saphenous vein is anastomosed to the left common femoral vein using 6/0 running polypropylene suture. A small catheter placed through the saphenous vein on the left is used for heparin perfusion perioperatively. (Reprinted with permission from the Mayo Foundation.)

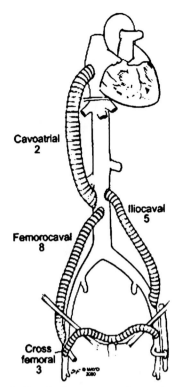

Fig. 3. Prosthetic reconstruction options for iliofemoral and caval obstructions in 18 patients. (Reprinted with permission from the Mayo Foundation.)

vein and the saphenofemoral junction under gentle pressure using heparinized papaverine-saline solution. The vein is then tunneled subcutaneously in the suprapubic space over to the contralateral side using an aortic clamp to ensure a large tunnel without any constriction of the graft whatsoever. Saphenous vein graft in morbidly obese patients is not recommended because of the high chance of external compression of the vein. The common femoral vein is cross clamped with small vascular clamps or bulldogs and the vein is opened longitudinally in a length of about 2 cm. The anastomosis between the saphenous vein and the femoral vein is performed with running 6/0 polypropylene suture. A vein at least 5 mm in diameter is required to achieve a satisfactory result and provide high venous flow to treat the basic problem in these patients: Poor venous emptying. For a smaller vein a temporary arteriovenous fistula can be added between the superficial femoral artery and the saphenous or common femoral vein using a 4- to 5-mm polytetrafluoroethylene (PTFE) graft or a large tributary of the saphenous vein. The Palma procedure, however, should not be performed with veins 4 mm or smaller.

Although few large series have been reported, overall patency of Palma grafts in nine series including 412 operations ranged between 70% and 83% at 3 to 5 years. Results were better in patients who had no or minimal infrainguinal venous disease in those with May-Thurner syndrome without previous deep vein thrombosis.

Crossover Femoral Venous Prosthetic Bypass

When the saphenous vein is small or not available, a crossover femoral venous prosthetic bypass with an 8- or 10-mm externally supported expanded PTFE (ePTFE) graft is a good alternative (Fig. 3). Similarly to the autologous femoral suprapubic bypass, the femoral veins are exposed bilaterally, the ePTFE graft is positioned in the subcutaneous suprapubic tunnel, and an end-to-side anastomosis is performed to the common femoral veins at each side. A distal arteriovenous fistula (AVF) on the affected side is routinely added to the procedure using a 4- to 5-mm PTFE graft for the fistula between the PTFE graft and the superficial femoral artery. Satturai recommended cutting out a small window rather than just making a longitudinal cut in cross-femoral graft at the hood of the femoral anastomosis to optimize inflow and decrease intimal hyperplasia of the AVF.

Variable patency rates of ePTFE grafts in this location have been reported and range between 0% and 100%, with data from one large series quoting a 100% (19 of 19) patency rate at long-term follow-up. In the authors' experience long-term patency is about 50% and preference still should be given to saphenous cross-over grafts.

Iliocaval and Femorocaval Bypass

Low-risk patients with bilateral iliac obstructions or with iliocaval obstruction that cannot be treated with stents should be considered for an in-line femorocaval (Fig. 4A–D) or iliocaval (Fig. 5) bypass. For in-line reconstruction of iliocaval or caval occlusions, an ePTFE graft with external support is the preferred conduit. Short, large-diameter (12-mm) grafts are used most frequently; a diameter of 12 to 14 mm is used for iliocaval bypasses and at least 10 mm for femorocaval bypass. The upper portion of the infrarenal IVC at and immediately distal to the renal veins is best approached transperitoneally through a midline incision, reflecting the ascending colon medially and mobilizing the duodenum using the Kocher maneuver. The low IVC just above the iliac bifurcation is well approachable through a right flank incision

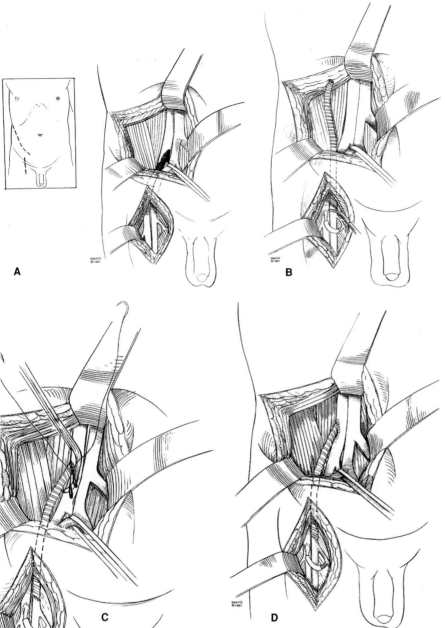

Fig. 4. A: Location of the incisions of a right femorocaval bypass. The common femoral vein and the proximal saphenous vein is exposed through a 6- to 8-cm vertical incision at the groin. The distal inferior vena cava is exposed retroperitoneally through a right oblique anterolateral flank incision, transecting the abdominal muscles and the transversalis fascia. The ureter is retracted medially. **B:** The femoral arteriovenous fistula is performed first in this case with a large tributary of the saphenous vein and the femoral artery. A silastic sheath is wrapped around the vein for easy late identification. The distal anastomosis is performed then in an end-to-end fashion between the common femoral vein and the 10-mm externally supported polytetrafluoroethylene graft. **C:** The anastomosis between the graft and the inferior vena cava is performed in an end-to-end fashion using 5/0 polypropylene suture. Air is carefully flushed from the graft before removing the clamp from the inferior vena. **D:** Completed femorocaval bypass with a saphenofemoral arteriovenous fistula. (Reprinted with permission from the Mayo Foundation.)

retroperitoneally (Fig. 4A). If the occlusion is limited to the right common iliac vein, the same incision is used to expose the external iliac vein for the distal anastomosis. The graft is tunneled under the ureter.

If a femorocaval graft is placed, a separate 8-cm long vertical groin incision is made on the affected side and the graft is tunneled under the inguinal ligament (Fig. 4A). To all grafts originating from the femoral vein and to most long iliocaval grafts, an arteriovenous fistula is added at the groin (Fig. 4B). To start local heparin therapy (500 units/hr), a 20-gauge catheter

is introduced through a tributary of the saphenous vein (Fig. 5) and advanced to the distal anastomosis. This catheter can be used for completion venography 24 to 48 hours after reconstruction and removed the third postoperative day, when full anticoagulation is started. Early clinical improvement can be expected in the majority of patients, but presence of coexisting femoropopliteal reflux can still be the cause of significant disability.

The use of autologous vein for femoroiliac or femorocaval reconstruction is also an option (Fig. 6). Because of a relatively small size, saphenous vein in this location can only rarely be used. If short segment of the common femoral or iliac vein has to be reconstructed, a better size match is a spiral saphenous vein graft, prepared using the contralateral saphenous vein (Fig. 7). The excised vein is opened longitudinally, the valves are excised, and the graft is wrapped around a 28- or 32-mm argyle chest tube. The edges are approximated with running 6/0 polypropylene sutures or with stainless steel nonpenetrating vascular clips. The internal or external jugular veins are other conduits that can be considered for venous reconstruction. The femoral vein is also an alternative for reconstruction of abdominal veins, although morbidity of removing this vein in many of these patients with underlying thrombophilia or postthrombotic syndrome is high and other options are recommended. Cryopreserved saphenous or femoral vein has also been reported for venous reconstruction, but long-term patency of these grafts for venous replacement in our experience has been poor.

Experience with femorocaval or iliocaval PTFE bypass grafts for benign disease has been limited; reported primary and secondary patency rates at 2 years were 37% and 54%, respectively. In one series, published by Satturai, long-term patency of 77% (10 of 13) was reported.

Cavoatrial Bypass

Patients with symptomatic short membranous occlusion of the IVC or longer congenital or acquired narrowing (caval coarctation) without or with hepatic venous outflow obstruction (Budd-Chiari syndrome) can be treated by cavoatrial bypass when attempts at percutaneous angioplasty or stenting have failed, or if transcardiac membranotomy is not feasible.

The suprahepatic inferior vena cava or right atrium is approached through an anterolateral right thoracotomy (Fig. 8A–D). The pericardium is opened anterior to the

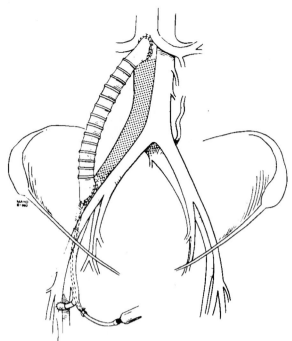

Fig. 5. Iliocaval polytetrafluoroethylene bypass between the right external iliac vein and the infrarenal inferior vena cava. Note the saphenofemoral arteriovenous fistula and placement of a 20-gauge pediatric central line into the saphenous vein and advanced up to the graft to perfuse heparin to prevent early thrombus formation on the graft surface. (Reprinted with permission from the Mayo Foundation.)

made more distally, a separate right subcostal or midline incision can be performed as previously described.

For a cavoatrial bypass an end-to-side anastomosis to the IVC is performed and the graft is routed under the liver parallel to the IVC. The graft is then anastomosed end to side to the suprarenal IVC or the lower portion of the right atrium. Partially occluding clamps are used to perform the anastomoses, and cardiopulmonary bypass is not needed. Traumatic or iatrogenic occlusions can also be managed by this technique. The use of a 16- to 20-mm externally supported PTFE graft is recommended.

The reported clinical success rate with cavoatrial grafts is about 77%, with a perioperative mortality of 3% and 2-, 5-, and 10-year patency rates of 86%, 78%, and 57%, respectively.

Inferior Vena Cava Reconstruction following Excision of Malignant Tumors

Primary venous leiomyosarcoma or secondary tumors invading the vena cava, such as hepatic tumors, retroperitoneal sarcomas, or adrenal tumors, are the most frequent indications. Most renal carcinomas that extend into the vena cava do not invade the wall of the vessel and the tumor thrombus can frequently be removed from the IVC without the need for venous reconstruction. Attention must be paid to avoid tumor embolization into the pulmonary arteries. Patients with extension of the tumor thrombus into the right

phrenic nerve. If the membranous occlusion is short and is located to this area, a short PTFE interposition graft can be performed from this exposure. If the occlusion extends distal to the hepatic veins, the abdomen is entered through the same

thoracotomy, transecting the diaphragm circumferentially and mobilizing the liver forward and medially. Division of the triangular and the right coronary ligament will help mobilization of the liver. The adrenal gland and the kidney are left in their bed and dissection is moved more medially. Excellent exposure of the suprarenal IVC can be achieved through this approach. If the distal anastomosis has to be

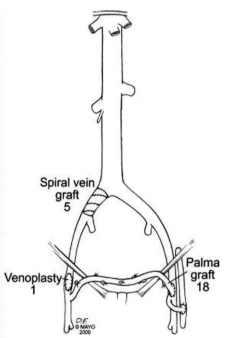

Fig. 6. Methods for reconstruction of the femoral and iliac veins with autologous vein in 24 patients. (Reprinted with permission from the Mayo Foundation.)

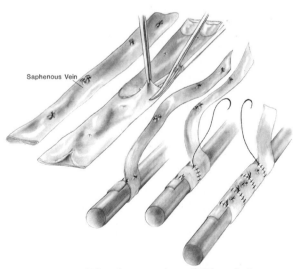

Fig. 7. Technique to prepare a spiral saphenous vein graft. The vein is cut open longitudinally, valves are excised, and the vein is wrapped around a 28- or 32-gauge argyle chest tube. The edges are approximated with running 6/0 polypropylene sutures, making interrupted stitches after each circle to minimize purse stringing. Alternatively, nonpenetrating vascular clips can be used for this purpose. (Reprinted with permission from the Mayo Foundation.)

Vascular Surgery

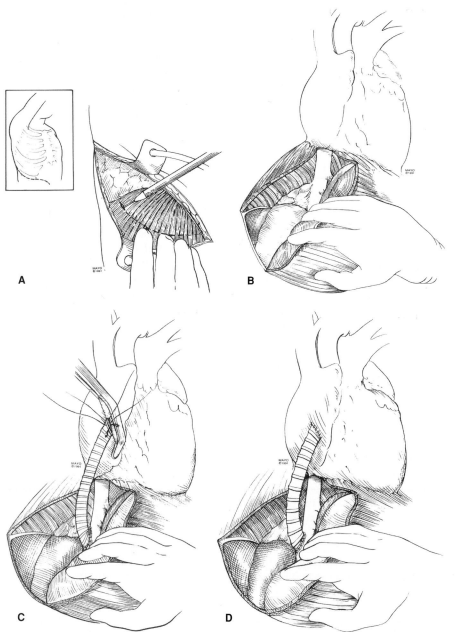

Fig. 8. A: For a cavoatrial bypass the thorax is entered through the eighth intercostal space performing an anterolateral thoracotomy. The costal arch is sharply divided through the eight and ninth ribs but the abdomen is not entered. The inferior pulmonary ligament is divided and the diaphragm is circumferentially incised and the abdomen is entered. (Reprinted with permission from the Mayo Foundation.) **B:** The triangular and right coronary ligament is divided and the right lobe of the liver is mobilized medially and anteriorly. (Reprinted with permission from the Mayo Foundation.) **C:** The suprarenal inferior vena cava is dissected and partially cross clamped. A 14- or 16-mm externally supported polytetrafluoroethylene (PTFE) graft is anastomosed first to the cava, then to the right atrium. Air is carefully flushed before opening up flow in the graft. **D:** Completed cavoatrial PTFE bypass. (Reprinted with permission from the Mayo Foundation.)

atrium need cardiopulmonary bypass to permit safe removal of the tumor.

The incision for resection of primary IVC tumors is transperitoneal, usually midline or right subcostal. Hepatic tumor resection may require a right thoracolaparotomy (Fig. 9A–D). The IVC is exposed by mobilizing the ascending colon and performing the Kocher maneuver to

mobilize the second portion of the duodenum medially, as described before. PTFE grafts (14 to 20 mm) with external support provide excellent patency of the reconstructed suprarenal or infrarenal inferior vena cava, since inflow is usually excellent and there is no associated iliac vein thrombosis. Short, 8- or 10-mm wide, externally supported PTFE grafts can also

be used to reconstruct the renal veins i[f] nephrectomy for treatment of the tumor does not have to be performed. For partial invasion of the IVC wide excision of the wall and direct suture or a PTFE or bovine pericardial patch are options for reconstruction.

A venovenous bypass between the IVC or iliac vein and the axillary or internal jugular vein using a mechanical (Biomedicus) pump is only needed in those patients with poor cardiac function who cannot maintain a systolic blood pressure above 100 mm Hg when both the IVC and the hepatic veins are occluded for an anastomosis. When resection of the retrohepatic suprarenal vena cava has to be performed, the proximal anastomosis is performed first to allow early restoration of hepatic venous outflow (Fig. 9C,D). A femoral AVF is usually not required because of the excellent venous inflow.

Perioperative complications are frequent (43%) and operative mortality because of the associated liver resection can be as high as 7%. Graft patency is 93% at 3 years. Early patency of caval reconstruction for malignant disease is excellent, but survival in many patients is limited due to recurrent local tumor or distant metastases. Nevertheless, aggressive surgical management may offer the only chance for cure or palliation of symptoms for patients with primary or secondary IVC tumors. Caval reconstruction may result in significant improvement of the quality of life in these patients even if their survival is limited due to the underlying malignant disease.

SPECIAL CONSIDERATIONS

Endophlebectomy

Postthrombotic femoral veins frequently have multiple lumens due to partial recanalization of the thrombus. Excision of the organized and usually fibrotic thrombus will enlarge the lumen, although the exposed collagen in the media of the vein wall is more thrombogenic than the intact venous wall. Still, careful endophlebectomy will improve inflow to a great extent; attention, however, must be paid to avoid injury to the thin residual venous wall. This procedure has long been performed combined with deep venous valve transplantation in patients with PTS, but it has become evident recently that it can be equally effective for treatment of venous obstruction as well. In patients who have localized high-grade stenosis of the common femoral vein, this

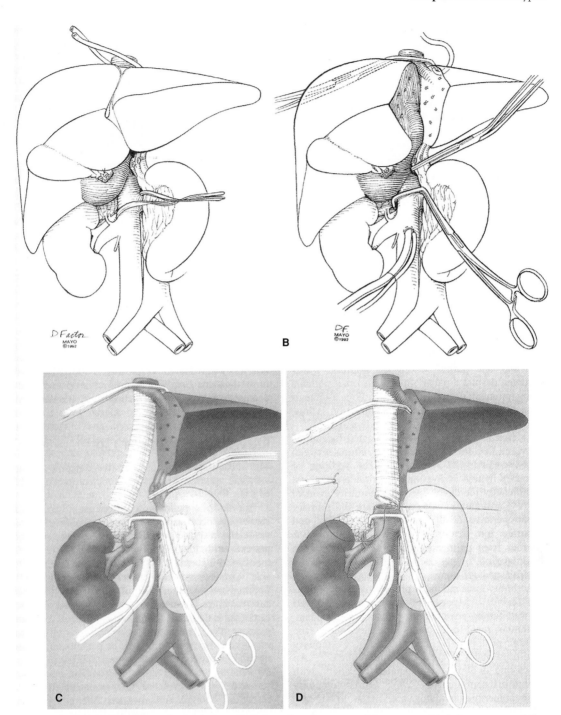

Fig. 9. Technique for polytetrafluoroethylene (PTFE) graft replacement of the suprarenal inferior vena cava following right hepatic lobectomy for a malignant tumor with caval invasion. **A:** Isolation of the suprahepatic and suprarenal segments of the vena cava and division of the right hepatic artery and portal vein branches. **B:** Hepatic vascular exclusion used to complete resection of the liver, tumor, and retrohepatic vena cava. If necessary, venovenous bypass via an infrarenal cannula is used. **C:** The upper caval anastomosis is performed first to minimize hepatic ischemia. **D:** The suprahepatic caval clamp is transferred across the graft after acid metabolites have been flushed from the liver. The lower caval anastomosis is completed. (From Bower TC, Nagorney DM, Toomey BJ, et al. Vena cava replacement for malignant disease: is there a role? *Ann Vasc Surg* 1993;7:51, with permission.)

operation alone is sufficient to improve venous outflow. The defect is closed with a patch using a segment of the saphenous vein or bovine pericardium. The endophlebectomized segment can also be used to improve inflow for iliocaval stenting or for a cross-femoral or femorocaval bypass. In a series of ten patients who underwent endophlebectomy alone, early results showed 77% patency of the operated segments at 8 months. Results of larger numbers of patients to assess long-term patency with this technique have not yet been reported.

ADJUNCTIVE PROCEDURES

With the exception of caval reconstructions or short iliocaval grafts, prosthetic bypasses used for venous outflow obstruction of the legs need an adjunctive temporary AVF to maintain patency. The best technique is a 4–

to 5-mm PTFE graft that is about 2 cm long and is placed between the superficial femoral artery and the lower portion of the PTFE venous graft. The authors use a tapered 4 × 7 mm PTFE graft to obtain a segment suitable for AVF. Both anastomoses are performed with 6/0 polypropylene sutures. A small silastic sheet is wrapped around the bypass to avoid healing and permit easy identification later when the fistula is closed. A 2/0 polypropylene suture is tied to the silastic sheath and positioned under the skin incision for easy identification. Patients who have saphenous Palma grafts undergo takedown of the fistula at 3 months. Patients who have PTFE grafts will keep the arteriovenous fistula longer, if possible. The AVF increases flow through the graft, decreases platelet and fibrin deposition, and contributes to improved patency. It also provides time for pannus formation over the anastomoses during the initial period when the graft surface is most thrombogenic. Potential side effects are a high cardiac output, functional outflow obstruction resulting in high distal venous pressures, and accelerated intimal hyperplasia.

PREVENTION OF COMPLICATIONS

In general, large vein reconstructions for benign disease are performed in good surgical candidates only, with a low risk of systemic complications. Of the local, nonvascular complications, wound infection and lymphatic leaks (fistula, lymphocele) are the most frequent, and atraumatic surgical technique, antibiotic prophylaxis, and standard surgical principles are helpful in prevention.

Intraoperative air embolism, especially during caval reconstruction, is a potentially fatal complication and may be prevented by meticulous flushing of the grafts before re-establishment of the circulation and passive Valsalva maneuver (30 mm Hg) as well as Trendelenburg position before release of the proximal clamp.

Deep venous thrombosis and pulmonary embolism are also serious systemic vascular complications. Perioperative anticoagulation with heparin and warfarin, the use of elastic stockings, intermittent pneumatic compression pumps, and early ambulation help prevent thromboembolic complications, which are fortunately rare. Local vascular complications are specific to venous reconstructions and include graft stenosis or thrombosis, perioperative bleeding, graft infection, and injury to the surrounding vascular and nonvascular structures.

ANTICOAGULATION

Grafts placed in the venous system have a higher rate of thrombosis than arterial grafts due to a low venous flow. Infrainguinal venous obstruction and valvular incompetence further decrease inflow to the graft, and it is a major contributing factor to failure. Thrombophilia is prevalent among patients undergoing venous reconstructions, and many patients have absent circulating anticoagulants such as protein factor C, protein factor S, and antithrombin III or have factor V Leiden mutation. The thrombogenic surface of any prosthetic graft also increases the risk of graft failure. For these reasons, perioperative anticoagulation is indicated in patients undergoing reconstructive venous surgery for deep venous obstruction.

The patient is fully heparinized during reconstruction and protamine is avoided at the completion of the procedure. Heparin in a dose of 500 units/hr is started in the operating room through a 20-gauge pediatric central line that is placed through the saphenous vein of the affected limb and advanced to the distal anastomosis of the prosthetic graft. Complete postoperative systemic heparinization is achieved by 48 hours, and full-dose low-molecular-weight heparin is continued subcutaneously for another 3 to 5 days, given simultaneously with warfarin. The incidence of postoperative bleeding has been between 5% and

10%, mainly as a result of anticoagulation. Warfarin is continued indefinitely in most patients with prosthetic grafts and in all with a known underlying coagulation abnormality.

FOLLOW-UP AND REINTERVENTIONS

Duplex scan on the first postoperative day or contrast venography is performed to confirm graft patency. Stenosis or thrombosis is corrected immediately after recognition. If thrombosis occurred in a graft without fistula, thrombectomy is done with addition of a fistula. Graft stenosis discovered during surveillance in the late postoperative period is treated first with angioplasty or venous stenting. Late graft thrombosis is treated with thrombolysis, angioplasty, and stenting. Surgical revision is usually limited to patch angioplasty of the stenotic portion of the graft, although occasionally aneurysmal dilation of the saphenous crossover graft may also need surgical correction.

SUGGESTED READING

Bower TC, Nagorney DM, Cherry KJ Jr., et al. Replacement of the inferior vena cava for malignancy: an update. *J Vasc Surg* 2000;31:270.

Gloviczki P. Clinical, hemodynamic, and anatomic predictors of long-term outcome of lower extremity venovenous bypasses. *J Vasc Surg* 1992;16:131.

Gloviczki P, Pairolero PC, Toomey BJ, et al. Reconstruction of large veins for nonmalignant venous occlusive disease. *J Vasc Surg* 1992;16:750.

Jost CJ, Gloviczki P, Cherry KJ Jr., et al. Surgical reconstruction of iliofemoral veins and the inferior vena cava for nonmalignant occlusive disease. *J Vasc Surg* 2001;33:320.

Sottiurai VS. Venous bypass and valve reconstruction: indication, technique and results. *Phlebol* 1997;25:183.

Xu PQ, Ma XX, Ye XX, et al. Surgical treatment of 1360 cases of Budd-Chiari syndrome: 20-year experience. *Hepatobiliary Pancreat Dis Int* 2004;3:391.

EDITOR'S COMMENT

Few centers have the extensive experience in major venous bypass surgery described in this excellent and comprehensive chapter by Gloviczki and Puggioni. In addition, few vascular surgeons have more than an anecdotal exposure to these challenging cases. Therefore, the techniques and management strategies described by the authors may

be considered definitive and authoritative. This chapter should be required reading for anyone embarking upon operative management of these patients.

The Palma procedure or crossover saphenous vein transposition is rarely successful in patients with postphlebitic syndrome from chronic occlu-

sion of the ileofemoral venous system. The ipsilateral femoral vein is frequently involved with recanalization changes that provide poor inflow to the bypass and may lead to thrombosis. Endophlebectomy with excision of multiple synechiae has not helped to improve patency in my experience. Because recurrent thrombosis of

(continued)

the femoral vein can result in worsening post-phlebitic symptoms, I have generally considered extensive scarring of the ipsilateral common femoral vein to be a relative contraindication for the Palma procedure. The best results are seen in patients with tumor compression or inflammatory entrapment of the iliac vein that spares the common femoral vein. Obviously, angioplasty and stenting should be attempted first.

Because of my interest and extensive experience in using the femoral-popliteal vein for arterial reconstructions, I have often been asked about

the feasibility of using the deep vein graft for venous reconstructions. We have successfully used this large-caliber vein graft for short-segment venous bypasses or replacements and the patency has been excellent (Hagino RT, et al. *J Vasc Surg* 1997;26:829). The femoral-popliteal vein graft works well for venous reconstructive surgery if it is in an environment in which it is not compressed. We have had good success with this vein graft for treatment of superior vena cava syndrome and much prefer this to creating a spiral vein graft. However, for iliofemoral and caval reconstructions, externally supported ePTFE works

much better because it resists compression of abdominal viscera.

We have also used the femoral-popliteal vein graft to reconstruct the superior mesenteric-portal vein when this structure is involved with tumor infiltration during pancreaticoduodenectomy (Fleming JB, et al. *Arch Surg* 2005;140:698). The size match is optimal and the patency superior in comparison to other venous grafts in this position. Prosthetic grafts in this position are contraindicated because of enteric contamination.

G.P.C.

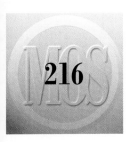

Autogenous Arteriovenous Hemodialysis Access

THOMAS S. HUBER

End-stage renal disease (ESRD) is a tremendous public health problem. In 2001, there were more than 400,000 individuals in the United States with ESRD, and it has been estimated that this number will increase to more than 500,000 by the year 2010. The corresponding costs totaled $12.3 billion in 2000 and have been projected to reach $28.3 billion by 2010. Indeed, the Medicare costs for ESRD alone represented 6% of the total budget in 2000. With approximately 75% of the patients with ESRD receiving hemodialysis, it is not surprising that maintaining hemodialysis access is a significant burden that is compounded by the limited functional patency rates for the various access options and the improving patient survival.

The National Kidney Foundation Kidney Disease Outcomes Quality Initiative (K/DOQI) has emphasized the importance of autogenous access. They recommended the autogenous radiocephalic and brachiocephalic accesses as their first and second choices, respectively, for permanent access. Furthermore, they have defined an autogenous access target of at least 50% for patients initiating dialysis and an overall prevalence of 40% for all patients receiving hemodialysis. The Center for Medicare and Medicaid Services recently initiated a 3-year program entitled the National Vascular Access Improvement Initiative or "Fistula First" (fistula: autogenous arteriovenous hemodialysis access) to achieve the K/DOQI targets, or specifically to "increase the proportion of hemodialysis patients who use arteriovenous fistulas (autogenous access) as the primary mode of vascular access."

The National Vascular Access Improvement Initiative is a multidisciplinary approach defined by 11 specific concepts designed to impact practice patterns (Table 1). Notably, a significant proportion of the Fistula First effort is targeted at access surgeons. Despite these national initiatives, the prevalence of autogenous access in the United States is less than 40% and dramatically less than the 80% prevalence reported from Europe (France, Germany, Italy, United Kingdom, Spain).

TABLE 1. FISTULA FIRST PRACTICE RECOMMENDATIONS

- Routine quality review for vascular access
- Timely referral to a nephrologist
- Early referral to a surgeon for AVF evaluation and timely placement
- Surgeon selection based on best outcomes, willingness, and ability to provide access services
- Full range of appropriate surgical approaches for AVF evaluation and placement
- Secondary AVF placement in patients with AV grafts
- AVF placement in patients with catheters when indicated
- Cannulation training for AVFs
- Monitoring and maintenance to ensure adequate access function
- Education for caregivers and patients
- Outcome feedback to guide practice

[a]AVF, autogenous arteriovenous hemodialysis access; AV grafts, prosthetic arteriovenous hemodialysis access.

The K/DOQI recommendations for autogenous accesses are based partly on the presumption that the patency rates for autogenous access are superior to their prosthetic counterparts. However, the data in the K/DOQI cited to justify the superiority of autogenous accesses are limited by evidence-based medicine standards and included retrospective case series and expert opinion. In a recent review of the literature designed to examine the evidence supporting the clinical decisions relevant to the hemodialysis access surgeon, we were unable to identify any randomized controlled trials or meta-analyses comparing autogenous and prosthetic accesses. However, our group has recently published a formal systematic review of the literature comparing the patency rates of upper extremity polytetrafluoroethylene (PTFE) and autogenous accesses in adults that represents the next level down (i.e., systematic review of observational studies) from a randomized, controlled trial in the hierarchy of evidence. Studies were considered acceptable for inclusion if patency was reported using either the life table or Kaplan-Meier methods, and included the number of patients at risk. Unfortunately, there were only 34 studies that satisfied the inclusion criteria, with the majority composed of cases series or non-randomized controlled studies with the data collected in a retrospective fashion. The primary annual patency rates for the autogenous and PTFE accesses were approximately 60% and 40%, respectively, and the corresponding secondary patency rates were 80% and 60% (Fig. 1). Notably, the annual secondary patency rate for the

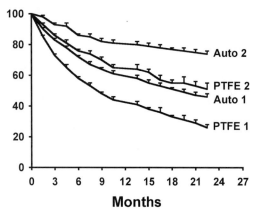

Fig. 1. The patency rates (percent patent) for the autogenous (Auto) and polytetrafluoroethylene (PTFE) upper extremity hemodialysis accesses are plotted against time (months) with the positive standard error bars. Both the primary (Auto 1, PTFE 1) and secondary (Auto 2, PTFE 2) patency rates for the two access types are shown. The patency rates for the autogenous accesses were better than their corresponding PTFE counterparts with the one exception of the initial (1.5 months) time point for the primary patency comparison. (From Huber TS, Carter JW, Carter RL, et al. Patency of autogenous and polytetrafluoroethylene upper extremity arteriovenous hemodialysis accesses: a systematic review. *J Vasc Surg* 2003;38:1005, with permission.)

PTFE accesses was below the cumulative 70% annual patency rate established by K/DOQI in their quality-of-care standards.

The K/DOQI also justified the use of autogenous accesses based on their lower complication rates, including conduit stenosis, infection, hand ischemia, and death. We were unable to determine accurate complication rates in our systematic review of the literature either because the complications were not described in the individual studies, the descriptions were not standardized, or the means of reporting were not amenable to meta-analysis. However, the results from the individual studies suggest that the perioperative mortality rate was essentially 0 (median, 0%; range, 0% to 1%) and the incidence of hand ischemia (median, 2%; range, 0% to 14%), access infection (median, 7%; range, 0% to 30%), and aneurysm/pseudo-aneurysm formation (median, 4%; range, 0% to 6%) were low for both autogenous and PTFE accesses. Not surprisingly, the overwhelming majority of the access infections were seen in the PTFE accesses.

The annual mortality rate associated with dialysis catheters and prosthetic accesses has been consistently shown to exceed those for autogenous accesses. Notably, Dhingra et al. reported from the United States Renal Data System that the relative mortality risk (reference group autogenous accesses) was 1.41 and 1.54 for diabetic patients dialyzed with prosthetic accesses and catheters, respectively, and the corresponding values were 1.08 and 1.70, respectively, among nondiabetics. Indeed, the annual unadjusted mortality rate for all hemodialysis patients across the United States was a staggering 21.7% in the Dialysis Outcomes and Practice Patterns Study and was significantly greater than those reported from Europe (15.6%) and Japan (6.6%). Although the mean patient age and the burden of co-morbidities were greater in the United States, the adjusted relative risk of mortality was 1.33 greater in the United States relative to Europe and 3.78 relative to Japan. It is likely that the discrepancy in the prevalence of the autogenous accesses between the three continents contributed.

There are a few distinct disadvantages to autogenous accesses. The obligatory period necessary to allow the autogenous access to mature usually exceeds the corresponding 4- to 6-week period required for incorporation of the prosthetic accesses. Indeed, Rayner et al. reported from the Dialysis Outcomes and Practice Patterns Study that the median duration from autogenous access creation to cannulation in the United States was 98 days. This obligatory period usually requires the use of dialysis catheters as a "bridge" and exposes the patients to all the potential catheter-related complications. Admittedly, the use of dialysis catheters in this setting may be reduced by early patient referral to an access surgeon prior to the initiation of dialysis. Furthermore, a significant proportion of the autogenous accesses fail to mature sufficiently for cannulation, with values ranging up to 40% depending on the specific type. Lastly, approximately 25% of the initial autogenous accesses need some type of remedial imaging or procedure to facilitate maturation.

Despite these limitations, the proverbial bottom line is that autogenous accesses are likely the optimal choice for permanent hemodialysis access as recommended by K/DOQI and National Vascular Access Improvement Initiative. The patency rates appear to be better and the incidence of complications appear lower. Autogenous accesses are associated with a requisite period for fistula maturation and likely require a higher incidence of remedial procedures to facilitate maturation, although these considerations can be minimized by timely referral to an access surgeon. We have attempted to optimize the use of autogenous access in our own practice, but would concede that an autogenous access is not possible and/or appropriate for all clinical settings. We currently use prosthesis for patients without autogenous options according to the preoperative imaging, those with limited life expectancy, and those with marginal autogenous access options who have had previous autogenous access attempts that have not matured sufficiently for cannulation.

DETERMINATION OF AUTOGENOUS ACCESS CONFIGURATION

General Principles

The overwhelming majority of patients presenting for permanent access are candidates for an autogenous access. Our approach, designed to optimize the use of autogenous upper extremity accesses, is predicated on the standard principles of vascular surgery including adequate arterial inflow, adequate venous outflow, and a suitable conduit. Furthermore, it is based on the use of dialysis catheters as a bridge or temporary access until the permanent access is suitable for cannulation, and an aggressive approach to "failing" or "nonmatured" accesses. Figure 2 shows our group's algorithm for permanent autogenous access.

History/Physical Examination

The initial evaluation of patents presenting for permanent hemodialysis access includes a focused history/physical examination. Special attention should be directed at documenting the access history, including procedures, revisions, and associated complications. This should include any history of central vein cannulation, arm or facial edema, and hand ischemia. Physical examination should include a detailed pulse examination with an Allen's test to determine

the clinical status of the patient, and the location/extent of the arterial lesion. Generically, the endovascular treatments tend to be safer, but not as durable, although their role in the various anatomic locations is being defined. Fortunately, the atherosclerotic lesions that affect the arterial inflow to the upper extremity commonly involve the origins of the innominate and subclavian arteries; both of these lesions are effectively treated with either balloon angioplasty alone or in combination with intraluminal stents.

Central Vein Stenosis/Occlusion

The presence of a significant central vein stenosis or occlusion is a relative contraindication to an ipsilateral permanent hemodialysis access because of the potential to develop significant venous hypertension and arm edema. Occasionally, however, a patient's only upper extremity access options are ipsilateral to a significant central vein lesion. The potential options in this setting include abandoning the upper extremities in favor of a lower extremity site, correcting the ipsilateral central vein lesion prior to placing the permanent access, or placing the permanent access and correcting the vein lesion if the patient develops significant, sustained arm edema. Our preferred approach is the latter, and we have been anecdotally impressed that only a small percentage of the patients with a central vein lesion develop significant edema after the procedure. The likely explanation for this finding is that a significant collateral network develops that reduces the venous hypertension, thereby preventing the edema. The invasive treatment options (endovascular or surgical) are the same whether they are performed before or after the access and are not particularly complicated by the procedure itself. Indeed, the high flow in the access may improve the initial patency after central vein angioplasty/stent so that there may be a theoretical advantage to performing these interventions postoperatively.

Unfortunately, the long-term durability of central vein angioplasty is only fair with primary patency rates ranging from 20% to 40% at 6 months. However, the majority of the lesions are amenable to remedial angioplasty procedures either alone or in combination with an intraluminal stent. Notably, the recurrent central vein stenoses after endovascular (or open surgical) revascularization may not necessarily translate into recurrent arm edema if additional collateral pathways develop. The open surgical options include jugular vein turndown, axillary/subclavian–jugular vein bypass, axillary/subclavian–contralateral axillary/subclavian vein bypass, axillary–common femoral vein bypass, and central vein–atrial bypass.

Multiple Prosthetic Access Failure

There is a subset of patients in whom prosthetic accesses will not stay open for a prolonged period of time despite the absence of an identifiable anatomic problem. A hypercoagulable condition may be contributory and should be investigated. Indeed, patients with repeated prosthetic access failures may benefit from long-term anticoagulation even in the absence a known hypercoagulable condition, although the improved patency may be at the expense of increased bleeding complications. The ideal solution for these patients is to construct an autogenous access and avoid further prostheses.

Obesity

Obese patients present a challenge because their superficial veins often run relatively deep to the skin and because they are at a higher risk for wound complications. Notably, a recent study reported that obese patients had a comparable number of access options as nonobese patients based on preoperative imaging. Because of their course deep to the skin, the standard autogenous radiocephalic and brachiocephalic accesses may not be able to be cannulated by the dialysis technologists even though they are sufficiently dilated. This potential problem can be overcome by transposing the "superficial" cephalic vein (forearm or arm segments) immediately deep to the dermis as previously outlined.

There is no obvious strategy to reduce the incidence of wound complications in obese patients. However, we have been somewhat circumspect about recommending a transposed brachiobasilic autogenous access in this subset of patients because of the extent of the necessary dissection. Furthermore, we have attempted to configure the respective accesses in such a fashion to assure that there is adequate soft tissue coverage over the anastomosis in the event that the skin breaks down.

Thin Skin

Patients with thin skin, such as elderly individuals and those on a chronic regimen of steroids, present a problem because any breakdown of the skin over the access can lead to a graft infection and/or bleeding. This is particularly a concern in the immediate postoperative period for the incision adjacent to the anastomosis. We have approached patients with thin skin using our same algorithm, but have attempted to tunnel the prosthetic grafts or autogenous vein as deep beneath the skin and subcutaneous tissue as possible. We have been anecdotally impressed that the repeated trauma from accessing the conduit can lead to fibrosis over the conduit that can be protective.

Human Immunodeficiency Virus (HIV)

The life expectancy for patients infected with HIV is quite good given the recent advances in medical therapy. Indeed, the decision to offer patients hemodialysis or permanent hemodialysis access is no longer relevant, given these advances. The patency rates for prosthetic accesses may be reduced among patients with HIV and the associated infectious complications may be increased. Because of these concerns, autogenous access is likely the most ideal choice for patients with HIV, and every option in the algorithm outlined here should be exhausted prior to considering a prosthetic access.

Prior Hand Ischemia

Patients with a previous episode of hand ischemia related to a permanent hemodialysis access are at a high risk for developing further episodes with each subsequent procedure. Despite these concerns, we have been willing to construct additional brachial artery-based access procedures in patients with a history of hand ischemia. However, a preoperative arteriogram with visualization of the arterial tree from the aortic arch to the wrist is mandatory, and all hemodynamically significant inflow lesions should be corrected. In the event that the patients develop recurrent hand ischemia, the treatment goals and strategies are the same as previously outlined.

Upper Extremity Access Precluded

There is a very small subset of patients in whom it is not possible to construct an upper extremity access. In our own practice, this includes patients with superior vena cava syndrome or refractory upper extremity edema and those with a history of bilateral hand ischemia refractory to remedial therapy. The options for permanent

Vascular Surgery

hemodialysis access in this setting include any number of lower extremity procedures with the arterial inflow based on one of the femoral arteries and the venous outflow being either the saphenous or one of the femoral veins. Although the published experience with lower extremity access procedures is somewhat limited, the graft patency rates may be lower than associated with the upper extremity procedures and the infectious complication rates appear to be significantly higher. Indeed, a recent publication suggested that infectious complication rates associated with femoral artery-based procedures were prohibitive and the authors concluded that tunneled catheters were a superior option. Furthermore, lower extremity arterial occlusive disease is relatively common among patients with end-stage renal disease and, thereby, complicates the choice of arterial inflow because of the increased likelihood of ischemic complications.

Our algorithm for lower extremity access procedures is comparable with the one outlined here with the lower extremity noninvasive arterial studies including ankle-brachial indices with segmental pressure measurements and velocity waveforms. The corresponding noninvasive venous studies include interrogation of the saphenous and deep systems for evidence of venous thrombosis in addition to assessment of their diameter. Invasive imaging includes an aortogram and lower extremity arterial runoff and venogram, although the noninvasive venous studies are usually sufficient to preclude the latter. Although the access options are often dictated by the distribution of arterial occlusive disease, we have attempted to site the anastomoses and tunnel the grafts away from the femoral triangle because of the potential infectious complications. Indeed, the distal superficial femoral artery and vein afford a nice alternative to the more proximal sites in patients without significant arterial occlusive disease.

Unfortunately, the autogenous options for the lower extremity are somewhat limited given the historic experience with the saphenous vein. A recent report documented a reasonable outcome using the ipsilateral superficial femoral/popliteal vein in the lower extremity, but the associated wound and ischemic complication rates were significant and similar to our own experience using it in the upper extremity. Cadaveric superficial femoral vein affords some theoretical appeal as a conduit for lower extremity access procedures because it may be more resistant to infection than the prosthetic alternatives,

although this potential advantage remains to be substantiated and it may preclude a subsequent kidney transplant because of allosensitization.

STRATEGIES TO MAINTAIN ACCESS

It is important to emphasize that maintaining adequate access is a lifelong process that requires a lifelong plan. Strategies should be designed to preserve all possible access options, select the access most likely to have the best long-term patency, and to sustain each individual access as long as is possible. Specifically, the cephalic and basilic veins should be preserved. They should not be used for blood draws, intravenous catheters, or conduits for lower extremity arterial bypass if at all possible. For the inpatients, we traditionally post a sign over the head of the bed, although it is likely more effective to counsel the patients about the importance of preserving these potential conduits and allow them to serve as their own advocate. The subclavian vein should not be used for dialysis access catheters, and, ideally, not for any other type of central vein catheter. Notably, subclavian vein dialysis catheters are associated with an approximately 30% incidence of subclavian vein stenosis or occlusion that precludes permanent hemodialysis access on the ipsilateral extremity.

Every effort should be made to construct autogenous accesses as emphasized by K/DOQI because of their better long-term patency rates. An aggressive surveillance protocol should be devised to identify "failing" accesses and appropriate remedial procedures performed. Admittedly, the ideal surveillance technique remains to be identified and it is likely that a variety of different ones are suitable. Lastly, attempts should be made to salvage all thrombosed accesses. The treatment algorithms have been worked out reasonably well for thrombosed prosthetic accesses, although the guidelines are less clear for thrombosed autogenous accesses. It has been our anecdotal impression that the same treatment options (i.e., chemical lyses, mechanical thrombectomy) are appropriate for thrombosed autogenous accesses and that the success rates are comparable if not superior to those for prosthetic accesses.

ALTERNATIVE STRATEGIES FOR RENAL REPLACEMENT THERAPY

Despite our aggressive algorithm, there is a very small subset of patients who are

not candidates for permanent hemodialysis access because of anatomic restrictions, limited life expectancy, or prohibitive co-morbidities. Fortunately, we have been able to obtain some type of access or use other strategies for renal replacement therapy in these patients with difficult situations. However, most nephrologists have had patients in their practices that have died because they were unable to obtain dialysis. We have used tunneled "temporary" catheters as the permanent hemodialysis access in this group of patients and believe that they likely represent better long-term solutions than some of the "heroic" permanent access options reported. Fortunately, the interventional radiologists at our institution have shared our dedication to these patients. Admittedly, these tunneled catheters are associated with significant complication rates and need to be changed frequently. Furthermore, we have aggressively explored the alternative options for renal replacement therapy including peritoneal dialysis and transplantation.

SUGGESTED READING

Benedetto B, Lipkowitz G, Madden R, et al. Use of cryopreserved cadaveric vein allograft for hemodialysis access precludes kidney transplantation because of allosensitization. *J Vasc Surg* 2001;34:139.

Cull JD, Cull DL, Taylor SM, et al. Prosthetic thigh arteriovenous access: outcome with SVS/AAVS reporting standards. *J Vasc Surg* 2004;39:381.

Dhingra RK, Young EW, Hulbert-Shearon TE, et al. Type of vascular access and mortality in U.S. hemodialysis patients. *Kidney Int* 2001;60:1443.

Feldman HI, Joffe M, Rosas SE, et al. Predictors of successful arteriovenous fistula maturation. *Am J Kidney Dis* 2003;42:1000.

Fistula First National Vascular Access Improvement Initiative. Available at: http://www.fistulafirst.org. Accessed 11/06.

Goodkin DA, Bragg-Gresham JL, Koenig KG, et al. Association of comorbid conditions and mortality in hemodialysis patients in Europe, Japan, and the United States: the Dialysis Outcomes and Practice Patterns Study (DOPPS). *J Am Soc Nephrol* 2003;14:3270.

Gradman WS, Laub J, Cohen W. Femoral vein transposition for arteriovenous hemodialysis access: improved patient selection and intraoperative measures reduce postoperative ischemia. *J Vasc Surg* 2005;41:279.

Huber TS, Buhler AG, Seeger JM. Evidence-based data for the hemodialysis access surgeon. *Semin Dial* 2004;17:217.

Huber TS, Carter JW, Carter RL, et al. Patency of autogenous and polytetrafluoroethylene upper extremity arteriovenous hemodialysis accesses: a systematic review. *J Vasc Surg* 2003;38:1005.

Huber TS, Ozaki CK, Flynn TC, et al. Prospective validation of an algorithm to maximize native arteriovenous fistulae for chronic hemodialysis access. *J Vasc Surg* 2002;36:452.

National Kidney Foundation. K/DOQI Clinical Practice Guidelines for Vascular Access, 2000. *Am J Kidney Dis* 2001;37:S137.

Owen WF, Jr. Patterns of care for patients with chronic kidney disease in the United States: dying for improvement. *J Am Soc Nephrol* 2003;14:S76.

Pisoni RL, Young EW, Dykstra DM, et al. Vascular access use in Europe and the United States: results from the DOPPS. *Kidney Int* 2002;61:305.

Rayner HC, Pisoni RL, Gillespie BW, et al. Creation, cannulation and survival of arteriovenous fistulae: data from the Dialysis Outcomes and Practice Patterns Study. *Kidney Int* 2003;63:323.

Szczech LA, Lazar IL. Projecting the United States ESRD population: issues regarding

treatment of patients with ESRD. *Kidney Int Suppl* 2004;S3-S7.

Vassalotti JA, Falk A, Cohl ED, et al. Obese and non-obese hemodialysis patients have a similar prevalence of functioning arteriovenous fistula using pre-operative vein mapping. *Clin Nephrol* 2002;58:211.

Xue JL, Ma JZ, Louis TA, et al. Forecast of the number of patients with end-stage renal disease in the United States to the year 2010. *J Am Soc Nephrol* 2001;12:2753.

EDITOR'S COMMENT

As Dr. Huber has pointed out, end-stage renal disease (ESRD) is an increasingly common and expensive health problem in the United States and worldwide, leading to more patients being maintained on chronic hemodialysis. Larger waiting lists for kidney transplantation results in patients waiting longer on hemodialysis for a transplant. Hemodialysis access is the lifeline for these patients and warrants careful surgical planning, meticulous surgical technique, and close follow-up to optimize patency rates and minimize complications. There are not, unfortunately, an unlimited number of sites and procedures for access, and access surgeons not uncommonly care for long-term hemodialysis patients who are running out of access sites or require complex procedures to maintain functional access.

Autogenous ateriovenous access procedures have the best patency rates and fewest complications compared PTFE grafts or catheters. The National Kidney Foundation Dialysis Outcome Quality Initiative (K/DOQI) has, therefore, appropriately emphasized the importance of autogenous arteriovenous access and has set a national target of 50% for patients beginning to undergo dialysis and

a prevalence rate of 40% for all patients receiving hemodialysis. However, as these guidelines were published in 2001, the expected increase in autogenous arteriovenous access placement seems to have stalled in many U.S. centers, compared with Europe, where the prevalence is now 80%.

This chapter appropriately focuses on best-practice recommendations for the creation of autogenous arteriovenous access, emphasizing that one must have the attitude that most patients are candidates for such procedures. Noninvasive imaging is emphasized as the "cornerstone of our algorithm." Dr. Huber presents a hierarchy for permanent access that differs somewhat from the K/DOQI that indicates a PTFE graft is a suitable third choice. He states that they have had good success with the autogenous brachiobasilic access. In fact, in their hierarchy there are four good autogenous choices before one considers a prosthetic graft. This careful attention to detail and technical expertise is what all access surgeons should aspire to.

It is worth emphasizing that patients requiring temporary catheter access while a fistula develops should have these catheters placed in the internal jugular vein, not subclavian vein, to avoid central ve-

nous stenosis that could compromise fistula development. Dr. Huber emphasizes the performance of an end of vein–side of artery anastomosis, but many surgeons prefer a side-to-side anastomosis. Admittedly there are no good data regarding outcomes between these two techniques. The descriptions of the procedures and the illustrations are excellent, as are the discussions of access problems and complications. Dr. Huber emphasizes the importance of continued follow-up and observation by the access surgeon before the access is cannulated for hemodialysis to prevent too early use and loss of the fistula. Furthermore, it is critical that more prospective data be collected on the outcomes of access procedures including such things as patency, revisions, thrombosis, and infection.

Finally, we must all work much harder, using techniques like those illustrated in this chapter, to exceed the K/DOQI standard and reach the 80% prevalence rate seen in other parts of the world. This can be achieved in this country as shown at one center recently (McGill RL, et al. *J Vasc Access* 2005;6:13).

D.W.H.

Vascular Surgery

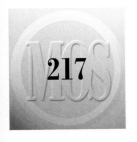

217

Prosthetic Bridge Grafts

MICHAEL S. HAYASHI AND SAMUEL E. WILSON

INTRODUCTION

Vascular surgery is an essential step for the provision of routine hemodialysis to the majority of the 300,000 patients in the United States living with end-stage renal disease (ESRD). Since 1943, when Kolff introduced dialysis as a means to support patients with end-stage renal disease, vascular access has proved difficult for both the patient and the physician. The ideal access would be easily accessible and provide long-term patency for hemodialysis. The autogenous fistula is currently the best solution as it is durable and obviates

the need for implantation of foreign material. Unfortunately, the hemodialysis patient frequently has co-morbidities that affect the vascular system, and whether due to peripheral vascular disease, previous cannulation of peripheral vessels, or intrinsically small veins, it is often not possible to construct an autogenous fistula. Alternatives to the autogenous fistula have included arteriovenous grafts made of materials such as bovine carotid artery, cryopreserved human umbilical vein, vein hemografts, and Dacron. Polytetrafluoroethylene (PTFE) grafts have, however, emerged as the material of choice in vas-

cular access due to their relatively low thrombogenicity, ease of handling, wide availability, and flexibility allowing various configurations. Constant modifications are ongoing to improve performance. Use of these prosthetic bridge grafts offer a vital solution to vascular access for the hemodialysis-dependent patient in whom it is not possible to construct a functioning arteriovenous fistula.

DEMOGRAPHICS

The 2004 U.S. Renal Data System (USRDS) annual report recorded 308,910 patients on dialysis and 122,374 with a functioning renal transplant in 2002. In this population, the most common primary diagnoses to which their renal failure was attributed were diabetes (45%), hypertension (30%), and glomerulonephritis (20%). The 2002 incidence rate for ESRD of 333 per million was almost quadruple the rate in 1980 and 36% higher than in 1992. Since the year 2000, these incidence rates continued to grow steadily between 0.2% and 1.4% per year. While patients aged 45 to 64 comprise 35% of the incident population and are expected to increase with the "baby boomer" generation, over 50% of new cases recorded were patients 65 years old and greater. The 65 to 74 and 75+ age groups have the highest incidence rates of 1,440 and 1,671 per million, respectively. Given that individuals 75 years or older already comprise 25% of our general population, the profile of the dialysis patient requiring vascular access is a fragile, elderly patient who has a major burden of co-morbidities associated with advanced age, including cardiovascular disease.

DISEASE OUTCOMES QUALITY INITIATIVE GUIDELINES

The National Kidney Foundation's Kidney Disease Outcomes Quality Initiative (K/DOQI) Clinical Practice Guidelines made "ex-cathedra" recommendations by committee, based on expert opinion and evidence from the literature, to help define standards for vascular access. Their current recommendations are for an autogenous fistula as the preferred type of vascular access with preference for a wrist (radial artery to cephalic vein) primary arteriovenous fistula first, followed by an elbow (brachial artery to cephalic vein) primary arteriovenous fistula. Third on the preference list is an arteriovenous graft of synthetic material or a transposed basilic vein fistula. The current DOQI guidelines target an incidence of 50% for autogenous access with a 40% overall prevalence rate. Expectations for a functioning arteriovenous fistula incidence are set to increase to 66%. These recommendations are based primarily on the experience that a forearm fistula offers a lower incidence of stenosis, infection, and vascular steal, as well as an improved performance over time and lower morbidity. Use of catheters as a permanent form of access is ideally limited to less than 10% of dialysis patients.

Guidelines related specifically to prosthetic grafts include evidence that PTFE grafts are preferred over other synthetic materials. The most recent opinion-based recommendations do not support the use of tapered versus nontapered, externally supported versus unsupported, thick versus thin walled, or elastic versus nonelastic prosthetic grafts. Use of straight, looped, or curved configurations is at the discretion of the surgeon to provide the greatest amount of surface area for cannulation. The preferred graft sites are straight or "U"-shaped forearm grafts and the upper arm curved graft (Fig. 1). Doppler imaging studies are recommended for any patient with a history of a subclavian catheter or a pacemaker, and to assist in identification of a suitable outflow tract. Arteriovenous graft surveillance for hemodynamically significant stenosis associated with increased venous pressure when followed by surgical or other correction is expected to improve patency and decrease the incidence of thrombosis. If flow is less than 1,000 mL/min, by Doppler, and has decreased by more than 25% over 4 months or is less than 600 mL/min, it is recommended that the patient be referred for a duplex ultrasound or a fistulogram. When these studies reveal a stenosis of greater than 50%, it is recommended that patients be treated with percutaneous transluminal angioplasty or surgical revision if associated with either previous thrombosis, elevated venous dialysis pres-

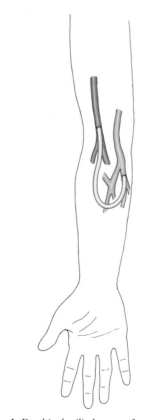

Fig. 1. Brachio-basilic loop graft.

sure, abnormal urea or other recirculation measurements, abnormal physical findings, or decreasing access flow. Following these guidelines, a 40% to 50% 6-month unassisted patency after outflow revision is expected. Overall, a synthetic graft is expected to have a 1-year primary patency of approximately 50% and a secondary patency rate of 70%, and last 3 to 5 years. The DOQI also recommends that prosthetic grafts be placed 3 to 6 weeks prior to use, although several reports indicate that earlier puncture with careful hemostasis is safe.

The Dialysis Outcomes and Practice Patterns Study (DOPPS) is an observational study of the international and domestic trends in vascular access. The most recent evaluation, which was the second in this series, examined trends from 2002 to 2003. Most ESRD patients in Europe and Japan have autogenous fistulas with few prosthetic grafts, findings that are contrary to results in the United States. Japan, Italy, Germany, Spain, and France all average more than 75% of patients using an autogenous fistula for hemodialysis access and less than 10% using prosthetic grafts. In the United States only 26.5% of patients have hemodialysis via an autogenous fistula and 44.6% via a prosthetic graft. While far from the DOQI proposed targets, when compared to data from the first DOPPS study in 1997 to 1999, domestic use of prosthetic grafts is down from 62.8% and use of fistulas are up from 20.7%. Unfortunately, catheter use is also up from 15.2% to 28.2% in this most recent audit, perhaps related to delays in fistula maturation. There are a number of reasons proposed to explain the unequal distribution of access methods including the preferential use of grafts by some hemodialysis centers because identification and puncture is easier. In addition, a significant number of patients present to a nephrologist immediately prior to requiring dialysis. If referred more than 30 days prior to starting dialysis, patients are more likely to have construction of a permanent type of access rather than insertion of a temporary catheter. These patients with early referrals are also more likely to have an autogenous fistula versus a prosthetic graft as a form of permanent access. The DOQI guidelines recommend referral for evaluation for a native fistula access when creatinine clearance is less than 25 mL/min, when serum creatinine is greater than 4mg/dL, or within 1 year of commencing dialysis.

A recent study questioned the validity of the DOQI guidelines and challenged them with evidence from published reports. While the data overall support the use of autogenous fistulas over prosthetic bridge grafts based on patency rates from various studies, there are no direct comparisons of the two forms of access and the studies available do not reveal with sufficient power the incidence and severity of associated complications for either access type. Furthermore, Huber et al. suggested that the primary patency rate and desired graft life targeted by the guidelines are unrealistic based on the actual outcomes consistently achieved. Also, the DOQI guidelines do not reflect recent evidence in the literature showing statistically significant improvements in outcomes for various graft modifications to be described later in this chapter. Finally, the data are slim in regard to outcomes of percutaneous angioplasty of failing grafts with more than 50% stenosis improving patency over no intervention, and routine use of intraluminal stents as an adjunct has not had a valid comparison with surgical outflow revision.

PROSTHETIC GRAFTS VERSUS AUTOGENOUS FISTULAS

Although there are no randomized controlled clinical trials in the literature that directly compare the performance of autogenous fistulas to prosthetic grafts, it is generally accepted that in most sites the autogenous fistula is superior to the prosthetic graft, especially in terms of patency. In 2003, Huber et al. conducted an extensive review of the literature to indirectly compare the performance of these two types of access. Their findings confirmed greater long-term patency of the autogenous fistula. Primary patency was found to be 72% for autogenous fistulas and 58% for PTFE grafts at 6 months; secondary patency for the same time interval was 86% and 76%, respectively. At 18 months, primary patency was 51% for autogenous fistulas and 33% for PTFE grafts with a respective secondary patency of 77% and 55%.

The retrospective study of a national database by Gibson et al. compared patency and revision rate for prosthetic grafts, autogenous fistulas, and brachio-basilic vein transpositions. Primary patency at 1 and 2 years was 56.1% and 39.8% for autogenous fistulas, 43.5% and 27.7% for brachio-basilic vein transposition, and 38.2% and 24.6% for prosthetic grafts, respectively. Secondary patency at 1 and 2 years was 73.2% and 64.2% for autogenous fistulas, 67.9% and 59.5% for brachio-basilic vein transposition, and 71.8% and 59.5% for prosthetic grafts, respectively. Across all demographic subgroups, autogenous fistulas were superior to prosthetic grafts in primary patency and need for revisions.

While the autogenous fistula is preferred, there are advantages to the use of prosthetic bridge grafts in selected clinical situations. Autogenous fistulas require a maturation period prior to use for routine hemodialysis and thus necessitate an early referral for vascular access during the predialysis phase. Even with early referral and successful construction of an autogenous fistula, there is still the risk that the fistula will not mature. In contrast, the bridge graft does not require any maturation period, although many delay hemodialysis for 2 to 3 weeks until incorporation into the surrounding tissues has occurred. Also, while patency is the major advantage to autogenous fistulas, once thrombosed, the bridge grafts can be revised and new conduits placed between previously used target vessels, allowing for increased flexibility and versatility of access options.

Performance of Prosthetic Grafts

With regard to PTFE performance during the first year of implantation, Cinat et al. sequentially examined the standard 6-mm expanded PTFE (ePTFE) graft. In this prospective study, primary and secondary patency rates at 1 year were 43% and 64%, respectively, and only 33% of patients were complication free at the end of this first year. Thrombosis was the most common complication, with about half occurring within the first 3 months after implantation. Following revision by thrombectomy with or without patch angioplasty, anastomotic revision, thrombolysis, or balloon angioplasty; the grafts benefited from an average of 6.6 months of additional patency. Thrombosis secondary to venous outflow stenosis accounted for 85% of the complications in forearm grafts versus 70% of complications in the upper arm grafts. Upper arm grafts, however, were more susceptible to other complications such as pseudoaneurysm, steal syndrome, and seroma formation. Grafts placed in the brachium generally have a longer patency than forearm grafts.

Performance of PTFE has been scrutinized for differences in patency between demographic groupings. In age group analysis, patients aged 60 or older had a statistically significant improvement in 1-year patency of 56% versus the 29% for persons younger than 60 years of age for PTFE grafts in one study. In another study, the secondary patency rates were equal for prosthetic grafts and autogenous fistula at age 50, and as patient age increased the secondary patency for the prosthetic grafts also increased. Primary access failure was 18% higher in women and 14% higher in African Americans vs. non–African Americans; however, both of these at-risk subgroups had a significantly lower number of autogenous fistulas created compared to their counterparts, and the differences observed cannot be solely attributable to either sex or race.

To predict graft failure, venous line pressures, blood flow rates, and recirculation values have been examined. Venous line pressures were found to increase over time, but there was no absolute value or percent increase over time that predicted graft failure. Blood flow rates were not found to be higher for grafts that remained patent, as compared to grafts that ultimately thrombosed. Also, recirculation values were found to be highly variable and not useful in predicting graft failure. Patients who require a graft revision appear to be at high risk for further complications, as retrospective analysis has shown an associated 1.8-fold increased risk of primary access failure, a 2.6-fold increase in secondary access failure, and a 1.8-fold increase in incidence for access revision.

Most physicians wait 1 to 2 weeks after insertion of a prosthetic bridge graft to allow incorporation of the graft into the surrounding tissue. However, this creates an interval in which a temporary form of access must be used for hemodialysis, and routine use of catheters is associated with complications including central venous stenosis and infection. Early cannulation of the PTFE bridge graft between 24 and 72 hours after placement has been compared with late cannulation at 14 days. All grafts were 6-mm PTFE grafts placed from the brachial artery to the axillary vein, and no significant differences were found in primary patency, infection, or bleeding between the two groups. Limiting the subcutaneous tunnel to a diameter of 7 mm was also found to decrease the incidence of hematoma formation. Accordingly, we recommend consideration of early graft cannulation to minimize central catheter use.

Modifications to the Standard Polytetrafluoroethylene Graft

One of the advantages of the prosthetic bridge graft is that the configuration design and resultant characteristics of the prosthetic graft can be tailored to the manufacturer's desired specifications. The various components used to construct the graft and alter its distinct individual properties undergo continuous modifications to improve its performance.

Standard-thickness (0.64 mm) stretch 6-mm ePTFE grafts have been compared to thin-wall (0.37 mm) 6-mm stretch ePTFE grafts to determine if the thin-wall, which had improved flexibility and easier handling, would outperform the standard-wall grafts. Primary patency, however, proved longer in the standard-wall group with 18.2 months versus 12.1 months in the thin-wall group. The primary patency trend at 6, 12, 18, and 30 months revealed rates of 62%, 49%, 40%, and 27% for the standard grafts and 39%, 35%, 31%, and 4% for the thin-walled grafts, respectively. Secondary patency was also higher in the standard-wall group, 22.2 months versus 15.2 months in the thin-walled grafts. The complication rates of 6% versus 5% for pseudoaneurysm formation, 2% versus 3% for infection, and 22% versus 19% for mortality in the standard- and thin-walled grafts, respectively, were not statistically different during the 3-year study. The thin-walled graft did not outperform the standard 0.64-mm thickness PTFE graft. Further, early cannulation of the thin-walled graft may cause tears.

The standard 6-mm straight ePTFE graft was also compared to the 4-mm to 7-mm tapered PTFE graft. It was thought that the tapered character would offer better patency and a lower risk of stenosis. At 1 year, the 46% primary patency for the tapered graft and 43% primary patency for the straight graft were not statistically different. Secondary patency was also not significantly different, with 87% for the tapered graft and 91% for the straight graft. There were also no differences in peak velocities or mean flow rates between the two groups. As far as stenoses, the two groups had an equal number of stenoses at 1 year with rates of 27% versus 20%. The tapered grafts were also hypothesized to decrease the risk of steal and high-output cardiac failure; however, no significant difference was found for these complications in the standard grafts compared to the tapered grafts. Diabetic, atherosclerotic disease restricting collateral arterial inflow remains the main causes of the steal phenomenon.

When ePTFE grafts made by different companies were compared, no differences in the grafts were found. No statistical difference could be found in the primary or secondary patency of the 6-mm grafts from Gore-Tex and Impra at 1 or 2 years. Also, there was no statistical difference in the occurrence of infection, steal syndrome, or

symptomatic venous hypertension between the two manufacturers' products.

To address the problem of intimal hyperplasia at the venous anastomosis, a venous cuff has been introduced to alter the flow dynamics and to attempt to improve patency. Results from this study showed that the cuffed ePTFE was associated with increased flow rates during hemodialysis and improved graft patency compared to the standard ePTFE grafts. While primary patency across the 2-year study was not significantly different between the two groups, the cuffed graft had a significantly improved secondary patency of 64% and 58% at 1 and 2 years versus 32% and 21% for the standard graft at 1 and 2 years, respectively. Also, the time to first intervention was longer in the cuffed group with an interval of 138 days versus 68 days. Furthermore, cuffed grafts maintained flow rates with 623 mL/min at 12 months and 531 mL/min at 24 months, which was statistically improved at both intervals versus standard grafts.

While ePTFE has long been the preferred graft material for vascular access, the standard 6-mm PTFE graft was recently compared to a graft made of polyurethaneurea. The polyurethaneurea graft is a self-sealing multilayered graft with a non-permeable middle layer that allows the graft wall to self-seal rapidly after needle puncture. Direct comparison logged a primary patency for the polyurethaneurea graft of 55% versus 47% for ePTFE at 6 months; at 12 months it was 44% versus 36%, respectively. The secondary patency for the polyurethaneurea of 87% versus 90% for PTFE grafts at 6 months, and 78% versus 80% at 12 months, respectively, showed no statistically significant difference as well. Additionally, no statistical difference in the number of complications between the two grafts was found except for kinking, which occurred in the polyurethaneurea group, each incidence of which required an intervention. Of note, bleeding time after dialysis cannulation between the two grafts was also compared. After 2 minutes of manual compression, 50% of the polyurethaneurea grafts had hemostasis versus 13% of PTFE grafts. At 5 minutes, 80% of the polyurethaneurea grafts were hemostatic versus 27% of PTFE grafts. Whether this can be directly extrapolated to less risk of bleeding into the subcutaneous graft tunnel, especially in new grafts, and obviate need for temporary dialysis catheters is under review. But at least for now, the performance of polyurethaneurea appears comparable to the standard PTFE graft. One can expect future evalua-

tion of a composite graft consisting of a polyurethaneurea segment useful for early access and a hooded PTFE venous end to promote patency.

 ## SURGICAL TECHNIQUE

The prosthetic bridge graft can be placed in the forearm, upper arm, or thigh between any artery and vein of adequate size. Most often, this is done under local anesthesia or with a regional block in the outpatient setting. Although the femoral vessels have traditionally offered a better patency rate, the upper extremity is the preferred site due to its decreased risk of infection, especially with incontinence or in the obese patient where skin folds and trapped moisture create an unfavorable environment for repeated percutaneous vascular access. Peripheral vascular disease is of concern as the majority of patients living with end-stage renal disease also suffer from diabetes and/or hypertension. Thigh grafts divert inflow from the lower extremity and amplify their underlying vascular insufficiency with decreased perfusion to the lower extremity (Fig. 2). Patients also express concern that the thigh graft interferes with sexual activity, although it does keep the upper extremities free for activities of daily living during hemodialysis.

Depending on the location of the anastomotic sites on the target artery and vein, the prosthetic bridge will take the

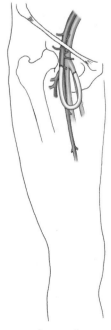

Fig. 2. Femoro-saphenous loop graft.

form of either a loop or U shape if the sites are in close proximity to one another, or a straight or C bridge if there is a large distance between the arterial and venous anastomoses. One intent of the graft configuration is to allow the greatest amount of graft surface area for the technologists to perform dialysis without repeated trauma to the same region of the graft. The grafts are anastomosed to the artery and vein in an end-to-side fashion.

Patients with end-stage renal disease can expect to undergo multiple vascular access procedures during their lifetime, and the vascular surgeon must plan accordingly. In the forearm, the radial artery may be accessed from the elbow to the wrist. A preoperative Allen test should be performed to confirm adequate collateral flow to the hand. The arterial anastomosis can be easily created proximal to a failed Brescia-Cimino fistula, or a proximal segment of the radial artery distal to the elbow crease will suffice. Distal to the elbow crease, a suitable basilic, cephalic, or antecubital vein can usually be identified as well. The venous anastomosis should be performed as distally as possible to allow, if necessary, for future revisions. During graft revision, if arterial inflow is adequate, the outflow obstruction can be resolved with patch angioplasty or a more proximal venous anastomosis, even on the same vein, as long as venous run-off is ad-

equate. In the upper arm, a brachial artery to basilic or axillary vein can be fashioned (Fig. 3). When suitable veins cannot be easily identified on preoperative physical examination, Doppler can image appropriate target veins for the bridge graft. This spares the need for intraoperative searching and unproductive incisions.

After the desired sites of anastomosis have been identified and approximately 2 to 3 cm of the target vessels has been dissected free, the subcutaneous tunnel is made with a graft tunneler such as the Kelly-Wick. The graft must be superficial enough to allow easy detection by the dialysis technologist yet provide enough soft tissue coverage to protect against infection from epidermal pathogens. A closely fitting tunnel will promote incorporation of the graft and reduces the risk of postoperative hematoma formation. For loop grafts, a counterincision at the apex of the loop is helpful to ensure the desired wide loop without twists and kinks in the graft. The ends of the graft are trimmed to size and cut obliquely to increase the anastomotic orifice. Lateral placement of the graft in the forearm allows the patient to be dialyzed without prolonged external rotation.

An intravenous dose of heparin (usually 2,500 to 5,000 U) is frequently administered prior to applying proximal and distal control to the anastomotic sites using small,

atraumatic vascular clamps. An incision is made longitudinally with a no. 11 blade scalpel and extended with Potts-Smith scissors to fit the graft. The anastomosis is performed with two 5-0 polypropylene cardiovascular sutures placed 180 degrees apart at the heel and toe of the anastomosis to avoid purse-stringing. This technique is used at both the arterial and venous anastomoses. Prior to securing the final stitches, the proximal and distal clamps are released, in turn, to flush out air and clots from the graft. At the completion of the anastomosis, a thrill should be readily palpable. Distal pulses and color of the digits should be inspected. If steal is suspected, Doppler examination can be used to evaluate distal flow and infrequently a surgical clip can be applied to the arterial end of the graft to decrease flow across the graft. A small amount of bleeding at the anastomoses can be addressed with pressure or use of local hemostatic agents. The incision should be closed in layers to provide soft tissue coverage for the graft and protection from superficial infection.

COMPLICATIONS

Thrombosis is the most common complication of the bridge graft. The majority of thrombotic events are due to progressive myointimal hyperplasia at the venous anastomosis that results in progressive venous outflow stenosis and eventual thrombosis. Turbulent blood flow, local wall shear stress, and endothelial injury are all thought to contribute to this by encouraging smooth muscle proliferation and upregulation of endothelial surface adhesion molecules. When a graft does thrombose, there are multiple options for revision after thrombectomy, including patch angioplasty and percutaneous angioplasty with or without stent. External beam radiation was recently examined as a modality to prevent anastomotic intimal hyperplasia. However, despite doses of 18 Gy given in two fractions of 9 Gy on the first and second postoperative days, there was no decrease in the incidence of thrombosis. A large study of clopidogrel and aspirin was performed in the Veterans Affairs hospital system to evaluate the effect of this combination of anticoagulants and graft thrombosis. This trial was stopped early as the treatment-group patients had a significantly increased risk of bleeding complications when on this combination of antiplatelet agents and no reduced risk of thrombosis. Currently, serial monitoring of venous pressures and/or flow rates is recommended, and if an abnormality is detected, imaging by

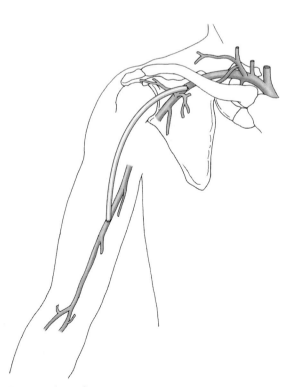

Fig. 3. Brachioaxillary straight graft.

Duplex scan is obtained. Venous outflow stenosis is corrected by patch angioplasty or a percutaneous transluminal angioplasty supported with a covered stent.

Infection is a difficult complication to manage with any implanted foreign material. When infected, the PTFE graft is less susceptible to the breakdown and early hemorrhage seen in biologic grafts. If identified early, local infection at a needle site and not involving an anastomosis can be managed aggressively with antibiotics and possibly incision and drainage in an attempt to retain the graft. However, when the subcutaneous tunnel along the graft is also involved, total graft excision is warranted. When excising an infected graft, it is reasonable to leave a 1- to 2-mm cuff of graft at the anastomotic site to allow closure of the arteriotomy without stenosis, as long as this site is not also infected. After an infected graft is removed, cellulitis, continued drainage, or bacteremia should be resolved prior to implantation of a new form of permanent access.

Other complications of grafts include pseudoaneurysm formation, steal syndrome, seroma formation, tissue necrosis, bleeding, and distal embolization. Large pseudoaneurysms of prosthetic bridge grafts should be treated with exclusion bypass or resection and insertion of an interposition graft if characterized by rapid expansion or if the overlying skin is threatened. Small pseudoaneurysms are best left alone, or at most repaired by a single suture closure of the opening in the graft. Steal syndrome can be anticipated by intraoperative evaluation of distal blood flow, for example, by direct palpation of the radial pulse or Doppler of digital arteries or arcades. Once steal is identified, it can be treated by applying clips or sutures to narrow the inflow sufficient to treat the symptoms. In some instances complete interruption of the graft will be required or in selected patients the distal revascularization and interval ligation (DRIL) procedure can be done. A recent study of the performance of autogenous fistulas and

PTFE grafts found no significant differences between the complication rates for hand ischemia (2%), infection (7%), and aneurysm or pseudoaneurysm (4%).

CONCLUSIONS

As physicians become more proficient in geriatric and critical care, an increasing number of patients will survive to develop end-stage renal disease. The number of available cadaveric kidneys has reached a plateau of approximately 9,000 organs per year, and an increasing number of renal transplants are from living related donors. Organ recipients often outlive their transplants and return to hemodialysis. This portends for sustained growth in the hemodialysis-dependent population. Based on clinical evidence, the autogenous fistula is still the best current form of vascular access; however, its construction is not always possible. Whether due to anatomic limitations, absence of suitable veins, or exhaustion of autogenous access sites, there will be an increasing need for alternative forms of access and the prosthetic bridge graft will continue to have an important role in vascular access. A broad-based effort to conserve the peripheral vasculature in all patients should begin at an early age to facilitate autogenous vascular access in the declining years.

SUGGESTED READING

Cinat ME, Hopkins J, Wilson SE. A prospective evaluation of PTFE graft patency and surveillance techniques in hemodialysis access. *Ann Vasc Surg* 1999;13:191.

Dammers R, Planken RN, Pouls KP, et al. Evaluation of 4-mm to 7-mm versus 6-mm prosthetic brachial-antecubial forearm loop access for hemodialysis: results of a randomized multicenter clinical trial. *J Vasc Surg* 2003;37:143.

Gibson K, Gillen DL, Caps MT, et al. Vascular access survival and incidence of revisions: a comparison of prosthetic grafts, simple autogenous fistulas, and venous transposition fistulas from the United States Renal Data

System Dialysis Morbidity and Mortality Study. *J Vasc Surg* 2001;34:694.

Hakaim AG, Scott TE. Durability of early prosthetic dialysis graft cannulation: results of a prospective, nonrandomized clinical trial. *J Vasc Surg* 1997;25:1002.

Huber TS, Buhler AG, Seeger JM. Evidence-based data for the hemodialysis access surgeon. *Semin Dial* 2004;17:217.

Huber TS, Carter JW, Carter RL, et al. Patency of autogenous and polytetrafluoroethylene upper extremity arteriovenous hemodialysis accesses: a systematic review. *J Vasc Surg* 2003;38:1005.

Hurlbert SN, Mattos MA, Henretta JP, et al. Long-term patency rates, complications and cost effectiveness for polytetrafluoroethylene (PTFE) grafts for hemodialysis access: a prospective study that compares Impra versus Gore-Tex grafts. *Cardiovasc Surg* 1998;6:652.

Kaufman JL, Garb JL, Berman JA, et al. A prospective comparison of two expanded polytetrafluoroethylene grafts for linear forearm hemodialysis access: does the manufacturer matter? *J Am Coll Surg* 1997;185:74.

Kaufman JS, O'Connor TZ, Zhang JH, et al. Randomized controlled trial of clopidogrel plus aspirin to prevent hemodialysis access graft thrombosis. *J Am Soc Nephrol* 2003; 14:2313.

Kolff WJ, Berk H, Welle N, et al. The artificial kidney, a dialyzer with great area. *Acta Med Scand* 1944;117:121.

Lenz BJ, Veldenz HC, Dennis JW, et al. A three-year follow-up on standard versus thin wall ePTFE grafts for hemodialysis. *J Vasc Surg* 1998;28:464.

National Kidney Foundation. National Kidney Foundation's Kidney Disease Outcomes Quality Initiative (NKF-K/DOQI) clinical practice guidelines for vascular access: update 2000. *Am J Kidney Dis* 2001;37: S137.

Rayner HC, Besarab A, Brown WW, et al. Vascular access results from the Dialysis Outcomes and Practice Patterns Study (DOPPS): performance against Kidney Disease Outcomes Quality Initiative (K/DOQI) clinical practice guidelines. *Am J Kidney Dis* 2004;44:S22.

Sorom AJ, Hughes CB, McCarthy JT, et al. Prospective, randomized evaluation of a cuffed expanded polytetrafluoroethylene graft for hemodialysis vascular access. *Surgery* 2002;132:135.

U.S. Renal Data System (USRDS). 2004 USRDS annual data report. Available at: www.usrds.org. Accessed.

EDITOR'S COMMENT

Successful placement of angioaccess for hemodialysis requires careful planning, a high level of surgical judgment, and meticulous technique. The NKF/DOQI was published in 1971 and has had major impact on the practice of angioaccess surgery. Many centers have embraced an "all autogenous" policy with 60% to 80% of procedures being arteriovenous fistulas (AVFs). Despite this, arteriovenous prosthetic grafts (AVGs) are required in many patients for the reasons discussed by Drs. Hayashi and Wilson. In addition to small superficial veins, delayed or lack of maturation of AVFs, and exhaustion of all superficial veins in the upper extremity after multiple access operations, we have found that obesity is an increasing reason to consider an AVG in preference to an AFV. Veins greater than 5 to 6 mm below the skin surface pose a challenge for venipuncture, and in this circumstance, we will often place an AVG. Because of the obesity epidemic in the United States and the associated increase in the incidence of type 2 diabetes mellitus, this will continue to pose problems for successful angioaccess placement.

Drs. Hayashi and Wilson have nicely reviewed the current literature on the different types of

(continued)

prosthetic AVGs. Most surgeons prefer ePTFE, and there is little difference in patency and overall complications when comparing thick versus thin, ringed versus unsupported, tapered versus nontapered, elastic versus nonelastic, and cuffed versus noncuffed ePTFE. In addition, there are no differences in outcomes when comparing ePTFE grafts from different manufacturers. The latter is an important point that we have used to our hospital's financial advantage in fostering competitive bidding among graft manufacturers.

In part, because of the DOQI initiative, brachial-basilic vein transposition has become an increasingly performed procedure. However, disappointing patency is reported by many centers, and the overall outcomes are only marginally better than AVGs. My preference is to place an upper extremity AVG before resorting to a brachial-basilic vein transposition because the high flow rates tend to dilate the upper extremity veins, and this may make subsequent brachial-basilic vein transposition more likely to be successful. In addition, a brachial-basilic vein transposition is almost always possible after failure of an AVG if the basilica vein is of adequate size. The converse, however, is not usually true. We have found the brachial-

basilic vein procedure most helpful in circumstances when all other upper extremity angioaccess options have been exhausted.

Not mentioned by Drs. Hayashi and Wilson is the axillary artery to ipsilateral or contralateral ("necklace" configuration) axillary vein AVG. This is an excellent option in patients with multiple failed AVGs and no other usable upper extremity vessels. Not only is the patency equivalent or superior to standard AVGs, but also patients have both upper extremities free during hemodialysis. Exposure for an axillary AVG is similar to the proximal dissection for a standard axillofemoral bypass. The AVG is tunneled just beneath the skin as described by Drs. Hayashi and Wilson in a gentle loop configuration that is facilitated with a short counterincision at the bottom aspect of the loop. In the "necklace" configuration, the contralateral axillary vein is used and no counterincision is necessary. The ipsilateral or contralateral internal jugular vein can be used if the axillary vein is thrombosed or stenotic. In patients with no other upper extremity options, the axillary AVG is a better choice than a femoral AVG because of the much lower incidence of infectious complications.

I find the noninvasive vascular laboratory to be indispensable in planning these operations. Location,

size, quality, and depth of vessels from the skin surface are important determinants of optimal AVG placement. Anatomic variations in arterial and venous anatomy can also be delineated. For example, the radial artery branches from the brachial artery high above the elbow in up to 15% of patients and can be confused for the brachial artery during dissection in the antecubital fossa. Anastomosis to this instead of the brachial artery may result in inadequate inflow for the AVG. Problems with upper extremity arterial inflow and venous outflow can also be readily assessed with noninvasive vascular testing. Many of these patients have had multiple central venous catheterizations as well as prior AVFs or AVGs, and arterial and venous abnormalities are common. If noninvasive testing is equivocal or indefinite, computed tomography or catheter-directed arteriography or venography is indicated. I also find it useful to be present when noninvasive testing is performed to direct the examinations to sites most likely to be amenable to optimal AVG placement. Marking precise sites for incisions with the aid of ultrasound imaging is also helpful, because it minimizes incision length and avoids unnecessary explorations in the operating room.

G.P.C.

Arterial and Venous Cannulation—Venous Catheters

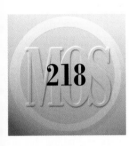

SHERRY D. SCOVELL AND SETH B. BLATTMAN

Percutaneous arterial and venous access is a basic and critical aspect in the care of general surgery, critical care, and vascular surgery patients. Although these procedures are simple in theory, cannulation of arteries and veins is a fundamental skill that is based on a firm knowledge of anatomy. In addition, care must be taken during these procedures to avoid the numerous complications that may arise with a haphazard approach, many of which may be associated with substantial morbidity. Percutaneous femoral, brachial, and radial arterial access as well as approaches to central venous access, including subclavian, internal jugular, and femoral vein access, will be delineated here. The importance of these procedures should not be underestimated.

In fact, these procedures have become the cornerstone of endovascular surgery. Recently, an ever-growing number of vascular procedures are being performed in a percutaneous manner. In a recent 20-year review of vascular surgery cases in the United States, the number of percutaneous procedures has increased from 0.1 procedures per 100,000 patients (125) in 1980 to 58.3 procedures per 100,000 pa-

tients (164,417) in 2000. If for no other reason, the shear numbers of these procedures compel surgeons to become familiar with and facile in their intricacies. In the world of vascular surgery today, these technical skills and endovascular procedures are essential in order to offer patients the full spectrum of care and that which is most appropriate for their overall medical condition.

This chapter will review the techniques of arterial and venous puncture, both for the general surgeon for the purpose of arterial pressure measurements in the intensive care setting and for the vascular surgeon in endovascular procedures. It will also review approaches to venous cannulation necessary for intravenous access.

GENERAL CONSIDERATIONS

Cannulation of arteries and central veins is an invasive procedure that requires sterile conditions, especially if an indwelling catheter is to be left in place. All of these procedures should be undertaken using strict sterile conditions with universal precautions.

The initial step in accessing any vessel is a review of the anatomic landmarks that are associated with those vessels. Bony landmarks as well as ligamentous structures and muscles are extremely helpful. Knowledge of the positioning of the vein in relation to the artery is critical. It is also helpful to acknowledge other vital structures in the general region of the site to be punctured, especially with respect to their avoidance. This is particularly significant in central venous punctures involving the veins near the thoracic outlet, as will be delineated later.

Patient positioning is also imperative before the procedure to adequately expose the vessel to be punctured. This positioning varies depending on the region to be accessed. All patients should begin in a supine position. The individual maneuvers will vary depending on the vessel to be cannulated.

In general, all percutaneous procedures may be performed using local anesthetic with or without the addition of conscious sedation. These medications are tailored to the individual patient and the pain threshold. Standard regimens of sedation are employed for endovascular procedures, which are also performed under local anesthesia with conscious sedation. At our institution, they include intravenous Versed and fentanyl. Typically, 1% lidocaine without epinephrine is used to infiltrate the region delineated for puncture.

ARTERIAL ACCESS

Arterial access may be obtained in by either an open cut-down method or, more commonly, a percutaneous method. Typically, arterial access is obtained for blood pressure monitoring in an intensive care unit or perioperative setting, or for the purpose of arteriography and intervention as in vascular surgical patients.

Before beginning any arterial procedure, it is prudent to carefully document arterial pulses distal to the region of intervention. In fact, this documentation should be undertaken both before and after the procedure with a comparison of the quality and strength of the pulses noted. This is especially critical because of the dreaded complication of arterial thrombosis that may occur following arterial cannulation.

These procedures are often considered elementary. However, if not preformed with due diligence, they can have catastrophic consequences. Laceration of the artery with the needle tip may result in substantial bleeding. Arterial dissection may be caused with the wire if it is advanced in a subintimal plane. This may lead to arterial thrombosis, which can be a surgical emergency. Arteriovenous fistulae may be created with careless cannulation of the artery. Failure to hold adequate pressure following removal of an arterial catheter as well may cause the development of a pseudoaneurysm, which may have to be managed operatively, especially in the case of rapid expansion. All of these complications can threaten both life and limb and underscore the fact that cannulation of arteries should be performed with the utmost of care and diligence.

APPROACHES TO ARTERIAL CANNULATION

There are three main arteries in which cannulation that should be mastered. These include the femoral artery, the brachial artery, and the radial artery. The best approach should be chosen based on the individual patient characteristics and the indication for cannulation.

Arterial cannulation is often used for patients undergoing vascular surgery for the purpose of arteriography in the case

of limb-threatening ischemia. For this purpose, cannulation of the arteries is undertaken in the interventional suite where fluoroscopy may be used. Fluoroscopy is often quite helpful in identifying bony landmarks in the region of the artery to be punctured, as will be discussed later.

Femoral Artery Access

The femoral artery is one of the most frequently cannulated arteries in the body. It is commonly used for arterial access for the purpose of arteriography in the vascular surgical patient. It is a large-caliber vessel that is appropriate for using the larger-profile devices for angioplasty and stenting of the peripheral vessels. It is also commonly used in cardiac catheterization for the purpose of imaging the coronary vessels, as well as for coronary interventions.

As previously mentioned, it is prudent to carefully document arterial pulses distal to the region of intervention prior to cannulation. For femoral arterial access, the femoral pulse as well as the popliteal, dorsalis pedis, and posterior tibial pulses should all be palpated and their presence or absence recognized. This is especially important if the leg becomes acutely ischemic as a result of arterial thrombosis following the procedure, one of the rare but dreaded complications of femoral arterial access, or if there should be any distal emboli following intervention.

Exposure is important prior to beginning the procedure. For femoral artery access, the patient should be placed in a supine position. In an obese patient, a large pannus may be a major impediment to groin access. A pannus should be retracted cephalad using 4-inch silk tape placed on its lower aspects. The tape is then retracted obliquely and bilaterally in a crossed pattern to gain the needed exposure.

Following routine sterile preparation and draping of the patient, assuming universal precautions, the procedure may be initiated. The initial step is localizing the appropriate site for arterial entry. For femoral arterial access, the puncture site should be intended for the common femoral artery. The common femoral artery, however, is only about 4 to 5 cm in length; therefore, localization using anatomic landmarks is critical.

The regional anatomic landmarks should be reviewed before each procedure. Anatomically, the external iliac artery becomes the common femoral artery as it crosses under the inguinal ligament. In every patient, the inguinal ligament should be identified and marked. This may

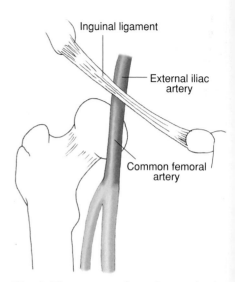

Fig. 1. The common femoral artery begins along the lower border of the inguinal ligament.

be accomplished by locating the anterior superior iliac spine and the pubic tubercle. A line connecting these two bony structures represents the inguinal ligament. This will serve to identify the upper extent of the common femoral artery (Fig. 1). If fluoroscopy is being used, the femoral artery is typically located over the medial third of the femoral head (Fig. 2).

A puncture site above the inguinal ligament, in the external iliac artery, is problematic. The external iliac artery is located in the retroperitoneal space, making this artery difficult, if not impossible, to compress and achieve postprocedure hemostasis. Not surprisingly, a puncture in this region if often associated with the potentially catastrophic complication of retroperitoneal hemorrhage.

A puncture site that is placed too distally, in either the superficial femoral artery or profunda femoris artery, will present problems as well. These arteries are sub-

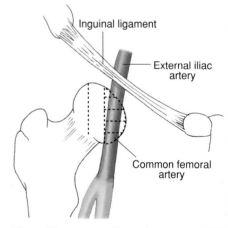

Fig. 2. The common femoral artery should lie over the medial third of the femoral head.

stantially smaller in caliber and have a higher incidence of postprocedure thrombosis. Additionally, the superficial femoral artery is often heavily diseased. There is also a higher incidence of pseudoaneurysm associated with distal puncture sites.

Using the groin crease in the identification of the common femoral artery is notoriously deceptive, especially in obese patients. The groin crease should not be used to identify the intended puncture site with respect to the common femoral artery. Once the inguinal ligament has been defined, the femoral artery may be identified in the inguinal region by its pulsation. It is important to recall that the femoral vein is located medial to the artery. The femoral nerve is located lateral to the artery.

Again, by inspection and palpation, the location of the inguinal ligament is confirmed. The position of the artery is typically located through palpation of the pulse below the ligament. An entry site should be positioned one to two fingerbreadths distal to the inguinal ligament over the pulse (Fig. 3). In the event that the pulse is weak or not easily palpable, the artery may typically be located along the medial third of the previously mentioned line. Again, the groin crease is unreliable in locating the ideal site of puncture and should not be used as a landmark.

Following administration of local anesthetic, the index and middle fingers are first used to palpate the femoral pulse with one finger on the pulse above the intended site of puncture and one finger below. The skin is held taunt. The needle is then advanced with the bevel facing up at a 45 degree angle to the skin. The needle is cautiously advanced through the skin and subcutaneous tissue until the artery is encountered. This is manifest via a pulsatile sensation that is transferred through the needle. At this point, gentle, firm pressure is applied to the needle until pulsatile blood return is noted (Fig. 3).

There are two methods of arterial wall puncture, the double-wall puncture and the single-wall puncture. As the name of the procedure indicates, the double-wall puncture involves penetrating both the anterior and posterior walls with the needle and then withdrawing the needle slowly until pulsatile blood flow is confirmed. This method is associated with a higher incidence of complications as the posterior wall of the artery is typically heavily calcified. With the single-wall puncture technique, only the anterior wall of the artery is punctured with the needle, which is confirmed by pulsatile blood flow through the needle. We recommend the single-wall puncture technique for all arterial punctures.

The artery may be approached in either a retrograde manner (against the direction of blood flow) or an antegrade manner (in the direction of blood flow). Retrograde access refers to placement of a sheath or catheter in a direction that is opposite from the flow of blood. This approach is often used in obtaining diagnostic arteriograms (Fig. 3). This method may be used for arterial interventions as well, in addition to placing arterial catheters for blood pressure monitoring. An antegrade approach may be required in other situations. The artery is cannulated in the direction of blood flow (Fig. 4). This technique is especially useful in arterial interventions in patients without the ability to access the contralateral femoral artery or in patients who have aortobifemoral bypass grafts. In this case, the aortobifemoral bypass graft limbs have a steep angulation at the bifurcation, which does not easily permit traversing from one limb into the other.

Once arterial flow has been confirmed, a wire is introduced through the lumen of the needle and advanced into the artery using the Seldinger technique. The wire should advance smoothly. Any resistance should prompt the operator to stop, remove the wire, and reconfirm flow through the needle. The wire should never be advanced if there is resistance because an arterial dissection may be created.

If one does not get the return of pulsatile blood flow and only has sluggish blood flow, most likely the lumen of the needle is not fully within the lumen of the vessel. If this happens, the needle should be withdrawn and pressure held. For the purpose of arterial line placement, the wire should not be advanced to avoid dissecting the artery.

If venous blood is encountered during an arterial access, the needle should be withdrawn and pressure applied. If this is not done, there is a higher incidence of a postprocedure arteriovenous fistula, which is associated with simultaneous cannulation of the artery and adjacent vein.

The needle typically used in a femoral arterial puncture is a 19-gauge needle, which is commonly used in conjunction with a 0.035-inch wire. There is, however, a micropuncture technique that employs a smaller 21-gauge needle and a 0.014-inch wire, which is especially useful for cannulation of smaller-caliber arteries such as the brachial artery. Once pulsatile blood flow is confirmed, a wire is advanced through the lumen of the needle. Again, advancement of the wire prior to obtaining pulsatile flow may lead to arterial dissection and should be avoided. Once the wire has advanced smoothly and is well seated in the artery, a small stab incision can be made in the skin with the tip of a No. 11 blade. With the index finger still below the needle and over the pulse, and the middle finger above the needle and over the pulse, pressure is applied to the artery. The needle is then removed by "walking" it over the wire. This entails holding the wire in a fixed position and slowly bringing the needle back to the point where the wire is fixed. The wire is then fixed in position further back, and

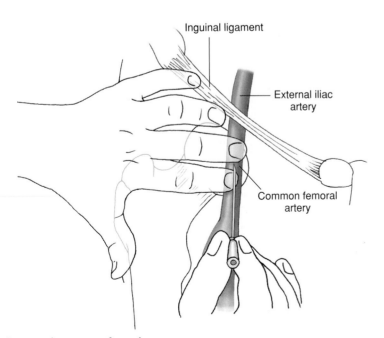

Fig. 3. Retrograde common femoral artery access.

Inguinal ligament

External iliac artery

Common femoral artery

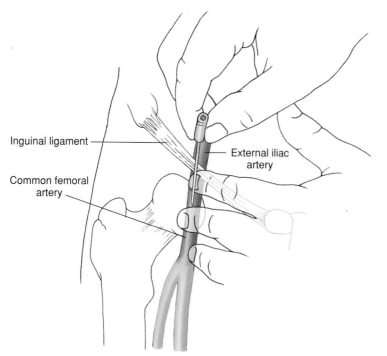

Fig. 4. Antegrade common femoral artery access.

the needle is again brought back to the point of fixation. This allows the needle to be removed without inadvertently pulling the wire out of the artery, thus losing arterial access.

Once the needle has been removed, a sheath may be placed over the wire and into the artery for arterial pressure monitoring. The sheath is loaded onto the wire, the wire is "pinned" or held in a fixed position, and the sheath advanced into the artery over the fixed wire. It is critical never to let go of the wire. Wires can be inadvertently advanced into the vessel completely, which would necessitate retrieval with the use of a snare or, less commonly, with the use of an open surgical procedure. Blood flow through the sheath should be confirmed to ensure that it is indeed intraluminal, and then it should be flushed with a heparinized saline solution followed by connection to a transducer.

Brachial Artery Access

There are times when the femoral artery is not favorable for puncture and an alternative site is needed. Specifically for the purpose of diagnostic and therapeutic arterial procedures, there will be times when the femoral artery is not able to be used, such as in patients with bilateral iliac artery occlusions or in patients with bypass grafts to both femoral arteries, which is a relative contraindication to puncture. In these cases, it is feasible and preferable

to use the upper extremity arteries as access, including the radial and brachial arteries. In the past, axillary arteries were used for this purpose, but not without a high rate of complications, including axillary sheath hematomas. We do not routinely recommend using the axillary artery for access for these reasons.

Prior to placement of a brachial artery catheter, clear documentation of a pulse examination should be completed as well as documenting blood pressures in both arms. When accessing the brachial artery for arterial pressure monitoring, either brachial artery may be used. However, when accessing the brachial artery for the purpose of arteriography, the left brachial artery is preferable. This is because a catheter will ultimately be placed into the aorta, which would necessitate crossing both carotid arteries if coming from the right brachial artery. Coming from the left brachial artery, the catheter would traverse the subclavian artery and enter the descending aorta without crossing the carotid arteries.

It is possible to access the brachial artery in a number of places; however, it is most advantageous to access the artery just above the antecubital fossa. This region is more easily compressed against the humerus and thus associated with a lower incidence of pseudoaneurysm. As this artery is quite delicate, the surgeon should have a low threshold for performing a cut-down method and open exposure of the artery for access.

Puncture of the brachial artery may be difficult because it may roll when the needle comes in contact with it. Therefore, it is easiest to palpate the artery with both the index and middle fingers of the nondominant hand and then pin it down (Fig. 5). The needle should be advanced into the artery at a more acute angle than for the femoral artery puncture. Again, because the caliber of this artery is smaller than the femoral artery, it is best to use the micropuncture technique with a 21-gauge needle and a 0.014 inch wire. Over this wire, several sheaths may be used to sequentially dilate the artery.

Radial Artery Access

More often in cardiac catheterizations, as well as in an intensive care setting, the radial artery is being cannulated (Figs. 6 and 7). The general considerations are similar to those of the brachial artery. However, prior to radial artery puncture, an Allen test must be done. An Allen test is used to determine the integrity of the blood flow to the hand. To perform this test, the hand

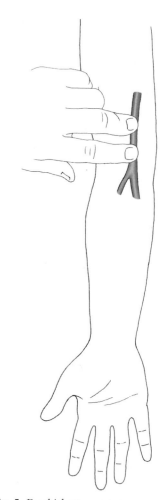

Fig. 5. Brachial artery access.

are usually accompanied by significant abnormalities on physical examination that are, in most cases, enough to make the diagnosis of neurogenic thoracic outlet syndrome without expensive, invasive testing.

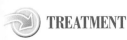 **TREATMENT**

Although decompression of the thoracic outlet is the mainstay of surgical treatment for TOS, there are a number of things to consider before proceeding with operative intervention. First, the variant of TOS is extremely important. While arterial and venous TOS tend to require a prompt surgical response, most experts recommend at least 6 weeks of conservative management with physical therapy for neurogenic TOS prior to considering surgical decompression. Second, the need for adjuvant therapy must be considered. Endovascular therapeutics such as thrombolysis and venoplasty play an important role in the treatment of venous TOS (Paget-Schroetter syndrome) and are used both before and after surgery depending on the clinical situation. Third, consideration must be given to the surgical approach and its effect on the vascular reconstructive options. While most experts would recommend the transaxillary approach to first rib resection and scalenectomy in uncomplicated TOS, the need for arterial reconstruction may necessitate another approach for proximal vascular control. In the following section each variant of thoracic outlet syndrome will be discussed separately, followed by a description of the operative approaches to decompression of the thoracic outlet.

Neurogenic Thoracic Outlet Syndrome

Because of the wide range of severity in the symptoms associated with neurogenic TOS, most patients with this form of the disease likely go undiagnosed and seek no medical intervention. Among those who are evaluated and diagnosed, the majority have substantial improvement without surgery. As has been stated previously, 6 weeks of physical therapy, designed to strengthen the muscles that open the thoracic outlet and relax the muscles that tighten it, is usually recommended prior to surgical intervention. The protocols that strengthen the trapezius, levator scapulae, and sternocleidomastoid while allowing the scalene, subclavius, and pectoralis muscles to relax can usually be undertaken with a combination of supervised and at-home exercises. In conjunction with physical therapy, some success has been reported with therapeutic (as opposed to diagnostic) scalene blocks. Although steroid injection has not been successful, electrophysiologic or fluoroscopic guided injection of botulinum toxin has met with some success. Some series have shown relief of symptoms for a mean duration of 88 days. This may allow for more aggressive physical therapy, lifestyle modifications, and/or changes in ergonomics at work. However, this procedure is not without its problems. First, there is a small but real risk of dysphagia with injection of botulinum toxin. Second, these injections can lead to scarring in the thoracic outlet that complicates operative intervention when needed.

Arterial Thoracic Outlet Syndrome

As has been mentioned previously, there are a number of different problems that are associated with arterial compression at the thoracic outlet. While cold intolerance, pain, and easy fatigability can be debilitating, these symptoms do not pose an immediate threat to the affected limb. On the other hand, complete thrombosis of the subclavian artery, aneurysm formation, and distal embolization from intraluminal lesions require a more expeditious approach to therapeutic intervention. It is the latter that poses the greatest threat to limb viability as ongoing embolization can obliterate the outflow vessels in the arm, severely limiting the options for revascularization. Acute limb-threatening ischemia must be addressed immediately and can be treated with a combination of standard open and endovascular therapies. Symptoms secondary to chronic ischemia can be addressed on a more elective basis. Again, the mainstay of treatment for arterial TOS is decompression of the thoracic outlet with the addition of arterial reconstruction when necessary. Decompression and arterial reconstruction can be undertaken as separate operations or as one combined procedure. In general, when staging the procedures or when revascularization is not necessary, a transaxillary approach to first rib resection and scalenectomy is preferred. This approach, however, does not provide adequate exposure for arterial reconstruction. For distal lesions a variety of supraclavicular and infraclavicular approaches can be used while proximal lesions may require a high thoracotomy (left) or median sternotomy (left or right) in order to obtain vascular control. Prosthetic material (polytetrafluoroethylene or Dacron) and vein and arterial grafts have all been used with success and rarely require anticoagulation. With adequate decompression of the thoracic outlet, patients tend to do well and rarely suffer from recurrent symptoms as the artery is no longer subject to trauma in the thoracic outlet.

Venous (Paget-Schroetter) Thoracic Outlet Syndrome

As with arterial TOS, presentation of acute axillosubclavian venous thrombosis should be treated aggressively. Current therapeutic protocols stress catheter-directed thrombolysis, maintenance of vein patency with systemic anticoagulation, and correction of the anatomic abnormality contributing to the thrombosis. Once the diagnosis is made (usually by physical examination and duplex evaluation), tissue plasminogen activator (tPA), urokinase, and streptokinase have all been employed to lyse the obstructing clot. Systemic anticoagulation is instituted after flow is re-established in order to maintain patency until surgical intervention can be undertaken to decompress the thoracic outlet. Traditional protocols mandated a 3-month period of oral anticoagulation with Coumadin (warfarin sodium) prior to first rib resection because immediate decompression following thrombolysis was thought to be high risk secondary to both recent administration of lytic agents and the inflammation seen with the acutely thrombosed axillosubclavian vein. This has, however, been challenged by some groups who have advocated early surgical decompression of the thoracic outlet following thrombolysis during a single hospital admission. Although there have been no randomized prospective trials to compare these two different treatment algorithms, a series published by Angle et al. reported excellent results with no increase in perioperative morbidity with early surgical decompression following thrombolysis.

For those patients presenting with chronic axillosubclavian venous thrombosis, it is often very difficult if not impossible to re-establish flow through the vein due to organized thrombus and severe scarring. In this subset of patients, decompression of the thoracic outlet should precede any attempt at recanalization or balloon angioplasty of the vein. Two weeks after first rib resection, the patients return for venography with thrombolysis and venoplasty, if necessary. Three months of oral anticoagulation is recommended in this setting after which patients can discontinue the Coumadin with only rare instances of recurrent or chronic symptoms.

Transaxillary First Rib Resection and Scalenectomy

In most instances of uncomplicated thoracic outlet syndrome, the transaxillary resection of the first rib and scalenectomy is the procedure of choice because of anatomic visualization of the area, effectiveness of decompression, and excellent published long-term results of this procedure. Induction of general anesthesia is undertaken with short-acting or no paralytics. The patient is positioned in a lateral decubitus position and the entire arm and chest wall are prepped and draped in a standard fashion. There are a number of devices available that can be used to elevate the arm in such a way as to expose the contents of the thoracic outlet. The authors prefer the Machleder retractor, which allows for easy lowering of the arm during the case to allow periods of increased blood flow and decreased tension on stretched nerves (Fig. 2). The retractor is attached to the operating room table and the arm positioned in the retractor such that it is abducted at a right angle to the chest wall. Care is taken to generously pad the forearm and antecubital fossa before securing the arm to the retractor with an elastic wrap. Incision is made approximately 1.0 cm below the hairline in the axilla between the border of the pectoralis and latissimus muscles and dissection of the subcutaneous tissues down to the chest wall is accomplished with electrocautery. In patients with long-standing venous occlusion, care must be taken to preserve the often large collateral veins during this dissection. Once the chest wall is reached, the retractor is raised on the vertical support toward the ceiling, providing an excellent view of the thoracic outlet. With minimal blunt dissection the vein can usually be identified medially while the subclavian artery and nerve roots can be located right behind the first rib. Once these structures are identified, the inferior aspect of the first rib is gently dissected from the surrounding connective tissue using a periosteal elevator. Care must be taken while freeing the underside of the rib as this can result in a pneumothorax (occurring in approximately 10% of patients). Next, a right-angle clamp is used to isolate the anterior scalene muscle and subclavius tendon from the artery and nerve (Fig. 3A). The muscle and tendon are then divided with scissors or a scalpel. Then the middle scalene is bluntly dissected off the rib with a periosteal elevator. The first rib is then divided with a bone cutter. At the costovertebral articulation no more than 2 to 4 mm of the rib is allowed to remain while at the costosternal junction the entire rib and costochondral cartilage are removed (Fig. 3B). If there are any compressive bands of tissue present after removal of the rib, they are divided prior to closure. The wound is irrigated and anesthesia is asked to give several large breaths to check for pneumothorax. A chest radiograph should also be obtained in the recovery room. The wound is then closed in two layers with absorbable sutures. Postoperatively, the arm is placed in a sling and pain managed overnight with intravenous narcotics administered by a patient-controlled analgesia (PCA) pump. Patients are routinely discharged on postoperative day 1 with oral analgesics. When systemic anticoagulation is necessary, as is usually the case with Paget-Schroetter syndrome, low-molecular-weight heparin (Lovenox) and Coumadin are instituted at home on postoperative day 3 because there is anecdotal evidence suggesting an increased risk of postoperative bleeding with immediate anticoagulation. As most of these patients have had preoperative experience with these medications, this protocol is well tolerated by patients without prolonging hospital stay or significantly increasing the incidence of postoperative bleeding.

Supraclavicular First Rib Resection and Scalenectomy

There are those who feel that the supraclavicular approach for decompression of the thoracic outlet is as effective and is safer than the transaxillary approach and therefore use this approach routinely. Moreover, there are several situations where this approach is preferred. First, when the patient's symptoms are particularly suggestive of upper brachial plexus involvement (as opposed to the more common lower plexus), it is reasonable to use a supraclavicular incision so that these nerves can be more directly decompressed. Second, for patients who have undergone inadequate transaxillary scalenectomy, the supraclavicular approach avoids the scar tissue usually present in the previous operative field. Third, when patients require vascular reconstruction such as is often the case with arterial TOS, this approach provides better access to the proximal vasculature for arterial control. Finally, anomalous anatomy such as cervical rib is dealt with more effectively with a supraclavicular approach.

While advocates of the supraclavicular approach believe that scalenectomy alone provides adequate decompression of the thoracic outlet, resection of the first rib can be accomplished through this incision. As with the transaxillary approach, short-acting or no paralytic is used on induction of anesthesia so that nerve function can be assessed during the procedure. The patient is placed in the semi-Fowler position, with the head turned away from the operative side (Fig. 4A). An incision is placed two fingerbreadths above the clavicle, extending from the external jugular vein to the sternocleidomastoid (SCM) muscle. The SCM is mobilized medially and the omohyoid muscle usually transected. The scalene fat pad is carefully divided, taking care to avoid the underlying phrenic nerve (Fig. 4B). Underlying the

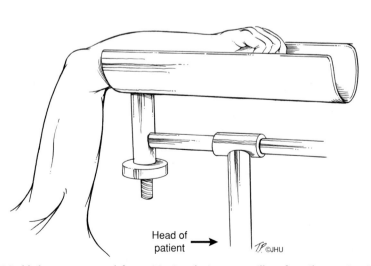

Fig. 2. Machleder retractor used for positioning during transaxillary first rib resection. The patient is placed in a decubitus position with the nonoperative side down. Ample sterile towels are used for padding (not shown) and the arm is secured in the retractor with a combination of gauze and elastic wraps (not shown). (Copyright Johns Hopkins University.)

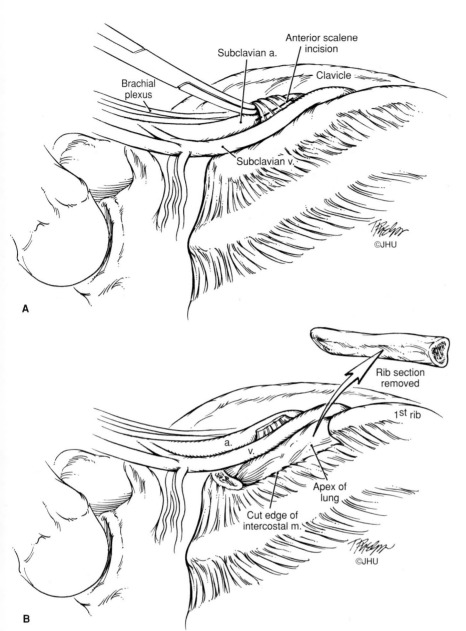

Fig. 3. A: Anatomic exposure during transaxillary first rib resection. Depicted is the right-angle clamp that is passed behind the anterior scalene muscle to protect the subclavian artery (a) and brachial plexus during division of the muscle. The subclavian vein (v) is also depicted medial to the anterior scalene muscle. **B:** Decompressed thoracic outlet with anterior scalene muscle transected and first rib removed. a, subclavian artery; v, subclavian vein; m, muscle. (A, B, copyright Johns Hopkins University.)

the same as with the transaxillary approach. A chest radiograph is obtained in the recovery room and patients are discharged on postoperative day 1 unless further medical therapy is required (e.g., anticoagulation).

RECURRENT THORACIC OUTLET SYNDROME

Published rates of recurrence for thoracic outlet syndrome range from 2% to 20%; recurrence is most often seen in patients presenting initially with neurogenic symptoms. With adequate decompression of the thoracic outlet and adequate adjuvant therapies (arterial reconstruction, thrombolysis, venoplasty), recurrence of the arterial and venous forms of TOS is exceedingly rare. With the neurogenic variant, the definition of recurrence can be difficult as it is sometimes unclear whether patients ever manifested any improvement postoperatively. Moreover, the cause of the recurrence is often not clear. There have been a variety of studies implicating long posterior first rib stumps, missed cervical ribs, and incomplete scalene resection, but none has shown good correlation with symptoms. Scar formation has also been implicated in persistent or recurrent neurogenic symptoms but there is no quantifiable measure that would allow for correlations to be drawn.

The workup and initial treatment for recurrent TOS are essentially the same as the initial workup of previously undiagnosed disease. Emphasis should be placed on ruling out other disease processes such as carpel tunnel syndrome, cervical arthritis, and tendonitis. Iatrogenic injury to the plexus must also be considered before any further surgical intervention is considered. Initial treatment should focus on physical therapy, although conservative treatment algorithms have proven to be far less successful when symptoms are recurrent.

When reoperation is deemed appropriate, there are a variety of ways to approach the postsurgical thoracic outlet. Although using the same incision can be done, most surgeons would elect to approach the thoracic outlet through a new incision and previously undissected tissues (e.g., supraclavicular incision if the initial operation was completed transaxillary). The first step is to identify the anatomy and any residual muscle or fibrous bands that need to be resected. If the first operation did not include a first rib resection, this procedure is also done at this time.

nerve is the anterior scalene muscle. This is divided inferiorly at its insertion on the first rib (Fig. 4C). Any adhesions between the muscle and the subclavian artery and brachial plexus must be lysed, and the proximal end of the muscle is divided medially to expose the C5 to C7 roots. The subclavius muscle is then divided exposing the area between the C7 root and the subclavian artery is next cleaned. At this point, the five roots should be completely cleared and tested using a nerve stimulator. If the operation is to include first rib

resection, the middle scalene muscle must also be divided. The rib is divided posteriorly and a finger used to dissect it from the pleura while elevating the divided end. The subclavian artery must be freed from the anterior portion of the rib before it is divided. As with the transaxillary procedure, the wound is filled with irrigation to assess for pleural leak. If present, a soft closed suction drain can be positioned so that the tip drains the pleural space. Otherwise, a drain placed in the wound is optional. The postoperative algorithm is

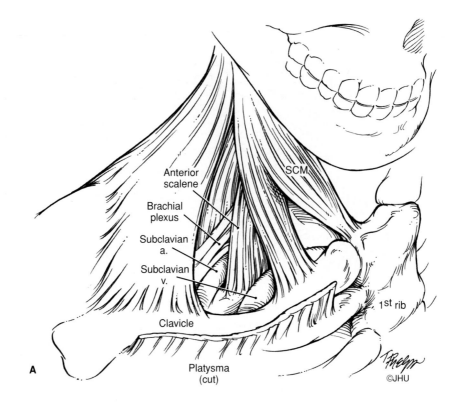

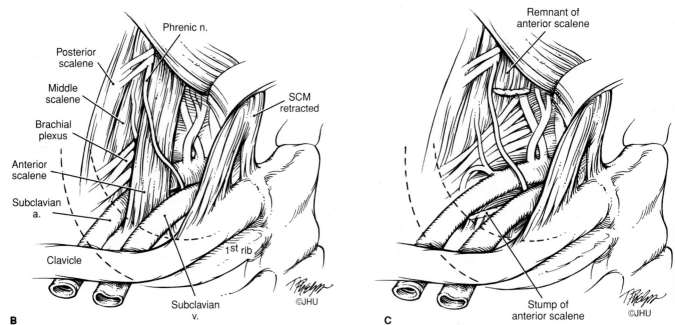

Fig. 4. A: Anatomy of the thoracic outlet from the supraclavicular approach. The patient is placed in the semi-Fowler position, with the head turned away from the operative side. An incision is placed two fingerbreadths above the clavicle, extending from the external jugular vein to the sternocleidomastoid (SCM) muscle. Depicted is the musculoskeletal anatomy with the scalene fat pad removed. a, artery; v, vein. **B:** View of the thoracic outlet with SCM mobilized medially. The scalene fat pad (not shown) is carefully divided, taking care to avoid the underlying phrenic nerve (n). Underlying the nerve is the anterior scalene muscle and the structures of the thoracic outlet as previously described. a, artery; v, vein. **C:** View of the decompressed thoracic outlet after resection of the anterior scalene muscle. The subclavian vein, artery, and nerve roots of the brachial plexus are all well visualized. The first rib is often left intact during this procedure; however, it can be resected if necessary from this approach. (A–C, copyright Johns Hopkins University.)